Inflammation, Oxidative Stress, and Cancer

Dietary Approaches for Cancer Prevention

Inflammation, Oxidative Stress, and Cancer

Dietary Approaches for Cancer Prevention

Edited by

Ah-Ng Tony Kong

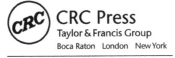

CRC Press
Taylor & Francis Group
Boca Raton London New York

CRC Press is an imprint of the
Taylor & Francis Group, an **informa** business

CRC Press
Taylor & Francis Group
6000 Broken Sound Parkway NW, Suite 300
Boca Raton, FL 33487-2742

First issued in paperback 2016

© 2014 by Taylor & Francis Group, LLC
CRC Press is an imprint of Taylor & Francis Group, an Informa business

No claim to original U.S. Government works

Version Date: 20130208

ISBN 13: 978-1-138-19984-2 (pbk)
ISBN 13: 978-1-4665-0370-0 (hbk)

Library of Congress Cataloging-in-Publication Data

Inflammation, oxidative stress, and cancer : dietary approaches for cancer prevention / editor, Ah-Ng Tony Kong.
     p. ; cm.
   Includes bibliographical references and index.
   ISBN 978-1-4665-0370-0 (haredcover : alk. paper)
   I. Kong, Ah-Ng Tony, editor of compilation.
   [DNLM: 1. Neoplasms--prevention & control. 2. Anti-Inflammatory Agents--pharmacology. 3. Antineoplastic Agents--pharmacology. 4. Inflammation--prevention & control. 5. Nutrition Therapy. 6. Oxidative Stress. QZ 266]
   RC271.C5
   616.99'4061--dc23

2013005011

Visit the Taylor & Francis Web site at
http://www.taylorandfrancis.com

and the CRC Press Web site at
http://www.crcpress.com

Dedication

For my father, Kong Yuk-Ming, and my mother,
Lai Lang-Kiew, for their love and support

My teachers and mentors for their guidance, mentorship, and friendship

My wife, Carolyn, and my children, Emily and Andrew,
for their love, support, and encouragement

Contents

SECTION I   Inflammation, Oxidative Stress, Nutritional Phytochemicals, and Cancer

SECTION II   Signal Transduction, Molecular Targets, and Biomarkers of Dietary Cancer-Preventive Phytochemicals

SECTION VI Flavonoids and Polyphenols

SECTION VII Garlic Organosulfur Compounds and Crucifer Glucusinolates

SECTION VIII Selenium, Herbal Medicines, Alpha Lipoic Acid, and Cancer Prevention

SECTION IX Epigenetics and Chronic Inflammation

Preface

The major impetus for this book stems from the recent explosion of research on nutritional/dietary phytochemicals—investigating their mechanisms of signaling/gene expression and their impact on diseases including cancer. The second impetus came from participating in a symposium titled "Diet, Inflammation and Cancer" for the American Institute Cancer Research (AICR) Annual Research Conference on Food, Nutrition, Physical Activity and Cancer, October 21 and 22, 2010, in Washington, DC, which triggered a lot of discussion.

Increasing scientific evidence suggests that a majority of diseases including cancer are driven by oxidative stress and inflammation, attributed to environmental factors (viruses, carcinogens, among others). These factors impinge on genetic materials, driving either genetic mutations and/or epigenetically modifying expression of key regulatory genes (DNAs, RNAs, enzymes, receptors, and cofactors, among others). These genetics/epigenetics events can occur as early as during gestational fetal development. The major questions remain as to how dietary phytochemical factors can biochemically interact with such genetic/epigenetic events.

The main purpose of this book was to assemble a group of internationally well-recognized scientific experts to examine and summarize the latest developments on the various dietary phytochemicals. As a result, this book is divided into nine subsections, beginning with the basic mechanisms of inflammation/oxidative stress–driven cancer initiation and development. This is followed by cellular signal transduction, molecular targets and biomarkers of dietary cancer-preventive phytochemicals, and their potential challenges with in vivo absorption and pharmacokinetics of these phytochemicals. Then the various classes/groups of phytochemicals are examined. These include vitamins A, D, and E; omega-3 and omega-6 fatty acids; flavonoids and polyphenols; garlic organosulfur compounds and cruciferous glucusinolates; and selenium, traditional Chinese herbal medicines, and alpha lipoic acid. The last section covers the latest developments in phyto-epigenomics and some future perspective on the development of phytochemicals in disease prevention and treatment.

The intended audience includes graduate students, postdoctoral fellows, and scientists working in the areas of nutrition, dietary phytochemicals, inflammation, oxidative stress, antioxidants in general, and cancer more specifically. Furthermore, the general public will benefit from the great overview, comprehensive analysis, and distillation of concepts discussed in this book.

Acknowledgments

I am deeply indebted to the contributing authors who are passionate and have done so much to advance the science of nutritional dietary phytochemicals and cancer chemoprevention as highlighted in the respective chapters of this book. I thank Ira Wolinsky who first contacted me regarding the idea of putting this book together. Several individuals at CRC Press–Taylor & Francis Group deserve special recognition for their efforts; Randy Brehm, Senior Editor, Chemical and Life Sciences Group, Taylor & Francis Group, who helped to work on the contents; Kari Budyk, Senior Project Coordinator, Editorial Project Development, CRC Press–Taylor & Francis Group, who helped to facilitate and coordinate all the chapters; Joette Lynch, Project Editor, Production Department, CRC Press–Taylor & Francis Group; and Amor Nanas, Manila Typesetting Company (MTC), who played a key role in the producing of this book. Last but not least, I am deeply indebted to my current and former laboratory members, many of whom are authors or coauthors in this book, and to Hui Pung and Douglas Pung who helped coordinate and manage the book, without whose help the completion of this book would not have been possible.

Editor

Ah-Ng "Tony" Kong, PhD, is a distinguished professor (PII), Glaxo Endowed Chair Professor of Pharmaceutics, and director of the Graduate Program in Pharmaceutical Sciences at Rutgers, the State University of New Jersey. He is also the director for the Center for Pharmacogenetics and Pharmacogenomics at Rutgers University. Professor Kong earned his BS in pharmacy from the University of Alberta, Canada; his PhD in pharmacokinetics and pharmacodynamics from the State University of New York at Buffalo; and his postdoctoral training in molecular genetics and cellular signaling at the National Institutes of Health (NIH). He is a fellow of the American Association of Pharmaceutical Scientists. He was on the faculty of Thomas Jefferson University Medical School and the University of Illinois at Chicago before joining Rutgers in early 2001. Dr. Kong has served on numerous NIH Study Section panels since 1999, and he has been continuously receiving funding support from the NIH since 1993.

Dr. Kong has trained more than 40 postdoctoral fellows, visiting professors, and PhD students. He has published more than 200 original research papers, review articles, and book chapters, and has chaired and given presentations at many national and international symposia and conferences. He is currently serving on the board of 15 international journals, including *Pharmaceutical Research; Carcinogenesis; Biopharmaceutics and Drug Disposition; Cancer Prevention Research (AACR); Molecular Carcinogenesis; Life Sciences; Pharmacological Research; Journal of Chinese Pharmaceutical Sciences; Oncology Letters; Archives of Pharmacal Research; Acta Pharmacologica Sinica; Cell Biosciences;* and *Journal of Traditional and Complementary Medicine*. His research areas are dietary phytochemicals (signaling and gene expression, nutrigenomics, cancer chemoprevention); animal tumor models of the prostate, colon, and skin; epigenetics/epigenomics; oxidative/redox/inflammatory stress response; Nrf2-mediated nuclear transactivation and signaling; and pharmacokinetics and pharmacodynamics of phytochemicals.

You can visit his website at http://pharmacy.rutgers.edu/content/faculty_profile_116.

Contributors

Rajesh Agarwal
Department of Pharmaceutical Sciences
Skaggs School of Pharmacy and
  Pharmaceutical Sciences
and
University of Colorado Cancer Center
University of Colorado Denver
Denver, Colorado

Aamir Ahmad
Department of Pathology
Barbara Ann Karmanos Cancer Institute
Wayne State University School of Medicine
Detroit, Michigan

Bin Bao
Department of Pathology
Barbara Ann Karmanos Cancer Institute
Wayne State University School of Medicine
Detroit, Michigan

Ann M. Bode
The Hormel Institute
University of Minnesota
Austin, Minnesota

Judy L. Bolton
Department of Medicinal Chemistry and
  Pharmacognosy
University of Illinois at Chicago
National Institutes of Health (UIC/NIH) Center
  for Botanical Dietary Supplements Research
University of Illinois at Chicago
Chicago, Illinois

Rodica P. Bunaciu
Department of Biomedical Sciences
Cornell University
Ithaca, New York

Scott Bussom
Department of Pharmacology
Yale University School of Medicine
New Haven, Connecticut

James Cardelli
Division of Basic and Translational Research
Feist-Weiller Cancer Center
and
Department of Microbiology
Louisiana State University Health Sciences
  Center
Shreveport, Louisiana

Barrie R. Cassileth
Integrative Medicine Service
Memorial Sloan–Kettering Cancer Center
New York, New York

Chi Chen
Department of Food Science and Nutrition
University of Minnesota
St. Paul, Minnesota

Xiaoxin Chen
Julius L. Chambers Biomedical/Biotechnology
  Research Institute
North Carolina Central University
Durham, North Carolina

Yong Q. Chen
Department of Cancer Biology
Wake Forest School of Medicine
Winston-Salem, North Carolina

and

State Key Laboratory of Food Science and
  Technology
School of Food Science and Technology
Jiangnan University
Wuxi, China

Yung-Chi Cheng
Department of Pharmacology
Yale University School of Medicine
New Haven, Connecticut

David Coleman
Department of Microbiology
Louisiana State University Health Sciences
    Center
Shreveport, Louisiana

Katherine D. Crew
Herber Irving Comprehensive Cancer Center
Columbia University Medical Center
New York, New York

Gagan Deep
Department of Pharmaceutical Sciences
Skaggs School of Pharmacy and
    Pharmaceutical Sciences
and
University of Colorado Cancer Center
University of Colorado Denver
Denver, Colorado

Birgit M. Dietz
Department of Medicinal Chemistry and
    Pharmacognosy
University of Illinois at Chicago
National Institutes of Health (UIC/NIH) Center
    for Botanical Dietary Supplements Research
University of Illinois at Chicago
Chicago, Illinois

Zigang Dong
The Hormel Institute
University of Minnesota
Austin, Minnesota

Fulan Guan
Department of Pharmacology
Yale University School of Medicine
New Haven, Connecticut

Tory M. Hagen
Linus Pauling Institute
and
Department of Biochemistry and Biophysics
Oregon State University
Corvallis, Oregon

Tabitha M. Hardy
Department of Biology
University of Alabama at Birmingham
Birmingham, Alabama

Ming Hu
Department of Pharmacological and
    Pharmaceutical Science
College of Pharmacy
University of Houston
Houston, Texas

Yoshihiko Ito
Department of Pharmacokinetics and
    Pharmacodynamics
School of Pharmaceutical Sciences
University of Shizuoka
Shizuoka, Japan

Cheng Jiang
Department of Biomedical Sciences
School of Pharmacy
Texas Tech University Health Sciences Center
Amarillo, Texas

Zaoli Jiang
Department of Pharmacology
Yale University School of Medicine
New Haven, Connecticut

Young-Sam Keum
Department of Biochemistry
College of Pharmacy
Dongguk University
Goyang, Republic of Korea

Naghma Khan
Department of Dermatology
University of Wisconsin
Madison, Wisconsin

Tin Oo Khor
Center for Cancer Prevention Research
and
Department of Pharmaceutics
Ernest Mario School of Pharmacy
Rutgers, State University of New Jersey
Piscataway, New Jersey

Kimberly Kline
Department of Nutritional Sciences
University of Texas at Austin
Austin, Texas

Ah-Ng Tony Kong
Center for Cancer Prevention Research
and
Department of Pharmaceutics
Ernest Mario School of Pharmacy
Rutgers, State University of New Jersey
Piscataway, New Jersey

Dejuan Kong
Department of Pathology
Barbara Ann Karmanos Cancer Institute
Wayne State University School of Medicine
Detroit, Michigan

Wing Lam
Department of Pharmacology
Yale University School of Medicine
New Haven, Connecticut

Ha-Na Lee
Tumor Microenvironment Global Core
    Research Center
College of Pharmacy
Seoul National University
Seoul, South Korea

Jong Hun Lee
Center for Cancer Prevention Research
and
Department of Pharmaceutics
Ernest Mario School of Pharmacy
Rutgers, State University of New Jersey
Piscataway, New Jersey

Yiwei Li
Department of Pathology
Barbara Ann Karmanos Cancer Institute
Wayne State University School of Medicine
Detroit, Michigan

Shwu-Huey Liu
PhytoCeutica Inc
Branford, Connecticut

Junxuan Lü
Department of Biomedical Sciences
School of Pharmacy
Texas Tech University Health Sciences Center
Amarillo, Texas

Yong Ma
Department of Pharmacological and
    Pharmaceutical Sciences
College of Pharmacy
University of Houston
Houston, Texas

Laura Marler
College of Pharmacy
University of Hawaii at Hilo
Hilo, Hawaii

Julie K. Mason
Department of Nutritional Sciences
Faculty of Medicine
University of Toronto
Toronto, Ontario, Canada

Regis F. Moreau
Department of Nutrition and Health Sciences
University of Nebraska
Lincoln, Nebraska

Marilyn E. Morris
Department of Pharmaceutical Sciences
School of Pharmacy and Pharmaceutical
    Sciences
University at Buffalo
State University of New York
Buffalo, New York

Hasan Mukhtar
Department of Dermatology
University of Wisconsin
Madison, Wisconsin

Hye-Kyung Na
Department of Food and Nutrition
Sungshin Women's University
Seoul, South Korea

Ximena Paredes-Gonzalez
Center for Cancer Prevention Research
and
Department of Pharmaceutics
Ernest Mario School of Pharmacy
Rutgers, State University of New Jersey
Piscataway, New Jersey

Dan Peiffer
Department of Medicine
Division of Hematology and Oncology
Medical College of Wisconsin
Milwaukee, Wisconsin

John M. Pezzuto
College of Pharmacy
University of Hawaii at Hilo
Hilo, Hawaii

Lucina C. Rouggly
Department of Surgery
and
Alvin J. Siteman Cancer Center
Washington University School of Medicine
St. Louis, Missouri

Bob G. Sanders
Section of Molecular Genetics and
    Microbiology
University of Texas at Austin
Austin, Texas

Fazlul H. Sarkar
Departments of Pathology and Oncology
Barbara Ann Karmanos Cancer Institute
Wayne State University School of Medicine
Detroit, Michigan

Constance Lay-Lay Saw
Center for Cancer Prevention Research
and
Department of Pharmaceutics
Ernest Mario School of Pharmacy
Rutgers, State University of New Jersey
Piscataway, New Jersey

Anuradha Sehrawat
Department of Pharmacology and Chemical
    Biology
and
University of Pittsburgh Cancer Institute
University of Pittsburgh School of Medicine
Pittsburgh, Pennsylvannia

Kate Petersen Shay
Linus Pauling Institute
Oregon State University
Corvallis, Oregon

Limin Shu
Center for Cancer Prevention Research
and
Department of Pharmaceutics
Ernest Mario School of Pharmacy
Rutgers, State University of New Jersey
Piscataway, New Jersey

Katrina M. Simmons
Department of Biomedical Sciences and Cancer
    Research Center
Environmental Health Sciences
University at Albany
Rensselaer, New York

Shivendra V. Singh
Department of Pharmacology and Chemical
    Biology
and
University of Pittsburgh Cancer Institute
University of Pittsburgh School of Medicine
Pittsburgh, Pennsylvannia

Amanda K. Smolarek
Department of Chemical Biology
Ernest Mario School of Pharmacy
and
Joint Graduate Program in Toxicology
Rutgers, State University of New Jersey
Piscataway, New Jersey

Na-Young Song
Tumor Microenvironment Global Core
    Research Center
College of Pharmacy
Seoul National University
Seoul, South Korea

Gary D. Stoner
Department of Medicine
Division of Hematology and Oncology
Medical College of Wisconsin
Milwaukee, Wisconsin

Zheng-Yuan Su
Center for Cancer Prevention Research
and
Department of Pharmaceutics
Ernest Mario School of Pharmacy
Rutgers, State University of New Jersey
Piscataway, New Jersey

Janel Suburu
Department of Cancer Biology
Wake Forest School of Medicine
Winston-Salem, North Carolina

Nanjoo Suh
Department of Chemical Biology
Ernest Mario School of Pharmacy
and
Joint Graduate Program in Toxicology
Rutgers, State University of New Jersey
Piscataway, New Jersey

and

The Cancer Institute of New Jersey
New Brunswick, New Jersey

Young-Joon Surh
Tumor Microenvironment Global Core
    Research Center
College of Pharmacy
Seoul National University
Seoul, South Korea

Martin P. R. Tenniswood
Department of Biomedical Sciences and Cancer
    Research Center
Environmental Health Sciences
University at Albany
Rensselaer, New York

Lilian U. Thompson
Department of Nutritional Sciences
Faculty of Medicine
University of Toronto
Toronto, Ontario, Canada

Richa Tiwary
Section of Molecular Genetics and Microbiology
University of Texas at Austin
Austin, Texas

Trygve O. Tollefsbol
Department of Biology
Center for Aging
Comprehensive Cancer Center
Nutrition Obesity Research Center
and
Comprehensive Diabetes Center
University of Alabama at Birmingham
Birmingham, Alabama

Alpna Tyagi
Department of Pharmaceutical Sciences
Skaggs School of Pharmacy and
    Pharmaceutical Sciences
University of Colorado Denver
Denver, Colorado

Wei-Lin W. Wang
Department of Biomedical Sciences and Cancer
    Research Center
Environmental Health Sciences
University at Albany
Rensselaer, New York

Yian Wang
Department of Surgery and Alvin J. Siteman
    Cancer Center
Washington University School of Medicine
St. Louis, Missouri

JoEllen Welsh
Cancer Research Center and Department of
    Environmental Health Sciences
University at Albany
Rensselaer, New York

Kathleen M. Wesa
Integrative Medicine Service
Memorial Sloan–Kettering Cancer Center
New York, New York

Ashleigh K. A. Wiggins
Department of Nutritional Sciences
Faculty of Medicine
University of Toronto
Toronto, Ontario, Canada

Shizuo Yamada
Department of Pharmacokinetics and
    Pharmacodynamics
School of Pharmaceutical Sciences
University of Shizuoka
Shizuoka, Japan

Chung S. Yang
Department of Chemical Biology
and
Center for Cancer Prevention Research
Ernest Mario School of Pharmacy
Rutgers, State University of New Jersey
Piscataway, New Jersey

Guang-Yu Yang
Department of Pathology
Feinberg School of Medicine
Northwestern University
Chicago, Illinois

Zhen Yang
Department of Pharmacological and
    Pharmaceutical Science
College of Pharmacy
University of Houston
Houston, Texas

Andrew Yen
Department of Biomedical Sciences
Cornell University
Ithaca, New York

Michael S. You
Department of Surgery
and
Alvin J. Siteman Cancer Center
Washington University School of Medicine
St. Louis, Missouri

Ming You
Medical College of Wisconsin Cancer Center
and
Department of Pharmacology and Toxicology
Medical College of Wisconsin
Milwaukee, Wisconsin

Weiping Yu
Section of Molecular Genetics and Microbiology
University of Texas at Austin
Austin, Texas

Chengyue Zhang
Department of Pharmaceutics
School of Pharmacy
Rutgers, State University of New Jersey
Piscataway, New Jersey

Jinhui Zhang
Department of Biomedical Sciences
School of Pharmacy
Texas Tech University Health Sciences Center
Amarillo, Texas

Wei Zhang
Department of Pharmacology
Yale University School of Medicine
New Haven, Connecticut

Noah P. Zimmerman
Department of Microbiology and Molecular
    Genetics
Medical College of Wisconsin
Milwaukee, Wisconsin

Section I

Inflammation, Oxidative Stress, Nutritional Phytochemicals, and Cancer

1 Overview on Oxidative Stress, Inflammation, Cancer Initiation/Progression, and How to Prevent Carcinogenesis/Cancer

Jong Hun Lee and Ah-Ng Tony Kong

CONTENTS

1.1 INTRODUCTION

Cancer is one of the major causes of mortality in the United States and other developed countries (WHO 2011; Xu 2010). In 1975, approximately 400 cases of age-adjusted cancer incidences per 100,000 people were reported in the United States. The rates of cancer incidence in the United States per 100,000 people in 1985, 1995, and 2005 were approximately 450, 475, and 465, respectively (Jemal et al. 2009). Although significant progress has been made in the diagnosis and treatment of human cancers, these malignancies remain a significant threat to human health.

The causes of most human cancers are complex and remain largely unknown. Carcinogenesis is an asymptomatic, long-term process, which typically takes several years to progress from initiation to advanced stages. Cancer can also occur in almost every anatomic part of the body and can arise from a variety of different causes.

Epidemiological data show that nutritional factors contribute to an average human cancer mortality rate of 35%. A broad range of substances, especially those found in processed foods, have been found to increase the risk of carcinogenesis. On the other hand, epidemiological studies suggest that increased consumption of fruits and vegetables reduces cancer risk at various sites in the body (Doll and Peto 1981; Giovannucci 1999). Many laboratory studies have reported that numerous natural compounds isolated from food and edible plants exert anticancer effects by modifying cancer-related cellular signaling pathways (Knasmuller et al. 2009; Surh 2003; Thomasset et al. 2007).

Wattenberg's classic theory of chemoprevention states that the administration of one or more chemical compounds can prevent the occurrence of cancer (Wattenberg 1966). Accumulating data demonstrating the effects of various dietary compounds on cancer prevention has modified the concept of chemoprevention. Currently, chemoprevention should be defined as an effective cancer preventive approach used to inhibit, retard, or reverse human carcinogenesis at early stages using nontoxic nutrients, phytochemicals, and synthetic pharmacological agents (Knasmuller et al. 2009). Increasing data from cancer epidemiology and experimental efforts supports the idea of chemoprevention as a promising new approach to prevent carcinogenesis. It is important to understand the molecular mechanisms of carcinogenesis because knowledge of these mechanisms enables us to identify novel agents for targeted cancer chemoprevention and effective routes of administration and to assay the bioavailability of currently available compounds.

Carcinogenesis is a long-term and multistage process that normally develops over more than 10 years and typically consists of three stages, known as initiation, promotion, and progression (Armitage 1985). In the initiation stage, initiators such as carcinogens and radiation either react with DNA directly or interact with intracellular macromolecules to form reactive molecules that cause DNA damage and promote the transformation of normal cell into precancerous cells (initiated cells). Once cells have unrepaired DNA damage, they are susceptible to progress into the promotion stage because any daughter cells derived from the damaged cells will inherit this alteration. Epigenetic alterations, including DNA methylation and histone modifications, are also important gene regulatory mechanisms, and they play essential roles both independently and cooperatively in tumor initiation and progression (Li, Carroll, and Dahiya 2005). In the promotion stage, the initiated cells develop into preneoplastic cells. Promoters interact with their specific receptors on the cell surface to induce the proliferation of preneoplastic cells through intracellular signaling pathways. During the progression stage, neoplastic transformation is advanced, and the growing tumors develop invasive and metastatic potential (Hanahan and Weinberg 2000; Moolgavkar 1978; Wattenberg 1985). Because reactive oxygen species (ROS) or electrophiles are believed to play a critical role in carcinogenesis, the nuclear factor (NF) erythroid-2 (NF-E2)–related factor 2 (Nrf2) and antioxidant and detoxifying enzymes acting downstream of Nrf2 have emerged as important and effective molecular targets for chemoprevention because they prevent the toxic effects of ROS and electrophiles (Arisawa et al. 2007; Braun et al. 2002). Various targets for chemoprevention have also been identified at each stage of carcinogenesis. It has been suggested that chemopreventive agents should be categorized into two groups, blocking agents and suppressing agents (Wattenberg 1985). Figure 1.1 describes the multistage carcinogenic model and the relevant chemoprevention strategies. Dietary phytochemicals obtained from daily foods and edible plants have received significant attention as emerging compounds for cancer prevention due to their relatively low toxicity, low cost, and ease of administration.

In this chapter, we will cover the various endogenous and exogenous carcinogenic factors that are currently known in the field of carcinogenesis. The relevant anticarcinogenic strategies and treatments, especially as they relate to chemopreventive dietary phytochemicals, will also be discussed.

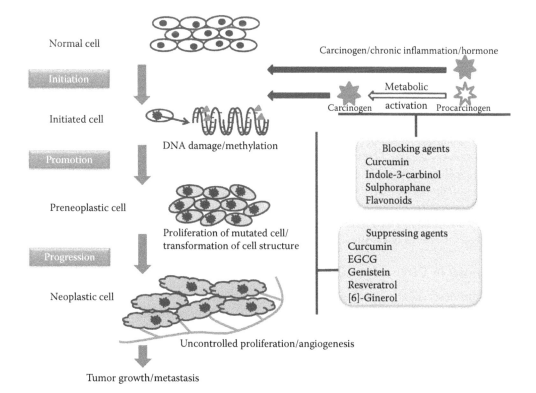

FIGURE 1.1 Dietary agents relevant for multistage carcinogenesis. The onset of carcinogenesis results from the interaction of exogenous/endogenous carcinogenic compounds with intracellular macromolecules in normal cells, either directly or after metabolic activation. This can cause DNA damage/methylation, which, if not repaired, can result in genetic and other cellular damage. These damaged cells develop into preneoplastic cells upon altered expression of oncogenes and tumor suppressor genes during the promotion stage, resulting in modified cell structure and proliferation. Finally, preneoplastic cells progress to neoplastic cells. This cascade of events offers various chemopreventive targets at every stage. Some chemopreventive phytochemicals block the initiation of carcinogenesis through inhibition of procarcinogen metabolic activation or of interaction of the carcinogen with cellular macromolecules. On the other hand, some agents suppress the malignant transformation of initiated cells during either the promotion or the progression stage. Some chemopreventive agents have both types of activity.

1.2 CHEMICAL CARCINOGENS AND THEIR METABOLIC ACTIVATION

Humans are exogenously exposed to various xenobiotic chemicals that possess carcinogenic or mutagenic properties. Chemical carcinogens can be categorized into two groups: direct-acting carcinogens and chemicals requiring activation. Due to their electrophilic properties and biologically and chemically reactive structures, direct-acting carcinogens can interact with nucleophilic centers in nucleic acids and proteins. In contrast, the majority of chemical carcinogens are biologically or chemically inert in the body. However, through metabolic activation, these procarcinogens can be converted into intermediate carcinogens and ultimately into electrophilic carcinogens. Because this conversion requires the participation of specific enzyme systems in various species and organs, procarcinogens have organ specificity for conversion and a wide variety of activities in the target organ (Williams 1977).

1.2.1 Metabolic Conversion of Chemical Carcinogens

Carcinogens or procarcinogens can be metabolized by a phase I system to form a series of metabolites. Phase I enzymes, especially cytochrome p450s (CYPs) and drug-metabolizing enzyme (DME), convert lipophilic procarcinogenic chemicals into electrophiles by oxidation, reduction, isomerization, or hydration of chemicals. This conversion results in the interaction of the electrophiles with intracellular macromolecules, such as DNA, RNA, and proteins (Shimada et al. 1996; Gonzalez and Gelboin 1994). Although a small fraction of procarcinogens are metabolically activated, these transformed products can act as carcinogens. Thus, compounds that can regulate either the transcription level or the activity of CYP could act as carcinogens (Danielson 2002; Wogan et al. 2004). As a result of a recent increase in attention to CYPs, a large amount of data have been accumulated demonstrating that metabolites formed by phase I CYPs can sometimes be reactive and damage DNA and other cellular biomolecules. The CYP family is one of the largest multigene families in the human genome; the CYPs are remarkable proteins because of the diversity of reactions they are involved in and the range of substrates they act upon (Maheo et al. 1997; Danielson 2002).

1.2.2 Classes of Carcinogenic Chemicals

Because of the concerns about human health risks, tremendous effort has been focused on identifying potential DNA-damaging and carcinogenic chemicals in human consumables, including food. Hazardous chemicals vary widely in their chemical structures, modes of action, sources, and the organs they affect. They are classified, mainly based on their functional groups, into the following classes: polycyclic aromatic hydrocarbons (PAHs), heterocyclic aromatic amines (HCAs), and N-nitrosamines (NAs) (Skog, Johansson, and Jagerstad 1998; Guengerich 1992).

1.2.2.1 Polycyclic Aromatic Hydrocarbons

PAHs are chemically inert and hydrophobic. However, CYP enzymes, particularly CYP1A1, metabolically activate PAHs to form diol epoxides that bind covalently to cellular macromolecules including DNA. These reactive metabolites cause mutations and/or errors in DNA replication and result in the initiation of carcinogenesis (Phillips 1983). The primary source of PAHs is the incomplete combustion of organic materials such as coal, petroleum, and cigarette smoke. Workers in heavily contaminated industrial areas, such as coal-tar production plants, iron foundries, coke ovens, and aluminum production plants, are exposed to PAHs. However, the most common sources of PAHs for humans are consumption of food that is contaminated by PAH particles and smoking. Several studies have been conducted to determine the levels of PAHs in human diets. Considerable levels of PAHs were detected in many types of uncooked food. In addition, cooking processes can generate PAHs in food (Gomaa et al. 1993; Phillips 1983, 1999; Meador et al. 1995).

Like most environmental carcinogens, once PAHs in the environment are deposited in plants or other low-level food sources, they enter the food chain and become concentrated as they accumulate at higher levels of the food chain (Meador et al. 1995). The generation of woodsmoke is an example of incomplete combustion, and PAHs are generated in the smoking process used to enrich flavor. In salmon, concentrations of five carcinogenic PAHs (benzo[a]pyrene (BaP), benz[a]anthracene, benzo[b]fluoranthene, dibenz[a,h]anthracene, and indeno[1,2,3-cd]pyrene) reached levels of 16.0 ppb (Gomaa et al. 1993). When meat is cooked in direct contact with an open flame, pyrolysis of the fats in the meat generates PAHs. Even if the meat is not in direct contact, fat dripping onto the flame or hot coals generates PAHs, which adhere to the outer crust of the meat. Using low-temperature cooking can reduce dietary exposure to PAHs (Phillips 1983, 1999). One cigarette contains 10–50 ng of BaP and 12–140 ng of benz[a]anthracene (Rustemeier et al. 2002). Certain types of PAHs, such as BaP and 7,12-dimethylbenzanthracene (7,12-DMBA), have been used frequently to induce carcinogenesis in laboratory rodents (Wattenberg 1977).

Early in the 1980s, Wattenberg et al. reviewed several nonnutrient constituents of food, including terpene, curcumin, flavones, and β-carotene, that protect against PAH-induced cancer formation in rodent models (Wattenberg 1992). They found that organic isothiocyanates blocked the production of PAH-induced tumors through the suppression of carcinogen activation by CYP and the induction of phase II detoxifying enzymes such as glutathione transferases and nicotinamide adenine dinucleotide phosphate NAD(P)H:quinone reductase (Zhang and Talalay 1994). It has been reported that the diol epoxides are substrates for glutathione S-transferases (GSTs), which conjugate them to glutathione (Jernstrom et al. 1996).

1.2.2.2 Heterocyclic Aromatic Amines

Since the Japanese scientist Takashi Sugimura discovered the mutagenicity of smoke from grilled fish, approximately 20 different HCAs have been identified (Sugimura et al. 2004). In a model system, a heated reaction of sugar and amino acids together with the major precursor creatine or creatinine generated mutagenic HCAs such as 2-amino-3-methylimidazo[4,5-f]quinolone (IQ), 2-amino-α-carboline (AαC), and 2-amino-1-methyl-6-phenylimidazo[4,5-b]pyridine (PhIP) (Jagerstad et al. 1991). HCAs are metabolized mainly by CYP1A2 in rodents and humans via the N-oxidation of the exocyclic primary amino group. The hydroxyamino group is subsequently catalyzed by N(O)-acetyltransferases (NATs). N-acetoxy metabolites of HCAs are spontaneously converted to arylnitrenium ions (R-NH$^+$) and react with DNA to form adducts at the 8-position carbon of the guanine base (Sugimura et al. 2004). Exposure of Fisher344 rats to PhIP, which is found in cooked meat, causes cancer in the rat ventral prostate by lobe-specific infiltration of mast cells and macrophages in response to PhIP (Nakai, Nelson, and De Marzo 2007).

Decreased consumption of fried meat, the reduction of frying temperature, and the usage of antioxidant-rich oil during cooking are ways to reduce the production and consumption of HCAs because HCA generation mainly depends on an increase in temperature and heating time and on dehydration of the meat (Knize et al. 2002). Treatment with Brussels sprout extract reduces DNA damage in PhIP-treated human lymphocytes by inhibiting sulfotransferase 1A1, which plays a key role in the activation of PhIP (Hoelzl et al. 2008). Indole-3-carbinol, which is present in cruciferous vegetables, was shown to suppress aberrant crypt foci (ACF) development caused by PhIP in IQ-treated rats (Dashwood 2002).

1.2.2.3 N-Nitrosamines

NAs are nitroso derivatives of secondary amines that occur in the human diet and environment and can be formed endogenously in the human digestive tract (Tricker and Preussmann 1991). NAs are metabolized by CYP2E1, which hydroxylates the α carbon atom to nitroso groups. The unstable intermediate produced easily releases a nitrogen molecule, leading to a reactive species. This highly reactive electrophile can contribute to the formation of protein and DNA adducts (Nouso, Thorgeirsson, and Battula 1992). The regulation of α-hyroxyalkylnitrosamine formation by CYP has been reported in animals and humans (Guengerich 1992; Yang et al. 1990).

Along with lifestyle modifications, such as reducing dietary exposure to NAs by decreasing consumption of cured meat that contains large amounts of NAs, the consumption of dietary polyphenol is another potential approach to reduce the risk of NA exposure. Various Chinese teas inhibit the endogenous formation of N-nitrosomorpholine in vitro and in vivo (Wu et al. 1993). The effect of vitamin A on 4-(methyl-nitrosamino)-1-(3-pyridyl)-1-butanone (NNK), a confirmed carcinogen in humans, was studied in a model of induced genotoxic damage in the rat liver. Compared with the group fed with a vitamin A–deficient diet, the vitamin A–supplemented group showed a significant decrease in the number of micronuclei. In isolated hepatocytes from vitamin A–fed rats, NNK was metabolized much less effectively, compared with cells from rats fed with a vitamin-deficient diet (Alaoui-Jamali, Rossignol, and Castonguay 1991).

1.3 ROS/REACTIVE NITROGEN SPECIES

ROS are byproducts of the mitochondrial respiratory chain that is responsible for most of the oxygen reduction and energy generation in cells; they are eliminated by protective mechanisms, including antioxidants, in normal conditions. Under sustained environmental stress, prolonged production of ROS may cause damages in cellular structure and induce somatic mutations and neoplastic transformation. Under hypoxic conditions, the mitochondrial respiratory chain also produces nitric oxide (NO), which can generate reactive nitrogen species (RNS). Thus, oxidative stress is an imbalance between the generation of ROS/RNS and the antioxidative stress defense systems (Poyton, Ball, and Castello 2009; Reuter et al. 2010; Valko et al. 2007). A large amount of evidence has demonstrated that oxidative stress contributes to most human diseases, including various types of cancers, Alzheimer's disease (AD), and Parkinson's disease (PD) (Emerit, Edeas, and Bricaire 2004; Cataldi 2010).

1.3.1 Defenses against Oxidative Stress

As introduced in Section 1.2, phase I enzymes, including CYP, are involved in the metabolic activation of procarcinogens. Phase II enzymes, also known as "detoxifying enzymes," can facilitate cellular protection. The induction of phase II detoxifying and antioxidant enzymes, such as GST, NAD(P)H quinone oxidoreductase 1 (NQO1), Uridine 5′-diphospho (UDP)-glucuronosyltransferase (UGT), and hemeoxigenase-1 (HO-1), has been proposed as an effective cytoprotective approach against oxidative stress, as well as the neoplastic process of carcinogenesis (Jeong, Jun, and Kong 2006). GST, UGT, and sulfotransferase modify electrophilic xenobiotics or metabolites of phase I enzymes with endogenous groups (glutathione, glucuronide, and sulfate, respectively) to reduce their toxicity and reactivity by increasing the solubility of these conjugates and excreting them. In addition to conjugating electrophiles and metabolites, phase II enzymes act as antioxidants by generating endogenous molecules such as glutathione (Jeong, Jun, and Kong 2006; Maheo et al. 1997; Paul et al. 2005; Pool-Zobel, Veeriah, and Bohmer 2005; Talalay 2000; Zhao et al. 2001).

1.3.2 Nrf2/Keap1 Complex

The expression of phase II enzymes at the transcriptional level is stimulated through antioxidant response elements (AREs), which are found in the regulatory regions of most phase II and antioxidant genes. Nrf2, a member of the NF-E2 family of nuclear basic leucine zipper (bZIP) transcription factors, and Kelch-like ECH-associated protein 1 (Keap1), a cytoplasmic protein homologous to the *Drosophila* actin-binding protein Kelch, play key roles in regulating ARE-mediated gene expression (Ramos-Gomez et al. 2001; Surh 2003). In both wild-type and heterozygous Nrf2 mutant mice, phenolic antioxidants markedly induced the expression of phase II enzymes such as GST and NQO1. However, in homozygous null mice, the expression of these enzymes was largely abolished. This result confirmed that Nrf2 plays an essential role in the transcriptional induction of phase II enzymes (Itoh et al. 1997). Wakabayashi et al. (2003) showed that homozygous Keap1 mutant mice died postnatally due to hyperkeratosis in their esophagus and forestomach, which led to starvation. This phenomenon was also observed in vitro in squamous cell epithelia. They also found that Nrf2 accumulates in the nuclei of homozygous *Keap1* mutant cells and that constitutive expression of Nrf2 target genes was markedly increased. These experiments demonstrated that Keap1 acts as an upstream regulator of Nrf2 in response to oxidative and xenobiotic stress (Wakabayashi et al. 2003).

1.3.3 Dietary Phytochemicals Targeting Nrf2/Keap1 Signaling

Isothiocyanates, including sulforaphane (SFN) and phenethyl isothiocyanate (PEITC), are present in cruciferous vegetables such as broccoli, watercress, and cabbage. These sulfur-containing compounds play a critical role in Nrf2/Keap1 signaling. Lin et al. (2008) compared the expression levels of various inflammatory markers to determine the effect of SFN on lipopolysaccharide (LPS)-induced macrophages. Pretreatment of Nrf2$^{+/+}$ macrophages with SFN inhibited LPS-induced messenger RNA (mRNA) expression, protein expression, and the production of tumor necrosis factor

(TNF)-alpha, interleukin (IL)-1β, cyclooxygenase-2 (COX-2), and inducible NO synthase (iNOS), whereas an attenuated anti-inflammatory response was observed in SFN-treated Nrf2$^{-/-}$ macrophages. The expression of HO-1, a detoxifying enzyme downstream of Nrf2, was significantly increased in LPS-induced Nrf2$^{+/+}$ macrophages by SFN. This result led to the conclusion that SFN exerts its anti-inflammatory activity primarily via the activation of Nrf2 in macrophages (Lin et al. 2008). Another isothiocyanate, PEITC, had a synergistic effect with curcumin in xenografted human PC-3 prostate cells. Combined intraperitoneal administration of PEITC and curcumin led to stronger growth-inhibitory effects, compared to PEITC and curcumin treatment alone. Immunohistochemistry and western blot analysis revealed that inhibition of the Akt and NF-κB signaling pathways contribute to the inhibition of cell proliferation and induction of apoptosis observed upon coadministration of PEITC and curcumin (Khor et al. 2006).

Resveratrol (3,4′,5-trihydroxystilbene), a phytoalexin found in the skin and seeds of grapes, has been reported to possess anti-inflammatory, anticarcinogenic, and antioxidant activities. Resveratrol treatment induces HO-1 expression through the transcriptional activation of Nrf2. In addition, PC12 cells treated with resveratrol exhibited transient activation of Akt/protein kinase B and Extracellular signal-regulated kinase (ERK1/2) (Chen et al. 2005). Table 1.1 lists various phytochemicals that regulate the Nrf2 pathway and inflammation.

TABLE 1.1
Chemopreventive Compounds Found in the Diet

Compound	Plant Source	Effects/Molecular Mechanisms	In Vivo Test
Caffeic acid/ chlorogenic acid	Coffee	Caffeic acid–modulated ceramide-induced signal transduction pathway and NF-κB activation via antioxidant and non-antioxidant mechanisms in U937 cells (Nardini et al. 2001). Pretreatment of JB6 cells with chlorogenic acid blocked UVB- or 12-O-tetradecanoylphorbol-13-acetate (TPA)-induced transactivation of AP-1 and NF-κB over the same dose range. Chlorogenic acid decreased the phosphorylation of MAPK was induced by UV-B/TPA (Feng et al. 2005).	
Curcumin	Curcuma longa	Curcumin inhibited NF-κB activation by repressing the degradation of its inhibitory unit, IκBα, which hampers subsequent nuclear translocation of active NF-κB, leading to inhibition of the expression of COX-2 and iNOS (Surh et al. 2001). Curcumin treatment led to decreased expression of NF-κB and COX-2. The tobacco-specific nitrosamine (NNK) is one of the carcinogenic components of smokeless tobacco extract. It was found that curcumin pretreatment abrogates NNK-induced activation of NF-κB and COX-2 expression (Sharma et al. 2006). Curcumin stimulates HO-1 and glutathione S-transferase pi (GSTP1) gene activity by causing dissociation of Nrf2 from Keap1, leading to increased Nrf2 binding to the resident HO-1 AREs in HepG2 cells (Balogun et al. 2003; Nishinaka et al. 2007).	Dietary curcumin caused an increase in Nrf2 protein levels and enhanced its nuclear translocation in the livers and lungs of BaP-treated mice (Garg, Gupta, and Maru 2008).

(continued)

TABLE 1.1 (Continued)
Chemopreventive Compounds Found in the Diet

Compound	Plant Source	Effects/Molecular Mechanisms	In Vivo Test
3,3′-diindolylmethane (DIM)	Cruciferous vegetables	DIM stimulated BRCA1 (breast cancer1) signaling by activating the antioxidant transcription factor Nrf2 in human mammary epithelial cells (Fan et al. 2009).	
(-)-Epogallocatechin gallate (EGCG)	Green tea	EGCG dose-dependently inhibited cell growth and induced apoptosis in A431 cells (Ahmad, Gupta, and Mukhtar 2000). EGCG inhibited COX-2 and iNOS expression by blocking improper activation of NF-κB (Surh et al. 2001). EGCG increased the nuclear accumulation, ARE binding, and transcriptional activity of Nrf2 via activation of PI3K and ERK in MCF10A cells (Na et al. 2008). The activation of AP-1 was attenuated by combined treatment with SFN and EGCG in PC-3 cells (Nair et al. 2010). EGCG abrogated p300-induced p65 acetylation and suppressed TNF-α–induced NF-κB activation, confirming that hyperacetylation is critical for NF-κB translocation and activity (Choi et al. 2009).	Nrf2-dependent gene expression was downregulated (3-fold to 35-fold) after combined administration of EGCG (100 mg/kg) and SFN (45 mg/kg) to Nrf2 knockout mice (Nair et al. 2010).
Genistein	Soy	The BTG3 tumor suppressor gene is epigenetically silenced in renal cell carcinoma but was shown to be reactivated by genistein-induced promoter demethylation and active histone modification in HEK-293 cells (Majid et al. 2009). Genistein treatment increased the acetylation of histones 3, 4, and H3/K4 at the p21 and p16 transcription start sites in LNCaP cells (Majid et al. 2008).	Feeding with genistein-enriched diets (2 g/kg) for more than 3 weeks significantly increased both the hepatic mRNA levels and the activity of NQO1 (Wiegand et al. 2009).
Lycopene	Tomato	Lycopene inhibited the inflammatory response of RAW 264.7 cells to LPS through inhibition of ERK, p38, and the NF-κB pathway (Feng, Ling, and Duan 2010). Activation of Nrf2 by apo-10′-lycopenoic acid, a metabolite of lycopene, induced the expression of phase II detoxifying/antioxidant enzymes including HO-1, NQO1, and GST in BEAS-2B cells (Lian and Wang 2008).	Lycopene caused DU145 cells to accumulate in the G(0)/G(1) phase and to undergo apoptosis in a dose-dependent manner in DU145 tumor xenografts in BALB/c male nude mice (Tang et al. 2005).

(continued)

TABLE 1.1 (Continued)
Chemopreventive Compounds Found in the Diet

Compound	Plant Source	Effects/Molecular Mechanisms	In Vivo Test
PEITC	Cruciferous vegetables	Combined treatment with PEITC and SFN decreased the expression of inflammatory markers, including TNF-α, IL-1, NO, and PGE$_2$. The synergism was most likely due to the synergistic induction of phase II/antioxidant enzymes including HO-1 and NQO1 (Cheung, Khor, and Kong 2009). PEITC induced the expression of HO-1 and increased ARE activity. PEITC also increased the phosphorylation of ERK1/2 and JNK1/2 and caused the release of Nrf2 from sequestration by Keap1 and its subsequent translocation into the nucleus in HepG2 cells (Xu et al. 2006).	A combination of curcumin and PEITC significantly reduced the growth of PC-3 xenografts. PEITC inhibited the Akt and NF-κB signaling pathways, leading to inhibition of proliferation and induction of apoptosis (Khor et al. 2006). Azoxymethane (AOM)/ Dextran sulfate sodium (DSS) mice fed a PEITC- or dopamine-beta-monooxygenase (DBM)-supplemented diet had lower tumor incidences, lower colon tumor multiplicities, and smaller polyps, as compared to mice fed with the standard AIN-76A diet (Cheung et al. 2010).
Resveratrol	Grapes, wine	Pretreatment with resveratrol attenuated hydrogen peroxide-induced cytotoxicity, DNA fragmentation, and intracellular accumulation of ROS via inhibition of the NF-κB pathway in PC12 cells (Jang and Surh 2001). Resveratrol inhibited TNF-α-induced NF-κB activation and inflammatory gene expression and attenuated monocyte adhesion to HCAECs (Csiszar et al. 2006). The treatment of resveratrol caused the release of cytosolic Nrf2, followed by the translocation of Nrf2 into the nucleus, leading to the transcriptional activation of NQO1 (Hsieh et al. 2006).	Resveratrol reduced lung tissue neutrophilia to a similar extent as treatment with budesonide in a rodent model of LPS-induced airway inflammation (Birrell et al. 2005).
SFN	Cruciferous vegetables	SFN and PEITC inhibited NF-κB, as well as expression of the NF-κB target genes VEGF, cyclin D1, and Bcl-X(L); it also decreased nuclear translocation of p65 in PC-3 cells (Xu et al. 2005). SFN reacts with the thiol groups of Keap1 to form thionoacyl adducts (Hong, Freeman, and Liebler 2005).	UV radiation–induced skin carcinogenesis was substantially inhibited by broccoli sprout extracts containing SFN (Dinkova-Kostova et al. 2006). SFN increased the expression of Nrf2-regulated proteins that directly detoxify exogenous toxins/carcinogens or endogenous ROS in Nrf2 knockout mice (Hu et al. 2006).

1.4 INFLAMMATION

The relationship between inflammation and cancer has been highlighted by cancer researchers as an exciting, promising area for exploration that could help to solve this global health concern (Bartsch and Nair 2006; Hussain, Hofseth, and Harris 2003). Approximately 18% of the 10 million new global cases of cancer in 2000 were related to chronic inflammation that was induced by persistent biological, chemical, and physical factors (Parkin 2001). If acute inflammation, the first defensive attempt of our body, fails to remove exogenous stimuli or lasts too long, it can become chronic and may serve as a cause of various diseases (Aggarwal et al. 2006). In chronic inflammation, activated inflammatory/immune cells, such as eosinophiles, dendritic cells, leukocytes, macrophages, mast cells, monocytes, natural killer cells, neutrophils, and phagocytes, release proinflammatory molecules, including cytokines, chemokines, matrix-remodeling proteases, ROS, and RNS, to eliminate pathogens and repair tissue damage. However, various proinflammatory cytokines, chemokines, ROS, and RNS can cause genetic changes or epigenetic alterations, such as DNA methylation and posttranslational modifications, in tumor suppressor genes (Hussain and Harris 2007).

Thus, due to the mechanistic relationship between cancer and inflammation, a better understanding of the molecular mechanisms of chronic inflammation could expand the scope of cancer prevention research. It has been reported that cytokines, NF-κB, iNOS, and COX2 play a pivotal role in inducing cancer (Lu, Ouyang, and Huang 2006).

1.4.1 Anti-Inflammatory Phytochemicals

Epigallocatechin-3-gallate (EGCG) is the most abundant catechin in green tea. Due to its strong antioxidant properties, EGCG is also one of the most widely studied polyphenolic compounds. In human chondrocytes, EGCG inhibited the activation of NF-κB by suppressing the degradation of IκBα in the cytoplasm, leading to reduced induction of iNOS and lower production of NO (Singh et al. 2002). EGCG also inhibited IL-1β-induced NO and prostaglandin E2 (PGE$_2$) production by regulating the expression and catalytic activity of iNOS and COX-2 (Ahmed et al. 2002). EGCG treatment inhibited ultraviolet (UV)-B–induced mitogen-activated protein kinase (MAPK) and NF-κB signaling in normal human epidermal keratinocytes in a dose-dependent manner (Afaq et al. 2003). EGCG not only acts as an anti-inflammatory modulator via effects on the NF-κB pathway but also regulates other anticancer effectors, including p53, Bcl-2, Bax, and the caspases. Lee et al. (2011) treated HT-1080 cells with fluorescein isothiocyanate (FITC)–conjugated EGCG (FITC-EGCG). The time-dependent internalization of FITC-EGCG into the cytosol of HT-1080 cells and its subsequent nuclear translocation were observed. The expression of p53, caspase-7, and caspase-9, as well as the ratio of the Bax/Bcl-2 protein, increased significantly in the EGCG-treated group, suggesting that EGCG may interrupt exogenous signals that are directed toward cancer-related genes (Lee et al. 2011). In fact, various inflammatory modulators are now believed to be connected to other carcinogenic mechanisms, such as apoptosis and metastasis. Various dietary phytochemicals also have multiple effects on these molecular targets. However, this review is focused on inflammation, antioxidant/detoxifying enzymes, and epigenetic modification.

Curcumin is a bright yellow powder present in the rhizome of turmeric (*Curcuma longa* L.) and is used as a food coloring and flavoring. Curcumin is extensively studied for its potential anticancer activity. Chen and Tan (1998) reported that curcumin inhibits the MEKK1-jun N-terminal kinase (JNK) pathway, suggesting a possible mechanism for the suppression of activator protein-1 (AP-1) and NF-κB signaling in various human cell lines. Oral administration of curcumin significantly attenuated histological damage and caused substantial reductions in myeloperoxidase activity and TNF-α. Curcumin also reduced the colonic nitrite levels and downregulated the expression of COX-2 and iNOS by decreasing p38 MAPK in a trinitrobenzenesulfonic acid–induced rat model (Camacho-Barquero et al. 2007). In a phase II trial of curcumin in patients with advanced pancreatic cancer, conjugated forms of curcumin were detected at very low levels in blood vessels. Some patients had tumor regression or stable disease without observed toxicity. In blood mononuclear cells from patients, curcumin decreased the expression of NF-κB, COX-2, and phosphorylated signal transducer and activator of transcription 3 (STAT3). This result demonstrated that oral administration of curcumin is well tolerated and, despite its limited absorption, has biological effects in some pancreatic cancer patients (Dhillon et al. 2008). As shown above, each phytochemical does not affect only one specific molecular target. Although the same compound was used for treatment in each case, numerous linked signaling pathways function in concert, thus leading to various results depending on cell type, dosage, and method of treatment. Various phytochemicals with in vitro and in vivo anti-inflammatory effects are summarized in Table 1.1.

In addition to Nrf2/Keap1, these compounds have multiple other biochemical targets. Interestingly, anti-inflammatory compounds also have significant effects on Nrf2 effects, which suggests that their cytoprotective mechanism is closely related to their anti-inflammatory reactions.

1.5 HORMONE-RELATED CANCERS

Hormone-related cancers, such as breast, uterine, ovary, prostate, thyroid, and osteosarcoma, are thought to share a unique mechanism of carcinogenesis. Both endogenous and exogenous hormones drive cell proliferation and increase the number of cell divisions. This proliferation leads to the increased probability of random genetic errors (Henderson et al. 1982; Henderson and Feigelson 2000). Random errors in DNA occur during cell division, and these mutations can cause a malignant phenotype. The hormonal stimulus for cell division continues in the latter stages of promotion and progression (Henderson et al. 1982; Ross et al. 1998; Henderson, Ross, and Pike 1991). Catechol estrogens (CEs) are the major metabolites of aromatase and estrone (Zhu et al. 1998). If these metabolites are oxidized to the electrophilic CE-quinone (CE-Q), they may react with DNA. In particular, the carcinogenic 4-hydroxyestrone (estradiol) [4-OHE$_1$ (E$_2$)] is oxidized to estrone (estradiol)-3,4-quinone [E$_1$ (E$_2$)-3,4-Q], which can react with DNA to form depurinating adducts (Cavalieri et al. 1997). The release of these adducts generates error-prone apurinic sites that may lead to cancer-initiating mutations. Finally, these mutations can initiate breast, prostate, and other types of cancer (Cavalieri et al. 2006). 17β-Estradiol is regarded as an endogenous tumor promoter, and it interacts with the estrogen receptors ERα and ERβ to stimulate cell growth and increase the risk of hormone-dependent tumors (Yager and Davidson 2006).

Modifying the endogenous levels of circulating hormones is a key therapeutic way to reduce the incidence of hormone-dependent cancers. However, in the absence of changes in exercise, diet, and smoking, the endogenous levels of a hormone are not easy to control. Using antihormonal therapies such as tamoxifen to block the hormonal stimuli that cause DNA damage can lead to a reduction in hormone-dependent cancers. It has been reported that tamoxifen reduces the risk of invasive breast cancer by 49% ($P < .00001$) and noninvasive breast cancer by 50% ($P < .002$) (Fisher et al. 1998). However, while tamoxifen reduces the risk of certain breast cancers and bone fractures, it increases the risk of endometrial cancer (Henderson and Feigelson 2000). Phytoestrogens such as lignans, isoflavones, and flavanones are plant-derived chemicals. Due to their structural homology with estrogens, phytoestrogens can mimic the effects of estrogen. Their estrogen-like activity may contribute to the chemoprotective effects of phytoestrogens by lowering the levels of circulating precursors. In addition, their antioxidant activity may prevent free-radical damage. However, the influence of phytoestrogens on hormone-dependent tumors is still controversial (Rice and Whitehead 2006).

1.6 PERSPECTIVE AND CONCLUSION

An urban lifestyle increases the risks of exposure to various toxins, including environmental pollutants, dietary mutagens, carcinogens, microorganisms, and solar radiation. Inflammation-induced oxidative stress on cellular macromolecules may downregulate the expression of tumor suppressor genes or lead to the transformation and activation of oncogenes (Coussens and Werb 2002; Shu et al. 2010). Preclinical and clinical trials, as well as laboratory research, have provided evidence that dietary phytochemicals have multiple chemopreventive effects during the initiation and progression of cancer. In this chapter, we reviewed promising dietary phytochemicals that possess potential chemopreventive effects on various carcinogenic factors, including inflammation, oxidative stress, chemical carcinogens, and endogenous hormones.

Although the beneficial effects of dietary phytochemicals on human carcinogenesis have been promising, effective, and safe, further studies on these natural dietary compounds will be required. It is necessary to elucidate which molecular targets in the signaling pathways are affected by phyto-chemicals to find more effective and efficient chemoprevention solutions.

The relatively low toxicity, ease of access, and low cost of a diverse number of phytochemicals encourage us to investigate their chemopreventive effects. Daily consumption of fresh vegetables and fruits containing beneficial phytochemicals could be a "quiet but strong" defense system that suppresses or prevents carcinogenesis.

ACKNOWLEDGMENTS

The authors' work cited in this review article was supported in part by institutional funds and by RO1-CA073674, RO1-CA094828, R01-CA118947, and R01-CA152826, which were awarded to Dr. Ah-Ng Tony Kong by the National Institutes of Health (NIH).

REFERENCES

Afaq, F., V. M. Adhami, N. Ahmad, and H. Mukhtar. 2003. Inhibition of ultraviolet B-mediated activation of nuclear factor kappa B in normal human epidermal keratinocytes by green tea Constituent (-)-epigallo-catechin-3-gallate. *Oncogene* 22 (7):1035–1044.

Aggarwal, B. B., S. Shishodia, S. K. Sandur, M. K. Pandey, and G. Sethi. 2006. Inflammation and cancer: How hot is the link? *Biochemical Pharmacology* 72 (11):1605–1621.

Ahmad, N., S. Gupta, and H. Mukhtar. 2000. Green tea polyphenol epigallocatechin-3-gallate differentially modulates nuclear factor kappa B in cancer cells versus normal cells. *Archives of Biochemistry and Biophysics* 376 (2):338–346.

Ahmed, S., A. Rahman, A. Hasnain, M. Lalonde, V. M. Goldberg, and T. M. Haqqi. 2002. Green tea polyphenol epigallocatechin-3-gallate inhibits the IL-1 beta-induced activity and expression of cyclooxygenase-2 and nitric oxide synthase-2 in human chondrocytes. *Free Radical Biology and Medicine* 33 (8):1097–1105.

Alaoui-Jamali, M. A., G. Rossignol, and A. Castonguay. 1991. Protective effects of vitamin A against the geno-toxicity of NNK, a nicotine-derived N-nitrosamine. *Carcinogenesis* 12 (3):379–384.

Arisawa, T., T. Tahara, T. Shibata, M. Nagasaka, M. Nakamura, Y. Kamiya, H. Fujita, S. Hasegawa, T. Takagi, F. Y. Wang, I. Hirata, and H. Nakano. 2007. The relationship between Helicobacter pylori infection and promoter polymorphism of the Nrf2 gene in chronic gastritis. *International Journal of Molecular Medicine* 19 (1):143–148.

Armitage, P. 1985. Multistage models of carcinogenesis. *Environmental Health Perspectives* 63:195–201.

Balogun, E., M. Hoque, P. F. Gong, E. Killeen, C. J. Green, R. Foresti, J. Alam, and R. Motterlini. 2003. Curcurnin activates the haem oxygenase-1 gene via regulation of Nrf2 and the antioxidant-responsive element. *Biochemical Journal* 371:887–895.

Bartsch, H., and J. Nair. 2006. Chronic inflammation and oxidative stress in the genesis and perpetuation of cancer: role of lipid peroxidation, DNA damage, and repair. *Langenbecks Arch Surg* 391 (5):499–510.

Birrell, M. A., K. McCluskie, S. Wong, L. E. Donnelly, P. J. Barnes, and M. G. Belvisi. 2005. Resveratrol, an extract of red wine, inhibits lipopolysaccharide induced airway neutrophilia and inflammatory mediators through an NF-kappaB-independent mechanism. *FASEB Journal* 19 (7):840–841.

Braun, S., C. Hanselmann, M. G. Gassmann, U. auf dem Keller, C. Born-Berclaz, K. Chan, Y. W. Kan, and S. Werner. 2002. Nrf2 transcription factor, a novel target of keratinocyte growth factor action which regulates gene expression and inflammation in the healing skin wound. *Molecular and Cell Biology* 22 (15):5492–5505.

Camacho-Barquero, L., I. Villegas, J. M. Sanchez-Calvo, E. Talero, S. Sanchez-Fidalgo, V. Motilva, and C. A. de la Lastra. 2007. Curcumin, a Curcuma longa constituent, acts on MAPK p38 pathway modulating COX-2 and NOS expression in chronic experimental colitis. *International Immunopharmacology* 7 (3):333–342.

Cataldi, A. 2010. Cell responses to oxidative stressors. *Current Pharmaceutical Design* 16 (12):1387–1395.

Cavalieri, E., D. Chakravarti, J. Guttenplan, E. Hart, J. Ingle, R. Jankowiak, P. Muti, E. Rogan, J. Russo, R. Santen, and T. Sutter. 2006. Catechol estrogen quinones as initiators of breast and other human cancers: implications for biomarkers of susceptibility and cancer prevention. *Biochimica et Biophysica Acta* 1766 (1):63–78.

Cavalieri, E. L., D. E. Stack, P. D. Devanesan, R. Todorovic, I. Dwivedy, S. Higginbotham, S. L. Johansson, K. D. Patil, M. L. Gross, J. K. Gooden, R. Ramanathan, R. L. Cerny, and E. G. Rogan. 1997. Molecular origin of cancer: catechol estrogen-3,4-quinones as endogenous tumor initiators. *Proceedings of the National Academy of Sciences of the United States of America* 94 (20):10937–10942.

Chen, C.-Y., J.-H. Jang, M.-H. Li, and Y.-J. Surh. 2005. Resveratrol upregulates heme oxygenase-1 expression via activation of NF-E2-related factor 2 in PC12 cells. *Biochemical and Biophysical Research Communications* 331 (4):993–1000.

Chen, Y. R., and T. H. Tan. 1998. Inhibition of the c-Jun N-terminal kinase (JNK) signaling pathway by curcumin. *Oncogene* 17 (2):173–178.

Cheung, K. L., T. O. Khor, M. T. Huang, and A. N. Kong. 2010. Differential in vivo mechanism of chemoprevention of tumor formation in azoxymethane/dextran sodium sulfate mice by PEITC and DBM. *Carcinogenesis* 31 (5):880–885.

Cheung, K. L., T. O. Khor, and A. N. Kong. 2009. Synergistic effect of combination of phenethyl isothiocyanate and sulforaphane or curcumin and sulforaphane in the inhibition of inflammation. *Pharmaceutical Research* 26 (1):224–231.

Choi, K. C., M. G. Jung, Y. H. Lee, J. C. Yoon, S. H. Kwon, H. B. Kang, M. J. Kim, J. H. Cha, Y. J. Kim, W. J. Jun, J. M. Lee, and H. G. Yoon. 2009. Epigallocatechin-3-gallate, a histone acetyltransferase inhibitor, inhibits EBV-induced B lymphocyte transformation via suppression of RelA acetylation. *Cancer Research* 69 (2):583–592.

Coussens, L. M., and Z. Werb. 2002. Inflammation and cancer. *Nature* 420 (6917):860–867.

Csiszar, A., K. Smith, N. Labinskyy, Z. Orosz, A. Rivera, and Z. Ungvari. 2006. Resveratrol attenuates TNF-alpha-induced activation of coronary arterial endothelial cells: role of NF-kB inhibition. *American Journal of Physiology-Heart and Circulatory Physiology* 291 (4):H1694–H1699.

Danielson, P. B. 2002. The cytochrome P450 superfamily: biochemistry, evolution and drug metabolism in humans. *Current Drug Metabolism* 3 (6):561–597.

Dashwood, R. H. 2002. Modulation of heterocyclic amine-induced mutagenicity and carcinogenicity: an 'A-to-Z' guide to chemopreventive agents, promoters, and transgenic models. *Mutation Research* 511 (2):89–112.

Dhillon, N., B. B. Aggarwal, R. A. Newman, R. A. Wolf, A. B. Kunnumakkara, J. L. Abbruzzese, C. S. Ng, V. Badmaev, and R. Kurzrock. 2008. Phase II trial of curcumin in patients with advanced pancreatic cancer. *Clinical Cancer Research* 14 (14):4491–4499.

Dinkova-Kostova, A. T., S. N. Jenkins, J. W. Fahey, L. Ye, S. L. Wehage, K. T. Liby, K. K. Stephenson, K. L. Wade, and P. Talalay. 2006. Protection against UV-light-induced skin carcinogenesis in SKH-1 high-risk mice by sulforaphane-containing broccoli sprout extracts. *Cancer Letters* 240 (2):243–252.

Doll, R., and R. Peto. 1981. The causes of cancer: quantitative estimates of avoidable risks of cancer in the United States today. *Journal of the National Cancer Institute* 66 (6):1191–1308.

Emerit, J., M. Edeas, and F. Bricaire. 2004. Neurodegenerative diseases and oxidative stress. *Biomedicine and Pharmacotherapy* 58 (1):39–46.

Fan, S., Q. Meng, T. Saha, F. H. Sarkar, and E. M. Rosen. 2009. Low concentrations of diindolylmethane, a metabolite of indole-3-carbinol, protect against oxidative stress in a BRCA1-dependent manner. *Cancer Research* 69 (15):6083–6091.

Feng, D., W.-H. Ling, and R.-D. Duan. 2010. Lycopene suppresses LPS-induced NO and IL-6 production by inhibiting the activation of ERK, p38MAPK, and NF-κB in macrophages. *Inflammation Research* 59 (2):115–121.

Feng, R., Y. Lu, L. L. Bowman, Y. Qian, V. Castranova, and M. Ding. 2005. Inhibition of activator protein-1, NF-κB, and MAPKs and induction of phase 2 detoxifying enzyme activity by chlorogenic acid. *Journal of Biological Chemistry* 280 (30):27888–27895.

Fisher, B., J. P. Costantino, D. L. Wickerham, C. K. Redmond, M. Kavanah, W. M. Cronin, V. Vogel, A. Robidoux, N. Dimitrov, J. Atkins, M. Daly, S. Wieand, E. Tan-Chiu, L. Ford, and N. Wolmark. 1998. Tamoxifen for prevention of breast cancer: report of the National Surgical Adjuvant Breast and Bowel Project P-1 Study. *Journal of the National Cancer Institute* 90 (18):1371–1388.

Garg, R., S. Gupta, and G. B. Maru. 2008. Dietary curcumin modulates transcriptional regulators of phase I and phase II enzymes in benzo pyrene-treated mice: mechanism of its anti-initiating action. *Carcinogenesis* 29 (5):1022–1032.

Giovannucci, E. 1999. Tomatoes, tomato-based products, lycopene, and cancer: review of the epidemiologic literature. *Journal of the National Cancer Institute* 91 (4):317–331.

Gomaa, E. A., J. I. Gray, S. Rabie, C. Lopez-Bote, and A. M. Booren. 1993. Polycyclic aromatic hydrocarbons in smoked food products and commercial liquid smoke flavourings. *Food Additives and Contaminants* 10 (5):503–521.

Gonzalez, F. J., and H. V. Gelboin. 1994. Role of human cytochromes P450 in the metabolic activation of chemical carcinogens and toxins. *Drug Metabolism Reviews* 26 (1–2):165–183.

Guengerich, F. P. 1992. Metabolic activation of carcinogens. *Pharmacology and Therapeutics* 54 (1):17–61.

Hanahan, D., and R. A. Weinberg. 2000. The hallmarks of cancer. *Cell* 100 (1):57–70.

Henderson, B. E., and H. S. Feigelson. 2000. Hormonal carcinogenesis. *Carcinogenesis* 21 (3):427–433.

Henderson, B. E., R. K. Ross, and M. C. Pike. 1991. Toward the primary prevention of cancer. *Science* 254 (5035):1131–1118.

Henderson, B. E., R. K. Ross, M. C. Pike, and J. T. Casagrande. 1982. Endogenous hormones as a major factor in human cancer. *Cancer Research* 42 (8):3232–3239.

Hoelzl, C., H. Glatt, W. Meinl, G. Sontag, G. Haidinger, M. Kundi, T. Simic, A. Chakraborty, J. Bichler, F. Ferk, K. Angelis, A. Nersesyan, and S. Knasmuller. 2008. Consumption of Brussels sprouts protects peripheral human lymphocytes against 2-amino-1-methyl-6-phenylimidazo[4,5-b]pyridine (PhIP) and oxidative DNA-damage: results of a controlled human intervention trial. *Mol Nutr Food Res* 52 (3):330–341.

Hong, F., M. L. Freeman, and D. C. Liebler. 2005. Identification of sensor cysteines in human Keap1 modified by the cancer chemopreventive agent sulforaphane. *Chemical Research in Toxicology* 18 (12):1917–1926.

Hsieh, T. C., X. Lu, Z. Wang, and J. M. Wu. 2006. Induction of quinone reductase NQO1 by resveratrol in human K562 cells involves the antioxidant response element ARE and is accompanied by nuclear translocation of transcription factor Nrf2. *Medicinal Chemistry* 2 (3):275–285.

Hu, R., C. J. Xu, G. X. Shen, M. R. Jain, T. O. Khor, A. Gopalkrishnan, W. Lin, B. Reddy, J. Y. Chan, and A. N. T. Kong. 2006. Gene expression profiles induced by cancer chemopreventive isothiocyanate sulforaphane in the liver of C57BL/6J mice and C57BL/6J/Nrf2 (−/−) mice. *Cancer Letters* 243 (2):170–192.

Hussain, S. P., and C. C. Harris. 2007. Inflammation and cancer: an ancient link with novel potentials. *International Journal of Cancer* 121 (11):2373–2380.

Hussain, S. P., L. J. Hofseth, and C. C. Harris. 2003. Radical causes of cancer. *Nature Reviews Cancer* 3 (4):276–285.

Itoh, K., T. Chiba, S. Takahashi, T. Ishii, K. Igarashi, Y. Katoh, T. Oyake, N. Hayashi, K. Satoh, I. Hatayama, M. Yamamoto, and Y. Nabeshima. 1997. An Nrf2/small Maf heterodimer mediates the induction of phase II detoxifying enzyme genes through antioxidant response elements. *Biochemical and Biophysical Research Communications* 236 (2):313–322.

Jagerstad, M., K. Skog, S. Grivas, and K. Olsson. 1991. Formation of heterocyclic amines using model systems. *Mutation Research* 259 (3–4):219–233.

Jang, J. H., and Y. J. Surh. 2001. Protective effects of resveratrol on hydrogen peroxide-induced apoptosis in rat pheochromocytoma (PC12) cells. *Mutation Research—Genetic Toxicology and Environmental Mutagenesis* 496 (1–2):181–190.

Jemal, A., R. Siegel, E. Ward, Y. Hao, J. Xu, and M. J. Thun. 2009. Cancer Statistics, 2009. *CA: A Cancer Journal for Clinicians* 59 (4):225–249.

Jeong, W. S., M. Jun, and A. N. Kong. 2006. Nrf2: a potential molecular target for cancer chemoprevention by natural compounds. *Antioxidants and Redox Signaling* 8 (1–2):99–106.

Jernstrom, B., M. Funk, H. Frank, B. Mannervik, and A. Seidel. 1996. Glutathione S-transferase A1-1-catalysed conjugation of bay and fjord region diol epoxides or polycyclic aromatic hydrocarbons with glutathione. *Carcinogenesis* 17 (7):1491–1498.

Khor, T. O., Y. S. Keum, W. Lin, J. H. Kim, R. Hu, G. Shen, C. Xu, A. Gopalakrishnan, B. Reddy, X. Zheng, A. H. Conney, and A. N. Kong. 2006. Combined inhibitory effects of curcumin and phenethyl isothiocyanate on the growth of human PC-3 prostate xenografts in immunodeficient mice. *Cancer Research* 66 (2):613–621.

Knasmuller, S., D. M. DeMarini, I. Johnson, and C. Gerhauser, eds. 2009. *Chemoprevention of Cancer and DNA Damage by Dietary Factors*. Wiley-Blackwell.

Knize, M. G., K. S. Kulp, C. P. Salmon, G. A. Keating, and J. S. Felton. 2002. Factors affecting human heterocyclic amine intake and the metabolism of PhIP. *Mutation Research* 506–507:153–162.

Lee, M., D.-W. Han, S.-H. Hyon, and J.-C. Park. 2011. Apoptosis of human fibrosarcoma HT-1080 cells by epigallocatechin-3-O-gallate via induction of p53 and caspases as well as suppression of Bcl-2 and phosphorylated nuclear factor-κB. *Apoptosis* 16 (1):75–85.

Li, L. C., P. R. Carroll, and R. Dahiya. 2005. Epigenetic changes in prostate cancer: Implication for diagnosis and treatment. *Journal of the National Cancer Institute* 97 (2):103–115.

Lian, F., and X. D. Wang. 2008. Enzymatic metabolites of lycopene induce Nrf2-mediated expression of phase II detoxifying/antioxidant enzymes in human bronchial epithelial cells. *International Journal of Cancer* 123 (6):1262–1268.

Lin, W., R. T. Wu, T. Wu, T.-O. Khor, H. Wang, and A.-N. Kong. 2008. Sulforaphane suppressed LPS-induced inflammation in mouse peritoneal macrophages through Nrf2 dependent pathway. *Biochemical Pharmacology* 76 (8):967–973.

Lu, H., W. Ouyang, and C. Huang. 2006. Inflammation, a key event in cancer development. *Molecular Cancer Research* 4 (4):221–233.

Maheo, K., F. Morel, S. Langouet, H. Kramer, E. Le Ferrec, B. Ketterer, and A. Guillouzo. 1997. Inhibition of cytochromes P-450 and induction of glutathione S-transferases by sulforaphane in primary human and rat hepatocytes. *Cancer Research* 57 (17):3649–3652.

Majid, S., A. A. Dar, A. E. Ahmad, H. Hirata, K. Kawakami, V. Shahryari, S. Saini, Y. Tanaka, A. V. Dahiya, G. Khatri, and R. Dahiya. 2009. BTG3 tumor suppressor gene promoter demethylation, histone modification and cell cycle arrest by genistein in renal cancer. *Carcinogenesis* 30 (4):662–670.

Majid, S., N. Kikuno, J. Nelles, E. Noonan, Y. Tanaka, K. Kawamoto, H. Hirata, L. C. Li, H. Zhao, S. T. Okino, R. F. Place, D. Pookot, and R. Dahiya. 2008. Genistein induces the p21WAF1/CIP1 and p16INK4a tumor suppressor genes in prostate cancer cells by epigenetic mechanisms involving active chromatin modification. *Cancer Research* 68 (8):2736–2744.

Meador, J. P., J. E. Stein, W. L. Reichert, and U. Varanasi. 1995. Bioaccumulation of polycyclic aromatic hydrocarbons by marine organisms. *Reviews of Environmental Contamination and Toxicology* 143:79–165.

Moolgavkar, S. H. 1978. The multistage theory of carcinogenesis and the age distribution of cancer in man. *Journal of the National Cancer Institute* 61 (1):49–52.

Na, H.-K., E.-H. Kim, J.-H. Jung, H.-H. Lee, J.-W. Hyun, and Y.-J. Surh. 2008. (-)-Epigallocatechin gallate induces Nrf2-mediated antioxidant enzyme expression via activation of PI3K and ERK in human mammary epithelial cells. *Archives of Biochemistry and Biophysics* 476 (2):171–177.

Nair, S., A. Barve, T.-O. Khor, G.-X. Shen, W. Lin, J. Y. Chan, L. Cai, and A.-N. Kong. 2010. Regulation of Nrf2- and AP-1-mediated gene expression by epigallocatechin-3-gallate and sulforaphane in prostate of Nrf2-knockout or C57BL/6J mice and PC-3 AP-1 human prostate cancer cells. *Acta Pharmacologica Sinica* 31 (9):1223–1240.

Nakai, Y., W. G. Nelson, and A. M. De Marzo. 2007. The dietary charred meat carcinogen 2-amino-1-methyl-6-phenylimidazo[4,5-b]pyridine acts as both a tumor initiator and promoter in the rat ventral prostate. *Cancer Research* 67 (3):1378–1384.

Nardini, M., F. Leonardi, C. Scaccini, and F. Virgili. 2001. Modulation of ceramide-induced NF-kappa B binding activity and apoptotic response by caffeic acid in U937 cells: Comparison with other antioxidants. *Free Radical Biology and Medicine* 30 (7):722–733.

Nishinaka, T., Y. Ichijo, M. Ito, M. Kimura, M. Katsuyama, K. Iwata, T. Miura, T. Terada, and C. Yabe-Nishimura. 2007. Curcumin activates human glutathione S-transferase P1 expression through antioxidant response element. *Toxicology Letters* 170 (3):238–247.

Nouso, K., S. S. Thorgeirsson, and N. Battula. 1992. Stable expression of human cytochrome P450IIE1 in mammalian cells: metabolic activation of nitrosodimethylamine and formation of adducts with cellular DNA. *Cancer Research* 52 (7):1796–1800.

Parkin, D. M. 2001. Global cancer statistics in the year 2000. *Lancet Oncology* 2 (9):533–543.

Paul, G., F. Bataille, F. Obermeier, J. Bock, F. Klebl, U. Strauch, D. Lochbaum, P. Rummele, S. Farkas, J. Scholmerich, M. Fleck, G. Rogler, and H. Herfarth. 2005. Analysis of intestinal haem-oxygenase-1 (HO-1) in clinical and experimental colitis. *Clinical and Experimental Immunology* 140 (3):547–555.

Phillips, D. H. 1999. Polycyclic aromatic hydrocarbons in the diet. *Mutation Research* 443 (1–2):139–147.

Phillips, D. H. 1983. Fifty years of benzo(a)pyrene. *Nature* 303 (5917):468–472.

Pool-Zobel, B., S. Veeriah, and F. D. Bohmer. 2005. Modulation of xenobiotic metabolising enzymes by anticarcinogens—focus on glutathione S-transferases and their role as targets of dietary chemoprevention in colorectal carcinogenesis. *Mutation Research* 591 (1–2):74–92.

Poyton, R. O., K. A. Ball, and P. R. Castello. 2009. Mitochondrial generation of free radicals and hypoxic signaling. *Trends in Endocrinology and Metabolism* 20 (7):332–340.

Ramos-Gomez, M., M. K. Kwak, P. M. Dolan, K. Itoh, M. Yamamoto, P. Talalay, and T. W. Kensler. 2001. Sensitivity to carcinogenesis is increased and chemoprotective efficacy of enzyme inducers is lost in nrf2 transcription factor-deficient mice. *Proceedings of the National Academy of Sciences of the United States of America* 98 (6):3410–3415.

Reuter, S., S. C. Gupta, M. M. Chaturvedi, and B. B. Aggarwal. 2010. Oxidative stress, inflammation, and cancer How are they linked? *Free Radical Biology and Medicine* 49 (11):1603–1616.

Rice, S., and S. A. Whitehead. 2006. Phytoestrogens and breast cancer—promoters or protectors? *Endocrine-Related Cancer* 13 (4):995–1015.

Ross, R. K., M. C. Pike, G. A. Coetzee, J. K. Reichardt, M. C. Yu, H. Feigelson, F. Z. Stanczyk, L. N. Kolonel, and B. E. Henderson. 1998. Androgen metabolism and prostate cancer: establishing a model of genetic susceptibility. *Cancer Research* 58 (20):4497–4504.

Rustemeier, K., R. Stabbert, H. J. Haussmann, E. Roemer, and E. L. Carmines. 2002. Evaluation of the potential effects of ingredients added to cigarettes. Part 2: Chemical composition of mainstream smoke. *Food and Chemical Toxicology* 40 (1):93–104.

Sharma, C., J. Kaur, S. Shishodia, B. B. Aggarwal, and R. Ralhan. 2006. Curcumin down regulates smokeless tobacco-induced NF-kappa B activation and COX-2 expression in human oral premalignant and cancer cells. *Toxicology* 228 (1):1–15.

Shimada, T., C. L. Hayes, H. Yamazaki, S. Amin, S. S. Hecht, F. P. Guengerich, and T. R. Sutter. 1996. Activation of chemically diverse procarcinogens by human cytochrome P-450 1B1. *Cancer Research* 56 (13):2979–2984.

Shu, L., K.-L. Cheung, T. Khor, C. Chen, and A.-N. Kong. 2010. Phytochemicals: cancer chemoprevention and suppression of tumor onset and metastasis. *Cancer and Metastasis Reviews* 29 (3):483–502.

Singh, R., S. Ahmed, N. Islam, V. M. Goldberg, and T. M. Haqqi. 2002. Epigallocatechin-3-gallate inhibits interleukin-1 beta-induced expression of nitric oxide synthase and production of nitric oxide in human chondrocytes—suppression of nuclear factor kappa B activation by degradation of the inhibitor of nuclear factor kappa B. *Arthritis and Rheumatism* 46 (8):2079–2086.

Skog, K. I., M. A. Johansson, and M. I. Jagerstad. 1998. Carcinogenic heterocyclic amines in model systems and cooked foods: a review on formation, occurrence and intake. *Food and Chemical Toxicology* 36 (9–10):879–896.

Sugimura, T., K. Wakabayashi, H. Nakagama, and M. Nagao. 2004. Heterocyclic amines: Mutagens/carcinogens produced during cooking of meat and fish. *Cancer Science* 95 (4):290–299.

Surh, Y. J., K. S. Chun, H. H. Cha, S. S. Han, Y. S. Keum, K. K. Park, and S. S. Lee. 2001. Molecular mechanisms underlying chemopreventive activities of anti-inflammatory phytochemicals: Down-regulation of COX-2 and iNOS through suppression of NF-kappa B activation. *Mutation Research—Fundamental and Molecular Mechanisms of Mutagenesis* 480:243–268.

Surh, Y.-J. 2003. Cancer chemoprevention with dietary phytochemicals. *Nature Reviews Cancer* 3 (10):768–780.

Talalay, P. 2000. Chemoprotection against cancer by induction of phase 2 enzymes. *Biofactors* 12 (1–4):5–11.

Tang, L. L., T. Y. Jin, X. B. Zeng, and J. S. Wang. 2005. Lycopene inhibits the growth of human androgen-independent prostate cancer cells in vitro and in BALB/c nude mice. *Journal of Nutrition* 135 (2):287–290.

Thomasset, S. C., D. P. Berry, G. Garcea, T. Marczylo, W. P. Steward, and A. J. Gescher. 2007. Dietary polyphenolic phytochemicals—promising cancer chemopreventive agents in humans? A review of their clinical properties. *International Journal of Cancer* 120 (3):451–458.

Tricker, A. R., and R. Preussmann. 1991. Carcinogenic N-nitrosamines in the diet: occurrence, formation, mechanisms and carcinogenic potential. *Mutation Research* 259 (3–4):277–289.

Valko, M., D. Leibfritz, J. Moncol, M. T. D. Cronin, M. Mazur, and J. Telser. 2007. Free radicals and antioxidants in normal physiological functions and human disease. *International Journal of Biochemistry & Cell Biology* 39 (1):44–84.

Wakabayashi, N., K. Itoh, J. Wakabayashi, H. Motohashi, S. Noda, S. Takahashi, S. Imakado, T. Kotsuji, F. Otsuka, D. R. Roop, T. Harada, J. D. Engel, and M. Yamamoto. 2003. Keap1-null mutation leads to postnatal lethality due to constitutive Nrf2 activation. *Nature Genetics* 35 (3):238–245.

Wattenberg, L. W. 1992. Inhibition of carcinogenesis by minor dietary constituents. *Cancer Research* 52 (7 Suppl):2085s–2091s.

Wattenberg, L. W. 1985. Chemoprevention of Cancer. *Cancer Research* 45 (1):1–8.

Wattenberg, L. W. 1977. Inhibition of carcinogenic effects of polycyclic hydrocarbons by benzyl isothiocyanate and related compounds. *Journal of the National Cancer Institute* 58 (2):395–398.

Wattenberg, L. W. 1966. Chemoprophylaxis of carcinogenesis: a review. *Cancer Research* 26 (7):1520–1526.

WHO, World Health Organization. 2011. *The 10 Leading Causes of Death by Broad Income Group (2008).* http://www.who.int/mediacentre/factsheets/fs310/en/

Wiegand, H., A. E. Wagner, C. Boesch-Saadatmandi, H. P. Kruse, S. Kulling, and G. Rimbach. 2009. Effect of dietary genistein on Phase II and antioxidant enzymes in rat liver. *Cancer Genomics Proteomics* 6 (2):85–92.

Williams, G. M. 1977. Detection of chemical carcinogens by unscheduled DNA synthesis in rat liver primary cell cultures. *Cancer Research* 37 (6):1845–1851.

Wogan, G. N., S. S. Hecht, J. S. Felton, A. H. Conney, and L. A. Loeb. 2004. Environmental and chemical carcinogenesis. *Seminars in Cancer Biology* 14 (6):473–486.

Wu, Y. N., H. Z. Wang, J. S. Li, and C. Han. 1993. The inhibitory effect of Chinese tea and its polyphenols on in vitro and in vivo N-nitrosation. *Biomedical and Environmental Sciences* 6 (3):237–258.

Xu, C., G. Shen, C. Chen, C. Gelinas, and A. N. Kong. 2005. Suppression of NF-kappaB and NF-kappaB-regulated gene expression by sulforaphane and PEITC through IkappaBalpha, IKK pathway in human prostate cancer PC-3 cells. *Oncogene* 24 (28):4486–4495.

Xu, C., X. Yuan, Z. Pan, G. Shen, J. H. Kim, S. Yu, T. O. Khor, W. Li, J. Ma, and A. N. Kong. 2006. Mechanism of action of isothiocyanates: The induction of ARE-regulated genes is associated with activation of ERK and JNK and the phosphorylation and nuclear translocation of Nrf2. *Molecular Cancer Therapeutics* 5 (8):1918–1926.

Xu, J., K. D. Kochanek, S. L. Murphy, B. Tejada-Vera. 2010. *Deaths: Final Data for 2007. National Vital Statistics Reports*, vol 58 no 19. Hyattsville, MD: National Center for Health Statistics.

Yager, J. D., and N. E. Davidson. 2006. Estrogen carcinogenesis in breast cancer. *New England Journal of Medicine* 354 (3):270–282.

Yang, Chung S., Jeong-Sook H. Yoo, Hiroyuki Ishizaki, and Junyan Hong. 1990. Cytochrome P450IIe1: Roles in nitrosamine metabolism and mechanisms of regulation. *Drug Metabolism Reviews* 22 (2–3):147–159.

Zhang, Y., and P. Talalay. 1994. Anticarcinogenic activities of organic isothiocyanates: chemistry and mechanisms. *Cancer Research* 54 (7 Suppl):1976s–1981s.

Zhao, Y., Y. Xue, T. D. Oberley, K. K. Kiningham, S. M. Lin, H. C. Yen, H. Majima, J. Hines, and D. St Clair. 2001. Overexpression of manganese superoxide dismutase suppresses tumor formation by modulation of activator protein-1 signaling in a multistage skin carcinogenesis model. *Cancer Research* 61 (16):6082–6088.

Zhu, B. T., D. P. Loder, M. X. Cai, C. T. Ho, M. T. Huang, and A. H. Conney. 1998. Dietary administration of an extract from rosemary leaves enhances the liver microsomal metabolism of endogenous estrogens and decreases their uterotropic action in CD-1 mice. *Carcinogenesis* 19 (10):1821–1827.

2 Overview of Obesity, Inflammation, and Cancer

Ximena Paredes-Gonzalez, Tin Oo Khor, Limin Shu, Constance Lay-Lay Saw, and Ah-Ng Tony Kong

CONTENTS

2.1 INTRODUCTION

Obesity has reached epidemic proportions and is recognized as a major cause of cancer worldwide (World Health Organization 2000, 2011). Obesity can be defined as an excess of body adiposity, which is evaluated according to the body weight. The body mass index (BMI) correlates weight and height (BMI = weight in kilograms divided by the square of the height in meters [kg/m^2]), and since 1980, BMI has been considered the standard measure for evaluating whether a person is obese. In general, an individual with a BMI between 25 and 30 is classified as overweight or pre-obese, while an individual with a BMI over 30 is classified as obese; different intervals are established according to the mortality risk (Table 2.1) (Caballero 2007; World Health Organization 2000).

Although data from the United States indicate that the incidence of obesity is increasing slowly or leveling off when compared to the past decade (Flegal et al. 2010, 2012), more than 1 billion people worldwide are overweight or obese (Deitel 2003). It has been estimated that 14% and 20% of all cancer deaths in men and women, respectively, can be attributed to excess body weight (Calle et al. 2003, 2004; Wolin et al. 2010). Obesity is associated with some types of cancer (Simard et al. 2012), such as colon, breast (postmenopausal), endometrial, kidney (renal cell), esophageal (adeno-carcinoma), pancreatic, colorectal, and, potentially, gall bladder carcinoma (Wiseman 2008; Vainio et al. 2002). In addition, a prospective study published in 2003 that considered more than 900,000

TABLE 2.1

International Classification of Underweight, Overweight, and Obese Adults According to BMI

Classification	BMI
Underweight	<18.50
Normal range	18.50–24.99
Overweight	≥25.00
Pre-obese	25.00–29.99
Obese	≥30.00
Class I	30.00–34.99
Class II	35.00–39.99
Class III	≥40.00

Sources: WHO, *Physical status: the use and interpretation of anthropometry, Report of a WHO Expert Committee. WHO Technical Report Series 854.* Geneva: World Health Organization, 1995. http://whqlibdoc. who.int/trs/WHO_TRS_854.pdf; World Health Organization. *Obesity: preventing and managing the global epidemic: report of a WHO consultation, WHO technical report series,* Geneva: World Health Organization, 2000, http://whqlibdoc.who.int/trs/WHO_TRS_894. pdf, WHO Expert Consultation, Appropriate body-mass index for Asian populations and its implications for policy and intervention strategies, *The Lancet* 157–163, 2004, http://www.ncbi.nlm.nih.gov/ pubmed/14726171?dopt=Abstract.

US adults found that non-Hodgkin's lymphoma, prostate cancer, and multiple myeloma are also associated with obesity (Calle et al. 2003).

If obesity can be controlled, the incidence and mortality of obesity-associated cancers may be reduced significantly with weight loss (Sedjo et al. 2007). The American Cancer Society (ACS) Board of Directors has proposed the ambitious and challenging goal of reducing cancer mortality by 50% and cancer incidence by 25% by the year 2015 (Byers et al. 1999; ACS 1996, 1998). Moreover, a better understanding of the relationship between cancer and obesity, beyond epidemiology and basic research, may lead to the development of new targeted therapies to prevent obesity-related cancers.

2.2   OBESITY AND CANCER RISK

An association between obesity and cancer was clearly observed in an experimental setting as early as the 1940–1950s, when overfed animals exhibited a higher incidence of neoplasia (Finkel et al. 1955). In 1949, Waxler and Brecher developed a novel obese murine model by injecting mice with a single dose of gold thioglucose, and in 1953, Waxler reported that these obese mice developed spontaneous mammary tumors earlier than nonobese controls (Brecher et al. 1949; Waxler et al. 1953). Lew and Garfinkel in 1979 published the first significant epidemiological evidence that excessive weight or obesity increases the risk of mortality from cancer (Lew et al. 1979). Since then, experimental and clinical studies have yielded a vast amount of information.

A meta-analysis of data from prospective studies published between 1966 and 1997 for six cancer types (breast, colon, endometrial, prostate, kidney, and gallbladder) reported that 3% and 6% of the attributable risks for men and women, respectively, were caused by excessive body mass (Bergstrom et al. 2001b). Other studies that included more types of cancers have confirmed these findings and reported a higher population-attributable risk in women (Renehan et al. 2008, 2010). In addition, for all cancers combined, the male and female populations with the highest BMI values (class III) have death rates that are 52% and 62% higher, respectively, than those of populations with normal weight (Calle et al. 2003). Therefore, it is now well established that being overweight or obese increases the risk of developing and dying from cancer (Calle et al. 1999, 2003; Berrington de Gonzalez et al. 2010; Lee et al. 2010; Parr et al. 2010; Samanic et al. 2004). A 5 kg/m² increase in BMI is significantly associated with esophageal adenocarcinoma in both sexes; thyroid, colon, and renal cancers in men; and endometrial, gallbladder, and renal cancers in women (Renehan et al. 2008).

Furthermore, it is not surprising that losing weight can reduce the probability of developing cancer; thus, gastric bypass has been found to decrease cancer risk by 24% and the risk of death from cancer by 46% (Adams et al. 2009). Interestingly, this impact is especially significant in women, for whom surgery decreases the overall risk of cancer by 42% (Sjostrom et al. 2009), with a large impact on breast and endometrial cancers (Ashrafian et al. 2011). As mentioned previously, weight gain has a larger effect on female cancer development than male cancer development; moreover, the Million Women Study developed in the United Kingdom, which included a 5.4-year follow-up for cancer incidence and a 7-year follow-up for cancer mortality, revealed a significant increase in cancer incidence and mortality risks with increasing BMI for 10 of 17 cancers that were examined in women 50 years of age or older (Reeves et al. 2007).

2.2.1 Breast Cancer

Although breast cancer incidence rates in the United States were stable in 2004–2008 (DeSantis et al. 2011), breast cancer still represents the most common cause of death among Hispanic women and the second most common cause of death among white, black, Asian/Pacific Islander, and American Indian/Alaska Native women (US Cancer Statistics 2010), with different epidemiological traits in premenopausal and postmenopausal women (Smigal et al. 2006; DeSantis et al. 2011). Obese women have an increased risk of cancer (Parker et al. 2003; Singh et al. 2011; Chlebowski 2012) and a poorer survival prognosis than lean women (Protani et al. 2010; Ewertz et al. 2011; Goodwin et al. 2002, 2012). Obesity has been associated with an increased risk of postmenopausal breast cancer (Renehan et al. 2008; Key et al. 2003; La Vecchia et al. 2011), but the effect of obesity on premenopausal women is controversial because some studies have demonstrated a negative relationship (Renehan et al. 2008; Fagherazzi et al. 2012; Michels et al. 2012; Vrieling et al. 2010; Baer et al. 2010).

Women older than 50 years of age, who are usually postmenopausal, constitute the majority of breast cancer diagnoses; until recently, the incidence of breast cancer has followed an increasing trend in this group. Among postmenopausal women, nulliparity and obesity are associated with a higher risk of breast cancer incidence and mortality, particularly in non–hormone therapy users (Ogden et al. 2006). Obesity has been associated with the production of increased levels of estrogen in adipose tissue (Cleary et al. 2009), which is positively correlated with tumors that express estrogen hormone receptors (ERs) and progesterone (PG) hormone receptors (Yang et al. 2011; Esfahlan et al. 2011).

In premenopausal women, who constitute approximately 35% of breast cancer diagnoses (Howlader 2011), the risk of breast cancer is more likely to be associated with genetic predisposition (Singletary 2003), and the effects of obesity are unclear. Nevertheless, epidemiological data from the Iowa Women's Health Study have suggested that weight gain between 18 years of age and menopause is consistently associated with a higher risk of developing breast cancer after menopause (Harvie et al. 2005), particularly hormone receptor–sensitive breast cancer (Suzuki et al. 2011). In addition, breast cancer survival may be reduced in premenopausal women (Abrahamson et al. 2006).

The relationship between obesity and breast cancer risk varies among different races and ethnicities. Some studies have shown that obesity plays an important role in breast cancer in Caucasian women but may not have an influence in Hispanic women (Sarkissyan et al. 2011; Abdel-Maksoud et al. 2012). In Hispanic women, breast cancer is increasingly diagnosed at a younger age, with a more advanced stage at diagnosis and worse prognosis than for non-Hispanic whites. In addition, this group is more likely to have estrogen receptor–negative tumors (Abdel-Maksoud et al.

2012). However, it remains unclear whether obesity plays a role in this trend. In African-American women, the link between obesity and cancer risk is controversial; despite higher rates of obesity, BMI differences do not explain the reduced breast cancer survival in this group (Eley et al. 1994; McCullough et al. 2005; Chlebowski et al. 2005). A recent case–control study found an important role for obesity in influencing adverse outcomes (development of distant metastases and death from breast cancer) in white but not black women with breast cancer (Lu et al. 2011). In Asian women, a stronger association between obesity and breast cancer has been observed for both postmenopausal and premenopausal women (Renehan et al. 2008; Parr et al. 2010).

2.2.2 Endometrial and Colorectal Cancers

Excess weight and obesity increase the risk of endometrial cancer by more than 40% (Renehan et al. 2008, 2010; Olsen et al. 2007) and are associated with a poor prognosis (Calle et al. 2003; von Gruenigen et al. 2006). There appears to be a linear weight–risk relationship between increased BMI and endometrial cancer risk (Schouten et al. 2004). This association appears to be independent of menopausal status but has a stronger effect in postmenopausal woman, particularly those who have never used hormone replacement therapy (Soliman et al. 2005; Friedenreich et al. 2007). Through the aromatization of estrogen precursors (Cauley et al. 1989) as well as inflammation and insulin resistance (Wang et al. 2011), excessive estrogen production by adipose tissue in obese women has been suggested to play a complex role in the relationship between obesity and endometrial cancer. Furthermore, obesity in combination with diabetes (Parazzini et al. 1999; Shoff et al. 1998; Anderson et al. 2001; Friberg, Orsini et al. 2007; Lindemann et al. 2008) and a lack of exercise (Friberg et al. 2006; Patel et al. 2008) has been associated with a poor predictive outcome (Lucenteforte et al. 2007; Friberg et al. 2007; Chia et al. 2007).

Obesity is associated with an increased risk of colorectal cancer in both men and women (Giovannucci et al. 1995; Larsson et al. 2006; Larsson and Wolk 2007b; Dai et al. 2007; Yamamoto et al. 2010; Hong et al. 2012), with a stronger association in men. Interestingly, compared to cancer in the proximal or distal colon, the distribution of fat may play a greater role in the increased risk of colorectal cancer, particularly in men, who more often develop abdominal obesity (Moore et al. 2004; Dai et al. 2007; Kim et al. 2009). The endocrine and paracrine effects of adipose tissue may lead to systemic alterations such as chronic inflammation and alterations in the levels of adipokines, sex steroids, insulin, insulin-related growth factor (including proinsulin and insulin-like growth factors [IGFs] 1 and 2), and vascular endothelial growth factor (VEGF), which may play an important effect in promoting colon cancer development (Donohoe et al. 2011; Lysaght et al. 2011).

2.2.3 Esophageal and Pancreatic Cancers

Like colorectal cancer, esophageal adenocarcinoma has been strongly associated with obesity (particularly abdominal obesity), through similar mechanisms; the incidence of esophageal adenocarcinoma is four times higher in obese patients (Lagergren et al. 1999; MacInnis et al. 2006; Renehan et al. 2008; Ogunwobi et al. 2008; Lysaght et al. 2011; Doyle et al. 2012; Donohoe et al. 2012), and men exhibit the strongest association between obesity and esophageal adenocarcinoma (Ryan et al. 2006; Kubo et al. 2006). Obesity may exacerbate esophageal inflammation, particularly in the presence of esophageal reflux (Hampel et al. 2005; Corley et al. 2006); however, the effect of obesity on Barrett's esophagus remains unclear (Corley et al. 2007; Cook et al. 2008; Seidel et al. 2009), as does the association between obesity and squamous carcinoma (Steffen et al. 2009; Samanic et al. 2006).

There is a slightly increased risk of pancreatic cancer in both men and women who are overweight or obese (Berrington de Gonzalez et al. 2003; Larsson et al. 2007; Jiao et al. 2010), particularly for individuals with abdominal obesity (Larsson et al. 2005; Luo et al. 2008). It has been suggested that obesity is correlated with an earlier age of disease in a dose–response manner (Genkinger et al. 2011), with lower overall survival in older patients (Li et al. 2009).

2.2.4 KIDNEY AND PROSTATE CANCERS

In 2008, Renehan et al. reported a strong association between obesity and renal cancer in both men and women, which has been confirmed by several studies (Lindblad et al. 1994; Chow et al. 2000; van Dijk et al. 2004; Bjorge et al. 2004; Flaherty et al. 2005; Lukanova et al. 2006; Pischon et al. 2006; Luo et al. 2007; Dal Maso et al. 2007; Adams et al. 2008; Ildaphonse et al. 2009; Mathew et al. 2009; Renehan et al. 2010). In renal cell carcinoma, which represents the majority of kidney cancers, this relationship appears to be stronger in obese women (Chow et al. 1996; Shapiro et al. 1999; Bergstrom et al. 2001a; Chiu et al. 2006). The mechanisms by which obesity may increase renal cell cancer risk and progression are poorly understood (Klinghoffer et al. 2009; Chow et al. 2010), but hormonal changes, such as increased levels of leptin and decreased levels of adiponectin, hyperinsulinemia and increases in related insulin growth factors, and increased levels of estrogen, lipid peroxidation, and defects in the immune response, may be responsible (Jiao et al. 2010; Moyad 2001; Pischon et al. 2006; Gago-Dominguez et al. 2006; Horiguchi et al. 2006; Spyridopoulos et al. 2007, 2009). Interestingly, in patients with renal cell carcinoma and melanoma, a mutation in small ubiquitin-like modifier (SUMO) on microphthalmia-associated transcription factor was identified, which could impair the adaptation of cells to stress and initiate tumor formation, thus increasing the risk of developing renal cell carcinoma, melanoma, or both fivefold (Bertolotto et al. 2011). However, the mechanism (if any) by which this genetic predisposition may be correlated with obesity remains to be elucidated.

The relationship between obesity and prostate cancer has been extensively studied but is not completely conclusive (De Nunzio et al. 2012). Obesity may cause stromal changes in sex steroid production and signaling pathways, which may affect prostate cancer growth via intracrine/paracrine mechanisms involving certain hormones and growth factors such as IGF-1 (Gross et al. 2009; Fowke et al. 2012). Three large, prospective cohort studies performed in the United States found that obesity is not associated with prostate cancer and may even reduce the risk of less aggressive tumors while increasing the risk of more aggressive tumors (Rodriguez et al. 2001, 2007; Gong et al. 2006), with a positive mortality association (Bassett et al. 2011; Cao et al. 2011; Parr et al. 2010). A recent meta-analysis suggests that obesity may have the dual effect of decreasing the risk for localized prostate cancer and increasing the risk for advanced prostate cancer (Discacciati et al. 2012).

This apparent paradox may be explained by the reduced detectability of prostate cancer among obese men with asymptomatic, clinically localized disease (Freedland et al. 2008). Parekh et al. (2010) analyzed three representative cross-sectional surveys in the United States (National Health and Nutrition Examination Survey [NHANES] III, NHANES 2001–2004, and National Health Interview Survey [NHIS] 2000) and concluded that the prostate-specific antigen (PSA)–driven biopsy rates are lower in men with BMIs above 30. In fact, overweight men may have more frequent PSA screening (Fontaine et al. 2005), but due to a possible hemodilution from their large plasma volume (Lopez Fontana et al. 2011), their PSA levels may appear normal, leading to lower biopsy rates in this group. Moreover, obesity is associated with a larger prostate size, which may also affect the early detection of prostate cancer (Kopp et al. 2011). Therefore, to clarify the relationship between obesity and prostate cancer, further studies considering all of these factors are needed.

2.2.5 OTHERS TYPES OF CANCER

Diverse meta-analyses reporting a positive correlation between excessive body weight and the risk of cancer have been published for gallbladder cancer (Larsson and Wolk 2007d), non-Hodgkin's lymphoma, Hodgkin's lymphoma (Larsson and Wolk 2007c; Larsson et al. 2011), leukemia (Larsson et al. 2008b), liver cancer (Larsson and Wolk 2007e), and, possibly, myeloma (Larsson and Wolk 2007a; Wallin et al. 2011). In addition, obesity may be involved in the development of nonalcoholic, fatty liver disease contributing to the development of hepatocellular carcinoma (Nair et al. 2002; Caldwell et al. 2004; Larsson et al. 2008a). The mechanisms involved are not well understood but may involve the same mechanisms previously discussed, such as increased levels of hormones, inflammation, and immunity impairment.

2.3 MOLECULAR PATHWAYS

The mechanism(s) by which obesity contributes to some or all of the hallmarks of cancer is an open question. Although the link between cancer and obesity has been clearly demonstrated by many epidemiological studies and several molecular pathways have been proposed (Khandekar et al. 2011), the interaction between obesity and cancer development and progression remains poorly understood. A cooperative mechanism involving increased insulin and IGF-1 axis signaling, chronic inflammation, changes in adipokine levels, increased availability of lipids and hormones, microenvironment changes, and immunity impairment, as well as genetic factors, may play a role in the conversion of normal epithelial cells to an invasive tumor.

2.3.1 INSULIN AND IGF-1

Weight gain induces progressive metabolic dysfunction, leading to insulin resistance, in which metabolic tissues (adipose tissue, liver, and muscle) are unable to respond to the anabolic actions of insulin. Thus, impaired glucose disposal in muscle and enhanced triglyceride lipolysis in adipose tissue results in hyperinsulinemia, hyperglycemia, and hyperlipidemia. As a compensatory mechanism, β-pancreatic cells subsequently increase the production of insulin, and the liver, which exhibits partial insulin resistance, performs lipogenesis but not gluconeogenesis. As a result, the β-cells become exhausted and contribute to sustained hyperglycemia and type 2 diabetes.

High levels of insulin and IGF-1 may promote tumor growth in a cooperative manner through a variety of pathways such as the phosphatidylinositol-3-kinase (PI3K) and serine/threonine protein kinase Akt (or protein kinase B [PKB]), Mammalian target of rapamycin (mTOR), S6 kinase, and mitogen-activated protein kinase pathways (Pollak et al. 2004). Insulin and insulin-related growth factors exert their effects after interacting with the tyrosine kinase receptors on the cell surface, which are homologous to the tyrosine kinase class oncogenes. The insulin receptor (INSR) exists in two variant isoforms, A and B. INSR isoform A interacts with insulin and IGF, whereas isoform B, which is more commonly expressed on tumors, interacts just with insulin. The IGF-1 receptor (IGF-1R) is a hybrid receptor that is able to interact with insulin as well as IGF-1 (Pollak 2012).

The downstream signaling pathways of insulin and IGF-1 are similar but not identical; insulin and IGF-1 can concurrently activate both the PI3K and mitogen-activated protein kinase (MAPK) pathways. After binding to its receptor, insulin induces extracellular signal–regulated kinase (ERK) activation through growth factor receptor bound 2/SHC-son of Sevenless (GRB2/SHC-SOS)–Ras–Raf and may also activate p38 and Jun kinase (JNK) with a regulatory role exerted by p85 (PI3K regulatory subunit), inducing cell cycle arrest and apoptosis (Moxham et al. 1996; Antonescu et al. 2005; Gehart et al. 2010). Insulin and IGF-1 can also recruit the PI3K to the plasma membrane, triggering its activation by increasing the production of phosphatidylinositol (3,4,5)-triphosphate (PIP3) from phosphatidylinositol (4,5)-bisphosphate (PIP2) (conversely, Phosphatase and tensin homolog [PTEN] converts PIP3 to PIP2) and promoting the phosphorylation of Akt on Thr308 by 3-phosphoinositide-dependent protein kinase-1 (PDK 1) and on Ser473 by the mammalian target of rapamycin complex 2 (mTORC2), also called PDK 2, through acetylation of Rictor (Glidden et al. 2012; Scheid et al. 2002; Sarbassov et al. 2005). These events produce the full activation of Akt, leading to cell growth and proliferation by a variety of downstream pathways that are involved in promoting cell survival and division. These pathways not only involve the activation of VEGF expression, which may be regulated by hypoxia-inducible factor (HIF), HIF-1α, signal transducer and activator of transcription 3 (STAT3), and peroxisome proliferator–activated receptor gamma (PPAR-γ) (Slomiany et al. 2004; He et al. 2011), but also include the activation of nuclear factor kappa B (NF-κB) (Mitsiades et al. 2002); the activation of the mTORC1 signaling pathway (Feng 2010; Chen 2011); the inhibition of p53 (Braun et al. 2011; He et al. 2011); the inhibition of Bcl-2-associated death promoter protein (BAD) and Bcl-2–associated X protein (BAX) (Datta et al. 1997; Matsuzaki et al. 1999) as well as the activation of cyclin D1 (Yang et al. 2007); and the inhibition of checkpoint kinase-1 (chK1) (King et al. 2004). Akt also phosphorylates forkhead box O (FOXO) transcription factors, resulting in nuclear exclusion and enhanced oxidative phosphorylation (Stitt et al. 2004).

The increase in insulin levels inhibits the production of insulin growth factor binding protein 1 (IGFBP-1) and IGFBP-2, leading to a decrease in the circulating levels of IGFBP-1 and IGFBP-2 as well as an increase in hepatic sensitivity (IGF-1 is mainly produced in the liver) (Brismar et al. 1994). These changes result in increased circulating levels of IGF-I (Sandhu et al. 2002). Due to their sequence homology, IGF-1 is able to interact with the same receptors as insulin; however, IGF-2, which is required for early development, can interact with its own receptor (IGF-2R) and with IGF-1R (Veronese et al. 2010). Cancer cells express IGF receptors on their surface and have increased expression of the insulin receptor (Pollak 2012), producing enhanced sensitivity to the circulating levels of IGF-1 as well as insulin levels which may lead to carcinogenesis by enhanced stimulation on the downstream signaling pathways

2.3.2 CHRONIC INFLAMMATION

Obese people often have chronic low-level, or "subacute," inflammation, which has been associated with an increased cancer risk due to the presence of proinflammatory cytokines that are released from phagocytes and other immune cells; these cytokines infiltrate adipose tissues and contribute to insulin resistance. Circulating blood monocytes migrate from the vasculature to the extravascular compartments, where they mature into tissue macrophages that infiltrate adipose tissue. Inflammatory factors such as interleukin 6 (IL-6), IL-17, IL-1β, plasminogen activator inhibitor 1 (PAI1), and tumor necrosis factor-alpha (TNF-α) are then released. These macrophages may possess a proinflammatory phenotype (Lumeng et al. 2008); infiltration by classically activated macrophages may coincide with the onset of insulin resistance, which may be produced through the inhibitor of NF-κB kinase β (IKK). Additionally, alternatively activated macrophages present in lean adipose tissue may play a crucial role in maintaining the insulin sensitivity of adipocytes via the secretion of IL-10 (Chawla et al. 2011).

These cytokines activate multiple signal pathways linked with carcinogenesis, such as PI3K/ Akt, MAPK, and STAT3. In hepatocellular carcinoma, high levels of TNF and cytokine IL-6, which are associated with obesity, can transform healthy cells into malignant cells through chronic low-grade inflammation (Park et al. 2010). TNF and cytokine IL-6 are considered master regulators of tumor-associated inflammation and tumorigenesis (Grivennikov et al. 2011). They can activate the Janus-family tyrosine kinases (JAK)–STAT3 and NF-κB pathway as well as the MAPK and PI3K/Akt pathways. TNF and cytokine IL-6 are also able to activate proliferation via cyclin D1 and cyclin-dependent kinase 2 (CDK2), which are known cell cycle regulators, thus inhibiting apoptosis and promoting proliferation and metastasis (Toffanin et al. 2010; Chawla et al. 2011). TNF-α, which is the best-known member of the TNF family, may contribute to insulin resistance by intervening in the intracellular insulin signaling cascade (Peraldi et al. 1996; Tzanavari et al. 2010).

Inflammatory cytokines can prevent apoptosis by activating inhibitors of apoptosis (IAPs) as well as B-cell lymphoma (BCL)-2 family factors. The increased expression of growth factors and of cell adhesion molecules such as vascular cell adhesion molecule 1 (VCAM1) and E-selectin (ELAM1) can stimulate metastasis. Furthermore, the expression of matrix metalloproteinases (MMPs), which can increase microenvironment remodeling phenomena (Khandekar et al. 2011; Chavey et al. 2003), is increased. PAI1 may also play a role through the increased production of adipose tissue (Wood 2009). As an inhibitor of tissue plasminogen activator (tPA) and urokinase (uPA), PAI1 may act to increase vascularization in a cooperative synergism with VEGF, which is induced by insulin and IGF (Gallagher et al. 2010).

2.3.3 LEPTIN, ADIPONECTIN, AND ESTROGEN

Adipocytes secrete the hormones leptin and adiponectin, which are common homeostatic components that act as feedback peripheral sensors for the hypothalamus in the control of appetite and energy expenditure. In the presence of weight gain, increased levels of the hormone leptin released from adipocytes affect the capacity to conduct negative feedback to the hypothalamus through their action on central leptin receptor (OBR). Leptin can also interact with peripheral receptors that are present at lower levels under normal conditions but are increased in breast, prostate, and colon cancer. Leptin can stimulate the IL-6 receptor, activating JAK/STAT signaling through STAT3 (an oncogenic transcription factor) and concomitantly activating the PI3K/Akt/mTOR axis, which results in the promotion of invasion and migration (Ghilardi et al. 1996; Li et al. 2008; Wang et al. 2012). Leptin can mediate tumorigenesis in endometrial cancer cells through the JAK2/STAT3, MAPK/ERK, and PI3K/Akt pathways, leading to the functional activation of cyclooxygenase-2 (COX-2) (Gao et al. 2009). In addition, leptin may act on the fat tissue, which produces excess amounts of estrogen. Leptin stimulates the expression and activity of aromatase and the transactivation of estrogen receptor-α in breast cancer cells, which has mitogenic and antiapoptotic effects. High levels of estrogen have been associated with an increased risk of postmenopausal breast and endometrial cancer; the main source of this estrogen is adipose tissue, through the aromatization of adrenal androgens (and decreased production of sex hormone–binding globulin) (Catalano et al. 2003, 2004).

The adipokine adiponectin appears to have an opposing role to leptin in cancer development. In obese individuals, adiponectin levels are usually decreased. Adiponectin may have a role in cancer due to its possible antiproliferative effects in prostate (Lu et al. 2012) and colon cancer cells (Kim et al. 2010). Adiponectin acts on a variety of tissues to regulate glucose and lipid metabolism by binding its receptors ADIPOR1 and ADIPOR2. Many of the effects of adiponectin are mediated by increasing the conversion of ceramide to sphingosine-1-phosphate (S1P); alterations in sphingolipid metabolism may modulate tumorigenesis through caspase 8 in a manner that is apparently independent of 5′ adenosine monophosphate activated protein kinase (AMP)-activated kinase (AMPK) signaling, which is a key regulator of proliferation in response to nutrient status (Holland et al. 2011); however, only a few studies have focused on the effects of adiponectin on cancer development.

2.3.4 MICROENVIRONMENT CHANGES

As the mass of adipose tissue is increased by the proliferation of adipocyte progenitors in the stromal–vascular fraction, angiogenesis increases to provide oxygen and nutrients. TNF-α contributes to this process by increasing the levels of endothelial-immune cell adhesion molecules and immune trafficking. Leptin secreted by adipocytes plays an important role through the overproduction and sensitivity of nitric oxide, which in turn leads to angiogenesis. Additionally, the chemokines released from macrophages, stromal cells, and adipocytes as well as changes in endothelial permeability or endothelial dysfunction and increased levels of hormones enhance the overall process. The infiltration of activated macrophages may contribute to tissue invasion, angiogenesis, and metastasis. Tumor-associated macrophages (TAMs) release macrophage chemoattractant protein 1 (MCP1), which enhances cell infiltration into the tissue; the presence of these factors has been associated with a poor outcome in some types of cancer (de Visser et al. 2006; Chawla et al. 2011; Lin et al. 2007).

The tumor microenvironment includes a variety of innate and adaptive immune cells that can communicate with each other in autocrine and paracrine manners to control tumor growth. Additionally, these immune cells can communicate with the surrounding stroma, which contains fibroblasts, endothelial cells, pericytes, and mesenchymal cells, which also appear to have an important role in tumorigenesis. The increased hypoxia induces fibrosis mediated by HIF-1α, leading to hypertrophy with abnormal deposition and accumulation of excess lipids. Hypertrophic adipocytes release free fatty acids (FFAs), which directly impair endothelial function by activating JNKs, which, in combination with the cytokines, enhance the production of reactive oxygen species (ROS) and activate stress signaling pathways, resulting in cell death. Cancer-associated fibroblasts (CAFs) and preadipocytes are important and also may enhance tumor growth and metastasis (Rutkowski et al. 2009; Chawla et al. 2011). Accordingly, Barone has proposed a bidirectional cross talk between cancer cells and CAFs in breast cancer through positive feedback between leptin and epidermal growth factor (EGF) that supports tumor progression, proliferation, migration, and invasiveness (Barone et al. 2012).

2.3.5 CHANGES IN LIPID AVAILABILITY

Decreased high-density lipoprotein levels, increased triglyceride levels, and other lipid abnormalities are common in obesity and may be key factors for tumor development and progression due to their functions in the production of new membrane structures and the regulation of growth factor receptors. In tumors and their precursor lesions, glycolysis and the de novo biogenesis of fatty acids (FAs) such as phosphatidylinositol, phosphatidyl serine, and phosphatidyl choline are increased independently of their circulating levels. These signaling lipids are known to be important factors that activate and mediate pathways such as PI3K/Akt, Ras, or Wnt (Fritz et al. 2010; Khandekar et al. 2011).

Adipose tissue is an important site of endogenous FA synthesis beyond the liver. By shifting from oxidative to glycolytic metabolism, tumor cells are able to catabolize glucose at a rate that exceeds their bioenergetic requirement, producing energy for tumors and the precursors for FA synthesis through the pentose phosphate pathway. In obesity, the upregulation of FA synthase (FASN) in adipocytes has been observed. The enhanced activity of FASN may provide the necessary support for the development of new membranes to promote tumor expansion. In hormonally responsive tumors, the overproduction of steroid hormones may have a role in regulating FASN gene expression and FASN biosynthesis, leading to proliferation (Menendez et al. 2007). The monoacylglycerol lipase (MAGL) pathway, which can control the production of FFAs, is also upregulated in some aggressive cancers that are associated with obesity. However, whether those pathways are important in tumor initiation and metastasis remains controversial (Menendez et al. 2007; Nomura et al. 2010). PPARα may play a role in tumor development via its ability to increase peroxisome-mediated FA oxidation, which increases the levels of ROS, which can drive mutagenesis and carcinogenesis (Chawla et al. 2011; Peters et al. 2012).

2.3.6 OTHER PATHWAYS

Novel genetic variants that are associated with obesity and/or BMI have been reported in recent years, such as single-nucleotide polymorphisms (SNPs) that are associated with the fat mass and obesity (FTO)–associated gene, melanocortin 4 receptor (MC4R), and other variants (Thorleifsson et al. 2009; Willer et al. 2009; Nock et al. 2011). Evidence of a correlation between these SNPs and obesity-related cancers is inconsistent for breast (Kaklamani et al. 2011; Kusinska et al. 2012), colorectal (Loos et al. 2008; Tarabra et al. 2012), and endometrial cancers (Gaudet et al. 2010; Zhang et al. 2012).

SNPs in obesity genes such as adiponectin (ADIPOQ), leptin (LEP), adiponectin receptor 1 (ADIPOR1), ADIPOR2, paraoxonase 1 (PON1), resistin (RETN), and leptin receptor (LEPR) have also been reported. SNPs in the ADIPOQ gene may play a role in endometrial cancer (Chen et al. 2012), and SNPs in LEP, LEPR, and PON1 genes may have roles in breast cancer (Snoussi et al. 2006; Han et al. 2007; Gallicchio et al. 2007; Okobia et al. 2008; Terrasi et al. 2009; Cleveland et al. 2010; Naidu et al. 2010; Liu et al. 2011; Hussein et al. 2011; He et al. 2012). LEP and LEPR SNPs have been linked with non-Hodgkin's lymphoma (Skibola et al. 2004; Willett et al. 2005), while SNPs in LEPR and ADIPOQ have been linked with colon and rectal cancers (Pechlivanis et al. 2009; Slattery et al. 2008; He et al. 2011). LEP and LEPR are associated with oral squamous cell carcinoma (Yapijakis et al. 2009) as well as prostate cancer (Kote-Jarai et al. 2003; Ribeiro et al. 2004), whereas LEP has been linked with increased susceptibility to non–small cell lung cancer (Ribeiro et al. 2006). Finally, correlations between microsatellite instability, obesity, and cancers have gained attention (Campbell et al. 2010).

2.4 PERSPECTIVES ON CHEMOPREVENTION

Although obesity may be influenced by genetic, biological, behavioral, and cultural factors, dietary and physical activity habits have been identified as the major risk factors for obesity (Martinez 2000). Therefore, the consumption of dietary compounds that have antiobesity properties, along with caloric restriction and physical activity, may be an effective strategy for the prevention of obesity-related cancers. A growing body of evidence indicates that natural dietary compounds may possess antiobesity/anticancer effects with minimal or no side effects (Murthy et al. 2009). Among the dietary compounds that have been reported to potentially possess antiobesity effects are curcumin (Shehzad et al. 2011), epigallocatechin gallate (EGCG) (Moon et al. 2007), soy isoflavone (Zhang et al. 2006; Ali et al. 2004; Deibert et al. 2004), bitter melon extracts (Huang et al. 2008; Chen et al. 2005; Chan et al. 2005), resveratrol (Shankar et al. 2007), pterostilbene (Rimando et al. 2005), eicosapentaenoic acid (EPA), docosahexaenoic acid (DHA) (Ruzickova et al. 2005), dibenzoylmethane (DBM) (Lin et al. 2001), oleanolic acid (Sung et al. 2010), capsiate (Masuda et al. 2003), and many traditional herbs (reviewed in Vermaak et al. 2011). Severe side effects have hindered the development of antiobesity drugs, and currently, only two Food and Drug Administration (FDA)–approved drugs, phentermine and orlistat, are available for the treatment of obesity (Powell et al. 2011). Therefore, the clinical development of natural dietary compounds for use as antiobesity drugs is an ideal strategy for the treatment of obesity and obesity-associated diseases.

REFERENCES

Abdel-Maksoud, M. F., B. C. Risendal, M. L. Slattery et al. 2012. Behavioral risk factors and their relationship to tumor characteristics in Hispanic and non-Hispanic white long-term breast cancer survivors. *Breast Cancer Res Treat* 131 (1):169–76.
Abrahamson, P. E., M. D. Gammon, M. J. Lund et al. 2006. General and abdominal obesity and survival among young women with breast cancer. *Cancer Epidemiol Biomarkers Prev* 15 (10):1871–7.
ACS, American Cancer Society Board of Directors. 1998. *ACS Challenge Goals for U.S. Cancer Incidence for the Year 2015. Proceedings of the Board of Directors.* Atlanta: American Cancer Society.
ACS, American Cancer Society Board of Directors. 1996. *ACS Challenge Goals for U.S. Cancer Mortality for the Year 2015. Proceeding of the Board of Directors.* Atlanta: American Cancer Society.
Adams, K. F., M. F. Leitzmann, D. Albanes et al. 2008. Body size and renal cell cancer incidence in a large US cohort study. *Am J Epidemiol* 168 (3):268–77.
Adams, T. D., A. M. Stroup, R. E. Gress et al. 2009. Cancer incidence and mortality after gastric bypass surgery. *Obesity (Silver Spring)* 17 (4):796–802.
Ali, A. A., M. T. Velasquez, C. T. Hansen, A. I. Mohamed, and S. J. Bhathena. 2004. Effects of soybean isoflavones, probiotics, and their interactions on lipid metabolism and endocrine system in an animal model of obesity and diabetes. *J Nutr Biochem* 15 (10):583–90.
Anderson, K. E., E. Anderson, P. J. Mink et al. 2001. Diabetes and endometrial cancer in the Iowa women's health study. *Cancer Epidemiol Biomarkers Prev* 10 (6):611–6.
Antonescu, C. N., C. Huang, W. Niu et al. 2005. Reduction of insulin-stimulated glucose uptake in L6 myotubes by the protein kinase inhibitor SB203580 is independent of p38MAPK activity. *Endocrinology* 146 (9):3773–81.
Ashrafian, H., K. Ahmed, S. P. Rowland et al. 2011. Metabolic surgery and cancer: protective effects of bariatric procedures. *Cancer* 117 (9):1788–99.
Baer, H. J., S. S. Tworoger, S. E. Hankinson, and W. C. Willett. 2010. Body fatness at young ages and risk of breast cancer throughout life. *Am J Epidemiol* 171 (11):1183–94.
Barone, I., S. Catalano, L. Gelsomino et al. 2012. Leptin mediates tumor-stromal interactions that promote the invasive growth of breast cancer cells. *Cancer Res* 72 (6):1416–27.
Bassett, J. K., G. Severi, L. Baglietto et al. 2012. Weight change and prostate cancer incidence and mortality. *Int J Cancer* 131 (7):1711–9.
Bergstrom, A., C. C. Hsieh, P. Lindblad et al. 2001a. Obesity and renal cell cancer—a quantitative review. *Br J Cancer* 131 (7):1711–9.

Bergstrom, A., P. Pisani, V. Tenet, A. Wolk, and H. O. Adami. 2001b. Overweight as an avoidable cause of cancer in Europe. *Int J Cancer* 91 (3):421–30.

Berrington de Gonzalez, A., P. Hartge, J. R. Cerhan et al. 2010. Body-mass index and mortality among 1.46 million white adults. *N Engl J Med* 363 (23):2211–9.

Berrington de Gonzalez, A., S. Sweetland, and E. Spencer. 2003. A meta-analysis of obesity and the risk of pancreatic cancer. *Br J Cancer* 89 (3):519–23.

Bertolotto, C., F. Lesueur, S. Giuliano et al. 2011. A SUMOylation-defective MITF germline mutation predisposes to melanoma and renal carcinoma. *Nature* 480 (7375):94–8.

Bjorge, T., S. Tretli, and A. Engeland. 2004. Relation of height and body mass index to renal cell carcinoma in two million Norwegian men and women. *Am J Epidemiol* 160 (12):1168–76.

Braun, S., K. Bitton-Worms, and D. LeRoith. 2011. The link between the metabolic syndrome and cancer. *Int J Biol Sci* 7 (7):1003–15.

Brecher, G., and S. H. Waxler. 1949. Obesity in albino mice due to single injections of goldthioglucose. *Proc Soc Exp Biol Med* 70 (3):498–501.

Brismar, K., E. Fernqvist-Forbes, J. Wahren, and K. Hall. 1994. Effect of insulin on the hepatic production of insulin-like growth factor-binding protein-1 (IGFBP-1), IGFBP-3, and IGF-I in insulin-dependent diabetes. *J Clin Endocrinol Metab* 79 (3):872–8.

Byers, T., J. Mouchawar, J. Marks et al. 1999. The American Cancer Society challenge goals. How far can cancer rates decline in the U.S. by the year 2015? *Cancer* 86 (4):715–27.

Caballero, B. 2007. The global epidemic of obesity: an overview. *Epidemiol Rev* 29:1–5.

Caldwell, S. H., D. M. Crespo, H. S. Kang, and A. M. Al-Osaimi. 2004. Obesity and hepatocellular carcinoma. *Gastroenterology* 127 (5 Suppl 1):S97–S103.

Calle, E. E., and R. Kaaks. 2004. Overweight, obesity and cancer: epidemiological evidence and proposed mechanisms. *Nat Rev Cancer* 4 (8):579–91.

Calle, E. E., C. Rodriguez, K. Walker-Thurmond, and M. J. Thun. 2003. Overweight, obesity, and mortality from cancer in a prospectively studied cohort of U.S. adults. *N Engl J Med* 348 (17):1625–38.

Calle, E. E., M. J. Thun, J. M. Petrelli, C. Rodriguez, and C. W. Heath, Jr. 1999. Body-mass index and mortality in a prospective cohort of U.S. adults. *N Engl J Med* 341 (15):1097–105.

Campbell, P. T., E. T. Jacobs, C. M. Ulrich et al. 2010. Case-control study of overweight, obesity, and colorectal cancer risk, overall and by tumor microsatellite instability status. *J Natl Cancer Inst* 102 (6):391–400.

Cao, Y., and J. Ma. 2011. Body mass index, prostate cancer-specific mortality, and biochemical recurrence: a systematic review and meta-analysis. *Cancer Prev Res (Phila)* 4 (4):486–501.

Catalano, S., L. Mauro, S. Marsico et al. 2004. Leptin induces, via ERK1/ERK2 signal, functional activation of estrogen receptor alpha in MCF-7 cells. *J Biol Chem* 279 (19):19908–15.

Catalano, S., S. Marsico, C. Giordano et al. 2003. Leptin enhances, via AP-1, expression of aromatase in the MCF-7 cell line. *J Biol Chem* 278 (31):28668–76.

Cauley, J. A., J. P. Gutai, L. H. Kuller, D. LeDonne, and J. G. Powell. 1989. The epidemiology of serum sex hormones in postmenopausal women. *Am J Epidemiol* 129 (6):1120–31.

Chan, L. L., Q. Chen, A. G. Go, E. K. Lam, and E. T. Li. 2005. Reduced adiposity in bitter melon (Momordica charantia)-fed rats is associated with increased lipid oxidative enzyme activities and uncoupling protein expression. *J Nutr* 135 (11):2517–23.

Chavey, C., B. Mari, M. N. Monthouel et al. 2003. Matrix metalloproteinases are differentially expressed in adipose tissue during obesity and modulate adipocyte differentiation. *J Biol Chem* 278 (14):11888–96.

Chawla, A., K. D. Nguyen, and Y. P. Goh. 2011. Macrophage-mediated inflammation in metabolic disease. *Nat Rev Immunol* 11 (11):738–49.

Chen, J. 2011. Multiple signal pathways in obesity-associated cancer. *Obes Rev* 12 (12):1063–70.

Chen, Q., and E. T. Li. 2005. Reduced adiposity in bitter melon (Momordica charantia) fed rats is associated with lower tissue triglyceride and higher plasma catecholamines. *Br J Nutr* 93 (5):747–54.

Chen, X., Y. B. Xiang, J. R. Long et al. 2012. Genetic polymorphisms in obesity-related genes and endometrial cancer risk. *Cancer* 118 (13):3356–64.

Chia, V. M., P. A. Newcomb, A. Trentham-Dietz, and J. M. Hampton. 2007. Obesity, diabetes, and other factors in relation to survival after endometrial cancer diagnosis. *Int J Gynecol Cancer* 17 (2):441–6.

Chiu, B. C., S. M. Gapstur, W. H. Chow et al. 2006. Body mass index, physical activity, and risk of renal cell carcinoma. *Int J Obes (Lond)* 30 (6):940–7.

Chlebowski, R. T. 2012. Obesity and breast cancer outcome: adding to the evidence. *J Clin Oncol* 30 (2):126–8.

Chlebowski, R. T., Z. Chen, G. L. Anderson et al. 2005. Ethnicity and breast cancer: factors influencing differences in incidence and outcome. *J Natl Cancer Inst* 97 (6):439–48.

Chow, W. H., L. M. Dong, and S. S. Devesa. 2010. Epidemiology and risk factors for kidney cancer. *Nat Rev Urol* 7 (5):245–57.

Chow, W. H., G. Gridley, J. F. Fraumeni, Jr., and B. Jarvholm. 2000. Obesity, hypertension, and the risk of kidney cancer in men. *N Engl J Med* 343 (18):1305–11.

Chow, W. H., J. K. McLaughlin, J. S. Mandel et al. 1996. Obesity and risk of renal cell cancer. *Cancer Epidemiol Biomarkers Prev* 5 (1):17–21.

Cleary, M. P., and M. E. Grossmann. 2009. Minireview: Obesity and breast cancer: the estrogen connection. *Endocrinology* 150 (6):2537–42.

Cleveland, R. J., M. D. Gammon, C. M. Long et al. 2010. Common genetic variations in the LEP and LEPR genes, obesity and breast cancer incidence and survival. *Breast Cancer Res Treat* 120 (3):745–52.

Cook, M. B., D. C. Greenwood, L. J. Hardie, C. P. Wild, and D. Forman. 2008. A systematic review and meta-analysis of the risk of increasing adiposity on Barrett's esophagus. *Am J Gastroenterol* 103 (2):292–300.

Corley, D. A., and A. Kubo. 2006. Body mass index and gastroesophageal reflux disease: a systematic review and meta-analysis. *Am J Gastroenterol* 101 (11):2619–28.

Corley, D. A., A. Kubo, T. R. Levin et al. 2007. Abdominal obesity and body mass index as risk factors for Barrett's esophagus. *Gastroenterology* 133 (1):34–41; quiz 311.

Dai, Z., Y. C. Xu, and L. Niu. 2007. Obesity and colorectal cancer risk: a meta-analysis of cohort studies. *World J Gastroenterol* 13 (31):4199–206.

Dal Maso, L., A. Zucchetto, A. Tavani et al. 2007. Renal cell cancer and body size at different ages: an Italian multicenter case-control study. *Am J Epidemiol* 166 (5):582–91.

Datta, S. R., H. Dudek, X. Tao et al. 1997. Akt phosphorylation of BAD couples survival signals to the cell-intrinsic death machinery. *Cell* 91 (2):231–41.

De Nunzio, C., W. Aronson, S. J. Freedland, E. Giovannucci, and J. K. Parsons. 2012. The correlation between metabolic syndrome and prostatic diseases. *Eur Urol* 61 (3):560–70.

de Visser, K. E., and L. M. Coussens. 2006. The inflammatory tumor microenvironment and its impact on cancer development. *Contrib Microbiol* 13:118–37.

Deibert, P., D. Konig, A. Schmidt-Trucksaess et al. 2004. Weight loss without losing muscle mass in pre-obese and obese subjects induced by a high-soy-protein diet. *Int J Obes Relat Metab Disord* 28 (10):1349–52.

Deitel, M. 2003. Overweight and obesity worldwide now estimated to involve 1.7 billion people. *Obes Surg* 13 (3):329–30.

DeSantis, C., R. Siegel, P. Bandi, and A. Jemal. 2011. Breast cancer statistics, 2011. *CA Cancer J Clin* 61 (6):409–18.

Discacciati, A., N. Orsini, and A. Wolk. 2012. Body mass index and incidence of localized and advanced prostate cancer—a dose-response meta-analysis of prospective studies. *Ann Oncol* 23 (7):1665–71.

Donohoe, C. L., S. L. Doyle, S. McGarrigle et al. 2012. Role of the insulin-like growth factor 1 axis and visceral adiposity in oesophageal adenocarcinoma. *Br J Surg* 99 (3):387–96.

Donohoe, C. L., S. L. Doyle, and J. V. Reynolds. 2011. Visceral adiposity, insulin resistance and cancer risk. *Diabetol Metab Syndr* 3:12.

Doyle, S. L., C. L. Donohoe, S. P. Finn et al. 2012. IGF-1 and its receptor in esophageal cancer: association with adenocarcinoma and visceral obesity. *Am J Gastroenterol* 107 (2):196–204.

Eley, J. W., H. A. Hill, V. W. Chen et al. 1994. Racial differences in survival from breast cancer. Results of the National Cancer Institute Black/White Cancer Survival Study. *JAMA* 272 (12):947–54.

Esfahlan, R. J., N. Zarghami, A. J. Esfahlan et al. 2011. The possible impact of obesity on androgen, progesterone and estrogen receptors (ERalpha and ERbeta) gene expression in breast cancer patients. *Breast Cancer (Auckl)* 5:227–37.

Ewertz, M., M. B. Jensen, K. A. Gunnarsdottir et al. 2011. Effect of obesity on prognosis after early-stage breast cancer. *J Clin Oncol* 29 (1):25–31.

Fagherazzi, G., N. Chabbert-Buffet, A. Fabre et al. 2012. Hip circumference is associated with the risk of premenopausal ER-/PR- breast cancer. *Int J Obes (Lond)* 36 (3):431–9.

Feng, Z. 2010. p53 regulation of the IGF-1/Akt/mTOR pathways and the endosomal compartment. *Cold Spring Harb Perspect Biol* 2 (2):a001057.

Finkel, M. P., and G. M. Scribner. 1955. Mouse cages and spontaneous tumors. *Br J Cancer* 9 (3):464–72.

Flaherty, K. T., C. S. Fuchs, G. A. Colditz et al. 2005. A prospective study of body mass index, hypertension, and smoking and the risk of renal cell carcinoma (United States). *Cancer Causes Control* 16 (9):1099–106.

Flegal, K. M., M. D. Carroll, B. K. Kit, and C. L. Ogden. 2012. Prevalence of obesity and trends in the distribution of body mass index among US adults, 1999–2010. *JAMA* 307 (5):491–7.

Flegal, K. M., M. D. Carroll, C. L. Ogden, and L. R. Curtin. 2010. Prevalence and trends in obesity among US adults, 1999-2008. *JAMA* 303 (3):235–41.

Fontaine, K. R., M. Heo, and D. B. Allison. 2005. Obesity and prostate cancer screening in the USA. *Public Health* 119 (8):694–8.

Fowke, J. H., S. S. Motley, R. S. Concepcion, D. F. Penson, and D. A. Barocas. 2012. Obesity, body composition, and prostate cancer. *BMC Cancer* 12:23.

Freedland, S. J., J. Wen, M. Wuerstle et al. 2008. Obesity is a significant risk factor for prostate cancer at the time of biopsy. *Urology* 72 (5):1102–5.

Friberg, E., C. S. Mantzoros, and A. Wolk. 2007. Diabetes and risk of endometrial cancer: a population-based prospective cohort study. *Cancer Epidemiol Biomarkers Prev* 16 (2):276–80.

Friberg, E., C. S. Mantzoros, and A. Wolk. 2006. Physical activity and risk of endometrial cancer: a population-based prospective cohort study. *Cancer Epidemiol Biomarkers Prev* 15 (11):2136–40.

Friberg, E., N. Orsini, C. S. Mantzoros, and A. Wolk. 2007. Diabetes mellitus and risk of endometrial cancer: a meta-analysis. *Diabetologia* 50 (7):1365–74.

Friedenreich, C., A. Cust, P. H. Lahmann et al. 2007. Anthropometric factors and risk of endometrial cancer: the European prospective investigation into cancer and nutrition. *Cancer Causes Control* 18 (4):399–413.

Fritz, V., and L. Fajas. 2010. Metabolism and proliferation share common regulatory pathways in cancer cells. *Oncogene* 29 (31):4369–77.

Gago-Dominguez, M., and J. E. Castelao. 2006. Lipid peroxidation and renal cell carcinoma: further supportive evidence and new mechanistic insights. *Free Radic Biol Med* 40 (4):721–33.

Gallagher, E. J., and D. LeRoith. 2010. The proliferating role of insulin and insulin-like growth factors in cancer. *Trends Endocrinol Metab* 21 (10):610–8.

Gallicchio, L., M. A. McSorley, C. J. Newschaffer et al. 2007. Body mass, polymorphisms in obesity-related genes, and the risk of developing breast cancer among women with benign breast disease. *Cancer Detect Prev* 31 (2):95–101.

Gao, J., J. Tian, Y. Lv et al. 2009. Leptin induces functional activation of cyclooxygenase-2 through JAK2/STAT3, MAPK/ERK, and PI3K/Akt pathways in human endometrial cancer cells. *Cancer Sci* 100 (3):389–95.

Gaudet, M. M., H. P. Yang, J. G. Bosquet et al. 2010. No association between FTO or HHEX and endometrial cancer risk. *Cancer Epidemiol Biomarkers Prev* 19 (8):2106–9.

Gehart, H., S. Kumpf, A. Ittner, and R. Ricci. 2010. MAPK signalling in cellular metabolism: stress or wellness? *EMBO Rep* 11 (11):834–40.

Genkinger, J. M., D. Spiegelman, K. E. Anderson et al. 2011. A pooled analysis of 14 cohort studies of anthropometric factors and pancreatic cancer risk. *Int J Cancer* 129 (7):1708–17.

Ghilardi, N., S. Ziegler, A. Wiestner et al. 1996. Defective STAT signaling by the leptin receptor in diabetic mice. *Proc Natl Acad Sci U S A* 93 (13):6231–5.

Giovannucci, E., A. Ascherio, E. B. Rimm et al. 1995. Physical activity, obesity, and risk for colon cancer and adenoma in men. *Ann Intern Med* 122 (5):327–34.

Glidden, E. J., L. G. Gray, S. Vemuru et al. 2012. Multiple site acetylation of Rictor stimulates mammalian target of rapamycin complex 2 (mTORC2)-dependent phosphorylation of Akt protein. *J Biol Chem* 287 (1):581–8.

Gong, Z., M. L. Neuhouser, P. J. Goodman et al. 2006. Obesity, diabetes, and risk of prostate cancer: results from the prostate cancer prevention trial. *Cancer Epidemiol Biomarkers Prev* 15 (10):1977–83.

Goodwin, P. J., M. Ennis, K. I. Pritchard et al. 2012. Insulin- and obesity-related variables in early-stage breast cancer: correlations and time course of prognostic associations. *J Clin Oncol* 30 (2):164–71.

Goodwin, P. J., M. Ennis, K. I. Pritchard et al. 2002. Fasting insulin and outcome in early-stage breast cancer: results of a prospective cohort study. *J Clin Oncol* 20 (1):42–51.

Grivennikov, S. I., and M. Karin. 2011. Inflammatory cytokines in cancer: tumour necrosis factor and interleukin 6 take the stage. *Ann Rheum Dis* 70 Suppl 1:i104–8.

Gross, M., C. Ramirez, D. Luthringer et al. 2009. Expression of androgen and estrogen related proteins in normal weight and obese prostate cancer patients. *Prostate* 69 (5):520–7.

Hampel, H., N. S. Abraham, and H. B. El-Serag. 2005. Meta-analysis: obesity and the risk for gastroesophageal reflux disease and its complications. *Ann Intern Med* 143 (3):199–211.

Han, C. Z., J. Shi, L. L. Du et al. 2007. [Association among lipids, leptin and leptin receptor polymorphisms with risk of breast cancer]. *Zhonghua Liu Xing Bing Xue Za Zhi* 28 (2):136–40.

Harvie, M., A. Howell, R. A. Vierkant et al. 2005. Association of gain and loss of weight before and after menopause with risk of postmenopausal breast cancer in the Iowa women's health study. *Cancer Epidemiol Biomarkers Prev* 14 (3):656–61.

He, B. S., Y. Q. Pan, Y. Zhang, Y. Q. Xu, and S. K. Wang. 2012. Effect of LEPR Gln223Arg polymorphism on breast cancer risk in different ethnic populations: a meta-analysis. *Mol Biol Rep* 39 (3):3117–22.

He, B., Y. Pan, Y. Zhang et al. 2011. Effects of genetic variations in the adiponectin pathway genes on the risk of colorectal cancer in the Chinese population. *BMC Med Genet* 12:94.

He, Q., Z. Gao, J. Yin et al. 2011. Regulation of HIF-1{alpha} activity in adipose tissue by obesity-associated factors: adipogenesis, insulin, and hypoxia. *Am J Physiol Endocrinol Metab* 300 (5):E877–85.

Holland, W. L., R. A. Miller, Z. V. Wang et al. 2011. Receptor-mediated activation of ceramidase activity initiates the pleiotropic actions of adiponectin. *Nat Med* 17 (1):55–63.

Hong, S., Q. Cai, D. Chen et al. 2012. Abdominal obesity and the risk of colorectal adenoma: a meta-analysis of observational studies. *Eur J Cancer Prev* 21 (6):523–31.

Horiguchi, A., M. Sumitomo, J. Asakuma et al. 2006. Increased serum leptin levels and over expression of leptin receptors are associated with the invasion and progression of renal cell carcinoma. *J Urol* 176 (4 Pt 1):1631–5.

Howlader, N., A. M. Noone, M. Krapcho et al., eds. 2011. *SEER Cancer Statistics Review, 1975–2009 (Vintage 2009 Populations)*. Bethesda, MD: National Cancer Institute.

Huang, H. L., Y. W. Hong, Y. H. Wong et al. 2008. Bitter melon (*Momordica charantia* L.) inhibits adipocyte hypertrophy and down regulates lipogenic gene expression in adipose tissue of diet-induced obese rats. *Br J Nutr* 99 (2):230–9.

Hussein, Y. M., A. F. Gharib, R. L. Etewa, and W. H. ElSawy. 2011. Association of L55M and Q192R polymorphisms in paraoxonase 1 (PON1) gene with breast cancer risk and their clinical significance. *Mol Cell Biochem* 351 (1–2):117–23.

Ildaphonse, G., P. S. George, and A. Mathew. 2009. Obesity and kidney cancer risk in men: a meta-analysis (1992–2008). *Asian Pac J Cancer Prev* 10 (2):279–86.

Jiao, L., A. Berrington de Gonzalez, P. Hartge et al. 2010. Body mass index, effect modifiers, and risk of pancreatic cancer: a pooled study of seven prospective cohorts. *Cancer Causes Control* 21 (8):1305–14.

Kaklamani, V., N. Yi, M. Sadim et al. 2011. The role of the fat mass and obesity associated gene (FTO) in breast cancer risk. *BMC Med Genet* 12:52.

Key, T. J., P. N. Appleby, G. K. Reeves et al. 2003. Body mass index, serum sex hormones, and breast cancer risk in postmenopausal women. *J Natl Cancer Inst* 95 (16):1218–26.

Khandekar, M. J., P. Cohen, and B. M. Spiegelman. 2011. Molecular mechanisms of cancer development in obesity. *Nat Rev Cancer* 11 (12):886–95.

Kim, A. Y., Y. S. Lee, K. H. Kim et al. 2010. Adiponectin represses colon cancer cell proliferation via AdipoR1- and -R2-mediated AMPK activation. *Mol Endocrinol* 24 (7):1441–52.

Kim, Y., and S. Lee. 2009. An association between colonic adenoma and abdominal obesity: a cross-sectional study. *BMC Gastroenterol* 9:4.

King, F. W., J. Skeen, N. Hay, and E. Shtivelman. 2004. Inhibition of Chk1 by activated PKB/Akt. *Cell Cycle* 3 (5):634–7.

Klinghoffer, Z., B. Yang, A. Kapoor, and J. H. Pinthus. 2009. Obesity and renal cell carcinoma: epidemiology, underlying mechanisms and management considerations. *Expert Rev Anticancer Ther* 9 (7):975–87.

Kopp, R. P., M. Han, A. W. Partin et al. 2011. Obesity and prostate enlargement in men with localized prostate cancer. *BJU Int* 108 (11):1750–6.

Kote-Jarai, Z., R. Singh, F. Durocher et al. 2003. Association between leptin receptor gene polymorphisms and early-onset prostate cancer. *BJU Int* 92 (1):109–12.

Kubo, A., and D. A. Corley. 2006. Body mass index and adenocarcinomas of the esophagus or gastric cardia: a systematic review and meta-analysis. *Cancer Epidemiol Biomarkers Prev* 15 (5):872–8.

Kusinska, R., P. Gorniak, A. Pastorczak et al. 2012. Influence of genomic variation in FTO at 16q12.2, MC4R at 18q22 and NRXN3 at 14q31 genes on breast cancer risk. *Mol Biol Rep* 39 (3):2915–9.

La Vecchia, C., S. H. Giordano, G. N. Hortobagyi, and B. Chabner. 2011. Overweight, obesity, diabetes, and risk of breast cancer: interlocking pieces of the puzzle. *Oncologist* 16 (6):726–9.

Lagergren, J., R. Bergstrom, and O. Nyren. 1999. Association between body mass and adenocarcinoma of the esophagus and gastric cardia. *Ann Intern Med* 130 (11):883–90.

Larsson, S. C., and A. Wolk. 2011. Body mass index and risk of non-Hodgkin's and Hodgkin's lymphoma: a meta-analysis of prospective studies. *Eur J Cancer* 47 (16):2422–30.

Larsson, S. C., and A. Wolk. 2008a. Excess body fatness: an important cause of most cancers. *Lancet* 371 (9612):536–7.

Larsson, S. C., and A. Wolk. 2008b. Overweight and obesity and incidence of leukemia: a meta-analysis of cohort studies. *Int J Cancer* 122 (6):1418–21.

Larsson, S. C., and A. Wolk. 2007a. Body mass index and risk of multiple myeloma: a meta-analysis. *Int J Cancer* 121 (11):2512–6.

Larsson, S. C., and A. Wolk. 2007b. Obesity and colon and rectal cancer risk: a meta-analysis of prospective studies. *Am J Clin Nutr* 86 (3):556–65.

Larsson, S. C., and A. Wolk. 2007c. Obesity and risk of non-Hodgkin's lymphoma: a meta-analysis. *Int J Cancer* 121 (7):1564–70.

Larsson, S. C., and A. Wolk. 2007d. Obesity and the risk of gallbladder cancer: a meta-analysis. *Br J Cancer* 96 (9):1457–61.

Larsson, S. C., and A. Wolk. 2007e. Overweight, obesity and risk of liver cancer: a meta-analysis of cohort studies. *Br J Cancer* 97 (7):1005–8.

Larsson, S. C., N. Orsini, and A. Wolk. 2007. Body mass index and pancreatic cancer risk: a meta-analysis of prospective studies. *Int J Cancer* 120 (9):1993–8.

Larsson, S. C., J. Rutegard, L. Bergkvist, and A. Wolk. 2006. Physical activity, obesity, and risk of colon and rectal cancer in a cohort of Swedish men. *Eur J Cancer* 42 (15):2590–7.

Larsson, S. C., J. Permert, N. Hakansson et al. 2005. Overall obesity, abdominal adiposity, diabetes and cigarette smoking in relation to the risk of pancreatic cancer in two Swedish population-based cohorts. *Br J Cancer* 93 (11):1310–5.

Lee, J. S., S. I. Cho, and H. S. Park. 2010. Metabolic syndrome and cancer-related mortality among Korean men and women. *Ann Oncol* 21 (3):640–5.

Lew, E. A., and L. Garfinkel. 1979. Variations in mortality by weight among 750,000 men and women. *J Chronic Dis* 32 (8):563–76.

Li, D., J. S. Morris, J. Liu et al. 2009. Body mass index and risk, age of onset, and survival in patients with pancreatic cancer. *JAMA* 301 (24):2553–62.

Li, L., Y. Gao, L. L. Zhang, and D. L. He. 2008. Concomitant activation of the JAK/STAT3 and ERK1/2 signaling is involved in leptin-mediated proliferation of renal cell carcinoma Caki-2 cells. *Cancer Biol Ther* 7 (11):1787–92.

Lin, C. C., C. T. Ho, and M. T. Huang. 2001. Mechanistic studies on the inhibitory action of dietary dibenzoylmethane, a beta-diketone analogue of curcumin, on 7,12-dimethylbenz[a]anthracene-induced mammary tumorigenesis. *Proc Natl Sci Counc Repub China B* 25 (3):158–65.

Lin, W. W., and M. Karin. 2007. A cytokine-mediated link between innate immunity, inflammation, and cancer. *J Clin Invest* 117 (5):1175–83.

Lindblad, P., A. Wolk, R. Bergstrom, I. Persson, and H. O. Adami. 1994. The role of obesity and weight fluctuations in the etiology of renal cell cancer: a population-based case-control study. *Cancer Epidemiol Biomarkers Prev* 3 (8):631–9.

Lindemann, K., L. J. Vatten, M. Ellstrom-Engh, and A. Eskild. 2008. Body mass, diabetes and smoking, and endometrial cancer risk: a follow-up study. *Br J Cancer* 98 (9):1582–5.

Liu, C., and L. Liu. 2011. Polymorphisms in three obesity-related genes (LEP, LEPR, and PON1) and breast cancer risk: a meta-analysis. *Tumour Biol* 32 (6):1233–40.

Loos, R. J., C. M. Lindgren, S. Li et al. 2008. Common variants near MC4R are associated with fat mass, weight and risk of obesity. *Nat Genet* 40 (6):768–75.

Lopez Fontana, C., M. E. Maselli, R. Perez Elizalde et al. 2011. Obesity modifies prostatic specific antigen in men over 45 years. *Arch Esp Urol* 64 (1):35–42.

Lu, J. P., Z. F. Hou, W. C. Duivenvoorden et al. 2012. Adiponectin inhibits oxidative stress in human prostate carcinoma cells. *Prostate Cancer Prostatic Dis* 15 (1):28–35.

Lu, Y., H. Ma, K. E. Malone et al. 2011. Obesity and survival among black women and white women 35 to 64 years of age at diagnosis with invasive breast cancer. *J Clin Oncol* 29 (25):3358–65.

Lucenteforte, E., C. Bosetti, R. Talamini et al. 2007. Diabetes and endometrial cancer: effect modification by body weight, physical activity and hypertension. *Br J Cancer* 97 (7):995–8.

Lukanova, A., O. Bjor, R. Kaaks et al. 2006. Body mass index and cancer: results from the Northern Sweden Health and Disease Cohort. *Int J Cancer* 118 (2):458–66.

Lumeng, C. N., J. B. DelProposto, D. J. Westcott, and A. R. Saltiel. 2008. Phenotypic switching of adipose tissue macrophages with obesity is generated by spatiotemporal differences in macrophage subtypes. *Diabetes* 57 (12):3239–46.

Luo, J., K. L. Margolis, H. O. Adami, A. LaCroix, and W. Ye. 2008. Obesity and risk of pancreatic cancer among postmenopausal women: the Women's Health Initiative (United States). *Br J Cancer* 99 (3):527–31.

Luo, J., K. L. Margolis, H. O. Adami et al. 2007. Body size, weight cycling, and risk of renal cell carcinoma among postmenopausal women: the Women's Health Initiative (United States). *Am J Epidemiol* 166 (7):752–9.

Lysaght, J., E. P. van der Stok, E. H. Allott et al. 2011. Pro-inflammatory and tumour proliferative properties of excess visceral adipose tissue. *Cancer Lett* 312 (1):62–72.

MacInnis, R. J., D. R. English, J. L. Hopper, and G. G. Giles. 2006. Body size and composition and the risk of gastric and oesophageal adenocarcinoma. *Int J Cancer* 118 (10):2628–31.

Martinez, J. A. 2000. Body-weight regulation: causes of obesity. *Proc Nutr Soc* 59 (3):337–45.

Masuda, Y., S. Haramizu, K. Oki et al. 2003. Upregulation of uncoupling proteins by oral administration of capsiate, a nonpungent capsaicin analog. *J Appl Physiol* 95 (6):2408–15.

Mathew, A., P. S. George, and G. Ildaphonse. 2009. Obesity and kidney cancer risk in women: a meta-analysis (1992–2008). *Asian Pac J Cancer Prev* 10 (3):471–8.

Matsuzaki, H., M. Tamatani, N. Mitsuda et al. 1999. Activation of Akt kinase inhibits apoptosis and changes in Bcl-2 and Bax expression induced by nitric oxide in primary hippocampal neurons. *J Neurochem* 73 (5):2037–46.

McCullough, M. L., H. S. Feigelson, W. R. Diver et al. 2005. Risk factors for fatal breast cancer in African-American women and White women in a large US prospective cohort. *Am J Epidemiol* 162 (8):734–42.

Menendez, J. A., and R. Lupu. 2007. Fatty acid synthase and the lipogenic phenotype in cancer pathogenesis. *Nat Rev Cancer* 7 (10):763–77.

Michels, K. B., K. L. Terry, A. H. Eliassen, S. E. Hankinson, and W. C. Willett. 2012. Adult weight change and incidence of premenopausal breast cancer. *Int J Cancer* 130 (4):902–9.

Mitsiades, C. S., N. Mitsiades, V. Poulaki et al. 2002. Activation of NF-kappaB and upregulation of intracellular anti-apoptotic proteins via the IGF-1/Akt signaling in human multiple myeloma cells: therapeutic implications. *Oncogene* 21 (37):5673–83.

Moon, H. S., H. G. Lee, Y. J. Choi, T. G. Kim, and C. S. Cho. 2007. Proposed mechanisms of (-)-epigallocatechin-3-gallate for anti-obesity. *Chem Biol Interact* 167 (2):85–98.

Moore, L. L., M. L. Bradlee, M. R. Singer et al. 2004. BMI and waist circumference as predictors of lifetime colon cancer risk in Framingham Study adults. *Int J Obes Relat Metab Disord* 28 (4):559–67.

Moxham, C. M., A. Tabrizchi, R. J. Davis, and C. C. Malbon. 1996. Jun N-terminal kinase mediates activation of skeletal muscle glycogen synthase by insulin in vivo. *J Biol Chem* 271 (48):30765–73.

Moyad, M. A. 2001. Obesity, interrelated mechanisms, and exposures and kidney cancer. *Semin Urol Oncol* 19 (4):270–9.

Murthy, N. S., S. Mukherjee, G. Ray, and A. Ray. 2009. Dietary factors and cancer chemoprevention: an overview of obesity-related malignancies. *J Postgrad Med* 55 (1):45–54.

Naidu, R., Y. C. Har, and N. A. Taib. 2010. Genetic polymorphisms of paraoxonase 1 (PON1) gene: association between L55M or Q192R with breast cancer risk and clinico-pathological parameters. *Pathol Oncol Res* 16 (4):533–40.

Nair, S., A. Mason, J. Eason, G. Loss, and R. P. Perrillo. 2002. Is obesity an independent risk factor for hepatocellular carcinoma in cirrhosis? *Hepatology* 36 (1):150–5.

Nock, N. L., S. J. Plummer, C. L. Thompson, G. Casey, and L. Li. 2011. FTO polymorphisms are associated with adult body mass index (BMI) and colorectal adenomas in African-Americans. *Carcinogenesis* 32 (5):748–56.

Nomura, D. K., J. Z. Long, S. Niessen et al. 2010. Monoacylglycerol lipase regulates a fatty acid network that promotes cancer pathogenesis. *Cell* 140 (1):49–61.

Ogden, C. L., M. D. Carroll, L. R. Curtin et al. 2006. Prevalence of overweight and obesity in the United States, 1999–2004. *JAMA* 295 (13):1549–55.

Ogunwobi, O. O., and I. L. Beales. 2008. Leptin stimulates the proliferation of human oesophageal adenocarcinoma cells via HB-EGF and Tgfalpha mediated transactivation of the epidermal growth factor receptor. *Br J Biomed Sci* 65 (3):121–7.

Okobia, M. N., C. H. Bunker, S. J. Garte et al. 2008. Leptin receptor Gln223Arg polymorphism and breast cancer risk in Nigerian women: a case control study. *BMC Cancer* 8:338.

Olsen, C. M., A. C. Green, D. C. Whiteman et al. 2007. Obesity and the risk of epithelial ovarian cancer: a systematic review and meta-analysis. *Eur J Cancer* 43 (4):690–709.

Parazzini, F., C. La Vecchia, E. Negri et al. 1999. Diabetes and endometrial cancer: an Italian case-control study. *Int J Cancer* 81 (4):539–42.

Parekh, N., Y. Lin, R. S. Dipaola, S. Marcella, and G. Lu-Yao. 2010. Obesity and prostate cancer detection: insights from three national surveys. *Am J Med* 123 (9):829–35.

Park, E. J., J. H. Lee, G. Y. Yu et al. 2010. Dietary and genetic obesity promote liver inflammation and tumorigenesis by enhancing IL-6 and TNF expression. *Cell* 140 (2):197–208.

Parker, E. D., and A. R. Folsom. 2003. Intentional weight loss and incidence of obesity-related cancers: the Iowa Women's Health Study. *Int J Obes Relat Metab Disord* 27 (12):1447–52.

Parr, C. L., G. D. Batty, T. H. Lam et al. 2010. Body-mass index and cancer mortality in the Asia-Pacific Cohort Studies Collaboration: pooled analyses of 424,519 participants. *Lancet Oncol* 11 (8):741–52.

Patel, A. V., H. S. Feigelson, J. T. Talbot et al. 2008. The role of body weight in the relationship between physical activity and endometrial cancer: results from a large cohort of US women. *Int J Cancer* 123 (8):1877–82.

Pechlivanis, S., J. L. Bermejo, B. Pardini et al. 2009. Genetic variation in adipokine genes and risk of colorectal cancer. *Eur J Endocrinol* 160 (6):933–40.

Peraldi, P., G. S. Hotamisligil, W. A. Buurman, M. F. White, and B. M. Spiegelman. 1996. Tumor necrosis factor (TNF)-alpha inhibits insulin signaling through stimulation of the p55 TNF receptor and activation of sphingomyelinase. *J Biol Chem* 271 (22):13018–22.

Peters, J. M., Y. M. Shah, and F. J. Gonzalez. 2012. The role of peroxisome proliferator-activated receptors in carcinogenesis and chemoprevention. *Nat Rev Cancer* 12 (3):181–95.

Pischon, T., P. H. Lahmann, H. Boeing et al. 2006. Body size and risk of renal cell carcinoma in the European Prospective Investigation into Cancer and Nutrition (EPIC). *Int J Cancer* 118 (3):728–38.

Pollak, M. 2012. The insulin and insulin-like growth factor receptor family in neoplasia: an update. *Nat Rev Cancer* 12 (3):159–69.

Pollak, M. N., E. S. Schernhammer, and S. E. Hankinson. 2004. Insulin-like growth factors and neoplasia. *Nat Rev Cancer* 4 (7):505–18.

Powell, A. G., C. M. Apovian, and L. J. Aronne. 2011. New drug targets for the treatment of obesity. *Clin Pharmacol Ther* 90 (1):40–51.

Protani, M., M. Coory, and J. H. Martin. 2010. Effect of obesity on survival of women with breast cancer: systematic review and meta-analysis. *Breast Cancer Res Treat* 123 (3):627–35.

Reeves, G. K., K. Pirie, V. Beral et al. 2007. Cancer incidence and mortality in relation to body mass index in the Million Women Study: cohort study. *BMJ* 335 (7630):1134.

Renehan, A. G., I. Soerjomataram, M. Tyson et al. 2010. Incident cancer burden attributable to excess body mass index in 30 European countries. *Int J Cancer* 126 (3):692–702.

Renehan, A. G., M. Tyson, M. Egger, R. F. Heller, and M. Zwahlen. 2008. Body-mass index and incidence of cancer: a systematic review and meta-analysis of prospective observational studies. *Lancet* 371 (9612):569–78.

Ribeiro, R., A. P. Araujo, A. Coelho et al. 2006. A functional polymorphism in the promoter region of leptin gene increases susceptibility for non-small cell lung cancer. *Eur J Cancer* 42 (8):1188–93.

Ribeiro, R., A. Vasconcelos, S. Costa et al. 2004. Overexpressing leptin genetic polymorphism (-2548 G/A) is associated with susceptibility to prostate cancer and risk of advanced disease. *Prostate* 59 (3):268–74.

Rimando, A. M., R. Nagmani, D. R. Feller, and W. Yokoyama. 2005. Pterostilbene, a new agonist for the peroxisome proliferator-activated receptor alpha-isoform, lowers plasma lipoproteins and cholesterol in hypercholesterolemic hamsters. *J Agric Food Chem* 53 (9):3403–7.

Rodriguez, C., S. J. Freedland, A. Deka et al. 2007. Body mass index, weight change, and risk of prostate cancer in the Cancer Prevention Study II Nutrition Cohort. *Cancer Epidemiol Biomarkers Prev* 16 (1):63–9.

Rodriguez, C., A. V. Patel, E. E. Calle et al. 2001. Body mass index, height, and prostate cancer mortality in two large cohorts of adult men in the United States. *Cancer Epidemiol Biomarkers Prev* 10 (4):345–53.

Rutkowski, J. M., K. E. Davis, and P. E. Scherer. 2009. Mechanisms of obesity and related pathologies: the macro- and microcirculation of adipose tissue. *FEBS J* 276 (20):5738–46.

Ruzickova, J., M. Rossmeisl, T. Prazak et al. 2004. Omega-3 PUFA of marine origin limit diet-induced obesity in mice by reducing cellularity of adipose tissue. *Lipids* 39 (12):1177–85.

Ryan, A. M., S. P. Rowley, A. P. Fitzgerald, N. Ravi, and J. V. Reynolds. 2006. Adenocarcinoma of the oesophagus and gastric cardia: male preponderance in association with obesity. *Eur J Cancer* 42 (8):1151–8.

Samanic, C., W. H. Chow, G. Gridley, B. Jarvholm, and J. F. Fraumeni, Jr. 2006. Relation of body mass index to cancer risk in 362,552 Swedish men. *Cancer Causes Control* 17 (7):901–9.

Samanic, C., G. Gridley, W. H. Chow et al. 2004. Obesity and cancer risk among white and black United States veterans. *Cancer Causes Control* 15 (1):35–43.

Sandhu, M. S., D. B. Dunger, and E. L. Giovannucci. 2002. Insulin, insulin-like growth factor-I (IGF-I), IGF binding proteins, their biologic interactions, and colorectal cancer. *J Natl Cancer Inst* 94 (13):972–80.

Sarbassov, D. D., D. A. Guertin, S. M. Ali, and D. M. Sabatini. 2005. Phosphorylation and regulation of Akt/PKB by the rictor-mTOR complex. *Science* 307 (5712):1098–101.

Sarkissyan, M., Y. Wu, and J. V. Vadgama. 2011. Obesity is associated with breast cancer in African-American women but not Hispanic women in South Los Angeles. *Cancer* 117 (16):3814–23.

Scheid, M. P., P. A. Marignani, and J. R. Woodgett. 2002. Multiple phosphoinositide 3-kinase-dependent steps in activation of protein kinase B. *Mol Cell Biol* 22 (17):6247–60.

Schouten, L. J., R. A. Goldbohm, and P. A. van den Brandt. 2004. Anthropometry, physical activity, and endometrial cancer risk: results from the Netherlands Cohort Study. *J Natl Cancer Inst* 96 (21):1635–8.

Sedjo, R. L., T. Byers, E. Barrera, Jr. et al. 2007. A midpoint assessment of the American Cancer Society challenge goal to decrease cancer incidence by 25% between 1992 and 2015. *CA Cancer J Clin* 57 (6):326–40.

Seidel, D., W. Muangpaisan, H. Hiro, A. Mathew, and G. Lyratzopoulos. 2009. The association between body mass index and Barrett's esophagus: a systematic review. *Dis Esophagus* 22 (7):564–70.

Shankar, S., G. Singh, and R. K. Srivastava. 2007. Chemoprevention by resveratrol: molecular mechanisms and therapeutic potential. *Front Biosci* 12:4839–54.

Shapiro, J. A., M. A. Williams, and N. S. Weiss. 1999. Body mass index and risk of renal cell carcinoma. *Epidemiology* 10 (2):188–91.

Shehzad, A., T. Ha, F. Subhan, and Y. S. Lee. 2011. New mechanisms and the anti-inflammatory role of curcumin in obesity and obesity-related metabolic diseases. *Eur J Nutr* 50 (3):151–61.

Shoff, S. M., and P. A. Newcomb. 1998. Diabetes, body size, and risk of endometrial cancer. *Am J Epidemiol* 148 (3):234–40.

Simard, E. P., E. M. Ward, R. Siegel, and A. Jemal. 2012. Cancers with increasing incidence trends in the United States: 1999 through 2008. *CA Cancer J Clin* 62 (2):118–28.

Singh, P., U. Kapil, N. Shukla, S. Deo, and S. Dwivedi. 2011. Association of overweight and obesity with breast cancer in India. *Indian J Community Med* 36 (4):259–62.

Singletary, S. E. 2003. Rating the risk factors for breast cancer. *Ann Surg* 237 (4):474–82.

Sjostrom, L., A. Gummesson, C. D. Sjostrom et al. 2009. Effects of bariatric surgery on cancer incidence in obese patients in Sweden (Swedish Obese Subjects Study): a prospective, controlled intervention trial. *Lancet Oncol* 10 (7):653–62.

Skibola, C. F., E. A. Holly, M. S. Forrest et al. 2004. Body mass index, leptin and leptin receptor polymorphisms, and non-Hodgkin lymphoma. *Cancer Epidemiol Biomarkers Prev* 13 (5):779–86.

Slattery, M. L., R. K. Wolff, J. Herrick, B. J. Caan, and J. D. Potter. 2008. Leptin and leptin receptor genotypes and colon cancer: gene-gene and gene-lifestyle interactions. *Int J Cancer* 122 (7):1611–7.

Slomiany, M. G., and S. A. Rosenzweig. 2004. IGF-1-induced VEGF and IGFBP-3 secretion correlates with increased HIF-1 alpha expression and activity in retinal pigment epithelial cell line D407. *Invest Ophthalmol Vis Sci* 45 (8):2838–47.

Smigal, C., A. Jemal, E. Ward et al. 2006. Trends in breast cancer by race and ethnicity: update 2006. *CA Cancer J Clin* 56 (3):168–83.

Snoussi, K., A. D. Strosberg, N. Bouaouina et al. 2006. Leptin and leptin receptor polymorphisms are associated with increased risk and poor prognosis of breast carcinoma. *BMC Cancer* 6:38.

Soliman, P. T., J. C. Oh, K. M. Schmeler et al. 2005. Risk factors for young premenopausal women with endometrial cancer. *Obstet Gynecol* 105 (3):575–80.

Spyridopoulos, T. N., E. T. Petridou, N. Dessypris et al. 2009. Inverse association of leptin levels with renal cell carcinoma: results from a case-control study. *Hormones (Athens)* 8 (1):39–46.

Spyridopoulos, T. N., E. T. Petridou, A. Skalkidou et al. 2007. Low adiponectin levels are associated with renal cell carcinoma: a case-control study. *Int J Cancer* 120 (7):1573–8.

Steffen, A., M. B. Schulze, T. Pischon et al. 2009. Anthropometry and esophageal cancer risk in the European prospective investigation into cancer and nutrition. *Cancer Epidemiol Biomarkers Prev* 18 (7):2079–89.

Stitt, T. N., D. Drujan, B. A. Clarke et al. 2004. The IGF-1/PI3K/Akt pathway prevents expression of muscle atrophy-induced ubiquitin ligases by inhibiting FOXO transcription factors. *Mol Cell* 14 (3):395–403.

Sung, H. Y., S. W. Kang, J. L. Kim et al. 2010. Oleanolic acid reduces markers of differentiation in 3T3-L1 adipocytes. *Nutr Res* 30 (12):831–9.

Suzuki, R., M. Iwasaki, M. Inoue et al. 2011. Body weight at age 20 years, subsequent weight change and breast cancer risk defined by estrogen and progesterone receptor status—the Japan public health center-based prospective study. *Int J Cancer* 129 (5):1214–24.

Tarabra, E., G. C. Actis, M. Fadda et al. 2012. The obesity gene and colorectal cancer risk: a population study in Northern Italy. *Eur J Intern Med* 23 (1):65–9.

Terrasi, M., E. Fiorio, A. Mercanti et al. 2009. Functional analysis of the -2548G/A leptin gene polymorphism in breast cancer cells. *Int J Cancer* 125 (5):1038–44.

Thorleifsson, G., G. B. Walters, D. F. Gudbjartsson et al. 2009. Genome-wide association yields new sequence variants at seven loci that associate with measures of obesity. *Nat Genet* 41 (1):18–24.

Toffanin, S., S. L. Friedman, and J. M. Llovet. 2010. Obesity, inflammatory signaling, and hepatocellular carcinoma-an enlarging link. *Cancer Cell* 17 (2):115–7.

Tzanavari, T., P. Giannogonas, and K. P. Karalis. 2010. TNF-alpha and obesity. *Curr Dir Autoimmun* 11:145–56.

US Cancer Statistics. 2010. United States Cancer Statistics: 1999–2007 Incidence and Mortality Web-based Report., ed C. f. D. C. a. P. Department of Health and Human Services, and National Cancer Institute. Atlanta (GA): U.S. Cancer Statistics Working Group. Available at http://www.cdc.gov/uscs, accessed May 15, 2012.

Vainio, H., R. Kaaks, and F. Bianchini. 2002. Weight control and physical activity in cancer prevention: international evaluation of the evidence. *Eur J Cancer Prev* 11 Suppl 2:S94–100.

van Dijk, B. A., L. J. Schouten, L. A. Kiemeney, R. A. Goldbohm, and P. A. van den Brandt. 2004. Relation of height, body mass, energy intake, and physical activity to risk of renal cell carcinoma: results from the Netherlands Cohort Study. *Am J Epidemiol* 160 (12):1159–67.

Vermaak, I., A. M. Viljoen, and J. H. Hamman. 2011. Natural products in anti-obesity therapy. *Nat Prod Rep* 28 (9):1493–533.

Veronese, A., L. Lupini, J. Consiglio et al. 2010. Oncogenic role of miR-483-3p at the IGF2/483 locus. *Cancer Res* 70 (8):3140–9.

von Gruenigen, V. E., C. Tian, H. Frasure et al. 2006. Treatment effects, disease recurrence, and survival in obese women with early endometrial carcinoma: a Gynecologic Oncology Group study. *Cancer* 107 (12):2786–91.

Vrieling, A., K. Buck, R. Kaaks, and J. Chang-Claude. 2010. Adult weight gain in relation to breast cancer risk by estrogen and progesterone receptor status: a meta-analysis. *Breast Cancer Res Treat* 123 (3):641–9.

Wallin, A., and S. C. Larsson. 2011. Body mass index and risk of multiple myeloma: a meta-analysis of prospective studies. *Eur J Cancer* 47 (11):1606–15.

Wang, D., J. Chen, H. Chen et al. 2012. Leptin regulates proliferation and apoptosis of colorectal carcinoma through PI3K/Akt/mTOR signalling pathway. *J Biosci* 37 (1):91–101.

Wang, T., T. E. Rohan, M. J. Gunter et al. 2011. A prospective study of inflammation markers and endometrial cancer risk in postmenopausal hormone nonusers. *Cancer Epidemiol Biomarkers Prev* 20 (5):971–7.

Waxler, S. H., P. Tabar, and L. R. Melcher. 1953. Obesity and the time of appearance of spontaneous mammary carcinoma in C3H mice. *Cancer Res* 13 (3):276–8.

WHO. Physical status: the use and interpretation of anthropometry. Report of a WHO Expert Committee. WHO Technical Report Series 854. Geneva: World Health Organization, 1995. http://whqlibdoc.who.int/trs/WHO_TRS_854.pdf.

World Health Organization. 2000. Obesity: preventing and managing the global epidemic: report of a WHO consultation, WHO technical report series. Geneva: World Health Organization. http://whqlibdoc.who.int/trs/WHO_TRS_894.pdf

WHO Expert Consultation. 2004. Appropriate body-mass index for Asian populations and its implications for policy and intervention strategies. *The Lancet.* 157–163.

Willer, C. J., E. K. Speliotes, R. J. Loos et al. 2009. Six new loci associated with body mass index highlight a neuronal influence on body weight regulation. *Nat Genet* 41 (1):25–34.

Willett, E. V., C. F. Skibola, P. Adamson et al. 2005. Non-Hodgkin's lymphoma, obesity and energy homeostasis polymorphisms. *Br J Cancer* 93 (7):811–6.

Wiseman, M. 2008. The second World Cancer Research Fund/American Institute for Cancer Research expert report. Food, nutrition, physical activity, and the prevention of cancer: a global perspective. *Proc Nutr Soc* 67 (3):253–6.

Wolin, K. Y., K. Carson, and G. A. Colditz. 2010. Obesity and cancer. *Oncologist* 15 (6):556–65.

Wood, P. A. 2009. Connecting the dots: obesity, fatty acids and cancer. *Lab Invest* 89 (11):1192–4.

World Health Organization. 2011. *A Prioritized Research Agenda for Prevention and Control of Noncommunicable Diseases.* Geneva: World Health Organization.

World Health Organization. 2000. *Obesity: Preventing and Managing the Global Epidemic: Report of a WHO Consultation, WHO Technical Report Series.* Geneva: World Health Organization.

Yamamoto, S., T. Nakagawa, Y. Matsushita et al. 2010. Visceral fat area and markers of insulin resistance in relation to colorectal neoplasia. *Diabetes Care* 33 (1):184–9.

Yang, W., Y. Zhang, Y. Li, Z. Wu, and D. Zhu. 2007. Myostatin induces cyclin D1 degradation to cause cell cycle arrest through a phosphatidylinositol 3-kinase/Akt/GSK-3 beta pathway and is antagonized by insulin-like growth factor 1. *J Biol Chem* 282 (6):3799–808.

Yang, X. R., J. Chang-Claude, E. L. Goode et al. 2011. Associations of breast cancer risk factors with tumor subtypes: a pooled analysis from the Breast Cancer Association Consortium studies. *J Natl Cancer Inst* 103 (3):250–63.

Yapijakis, C., M. Kechagiadakis, E. Nkenke et al. 2009. Association of leptin -2548G/A and leptin receptor Q223R polymorphisms with increased risk for oral cancer. *J Cancer Res Clin Oncol* 135 (4):603–12.

Zhang, H. M., S. W. Chen, L. S. Zhang, and X. F. Feng. 2006. [Effects of soy isoflavone on low-grade inflammation in obese rats]. *Zhong Nan Da Xue Xue Bao Yi Xue Ban* 31 (3):336–9.

Zhang, Z., D. Zhou, Y. Lai et al. 2012. Estrogen induces endometrial cancer cell proliferation and invasion by regulating the fat mass and obesity-associated gene via PI3K/Akt and MAPK signaling pathways. *Cancer Lett* 319 (1):89–97.

3 Inflammation-Induced Esophageal and Colon Adenocarcinoma Formation in Animal Models
Mechanisms of Carcinogenesis and Prevention

Chung S. Yang, Xiaoxin Chen, and Guang-Yu Yang

CONTENTS

3.1 INTRODUCTION

Inflammation is an adaptive host defense against infection and injury and is primarily a self-limiting process; however, inadequate resolution of inflammation could often lead to different chronic diseases, including cancer (Ullman et al. 2011; Kundu and Surh 2008; Schottenfeld and Beebe-Dimmer 2006; Jackson and Evers 2006). It has been estimated that approximately 25% of human cancers are associated with chronic infection and inflammation (Hussain and Harris 2007). For example, the development of stomach cancer is strongly associated with *Helicobacter pylori*–induced gastric inflammation (Peek and Blaser 2002). The development of liver cancer is strongly associated with hepatitis B or hepatitis C virus–induced chronic hepatic inflammation (Matsuzaki et al. 2007). The development of esophageal adenocarcinoma (EAC) is strongly associated with gastroesophageal reflux inflammation of the esophagus (Kruse et al. 1993; Altorki et al. 1997). Inflammatory bowel disorders such as ulcerative colitis (UC) and Crohn's disease predispose individuals to the development of colorectal cancer (Ullman et al. 2011; Seril et al. 2003). Several lines of evidence from laboratory studies also suggest an important role of inflammation in carcinogenesis (Kundu and Surh 2008; Hussain and Harris 2007; Chen and Yang 2001; Seril et al. 2003).

In this chapter, we will discuss two experimental models in which EAC and colorectal carcinoma (CRC) are induced by inflammation, without the presence of a carcinogen or genetic manipulations. In the esophageal cancer model, adenocarcinoma formation is induced in rats by a surgical procedure, esophagogastroduodenal anastomosis (EGDA), which produces gastroesophageal reflux and inflammation of the lower esophagus. In the UC-associated CRC model, the inflammation and carcinogenesis are induced in mice by 15 cycles of inflammation, produced by treatment with dextran sulfate sodium (DSS). In both experimental systems, carcinogenesis is enhanced by iron supplementation, which increased oxidative stress. Reactive oxygen and nitrogen species (RONS) produced by inflammation as well as overproduction of prostaglandin E_2 (PGE_2) have been shown to be the major driving forces for carcinogenesis. These events are proposed to produce both genetic and epigenetic changes that lead to the formation of adenocarcinomas. In these model systems, carcinogenesis has been shown to be inhibited by some antioxidants, anti-inflammatory agents, and other agents. The inflammation mechanisms of carcinogenesis and its prevention, as well as implications to human esophageal and colorectal adenocarcinomas, are discussed in this chapter.

3.2 HUMAN EAC

Esophageal squamous cell carcinoma has historically been the major form of esophageal cancer worldwide and is still the major form of esophageal cancer in many developing countries. Between 1976 and 1990, the incidence rate of EAC in the United States tripled, with a yearly increase of ~10%, displaying the fastest increase of all types of cancers (Devesa et al. 1998). Now EAC is the predominant form of esophageal cancer in the United States and other Western countries (Brown et al. 2008). It is known that most EACs develop from columnar-lined esophagus (CLE), also known as Barrett's esophagus (BE). BE, a common medical condition afflicting the human esophagus, is characterized by the replacement of the squamous epithelium in the lower esophagus by columnar epithelium (Kruse et al. 1993).

BE is mainly caused by gastroesophageal reflux, which is a commonly seen clinical entity in Western countries and known as gastroesophageal reflux disease (GERD). About 10% of GERD patients will eventually develop BE (Altorki et al. 1997). BE was originally believed to be congenital, and there is evidence for the genetic predisposition to the development of BE in families of BE and EAC patients (Romero et al. 1997). More and more evidence, however, has shown that BE is an acquired disease. Among the many risk factors described for the development of BE and EAC, GERD is by far the most important etiological factor. For example, a recent epidemiological study conducted in Sweden showed that, in patients with recurrent symptoms of reflux, the odds ratio for EAC was 7.7; among patients with long-standing and severe symptoms of reflux, the odds ratio was 43.4 (Lagergren et al. 1999). The prevalence of EAC increases with age, reaching a plateau by the seventh decade (Cameron and Lomboy 1992). Other risk factors included high intake of red meat and polyunsaturated fat; low consumption of fruit, vegetables, fish, vitamin A, vitamin C, vitamin E, β-carotene, and crude fibers; high body iron store; obesity; cigarette smoking; and alcohol consumption (Gammon et al. 1997; Vial et al. 2010; Edelstein et al. 2007; Cook et al. 2010; El-Serag and Lagergren 2009; Thompson et al. 2009; Cross et al. 2011).

At the molecular level, development of BE is complex and involves squamous transcription factors, intestinal transcription factors, signaling pathways, microRNAs, epigenetics, and many other factors (Chen et al. 2011). A recent genome-wide analysis of DNA methylation and copy number and transcriptome in human BE found that many genes were overexpressed, amplified, or hypomethylated (Alvarez et al. 2011). Although a molecular network has started to emerge, the mechanisms by which gastroesophageal reflux induces intestinal metaplasia in the esophagus are not fully understood. Nevertheless, loss of *p63*, activation of nuclear factor kappaB (NF-κB) pathway, and expression of *Cdx2* appear to be the most important events. Loss of *p63* is essential for squamous epithelial cells to silence the squamous differentiation program. Activation of the NF-κB pathway, either directly by reflux or indirectly by reflux-induced inflammation, is critical in activating *Cdx2* and/or *Cdx1* (Chen et al. 2011; Quante et al. 2012). *p53* is the most extensively studied gene in EAC. Approximately 50% of EAC cases have *p53* mutations, whereas in BE and BE with dysplasia, *p53* mutations are less frequent (Altorki et al. 1997). Transition mutations, especially G:C to A:T mutations, are the most frequent type observed. As will be discussed later, these events may be closely related to inflammation and RONS.

In studying the clonal ordering of neoplastic lineages in human EAC, *p53* gene mutation, *p16^{INKa}* gene mutation, nonrandom loss of heterozygosity, *p16^{INKa}* methylation, and ploidy were analyzed, and many intermediate clones with cancer-developing tendencies were detected (Barrett et al. 1999). The results suggest multiple pathways leading to EAC: some of these clones persisted and developed into EAC, whereas others had no progression or were delayed in their progression. Such studies of the genetic events in carcinogenesis may improve our understanding of BE and EAC, help in identifying high-risk patients, and thus lead to more efficient strategies for prevention and treatment.

3.3 ANIMAL MODELS FOR EAC

Several animal models have been developed to study EAC, and the most effective approach is to use surgery to induce gastroesophageal reflux. Attwood et al. (1992) used duodenoesophagostomy (side to side and end to side), also known as esophagoduodenal anastomosis (EDA), to induce EAC in rats (Figure 3.1a). The addition of 2,6-dimethylnitrosomorphine or methyl-*n*-amylnitrosamine treatment to the model promoted the formation of tumors, showing both squamous cell carcinoma and EAC characteristics. Only a small percentage of tumors were pure, well-differentiated EAC (Pera et al. 1989; Clark et al. 1994). We have adapted the EDA rat model in our laboratory (Goldstein et al. 1997, 1998) and found that the animals developed EAC at a low incidence rate (~10%) at 30 weeks after surgery, but the incidence was enhanced to 73% with iron supplementation (50 mg Fe/kg/month, administered as iron dextran i.p.). The EDA model, however, has inherent problems due to partial loss of stomach function, resulting in malabsorption of certain nutrients and nutritional deficiencies. The EDA rats have lower body weight, lower iron nutritional status, lower serum albumin levels, and lower levels of fat-soluble vitamins than the nonoperated control rats (Chen et al. 2000). In order to avoid these problems, we developed a new procedure, EGDA, by making an anastomosis

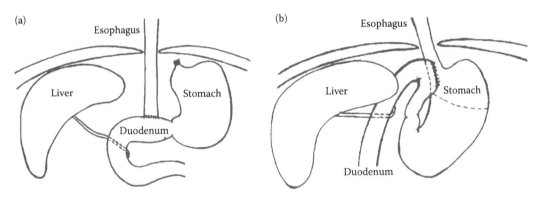

FIGURE 3.1 Surgical models of EAC. (a) EDA: the gastroesophageal junction is ligated flush with the stomach and the distal esophagus transected proximal to the ligature. An enterotomy is made 1 cm distal to the pylorus on the antimesenteric border. The distal esophagus was then anastomosed to the duodenal enterotomy with accurate mucosal-to-mucosal opposition. (b) EGDA: two 1.5 cm incisions were made, each on the gastroesophageal junction and the duodenum on the antimesenteric border, and then were anastomosed together with accurate mucosal-to-mucosal opposition. (From Chen, X., and C. S. Yang, *Carcinogenesis* 22 (8):1119–29, 2001.)

between the gastroesophageal junction and the duodenum (Figure 3.1b). This procedure produced CLE and EAC without severe, large-area esophagitis and major nutritional complications (Chen et al. 1999). The EGDA model mimics the two essential features for the development of human EAC: the duodenogastroesophageal reflux and the presence of intestinal or "specialized" columnar epithelium in the esophagus. Continuity of the duodenal epithelium to CLE in all cases suggests that specialized columnar cells come from creeping substitution after EGDA. Compared with the other existing animal models for EAC, the EGDA model has the following advantages: (1) it allows food to pass through the normal alimentary tract, and the rats have close to normal stomach functions and nutritional status; (2) there is substantial reflux of both gastric and duodenal contents of the esophagus, both of which are needed to induce CLE and EACs; and (3) recirculation of bile through the stomach raises the antral pH, thus resulting in gastrin release by the antral G cells. Gastrin is known to have a trophic effect in the gastrointestinal epithelium by encouraging the growth of esophageal carcinoma (Van Nieuwenhove et al. 1998).

In collaboration with Dr. Goyal and his associates, we compared the morphology and phenotypic features of CLE and EAC in the rat EDGA model with the corresponding lesions in human BE and EAC (Su et al. 2004). The esophagi of EGDA rats showed esophagitis, islands of multilayered epithelium (MLE), CLE, dysplasia, and EAC. The CLE had features of specialized intestinal metaplasia. MLE frequently occurred at the new squamocolumnar junction and occasionally in the mid-esophagus in isolated foci. Scattered mucinous cells in esophageal squamous epithelium were also found. The CLE and MLE in EGDA rats also resembled the lesions in human BE in morphology, mucin features, and expression of differentiation markers, such as CK7, CK20, Das-1, villin, and pS2/TFF1. In the EGDA rat model, the invasive EAC was of the well-differentiated mucinous type, which is different from the variably differentiated glandular type of adenocarcinoma in human BE. *p53*, c-myc, and cyclooxygenase 2 (Cox2) were expressed in both the rat and human specialized intestinal metaplasia and EAC. These results indicate that, although there are small differences, the metaplasia and EAC induced in EGDA rats are similar to the corresponding lesions in human BE and EAC (Su et al. 2004). We believe that EGDA rats can serve as a useful model to study the pathogenesis, molecular biology, and chemoprevention of human BE and EAC.

In order to further characterize the molecular changes in the EGDA model, we compared the protein expression pattern between rat EAC and normal tissues by two-dimensional protein gel electrophoresis (Chen, Ding et al. 2002). The overexpressed protein spots of the tumor sample were cut out and analyzed by matrix-assisted laser desorption/ionization mass spectrometry. Several stress proteins (Grp94, Grp78, calnexin, Hsp90β, and ER61), as well as leukotriene A_4 hydrolase (LTA$_4$H), were identified by this method. Western blotting and reverse transcriptase polymerase chain reaction (RT–PCR) further confirmed overexpression of Grp94 in rat EAC. Immunohistochemical staining also demonstrated expression of Grp94 in the epithelial cells of CLE and EAC. Similar to the rat model, well-differentiated human EAC and gastric cardia adenocarcinomas were also found to overexpress Grp94, but esophageal squamous cell carcinomas were not. We also observed increased levels of oxidative DNA damage, apoptosis, and cell proliferation in the rat CLE and EAC. Grp94 is known to inhibit apoptosis by maintaining intracellular Ca^{2+} homeostasis; however, an inverse correlation between Grp94 overexpression and apoptosis was not observed (Chen, Ding et al. 2002).

In both the EDA and EGDA rat models, we demonstrated that long-term iron supplementation promoted the formation of EAC. Esophageal iron overload might result from transient increase in blood iron after i.p. injection and the overexpression of transferring receptor in the premalignant CLE cells. Iron was found deposited in the esophageal epithelium after iron administration and significantly enhanced oxidative stress in rats with gastroesophageal reflux due to surgery. Overexpression of inducible nitric oxide synthase (iNOS) and the presence of nitrotyrosine were observed immunohistochemically, and these markers were correlated with inflammation and cell proliferation (Goldstein et al. 1997, 1998). Oxidative damage to DNA, protein, and lipids in the esophagus was significantly higher in treated rats than in the nonoperated controls. The overexpression of heme oxygenase 1 and metallothionein in CLE cells suggested that these cells were under oxidative stress (Goldstein et al. 1998). Supplementation of vitamin E in the diet (10-fold the amount in the AIN93M) maintained the normal plasma level of alpha-tocopherol in the EDA rats and inhibited esophageal adenocarcinogenesis (Chen, Mikhail et al. 2000).

Aberrant arachidonic acid metabolism was demonstrated in studies with mass spectrometry (Chen, Li et al. 2002). PGE_2, leukotriene B_4 (LTB_4), 15-hydroeicosatetraenoic acid (HETE), 12-HETE, 8-HETE, and 5-HETE all increased at the esophagoduodenal junction after EGDA, as compared with the proximal esophagus. PGE2 was the major metabolite. Consistent with this profile, Cox2 was overexpressed in the basal cell layer of esophageal squamous epithelium, CLE cells, and EAC tumor cells of the EGDA rats, as compared with the normal esophageal epithelium. In a short-term study (for 4 weeks after surgery), dietary administration of a Cox inhibitor, sulindac (300 and 600 ppm); a lipoxygenase inhibitor, nordihydroguaiaretic acid (NDGA) (100 ppm) effectively reduced the EGDA-induced inflammation (Chen et al. 2002).

LTA_4H is a rate-limiting enzyme in the biosynthesis of LTB_4 and a potent inflammatory mediator. We discovered the overexpression of LTA_4H in EAC by two-dimensional protein gel electrophoresis proteomics and further investigated this enzyme in rat and human EACs (Chen et al. 2003). LTA_4H was overexpressed in all 10 rat EACs examined, as compared with its level in normal rat tissue. It was also overexpressed in four of six human EAC tumor samples, as compared with its level in adjacent nontumor tissue. In tissue sections from 20 EGDA rats and 92 patients (86 with EAC, 1 with dysplasia, and 5 with BE), LTA_4H was expressed in infiltrating inflammatory cells and overexpressed in the columnar cells of preinvasive lesions and cancers, especially in well-differentiated EACs, as compared with the basal cells of the normal esophageal squamous epithelium. An LTA_4H inhibitor, bestatin, significantly inhibited LTB_4 biosynthesis in the esophageal tissues of EGDA rats (4.68 vs. 8.28 ng/mg of protein in the control) (Chen et al. 2003).

3.4 MECHANISTIC CONSIDERATIONS AND PREVENTION OF EAC FORMATION

Based on our understanding of esophageal adenocarcinogenesis, a hypothesis for a chronic inflammation-driven mechanism has been proposed (Chen and Yang 2001) (Figure 3.2). The pathogenesis starts with surgery-induced reflux in animal models or GERD in humans. Gastric acid, bile acids, and digestive enzymes induce irritation and inflammation in the esophagus. The squamous epithelium of the esophagus responds with inflammatory cell infiltration, hyperkeratinization, basal cell hyperproliferation, and even sloughing or ulceration of the epithelium. Two categories of inflammatory mediators produced by the inflammatory cells in the esophagus, eicosanoids (such as PGE_2 and LTB_4) and RONS, are of particular importance. They exert feedforward effects on the inflammatory cells and direct effects on cells expressing respective receptors, such as the goblet cells expressing receptors for PGE_2. RONS, on the other hand, may cause DNA strand breaks, DNA base modification, lipid peroxidation, and protein oxidation. In the surgical animal models, both eicosanoids and RONS may stimulate the growth of columnar epithelium at the squamocolumnar junction, to induce creeping substitution of the squamous epithelium in the esophagus by columnar epithelium. In human patients with GERD, metaplasia of the stem cells in the esophagus or creeping substitution by the intestinalized cardia epithelium may be induced. Persistent stimulation of the columnar cells by these inflammatory mediators will result in a series of genetic and epigenetic changes, such as gene mutation and allelic loss, genomic instability, gene amplification, hyperproliferation, altered gene expression and cell cycle control, and altered apoptosis. This hypothesis may help us identify targets and design strategies for the chemoprevention of EAC.

We have conducted two prevention studies with antioxidants. In the first study, α-tocopheryl acetate (750 IU/kg diet) and sodium selenite (1.7 mg Se/kg diet) were given, in a two-by-two design, to rats that received EDA surgery plus iron supplementation (12 mg/kg/week). At 40 weeks after surgery, α-tocopheryl acetate supplementation maintained the normal plasma concentrations of

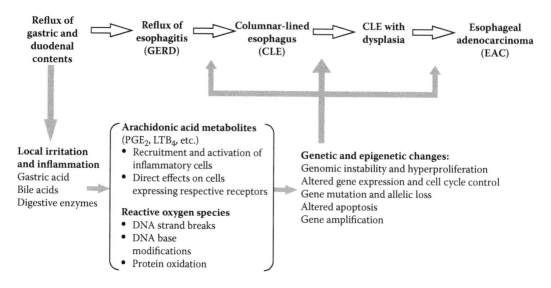

FIGURE 3.2 Proposed histopathological and molecular events leading to esophageal adenocarcinogenesis. Gastroduodenoesophageal reflux causes irritation and inflammation. RONS and inflammatory mediators (especially arachidonic acid metabolites) are proposed to induce genetic and epigenetic changes leading to CLE, CLE with dysplasia, and EAC. This hypothesis, developed on the basis of the animal models, may also be applicable to humans. (From Chen, X., and C. S. Yang, *Carcinogenesis* 22 (8):1119–29, 2001.)

α-tocopherol, but decreased γ-tocopherol levels. Selenium supplementation increased the serum and tumor selenium contents of the rats. Surprisingly, selenium supplementation increased the incidence of EAC and tumor volume. α-Tocopheryl acetate, however, inhibited tumorigenesis, especially in the selenium-supplemented group. The reason for the unexpected cancer promotion effect of selenium is not known, but may be due to the high concentration of inorganic selenium used in rats experiencing inflammation and oxidative stress. The inhibitory effect of α-tocopheryl acetate was lower than expected. In a second study, the inhibitory effects of α-tocopheryl acetate and other agents were studied in the EGDA rats at 40 weeks after surgery (Hao et al. 2009). α-Tocopheryl acetate (778 IU/kg diet) significantly decreased the incidence of EAC. The combination of α-tocopheryl acetate (389 IU/kg diet) and *N*-acetylcysteine (NAC, 500 ppm) appeared to have higher inhibitory activity, even though 500 and 1000 ppm NAC did not significantly decrease EAC incidence. The commonly used antiacid agent, omeprazole (at 1400 ppm), showed only a nonsignificant inhibitory effect (Hao et al. 2009).

LTA$_4$H overexpression appears to be an early event in esophageal adenocarcinogenesis and is a potential target for the chemoprevention of EAC (Chen et al. 2003). An inhibitor of LTA$_4$H, bestatin, was shown to reduce the incidence of EAC in the EGDA rats from 57.7% (15 of 26 rats) to 26.1% (6 of 23 rats) (difference = 31.6%, 95% confidence interval = 0.3% to 56.2%; $P = .042$). The possible inhibitory actions of sulindac (a Cox inhibitor), NDGA (a lipoxygenase inhibitor), and α-difluoromethylornithine (DFMO, an ornithine decarboxylase inhibitor) against the formation of EAC were investigated in the rat EGDA model (Chen, Li et al. 2002). Rats were treated with chemopreventive agents for 40 weeks after surgery; 300 ppm sulindac, alone or in combination with 100 ppm NDGA or 0.5% DFMO, decreased the tumor incidence from 57.7% to 26.9%, or 16.7% or 20%, respectively ($P < .05$). NDGA alone (100 and 200 ppm) slightly decreased the tumor incidence to 52.4% and 37%, respectively, although the difference was not statistically significant. DFMO alone did not show significant effects on tumor incidence. Inhibition of tumor formation by sulindac was correlated with lowered levels of PGE$_2$. The results suggested that sulindac exerted its chemopreventive effect against the formation of EAC in the rat EGDA model, possibly through its inhibition of Cox activity.

3.5 UC-ASSOCIATED COLORECTAL CANCER IN HUMANS

UC is an idiopathic disease characterized by mucosal inflammation of the large bowel, with an incidence rate of approximately 10 per 100,000 per year (Russel and Stockbrugger 1996). It is predominately a disease of late adolescence and early adulthood, with the peak of incidence occurring in the third decade of life (Ekbom et al. 1991). The incidence of UC varies depending on geography and is more common in the Western countries and among Caucasians. The susceptibility of certain ethnic groups to UC suggests a genetic contribution to this disease, and environmental factors are clearly known to play important roles (Fiocchi 1998). Many factors have been proposed to be involved in the initiation and propagation of the chronic inflammatory response in UC. These factors suggest that UC is an aberrant response to commonly encountered environmental stimuli and/or UC arises as a normal immune response to a persistent infection or altered colonic microflora (Fiocchi 1998). Chronic UC is associated with an increased risk of developing CRC. The relative risk of CRC development in UC patients is 10-fold greater than in the general population (Ekbom et al. 1990). The risk of developing cancer increases exponentially with the duration of the disease, and surveillance for dysplasia and cancer is recommended for patients with UC for more than 10 years (Collins et al. 1987). Individuals with pancolitis (UC involving the entire colon) are more likely to develop colorectal cancer than those with left-sided disease only (Ekbom et al. 1990). The histopathogenesis of UC-associated colorectal carcinogenesis is known to involve a stepwise progression from inflamed and hyperplastic epithelia to flat dysplasia and, finally, adenocarcinoma (Riddell et al. 1983). The adenocarcinoma is presumed to arise from an accumulation of genetic alterations in tumor suppressor genes, oncogenes, and genes encoding DNA repair proteins, as well as an overall loss of genomic stability. Comparisons of the molecular alteration profiles of sporadic and UC-associated CRCs have indicated that the two types of colorectal cancer share alterations in many of the same genes and overall processes. However, the timing and frequency of the molecular genetic alterations in UC-associated cancers are different.

The more characteristic difference is that *p53* mutation and hypermethylation-related silencing of *p16^{INK4a}* and *p14^{ARF}* occur early and frequently in UC-associated CRC (Lashner et al. 1999; Yin et al. 1993; Holzmann et al. 1998; Hsieh et al. 1998; Sato et al. 2002), whereas in sporadic CRC, these events occur less frequently and often at later stages of cancer development. On the other hand, *APC* gene mutation and activating mutations of the *K-Ras* oncogene, which are common in early stages of sporadic colorectal carcinogenesis, occur less frequently in UC-associated CRC (Redston et al. 1995; Burmer et al. 1990). The early occurrence of *p53* mutation and gene silencing by hypermethylation may be caused by the inflammation and oxidative stress. For example, the *p53* mutations found in UC-associated CRC are predominately transition mutations (Holzmann et al. 1998; Yin et al. 1993). They can be induced by G-to-A mutation caused by lipid peroxidation products, by C-to-T transitions caused by the formation of 5-hydroxycytosine, or by the spontaneous or nitric oxide–induced deamination of 5-methylcytosine at CpG sites (Greenblatt et al. 1994). Hypermethylation of the CpG islands at the promoter region is often associated with inflammation (Issa et al. 2001; Schulmann et al. 2005; Kundu and Surh 2008).

3.6 ANIMAL MODELS FOR UC-ASSOCIATED COLORECTAL CANCER

As reviewed previously (Seril et al. 2003), several genetic modification and chemically induced models for UC have been developed. The DSS model has been among the most widely used models of chemically induced colitis and, more recently, UC-associated colorectal cancer development. DSS is a synthetic, sulfated polysaccharide that induces colitis in rodents and is clinically and histologically reminiscent of human UC. The DSS model in mice is characterized by both acute and chronic UC (Okayasu et al. 1990) and may result from altered colonic microflora or macrophage activity (Ohkusa et al. 1995). DSS has also been shown to be directly toxic to crypt cells, and colonic crypt loss may precede the onset of an immune response (Cooper et al. 1993). Susceptibility to DSS-induced UC varies between species and strains (Mahler et al. 1998), indicating a strong interplay within the model between causative factors and background genetics.

We and others have been studying the colitis-associated carcinogenesis process using the DSS model in mice (Seril et al. 2003). Typically, it involves cyclic DSS treatment, in which DSS is administered via the drinking fluid at doses of 1%–3% for 3 to 7 days, followed by water administration for 1 to 2 weeks to permit healing of the colonic mucosa (Okayasu et al. 1990). The animals are subjected to several such DSS "cycles" to simulate the course of UC observed in humans, which is characterized by periods of active inflammation (flare-ups), separated by periods of disease inactivity. Cooper et al. (2000) analyzed the relationship between the severity of DSS-induced inflammation and colorectal carcinogenesis and found that (1) higher inflammation scores correlated with a greater occurrence of dysplasia or cancer and (2) dysplasia-associated lesions or masses occurred in settings of mild inflammation, whereas flat lesions were associated with colitis of greater severity. Dysplasia-associated lesions or masses, but not flat lesions, were characterized by β-catenin accumulation in the cytoplasm and nucleus, indicative of *Apc* pathway alteration. Neither type of lesion in the DSS model seems to be associated with *p53* alteration (Cooper et al. 2000), not unlike many other murine models of cancer.

The DSS model of chronic UC in mice has also been used to study the mechanistic roles of genes and processes thought to be involved in human UC-associated carcinogenesis. Cyclic DSS treatment promotes colorectal tumorigenesis in the $Apc^{Min/+}$ mouse, with loss of function of the remaining *Apc* allele by mutation (Cooper et al. 2001). This is similar to human studies, which have indicated that *APC* alteration is involved in a subset of UC-associated cancers. Cyclic DSS treatment also promotes colorectal tumor development initiated by the carcinogen azoxymethane (AOM) (Okayasu et al. 1996). Tumorigenesis in the AOM model is known to involve loss of *Apc* function.

We have been studying UC-associated colorectal carcinogenesis in mice and the role of inflammation. In our studies, C57BL/6J mice, which are not susceptible to spontaneous colorectal tumor development and moderately sensitive to DSS treatment (Mahler et al. 1998), were subjected to 12 to 15 consecutive DSS cycles consisting of 7 days of low-dose DSS treatment (0.7% in drinking water) followed by 10 days of tap water administration. Invasive colorectal adenocarcinoma and anal squamous cell carcinoma, as well as dysplasia, occurred at rates of approximately 30% in a setting of moderately severe inflammation (Seril et al. 2002). The majority of the tumors observed in this model were well-differentiated, mucinous adenocarcinomas, the most commonly observed type of carcinoma in UC patients (Heimann et al. 1992).

UC patients frequently experience iron deficiency anemia due to chronic disease and colonic blood loss, and these individuals are often recommended to take iron supplementation to prevent anemia. In order to assess the role of iron supplementation in the UC-associated carcinogenesis process, we administered a diet containing 90 mg iron per kilogram diet (versus 45 mg/kg iron in the AIN76A diet) to DSS-treated mice (Seril et al. 2002). The consumption of a high-iron diet significantly increased colorectal tumor development; the adenocarcinoma incidence increased from approximately 30% in mice on the AIN76A diet to greater than 80% with a high-iron diet. In short-term studies, elevated dietary iron increased local iron deposition, the levels of iNOS and nitrotyrosine, and DSS-induced UC index (Seril et al. 2002). In a subsequent study, we analyzed the effect of NAC administration on cancer development in this murine model. Colorectal tumor incidence and tumor multiplicity were significantly decreased in mice consuming the 2000 ppm NAC in the diet during the water recovery period, as compared to positive controls. Dietary NAC also decreased inflammation-driven epithelial cell proliferation, nitrotyrosine staining, and iNOS-positive macrophage involvement (Seril et al. 2002). These results suggest that oxidative stress and inflammation play important roles in the development of CRC in UC patients. Iron supplementation may contribute to the carcinogenesis process by augmenting oxidative damage and inflammation-caused epithelial proliferation. NAC may inhibit these processes by way of antioxidant activities.

3.7 MECHANISTIC CONSIDERATION AND PREVENTION STUDIES OF UC-ASSOCIATED COLORECTAL CARCINOGENESIS

Inflammation and oxidative cellular damage are hallmarks of UC and likely play key roles in the pathogenesis of UC-associated CRC (Seril et al. 2003; Ullman et al. 2011). The activities of phago-cytic leukocytes are greatly increased in the colons of UC patients, resulting in enhanced genera-tion of pro-oxidative molecules (Schreiber et al. 1991; Babbs 1992; Grisham 1994). UC manifests deficiencies in antioxidant defenses, presumably due to excessive inflammation (Buffinton and Doe 1995; Lih-Brody et al. 1996; Holmes et al. 1998). Cellular damage caused by oxidative stress may provide a mechanistic basis for many of the events thought to drive UC-associated carcinogenesis in humans and animal models, including specific gene alterations, genetic instability, and aber-rant methylation. RONS can covalently modify DNA bases, and failure to remove these lesions leads to base substitutions, deletions, and insertions (Wang et al. 1998; Marnett 2000). The Ogg DNA repair enzyme recognizes and excises 8-oxo-dG from GC base pairs. We have demonstrated that DSS-induced UC-associated colon carcinogenesis was enhanced in Ogg knockout mice (Liao et al. 2008).

In active UC patients, the nitrite levels and iNOS activity in UC biopsies as well as serum nitrite levels were increased, suggesting the involvement of reactive nitrogen species (Oudkerk Pool et al. 1995; Rachmilewitz, Stamler et al. 1995). The involvement of RONS in the pathogenesis of colitis is also supported by the observation that radical scavengers, superoxide dismutase, catalase, and iNOS inhibitors are protective in chemically induced models of colon inflammation, including the DSS model (Rachmilewitz, Karmeli et al. 1995; Naito et al. 2001). Intrarectal administration of per-oxynitrite induces colonic inflammation in rats (Rachmilewitz et al. 1993). Genetic iNOS knockout, however, did not affect colon tumorigenesis in mice that were subjected to 15 cycles of DSS-induced inflammation in our UC model (Seril et al. 2007). Nitrotyrosine, an indicator of peroxynitrite-caused protein modification, however, was detected by IHC in inflammatory cells and epithelial cells in the colons of both the iNOS knockout and wild-type mice. The results suggest that other forms of NOS, such as endothelial nitric oxide synthase (eNOS), may play a role in generating nitric oxidase in UC (Seril et al. 2007). Telomere shortening is observed in the colonic epithelial cells of UC patients, and telomere length progressively decreases from inflamed epithelia to dysplasia and carcinoma (Kinouchi et al. 1998). This shortening and breakage of the chromosomal ends may cause DNA translocations, deletions, and amplifications. Telomere dysfunction can also lead to loss or gain of whole chromosomes (Artandi and DePinho 2000; Cottliar et al. 2000).

Mesalamine is a mainstay therapeutic agent for chronic UC; it reverses crypt architectural changes and reduces UC-associated CRC, and its activity has been attributed, in part, to iron-chelating and radical-scavenging effects (Yamada et al. 1990). Recently, mesalamine has been shown to reduce Akt phosphorylation and β-catenin activation in the middle and upper crypt in interleukin (IL)-10 knockout and human colitis samples (Brown et al. 2010). In IL-10 knockout mice, mesalamine-reduced colitis-induced dysplasia was associated with inhibition of crypt Akt and β-catenin signaling. As discussed previously, in the DSS-induced UC model, NAC has been shown to reduce RONS and inhibit tumorigenesis (Seril et al. 2002). Myoinositol was also shown to inhibit UC-associated CRC (Liao et al. 2007). In this study, myoinositol was administered at a dose of 1% in drinking water throughout the experiment, and the tumor incidence, multiplicity, and volume were inhibited by 41%, 60%, and 80%, respectively. In comparison, phytic acid (inositol hexaphosphate [IP6]) at 1.0% reduced tumor volume, but not tumor incidence and multiplicity. This is possibly due to the low amount of inositol used; in the 1% solution of IP6, the myoinositol con-centration is 0.27% (Liao et al. 2007). In another study, freeze-dried black raspberry powder (5% or 10% in the diet) was found to reduce DSS-induced colon injury (Montrose et al. 2011). The black raspberry powder–treated mice had lower tissue levels of tumor necrosis factor α and interleukin 1β as well as phosphor-1κBα and Cox2.

3.8 CONCLUDING REMARKS ON INFLAMMATION-INDUCED ESOPHAGEAL AND COLORECTAL ADENOCARCINOMAS

As demonstrated in the EGDA-induced EAC and DSS-induced UC-associated CRC models, carcinomas can be induced by inflammation in the absence of any added carcinogen without any genetic manipulations. Inflammation appears to be the sole driving force for carcinogenesis. RONS are involved in both EAC and UC-associated CRC formation. RONS can cause DNA base oxidation and strand breaks. In inflamed mucosa and cancer samples from EAC and UC patients, the *p53* mutation spectra are dominated by base transitions that may be caused by oxidative base modification (Hussain and Harris 1998). The products of lipid peroxidation may cause the formation of etheno- and propano-DNA adducts, leading to base transition mutations (Nair et al. 1999). Nitric oxide–mediated nitration of 5-methylcytosine and subsequent base deamination may lead to C-to-T transition (Greenblatt et al. 1994). Nitric oxide has also been found to inhibit the function of DNA repair proteins and may thereby act to impair the removal of DNA lesions (Wink et al. 1998). Other cancer-related genes may also be altered by the action of RONS in the setting of chronic UC. Repair of these DNA breaks by illegitimate recombination can form mutations and DNA rearrangements, and unrepaired breaks can lead to chromosomal breakage, fragmentation, and translocation (Morgan et al. 1998). It has been suggested that inflammation can contribute to the hypermethylation of many tumor suppressor genes (Kundu and Surh 2008; Issa et al. 2001; Schulmann et al. 2005), and specifically, inflammation-mediated halogenated cytosine products have been proposed to mimic 5-methylcytosine in causing epigenetic alterations (Valinluck and Sowers 2007).

These inflammation-caused genetic and epigenetic events are expected to take place in the esophagus and colon in both animal models and humans, even though the specific genes involved in the different systems are known to be different. Another feature is the overproduction of PGE_2 and LTB_4, which has been demonstrated in the gastroesophageal reflux-induced inflammation in animal models as well as human BE and EAC (Chen, Li et al. 2002; Chen et al. 2003). These events are also expected to be important in UC-associated CRC. Based on these considerations, certain anti-inflammatory agents and selected antioxidants may be useful chemopreventive agents. However, cautions need to be applied; for example, Cox2 inhibitors are not suitable for UC patients, because PGE_2 is needed for normal colon epithelial turnover. Myo-inositol may be a better agent. Some other chemopreventive agents, such as green tea polyphenols, which are thought to have anti-inflammatory activity, may aggravate the colitis situation (Yang, C. S., unpublished results).

ACKNOWLEDGMENTS

This work was supported by grants from the US National Institutes of Health (CA122474 and CA133021) and the John L. Colaizzi chair endowment fund to C. S. Yang as well as Grants CA156735 and DK63650 to X. Chen.

REFERENCES

Altorki, N. K., S. Oliveria, and D. S. Schrump. 1997. Epidemiology and molecular biology of Barrett's adenocarcinoma. *Semin Surg Oncol* 13 (4):270–80.
Alvarez, H., J. Opalinska, L. Zhou et al. 2011. Widespread hypomethylation occurs early and synergizes with gene amplification during esophageal carcinogenesis. *PLoS Genet* 7 (3):e1001356.
Artandi, S. E., and R. A. DePinho. 2000. A critical role for telomeres in suppressing and facilitating carcinogenesis. *Curr Opin Genet Dev* 10 (1):39–46.
Attwood, S. E., T. C. Smyrk, T. R. DeMeester et al. 1992. Duodenoesophageal reflux and the development of esophageal adenocarcinoma in rats. *Surgery* 111 (5):503–10.
Babbs, C. F. 1992. Oxygen radicals in ulcerative colitis. *Free Radic Biol Med* 13 (2):169–81.
Barrett, M. T., C. A. Sanchez, L. J. Prevo et al. 1999. Evolution of neoplastic cell lineages in Barrett oesophagus. *Nat Genet* 22 (1):106–9.

Brown, J. B., G. Lee, E. Managlia et al. 2010. Mesalamine inhibits epithelial beta-catenin activation in chronic ulcerative colitis. *Gastroenterology* 138 (2):595–605, 605 e1–3.

Brown, L. M., S. S. Devesa, and W. H. Chow. 2008. Incidence of adenocarcinoma of the esophagus among white Americans by sex, stage, and age. *J Natl Cancer Inst* 100 (16):1184–7.

Buffinton, G. D., and W. F. Doe. 1995. Depleted mucosal antioxidant defences in inflammatory bowel disease. *Free Radic Biol Med* 19 (6):911–8.

Burmer, G. C., D. S. Levine, B. G. Kulander et al. 1990. c-Ki-ras mutations in chronic ulcerative colitis and sporadic colon carcinoma. *Gastroenterology* 99 (2):416–20.

Cameron, A. J., and C. T. Lomboy. 1992. Barrett's esophagus: age, prevalence, and extent of columnar epithelium. *Gastroenterology* 103 (4):1241–5.

Chen, H., Y. Fang, W. Tevebaugh et al. 2011. Molecular mechanisms of Garrett's esophagus. *Dig Dis Sci* 56:3405–20.

Chen, X., Y. Ding, C. G. Liu, S. Mikhail, and C. S. Yang. 2002. Overexpression of glucose-regulated protein 94 (Grp94) in esophageal adenocarcinomas of a rat surgical model and humans. *Carcinogenesis* 23 (1):123–30.

Chen, X., Y. W. Ding, G. Yang et al. 2000. Oxidative damage in an esophageal adenocarcinoma model with rats. *Carcinogenesis* 21 (2):257–63.

Chen, X., N. Li, S. Wang et al. 2002. Aberrant arachidonic acid metabolism in esophageal adenocarcinogenesis, and the effects of sulindac, nordihydroguaiaretic acid, and alpha-difluoromethylornithine on tumorigenesis in a rat surgical model. *Carcinogenesis* 23 (12):2095–102.

Chen, X., N. Li, S. Wang et al. 2003. Leukotriene A4 hydrolase in rat and human esophageal adenocarcinomas and inhibitory effects of bestatin. *J Natl Cancer Inst* 95 (14):1053–61.

Chen, X., S. S. Mikhail, Y. W. Ding et al. 2000. Effects of vitamin E and selenium supplementation on esophageal adenocarcinogenesis in a surgical model with rats. *Carcinogenesis* 21 (8):1531–6.

Chen, X., and C. S. Yang. 2001. Esophageal adenocarcinoma: a review and perspectives on the mechanism of carcinogenesis and chemoprevention. *Carcinogenesis* 22 (8):1119–29.

Chen, X., G. Yang, W. Y. Ding et al. 1999. An esophagogastroduodenal anastomosis model for esophageal adenocarcinogenesis in rats and enhancement by iron overload. *Carcinogenesis* 20 (9):1801–8.

Clark, G. W., T. C. Smyrk, S. S. Mirvish et al. 1994. Effect of gastroduodenal juice and dietary fat on the development of Barrett's esophagus and esophageal neoplasia: an experimental rat model. *Ann Surg Oncol* 1 (3):252–61.

Collins, R. H., Jr., M. Feldman, and J. S. Fordtran. 1987. Colon cancer, dysplasia, and surveillance in patients with ulcerative colitis. A critical review. *N Engl J Med* 316 (26):1654–8.

Cook, M. B., F. Kamangar, D. C. Whiteman et al. 2010. Cigarette smoking and adenocarcinomas of the esophagus and esophagogastric junction: a pooled analysis from the international BEACON consortium. *J Natl Cancer Inst* 102 (17):1344–53.

Cooper, H. S., L. Everley, W. C. Chang et al. 2001. The role of mutant Apc in the development of dysplasia and cancer in the mouse model of dextran sulfate sodium-induced colitis. *Gastroenterology* 121 (6):1407–16.

Cooper, H. S., S. Murthy, K. Kido, H. Yoshitake, and A. Flanigan. 2000. Dysplasia and cancer in the dextran sulfate sodium mouse colitis model. Relevance to colitis-associated neoplasia in the human: a study of histopathology, B-catenin and p53 expression and the role of inflammation. *Carcinogenesis* 21 (4):757–68.

Cooper, H. S., S. N. Murthy, R. S. Shah, and D. J. Sedergran. 1993. Clinicopathologic study of dextran sulfate sodium experimental murine colitis. *Lab Invest* 69 (2):238–49.

Cottliar, A., A. Fundia, L. Boerr et al. 2000. High frequencies of telomeric associations, chromosome aberrations, and sister chromatid exchanges in ulcerative colitis. *Am J Gastroenterol* 95 (9):2301–7.

Cross, A. J., N. D. Freedman, J. Ren et al. 2011. Meat consumption and risk of esophageal and gastric cancer in a large prospective study. *Am J Gastroenterol* 106 (3):432–42.

Devesa, S. S., W. J. Blot, and J. F. Fraumeni, Jr. 1998. Changing patterns in the incidence of esophageal and gastric carcinoma in the United States. *Cancer* 83 (10):2049–53.

Edelstein, Z. R., D. C. Farrow, M. P. Bronner, S. N. Rosen, and T. L. Vaughan. 2007. Central adiposity and risk of Barrett's esophagus. *Gastroenterology* 133 (2):403–11.

Ekbom, A., C. Helmick, M. Zack, and H.-O. Adami. 1990. Ulcerative colitis and colorectal cancer. A population-based study. *N Engl J Med* 323:1229–33.

Ekbom, A., C. Helmick, M. Zack, and H. O. Adami. 1991. The epidemiology of inflammatory bowel disease: a large, population-based study in Sweden. *Gastroenterology* 100 (2):350–8.

El-Serag, H. B., and J. Lagergren. 2009. Alcohol drinking and the risk of Barrett's esophagus and esophageal adenocarcinoma. *Gastroenterology* 136 (4):1155–7.

Fiocchi, C. 1998. Inflammatory bowel disease: etiology and pathogenesis. *Gastroenterology* 115 (1):182–205.

Gammon, M. D., J. B. Schoenberg, H. Ahsan et al. 1997. Tobacco, alcohol, and socioeconomic status and adenocarcinomas of the esophagus and gastric cardia. *J Natl Cancer Inst* 89 (17):1277–84.

Goldstein, S. R., G. Y. Yang, X. Chen, S. K. Curtis, and C. S. Yang. 1998. Studies of iron deposits, inducible nitric oxide synthase and nitrotyrosine in a rat model for esophageal adenocarcinoma. *Carcinogenesis* 19 (8):1445–9.

Goldstein, S. R., G. Y. Yang, S. K. Curtis et al. 1997. Development of esophageal metaplasia and adenocarcinoma in a rat surgical model without the use of a carcinogen. *Carcinogenesis* 18 (11):2265–70.

Greenblatt, M. S., W. P. Bennett, M. Hollstein, and C. C. Harris. 1994. Mutations in the p53 tumor suppressor gene: clues to cancer etiology and molecular pathogenesis. *Cancer Res* 54 (18):4855–78.

Grisham, M. B. 1994. Oxidants and free radicals in inflammatory bowel disease. *Lancet* 344 (8926):859–61.

Hao, J., B. Zhang, B. Liu et al. 2009. Effect of alpha-tocopherol, N-acetylcysteine and omeprazole on esophageal adenocarcinoma formation in a rat surgical model. *Int J Cancer* 124 (6):1270–5.

Heimann, T. M., S. C. Oh, G. Martinelli et al. 1992. Colorectal carcinoma associated with ulcerative colitis: a study of prognostic indicators. *Am J Surg* 164 (1):13–7.

Holmes, E. W., S. L. Yong, D. Eiznhamer, and A. Keshavarzian. 1998. Glutathione content of colonic mucosa: evidence for oxidative damage in active ulcerative colitis. *Dig Dis Sci* 43 (5):1088–95.

Holzmann, K., B. Klump, F. Borchard et al. 1998. Comparative analysis of histology, DNA content, p53 and Ki-ras mutations in colectomy specimens with long-standing ulcerative colitis. *Int J Cancer* 76 (1):1–6.

Hsieh, C. J., B. Klump, K. Holzmann et al. 1998. Hypermethylation of the p16INK4a promoter in colectomy specimens of patients with long-standing and extensive ulcerative colitis. *Cancer Res* 58 (17):3942–5.

Hussain, S. P., and C. C. Harris. 1998. Molecular epidemiology of human cancer: contribution of mutation spectra studies of tumor suppressor genes. *Cancer Res* 58 (18):4023–37.

Hussain, S. P., and C. C. Harris. 2007. Inflammation and cancer: an ancient link with novel potentials. *Int J Cancer* 121 (11):2373–80.

Issa, J. P., N. Ahuja, M. Toyota, M. P. Bronner, and T. A. Brentnall. 2001. Accelerated age-related CpG island methylation in ulcerative colitis. *Cancer Res* 61 (9):3573–7.

Jackson, L., and B. M. Evers. 2006. Chronic inflammation and pathogenesis of GI and pancreatic cancers. *Cancer Treat Res* 130:39–65.

Kinouchi, Y., N. Hiwatashi, M. Chida et al. 1998. Telomere shortening in the colonic mucosa of patients with ulcerative colitis. *J Gastroenterol* 33 (3):343–8.

Kruse, P., S. Boesby, I. T. Bernstein, and I. B. Andersen. 1993. Barrett's esophagus and esophageal adenocarcinoma. Endoscopic and histologic surveillance. *Scand J Gastroenterol* 28 (3):193–6.

Kundu, J. K., and Y. J. Surh. 2008. Inflammation: gearing the journey to cancer. *Mutat Res* 659 (1–2):15–30.

Lagergren, J., R. Bergstrom, A. Lindgren, and O. Nyren. 1999. Symptomatic gastroesophageal reflux as a risk factor for esophageal adenocarcinoma. *N Engl J Med* 340 (11):825–31.

Lashner, B. A., B. D. Shapiro, A. Husain, and J. R. Goldblum. 1999. Evaluation of the usefulness of testing for p53 mutations in colorectal cancer surveillance for ulcerative colitis. *Am J Gastroenterol* 94 (2):456–62.

Liao, J., D. N. Seril, G. G. Lu et al. 2008. Increased susceptibility of chronic ulcerative colitis-induced carcinoma development in DNA repair enzyme Ogg1 deficient mice. *Mol Carcinog* 47 (8):638–46.

Liao, J., D. N. Seril, A. L. Yang, G. G. Lu, and G. Y. Yang. 2007. Inhibition of chronic ulcerative colitis associated adenocarcinoma development in mice by inositol compounds. *Carcinogenesis* 28 (2):446–54.

Lih-Brody, L., S. R. Powell, K. P. Collier et al. 1996. Increased oxidative stress and decreased antioxidant defenses in mucosa of inflammatory bowel disease. *Dig Dis Sci* 41 (10):2078–86.

Mahler, M., I. J. Bristol, E. H. Leiter et al. 1998. Differential susceptibility of inbred mouse strains to dextran sulfate sodium-induced colitis. *Am J Physiol* 274 (3 Pt 1):G544–51.

Marnett, L. J. 2000. Oxyradicals and DNA damage. *Carcinogenesis* 21 (3):361–70.

Matsuzaki, K., M. Murata, K. Yoshida et al. 2007. Chronic inflammation associated with hepatitis C virus infection perturbs hepatic transforming growth factor beta signaling, promoting cirrhosis and hepatocellular carcinoma. *Hepatology* 46 (1):48–57.

Montrose, D. C., N. A. Horelik, J. P. Madigan et al. 2011. Anti-inflammatory effects of freeze-dried black raspberry powder in ulcerative colitis. *Carcinogenesis* 32 (3):343–50.

Morgan, W. F., J. Corcoran, A. Hartmann et al. 1998. DNA double-strand breaks, chromosomal rearrangements, and genomic instability. *Mutat Res* 404 (1–2):125–8.

Nair, J., A. Barbin, I. Velic, and H. Bartsch. 1999. Etheno DNA-base adducts from endogenous reactive species. *Mutat Res* 424 (1–2):59–69.

Naito, Y., T. Takagi, T. Ishikawa et al. 2001. The inducible nitric oxide synthase inhibitor ONO-1714 blunts dextran sulfate sodium colitis in mice. *Eur J Pharmacol* 412 (1):91–9.

Ohkusa, T., I. Okayasu, S. Tokoi, A. Araki, and Y. Ozaki. 1995. Changes in bacterial phagocytosis of macrophages in experimental ulcerative colitis. *Digestion* 56 (2):159–64.

Okayasu, I., S. Hatakeyama, M. Yamada et al. 1990. A novel method in the induction of reliable experimental acute and chronic ulcerative colitis in mice. *Gastroenterology* 98 (3):694–702.

Okayasu, I., T. Ohkusa, K. Kajiura, J. Kanno, and S. Sakamoto. 1996. Promotion of colorectal neoplasia in experimental murine ulcerative colitis. *Gut* 39 (1):87–92.

Oudkerk Pool, M., G. Bouma, J. J. Visser et al. 1995. Serum nitrate levels in ulcerative colitis and Crohn's disease. *Scand J Gastroenterol* 30 (8):784–8.

Peek, R. M., Jr., and M. J. Blaser. 2002. Helicobacter pylori and gastrointestinal tract adenocarcinomas. *Nat Rev Cancer* 2 (1):28–37.

Pera, M., A. Cardesa, J. A. Bombi et al. 1989. Influence of esophagojejunostomy on the induction of adenocarcinoma of the distal esophagus in Sprague-Dawley rats by subcutaneous injection of 2,6-dimethylnitrosomorpholine. *Cancer Res* 49 (23):6803–8.

Quante, M., G. Bhagat, J. A. Abrams et al. 2012. Bile acid and inflammation activate gastric cardia stem cells in a mouse model of Barrett-like metaplasia. *Cancer Cell* 21:36–51.

Rachmilewitz, D., F. Karmeli, E. Okon, and M. Bursztyn. 1995. Experimental colitis is ameliorated by inhibition of nitric oxide synthase activity. *Gut* 37 (2):247–55.

Rachmilewitz, D., J. S. Stamler, D. Bachwich et al. 1995. Enhanced colonic nitric oxide generation and nitric oxide synthase activity in ulcerative colitis and Crohn's disease. *Gut* 36 (5):718–23.

Rachmilewitz, D., J. S. Stamler, F. Karmeli et al. 1993. Peroxynitrite-induced rat colitis—a new model of colonic inflammation. *Gastroenterology* 105 (6):1681–8.

Redston, M. S., N. Papadopoulos, C. Caldas, K. W. Kinzler, and S. E. Kern. 1995. Common occurrence of APC and K-ras gene mutations in the spectrum of colitis-associated neoplasias. *Gastroenterology* 108 (2):383–92.

Riddell, R. H., H. Goldman, D. F. Ransohoff et al. 1983. Dysplasia in inflammatory bowel disease: standardized classification with provisional clinical applications. *Hum Pathol* 14 (11):931–68.

Romero, Y., A. J. Cameron, G. R. Locke, 3rd et al. 1997. Familial aggregation of gastroesophageal reflux in patients with Barrett's esophagus and esophageal adenocarcinoma. *Gastroenterology* 113 (5):1449–56.

Russel, M. G., and R. W. Stockbrugger. 1996. Epidemiology of inflammatory bowel disease: an update. *Scand J Gastroenterol* 31 (5):417–27.

Sato, F., N. Harpaz, D. Shibata et al. 2002. Hypermethylation of the p14(ARF) gene in ulcerative colitis-associated colorectal carcinogenesis. *Cancer Res* 62 (4):1148–51.

Schottenfeld, D., and J. Beebe-Dimmer. 2006. Chronic inflammation: a common and important factor in the pathogenesis of neoplasia. *CA Cancer J Clin* 56 (2):69–83.

Schreiber, S., R. P. MacDermott, A. Raedler et al. 1991. Increased activation of isolated intestinal lamina propria mononuclear cells in inflammatory bowel disease. *Gastroenterology* 101 (4):1020–30.

Schulmann, K., A. Sterian, A. Berki et al. 2005. Inactivation of p16, RUNX3, and HPP1 occurs early in Barrett's-associated neoplastic progression and predicts progression risk. *Oncogene* 24 (25):4138–48.

Seril, D. N., J. Liao, K. L. Ho et al. 2002. Dietary iron supplementation enhances DSS-induced colitis and associated colorectal carcinoma development in mice. *Dig Dis Sci* 47 (6):1266–78.

Seril, D. N., J. Liao, K. L. Ho, C. S. Yang, and G. Y. Yang. 2002. Inhibition of chronic ulcerative colitis-associated colorectal adenocarcinoma development in a murine model by N-acetylcysteine. *Carcinogenesis* 23 (6):993–1001.

Seril, D. N., J. Liao, and G. Y. Yang. 2007. Colorectal carcinoma development in inducible nitric oxide synthase-deficient mice with dextran sulfate sodium-induced ulcerative colitis. *Mol Carcinog* 46 (5):341–53.

Seril, D. N., J. Liao, G. Y. Yang, and C. S. Yang. 2003. Oxidative stress and ulcerative colitis-associated carcinogenesis: studies in humans and animal models. *Carcinogenesis* 24 (3):353–62.

Su, Y., X. Chen, M. Klein et al. 2004. Phenotype of columnar-lined esophagus in rats with esophagogastroduodenal anastomosis: similarity to human Barrett's esophagus. *Lab Invest* 84 (6):753–65.

Thompson, O. M., S. A. Beresford, E. A. Kirk, and T. L. Vaughan. 2009. Vegetable and fruit intakes and risk of Barrett's esophagus in men and women. *Am J Clin Nutr* 89 (3):890–6.

Ullman, T. A., and S. H. Itzkowitz. 2011. Intestinal inflammation and cancer. *Gastroenterology* 140 (6):1807–16.

Valinluck, V., and L. C. Sowers. 2007. Inflammation-mediated cytosine damage: a mechanistic link between inflammation and the epigenetic alterations in human cancers. *Cancer Res* 67 (12):5583–6.

Van Nieuwenhove, Y., T. De Backer, D. Chen, R. Hakanson, and G. Willems. 1998. Gastrin stimulates epithelial cell proliferation in the oesophagus of rats. *Virchows Arch* 432 (4):371–5.

Vial, M., L. Grande, and M. Pera. 2010. Epidemiology of adenocarcinoma of the esophagus, gastric cardia, and upper gastric third. *Recent Results Cancer Res* 182:1–17.

Wang, D., D. A. Kreutzer, and J. M. Essigmann. 1998. Mutagenicity and repair of oxidative DNA damage: insights from studies using defined lesions. *Mutat Res* 400 (1–2):99–115.

Wink, D. A., Y. Vodovotz, J. Laval et al. 1998. The multifaceted roles of nitric oxide in cancer. *Carcinogenesis* 19 (5):711–21.

Yamada, T., C. Volkmer, and M. B. Grisham. 1990. Antioxidant properties of 5-ASA: potential mechanism for its anti-inflammatory activity. *Canadian J. Gastroenterology* 4:295–302.

Yin, J., N. Harpaz, Y. Tong et al. 1993. p53 point mutations in dysplastic and cancerous ulcerative colitis lesions. *Gastroenterology* 104 (6):1633–9.

4 Overview of Common Dietary Phytochemicals Possessing Antioxidant Properties through Nrf2

Limin Shu, Chengyue Zhang, and Ah-Ng Tony Kong

CONTENTS

4.1 INTRODUCTION

4.1.1 BENEFITS OF NUTRITIONAL PHYTOCHEMICALS IN HEALTH IMPROVEMENT

Our daily food affords us the nutritional value we need. However, the philosophy that the health-promoting role of food may afford us more than just that its nutritional value has been recognized among the scientific community, in which many dietary components have been found to be beneficial for disease prevention and treatment (Reddy 1996). Epidemiological studies suggest that a reduced risk of cancer is associated with high consumption of vegetables and fruits, which are major sources of phytochemicals and micronutrients (Reddy, Wang et al. 1997). Several phytochemicals and micronutrients present in fruits and vegetables are known to exert cancer chemopreventive effects. Monoterpenes such as D-limonene and perillyl alcohol derived from orange peels and lavender, respectively, have been shown to possess chemopreventive properties against mammary, liver, and/or lung carcinogenesis (Reddy, Wang et al. 1997).

There is a long history of the application of herbs and their extracts for treatment of various kinds of diseases, including cancer, in the world, especially in Asia, where it was referred to as traditional Chinese medicine (TCM), Japanese–Chinese medicine (kampo), Korean–Chinese medicine, jamu (Indonesia), and ayurvedic medicine (India) (Itokawa, Morris-Natschke et al. 2008). In Europe and America, it has been accepted as "alternative medicine" or "integrative medicine," because of the potential synergistic effect of the combination therapy (Itokawa, Morris-Natschke et al. 2008; Lu, Li et al. 2008). In the United States, for example, it was estimated that one-third of adults use dietary herbal supplements on a regular basis (Jiang and Hu 2009). However, when the botanicals were introduced into the disease therapy, some herbal supplements and botanicals might have possessed adverse effects or caused a drug–botanicals interaction, although some of those herbal supplements have shown potent pharmacological activity (Kumar, Allen et al. 2005; Shord, Shah et al. 2009). Therefore, detailed chemical and health benefit analysis of those botanical medicines is becoming important to establish safe and effective clinical practice. Meanwhile, the inner mechanistic investigation of the molecular events triggered by those supplements is also highly required. So far, a number of molecular pathways influenced by those botanical extracts including antioxidants and inhibition of cancer cell proliferation in vitro or in animal experiments are under exploration (Shu, Cheung et al. 2010).

4.1.2 APPLICATION OF NUTRITIONAL PHYTOCHEMICALS ON CHEMOPREVENTION

Chemoprevention refers to the use of natural or laboratory-made substances to prevent diseases such as cancer (Sporn, Dunlop et al. 1976; Kucuk 2002). Phytochemicals are a wide variety of compounds produced from plants. Many of them have been tested in cancer chemoprevention studies and were considered as a large source of chemopreventive agents and therapeutic agents for cancer (Surh 2003; Johnson, Wang et al. 2009). Among them, some are produced from dietary food, for example, phenethyl isothiocyanate (PEITC) from broccoli, selenium from garlic, and genistein from soy products; they have been shown to have protective effects against some types of tumor development in animal experiments (Ganther 1999; Sarkar and Li 2002; Cheung, Khor et al. 2010). Some phytochemicals from nondietary plants such as herbs, which have historic usage, could be introduced into modern medicine as potential anticancer remedies (Chin, Balunas et al. 2006). Current clinically used phytochemicals can be classified into four main classes of phytochemicals based on their structure and functions: vinca (or *Catharanthus*) alkaloids, epipodophyllotoxins, taxanes, and camptothecins (van Der Heijden, Jacobs et al. 2004). These phytochemicals may function as inhibitors of signal transduction pathways essential for cancer cell proliferation, tumor growth, invasion, and metastasis, or potentiate the response of cancer cells to radiotherapy and reduce radiation-induced toxicity to normal surrounding tissues, thereby demonstrating synergistic anticancer effects (Raffoul, Sarkar et al. 2007).

Interest in dietary phytochemicals for potential cancer chemoprevention has increased substantially. Among numerous nutritional phytochemicals, many of them have been shown to be promising chemoprevention agents. Some lead compounds identified were listed as follows: genistein (from soybeans); lycopene (from tomatoes); brassinin (from cruciferous vegetables); sulforaphane (from asparagus); indole-3-carbinol (from broccoli); curcumin (from turmeric); resveratrol (from red grapes, peanuts, and berries); diallyl sulfide (allium); S-allyl cysteine (allium); allicin (from garlic); capsaicin (from red chili); diosgenin (from fenugreek); 6-gingerol (from ginger); ellagic acid (from pomegranate); ursolic acid (from apple, pears, and prunes); silymarin (from milk thistle); anethol (from anise, camphor, and fennel); catechins (from green tea); eugenol (from cloves); limonene (from citrus fruits); beta-carotene (from carrots); and dietary fiber, withanolides (from tomatillos), and some others, such as vitamin E and selenium. Currently, many of them are in preclinical or clinical trials for cancer chemoprevention (Park and Pezzuto 2002; Aggarwal and Shishodia 2006; Gullett, Ruhul Amin et al. 2010). Due to the concept difference between cancer therapy and cancer prevention and the complex of individual dietary style, few of them have gotten very ideal clinical test effects in various types of cancers and been approved by the United States Food and Drug Administration (Tan, Konczak et al. 2011). Nevertheless, inclusion of appropriate biomarkers in the clinical trials have been shown to be beneficial in investigating the mechanisms by which genetic and epigenetic pathways of carcinogenesis are modulated by nutrients and phytochemicals (Kucuk 2002).

4.2 ANTIOXIDANT SIGNALING PATHWAY AND CHEMOPREVENTION

4.2.1 Carcinogenesis and Chemoprevention

Cancer development was recognized as a multiple-stage process, which includes the initiation, promotion, and progression stage (Armitage 1985; Boyd and Barrett 1990; Ottini, Falchetti et al. 2006; Fimognari, Lenzi et al. 2008). Correspondingly, based on the inhibition stage of cancer development, the chemopreventive agents have been classified into two categories: blocking agents and suppressing agents (Wattenberg 1985). Blocking agents act by scavenging or blocking the carcinogens at initiation stage; they prevent carcinogens from reaching the target sites, subsequently interacting with crucial macromolecules such as DNA, RNA, and proteins. Suppressing agents, on the other hand, function at both the promotion and the progression stages; they are able to inhibit the malignant transformation of initiated cells. Some agents may be classified into both categories, since they may work on all three stages of carcinogenesis (Sporn, Dunlop et al. 1976). For both strategies, the chemoprevention agents would trigger tremendous improvements of the defense systems of the body. To prevent cancer initiation, the phytochemicals are used to induce protective enzymes to target carcinogen metabolism and enhance the detoxification and free-radical scavenging of the body; to prevent tumor promotion and progression, the phytochemicals are used to inhibit the proliferation, angiogenesis, and inflammation and to induce cell apoptosis and differentiation (Greenwald 2002; Tsao, Kim et al. 2004).

Oxidative stress, inflammation, and the evasion of apoptosis are known to be critical triggers for the development of carcinogenesis and contribute to genomic instability, defects in repair of DNA damage, and subsequent incorrect chromosomal segregation during mitosis and further transformation of premalignant cells (Tan, Konczak et al. 2011). Therefore, antioxidant, anti-inflammatory, and proapoptotic activities would represent anticancer mechanisms for preventing, suppressing, or reversing this process. Those activities provide a useful basis for evaluation of the phytochemical effects in the screen approach (Tan, Konczak et al. 2011). Some intensively investigated phytochemical compounds, their structures and related anticancer mechanisms are listed in Table 4.1.

4.2.2 Reactive Oxygen/Nitrogen Species and the Body Defense of Human Diseases

During the metabolism of oxygen in normal cells, a hydroxyl radical is produced as a byproduct. Hydrogen peroxide, superoxide, and hydroxyl radicals are more generally known as reactive oxygen species (ROS), while byproducts of the metabolism of nitric oxide (NO), nitrite, nitrate, and peroxynitrite, are referred as reactive nitrogen species (RNS) (Darley-Usmar and Halliwell 1996). ROS and RNS are generated through various processes, such as mitochondria-catalyzed electron transport reactions, irradiation by ultraviolet (UV) light, x-rays and gamma rays, inflammatory processes, lipid peroxidation, and environmental pollutants (Yu 1994). The reactive species may play both a deleterious and beneficial role in the dynamic interactions between the body and environmental stimulus (Azad, Iyer et al. 2010). ROS and RNS are important intracellular signaling molecules and trigger various physiological processes, including cellular senescence and apoptosis, and therefore function as beneficial antitumorigenic species (Valko, Rhodes et al. 2006; Tan, Konczak et al. 2011). However, when produced ROS and RNS accumulate and fail to be counteracted by the antioxidative defense system, oxidative stress is formed (Beckman and Ames 1998; Halliwell and Gutteridge 1999).

TABLE 4.1
Anticancer Effect and Mechanisms of Some Phytochemicals

Compound(s)	Plant	Cancer Cell Lines	Effects/Molecular Targets (References)	In Vivo Test
Curcumin	Curcuma longa	HCT116; prostate cancer; gastrointestinal cancers; etc.	Increased Nrf2 expression; induced apoptosis; exerted anti-inflammatory effect; inhibited NF-κB by blocking IκB degradation; inhibited phosphorylation of Akt and ERK (Chun, Keum et al. 2003; Reuter, Eifes et al. 2008); inhibited activity of AP-1; downregulated the cytokine TNF-α; down-regulated endogenous bCL-2 and Bcl-xL; enhanced cell death in LNCaP cells in combination with TNF-related apoptosis-inducing ligand (TRAIL) (Aggarwal, Kumar et al. 2003; Deeb, Xu et al. 2003)	Decreased incidence of prostate tumor formation in PC3-implanted nude mice (Barve, Khor et al. 2008)
(-)-Epigallocatechingallate (EGCG)	Green tea	HT-29; DU145; PC3; etc.	Induced G0/G1 cell cycle arrest; inhibited NF-κB activity; inhibited COX2 (Khan, Adhami et al. 2009); inhibited DNA methyltransferase 1 (DNMT1) (Pandey and Gupta 2009); acted as inhibitor of matrix metalloproteinase-2; blocked induction of vascular endothelial growth factor (VEGF); inhibited angiogenesis via blocking of ERK-1/2; modulated NF-κB and AP-1; induced cytochrome C release; regulated VCAM-1; inhibited the expression of p38 MAPK, (Jeong, Kim et al. 2004; Jagtap, Meganathan et al. 2009)	Reduced tumor size and abrogated tumors in both androgen-repressed LNCaP 104-R and the androgen-refractory PC3 tumor xenograft in athymic nude mice (Liao and Hiipakka 1995)

6-Gingerol	Ginger	JB-6	Enhanced TRAIL-induced apoptosis; inhibited 12-O-tetradecanoyl-phorbal-13-acetate (TPA)-induced phosphorylation of p65 and p38 MAPK (Kim, Kundu et al. 2005; Ishiguro, Ando et al. 2007); decreased iNOS and TNF-α); suppressed I-κBα phosphorylation; increased apoptotic protease-activating factor-1 (Apaf-1) (Oyagbemi, Saba et al. 2010); decreased the expression of Bcl-2 and Survivin; increased in apoptotic protease-activating factor-1 (Apaf-1) (Nigam, George et al. 2010)	Topical application onto shaven backs of female ICR mice inhibited 7,12-dimethylbenz[a] anthracene–induced skin papillomagenesis (Park, Chun et al. 1998)
Phenethylisothiocyanate (PEITC)	Cruciferous vegetables	HT-29; PC3; LNCaP; HeLa; SKOV3	Increased Nrf2 expression; induced apoptosis through caspase-3 (Yu, Mandlekar et al. 1998); upregulated p53 and bax; downregulated expression of X-linked inhibitor of apoptosis protein (XIAP), Bcl-2, Bcl-xL, and Mcl-1 (Wu, Ng et al. 2005); increased ROS generation; sensitized cells to PEITC (Trachootham, Zhou et al. 2006); upregulated CYP1A1 and CYP1A2 and phase II genes; decreased iNOS and COX2; inhibited NF-κB transcriptional activity (Cheung and Kong 2010); inhibited MAPK (Cheung, Khor et al. 2009); decreased DNA and hemoglobin adduct formation induced by nicotine-derived nitrosamine ketone (NNK) (Hecht 1995)	Inhibited intestinal carcinogenesis in Apc(Min/+) mice (Cheung, Khor et al. 2010); retarded the growth of PC3 xenografts (Khor, Keum et al. 2006); inhibited NNK-induced lung carcinogenesis (Hecht 1999)

(continued)

TABLE 4.1 (Continued)
Anticancer Effect and Mechanisms of Some Phytochemicals

Compound(s)	Plant	Cancer Cell Lines	Effects/Molecular Targets (References)	In Vivo Test
Sulforaphane (SFN)	Cruciferous vegetables	HeLa; HepG2; T24; LNCaP; C4-2; HT-29	Induced cell cycle arrest and apoptosis; induced phase II enzymes; promoted the mitochondrial formation of ROS and induced DNA breakage (Sestili, Paolillo et al. 2010); suppressed phosphorylation of Akt (Ser-473) and then inhibited phosphorylation of human telomerase reverse transcriptase (hTERT) (Moon, Kang et al. 2010); acted as a histone deacetylase (HDAC); enhanced histone acetylation (Ho, Clarke et al. 2009); decreased the expression and phosphorylation of (Kim and Singh 2009); increased expression and phosphorylation of p38 (Shan, Wu et al. 2009); upregulated TRAIL-R1/DR4 and TRAIL-R2/DR5 (Shankar, Ganapathy et al. 2008)	Retarded prostate tumor growth in TRAMP mouse (Keum, Khor et al. 2009); suppressed the growth of PC3 in nude mice (Myzak, Tong et al. 2007)
Genistein		Prostate cancer cells (LNCaP and PC3, DU-145; ovarian cancer cells (AS4 and NEO)	Inhibited angiogenesis and downregulation of TGF-β and EGF (Banerjee, Li et al. 2008; Zhao, Xiang et al. 2009); increased GPX1 (Perabo, Von Low et al. 2008); inhibited 5-α-reductase or aromatase; inhibited prostate specific antigen (PSA) expression; increased p21; blocked cell cycle progression at G1; inhibited activation of p38 MAPK and FAK (promotility proteins) in vivo, blocking cell motility (Lakshman, Xu et al. 2008); decreased UGT activities and decreased liver GST in female mice (Froyen, Reeves et al. 2009); decreased COX2	Reduction tissue p-EGFR staining in bladder cancer tissue when treated with lower dose (300 mg) but not with 600-mg (Messing, Gee et al. 2012)

(Swami, Krishnan et al. 2009); inhibited estrogen receptor-alpha and activated BARD1; induced estrogen receptor-beta and FAS in presence of BRCA1 (Thasni, Rojini et al. 2008); downregulated AR in prostate cancer cells (Bektic, Berger et al. 2004)

Resveratrol	Red grapes	Breast cancer (MCF-7, MDA-MB-231); prostate cancer (LNCap, PC3, DU145); colon cancer (HT-29, DLD1, HCT116); ovarian cancer cell lines (A-2780, SKOV-3); hepatocellular carcinoma (Huh-7)	Suppressed IGF-1R; attenuated Akt/Wnt signaling (Vanamala, Reddivari et al. 2010); downregulated cyclin E, cyclin A, and cyclin-dependent kinase 2; downregulated phospho-ERK and phospho-p38 expression (Liao, Ng et al. 2010); activated caspases 9 and 3 (Benitez, Pozo-Guisado et al. 2007); upregulated proapoptotic Bax, Apaf-1, and p53 and p21 (Dong 2003; Piotrowska, Myszkowski et al. 2012); decreased Bcl-2 and Bcl-2110; decreased CYP1A1 and CYP1B1 (Piotrowska, Myszkowski et al. 2012); sensitized breast cancer cell to cell death; increased the levels of p-Chk2 (Casanova, Quarti et al. 2012), inhibited p-glycoprotein efflux activity (Al-Abd, Mahmoud et al. 2011); promoted interaction between Bax and XIAP) (Gogada, Prabhu et al. 2011); decreased SIRT1 content (Pizarro, Verdaguer et al. 2011)

Oxidative stress may cause oxidative damage to large biomolecules such as lipids, proteins, and DNA and eventually may lead to mutations and final formation of cancer. Population analysis revealed that a chronic oxidative condition caused by some chemical agents, such as alcohol and cigarette smoke, and physical agents, such as radiation, burns, and virus infection, is associated with high incidence of cancer (Tan, Konczak et al. 2011). Oxidative stress has also been linked to many other chronic diseases such as neurodegenerative diseases (Alzheimer's disease [AD], Parkinson's disease [PD], and amyotrophic lateral sclerosis [ALS]), cardiovascular disease, diabetes, and inflammatory diseases (Emerit, Edeas et al. 2004; Cataldi 2010; Tan, Konczak et al. 2011).

4.2.3 Antioxidant Regulation in the Health System

Antioxidants are enzymes or some organic substances that are capable of counteracting the damaging effects of oxidation, and they may be characterized as inhibiting the generation of ROS or directly scavenging free radicals (Tan, Konczak et al. 2011). In living organisms, the effects of ROS/RNS are balanced by these enzymatic and nonenzymatic antioxidants, which maintain the intracellular redox and status (Reddy 2008). Vitamin C (L-ascorbate), vitamin E, carotenoids, selenium, flavonoids, and thiol antioxidants such as glutathione (GSH), thioredoxin (TRX), and lipoic acid are characterized as nonenzymatic antioxidants (Valko, Izakovic et al. 2004; Valko, Rhodes et al. 2006; Jomova, Vondrakova et al. 2010). However, some of them, such as vitamin C, can act as a prooxidant to promote the ROS level when the concentration is high (Mamede, Tavares et al. 2011). A similar observation has been reported for vitamin E, which serves as both antioxidant and prooxidant, with different mechanisms (Mamede, Tavares et al. 2011).

The enzymatic antioxidants include superoxide dismutase (SOD), catalase, and GSH peroxidase (Kojo 2004). SODs are the major antioxidant defense systems against $\left(O_2^-\right)$; there are three isoforms, SOD1–SOD3, in mammals, and all of them require catalytic metal (Cu or Mn) for their activation (Fukai and Ushio-Fukai 2011). Catalase is an enzyme that degrades hydrogen peroxide, reduces H_2O_2 to water, and oxidizes it to molecular oxygen (Nishikawa, Hashida et al. 2009); GSH peroxidases (GPXs), are important in protecting living organisms from free radical–induced oxidative damage (Jung and Kwak 2010; Limon-Pacheco and Gonsebatt 2010).

In addition to the above enzymes, two families of enzymes related to xenobiotic metabolism are also involved in antioxidant actions: phase I and phase II enzymes. Phase I drug metabolism enzymes, which belong to the larger cytochrome P450 enzyme family, catalyze reaction through oxidation, reduction, hydrolysis, cyclization, decyclization, and addition of oxygen or removal of hydrogen (Mansuy 2011). Phase II conjugating enzymes inactivate and detoxify potentially dangerous substrates, typically through a conjugation reaction with substances such as glucuronic acid, sulfation, and GSH, increasing their solubility and facilitating excretion (Boddupalli, Mein et al. 2012). Phase II enzymes play crucial cytoprotective roles against carcinogens and ROS (Giudice and Montella 2006). Most polyphenolic antioxidants are monofunctional inducers, primarily exerting their activity through phase II enzymes (Giudice and Montella 2006). The expression of many phase II enzymes, such as GST, γ-glutamate cysteine ligase (γ– glutamate–cysteine ligase catalytic subunit [GCLC] and gamma-glutamylcysteine synthetase [γ-GCLM]), heme oxygenase 1 (HO-1), and NAD(P)H:quinone oxidoreductase (NQO1), is inducible and can be activated by the redox-sensitive transcription factors (Lau, Villeneuve et al. 2008).

4.3 NRF2, A CENTRAL MEDIATOR OF ANTIOXIDANT RESPONSE

Under alteration of the cellular redox status of cells by ROS/RNS, many protein conformations and functions, activities of various transcription factors, and gene expression are modified. In response to oxidative/redox conditions, ROS/RNS-sensitive regulatory transcription factors would be subject to various modifications and lead to downstream gene expression change. Nuclear factor-erythroid

2 p45 (NF-E2)–related factor 2 (Nrf2), nuclear factor kappaB (NF-κB), and hypoxia-inducible factor-1 alpha (HIF-1α) are among the list of transcription factors that can be directly influenced by reactive species and proinflammatory signals (Darley-Usmar and Halliwell 1996).

4.3.1 Nrf2 and Antioxidant Regulation

Many detoxifying and antioxidant enzymes such as GST, uridine diphosphate glucuronyltransferase (UDP)-glucuronosyltransferase, HO-1, NQO1, and glutamate cysteine ligase (gamma glutamylcysteine synthetase) are regulated by this transcription factor. In the promoters of these drug-metabolizing and detoxifying enzyme genes, there exist xenobiotic response elements (XRE) and antioxidant response elements (ARE) (Rushmore and Pickett 1993; McMahon, Itoh et al. 2001; Miao, Hu et al. 2005; Hu, Saw et al. 2010). AREs referred a conservative sequence as 5_A/G TGA C/T NNNGC A/G_3, and they are found in the promoter regions of a wide spectrum of more than 200 genes. Under stress conditions, the above detoxifying genes are transactivated by the basic leucine zipper transcription factor Nrf2, which plays a crucial role in the mediation of detoxifying and antioxidant enzymes (Rushmore, Morton et al. 1991; Chan, Han et al. 2001; McMahon, Itoh et al. 2001; Li, Khor et al. 2008).

4.3.2 Nrf2 Regulation by Keap1

Nrf2 has emerged as a master regulator of an intracellular antioxidant response through transcriptional activation of a number of genes, including phase II detoxifying enzymes, antioxidants, and transporters that protect cells from toxic and carcinogenic chemicals (Zhang 2006; Kensler, Wakabayashi et al. 2007; Shen and Kong 2009). The importance of Nrf2 was exemplified by Nrf2 knockout mice, since those mice possess a much lower level of detoxifying enzymes than wild-type mice and are susceptible to xenobiotics (Chen and Kong 2005). The Nrf2 knockout mice were also shown to be more highly susceptible to carcinogenesis and to have diminished ability of induction response to chemoprotective agents (Chen and Kong 2005; Kwon, Barve et al. 2007). Under homeostatic conditions, Nrf2 protein is retained in the cytosol by Kelch-like ECH-associating protein 1 (Keap1), which serves also as an adaptor that bridges Nrf2 to Cul 3 for protein ubiquitination (Cullinan, Gordan et al. 2004). The Keap1–Nrf2 complex itself has been identified as an intracellular sensor. Keap1 contains several cysteinethiol (sulfhydyl) residues, which are thought to be critical in regulating the interaction between Keap1 and Nrf2, and they are sensitive to electrophile- and ROS-caused cellular redox status changes (Dinkova-Kostova, Holtzclaw et al. 2002, 2005). Therefore, in the Keap1–Nrf2 antioxidant axis, Keap1 was recognized as a primary redox sensor Dinkova-Kostova 2002, 2005). However, Nrf2 itself may also work as a redox sensor because of its nuclear exporting signal in the transactivation domain (NES$_{TA}$) motif, which also plays a role in the subcellular localization of Nrf2 (Li and Kong 2009).

Nrf2 protein is conservative among different species and contains six highly conserved domains called Nrf2-ECH homology (Neh) domains (Zhang 2006). The Neh2 domains of Nrf2 are located at the very N-terminal, and it contains two conservative [29]DLG[31] and [79]ETGE[82] motifs, through which Nrf2 binds to the double glycine repeat (DGR) domain of Keap1 (Zhang 2006; Copple, Goldring et al. 2010). A "hinge and latch" model was raised to recapture this two-site substrate recognition pattern. The [79]ETGE[82] motif serves as the "hinge" and provides the high binding affinity, which is a major contributor for the binding, while [29]DLG[3] serves as the "latch" and provides concomitant lower affinity for the binding, which allows Keap1 to bind Nrf2 tightly and enables optimal positioning of target lysine for conjugation with ubiquitin (Tong, Kobayashi et al. 2006; Copple, Goldring et al. 2010). The Neh1 domain contains the conserved CNC and bZip motifs, which are required for DNA binding and dimerization with small Maf proteins (MafG and MafK), while the Neh4 and Neh5 domains are involved in the recruitment of transcriptional coactivators (Lin, Shen et al. 2006). Upon oxidative stress, the cysteine residues, such as C151, C273, or C288 in the BTB or linker domain, would be modified, thereby causing a conformational change and subsequent disruption of the Kelch–[29]DLG[31] binding, resulting in diminished Nrf2 ubiquitination and increased Nrf2 expression level (McMahon, Thomas et al. 2006; Tong, Katoh et al. 2006; Chen, Sun et al. 2009).

4.3.3 Nrf2 Regulation under Kinase Signaling

Although many agents including phytochemicals can activate Nrf2, the detailed molecular events are still not very clear. It is known that Nrf2 can be regulated directly, by several kinases such as mitogen-activated protein kinase (MAPK), phosphatidylinositol 3-kinase (PI3-K), or protein kinase C (PKC) (Huang, Nguyen et al. 2002; Nakaso, Yano et al. 2003; Nguyen, Sherratt et al. 2003; Zipper and Mulcahy 2003), or indirectly, through affecting its coactivators such as CREB-binding protein (CBP) (Zipper and Mulcahy 2000). The MAPKs include extracellular signal–regulated kinases (ERKs), c-Jun amino-terminal kinases (JNKs), and protein 38 (p38). Different MAPKs may have different regulation on Nrf2 signaling. Many studies revealed that ERK and JNK have a positive effect on ARE-mediated activities and Nrf2 transactivation (Kong, Yu et al. 2001; Shen, Hebbar et al. 2004; Hu, Shen et al. 2006; Tan, Konczak et al. 2011), while phosphorylation of Nrf2 by p38 may inhibit Nrf2 activation by increasing Keap1/Nrf2 binding (Keum, Yu et al. 2006). PKC can be directly phosphorylated at serine 40 (Huang, Nguyen et al. 2000, 2002; Bloom and Jaiswal 2003; Numazawa, Ishikawa et al. 2003). PI3-K signaling is able to increase Nrf2 nuclear translocation (Lee, Hanson et al. 2001; Kang, Choi et al. 2002; Kang, Lee et al. 2002; Nakaso, Yano et al. 2003). These three pathways may all act simultaneously, with significant cross-reactions between them, and different tissues or cell types may involve different mechanisms and signaling pathways (Tan, Konczak et al. 2011). However, in the Keap1–Nrf2 antioxidant axis, Keap1 may be a major effector, since it is also reported that direct phosphorylation of Nrf2 by MAPKs has only a slight effect on Nrf2 translocation and activity (Sun, Huang et al. 2009).

4.4 INFLAMMATION AND NF-κB REGULATION

4.4.1 Inflammation and Cancer Development

Inflammation is associated with the alteration of genetic instability and malignant cell transformation (Mantovani, Allavena et al. 2008). It has been estimated that approximately 20% of all human cancers are due to chronic inflammation (De Marzo, Platz et al. 2007). Persistent inflammation in the tumor microenvironment promotes proliferation and survival of malignant cells, angiogenesis, and metastasis (Colotta, Allavena et al. 2009; Mantovani 2010). NF-κB is a key orchestrator of innate immunity/inflammation responses, and it may be involved in tumor initiation and progression (Sen and Baltimore 1986a). The NF-κB pathway is important in driving cancer-related inflammation, which has been reported in gastrointestinal and liver cancer (Greten, Eckmann et al. 2004; Luedde, Beraza et al. 2007). When IKK-β (inhibitor of NF-κB kinase subunit β), an upstream regulator of NF-κB, is deleted, there is a dramatic decrease in tumor incidence in a colitis-associated cancer model (Greten, Eckmann et al. 2004). In addition, aberrant activation of NF-κB is frequently observed in many cancers, and suppression of NF-κB inhibits the proliferation of cancer cells (Garg and Aggarwal 2002; Sethi, Sung et al. 2008).

4.4.2 NF-κB Cascade

All NF-κB proteins contain a conserved Rel homology domain responsible for dimerization and DNA binding to the consensus sequence GGGRNNYYCC (R = purine, N = any base, Y = pyrimidine) (Sen and Baltimore 1986b). The Rel/NF-κB family contains six family members: NF-κB1 (p50/p105, p50 and its precursor p105), NF-κB2 (p52/p100, p52 and its precursor p100), RelA (p65), RelB (p68), c-Rel (p75), and v-Rel. RelA (p65). RelB and c-Rel contain transactivation domains, whereas p50 and p52 do not, and they form heterodimers with Rel proteins to activate transcription. IκB (inhibitor κB) is a negative regulator of NF-κB; it associates with and conceals the nuclear localization sequence or DNA-binding domain of NF-κB and prevents the nuclear translocation and transcription activation (Zabel and Baeuerle 1990; Thompson, Phillips et al. 1995). NF-κB activation usually goes through the IκB protein phosphorylation pathway. Under various sources of stimulation, including TNF-α, IL-1, H_2O_2, lipopoly-saccharide (LPS), or microbial infection, IκB proteins will be phosphorylated at serine and threonine by the upstream IκB kinase (IKK) complex containing IKKs (Inoue, Kerr et al. 1992; Pahl 1999) or IKK-associated protein 1 (IKKAP1) (Jacobs and Harrison 1998), followed by proteasome-mediated degradation. The degradation of IκBs leads to translocation of NF-κB into the nucleus (Traenckner, Pahl et al. 1995; Karin and Ben-Neriah 2000; Bonizzi and Karin 2004).

More than 150 target genes have been reported to be activated by NF-κB, including different inflammatory cytokines and chemokines; immunoreceptors; adhesion molecules; enzymes in the prostaglandin synthase pathway, such as cyclooxygenase 2 (COX2) and NO synthase; angiogenic factors; as well as various stress response genes (Pahl 1999). This signaling pathway has an extensive effect on the cellular events, including inflammation, immune response, apoptosis, development, and cell growth (Pikarsky and Ben-Neriah 2006).

4.5 CROSS TALK BETWEEN THE ANTIOXIDANT AND INFLAMMATION SIGNALING

Based on the transcription control, the function of downstream target proteins, and their self-regulation, Nrf2 and NF-κB may have a potential interface and significant cross talk. The indicative evidence can be found using Nrf2 KO mice. The anti-inflammation effect of the primary peritoneal macrophages was attenuated compared with Nrf2 wild-type macrophage upon LPS stimulation when pretreated with sulforaphane (SFN), TNF, IL-1, COX2, and inducible nitric oxide synthase (iNOS); these inflammation-related signals have much less expression in Nrf2 wild-type macrophages (Heiss, Herhaus et al. 2001; Lin, Wu et al. 2008). In addition, Nrf2-deficient mice are more sensitive to dextran sulfate sodium (DSS)–induced colitis and colorectal carcinogenesis, and the expression level of proinflammatory cytokines/biomarkers was reverse-associated with the downstream detoxifying and phase II enzymes (Li, Khor et al. 2008). Several other chemicals and phytochemical compounds, such as curcumin (Pan, Lin-Shiau et al. 2000; Shen, Xu et al. 2006), epigallocatechin-3-gallate (EGCG) (Sriram, Kalayarasan et al. 2009; Lambert, Sang et al. 2010), chalcone (Liu, Hsieh et al. 2007), and synthetic triterpenoid methyl-2-cyano-3,12-dioxooleana-1,9-dien-28-oic acid (CDDO-Me) (Ahmad, Raina et al. 2006; Shin, Wakabayashi et al. 2009), can induce Nrf2 expression and concomitantly inhibit the activation of NF-κB, although the inner mechanisms involved could be different.

There exist intricate interactions between these two signaling cascade members. First, under constitutive expression of NF-κB subunit p65 and Nrf2, S276 phosphorylated p65 can antagonize Nrf2 transcription activity and suppress the expression of its downstream target such as HO-1, which may, through the competitive binding to CBP, a coactivator of Nrf2, or through promoting recruitment of histone deacetylase (HDAC3), a corepressor to ARE, facilitate the interaction between HDAC3 and CBP or Mafk, resulting in local histone hypoacetylation (Liu, Qu et al. 2008; Wakabayashi, Slocum et al. 2010). In addition, p65 may regulate Nrf2 ubiquitination and Nrf2–ARE binding through direct interaction with Keap1; it was demonstrated that p65 can bind to Keap1 both in vivo and in vitro. However, the detailed mechanism is under further exploration (Yu, Li et al. 2011).

Secondly, Nrf2 may decrease the phosphorylation of IκB and thereby promote the degradation of NF-κB, since a higher level of phosphorylated IκB and greater IKK kinase activity were observed in Nrf2$^{-/-}$ mouse embryonic fibroblasts (MEFs) after challenge with LPS or TNF-α (Thimmulappa, Lee et al. 2006). However, in some tests, there were controversial observations obtained; overexpression of Nrf2 did not change the expression level of NF-κB or IκB but decreased the expression level of some NF-κB downstream genes (Chen, Varner et al. 2003;

Levonen, Inkala et al. 2007). These may be because the loss of Nrf2 has some essential effect on cellular environment, which is out of the range that is explainable when the Nrf2 is at normal or overexpressed levels (Wakabayashi, Slocum et al. 2010). GCLC is an important enzyme catalyzing GSH biosynthesis; human GCLC contains ARE in the promoter region, but mouse GCLC does not. However, in the livers of Nrf2$^{-/-}$ mice, GCLC level is also lower compared with the wild type; meanwhile a lower c-Jun and p65 expression were also detected in these mice, indicating that Nrf2 may regulate mouse GCLC through AP-1 and NF-κB family members (Yang, Magilnick et al. 2005). Under stimulation of TNF-α or LPS, Nrf2$^{-/-}$ fibroblasts had increased activation of NF-κB (Thimmulappa, Lee et al. 2006). Thus, enhancement of NF-κB by loss of Nrf2 may be coordinated in a subset of the NF-κB family members to drive expression of specific genes (Wakabayashi, Slocum et al. 2010).

Thirdly, there is an intricate regulation between downstream targets of these two pathways. HO-1 (Alam, Stewart et al. 1999), NQO1 (McMahon, Itoh et al. 2001), and TRX (Ishii, Itoh et al. 1999) are among the typical targets of Nrf2. HO-1 is able to inhibit RelA (p65) phosphorylation at Ser(276), a critical phosphorylation site to sustain TNF-driven NF-κB activity. HO-1 catalyzes the degradation of free heme into biliverdin via a reaction that releases iron (Fe) and carbon monoxide. The endothelial cells (ECs) from HO-1$^{-/-}$ mice have higher levels of intracellular labile Fe and ROS and higher expression of vascular cell adhesion molecule 1 (VCAM 1), intercellular cell adhesion molecule 1 (ICAM-1), and E-selectin compared with EC from wild type in the basal and TNF-induced expressions, while Fe chelation inhibits TNF-driven transcription of VCAM-1, ICAM-1, and E-selectin (Seldon, Silva et al. 2007). It was also observed that in HT-29 cells and colonic mucosa, inhibition of HO-1 increases p65 activity, whereas induction of HO-1 can inhibit IκB degradation after treatment with TNF-α or IL-1ß (Jun, Kim et al. 2006). NQO1 is also involved in immune response regulation; NQO1-null mice showed altered intracellular redox status and decreased expression and activation of NF-κB as well under basal or LPS-treated conditions (Iskander, Li et al. 2006), whereas in THP-1 cells, NQO1 overexpression reduced LPS-induced inflammatory genes TNF-α and IL-1 (Rushworth, MacEwan et al. 2008). Because NF-κB is also a redox-sensitive transcription factor, TRX modulates NF-κB activity and nuclear translocation through the reduction of cysteine residues (Matthews, Wakasugi et al. 1992; Hayashi, Ueno et al. 1993; Freemerman, Gallegos et al. 1999). Overexpression of human TRX caused activation of NF-κB and degradation of IκB (Das 2001). On the other hand, some antioxidant/detoxifying enzymes downstream of Nrf2 can also be regulated by the molecules in the NF-κB signaling. For example, IL-10, which is an NF-κB target, has been shown to induce HO-1 in murine macrophages and in vivo (Lee and Chau 2002). Expression of iNOS leads to overproduction of NO and subsequent HO-1 induction (Foresti, Clark et al. 1997; Immenschuh, Tan et al. 1999). As a negative feedback loop, HO-1 is able to inhibit iNOS through the action of free iron (Weiss, Werner-Felmayer et al. 1994) and CO (Sarady, Zuckerbraun et al. 2004). COX2 metabolizes arachidonic acid to prostaglandin H2, the precursor of thromboxane and prostaglandins. Induction of COX2 may contribute to the resolution of inflammation by producing cyclopentenone prostaglandins, including 15-deoxy-Δ12,14-prostaglandin J2 (15d-PGJ2) (Gilroy, Colville-Nash et al. 1999). Nrf2 and transactivation of its downstream targets have been reported to be regulated by COX2 and 15d-PGJ2 by directly binding to Keap1 and subsequent Nrf2 translocation in vitro and in Nrf2$^{-/-}$ mice (Itoh, Mochizuki et al. 2004; Mochizuki, Ishii et al. 2005).

4.6 NRF2 MEDIATION ON CARCINOGENESIS

4.6.1 Nrf2-Mediated Antioxidants in Cancer Prevention

As previously described, oxidative stress has been implicated in the etiology of many acute and chronic diseases linked to exposures to environmental toxicants. As a pivotal regulator of cytoprotective antioxidant response, Nrf2 has been shown to be of great importance in both in vitro cell lines and different mouse test models (Osburn and Kensler 2008).

In constitutively overexpressing the cytochrome P450 2E1 (CYP2E1) E47 cell, a variant of the HepG2 human liver cell line, knockdown of Nrf2 resulted in decreased cell viability and markedly decreased expression of antioxidative enzymes and corresponding increased oxidative damage biomarkers, compared with knockdown in the normal HepG2 cells (Gong and Cederbaum 2006). Because CYP2E1 could metabolize and activate toxicologically important substrates into more toxic products and produce higher ROS damage (Guengerich, Kim et al. 1991), suggesting that Nrf2 has a distinct role in oxidative stress regulation (Osburn and Kensler 2008). 4-Hydroxynonenal (HNE) is an end product of lipoperoxidation with antiproliferative and proapoptotic properties in various tumors, and it was considered as a second messenger of oxidative damage that can contribute in controlling cancer cell growth (Cipak, Mrakovcic et al. 2010). In DU145, PC3, and LNCaP human prostate cancer cell lines, Nrf2 knockdown resulted in a reduction in expression of GST A4, an isoform of GST enzyme and glutathione–HNE formation, and sensitized DU145 cells to HNE-mediated antiproliferative and proapoptotic activity, suggesting that Nrf2 plays a crucial role in controlling HNE metabolism (Pettazzoni, Ciamporcero et al. 2011). In prostate tumors of TRAMP (transgenic adenocarcinoma of mouse prostate) mice, Nrf2 expression is suppressed. Similarly, examined expression of Nrf2 and NQO1 is also substantially suppressed in tumorigenic TRAMP C1 cells but not in nontumorigenic TRAMP C3 cells, and the expression of Nrf2 is epigenetically modulated by the DNA methylation of the promoter region (Yu, Khor et al. 2010).

Further evidence of the role of Nrf2 on chemoprevention comes from Nrf2$^{-/-}$ mice. Although Nrf2 is dispensable for mouse development (Chan, Lu et al. 1996), it was shown that some phase II gene induction was largely eliminated in the Nrf2-deficient mice when induced by a phenolic antioxidant, suggesting that it could be an ideal model for the in vivo analysis of chemical carcinogenesis and resistance to anticancer drugs (Itoh, Chiba et al. 1997). Nrf2 knockout mice are greatly predisposed to chemical-induced DNA damage and exhibit higher susceptibility toward cancer development in several models of chemical carcinogenesis. Nrf2 also mediates protection against oxidative stress and influences inflammatory processes, both of which contribute to carcinogenesis (Yu and Kensler 2005). Following exposure to hyperoxic oxygen, the wild-type mice showed increased expression of GSH peroxidase 2 (GPX2) and HO-1, indicating a protective role of Nrf2 on induced oxidative stress (Cho, Jedlicka et al. 2002). In the azoxymethane (AOM)– and DSS-induced colorectal cancer mouse models, following 1 week of AOM/DSS treatment, Nrf2-deficient mice showed reduced length of colon and increased severity of colitis, while following 20 weeks of AOM/DSS treatment, Nrf2-deficient mice showed 40% higher incidence of colonic tumors (Khor, Huang et al. 2006, 2008). In the MEFs from wild-type and Nrf2-deficient mice, although the basal expressions of antioxidative enzymes and oxidative damage biomarkers are similar, the MEF from Nrf2-deficient mice produced higher levels of ROS and oxidative damage biomarkers when exposed to diquat dibromide (DQ), a nonelectrophilic redox cycling bipyridylium herbicide (Osburn et al. 2006).

4.6.2　Nrf2 Expression in Advanced Cancers

Nrf2 would be expected to be anticarcinogenic by reducing levels of ROS-derived DNA adducts and redox-sensitive signaling of tumor promotion. However, it is kind of embarrassing when it was reported that in some cancer types, such as head and neck squamous cell carcinoma (HNSCC) patients, Nrf2 and TRX had significant increased expression (Stacy et al. 2006). Following that, in non–small-cell lung cancer (NSCLC) cell lines and patients, mutation of Keap1 and nuclear accumulation of Nrf2 were observed with a high frequency (Singh, Misra et al. 2006; Ohta, Iijima et al. 2008). Similar observations were obtained in gallbladder cancer (Shibata, Kokubu et al. 2008). Nrf2 mutations and increased Nrf2 expression were also reported in esophageal and skin cancers (Kim, Oh et al. 2010). It was reported that Nrf2 was highly expressed in endometrial serous carcinoma (ESC), whereas complex hyperplasia and endometrial endometrioid carcinoma (EEC) had no or marginal expression of Nrf2 (Jiang, Chen et al. 2010).

These observations caused a reexamination of the role of Nrf2 in cancer progression, which revealed a dark side, a cancer-promoting effect of Nrf2. The dark side of Nrf2 is attributed to the following:

(1) Nrf2 activation provides cancer cells with microenvironment adapted protection. The malignant cells produce an inherently stressed microenvironment from the high rate of proliferation, while the ability of Nrf2 on detoxification and antioxidative regulation was acknowledged by cancer cells, giving cancer cells an advantage for survival and growth (Shibata, Ohta et al. 2008; Lau, Villeneuve et al. 2008).

(2) The high constitutive level of Nrf2 in the tumor cells is responsible for acquired chemoresistance and radioresistance (Zhang 2010). Nrf2 can regulate the expression of the multidrug resistance protein family, including multidrug-resistant protein-3 (MRP3), which facilitates detoxification by transporting toxic chemicals, including chemotherapeutic drugs, out of cells (Mahaffey, Zhang et al. 2009). Silencing Nrf2 by small interfering RNA (siRNA) or Keap1 overexpression rendered cancer cells more susceptible to the chemotherapeutic agents such as cisplatin, doxorubicin, and etoposide, while treatment with tert-butylhydroquinone (tBHQ) to increase the expression of Nrf2 enhanced the resistance of cancer cells (Wang, Sun et al. 2008; Jiang, Chen et al. 2010). Brusatol was found to selectively reduce the expression of Nrf2 through enhanced ubiquitination and degradation of Nrf2. In A549 xenografts, cisplatin cotreated with brusatol caused a more dramatic effect on induction of cell apoptosis, reduction of cell proliferation, and inhibition of tumor growth compared with cisplatin alone, which is Nrf2 dependent (Ren, Villeneuve et al. 2011).

(3) Nrf2 is able to interact and enhance Notch 1 expression, which may contribute to the increased proliferation rate and malignant phenotype (Wakabayashi, Shin et al. 2010). Therefore, Nrf2 appears to be an important consideration in cancer therapy.

4.6.3 Nrf2-Mediated Antioxidant Regulation in Other Diseases

In addition to cancer, disruption of redox homeostasis is associated with the toxic effects of many environmental insults and pathogenesis of neurodegenerative disorders (Sun, Huang et al. 2009). Because of the high oxygen consumption rate and enrichment in polyunsaturated fatty acids, the brain and the rest of the central nervous system (CNS) are vulnerable to oxidative damage (Scapagnini, Vasto et al. 2011). Oxidative stress injury has been implicated in the pathogenesis of neurogenerative disorders, such as AD, PD, and Huntington's disease (HD) (de Vries, Witte et al. 2008). In the CNS, HO-1 has been reported to be very active, and its modulation seems to play a crucial role in the pathogenesis of neurodegenerative disorders (Pappolla, Chyan et al. 1998; Stocker 2004; Droge and Schipper 2007; Venkateshappa, Harish et al. 2012). Curcumin is the active antioxidant from *Curcuma longa*; it is able to increase HO-1 in brain cells, with the potential to inhibit lipid peroxidation and neutralization of ROS and RNS (Butterfield, Castegna et al. 2002; Scapagnini, Colombrita et al. 2006). The presence of curcumin and other dietary phytochemicals such as acetyl-L-carnitine and carnosine has been demonstrated through the activation of these redox-sensitive intracellular pathways (Calabrese, Cornelius et al. 2008). The Nrf2 antioxidant response has also been shown to protect against other aging-related diseases, such as diabetes (Cheng, Siow et al. 2011), skin photooxidative stress (Wondrak, Cabello et al. 2008), cardiovascular disease (Koenitzer and Freeman 2010), and some others (Villeneuve, Lau et al. 2010).

4.7 CONCLUSION AND REMARKS

Phytochemicals have emerged as an important resource for cancer prevention (Johnson, Wang et al. 2009). Among the many common anticancer mechanisms, antioxidant and antiinflammatory regulations play pivotal roles (Shu, Cheung et al. 2010). They have dramatic effects on cellular proliferation and apoptosis regulation. Furthermore, there exist extensive interactions between these two signaling pathways. Nrf2-mediated antioxidant response has been shown in the prevention of many age-related diseases, including cancer. Although Nrf2 did not show enough intelligence in telling the normal cells from the malignant tissues, we can take advantage of its cell protection characteristics, regulate its expression in various situations, and merge this into our strategy of cancer prevention and therapy. It is still promising that we can make great discovery of effective anticancer compounds from the dietary and herbal phytochemicals.

REFERENCES

Aggarwal, B. B. and S. Shishodia (2006). "Molecular targets of dietary agents for prevention and therapy of cancer." *Biochem Pharmacol* 71(10): 1397–1421.

Aggarwal, B. B., A. Kumar et al. (2003). "Anticancer potential of curcumin: preclinical and clinical studies." *Anticancer Res* 23(1A): 363–398.

Ahmad, R., D. Raina et al. (2006). "Triterpenoid CDDO-Me blocks the NF-kappaB pathway by direct inhibition of IKKbeta on Cys-179." *J Biol Chem* 281(47): 35764–35769.

Al-Abd, A. M., A. M. Mahmoud et al. (2011). "Resveratrol enhances the cytotoxic profile of docetaxel and doxorubicin in solid tumour cell lines in vitro." *Cell Prolif* 44(6): 591–601.

Alam, J., D. Stewart et al. (1999). "Nrf2, a Cap'n'Collar transcription factor, regulates induction of the heme oxygenase-1 gene." *J Biol Chem* 274(37): 26071–26078.

Armitage, P. (1985). "Multistage models of carcinogenesis." *Environ Health Perspect* 63: 195–201.

Azad, N., A. Iyer et al. (2010). "Role of oxidative/nitrosative stress-mediated Bcl-2 regulation in apoptosis and malignant transformation." *Ann N Y Acad Sci* 1203: 1–6.

Banerjee, S., Y. Li et al. (2008). "Multi-targeted therapy of cancer by genistein." *Cancer Lett* 269(2): 226–242.

Barve, A., T. O. Khor et al. (2008). "Murine prostate cancer inhibition by dietary phytochemicals—curcumin and phenethylisothiocyanate." *Pharm Res* 25(9): 2181–2189.

Beckman, K. B. and B. N. Ames (1998). "The free radical theory of aging matures." *Physiol Rev* 78(2): 547–581.

Bektic, J., A. P. Berger et al. (2004). "Androgen receptor regulation by physiological concentrations of the isoflavonoid genistein in androgen-dependent LNCaP cells is mediated by estrogen receptor beta." *Eur Urol* 45(2): 245–251; discussion 251.

Benitez, D. A., E. Pozo-Guisado et al. (2007). "Mechanisms involved in resveratrol-induced apoptosis and cell cycle arrest in prostate cancer-derived cell lines." *J Androl* 28(2): 282–293.

Bloom, D. A. and A. K. Jaiswal (2003). "Phosphorylation of Nrf2 at Ser40 by protein kinase C in response to antioxidants leads to the release of Nrf2 from INrf2, but is not required for Nrf2 stabilization/accumulation in the nucleus and transcriptional activation of antioxidant response element-mediated NAD(P)H:quinone oxidoreductase-1 gene expression." *J Biol Chem* 278(45): 44675–44682.

Boddupalli, S., J. R. Mein et al. (2012). "Induction of phase 2 antioxidant enzymes by broccoli sulforaphane: perspectives in maintaining the antioxidant activity of vitamins a, C, and e." *Front Genet* 3: 7.

Bonizzi, G. and M. Karin (2004). "The two NF-kappaB activation pathways and their role in innate and adaptive immunity." *Trends Immunol* 25(6): 280–288.

Boyd, J. A. and J. C. Barrett (1990). "Genetic and cellular basis of multistep carcinogenesis." *Pharmacol Ther* 46(3): 469–486.

Butterfield, D., A. Castegna et al. (2002). "Nutritional approaches to combat oxidative stress in Alzheimer's disease." *J Nutr Biochem* 13(8): 444.

Calabrese, V., C. Cornelius et al. (2008). "Cellular stress response: a novel target for chemoprevention and nutritional neuroprotection in aging, neurodegenerative disorders and longevity." *Neurochem Res* 33(12): 2444–2471.

Casanova, F., J. Quarti et al. (2012). "Resveratrol chemosensitizes breast cancer cells to melphalan by cell cycle arrest." *J Cell Biochem* 113(8): 2586–2596.

Cataldi, A. (2010). "Cell responses to oxidative stressors." *Curr Pharm Des* 16(12): 1387–1395.

Chan, K., X. D. Han et al. (2001). "An important function of Nrf2 in combating oxidative stress: detoxification of acetaminophen." *Proc Natl Acad Sci U S A* 98(8): 4611–4616.

Chan, K., R. Lu et al. (1996). "Nrf2, a member of the NFE2 family of transcription factors, is not essential for murine erythropoiesis, growth, and development." *Proc Natl Acad Sci U S A* 93(24): 13943–13948.

Chen, C. and A. N. Kong (2005). "Dietary cancer-chemopreventive compounds: from signaling and gene expression to pharmacological effects." *Trends Pharmacol Sci* 26(6): 318–326.

Chen, W., Z. Sun et al. (2009). "Direct interaction between Nrf2 and p21(Cip1/WAF1) upregulates the Nrf2-mediated antioxidant response." *Mol Cell* 34(6): 663–673.

Cheng, X., R. C. Siow et al. (2011). "Impaired redox signaling and antioxidant gene expression in endothelial cells in diabetes: a role for mitochondria and the nuclear factor-E2-related factor 2-Kelch-like ECH-associated protein 1 defense pathway." *Antioxid Redox Signal* 14(3): 469–487.

Chen, X. L., S. E. Varner et al. (2003). "Laminar flow induction of antioxidant response element-mediated genes in endothelial cells. A novel anti-inflammatory mechanism." *J Biol Chem* 278(2): 703–711.

Cheung, K. L. and A. N. Kong (2010). "Molecular targets of dietary phenethyl isothiocyanate and sulforaphane for cancer chemoprevention." *AAPS J* 12(1): 87–97.

Cheung, K. L., T. O. Khor et al. (2010). "Differential in vivo mechanism of chemoprevention of tumor formation in azoxymethane/dextran sodium sulfate mice by PEITC and DBM." *Carcinogenesis* 31(5): 880–885.

Cheung, K. L., T. O. Khor et al. (2009). "Synergistic effect of combination of phenethyl isothiocyanate and sulforaphane or curcumin and sulforaphane in the inhibition of inflammation." *Pharm Res* 26(1): 224–231.

Chin, Y. W., M. J. Balunas et al. (2006). "Drug discovery from natural sources." *AAPS J* 8(2): E239–E253.

Cho, H. Y., A. E. Jedlicka et al. (2002). "Role of Nrf2 in protection against hyperoxic lung injury in mice." *Am J Respir Cell Mol Biol* 26(2): 175–182.

Chun, K. S., Y. S. Keum et al. (2003). "Curcumin inhibits phorbol ester-induced expression of cyclooxygenase-2 in mouse skin through suppression of extracellular signal-regulated kinase activity and NF-kappaB activation." *Carcinogenesis* 24(9): 1515–1524.

Cipak, A., L. Mrakovcic et al. (2010). "Growth suppression of human breast carcinoma stem cells by lipid peroxidation product 4-hydroxy-2-nonenal and hydroxyl radical-modified collagen." *Acta Biochim Pol* 57(2): 165–171.

Colotta, F., P. Allavena et al. (2009). "Cancer-related inflammation, the seventh hallmark of cancer: links to genetic instability." *Carcinogenesis* 30(7): 1073–1081.

Copple, I. M., C. E. Goldring et al. (2010). "The keap1-nrf2 cellular defense pathway: mechanisms of regulation and role in protection against drug-induced toxicity." *Handb Exp Pharmacol* (196): 233–266.

Cullinan, S. B., J. D. Gordan et al. (2004). "The Keap1-BTB protein is an adaptor that bridges Nrf2 to a Cul3-based E3 ligase: oxidative stress sensing by a Cul3-Keap1 ligase." *Mol Cell Biol* 24(19): 8477–8486.

Darley-Usmar, V. and B. Halliwell (1996). "Blood radicals: reactive nitrogen species, reactive oxygen species, transition metal ions, and the vascular system." *Pharm Res* 13(5): 649–662.

Das, K. C. (2001). "c-Jun NH2-terminal kinase-mediated redox-dependent degradation of IkappaB: role of thioredoxin in NF-kappaB activation." *J Biol Chem* 276(7): 4662–4670.

De Marzo, A. M., E. A. Platz et al. (2007). "Inflammation in prostate carcinogenesis." *Nat Rev Cancer* 7(4): 256–269.

de Vries, H. E., M. Witte et al. (2008). "Nrf2-induced antioxidant protection: a promising target to counteract ROS-mediated damage in neurodegenerative disease?" *Free Radic Biol Med* 45(10): 1375–1383.

Deeb, D., Y. X. Xu et al. (2003). "Curcumin (diferuloyl-methane) enhances tumor necrosis factor-related apoptosis-inducing ligand-induced apoptosis in LNCaP prostate cancer cells." *Mol Cancer Ther* 2(1): 95–103.

Dinkova-Kostova, A. T., W. D. Holtzclaw et al. (2002). "Direct evidence that sulfhydryl groups of Keap1 are the sensors regulating induction of phase 2 enzymes that protect against carcinogens and oxidants." *Proc Natl Acad Sci U S A* 99(18): 11908–11913.

Dinkova-Kostova, A. T., W. D. Holtzclaw et al. (2005). "Keap1, the sensor for electrophiles and oxidants that regulates the phase 2 response, is a zinc metalloprotein." *Biochemistry* 44(18): 6889–6899.

Dong, Z. (2003). "Molecular mechanism of the chemopreventive effect of resveratrol." *Mutat Res* 523–524: 145–150.

Droge, W. and H. M. Schipper (2007). "Oxidative stress and aberrant signaling in aging and cognitive decline." *Aging Cell* 6(3): 361–370.

Emerit, J., M. Edeas et al. (2004). "Neurodegenerative diseases and oxidative stress." *Biomed Pharmacother* 58(1): 39–46.

Fimognari, C., M. Lenzi et al. (2008). "Chemoprevention of cancer by isothiocyanates and anthocyanins: mechanisms of action and structure-activity relationship." *Curr Med Chem* 15(5): 440–447.

Foresti, R., J. E. Clark et al. (1997). "Thiol compounds interact with nitric oxide in regulating heme oxygenase-1 induction in endothelial cells. Involvement of superoxide and peroxynitrite anions." *J Biol Chem* 272(29): 18411–18417.

Freemerman, A. J., A. Gallegos et al. (1999). "Nuclear factor kappaB transactivation is increased but is not involved in the proliferative effects of thioredoxin overexpression in MCF-7 breast cancer cells." *Cancer Res* 59(16): 4090–4094.

Froyen, E. B., J. L. Reeves et al. (2009). "Regulation of phase II enzymes by genistein and daidzein in male and female Swiss Webster mice." *J Med Food* 12(6): 1227–1237.

Fukai, T. and M. Ushio-Fukai (2011). "Superoxide dismutases: role in redox signaling, vascular function, and diseases." *Antioxid Redox Signal* 15(6): 1583–1606.

Ganther, H. E. (1999). "Selenium metabolism, selenoproteins and mechanisms of cancer prevention: complexities with thioredoxin reductase." *Carcinogenesis* 20(9): 1657–1666.

Garg, A. and B. B. Aggarwal (2002). "Nuclear transcription factor-kappaB as a target for cancer drug development." *Leukemia* 16(6): 1053–1068.

Gilroy, D. W., P. R. Colville-Nash et al. (1999). "Inducible cyclooxygenase may have anti-inflammatory properties." *Nat Med* 5(6): 698–701.

Giudice, A. and M. Montella (2006). "Activation of the Nrf2-ARE signaling pathway: a promising strategy in cancer prevention." *Bioessays* 28(2): 169–181.

Gogada, R., V. Prabhu et al. (2011). "Resveratrol induces p53-independent, X-linked inhibitor of apoptosis protein (XIAP)-mediated Bax protein oligomerization on mitochondria to initiate cytochrome c release and caspase activation." *J Biol Chem* 286(33): 28749–28760.

Gong, P. and A. I. Cederbaum (2006). "Nrf2 is increased by CYP2E1 in rodent liver and HepG2 cells and protects against oxidative stress caused by CYP2E1." *Hepatology* 43(1): 144–153.

Greenwald, P. (2002). "Cancer chemoprevention." *BMJ* 324(7339): 714–718.

Greten, F. R., L. Eckmann et al. (2004). "IKKbeta links inflammation and tumorigenesis in a mouse model of colitis-associated cancer." *Cell* 118(3): 285–296.

Guengerich, F. P., D. H. Kim et al. (1991). "Role of human cytochrome P-450 IIE1 in the oxidation of many low molecular weight cancer suspects." *Chem Res Toxicol* 4(2): 168–179.

Gullett, N. P., A. R. Ruhul Amin et al. (2010). "Cancer prevention with natural compounds." *Semi Oncol* 37: 258–281.

Halliwell, B. and J. Gutteridge (1999). *Free Radicals in Biology and Medicine*, Oxford University Press, Oxford, UK.

Hayashi, T., Y. Ueno et al. (1993). "Oxidoreductive regulation of nuclear factor kappa B. Involvement of a cellular reducing catalyst thioredoxin." *J Biol Chem* 268(15): 11380–11388.

Hecht, S. S. (1995). "Chemoprevention by isothiocyanates." *J Cell Biochem Suppl* 22: 195–209.

Hecht, S. S. (1999). "Chemoprevention of cancer by isothiocyanates, modifiers of carcinogen metabolism." *J Nutr* 129(3): 768S–774S.

Heiss, E., C. Herhaus et al. (2001). "Nuclear factor kappa B is a molecular target for sulforaphane-mediated anti-inflammatory mechanisms." *J Biol Chem* 276(34): 32008–32015.

Ho, E., J. D. Clarke et al. (2009). "Dietary sulforaphane, a histone deacetylase inhibitor for cancer prevention." *J Nutr* 139(12): 2393–2396.

Hu, R., C. L. Saw et al. (2010). "Regulation of NF-E2-related factor 2 signaling for cancer chemoprevention: antioxidant coupled with antiinflammatory." *Antioxid Redox Signal* 13(11): 1679–1698.

Hu, R., G. Shen et al. (2006). "In vivo pharmacokinetics, activation of MAPK signaling and induction of phase II/III drug metabolizing enzymes/transporters by cancer chemopreventive compound BHA in the mice." *Arch Pharm Res* 29(10): 911–920.

Huang, H. C., T. Nguyen et al. (2000). "Regulation of the antioxidant response element by protein kinase C-mediated phosphorylation of NF-E2-related factor 2." *Proc Natl Acad Sci U S A* 97(23): 12475–12480.

Huang, H. C., T. Nguyen et al. (2002). "Phosphorylation of Nrf2 at Ser-40 by protein kinase C regulates antioxidant response element-mediated transcription." *J Biol Chem* 277(45): 42769–42774.

Immenschuh, S., M. Tan et al. (1999). "Nitric oxide mediates the lipopolysaccharide dependent upregulation of the heme oxygenase-1 gene expression in cultured rat Kupffer cells." *J Hepatol* 30(1): 61–69.

Inoue, J., L. D. Kerr et al. (1992). "I kappa B gamma, a 70 kd protein identical to the C-terminal half of p110 NF-kappa B: a new member of the I kappa B family." *Cell* 68(6): 1109–1120.

Ishiguro, K., T. Ando et al. (2007). "Ginger ingredients reduce viability of gastric cancer cells via distinct mechanisms." *Biochem Biophys Res Commun* 362(1): 218–223.

Ishii, T., K. Itoh et al. (1999). "Oxidative stress-inducible proteins in macrophages." *Free Radic Res* 31(4): 351–355.

Iskander, K., J. Li et al. (2006). "NQO1 and NQO2 regulation of humoral immunity and autoimmunity." *J Biol Chem* 281(41): 30917–30924.

Itoh, K., T. Chiba et al. (1997). "An Nrf2/small Maf heterodimer mediates the induction of phase II detoxifying enzyme genes through antioxidant response elements." *Biochem Biophys Res Commun* 236(2): 313–322.

Itoh, K., M. Mochizuki et al. (2004). "Transcription factor Nrf2 regulates inflammation by mediating the effect of 15-deoxy-Delta(12,14)-prostaglandin j(2)." *Mol Cell Biol* 24(1): 36–45.

Itokawa, H., S. L. Morris-Natschke et al. (2008). "Plant-derived natural product research aimed at new drug discovery." *J Nat Med* 62(3): 263–280.

Jacobs, M. D. and S. C. Harrison (1998). "Structure of an IkappaBalpha/NF-kappaB complex." *Cell* 95(6): 749–758.

Jagtap, S., K. Meganathan et al. (2009). "Chemoprotective mechanism of the natural compounds, epigallocatechin-3-O-gallate, quercetin and curcumin against cancer and cardiovascular diseases." *Curr Med Chem* 16(12): 1451–1462.

Jeong, W. S., I. W. Kim et al. (2004). "Modulation of AP-1 by natural chemopreventive compounds in human colon HT-29 cancer cell line." *Pharm Res* 21(4): 649–660.

Jiang, J. and C. Hu (2009). "Evodiamine: a novel anti-cancer alkaloid from Evodia rutaecarpa." *Molecules* 14(5): 1852–1859.

Jiang, T., N. Chen et al. (2010). "High levels of Nrf2 determine chemoresistance in type II endometrial cancer." *Cancer Res* 70(13): 5486–5496.

Johnson, S. M., X. Wang et al. (2011). "Triptolide inhibits proliferation and migration of colon cancer cells by inhibition of cell cycle regulators and cytokine receptors." *J Surg Res* 168(2): 197–205.

Jomova, K., D. Vondrakova et al. (2010). "Metals, oxidative stress and neurodegenerative disorders." *Mol Cell Biochem* 345(1–2): 91–104.

Jun, C. D., Y. Kim et al. (2006). "Gliotoxin reduces the severity of trinitrobenzene sulfonic acid-induced colitis in mice: evidence of the connection between heme oxygenase-1 and the nuclear factor-kappaB pathway in vitro and in vivo." *Inflamm Bowel Dis* 12(7): 619–629.

Jung, K. A. and M. K. Kwak (2010). "The Nrf2 system as a potential target for the development of indirect antioxidants." *Molecules* 15(10): 7266–7291.

Kang, K. W., S. H. Choi et al. (2002). "Peroxynitrite activates NF-E2-related factor 2/antioxidant response element through the pathway of phosphatidylinositol 3-kinase: the role of nitric oxide synthase in rat glutathione S-transferase A2 induction." *Nitric Oxide* 7(4): 244–253.

Kang, K. W., S. J. Lee et al. (2002). "Phosphatidylinositol 3-kinase regulates nuclear translocation of NF-E2-related factor 2 through actin rearrangement in response to oxidative stress." *Mol Pharmacol* 62(5): 1001–1010.

Karin, M. and Y. Ben-Neriah (2000). "Phosphorylation meets ubiquitination: the control of NF-[kappa]B activity." *Annu Rev Immunol* 18: 621–663.

Kensler, T. W., N. Wakabayashi et al. (2007). "Cell survival responses to environmental stresses via the Keap1-Nrf2-ARE pathway." *Annu Rev Pharmacol Toxicol* 47: 89–116.

Keum, Y. S., T. O. Khor et al. (2009). "Pharmacokinetics and pharmacodynamics of broccoli sprouts on the suppression of prostate cancer in transgenic adenocarcinoma of mouse prostate (TRAMP) mice: implication of induction of Nrf2, HO-1 and apoptosis and the suppression of Akt-dependent kinase pathway." *Pharm Res* 26(10): 2324–2331.

Keum, Y. S., S. Yu et al. (2006). "Mechanism of action of sulforaphane: inhibition of p38 mitogen-activated protein kinase isoforms contributing to the induction of antioxidant response element-mediated heme oxygenase-1 in human hepatoma HepG2 cells." *Cancer Res* 66(17): 8804–8813.

Khan, N., V. M. Adhami et al. (2009). "Review: green tea polyphenols in chemoprevention of prostate cancer: preclinical and clinical studies." *Nutr Cancer* 61(6): 836–841.

Khor, T. O., Y. S. Keum et al. (2006). "Combined inhibitory effects of curcumin and phenethyl isothiocyanate on the growth of human PC-3 prostate xenografts in immunodeficient mice." *Cancer Res* 66(2): 613–621.

Khor, T. O., M. T. Huang et al. (2006). "Nrf2-deficient mice have an increased susceptibility to dextran sulfate sodium-induced colitis." *Cancer Res* 66(24): 11580–11584.

Khor, T. O., M. T. Huang et al. (2008). "Increased susceptibility of Nrf2 knockout mice to colitis-associated colorectal cancer." *Cancer Prev Res (Phila)* 1(3): 187–191.

Kim, S. H. and S. V. Singh (2009). "D,L-Sulforaphane causes transcriptional repression of androgen receptor in human prostate cancer cells." *Mol Cancer Ther* 8(7): 1946–1954.

Kim, S. O., J. K. Kundu et al. (2005). "[6]-Gingerol inhibits COX-2 expression by blocking the activation of p38 MAP kinase and NF-kappaB in phorbol ester-stimulated mouse skin." *Oncogene* 24(15): 2558–2567.

Kim, Y. R., J. E. Oh et al. (2010). "Oncogenic Nrf2 mutations in squamous cell carcinomas of oesophagus and skin." *J Pathol* 220(4): 446–451.

Koenitzer, J. R. and B. A. Freeman (2010). "Redox signaling in inflammation: interactions of endogenous electrophiles and mitochondria in cardiovascular disease." *Ann N Y Acad Sci* 1203: 45–52.

Kojo, S. (2004). "Vitamin C: basic metabolism and its function as an index of oxidative stress." *Curr Med Chem* 11(8): 1041–1064.

Kong, A. N., R. Yu et al. (2001). "Signal transduction events elicited by cancer prevention compounds." *Mutat Res* 480–481: 231–241.

Kucuk, O. (2002). "Chemoprevention of prostate cancer." *Cancer Metastasis Rev* 21(2): 111–124.

Kumar, N. B., K. Allen et al. (2005). "Perioperative herbal supplement use in cancer patients: potential implications and recommendations for presurgical screening." *Cancer Control* 12(3): 149–157.

Kwon, K. H., A. Barve et al. (2007). "Cancer chemoprevention by phytochemicals: potential molecular targets, biomarkers and animal models." *Acta Pharmacol Sin* 28(9): 1409–1421.

Lakshman, M., L. Xu et al. (2008). "Dietary genistein inhibits metastasis of human prostate cancer in mice." *Cancer Res* 68(6): 2024–2032.

Lambert, J. D., S. Sang et al. (2010). "Anticancer and anti-inflammatory effects of cysteine metabolites of the green tea polyphenol, (-)-epigallocatechin-3-gallate." *J Agric Food Chem* 58(18): 10016–10019.

Lau, A., N. F. Villeneuve et al. (2008). "Dual roles of Nrf2 in cancer." *Pharmacol Res* 58(5–6): 262–270.

Lee, J. M., J. M. Hanson et al. (2001). "Phosphatidylinositol 3-kinase, not extracellular signal-regulated kinase, regulates activation of the antioxidant-responsive element in IMR-32 human neuroblastoma cells." *J Biol Chem* 276(23): 20011–20016.

Lee, T. S. and L. Y. Chau (2002). "Heme oxygenase-1 mediates the anti-inflammatory effect of interleukin-10 in mice." *Nat Med* 8(3): 240–246.

Levonen, A. L., M. Inkala et al. (2007). "Nrf2 gene transfer induces antioxidant enzymes and suppresses smooth muscle cell growth in vitro and reduces oxidative stress in rabbit aorta in vivo." *Arterioscler Thromb Vasc Biol* 27(4): 741–747.

Li, W. and A. N. Kong (2009). "Molecular mechanisms of Nrf2-mediated antioxidant response." *Mol Carcinog* 48(2): 91–104.

Li, W., T. O. Khor et al. (2008). "Activation of Nrf2-antioxidant signaling attenuates NFkappaB-inflammatory response and elicits apoptosis." *Biochem Pharmacol* 76(11): 1485–1489.

Liao, P. C., L. T. Ng et al. (2010). "Resveratrol arrests cell cycle and induces apoptosis in human hepatocellular carcinoma Huh-7 cells." *J Med Food* 13(6): 1415–1423.

Liao, S. and R. A. Hiipakka (1995). "Selective inhibition of steroid 5 alpha-reductase isozymes by tea epicatechin-3-gallate and epigallocatechin-3-gallate." *Biochem Biophys Res Commun* 214(3): 833–838.

Limon-Pacheco, J. H. and M. E. Gonsebatt (2010). "The glutathione system and its regulation by neurohormone melatonin in the central nervous system." *Cent Nerv Syst Agents Med Chem* 10(4): 287–297.

Lin, W., R. T. Wu et al. (2008). "Sulforaphane suppressed LPS-induced inflammation in mouse peritoneal macrophages through Nrf2 dependent pathway." *Biochem Pharmacol* 76(8): 967–973.

Lin, W., G. Shen et al. (2006). "Regulation of Nrf2 transactivation domain activity by p160 RAC3/SRC3 and other nuclear co-regulators." *J Biochem Mol Biol* 39(3): 304–310.

Liu, G. H., J. Qu et al. (2008). "NF-kappaB/p65 antagonizes Nrf2-ARE pathway by depriving CBP from Nrf2 and facilitating recruitment of HDAC3 to MafK." *Biochim Biophys Acta* 1783(5): 713–727.

Liu, Y. C., C. W. Hsieh et al. (2007). "Chalcone inhibits the activation of NF-kappaB and STAT3 in endothelial cells via endogenous electrophile." *Life Sci* 80(15): 1420–1430.

Lu, Y., C. S. Li et al. (2008). "Chinese herb related molecules of cancer-cell-apoptosis: a minireview of progress between Kanglaite injection and related genes." *J Exp Clin Cancer Res* 27: 31.

Luedde, T., N. Beraza et al. (2007). "Deletion of NEMO/IKKgamma in liver parenchymal cells causes steatohepatitis and hepatocellular carcinoma." *Cancer Cell* 11(2): 119–132.

Mahaffey, C. M., H. Zhang et al. (2009). "Multidrug-resistant protein-3 gene regulation by the transcription factor Nrf2 in human bronchial epithelial and non-small-cell lung carcinoma." *Free Radic Biol Med* 46(12): 1650–1657.

Mamede, A. C., S. D. Tavares et al. (2011). "The role of vitamins in cancer: a review." *Nutr Cancer* 63(4): 479–494.

Mansuy, D. (2011). "Brief historical overview and recent progress on cytochromes P450: adaptation of aerobic organisms to their chemical environment and new mechanisms of prodrug bioactivation." *Ann Pharm Fr* 69(1): 62–69.

Mantovani, A. (2010). "Molecular pathways linking inflammation and cancer." *Curr Mol Med* 10(4): 369–373.

Mantovani, A., P. Allavena et al. (2008). "Cancer-related inflammation." *Nature* 454(7203): 436–444.

Matthews, J. R., N. Wakasugi et al. (1992). "Thioredoxin regulates the DNA binding activity of NF-kappa B by reduction of a disulphide bond involving cysteine 62." *Nucleic Acids Res* 20(15): 3821–3830.

McMahon, M., K. Itoh et al. (2001). "The Cap'n'Collar basic leucine zipper transcription factor Nrf2 (NF-E2 p45-related factor 2) controls both constitutive and inducible expression of intestinal detoxification and glutathione biosynthetic enzymes." *Cancer Res* 61(8): 3299–3307.

McMahon, M., N. Thomas et al. (2006). "Dimerization of substrate adaptors can facilitate cullin-mediated ubiquitylation of proteins by a "tethering" mechanism: a two-site interaction model for the Nrf2-Keap1 complex." *J Biol Chem* 281(34): 24756–24768.

Messing, E., J. R. Gee et al. (2012). "A phase 2 cancer chemoprevention biomarker trial of isoflavone G-2535 (genistein) in presurgical bladder cancer patients." *Cancer Prev Res (Phila)* 5(4): 621–630.

Miao, W., L. Hu et al. (2005). "Transcriptional regulation of NF-E2 p45-related factor (Nrf2) expression by the aryl hydrocarbon receptor-xenobiotic response element signaling pathway: direct cross-talk between phase I and II drug-metabolizing enzymes." *J Biol Chem* 280(21): 20340–20348.

Mochizuki, M., Y. Ishii et al. (2005). "Role of 15-deoxy delta(12,14) prostaglandin J2 and Nrf2 pathways in protection against acute lung injury." *Am J Respir Crit Care Med* 171(11): 1260–1266.

Moon, D. O., S. H. Kang et al. (2010). "Sulforaphane decreases viability and telomerase activity in hepatocellular carcinoma Hep3B cells through the reactive oxygen species-dependent pathway." *Cancer Lett* 295(2): 260–266.

Myzak, M. C., P. Tong et al. (2007). "Sulforaphane retards the growth of human PC-3 xenografts and inhibits HDAC activity in human subjects." *Exp Biol Med (Maywood)* 232(2): 227–234.

Nakaso, K., H. Yano et al. (2003). "PI3K is a key molecule in the Nrf2-mediated regulation of antioxidative proteins by hemin in human neuroblastoma cells." *FEBS Lett* 546(2–3): 181–184.

Nguyen, T., P. J. Sherratt et al. (2003). "Increased protein stability as a mechanism that enhances Nrf2-mediated transcriptional activation of the antioxidant response element. Degradation of Nrf2 by the 26 S proteasome." *J Biol Chem* 278(7): 4536–4541.

Nigam, N., J. George et al. (2010). "Induction of apoptosis by [6]-gingerol associated with the modulation of p53 and involvement of mitochondrial signaling pathway in B[a]P-induced mouse skin tumorigenesis." *Cancer Chemother Pharmacol* 65(4): 687–696.

Nishikawa, M., M. Hashida et al. (2009). "Catalase delivery for inhibiting ROS-mediated tissue injury and tumor metastasis." *Adv Drug Deliv Rev* 61(4): 319–326.

Numazawa, S., M. Ishikawa et al. (2003). "Atypical protein kinase C mediates activation of NF-E2-related factor 2 in response to oxidative stress." *Am J Physiol Cell Physiol* 285(2): C334–C342.

Ohta, T., K. Iijima et al. (2008). "Loss of Keap1 function activates Nrf2 and provides advantages for lung cancer cell growth." *Cancer Res* 68(5): 1303–1309.

Osburn, W. O. and T. W. Kensler (2008). "Nrf2 signaling: an adaptive response pathway for protection against environmental toxic insults." *Mutat Res* 659(1–2): 31–39.

Osburn, W. O., N. Wakabayashi et al. (2006). "Nrf2 regulates an adaptive response protecting against oxidative damage following diquat-mediated formation of superoxide anion." *Arch Biochem Biophys* 454(1): 7–15.

Ottini, L., M. Falchetti et al. (2006). "Patterns of genomic instability in gastric cancer: clinical implications and perspectives." *Ann Oncol* 17 Suppl 7: vii97–102.

Oyagbemi, A. A., A. B. Saba et al. (2010). "Molecular targets of [6]-gingerol: its potential roles in cancer chemoprevention." *Biofactors* 36(3): 169–178.

Pahl, H. L. (1999). "Activators and target genes of Rel/NF-kappaB transcription factors." *Oncogene* 18(49): 6853–6866.

Pan, M. H., S. Y. Lin-Shiau et al. (2000). "Comparative studies on the suppression of nitric oxide synthase by curcumin and its hydrogenated metabolites through down-regulation of IkappaB kinase and NFkappaB activation in macrophages." *Biochem Pharmacol* 60(11): 1665–1676.

Pandey, M. and S. Gupta (2009). "Green tea and prostate cancer: from bench to clinic." *Front Biosci (Elite Ed)* 1: 13–25.

Pappolla, M. A., Y. J. Chyan et al. (1998). "Evidence of oxidative stress and in vivo neurotoxicity of beta-amyloid in a transgenic mouse model of Alzheimer's disease: a chronic oxidative paradigm for testing antioxidant therapies in vivo." *Am J Pathol* 152(4): 871–877.

Park, E. J. and J. M. Pezzuto (2002). "Botanicals in cancer chemoprevention." *Cancer Metastasis Rev* 21(3–4): 231–255.

Park, K. K., K. S. Chun et al. (1998). "Inhibitory effects of [6]-gingerol, a major pungent principle of ginger, on phorbol ester-induced inflammation, epidermal ornithine decarboxylase activity and skin tumor promotion in ICR mice." *Cancer Lett* 129(2): 139–144.

Perabo, F. G., E. C. Von Low et al. (2008). "Soy isoflavone genistein in prevention and treatment of prostate cancer." *Prostate Cancer Prostatic Dis* 11(1): 6–12.

Pettazzoni, P., E. Ciamporcero et al. (2011). "Nuclear factor erythroid 2-related factor-2 activity controls 4-hydroxynonenal metabolism and activity in prostate cancer cells." *Free Radic Biol Med* 51(8): 1610–1618.

Pikarsky, E. and Y. Ben-Neriah (2006). "NF-kappaB inhibition: a double-edged sword in cancer?" *Eur J Cancer* 42(6): 779–784.

Piotrowska, H., K. Myszkowski et al. (2012). "Resveratrol analogue 3,4,4′,5-tetramethoxystilbene inhibits growth, arrests cell cycle and induces apoptosis in ovarian SKOV-3 and A-2780 cancer cells." *Toxicol Appl Pharmacol* 263(1): 53–60.

Pizarro, J. G., E. Verdaguer et al. (2011). "Resveratrol inhibits proliferation and promotes apoptosis of neuroblastoma cells: role of sirtuin 1." *Neurochem Res* 36(2): 187–194.

Raffoul, J. J., F. H. Sarkar et al. (2007). "Radiosensitization of prostate cancer by soy isoflavones." *Curr Cancer Drug Targets* 7(8): 759–765.

Reddy, B. S. (1996). "Chemoprevention of colon cancer by minor dietary constituents and their synthetic analogues." *Prev Med* 25(1): 48–50.

Reddy, B. S., C. X. Wang et al. (1997). "Chemoprevention of colon carcinogenesis by dietary perillyl alcohol." *Cancer Res* 57(3): 420–425.

Reddy, S. P. (2008). "The antioxidant response element and oxidative stress modifiers in airway diseases." *Curr Mol Med* 8(5): 376–383.

Ren, D., N. F. Villeneuve et al. (2011). "Brusatol enhances the efficacy of chemotherapy by inhibiting the Nrf2-mediated defense mechanism." *Proc Natl Acad Sci U S A* 108(4): 1433–1438.

Reuter, S., S. Eifes et al. (2008). "Modulation of anti-apoptotic and survival pathways by curcumin as a strategy to induce apoptosis in cancer cells." *Biochem Pharmacol* 76(11): 1340–1351.

Rushmore, T. H. and C. B. Pickett (1993). "Glutathione S-transferases, structure, regulation, and therapeutic implications." *J Biol Chem* 268(16): 11475–11478.

Rushmore, T. H., M. R. Morton et al. (1991). "The antioxidant responsive element. Activation by oxidative stress and identification of the DNA consensus sequence required for functional activity." *J Biol Chem* 266(18): 11632–11639.

Rushworth, S. A., D. J. MacEwan et al. (2008). "Lipopolysaccharide-induced expression of NAD(P)H:quinone oxidoreductase 1 and heme oxygenase-1 protects against excessive inflammatory responses in human monocytes." *J Immunol* 181(10): 6730–6737.

Sarady, J. K., B. S. Zuckerbraun et al. (2004). "Carbon monoxide protection against endotoxic shock involves reciprocal effects on iNOS in the lung and liver." *FASEB J* 18(7): 854–856.

Sarkar, F. H. and Y. Li (2002). "Mechanisms of cancer chemoprevention by soy isoflavone genistein." *Cancer Metastasis Rev* 21(3–4): 265–280.

Scapagnini, G., S. Vasto et al. (2011). "Modulation of Nrf2/ARE pathway by food polyphenols: a nutritional neuroprotective strategy for cognitive and neurodegenerative disorders." *Mol Neurobiol* 44(2): 192–201.

Scapagnini, G., C. Colombrita et al. (2006). "Curcumin activates defensive genes and protects neurons against oxidative stress." *Antioxid Redox Signal* 8(3–4): 395–403.

Seldon, M. P., G. Silva et al. (2007). "Heme oxygenase-1 inhibits the expression of adhesion molecules associated with endothelial cell activation via inhibition of NF-kappaB RelA phosphorylation at serine 276." *J Immunol* 179(11): 7840–7851.

Sen, R. and D. Baltimore (1986a). "Inducibility of kappa immunoglobulin enhancer-binding protein Nf-kappa B by a posttranslational mechanism." *Cell* 47(6): 921–928.

Sen, R. and D. Baltimore (1986b). "Multiple nuclear factors interact with the immunoglobulin enhancer sequences." *Cell* 46(5): 705–716.

Sestili, P., M. Paolillo et al. (2010). "Sulforaphane induces DNA single strand breaks in cultured human cells." *Mutat Res* 689(1–2): 65–73.

Sethi, G., B. Sung et al. (2008). "Nuclear factor-kappaB activation: from bench to bedside." *Exp Biol Med (Maywood)* 233(1): 21–31.

Shan, Y., K. Wu et al. (2009). "Sulforaphane down-regulates COX-2 expression by activating p38 and inhibiting NF-kappaB-DNA-binding activity in human bladder T24 cells." *Int J Oncol* 34(4): 1129–1134.

Shankar, S., S. Ganapathy et al. (2008). "Sulforaphane enhances the therapeutic potential of TRAIL in prostate cancer orthotopic model through regulation of apoptosis, metastasis, and angiogenesis." *Clin Cancer Res* 14(21): 6855–6866.

Shen, G., V. Hebbar et al. (2004). "Regulation of Nrf2 transactivation domain activity. The differential effects of mitogen-activated protein kinase cascades and synergistic stimulatory effect of Raf and CREB-binding protein." *J Biol Chem* 279(22): 23052–23060.

Shen, G. and A. N. Kong (2009). "Nrf2 plays an important role in coordinated regulation of Phase II drug metabolism enzymes and Phase III drug transporters." *Biopharm Drug Dispos* 30(7): 345–355.

Shen, G., C. Xu et al. (2006). "Modulation of nuclear factor E2-related factor 2-mediated gene expression in mice liver and small intestine by cancer chemopreventive agent curcumin." *Mol Cancer Ther* 5(1): 39–51.

Shibata, T., A. Kokubu et al. (2008). "Genetic alteration of Keap1 confers constitutive Nrf2 activation and resistance to chemotherapy in gallbladder cancer." *Gastroenterology* 135(4): 1358–1368, 1368 e1351–e1354.

Shibata, T., T. Ohta et al. (2008). "Cancer related mutations in Nrf2 impair its recognition by Keap1-Cul3 E3 ligase and promote malignancy." *Proc Natl Acad Sci U S A* 105(36): 13568–13573.

Shin, S., J. Wakabayashi et al. (2009). "Role of Nrf2 in prevention of high-fat diet-induced obesity by synthetic triterpenoid CDDO-imidazolide." *Eur J Pharmacol* 620(1–3): 138–144.

Shord, S. S., K. Shah et al. (2009). "Drug-botanical interactions: a review of the laboratory, animal, and human data for 8 common botanicals." *Integr Cancer Ther* 8(3): 208–227.

Shu, L., K. L. Cheung et al. (2010). "Phytochemicals: cancer chemoprevention and suppression of tumor onset and metastasis." *Cancer Metastasis Rev* 29(3): 483–502.

Singh, A., V. Misra et al. (2006). "Dysfunctional KEAP1-Nrf2 interaction in non-small-cell lung cancer." *PLoS Med* 3(10): e420.

Sporn, M. B., N. M. Dunlop et al. (1976). "Prevention of chemical carcinogenesis by vitamin A and its synthetic analogs (retinoids)." *Fed Proc* 35(6): 1332–1338.

Sriram, N., S. Kalayarasan et al. (2009). "Epigallocatechin-3-gallate augments antioxidant activities and inhibits inflammation during bleomycin-induced experimental pulmonary fibrosis through Nrf2-Keap1 signaling." *Pulm Pharmacol Ther* 22(3): 221–236.

Stacy, D. R., K. Ely et al. (2006). "Increased expression of nuclear factor E2 p45-related factor 2 (Nrf2) in head and neck squamous cell carcinomas." *Head Neck* 28(9): 813–818.

Stocker, R. (2004). "Antioxidant activities of bile pigments." *Antioxid Redox Signal* 6(5): 841–849.

Sun, Z., Z. Huang et al. (2009). "Phosphorylation of Nrf2 at multiple sites by MAP kinases has a limited contribution in modulating the Nrf2-dependent antioxidant response." *PLoS One* 4(8): e6588.

Surh, Y. J. (2003). "Cancer chemoprevention with dietary phytochemicals." *Nat Rev Cancer* 3(10): 768–780.

Swami, S., A. V. Krishnan et al. (2009). "Inhibition of prostaglandin synthesis and actions by genistein in human prostate cancer cells and by soy isoflavones in prostate cancer patients." *Int J Cancer* 124(9): 2050–2059.

Tan, A. C., I. Konczak et al. (2011). "Molecular pathways for cancer chemoprevention by dietary phytochemicals." *Nutr Cancer* 63(4): 495–505.

Thasni, K. A., G. Rojini et al. (2008). "Genistein induces apoptosis in ovarian cancer cells via different molecular pathways depending on Breast Cancer Susceptibility gene-1 (BRCA1) status." *Eur J Pharmacol* 588(2–3): 158–164.

Thimmulappa, R. K., H. Lee et al. (2006). "Nrf2 is a critical regulator of the innate immune response and survival during experimental sepsis." *J Clin Invest* 116(4): 984–995.

Thompson, J. E., R. J. Phillips et al. (1995). "I kappa B-beta regulates the persistent response in a biphasic activation of NF-kappa B." *Cell* 80(4): 573–582.

Tong, K. I., Y. Katoh et al. (2006). "Keap1 recruits Neh2 through binding to ETGE and DLG motifs: characterization of the two-site molecular recognition model." *Mol Cell Biol* 26(8): 2887–2900.

Tong, K. I., A. Kobayashi et al. (2006). "Two-site substrate recognition model for the Keap1-Nrf2 system: a hinge and latch mechanism." *Biol Chem* 387(10–11): 1311–1320.

Trachootham, D., Y. Zhou et al. (2006). "Selective killing of oncogenically transformed cells through a ROS-mediated mechanism by beta-phenylethyl isothiocyanate." *Cancer Cell* 10(3): 241–252.

Traenckner, E. B., H. L. Pahl et al. (1995). "Phosphorylation of human I kappa B-alpha on serines 32 and 36 controls I kappa B-alpha proteolysis and NF-kappa B activation in response to diverse stimuli." *EMBO J* 14(12): 2876–2883.

Tsao, A. S., E. S. Kim et al. (2004). "Chemoprevention of cancer." *CA Cancer J Clin* 54(3): 150–180.

Valko, M., M. Izakovic et al. (2004). "Role of oxygen radicals in DNA damage and cancer incidence." *Mol Cell Biochem* 266(1–2): 37–56.

Valko, M., C. J. Rhodes et al. (2006). "Free radicals, metals and antioxidants in oxidative stress-induced cancer." *Chem Biol Interact* 160(1): 1–40.

van Der Heijden, R., D. I. Jacobs et al. (2004). "The Catharanthus alkaloids: pharmacognosy and biotechnology." *Curr Med Chem* 11(5): 607–628.

Vanamala, J., L. Reddivari et al. (2010). "Resveratrol suppresses IGF-1 induced human colon cancer cell proliferation and elevates apoptosis via suppression of IGF-1R/Wnt and activation of p53 signaling pathways." *BMC Cancer* 10: 238.

Venkateshappa, C., G. Harish et al. (2012). "Increased oxidative damage and decreased antioxidant function in aging human substantia nigra compared to striatum: implications for Parkinson's disease." *Neurochem Res* 37(2): 358–369.

Villeneuve, N. F., A. Lau et al. (2010). "Regulation of the Nrf2-Keap1 antioxidant response by the ubiquitin proteasome system: an insight into cullin-ring ubiquitin ligases." *Antioxid Redox Signal* 13(11): 1699–1712.

Wakabayashi, N., S. Shin et al. (2010). "Regulation of notch1 signaling by nrf2: implications for tissue regeneration." *Sci Signal* 3(130): ra52.

Wakabayashi, N., S. L. Slocum et al. (2010). "When Nrf2 talks, who's listening?" *Antioxid Redox Signal* 13(11): 1649–1663.

Wang, X. J., Z. Sun et al. (2008). "Nrf2 enhances resistance of cancer cells to chemotherapeutic drugs, the dark side of Nrf2." *Carcinogenesis* 29(6): 1235–43.

Wattenberg, L. W. (1985). "Chemoprevention of cancer." *Cancer Res* 45(1): 1–8.

Weiss, G., G. Werner-Felmayer et al. (1994). "Iron regulates nitric oxide synthase activity by controlling nuclear transcription." *J Exp Med* 180(3): 969–976.

Wondrak, G. T., C. M. Cabello et al. (2008). "Cinnamoyl-based Nrf2-activators targeting human skin cell photo-oxidative stress." *Free Radic Biol Med* 45(4): 385–395.

Wu, S. J., L. T. Ng et al. (2005). "Effects of antioxidants and caspase-3 inhibitor on the phenylethyl isothiocyanate-induced apoptotic signaling pathways in human PLC/PRF/5 cells." *Eur J Pharmacol* 518(2–3): 96–106.

Yang, H., N. Magilnick et al. (2005). "Nrf1 and Nrf2 regulate rat glutamate-cysteine ligase catalytic subunit transcription indirectly via NF-kappaB and AP-1." *Mol Cell Biol* 25(14): 5933–5946.

Yu, B. P. (1994). "Cellular defenses against damage from reactive oxygen species." *Physiol Rev* 74(1): 139–162.

Yu, M., H. Li et al. (2011). "Nuclear factor p65 interacts with Keap1 to repress the Nrf2-ARE pathway." *Cell Signal* 23(5): 883–892.

Yu, R., S. Mandlekar et al. (1998). "Chemopreventive isothiocyanates induce apoptosis and caspase-3-like protease activity." *Cancer Res* 58(3): 402–408.

Yu, S., T. O. Khor et al. (2010). "Nrf2 expression is regulated by epigenetic mechanisms in prostate cancer of TRAMP mice." *PLoS One* 5(1): e8579.

Yu, X. and T. Kensler (2005). "Nrf2 as a target for cancer chemoprevention." *Mutat Res* 591(1–2): 93–102.

Zabel, U. and P. A. Baeuerle (1990). "Purified human I kappa B can rapidly dissociate the complex of the NF-kappa B transcription factor with its cognate DNA." *Cell* 61(2): 255–265.

Zhang, D. D. (2006). "Mechanistic studies of the Nrf2-Keap1 signaling pathway." *Drug Metab Rev* 38(4): 769–789.

Zhang, D. D. (2010). "The Nrf2-Keap1-ARE signaling pathway: the regulation and dual function of Nrf2 in cancer." *Antioxid Redox Signal* 13(11): 1623–1626.

Zhao, R., N. Xiang et al. (2009). "Effects of selenite and genistein on G2/M cell cycle arrest and apoptosis in human prostate cancer cells." *Nutr Cancer* 61(3): 397–407.

Zipper, L. M. and R. T. Mulcahy (2003). "Erk activation is required for Nrf2 nuclear localization during pyrrolidine dithiocarbamate induction of glutamate cysteine ligase modulatory gene expression in HepG2 cells." *Toxicol Sci* 73(1): 124–134.

Zipper, L. M. and R. T. Mulcahy (2000). "Inhibition of ERK and p38 MAP kinases inhibits binding of Nrf2 and induction of GCS genes." *Biochem Biophys Res Commun* 278(2): 484–492.

Section II

Signal Transduction, Molecular Targets, and Biomarkers of Dietary Cancer-Preventive Phytochemicals

5 Signal Transduction and Molecular Targets of Dietary Cancer-Preventive Phytochemicals

Ann M. Bode and Zigang Dong

CONTENTS

5.1 INTRODUCTION

Carcinogenesis is a complex, multistage process that impacts hundreds of genes and gene products that are critical in the regulation of a multitude of cellular functions. A major focus of much of our work over the past decade has been the elucidation of molecular and cellular mechanisms and targets essential in cancer prevention. An important outcome of these investigations is the clarification of signal transduction pathways induced by a variety of tumor promoters in cancer development. A prevailing idea today is that cancer might be prevented (Bode et al. 2009a) or treated by using small molecules to target specific and, perhaps, multiple cancer genes, signaling proteins, and transcription factors. Each stage of cancer development could be a potential target for anticancer agents, especially the promotion stage. Importantly, new cutting-edge technologies, including supercomputer *in silico* screening and protein simulation and modeling, not only are rapidly clarifying the molecular mechanisms explaining how normal cells undergo neoplastic transformation induced by tumor promoters but also have been key in identifying the mechanisms of action and molecular targets of small-molecule anticancer agents.

Protein kinases and their inhibitory phosphatases are vital regulators of normal cellular processes including proliferation, migration, metabolism, differentiation, and survival. However, their abnormal activation can drive oncogenesis. Many kinases are aberrantly expressed in various cancers (Weir et al. 2004). In particular, the receptor tyrosine kinases (RTKs) are transmembrane protein receptors that exhibit intrinsic, ligand-controlled tyrosine kinase activity. In quiescent cells, RTK activity is also quiet, whereas in many types of cancer cells, the RTKs can become incongruously phosphorylated. Among the RTKs, the inappropriate phosphorylation and activation of the Human Growth Factor Receptor (HER)/*erb*B family have been observed in many cancers (Ciardiello and Tortora 2008), including breast, colorectal, and non–small-cell lung carcinomas.

Epidermal growth factor receptor (EGFR) activation triggers three main signaling pathways, the rat sarcoma (RAS)–rapidly accelerated fibrosarcoma (RAF)–mitogen-activated protein kinase kinase (MKK)–mitogen-activated protein kinase (MAPK) pathway; the phosphoinositide 3-kinase (PI3-K)–phosphatase and tensin homolog (PTEN)–protein kinase B (Akt)–mammalian target of rapamycin (mTOR) pathway; and the signal transducer and activator of transcription (STAT) signal cascade (Baselga 2001; Di Nicolantonio et al. 2008; De Luca et al. 2008; Hynes and Lane 2005; Jimeno and Hidalgo 2006). These signaling pathways ultimately lead to increased proliferation, angiogenesis, metastasis, survival, and motility and decreased apoptosis (Mosesson and Yarden 2004). In particular, the MAPK signaling pathways are activated differentially by various tumor promoters (reviewed in Bode et al. 2010; Bode and Dong 2000, 2002, 2003a,b, 2004a,b,c,d, 2005, 2006, 2007a,b, 2009a,b,c,d, 2011a,b, 2012). MAPKs are activated by translocation to the nucleus, where they phosphorylate a variety of target transcription factors important in tumor development, including activator protein-1 (AP-1) and nuclear factor kappaB (NF-κB) (Davis 1994; Angel et al. 1988; Kallunki et al. 1994; Sanchez et al. 1994), which in turn may activate transcription of a variety of cancer-related genes such as *cyclooxygenase 2*. AP-1 is a well-characterized transcription factor composed of homodimers and/or heterodimers of the *jun* and *fos* gene families (Angel et al. 1991). AP-1 regulates the transcription of various genes that govern cellular processes including inflammation, proliferation, and apoptosis (Angel and Karin 1991). This transcription factor plays a major role in tumor promotion (Dong et al. 1994, 1995), and blocking tumor promoter–induced AP-1 activity abolishes neoplastic cell transformation (Dong et al. 1994). NF-κB is a stress-responsive transcription factor that is rapidly induced and functions to intensify the transcription of a variety of genes leading to expression of cytokines, growth factors, cyclooxygenase 2 (COX2) and other acute response proteins (Baldwin 1996). Its activation is strongly linked to MAPK signaling pathways (Schulze-Osthoff et al. 1997). Initiation or acceleration of tumorigenesis is strongly associated with NF-κB activation (Gilmore 1997), and inhibition of NF-κB activation blocks tumor promoter–induced malignant cell transformation (Gilmore 1997). COX enzymes or prostaglandin-endoperoxide synthases catalyze the conversion of arachidonic acid into prostaglandins and are important transcriptional targets of AP-1 and NF-κB. COX has two well-known isoforms, denoted COX1 and COX2. COX1 is constitutively expressed in almost every cell type, whereas COX2 is induced by stresses, including inflammation. Overexpression of COX2 has been implicated in cancer development (Turini and DuBois 2002; Subbaramaiah and Dannenberg 2003; Prescott and Fitzpatrick 2000), including cancers of the colon (Sano et al. 1995; Eberhart et al. 1994; Kutchera et al. 1996), breast (Hwang et al. 1998; Subbaramaiah et al. 1996), lung (Wolff et al. 1998; Hida et al. 1998), stomach (van Rees et al. 2002) and gastric system (Ristimaki et al. 1997), head and neck (Chan et al. 1999; Gallo et al. 2001; Mestre et al. 1999), pancreas (Tucker et al. 1999), uterus (Tong et al. 2000), cervix (Gaffney et al. 2001), urinary bladder (Grubbs et al. 2000), gall bladder (Grossman et al. 2000), and skin (Denkert et al. 2001; Buckman et al. 1998; Lee et al. 2003; An et al. 2002; Athar et al. 2001). Studies utilizing mice deficient in COX1 or 2 develop fewer tumors when subjected to the two-stage 7,12-dimethylbenz(a)anthracene (DMBA)/12-*O*-tetradecanoylphorbol-13-acetate

(TPA) mouse skin tumorigenesis protocol (Tiano et al. 2002). On the other hand, overexpression of COX2 in mouse skin also led to fewer tumors in a similar protocol (Bol et al. 2002). These types of conflicting results are difficult to rationalize. However, research findings generally suggest that development of compounds, which can block COX2 expression preferably without affecting COX1, is highly interesting to cancer researchers.

Many natural or dietary compounds are believed to have potent anticancer activity, have low toxicity, and cause very few adverse side effects. Accumulating research evidence suggests that many of these compounds may be used alone or in combination with traditional chemotherapeutic agents to prevent or treat cancer (reviewed in Bode and Dong 2000, 2002, 2003a,b, 2004a,b,c,d, 2005, 2006, 2009a,b,c,d, 2011a,b, 2012). Our work has focused on elucidating the effects of various dietary components and other natural compounds on cancer cells and tumor growth, discovering mechanisms to explain the effects, and identifying the specific cellular and molecular targets of these compounds (reviewed in K.W. Lee et al. 2011). Precisely defining the mechanisms of action based on molecular target identification can be linked to successful drug discovery. Our overall strategy for discovering specific molecular targets of dietary factors involves the extensive use of supercomputer technology combined with protein crystallography, molecular biology, and experimental laboratory verification. Computer modeling and biological simulation are increasingly being used as highly effective tools in cancer research. Protein kinases and their target transcription factors are strategic targets for drug screening. Our overall approach involves the virtual screening (McInnes 2007) of various ligand databases such as the ZINC (i.e., ZINC is not commercial) free database of commercially available compounds (http://zinc.docking.org) (Irwin and Shoichet 2005) for virtual screening and the Research Collaboratory for Structural Bioinformatics (RCSB) Protein Data Bank (PDB; http://www.pdb.org/pdb/home/home.do) (Bernstein et al. 1977) for available protein crystal structures. If a protein crystal structure with a resolution average of about 2.0 Å does not exist or the structure has not been solved, homology-modeling methods are used to create a suitable structure with which to work. Homology modeling between proteins requires that the two proteins possess a minimum protein sequence identity of 30% (Xiang 2006), and the European Molecular Biology Laboratory–European Bioinformatics Institute (EMBL-EBI) Web service (http://www.ebi.ac.uk/embl/) provides many of the tools necessary for protein sequence searching and alignments (McWilliam et al. 2009). In addition, the National Center for Biotechnology Information provides databases on protein structures and sequences (http:// www.ncbi.nlm.nih.gov/). The *in silico* screening is followed by experimental verification of the newly identified compound's effect on a predetermined target protein or the effect of a predetermined compound on a newly *in silico*–identified protein target. Finally, we can synthesize or chemically modify a potential candidate compound to possibly enhance the verified effectiveness of the *in silico*–identified or predetermined compound on the target protein.

Using this strategy, we have studied the anticancer activities and elucidated the role and molecular targets for tea, coffee, and cocoa components; resveratrol; [6]-gingerol; and a large number of flavonoids found in our everyday diet. The remainder of this chapter will highlight our major findings regarding the specific molecular mechanisms and protein-binding targets of a select few of these dietary components as effective anticancer agents. The main emphasis will be on the protein targets that have been identified for these compounds.

5.2   TEA, COFFEE, AND COCOA AS ANTICANCER AGENTS

5.2.1   Protein Targets of Epigallocatechin Gallate

One of the most well-studied green tea catechins is (-)-epigallocatechin gallate (EGCG) (Table 5.1) (Suzuki and Isemura 2001; Tachibana et al. 2004; Bode and Dong 2009b,c,d). This polyphenol reportedly prevents various cancers, obesity, diabetes, and cardiovascular disease. As for many natural food compounds, elucidating a specific mechanism of action has been challenging. Thus,

TABLE 5.1
Molecular Targets of Dietary Compounds

Dietary Compound	Chemical or International Union of Pure and Applied Chemistry (IUPAC) Name	Chemical Structure	Reported Molecular Target	Reference
EGCG	(2R,3R)-5,7-dihydroxy-2-(3,4,5-trihydroxyphenyl)-3,4-dihydro-2H-1-benzopyran-3-yl 3,4,5-trihydroxybenzoate (-)-Epigallocatechin gallate	(chemical structure)	-Fibronectin	(Sazuka et al. 1998)
			-Fibrinogen	
			-Histidine-rich glycoprotein	
			Apoptotic Fas	(Hayakawa et al. 2001)
			-Laminin	(Hayakawa et al. 2001; Tachibana et al. 2004)
			-67 kDa laminin receptor	(Tian 2006)
			Fatty acid synthase	(Palermo et al. 2005; Yin et al. 2009)
			Heat shock protein 90	(Williamson et al. 2006)
			T-cell receptor CD4	(Ermakova et al. 2005)
			Vimentin	(Ermakova et al. 2006)
			GRP78	(Li et al. 2007)
			IGF-IR	(He et al. 2008)
			SH2 domain Fyn	(Shim et al. 2008)
			ZAP-70	(Shim et al. 2010)
			G3BP1	(Urusova et al. 2011)
			Pin1	(Kang et al. 2009)
			Fyn	(Kang et al. 2011)
Caffeic acid	3,4-dihydroxycinnamic acid	(chemical structure)	-Mitogen-activated protein kinase kinase (MKK1)	
			-Lymphokine-activated killer TOPK	
Decaffeinated coffee extract			- MKK1	(Kang et al. 2011)
			-Lymphokine-activated killer TOPK	

- CPF -Procyanidin B2	(−)-Epicatechin-(4β → 8)-(−)-epicatechin	MKK1	(Kang et al. 2008b)
Resveratrol	3,5,4′-trihydroxy-trans-stilbene	αVβ3 integrin receptor Ref-1 COX2 LTA$_4$H	(Lin et al. 2006) (Yang et al. 2005) (Zykova et al. 2008) (Oi et al. 2010)
RSVL2	3,5,3′,4′,5′-pentahydroxy-trans-stilbene	COX2 MKK1	(Zykova et al. 2008) (Lee et al. 2008b)
[6]-Gingerol	1-[4′-hydroxy-3′-methoxyphenyl]-5-hydroxy-3-decanone	LTA$_4$H	(Jeong et al. 2009)

(continued)

TABLE 5.1 (Continued)
Molecular Targets of Dietary Compounds

Dietary Compound	Chemical or International Union of Pure and Applied Chemistry (IUPAC) Name	Chemical Structure	Reported Molecular Target	Reference
Kaempferol	3,5,7-trihydroxy-2-(4-hydroxyphenyl)-4H-chromen-4-one		RSK2 Src	(Cho et al. 2009) (Lee et al. 2010b)
5-Deoxykaempferol			-Src - PI3-K -RSK2	(Lee et al. 2010a)
Eriodictyol	(2S)-2-(3,4-dihydroxyphenyl)-5,7-dihydroxy-4-chromanone		RSK2	(Liu et al. 2011)
-Quercetin -Red wine extract	2-(3,4-dihydroxyphenyl)-3,5,7-trihydroxy-4H-chromen-4-one		-MKK1 -Raf1 PI3-K	(Lee et al. 2008a) (Hwang et al. 2009)

Name	Chemical name	Structure	Targets	References
Quercetin-3-methyl ether	3',4',5,7-tetrahydroxy-3-methoxyflavone		ERKs	(Li et al. 2012b)
Myricetin	3,5,7-trihydroxy-2-(3,4,5-trihydroxyphenyl)-4-chromenone		MKK1 Raf1 MKK4 Fyn Akt PI3-K -JAK1 -STAT3	(Lee et al. 2007) (Jung et al. 2010) (Kim et al. 2009) (Jung et al. 2008) (Kumamoto et al. 2009a) (Jung et al. 2009) (Kumamoto et al. 2009b)
Equol	(3S)-3-(4-hydroxyphenyl)-7-chromanol		MKK1	(Kang et al. 2007)
7,3',4'-trihydroxy-isoflavone			-Cot -MKK4 -Cdk2 -Cdk4 -PI3-K	(Lee et al. 2010) (Lee et al. 2011a)

(continued)

TABLE 5.1 (Continued)
Molecular Targets of Dietary Compounds

Dietary Compound	Chemical or International Union of Pure and Applied Chemistry (IUPAC) Name	Chemical Structure	Reported Molecular Target	Reference
6,7,4′-trihydroxy-isoflavone			-Cdk1 -Cdk2	(Lee et al. 2011b)
Luteolin	2-(3,4-dihydroxyphenyl)-5,7-dihydroxy-4-chromenone		- PKCε -Src	(Byun et al. 2010)
Isorhamnetin	3,5,7-trihydroxy-2-(4-hydroxy-3-methoxyphenyl) chromen-4-one		-MKK1 -PI3-K	(J.E. Kim et al. 2011)

Delphinidin	2-(3,4,5-trihydroxyphenyl)-chromenylium-3,5,7-triol		-Raf -MKK -PI3-K -MKK	(Kang et al. 2008a) (Kwon et al. 2009)
(3-Chloroacetyl)-indole			-Akt1 -Akt2	(D.J. Kim et al. 2011)
Norathyriol			-ERK2	(Li et al. 2012a)

our goal has been to identify "receptors" or high-affinity proteins that specifically bind compounds such as EGCG. We believe this to be a fundamental first step in understanding the molecular and biochemical mechanisms of the anticancer effects of natural food compounds, including tea polyphenols. Over the past decade, several proteins that directly bind with EGCG have been identified and include plasma proteins, fibronectin, fibrinogen, and histidine-rich glycoprotein (Sazuka et al. 1998); apoptotic Fas (Hayakawa et al. 2001); laminin and the 67 kDa laminin receptor (Hayakawa et al. 2001; Tachibana et al. 2004); fatty acid synthase (Tian 2006), heat shock protein 90 (Palermo et al. 2005; Yin et al. 2009); and T-cell receptor cluster of differentiation 4 (CD4) (Williamson et al. 2006). Even though these targets of tea polyphenols have been identified, the biologic and physiologic significance of their role in the anticancer effects of tea polyphenols is still not totally clear. Part of the challenge in these and other studies is whether EGCG or other tea compounds can reach a level that is physiologically achievable and the extent to which these compounds can penetrate the cell membrane.

Identification of novel high-affinity EGCG-binding proteins could facilitate the design of new strategies to prevent cancer. We first used JB6 Cl41 cell lysates and EGCG-conjugated Sepharose 4B beads followed by two-dimensional electrophoresis and matrix-assisted laser desorption/ionization–time-of-flight (MALDI-TOF) analysis to identify the intermediate filament protein, vimentin (Ermakova et al. 2005), and glucose-regulated protein 78 (GRP78) (Ermakova et al. 2006) as novel EGCG-binding proteins. EGCG bound to and inhibited phosphorylation of vimentin (Ser50/55), and the binding was associated with decreased breast cancer cell proliferation. Notably, the binding affinity of vimentin and [^{3}H]-labeled EGCG exhibited a K_d value of 3.3 nM, which is clearly achievable physiologically. GRP78 is associated with the multidrug resistance phenotype of many types of cancer cells, and EGCG binding caused the conversion of GRP78 from its active monomer to the inactive dimer and oligomer forms (Ermakova et al. 2006). The binding of EGCG interfered with the formation of the antiapoptotic GRP78–caspase-7 complex, which resulted in an increased etoposide-induced apoptosis in cancer cells (Ermakova et al. 2006).

We also used EGCG-conjugated Sepharose 4B affinity beads and found that EGCG directly binds with the insulin-like growth factor-I receptor (IGF-IR) and acts as a small-molecule inhibitor of IGF-IR activity (IC$_{50}$ of 14 μM) (Li et al. 2007). IGF-IR has been implicated in cancer pathophysiology, and suppressing IGF-IR signaling in various cancer cell lines causes inhibition of the transformed phenotype, as shown by the attenuation of colony formation in soft agar and the reduction of tumor formation in athymic nude mice. To confirm the EGCG and IGF-1R *in vitro* binding assay results in cells, we used IGF-IR kinase domain mutant (Y1131F, Y1135F, and Y1136F) cells (YF3) to compare binding with wild-type IGF-IR–expressing cells. Results indicated that mutant IGF-IR could not bind with EGCG–Sepharose 4B beads (Li et al. 2007). We constructed a docking model of the IGF-IR, and the model predicted that EGCG could bind within the ATP pocket of the IGF-1R and interact with Gln977, Lys1003, Met1052, Thr1053, and Asp1123 (Li et al. 2007). Cell-based experiments confirmed that EGCG competed with ATP for binding and that Lys1003 and Asp1123 were the most important for the interaction of EGCG with IGF-IR. Besides the IGF-IR, we also found that EGCG could bind with Fyn, a member of the nonreceptor protein tyrosine kinase family, at its Src Homology (SH2) domain but not at its SH3 domain (K_d 0.37 μM and Bmax 1.35 nmol/mg) (He et al. 2008). The binding was associated with decreased epidermal growth factor (EGF)–induced cell transformation mediated by Fyn kinase activity and phosphorylation. In addition, knockdown of Fyn or EGCG inhibited phosphorylation of p38, activating transcription factor 2 (ATF2), and STAT1 and decreased the DNA-binding ability of AP-1, STAT1, and ATF 2 (He et al. 2008).

The zeta chain–associated protein of 70 kDa (ZAP-70) tyrosine kinase plays a critical role in T-cell receptor–mediated signal transduction and the immune response, and a high level of ZAP-70 expression is observed in leukemia. Cell-based studies suggested that EGCG could suppress ZAP-70 activity, and therefore, we performed molecular docking studies with EGCG and ZAP-70 using the Maestro software suite (Maestro, version 7.5, Schrödinger, New York, NY) (Shim et al. 2008). The ZAP-70 crystal structure complexed with staurosporine (PDB code 1u59) was prepared for docking following the Glide standard procedure (Friesner et al. 2004). The results of the molecular docking studies were supported by *in vitro* and *ex vivo* laboratory experiments, which showed that EGCG could form numerous intermolecular hydrogen bonds and hydrophobic interactions within the ATP binding domain of ZAP-70 (Shim et al. 2008). The binding of EGCG with ZAP-70 occurred with high affinity ($K_d = 0.6207$ µM) and was associated with decreases in ZAP-70 activity and AP-1 activation along with an induction of caspase-mediated apoptosis in leukemia cells expressing ZAP-70 but not in ZAP-70 deficient cells (Shim et al. 2008). All of these results suggest that EGCG seems to interact with many proteins to suppress their activities. However, we also determined that EGCG did not bind to other tyrosine kinases, including Abelson murine leukemia viral oncogene homolog (Abl), platelet-derived growth factor receptor (PDGFR), c-Src, bone marrow X (Bmx), or Yes (Li et al. 2007).

Most recently, we found that EGCG interacted with the Ras-GTPase–activating protein SH3 domain–binding protein 1 (G3BP1) with good binding affinity ($K_d = 0.4$ µM). H1299 and CL13 lung cancer cells highly express G3BP1 and EGCG effectively suppressed anchorage-independent growth of these cells (Shim et al. 2010). In contrast, EGCG was much less effective in retarding the growth of H460 lung cancer cells, which express much lower levels of G3BP1, and similar effects were also observed in H1299 cells expressing small hairpin G3BP1 (Shim et al. 2010). Finally, we (Urusova et al. 2011) found that EGCG binds with the human peptidyl prolyl *cis/trans*-isomerase (Pin1), which plays a critical role in oncogenic signaling (Dominguez-Sola and Dalla-Favera 2004; Sears 2004). In this case, we were able to combine crystallography, computational biology, and cell- and animal-based studies to identify Pin1 as a novel binding protein of EGCG. Pin 1 comprises two distinct functional domains, the protein–protein interaction N-terminal WW domain (1–39 amino acids [aa]), a protein domain with two highly conserved tryptophans (W) that binds proline-rich peptide motifs, and the isomerization catalysis peptidylprolylisomerase (PPI) domain (45–168 aa) connected by a flexible linker region (40–44 aa) (Ranganathan et al. 1997). This protein is very likely required for the full activation of multiple signal transduction pathways including NF-κB, AP-1, β-catenin, and nuclear factor of activated T cells (NFAT) (Wulf et al. 2001, 2005; Ryo et al. 2001). We solved the x-ray crystal structure of the Pin1/EGCG complex resolved at 1.9 Å resolution, and the structure revealed the presence of EGCG in both the WW and PPIase domains of Pin1. Direct binding between Pin1 and EGCG was confirmed and resulted in the inhibition of Pin1 PPIase activity, growth of Pin1-expressing cells, and xenograft tumor growth (Urusova et al. 2011). Importantly, the binding of EGCG with Arg17 in the WW domain prevented the binding of c-Jun, a well-known Pin1 substrate. Finally, EGCG treatment corresponded with a decreased abundance of cyclin D1 and attenuation of TPA-induced *AP-1* or *NF-κB* promoter activity in cells expressing Pin1 (Urusova et al. 2011). Notably, this work was the subject of a "Perspective," in which the authors indicated, "The data provide a glimpse of the mechanism of action of EGCG and set a new bar for the future study of natural products with chemopreventive activity" (Rouzer and Marnett 2011).

5.2.2 ANTICANCER ACTIVITIES AND MOLECULAR TARGETS OF COFFEE AND COCOA PHYTOCHEMICALS

Epidemiological studies suggest that drinking coffee might reduce the risk of cancers, such as colon cancer. Caffeic acid (3,4-dihydroxycinnamic acid) (Table 5.1) is a well-known phenolic phytochemical present in many foods, including coffee. We reported that caffeic acid directly binds with the non-RTK, Fyn, noncompetitively with ATP (Kang et al. 2009). Fyn is required for ultraviolet B (UVB)–induced COX2 expression, and caffeic acid suppressed UVB-induced skin carcinogenesis by directly inhibiting Fyn kinase activity (Kang et al. 2009). We also reported that a decaffein-ated coffee extract or caffeic acid reduced CT-26 colon cancer cell–induced lung metastasis by blocking phosphorylation of extracellular signal–regulated kinases (ERKs) through direct binding with MKK1 or lymphokine-activated killer T-cell–originated protein kinase (TOPK) in an ATP-noncompetitive manner (Kang et al. 2011). Coffee or caffeic acid also reduced AP-1 and NF-κB transactivation and subsequently attenuated TPA-, EGF-, and H-Ras-induced neoplastic transfor-mation of JB6 promotion-sensitive (P+) mouse epidermal skin cells. We further found that coffee consumption was associated with a significant diminution of ERK phosphorylation in colon cancer patients (Kang et al. 2011).

Besides coffee and tea components, constituents of cocoa have been shown to inhibit cancer cell growth and chemically induced carcinogenesis in animals. We found that a cocoa procyanidin fraction (CPF) and procyanidin B2 (Table 5.1) inhibited EGF- or H-Ras-induced neoplastic cell transformation by directly binding with and suppressing the phosphorylation and kinase activity of MKK (Kang et al. 2008b). The inhibition of MKK was associated with decreased TPA-induced *cox2* promoter activity and protein expression and attenuated phosphorylation of ERKs and ribosomal S6 kinase (RSK). Procyanidin B2 exerted stronger inhibitory effects compared to PD098059, a well-known pharmacological inhibitor of MKK (Kang et al. 2008b).

5.3   MOLECULAR TARGETS OF RESVERATROL

Resveratrol (3,5,4′-trihydroxy-*trans*-stilbene) (Table 5.1) is a phytoalexin, one of a group of compounds that is produced in plants during environmental stress or pathogenic attack. This compound has been extensively studied and reviewed (Athar et al. 2009; Baxter 2008; Bishayee 2009; Bishayee and Dhir 2009; Bode and Dong 2004c; Brisdelli et al. 2009; Gatz et al. 2008; Goswami and Das 2009; Guerrero et al. 2009; Harikumar and Aggarwal 2008; Kundu and Surh 2008; Pervaiz and Holme 2009; Pirola and Frojdo 2008; Reagan-Shaw et al. 2008; Saiko et al. 2008a,b) since it was first reported (Jang et al. 1997) to possess potent chemopreventive effects. One group reported the αVβ3 integrin receptor in breast cancer cells as a protein-binding target of resveratrol (Lin et al. 2006). The binding apparently triggers the downstream activation of the ERK1/2 pathway, leading to p53 phosphorylation at Ser15, culminating in apoptosis (Lin et al. 2006). The modeling of resveratrol and redox factor-1 (Ref-1) also showed the possibility that resveratrol can bind to Ref-1 and regulate its activity (Yang et al. 2005).

In some of our earlier work, we found that resveratrol suppresses tumor promoter–induced cell transformation and induces apoptosis, transactivation of p53 activity, and expression of the p53 protein (Huang et al. 1999). Resveratrol-induced apoptosis occurred only in cells expressing wild type p53. These results suggested that resveratrol primarily acted as an anticancer agent by inducing apoptosis (Huang et al. 1999). We also found that resveratrol activated ERKs, c-Jun NH$_2$-terminal kinases (JNKs), and p38 and induced serine 15 phosphorylation of p53 (She et al. 2001). ERKs and p38 formed a complex with p53 after treatment with resveratrol; resveratrol-activated ERKs and p38, but not JNKs, phosphorylated p53 at serine 15 and induced apoptosis (She et al. 2001).

We went on to develop three structural analogs of resveratrol and found that at least one analog resveratrol 2 (RSVL2) (Table 5.1) was a more potent inhibitor of EGF-induced cell transformation than the parent resveratrol compound and was less toxic to normal nontransformed cells (She et al. 2003). Notably, this compound appeared to act by causing G1 cell cycle phase arrest but did not affect p53 or induce apoptosis. Rather, it appeared to attenuate the activity of the PI3-K/Akt signaling pathway (She et al. 2003). A second analog, RSVL1, had no effect on any parameter measured (She et al. 2003). We subsequently reported that resveratrol directly binds with COX2 and this binding was required for resveratrol's inhibition of human colon adenocarcinoma HT-29 cell growth in soft agar (Zykova et al. 2008). HT-29 cells express high levels of COX2. We again compared resveratrol and two of its analogs (RSVL2 and 3) in terms of their ability to bind COX2 and found that COX2 could bind with RSVL2 more strongly than with resveratrol, but it did not bind with RSVL3. Both resveratrol and RSVL2 inhibited COX2-mediated prostaglandin E2 (PGE$_2$) production, but the effect of RSVL2 was more potent compared to the parent compound (Zykova et al. 2008). We also found that RSVL2, but not resveratrol, directly binds with MKK1 (Lee et al. 2008b), but similar to other MKK1-selective small-molecule inhibitors (i.e., PD318088, PD184352, PD098059, U0126), RSVL2 did not compete with ATP for binding with MKK1 (Alessi et al. 1995; Duncia et al. 1998; Favata et al. 1998;

Ohren et al. 2004). The effect of RSVL2 was specific against MKK1 because RSVL2 inhibited MKK1 kinase activity but had no effect on Raf1 or ERK2 kinase activity (Lee et al. 2008b). The net result of the binding was reduced cell transformation mediated through inhibition of AP-1 transactivation and c-Fos activation. RSVL2 was more potent than the MKK inhibitor, PD098059, or resveratrol (Lee et al. 2008b). These data are significant because they provide evidence that more potent anticancer agents can be developed that are based on a parent compound such as resveratrol. Importantly, the analogs can act by different mechanisms, thus making their combination with the parent compound highly feasible for producing a more effective and potent anticancer activity.

Most recently, in our search to find novel protein targets for resveratrol, we conducted an extensive *in silico* screening using a shape-similarity approach (Oi et al. 2010). Resveratrol was screened against all crystallized ligands available from the PDB (Bernstein et al. 1977). Screening results showed that resveratrol was similar to 2-amino-N-[4-(phenylmethoxy)phenyl]-acetamide, a well-known leukotriene A4 hydrolase (LTA$_4$H) inhibitor, implying that LTA$_4$H might also be a possible molecular target for resveratrol. To test the results of the shape-similarity search for resveratrol, we performed *in vitro* and *ex vivo* pull-down assays using resveratrol- or RSVL3-conjugated (as a control) Sepharose 4B beads. Our data showed that recombinant LTA$_4$H or endogenous LTA$_4$H in MIA PaCa-2 pancreatic cancer cells bound to resveratrol-conjugated Sepharose 4B beads, but not to RSVL3-conjugated beads (Oi et al. 2010). Resveratrol also effectively suppressed pancreatic cancer cell growth both in culture and in a xenograft mouse model (Oi et al. 2010).

5.4 PROTEIN TARGETS OF [6]-GINGEROL

One of the most popular and highly consumed dietary substances in the world is derived from the plants of the ginger (*Zingiber officinable* Roscoe, *Zingiberaceae*) family (Surh et al. 1999). The oleoresin or oil from ginger root contains [6]-gingerol (1-[4′-hydroxy-3′-methoxyphenyl]-5-hydroxy-3-decanone) (Table 5.1), which is the major pharmacologically active component. The medicinal, chemical, and pharmacological properties of ginger have been extensively reviewed (Afzal et al. 2001; Bode and Dong 2004d, 2011b; Grant and Lutz 2000; Langner et al. 1998). Numerous research studies have reported that components of ginger suppress cancer cell growth (Bode et al. 2001; Lee et al. 1998; Lee and Surh 1998; Surh et al. 1998) and tumor growth in mice (Katiyar et al. 1996; Park et al. 1998; Chung et al. 2001; Kim et al. 2004). Reported targets of [6]-gingerol and related compounds include AP-1 (Bode et al. 2001), COX2, p38, NF-κB (Kim et al. 2004, 2005), and cyclic adenosine monophosphate (cAMP) response element–binding (CREB) (Kim et al. 2005) to name a few. However, specific binding or mechanistic data were not obtained until recently (Jeong et al. 2009).

Some investigators suggested that the effectiveness of ginger might be related to its ability to inhibit prostaglandin and leukotriene biosynthesis (Srivastava and Mustafa 1992). Others showed that gingerol actively inhibits arachidonate 5-lipoxygenase, an enzyme of leukotriene biosynthesis (Kiuchi et al. 1992). The LTA$_4$H protein is regarded as a relevant target for cancer therapy, and our *in silico* prediction using a reverse-docking approach revealed that LTA$_4$H was also a potential protein target of [6]-gingerol (Jeong et al. 2009). In this work, [6]-gingerol was docked to each target protein in the protein database using a reverse-docking tool, TarFisDock (Li et al. 2006). To define the specific protein-binding mode, the LTA$_4$H crystal structure (PDB code 1HS6) was applied for additional docking studies using the quantum mechanical (QM)-Polarized Ligand Docking program (Schrödinger 2006). Cell- and animal-based studies revealed that [6]-gingerol did indeed bind to LTA$_4$H to suppress its activity and growth of colon cancer cells both in culture and in a xenograft mouse model (Jeong et al. 2009). Collectively, these findings indicate a crucial role of LTA$_4$H in cancer and also support the anticancer efficacy of [6]-gingerol's targeting of LTA$_4$H for the prevention of colorectal cancer (Jeong et al. 2009). Notably, these were the first results to identify a direct target of [6]-gingerol to explain its anticancer activity.

5.5 ANTICANCER TARGETS OF SELECTED FLAVONOIDS AND OTHER POLYPHENOL COMPOUNDS

Flavonoids comprise a large family of polyphenol compounds that are found in numerous and various edible plants, and many have been reported to exert potent anticancer and other activities *in vitro, ex vivo,* and *in vivo.* The likelihood exists that most of these compounds also target multiple cellular and molecular targets to exert their anticancer effects. Nontoxic small molecules that affect multiple cellular targets are believed to have potential in cancer prevention. However, the possibility of different target specificities also exists allowing for the combination of compounds for more effective anticancer activity.

5.5.1 KAEMPFEROL AND 5-DEOXYKAEMPFEROL

Kaempferol (3,4′,5,7-tetrahydroxyflavone) (Table 5.1) is a flavonol present in various natural sources, especially in onion leaves (832.0 mg/kg) (Miean and Mohamed 2001). We found that kaempferol inhibited proliferation of malignant human cancer cell lines, including A431 epithelial carcinoma, SK-MEL-5 and SK-MEL-28 melanoma cells, and HCT116 colon cancer cells (Cho et al. 2009). The mechanism of inhibition was through the direct binding to RSK2, which is a member of the p^{90}RSK (RSK) family of proteins. RSK2 is a widely expressed serine/threonine kinase that is activated by ERKs and phosphoinositide-dependent kinase 1 (PDK1) in response to growth factors, and its activation enhances cell survival. RSK2 is a key regulator for tumor promoter–induced cell transformation, and its high expression increases proliferation as well as anchorage-independent transformation of JB6 Cl41 skin cells and foci formation in NIH3T3 cells (Cho et al. 2007). The RSK2 protein level is markedly higher in cancer cell lines as well as cancer tissues compared with nonmalignant cell lines or normal tissues. We have solved and reported the crystal structure for the NH_2-terminal kinase domain (NTD) (Malakhova et al. 2009) and the COOH-terminal kinase domain (CTD) (Malakhova et al. 2008). We provided evidence showing that the NTD activation of RSK2 is required for the activation of the ERK-mediated CTD. Computational modeling predicted that kaempferol binds with the NTD but not the CTD (Cho et al. 2009). We conducted mutagenesis experiments and clearly showed that Val82 and Lys100 are critical amino acids for kaempferol binding and RSK2 activity (Cho et al. 2009). We recently found that kaempferol suppressed UVB-induced COX2 protein expression in mouse skin epidermal JB6 P+ cells and attenuated the UVB-induced transcriptional activities of COX2 and AP-1 (Lee et al. 2010b). In addition, kaempferol reduced UVB-induced phosphorylation of ERKs, p38, and JNKs and also inhibited the upstream Src kinase activity. Pull-down assays and computer docking data indicated that kaempferol competes with ATP for direct binding with Src in the RSK2 ATP-binding site (Lee et al. 2010b). We further found that an analog of kaempferol, 5-deoxykaempferol (Table 5.1), also suppressed UVB-induced COX2 expression along with vascular endothelial growth factor (VEGF) expression (Lee et al. 2010a). This compound had effects on multiple proteins but directly bound to Src, PI3-K, and RSK2 competitively with ATP to exert those effects. The next result was an inhibition of UVB-induced mouse skin carcinogenesis (Lee et al. 2010a).

5.5.2 ERIODICTYOL

Eriodictyol (Table 5.1) is a flavanone found in various fruits, and we discovered that it also binds to the NTD of RSK2 to inhibit RSK2 N-terminal kinase activity (Liu et al. 2011). In this same study, we found that ATF1 is a novel substrate of RSK2 and that RSK2-ATF1 signaling plays an important role in EGF-induced neoplastic cell transformation. RSK2 phosphorylated ATF1 at Ser63 and enhanced ATF1 transcriptional activity and tumor promoter–induced JB6 cell transormation. The phosphorylation of ATF1 by RSK2 and its subsequent cellular effects were abolished by eriodictyol treatment (Liu et al. 2011).

5.5.3 Quercetin and Quercetin Methyl Ether

Quercetin (Table 5.1) is another flavanoid compound found at high levels in various foods, including red wine. It has been reported to inhibit the proliferation of cancer cells but with no effect on normal cells, and it also suppressed TPA-promoted mouse skin cancer (Soleas et al. 2002). We reported that red wine extract (RWE) or quercetin reduced TPA-induced neoplastic JB6 cell transformation, which was associated with decreased AP-1 and NF-κB activation (Lee et al. 2008a). Pull-down assay results indicated that RWE or quercetin directly bound with either MKK1 or Raf1, and docking data indicated that quercetin hydrogen-bonded with the backbone amide group of Ser212 on MKK1, which is a key interaction for stabilizing the inactive conformation of the activation loop of MKK1 (Lee et al. 2008a). RWE and quercetin also were found to decrease the tumor necrosis factor (TNF)-α–induced upregulation of matrix metallopeptidase 9 (MMP-9) and cell migration that was mediated by suppression of Akt phosphorylation and AP-1 or NF-κB transactivation (Hwang et al. 2009). In this case, quercetin and RWE were discovered to interact with and inhibit PI3-K activity (Hwang et al. 2009). Overall, the computational and experimental evidence suggests that quercetin targets Raf1, MKK1, and PI3-K to exert its anticancer activities. Raf and/or Ras are constitutively activated in several tumor cell lines, and MKK generally plays a critical role in transmitting signals initiated by various tumor promoters, such as TPA or EGF. Constitutive activation of MKK1 causes cell transformation, and inhibiting MKK activity can suppress transformation and tumor growth *in vivo* (Cowley et al. 1994; Sebolt-Leopold et al. 1999).

Quercetin-3-methyl ether, a naturally occurring compound present in various plants including the edible prickly pear cactus, reportedly has potent anticancer activity. We found that quercetin-3-methyl ether could control the growth of breast cancer cells that were sensitive or resistant to the RTK inhibitor, lapatinib (Li et al. 2011). Quercetin-3-methyl ether appeared to act mainly by inducing cell cycle arrest and apoptosis in either cell type (Li et al. 2011). We also found that quercetin-3-methyl ether inhibited proliferation of mouse skin epidermal JB6 P+ cells in a dose- and time-dependent manner by inducing cell cycle interphase/mitosis (G2/M) phase accumulation and decreasing AP-1 activation and ERKs phosphorylation. The net result was suppression of TPA-induced JB6 neoplastic cell transformation. Pull-down assays revealed that quercetin-3-methyl ether directly binds with ERKs to exert its potent chemopreventive activity (Li et al. 2012b).

5.5.4 Myricetin

Myricetin (3,3′,4′,5,5′,7-hexahydroxyflavone) (Table 5.1) is a major flavonol found in numerous foods, including onions, berries, and grapes as well as red wine (German and Walzem 2000; Hakkinen et al. 1999). Its anticancer activities include inhibition of two-stage skin tumorigenesis (Mukhtar et al. 1988), reduction of A549 lung cancer cell growth (Lu et al. 2006), and attenuation of invasion associated with decreased MMP-2 protein expression and enzyme activity in colorectal carcinoma cells (Ko et al. 2005). Thus, myricetin appears to be an effective chemopreventive agent against carcinogenesis, but its specific protein targets have not been identified until recently. Others and we have found that myricetin binds with various protein kinases both competitively and noncompetitively with ATP to exert its anticancer activities.

We first demonstrated that myricetin suppressed TPA- or EGF-induced transformation of JB6 P+ cells coinciding with a decreased activation of c-Fos or AP-1 (Lee et al. 2007). Myricetin directly bound to and inhibited MKK1 kinase activity noncompetitively with ATP, resulting in decreased phosphorylation of MKK downstream targets, ERKs, or RSK. Notably, myricetin inhibited H-Ras–induced cell transformation more effectively than the well-known MKK inhibitor, PD098059 (Lee et al. 2007). We also found that myricetin bound to and inhibited UVB-induced Raf kinase activity, also in an ATP-noncompetitive manner (Jung et al. 2010). In this case, the inhibition resulted in decreased UVB-induced wrinkle formation and epidermal thickening mediated through MMP-9 (Jung et al. 2010). Additional work showed that myricetin inhibited TNF-α–induced VEGF expression by binding directly to MAPK kinase 4 (MKK4) in an ATP-competitive manner to suppress its kinase activity, resulting in decreased JNKs and ERKs phosphorylation (Kim et al. 2009). Similarly, myricetin was shown to directly bind with Fyn and suppress Fyn kinase activity, also in an ATP-competitive manner (Jung et al. 2008). Docking data revealed that myricetin docked to the ATP binding site of Fyn, located between the N- and C-lobes of the kinase domain. The binding of myricetin with Fyn corresponded with reduction of UVB-induced COX2 expression and decreased activation of AP-1 and NF-κB in JB6 P+ cells (Jung et al. 2008). Myricetin effectively suppressed Fyn kinase activity directly to reduce UVB-induced COX2 expression and UVB-induced skin tumor incidence in a dose-dependent manner (Jung et al. 2008).

Finally, Akt, a serine/threonine kinase, is a critical regulator in many cellular processes including cell growth, proliferation, and apoptosis, and myricetin was reported to bind to it and inhibit its phosphorylation and activity in an ATP-competitive manner (Kumamoto et al. 2009a). We also reported that topical treatment with myricetin reduced UVB-induced neovascularization in SKH-1 (mouse strain designation) hairless mouse skin and suppressed UVB-induced VEGF, MMP-9, and MMP-13 expression and PI3-K activity (Jung et al. 2009). Myricetin directly bound to PI3-K, resulting in the subsequent attenuation of the UVB-induced phosphorylation of Akt/p70S6 kinase in mouse skin (Jung et al. 2009). Finally, the Janus kinase (JAK1)/STAT3 pathway has been suggested to play a role in cell transformation and carcinogenesis, and myricetin was reported to directly bind to JAK1 and STAT3 to inhibit EGF-induced transformation of JB6 P+ cells (Kumamoto et al. 2009b). Data revealed that myricetin inhibited DNA-binding and transcriptional activity of STAT3 and suppressed phosphorylation of JAK1 and STAT3 at Tyr705 and Ser727 (Kumamoto et al. 2009b).

5.5.5 SOY COMPOUNDS—TRIHYDROXYISOFLAVONES AND EQUOL

A subfamily of flavonoid compounds are the isoflavones, which act as weak estrogen-active compounds and thus are referred to as phytoestrogens (Harris et al. 2005; Kuiper et al. 1998). The isoflavones are believed to be the soy ingredients responsible for observed biological effects (Craig 1997; Messina 1999). Daidzein (4',7-dihydroxyisoflavone), genistein (4',5,7-trihydroxyisoflavone), and glycitein (4',7-dihydroxy-6-methoxyisoflavone) are the major isoflavone phytoestrogens found in soybean products, which are commonly consumed in vegetarian and Asian diets. Enzymes of the colonic microbiotics convert soy isoflavones to numerous metabolites such as equol (4',7-isoflavandiol) formed from daidzein (Joannou et al. 1995; Kelly et al. 1993) and to various other compounds including 6,7,4'-trihydroxyisoflavone (6,7,4'THIF) (Kulling et al. 2001) and 7,3',4'-trihydroxyisoflavone (7,3'4'-THIF) (Kulling et al. 2000, 2001; Table 5.1). Various epidemiological and animal studies suggest that soy foods and isoflavones may have beneficial effects on preventing cancers; however, tumor-promoting effects were observed in some human and animal studies as well. Thus, elucidating the underlying molecular targets and mechanisms of the chemopreventive activities of daidzein and its metabolites, equol, 6,7,4'-THIF, and 7,3',4'-THIF, is highly significant and critical in understanding the apparent contradictory effects of soy consumption.

Equol was shown to protect against UV-induced skin cancer in the hairless mouse model (Widyarini et al. 2005). We compared the effects of equol and daidzein on TPA-induced AP-1 activity and cell transformation in JB6 P+ cells, and results indicated that equol, but not daidzein, was a potent inhibitor of MKK activity and subsequently inhibited c-Fos activation and AP-1 transactivation and cell transformation (Kang et al. 2007). Equol inhibited MKK1, but not Raf1, kinase activity. Importantly, equol specifically bound to MKK noncompetitively with ATP to inhibit MKK activity (Kang et al. 2007).

We also found that 7,3',4'-THIF effectively inhibits UVB-induced COX2 expression through the inhibition of NF-κB transcription activity in mouse skin epidermal JB6 P+ cells (Lee et al. 2010). In contrast, daidzein had no effect on COX2 expression levels. 7,3',4'-THIF directly bound to and inhibited Cot (MKKK8) and MKK4 activity, thereby suppressing UVB-induced phosphorylation of MAPKs. Topical application of 7,3′,4′-THIF clearly suppressed the incidence and multiplicity of UVB-induced tumors in hairless mouse skin by directly inhibiting Cot or MKK4 kinase activity. A docking study revealed that 7,3′,4′-THIF, but not daidzein, easily docked to the ATP binding site of Cot and MKK4, which is located between the N- and C-lobes of the kinase domain (Lee et al. 2010). Further studies indicated that 7,3′,4′-THIF prevented EGF-induced neoplastic transformation and proliferation of JB6 P+ mouse epidermal cells. It significantly blocked cell cycle progression of EGF-stimulated cells at the G1 phase and suppressed the phosphorylation of retinoblastoma protein at Ser795 and Ser807/Ser811, which are the specific sites of phosphorylation by cyclin-dependent kinase 4 (Cdk4). Furthermore, it also inhibited the expression of G1 phase-regulatory proteins, including cyclin D1, Cdk4, cyclin E, and Cdk2. In addition to regulating the expression of cell cycle–regulatory proteins, 7,3′,4′-THIF bound to Cdk4 and Cdk2 and strongly inhibited their kinase activities. It also bound to PI3-K, markedly inhibiting its kinase activity and thereby suppressing the Akt/glycogen synthase kinase-3 beta (GSK-3β)/AP-1 pathway and subsequently attenuating the expression of cyclin D1 (Lee et al. 2011a). We investigated the biological activity of 6,7,4′-THIF in *in vitro* and *in vivo* models of human colon cancer. 6,7,4′-THIF suppressed anchorage-dependent and -independent growth of HCT116 and DLD1 human colon cancer cells more effectively than daidzein. In addition, 6,7,4′-THIF induced cell cycle arrest at the S (synthesis) and G2/M phases in HCT116 human colon cancer cells and effectively suppressed the expression of Cdk2, but it had no effect on other S- or G2/M-phase regulatory proteins such as cyclin A, cyclin B1, or Cdk1. Daidzein did not affect the expression of any of these proteins. 6,7,4′-THIF, but not daidzein, inhibited Cdk1 and Cdk2 activities in HCT116 cells by directly interacting with Cdk1 and Cdk2. 6,7,4′-THIF significantly decreased tumor growth, volume, and weight of HCT116 xenograft tumors and bound directly to Cdk1 and Cdk2 *in vivo*, resulting in the suppression of Cdk1 and Cdk2 activity in tumors, corresponding with our *in vitro* results (Lee et al. 2011b).

5.5.6 LUTEOLIN

Luteolin (Table 5.1) is another flavonoid present in various vegetables including onion and broccoli, and it also has been reported to possess anticancer activities. We found that luteolin suppressed UVB-induced COX2 expression and AP-1 and NF-κB activity in JB6 P+ cells. This was likely related to the direct binding of luteolin to protein kinase Cε (PKCε) and Src in an ATP-competitive manner (Byun et al. 2010). Other effects included an inhibition of UVB-induced Akt phosphorylation, TNF-α, and proliferating cell nuclear antigen (PCNA). Notably, luteolin reduced tumor incidence, multiplicity, and overall tumor size in SKH-1 hairless mice exposed to chronic UVB (Byun et al. 2010). Further analysis using skin lysates confirmed that luteolin inhibited PKCε and Src kinase activities *in vivo* (Byun et al. 2010).

5.5.7 ISORHAMNETIN

Isorhamnetin (3′-methoxy-3,4′,5,7-tetrahydroxyflavone) (Table 5.1) is a plant flavonoid that is found in various fruits and medicinal herbs. We found that isorhamnetin inhibited EGF-induced neoplastic cell transformation of JB6 cells and suppressed anchorage-dependent and -independent growth of A431 human epithelial carcinoma cells (Kim et al. 2011). Isorhamnetin attenuated EGF-induced COX2 expression in JB6 and A431 cells and reduced A431 tumor growth and COX2 expression in a xenograft mouse model. EGF induced phosphoryaltion of ERKs, RSK, p70S6 kinase, and Akt, and isorhamnetin effectively suppressed that phosphorylation. Binding assay results indicated that isorhamnetin directly binds to MKK1 in an ATP-noncompetitive manner and to PI3-K in an ATP-competitive manner to suppress their respective activities (Kim et al. 2011).

5.5.8 DELPHINIDIN

Anthocyanidins are reported to display anticancer activities, and delphinidin (Table 5.1) is an antho-cyanidin found in many fruits and vegetables. We determined that it inhibits EGF-induced or H-Ras–induced transformation and COX2 expression in JB6 P+ cells by directly binding to Raf and MKK and suppressing their kinase activity (Kang et al. 2008a). The activation of AP-1 and NF-κB induced by TPA was dose dependently inhibited by delphinidin treatment. The inhibition of Raf and MKK by delphinidin resulted in the subsequent attenuation of TPA-induced phosphorylation of MKK, ERKs, and RSK (Kang et al. 2008a). We also found that delphinidin suppressed UVB-induced COX2 expression in JB6 P+ mouse epidermal cells. COX2 promoter activity and PGE_2 production were also inhibited by delphinidin treatment (Kwon et al. 2009). Delphinidin attenuated the activation of AP-1 and NF-κB, which are critical transcription factors involved in COX2 expression. In addition, UVB-induced phosphorylation of JNKs, p38, and Akt and kinase activities of MKK4 and PI3-K were decreased by delphinidin treatment. MKK4 and PI3-K were identified as direct binding targets of delphinidin *in vitro,* in cells, and *in vivo* (Kwon et al. 2009).

5.5.9 (3-CHLOROACETYL)-INDOLE

Indole-3-carbinol (I3C) is produced in Brassica vegetables such as broccoli and cabbage, has been shown to inhibit proliferation, and at high doses, can induce apoptosis in various cancer cell lines. Our goal was to develop a more potent antitumor agent by modifying the structure of I3C, and therefore, we created I3C derivatives and found that (3-chloroacetyl)-indole (3CAI) (Table 5.1) more strongly inhibited colon cancer cell growth than the parent I3C (D.J. Kim et al. 2011). Additional screening of kinases in a competitive kinase assay identified 3CAI as a specific Akt inhibitor. Akt is a serine/threonine kinase that can promote transformation and chemoresistance by inducing pro-liferation and inhibiting apoptosis. 3CAI directly binds to Akt1 or Akt2 in an ATP-noncompetitive manner, resulting in a substantial inhibition of Akt and its direct downstream targets such as mTOR and GSK3β. The effects included growth inhibition and apoptosis of colon cancer cells and suppres-sion of colon cancer cell growth in an *in vivo* xenograft mouse model (D.J. Kim et al. 2011).

5.5.10 NORATHYRIOL

UV irradiation is the leading factor in the development of skin cancer, prompting great interest in chemopreventive agents to prevent this disease. Norathyriol (Table 5.1) is a metabolite of mangiferin found in mango and reportedly possesses anticancer activity. We found that norathyriol inhibits ERK activity and confirmed the direct and specific binding of norathyriol with the ATP pocket of ERK2 through a co-crystal structural analysis (Li et al. 2012a). The inhibition of ERK2 by norathyriol caused decreased ERK-dependent activity of transcriptional factors AP-1 and NF-κB, which resulted in a significant attenuation of solar UV-induced skin carcinogenesis *in vivo* (Li et al. 2012a).

5.6 SUMMARY AND CONCLUSIONS

The influence of diet on health is indisputable. This statement is based on accumulating epidemio-logical and experimental data indicating that diet has a dramatic effect on the risk for developing certain diseases, especially cancer and heart disease. However, one of our greatest challenges is to reduce the overabundance of myth and misinformation reported in the popular media regarding the health benefits of certain foods or food supplements. The use of food or food supplements is not new, but interest in their use has increased dramatically because of perceived health benefits, presumably without unwanted or unpleasant side effects (Hardy et al. 2002). This is especially true in cancer prevention and treatment. A critical need exists (1) to identify food components that can act as cancer-preventive agents and effectively inhibit cancer development, and importantly, (2) to determine the molecular targets within cancer cells that are modulated by specific food factors.

One could suggest that food or other natural compounds with multiple molecular targets might be the most effective chemopreventive agents because they can be combined with traditional chemotherapeutic agents to overcome drug resistance by targeting multiple upstream or downstream molecules. They might also be used at lower concentrations in combination with each other or other anticancer agents. The apparent promiscuity of compounds such as EGCG, resveratrol, and the flavonoids actually might provide at least a partial explanation in support of the epidemiological evidence suggesting that consumption of green tea or fruits and vegetables reduces cancer risk. Many food components, like resveratrol, EGCG, genistein, and most of the flavonoid compounds are sold as supplements. However, the beneficial effects of supplements have not been supported in controlled human studies. In spite of the interest in food-derived compounds as supplements, research on most of them is still in its infancy, and the effects of long-term supplementation in humans are not known.

ACKNOWLEDGMENTS

This work is supported by The Hormel Foundation; Pediatric Pharmaceuticals and grants from the American Institute for Cancer Research; and National Institutes of Health grants CA077646, CA027502, CA120388, R37 CA081064, and ES016548.

REFERENCES

Afzal, M., D. Al-Hadidi, M. Menon, J. Pesek, and M. S. Dhami. 2001. Ginger: an ethnomedical, chemical and pharmacological review. *Drug Metabol Drug Interact* 18 (3–4):159–90.

Alessi, D. R., A. Cuenda, P. Cohen, D. T. Dudley, and A. R. Saltiel. 1995. PD 098059 is a specific inhibitor of the activation of mitogen-activated protein kinase kinase in vitro and in vivo. *J Biol Chem* 270 (46):27489–94.

An, K. P., M. Athar, X. Tang et al. 2002. Cyclooxygenase-2 expression in murine and human nonmelanoma skin cancers: implications for therapeutic approaches. *Photochem Photobiol* 76 (1):73–80.

Angel, P., K. Hattori, T. Smeal, and M. Karin. 1988. The jun proto-oncogene is positively autoregulated by its product, Jun/AP-1. *Cell* 55 (5):875–85.

Angel, P., and M. Karin. 1991. The role of Jun, Fos and the AP-1 complex in cell-proliferation and transformation. *Biochim Biophys Acta* 1072 (2–3):129–57.

Athar, M., K. P. An, K. D. Morel et al. 2001. Ultraviolet B(UVB)-induced cox-2 expression in murine skin: an immunohistochemical study. *Biochem Biophys Res Commun* 280 (4):1042–7.

Athar, M., J. H. Back, L. Kopelovich, D. R. Bickers, and A. L. Kim. 2009. Multiple molecular targets of resveratrol: anti-carcinogenic mechanisms. *Arch Biochem Biophys* 486 (2):95–102.

Baldwin, A. S., Jr. 1996. The NF-kappa B and I kappa B proteins: new discoveries and insights. *Annu Rev Immunol* 14:649–83.

Baselga, J. 2001. The EGFR as a target for anticancer therapy—focus on cetuximab. *Eur J Cancer* 37 Suppl 4:S16–22.

Baxter, R. A. 2008. Anti-aging properties of resveratrol: review and report of a potent new antioxidant skin care formulation. *J Cosmet Dermatol* 7 (1):2–7.

Bernstein, F. C., T. F. Koetzle, G. J. Williams et al. 1977. The Protein Data Bank: a computer-based archival file for macromolecular structures. *J Molec Biol* 112 (3):535–42.

Bishayee, A. 2009. Cancer prevention and treatment with resveratrol: from rodent studies to clinical trials. *Cancer Prev Res (Phila Pa)* 2 (5):409–18.

Bishayee, A., and N. Dhir. 2009. Resveratrol-mediated chemoprevention of diethylnitrosamine-initiated hepatocarcinogenesis: inhibition of cell proliferation and induction of apoptosis. *Chem Biol Interact* 179 (2–3):131–44.

Bode, A. M., Y. Cao, and Z. Dong. 2010. Update on cancer prevention research in the United States and China: the 2009 China—U.S. forum on frontiers of cancer research. *Cancer Prev Res (Phila)* 3 (12):1630–7.

Bode, A. M., and Z. Dong. 2000. Signal transduction pathways: targets for chemoprevention of skin cancer. *Lancet Oncol* 1:181–8.

Bode, A. M., and Z. Dong. 2002. Signal transduction pathways: Targets for green and black tea polyphenols. In *Recent Research Developments in Cancer*, edited by S. G. Pandalai. Fort P.O., Trivandrum-696 023, India: Transworld Research Network.

Bode, A. M., and Z. Dong. 2003a. Mitogen-activated protein kinase activation in UV-induced signal transduction. *Sci STKE* 2003 (167):RE2.

Bode, A. M., and Z. Dong. 2003b. Signal transduction pathways: targets for green and black tea polyphenols. *J Biochem Mol Biol* 36 (1):66–77.

Bode, A. M., and Z. Dong. 2004a. Cancer prevention by food factors through targeting signal transduction pathways. *Nutrition* 20 (1):89–94.

Bode, A. M., and Z. Dong. 2004b. Targeting signal transduction pathways by chemopreventive agents. *Mutat Res* 555 (1–2):33–51.

Bode, A. M., and Z. Dong. 2004c. Beneficial effects of resveratrol. *Phytochem Health Dis* 12:257–84.

Bode, A. M., and Z. Dong. 2004d. Ginger. *Herbal Trad Med Molec Aspects Health*:165–77.

Bode, A. M., and Z. Dong. 2005. Signal transduction pathways in cancer development and as targets for cancer prevention. *Prog Nucleic Acid Res Mol Biol* 79:237–97.

Bode, A. M., and Z. Dong. 2006. Molecular and cellular targets. *Mol Carcinog* 45 (6):422–30.

Bode, A. M., and Z. Dong. 2007a. The enigmatic effects of caffeine in cell cycle and cancer. *Cancer Lett* 247 (1):26–39.

Bode, A. M., and Z. Dong. 2007b. The functional contrariety of JNK. *Mol Carcinog* 46 (8):591–8.

Bode, A. M., and Z. Dong. 2009a. Cancer prevention research—then and now. *Nat Rev Cancer* 9 (7):508–16.

Bode, A. M., and Z. Dong. 2009b. Epigallocatechin 3-gallate and green tea catechins: United they work, divided they fail. *Cancer Prev Res (Phila Pa)* 2 (6):514–7.

Bode, A. M., and Z. Dong. 2009c. Signal transduction molecules as targets for cancer prevention. *Sci Signal* 2 (59):mr2.

Bode, A. M., and Z. Dong. 2009d. Modulation of cell signal transduction by tea and ginger. In *Dietary Modulation of Cell Signaling Pathways*, edited by Y.-J. Surh, E. Cadenas, Z. Dong and L. Packer. New York: CRC Press—Taylor & Francis Group.

Bode, A. M., and Z. Dong. 2011a. The two faces of capsaicin. *Cancer Res* 71 (8):2809–14.

Bode, A. M., and Z. Dong. 2011b. The amazing and mighty ginger. In *Herbal Medicine—Biomolecular and Clinical Aspects*, edited by I. F. F. Benzie and S. Wachtel-Galor. New York: CRC Press—Taylor and Francis Group.

Bode, A. M., and Z. Dong. 2012. Effects of dietary effectors on signal transduction pathways related to cancer prevention. In *Nutritional Genomics—The Impact of Dietary Regulation of Gene Function on Human Disease*, edited by W. R. Bidlack and R. L. Rodriguez. New York: CRC Press.

Bode, A. M., W. Y. Ma, Y. J. Surh, and Z. Dong. 2001. Inhibition of epidermal growth factor-induced cell transformation and activator protein 1 activation by [6]-gingerol. *Cancer Res* 61 (3):850–3.

Bol, D. K., R. B. Rowley, C. P. Ho et al. 2002. Cyclooxygenase-2 overexpression in the skin of transgenic mice results in suppression of tumor development. *Cancer Res* 62 (9):2516–21.

Brisdelli, F., G. D'Andrea, and A. Bozzi. 2009. Resveratrol: a natural polyphenol with multiple chemopreventive properties. *Curr Drug Metab* 10 (6):530–46.

Buckman, S. Y., A. Gresham, P. Hale et al. 1998. COX-2 expression is induced by UVB exposure in human skin: implications for the development of skin cancer. *Carcinogenesis* 19 (5):723–9.

Byun, S., K. W. Lee, S. K. Jung et al. 2010. Luteolin inhibits protein kinase C(epsilon) and c-Src activities and UVB-induced skin cancer. *Cancer Res* 70 (6):2415–23.

Chan, G., J. O. Boyle, E. K. Yang et al. 1999. Cyclooxygenase-2 expression is up-regulated in squamous cell carcinoma of the head and neck. *Cancer Res* 59 (5):991–4.

Cho, Y. Y., K. Yao, H. G. Kim et al. 2007. Ribosomal S6 kinase 2 is a key regulator in tumor promoter induced cell transformation. *Cancer Res* 67 (17):8104–12.

Cho, Y. Y., K. Yao, A. Pugliese et al. 2009. A regulatory mechanism for RSK2 NH(2)-terminal kinase activity. *Cancer Res* 69 (10):4398–406.

Chung, W. Y., Y. J. Jung, Y. J. Surh, S. S. Lee, and K. K. Park. 2001. Antioxidative and antitumor promoting effects of [6]-paradol and its homologs. *Mutat Res* 496 (1–2):199–206.

Ciardiello, F., and G. Tortora. 2008. EGFR antagonists in cancer treatment. *N Engl J Med* 358 (11):1160–74.

Cowley, S., H. Paterson, P. Kemp, and C. J. Marshall. 1994. Activation of MAP kinase kinase is necessary and sufficient for PC12 differentiation and for transformation of NIH 3T3 cells. *Cell* 77 (6):841–52.

Craig, W. J. 1997. Phytochemicals: guardians of our health. *J Am Dietetic Assoc* 97 (10 Suppl 2):S199–S204.

Davis, R. J. 1994. MAPKs: new JNK expands the group. *Trends Biochem Sci* 19 (11):470–3.

De Luca, A., A. Carotenuto, A. Rachiglio et al. 2008. The role of the EGFR signaling in tumor microenvironment. *J Cellular Physiol* 214 (3):559–67.

Denkert, C., M. Kobel, S. Berger et al. 2001. Expression of cyclooxygenase 2 in human malignant melanoma. *Cancer Res* 61 (1):303–8.

Di Nicolantonio, F., M. Martini, F. Molinari et al. 2008. Wild-type BRAF is required for response to panitumumab or cetuximab in metastatic colorectal cancer. *J Clin Oncol* 26 (35):5705–12.

Dominguez-Sola, D., and R. Dalla-Favera. 2004. PINning down the c-Myc oncoprotein. *Nature Cell Biol* 6 (4):288–9.

Dong, Z., M. J. Birrer, R. G. Watts, L. M. Matrisian, and N. H. Colburn. 1994. Blocking of tumor promoter-induced AP-1 activity inhibits induced transformation in JB6 mouse epidermal cells. *Proc Natl Acad Sci U S A* 91 (2):609–13.

Dong, Z., R. Watts, Y. Sun, S. Zhan, and N. Colburn. 1995. Progressive elevation of ap-1 activity during pre-neoplastic-to-neoplastic progression as modeled in mouse jb6 cell variants. *Intl J Oncol* 7 (2):359–64.

Duncia, J. V., J. B. Santella, 3rd, C. A. Higley et al. 1998. MEK inhibitors: the chemistry and biological activity of U0126, its analogs, and cyclization products. *Bioorg Med Chem Lett* 8 (20):2839–44.

Eberhart, C. E., R. J. Coffey, A. Radhika et al. 1994. Up-regulation of cyclooxygenase 2 gene expression in human colorectal adenomas and adenocarcinomas. *Gastroenterology* 107 (4):1183–8.

Ermakova, S., B. Y. Choi, H. S. Choi et al. 2005. The intermediate filament protein vimentin is a new target for epigallocatechin gallate. *J Biol Chem* 280 (17):16882–90.

Ermakova, S. P., B. S. Kang, B. Y. Choi et al. 2006. (-)-Epigallocatechin gallate overcomes resistance to etoposide-induced cell death by targeting the molecular chaperone glucose-regulated protein 78. *Cancer Res* 66 (18):9260–9.

Favata, M. F., K. Y. Horiuchi, E. J. Manos et al. 1998. Identification of a novel inhibitor of mitogen-activated protein kinase kinase. *J Biol Chem* 273 (29):18623–32.

Friesner, R. A., J. L. Banks, R. B. Murphy et al. 2004. Glide: a new approach for rapid, accurate docking and scoring. 1. Method and assessment of docking accuracy. *J Med Chem* 47 (7):1739–49.

Gaffney, D. K., J. Holden, M. Davis et al. 2001. Elevated cyclooxygenase-2 expression correlates with diminished survival in carcinoma of the cervix treated with radiotherapy. *Intl J Radiat Oncol Biol Phys* 49 (5):1213–7.

Gallo, O., A. Franchi, L. Magnelli et al. 2001. Cyclooxygenase-2 pathway correlates with VEGF expression in head and neck cancer. Implications for tumor angiogenesis and metastasis. *Neoplasia* 3 (1):53–61.

Gatz, S. A., M. Keimling, C. Baumann et al. 2008. Resveratrol modulates DNA double-strand break repair pathways in an ATM/ATR-p53- and -Nbs1-dependent manner. *Carcinogenesis* 29 (3):519–27.

German, J. B., and R. L. Walzem. 2000. The health benefits of wine. *Annu Rev Nutr* 20:561–93.

Gilmore, T. D. 1997. Clinically relevant findings. *J Clin Invest* 100 (12):2935–6.

Goswami, S. K., and D. K. Das. 2009. Resveratrol and chemoprevention. *Cancer Lett* 284 (1):1–6.

Grant, K. L., and R. B. Lutz. 2000. Ginger. *Am J Health Syst Pharm* 57 (10):945–7.

Grossman, E. M., W. E. Longo, N. Panesar, J. E. Mazuski, and D. L. Kaminski. 2000. The role of cyclooxygenase enzymes in the growth of human gall bladder cancer cells. *Carcinogenesis* 21 (7):1403–9.

Grubbs, C. J., R. A. Lubet, A. T. Koki et al. 2000. Celecoxib inhibits N-butyl-N-(4-hydroxybutyl)-nitrosamine-induced urinary bladder cancers in male B6D2F1 mice and female Fischer-344 rats. *Cancer Res* 60 (20):5599–602.

Guerrero, R. F., M. C. Garcia-Parrilla, B. Puertas, and E. Cantos-Villar. 2009. Wine, resveratrol and health: a review. *Nat Prod Commun* 4 (5):635–58.

Hakkinen, S. H., S. O. Karenlampi, I. M. Heinonen, H. M. Mykkanen, and A. R. Torronen. 1999. Content of the flavonols quercetin, myricetin, and kaempferol in 25 edible berries. *J Agric Food Chem* 47 (6):2274–9.

Hardy, G., I. Hardy, and B. McElroy. 2002. Nutraceuticals: a pharmaceutical viewpoint: I. *Curr Opin Clin Nutr Metab Care* 5 (6):671–7.

Harikumar, K. B., and B. B. Aggarwal. 2008. Resveratrol: a multitargeted agent for age-associated chronic diseases. *Cell Cycle* 7 (8).

Harris, D. M., E. Besselink, S. M. Henning, V. L. Go, and D. Heber. 2005. Phytoestrogens induce differential estrogen receptor alpha- or beta-mediated responses in transfected breast cancer cells. *Exp Biol Med* 230 (8):558–68.

Hayakawa, S., K. Saeki, M. Sazuka et al. 2001. Apoptosis induction by epigallocatechin gallate involves its binding to Fas. *Biochem Biophys Res Commun* 285 (5):1102–6.

He, Z., F. Tang, S. Ermakova et al. 2008. Fyn is a novel target of (-)-epigallocatechin gallate in the inhibition of JB6 Cl41 cell transformation. *Mol Carcinog* 47 (3):172–83.

Hida, T., Y. Yatabe, H. Achiwa et al. 1998. Increased expression of cyclooxygenase 2 occurs frequently in human lung cancers, specifically in adenocarcinomas. *Cancer Res* 58 (17):3761–4.

Huang, C., W. Y. Ma, A. Goranson, and Z. Dong. 1999. Resveratrol suppresses cell transformation and induces apoptosis through a p53-dependent pathway. *Carcinogenesis* 20 (2):237–42.

Hwang, D., D. Scollard, J. Byrne, and E. Levine. 1998. Expression of cyclooxygenase-1 and cyclooxygenase-2 in human breast cancer. *J Natl Cancer Inst* 90 (6):455–60.

Hwang, M. K., N. R. Song, N. J. Kang, K. W. Lee, and H. J. Lee. 2009. Activation of phosphatidylinositol 3-kinase is required for tumor necrosis factor-alpha-induced upregulation of matrix metalloproteinase-9: its direct inhibition by quercetin. *Int J Biochem Cell Biol* 41 (7):1592–600.

Hynes, N. E., and H. A. Lane. 2005. ERBB receptors and cancer: the complexity of targeted inhibitors. *Nat Rev. Cancer* 5 (5):341–54.

Irwin, J. J., and B. K. Shoichet. 2005. ZINC—a free database of commercially available compounds for virtual screening. *J Chem Inform Model* 45 (1):177–82.

Jang, M., L. Cai, G. O. Udeani et al. 1997. Cancer chemopreventive activity of resveratrol, a natural product derived from grapes. *Science* 275 (5297):218–20.

Jeong, C. H., A. M. Bode, A. Pugliese et al. 2009. [6]-Gingerol suppresses colon cancer growth by targeting leukotriene A4 hydrolase. *Cancer Res* 69 (13):5584–91.

Jimeno, A., and M. Hidalgo. 2006. Pharmacogenomics of epidermal growth factor receptor (EGFR) tyrosine kinase inhibitors. *Biochim Biophys Acta* 1766 (2):217–29.

Joannou, G. E., G. E. Kelly, A. Y. Reeder, M. Waring, and C. Nelson. 1995. A urinary profile study of dietary phytoestrogens. The identification and mode of metabolism of new isoflavonoids. *J Steroid Biochemi Molec Biol* 54 (3–4):167–84.

Jung, S. K., K. W. Lee, S. Byun et al. 2008. Myricetin suppresses UVB-induced skin cancer by targeting Fyn. *Cancer Res* 68 (14):6021–9.

Jung, S. K., K. W. Lee, S. Byun et al. 2010. Myricetin inhibits UVB-induced angiogenesis by regulating PI-3 kinase in vivo. *Carcinogenesis* 31 (5):911–7.

Jung, S. K., K. W. Lee, H. Y. Kim et al. 2010. Myricetin suppresses UVB-induced wrinkle formation and MMP-9 expression by inhibiting Raf. *Biochem Pharmacol* 79 (10):1455–61.

Kallunki, T., B. Su, I. Tsigelny et al. 1994. JNK2 contains a specificity-determining region responsible for efficient c-Jun binding and phosphorylation. *Genes Dev* 8 (24):2996–3007.

Kang, N. J., K. W. Lee, E. A. Rogozin et al. 2007. Equol, a metabolite of the soybean isoflavone daidzein, inhibits neoplastic cell transformation by targeting the MEK/ERK/p90RSK/activator protein-1 pathway. *J Biol Chem* 282 (45):32856–66.

Kang, N. J., K. W. Lee, J. Y. Kwon et al. 2008a. Delphinidin attenuates neoplastic transformation in JB6 Cl41 mouse epidermal cells by blocking Raf/mitogen-activated protein kinase kinase/extracellular signal-regulated kinase signaling. *Cancer Prev Res (Phila Pa)* 1 (7):522–31.

Kang, N. J., K. W. Lee, D. E. Lee et al. 2008b. Cocoa procyanidins suppress transformation by inhibiting mitogen-activated protein kinase kinase. *J Biol Chem* 283 (30):20664–73.

Kang, N. J., K. W. Lee, B. J. Shin et al. 2009. Caffeic acid, a phenolic phytochemical in coffee, directly inhibits Fyn kinase activity and UVB-induced COX-2 expression. *Carcinogenesis* 30 (2):321–30.

Kang, N. J., K. W. Lee, B. H. Kim et al. 2011. Coffee phenolic phytochemicals suppress colon cancer metastasis by targeting MEK and TOPK. *Carcinogenesis* 32 (6):921–8.

Katiyar, S. K., R. Agarwal, and H. Mukhtar. 1996. Inhibition of tumor promotion in SENCAR mouse skin by ethanol extract of Zingiber officinale rhizome. *Cancer Res* 56 (5):1023–30.

Kelly, G. E., C. Nelson, M. A. Waring, G. E. Joannou, and A. Y. Reeder. 1993. Metabolites of dietary (soya) isoflavones in human urine. *Clin Chim Acta* 223 (1–2):9–22.

Kim, D. J., K. Reddy, M. O. Kim et al. 2011. (3-Chloroacetyl)-indole, a novel allosteric AKT inhibitor, suppresses colon cancer growth in vitro and in vivo. *Cancer Prev Res* 4 (11):1842–51.

Kim, J. E., J. Y. Kwon, D. E. Lee et al. 2009. MKK4 is a novel target for the inhibition of tumor necrosis factor-alpha-induced vascular endothelial growth factor expression by myricetin. *Biochem Pharmacol* 77 (3):412–21.

Kim, J. E., D. E. Lee, K. W. Lee et al. 2011. Isorhamnetin suppresses skin cancer through direct inhibition of MEK1 and PI3-K. *Cancer Prev Res (Phila)* 4 (4):582–91.

Kim, S. O., K. S. Chun, J. K. Kundu, and Y. J. Surh. 2004. Inhibitory effects of [6]-gingerol on PMA-induced COX-2 expression and activation of NF-kappaB and p38 MAPK in mouse skin. *Biofactors* 21 (1–4):27–31.

Kim, S. O., J. K. Kundu, Y. K. Shin et al. 2005. [6]-Gingerol inhibits COX-2 expression by blocking the activation of p38 MAP kinase and NF-kappaB in phorbol ester-stimulated mouse skin. *Oncogene* 24 (15):2558–67.

Kiuchi, F., S. Iwakami, M. Shibuya, F. Hanaoka, and U. Sankawa. 1992. Inhibition of prostaglandin and leuko-triene biosynthesis by gingerols and diarylheptanoids. *Chem Pharm Bull (Tokyo)* 40 (2):387–91.

Ko, C. H., S. C. Shen, T. J. Lee, and Y. C. Chen. 2005. Myricetin inhibits matrix metalloproteinase 2 protein expression and enzyme activity in colorectal carcinoma cells. *Molec Cancer Ther* 4 (2):281–90.

Kuiper, G. G., J. G. Lemmen, B. Carlsson et al. 1998. Interaction of estrogenic chemicals and phytoestrogens with estrogen receptor beta. *Endocrinology* 139 (10):4252–63.

Kulling, S. E., D. M. Honig, T. J. Simat, and M. Metzler. 2000. Oxidative in vitro metabolism of the soy phy-toestrogens daidzein and genistein. *J Agric Food Chem* 48 (10):4963–72.

Kulling, S. E., D. M. Honig, and M. Metzler. 2001. Oxidative metabolism of the soy isoflavones daidzein and genistein in humans in vitro and in vivo. *J Agric Food Chem* 49 (6):3024–33.

Kumamoto, T., M. Fujii, and D. X. Hou. 2009a. Akt is a direct target for myricetin to inhibit cell transformation. *Mol Cell Biochem* 332 (1–2):33–41.

Kumamoto, T., M. Fujii, and D. X. Hou. 2009b. Myricetin directly targets JAK1 to inhibit cell transformation. *Cancer Lett* 275 (1):17–26.

Kundu, J. K., and Y. J. Surh. 2008. Cancer chemopreventive and therapeutic potential of resveratrol: mechanis-tic perspectives. *Cancer Lett* 269 (2):243–61.

Kutchera, W., D. A. Jones, N. Matsunami et al. 1996. Prostaglandin H synthase 2 is expressed abnormally in human colon cancer: evidence for a transcriptional effect. *Proc Natl Acad Sci U S A* 93 (10):4816–20.

Kwon, J. Y., K. W. Lee, J. E. Kim et al. 2009. Delphinidin suppresses ultraviolet B-induced cyclooxygenases-2 expression through inhibition of MAPKK4 and PI-3 kinase. *Carcinogenesis* 30 (11):1932–40.

Langner, E., S. Greifenberg, and J. Gruenwald. 1998. Ginger: history and use. *Adv Ther* 15 (1):25–44.

Lee, D. E., K. W. Lee, N. R. Song et al. 2010. 7,3′,4′-Trihydroxyisoflavone inhibits epidermal growth factor-induced proliferation and transformation of JB6 P+ mouse epidermal cells by suppressing cyclin-dependent kinases and phosphatidylinositol 3-kinase. *J Biol Chem* 285 (28):21458–66.

Lee, D. E., K. W. Lee, S. Byun et al. 2011a. 7,3′,4′-Trihydroxyisoflavone, a metabolite of the soy isofla-vone daidzein, suppresses ultraviolet B-induced skin cancer by targeting Cot and MKK4. *J Biol Chem* 286 (16):14246–56.

Lee, D. E., K. W. Lee, S. K. Jung et al. 2011b. 6,7,4′-trihydroxyisoflavone inhibits HCT-116 human colon can-cer cell proliferation by targeting CDK1 and CDK2. *Carcinogenesis* 32 (4):629–35.

Lee, E., and Y. J. Surh. 1998. Induction of apoptosis in HL-60 cells by pungent vanilloids, [6]-gingerol and [6]-paradol. *Cancer Lett* 134 (2):163–8.

Lee, E., K. K. Park, J. M. Lee et al. 1998. Suppression of mouse skin tumor promotion and induction of apop-tosis in HL-60 cells by Alpinia oxyphylla Miquel (Zingiberaceae). *Carcinogenesis* 19 (8):1377–81.

Lee, J. L., H. Mukhtar, D. R. Bickers, L. Kopelovich, and M. Athar. 2003. Cyclooxygenases in the skin: phar-macological and toxicological implications. *Toxicology and applied pharmacology* 192 (3):294–306.

Lee, K. W., N. J. Kang, E. A. Rogozin et al. 2007. Myricetin is a novel natural inhibitor of neoplastic cell transformation and MEK1. *Carcinogenesis* 28 (9):1918–27.

Lee, K. W., N. J. Kang, Y. S. Heo et al. 2008a. Raf and MEK protein kinases are direct molecular targets for the chemopreventive effect of quercetin, a major flavonol in red wine. *Cancer Res* 68 (3):946–55.

Lee, K. W., N. J. Kang, E. A. Rogozin et al. 2008b. The resveratrol analogue 3,5,3′,4′,5′-pentahydroxy-trans-stilbene inhibits cell transformation via MEK. *Int J Cancer* 123 (11):2487–96.

Lee, K. M., K. W. Lee, S. Byun et al. 2010a. 5-deoxykaempferol plays a potential therapeutic role by targeting multiple signaling pathways in skin cancer. *Cancer Prev Res (Phila Pa)* 3 (4):454–65.

Lee, K. M., K. W. Lee, S. K. Jung et al. 2010b. Kaempferol inhibits UVB-induced COX-2 expression by sup-pressing Src kinase activity. *Biochem Pharmacol* 80 (12):2042–9.

Lee, K. W., A. M. Bode, and Z. Dong. 2011. Molecular targets of phytochemicals for cancer prevention. *Nat Rev Cancer* 11 (3):211–8.

Li, H., Z. Gao, L. Kang et al. 2006. TarFisDock: a web server for identifying drug targets with docking approach. *Nucleic Acids Res* 34 (Web Server issue):W219–W224.

Li, J., M. Malakhova, M. Mottamal et al. 2012a. Norathyriol suppresses skin cancers induced by solar ultravio-let radiation by targeting ERK kinases. *Cancer Res* 72 (1):260–70.

Li, J., M. Mottamal, H. Li et al. 2012b. Quercetin-3-methyl ether suppresses proliferation of mouse epidermal JB6 P+ cells by targeting ERKs. *Carcinogenesis* 33 (2):459–65.

Li, J., F. Zhu, R. A. Lubet et al. 2013. Quercetin-3-methyl ether inhibits lapatinib-sensitive and -resistant breast cancer cell growth by inducing G(2)/M arrest and apoptosis. *Molecular Carcinogen* 52 (2):134–43.

Li, M., Z. He, S. Ermakova et al. 2007. Direct inhibition of insulin-like growth factor-I receptor kinase activ-ity by (-)-epigallocatechin-3-gallate regulates cell transformation. *Cancer Epidemiol Biomark Prev* 16 (3):598–605.

Lin, H. Y., L. Lansing, J. M. Merillon et al. 2006. Integrin alphaVbeta3 contains a receptor site for resveratrol. *FASEB J* 20 (10):1742–4.

Liu, K., Y. Y. Cho, K. Yao et al. 2011. Eriodictyol inhibits RSK2-ATF1 signaling and suppresses EGF-induced neoplastic cell transformation. *J Biol Chem* 286 (3):2057–66.

Lu, J., L. V. Papp, J. Fang et al. 2006. Inhibition of mammalian thioredoxin reductase by some flavonoids: implications for myricetin and quercetin anticancer activity. *Cancer Res* 66 (8):4410–8.

Malakhova, M., V. Tereshko, S. Y. Lee et al. 2008. Structural basis for activation of the autoinhibitory C-terminal kinase domain of p90 RSK2. *Nat Struct Mol Biol* 15 (1):112–3.

Malakhova, M., I. Kurinov, K. Liu et al. 2009. Structural diversity of the active N-terminal kinase domain of p90 ribosomal S6 kinase 2. *PLoS One* 4 (11):e8044.

McInnes, C. 2007. Virtual screening strategies in drug discovery. *Curr Opin Chem Biol* 11 (5):494–502.

McWilliam, H., F. Valentin, M. Goujon et al. 2009. Web services at the European Bioinformatics Institute-2009. *Nucleic Acids Res* 37 (Web Server issue):W6–10.

Messina, M. J. 1999. Legumes and soybeans: overview of their nutritional profiles and health effects. *Am J Clin Nutr* 70 (3 Suppl):439S–50S.

Mestre, J. R., G. Chan, F. Zhang et al. 1999. Inhibition of cyclooxygenase-2 expression. An approach to preventing head and neck cancer. *Ann N Y Acad Sci* 889:62–71.

Miean, K. H., and S. Mohamed. 2001. Flavonoid (myricetin, quercetin, kaempferol, luteolin, and apigenin) content of edible tropical plants. *J Agric Food Chem* 49 (6):3106–12.

Mosesson, Y., and Y. Yarden. 2004. Oncogenic growth factor receptors: implications for signal transduction therapy. *Semin Cancer Biol* 14 (4):262–70.

Mukhtar, H., M. Das, W. A. Khan et al. 1988. Exceptional activity of tannic acid among naturally occurring plant phenols in protecting against 7,12-dimethylbenz(a)anthracene-, benzo(a)pyrene-, 3-methylcholanthrene-, and N-methyl-N-nitrosourea-induced skin tumorigenesis in mice. *Cancer research* 48 (9):2361–5.

Ohren, J. F., H. Chen, A. Pavlovsky et al. 2004. Structures of human MAP kinase kinase 1 (MEK1) and MEK2 describe novel noncompetitive kinase inhibition. *Nat Struct Molec Biol* 11 (12):1192–7.

Oi, N., C. H. Jeong, J. Nadas et al. 2010. Resveratrol, a red wine polyphenol, suppresses pancreatic cancer by inhibiting leukotriene a4 hydrolase. *Cancer Res* 70 (23):9755–64.

Palermo, C. M., C. A. Westlake, and T. A. Gasiewicz. 2005. Epigallocatechin gallate inhibits aryl hydrocarbon receptor gene transcription through an indirect mechanism involving binding to a 90 kDa heat shock protein. *Biochemistry* 44 (13):5041–52.

Park, K. K., K. S. Chun, J. M. Lee, S. S. Lee, and Y. J. Surh. 1998. Inhibitory effects of [6]-gingerol, a major pungent principle of ginger, on phorbol ester-induced inflammation, epidermal ornithine decarboxylase activity and skin tumor promotion in ICR mice. *Cancer Lett* 129 (2):139–44.

Pervaiz, S., and A. L. Holme. 2009. Resveratrol: its biologic targets and functional activity. *Antioxid Redox Signal* 11 (11):2851–97.

Pirola, L., and S. Frojdo. 2008. Resveratrol: one molecule, many targets. *IUBMB Life* 60 (5):323–32.

Prescott, S. M., and F. A. Fitzpatrick. 2000. Cyclooxygenase-2 and carcinogenesis. *Biochim Biophys Acta* 1470 (2):M69–78.

Ranganathan, R., K. P. Lu, T. Hunter, and J. P. Noel. 1997. Structural and functional analysis of the mitotic rotamase Pin1 suggests substrate recognition is phosphorylation dependent. *Cell* 89 (6):875–86.

Reagan-Shaw, S., H. Mukhtar, and N. Ahmad. 2008. Resveratrol imparts photoprotection of normal cells and enhances the efficacy of radiation therapy in cancer cells. *Photochem Photobiol* 84 (2):415–21.

Ristimaki, A., N. Honkanen, H. Jankala, P. Sipponen, and M. Harkonen. 1997. Expression of cyclooxygenase-2 in human gastric carcinoma. *Cancer Res* 57 (7):1276–80.

Rouzer, C. A., and L. J. Marnett. 2011. Green tea gets molecular. *Cancer Prev Res* 4 (9):1343–5.

Ryo, A., M. Nakamura, G. Wulf, Y. C. Liou, and K. P. Lu. 2001. Pin1 regulates turnover and subcellular localization of beta-catenin by inhibiting its interaction with APC. *Nat Cell Biol* 3 (9):793–801.

Saiko, P., M. Pemberger, Z. Horvath et al. 2008a. Novel resveratrol analogs induce apoptosis and cause cell cycle arrest in HT29 human colon cancer cells: inhibition of ribonucleotide reductase activity. *Oncol Rep* 19 (6):1621–6.

Saiko, P., A. Szakmary, W. Jaeger, and T. Szekeres. 2008b. Resveratrol and its analogs: defense against cancer, coronary disease and neurodegenerative maladies or just a fad? *Mutat Res* 658 (1–2):68–94.

Sanchez, I., R. T. Hughes, B. J. Mayer et al. 1994. Role of SAPK/ERK kinase-1 in the stress-activated pathway regulating transcription factor c-Jun. *Nature* 372 (6508):794–8.

Sano, H., Y. Kawahito, R. L. Wilder et al. 1995. Expression of cyclooxygenase-1 and -2 in human colorectal cancer. *Cancer Res* 55 (17):3785–9.

Sazuka, M., M. Isemura, and S. Isemura. 1998. Interaction between the carboxyl-terminal heparin-binding domain of fibronectin and (-)-epigallocatechin gallate. *Biosci Biotechnol Biochem* 62 (5):1031–2.

Schrödinger Suite. 2006. QM-Polarized Ligand Docking Protocol 2005. L.L.C., New York.

Schulze-Osthoff, K., D. Ferrari, K. Riehemann, and S. Wesselborg. 1997. Regulation of NF-kappa B activation by MAP kinase cascades. *Immunobiology* 198 (1–3):35–49.

Sears, R. C. 2004. The life cycle of C-myc: from synthesis to degradation. *Cell Cycle* 3 (9):1133–7.

Sebolt-Leopold, J. S., D. T. Dudley, R. Herrera et al. 1999. Blockade of the MAP kinase pathway suppresses growth of colon tumors in vivo. *Nat Med* 5 (7):810–6.

She, Q. B., A. M. Bode, W. Y. Ma, N. Y. Chen, and Z. Dong. 2001. Resveratrol-induced activation of p53 and apoptosis is mediated by extracellular-signal-regulated protein kinases and p38 kinase. *Cancer Res* 61 (4):1604–10.

She, Q. B., W. Y. Ma, M. Wang et al. 2003. Inhibition of cell transformation by resveratrol and its derivatives: differential effects and mechanisms involved. *Oncogene* 22 (14):2143–50.

Shim, J. H., H. S. Choi, A. Pugliese et al. 2008. (-)-Epigallocatechin gallate regulates CD3-mediated T cell receptor signaling in leukemia through the inhibition of ZAP-70 kinase. *J Biol Chem* 283 (42):28370–9.

Shim, J. H., Z. Y. Su, J. I. Chae et al. 2010. Epigallocatechin gallate suppresses lung cancer cell growth through Ras-GTPase-activating protein SH3 domain-binding protein 1. *Cancer Prev Res (Phila)* 3 (5):670–9.

Soleas, G. J., L. Grass, P. D. Josephy, D. M. Goldberg, and E. P. Diamandis. 2002. A comparison of the anticarcinogenic properties of four red wine polyphenols. *Clin Biochem* 35 (2):119–24.

Srivastava, K. C., and T. Mustafa. 1992. Ginger (*Zingiber officinale*) in rheumatism and musculoskeletal disorders. *Med Hypotheses* 39 (4):342–8.

Subbaramaiah, K., and A. J. Dannenberg. 2003. Cyclooxygenase 2: a molecular target for cancer prevention and treatment. *Trends Pharmacol Sci* 24 (2):96–102.

Subbaramaiah, K., N. Telang, J. T. Ramonetti et al. 1996. Transcription of cyclooxygenase-2 is enhanced in transformed mammary epithelial cells. *Cancer Res* 56 (19):4424–9.

Surh, Y. J., E. Lee, and J. M. Lee. 1998. Chemoprotective properties of some pungent ingredients present in red pepper and ginger. *Mutat Res* 402 (1–2):259–67.

Surh, Y. J., K. K. Park, K. S. Chun et al. 1999. Anti-tumor-promoting activities of selected pungent phenolic substances present in ginger. *J Environ Pathol Toxicol Oncol* 18 (2):131–9.

Suzuki, Y., and M. Isemura. 2001. Inhibitory effect of epigallocatechin gallate on adhesion of murine melanoma cells to laminin. *Cancer Lett* 173 (1):15–20.

Tachibana, H., K. Koga, Y. Fujimura, and K. Yamada. 2004. A receptor for green tea polyphenol EGCG. *Nat Struct Molec Biol* 11 (4):380–1.

Tian, W. X. 2006. Inhibition of fatty acid synthase by polyphenols. *Curr Med Chem* 13 (8):967–77.

Tiano, H. F., C. D. Loftin, J. Akunda et al. 2002. Deficiency of either cyclooxygenase (COX)-1 or COX-2 alters epidermal differentiation and reduces mouse skin tumorigenesis. *Cancer Res* 62 (12):3395–401.

Tong, B. J., J. Tan, L. Tajeda et al. 2000. Heightened expression of cyclooxygenase-2 and peroxisome proliferator-activated receptor-delta in human endometrial adenocarcinoma. *Neoplasia* 2 (6):483–90.

Tucker, O. N., A. J. Dannenberg, E. K. Yang et al. 1999. Cyclooxygenase-2 expression is up-regulated in human pancreatic cancer. *Cancer Res* 59 (5):987–90.

Turini, M. E., and R. N. DuBois. 2002. Cyclooxygenase-2: a therapeutic target. *Annu Rev Med* 53:35–57.

Urusova, D. V., J. H. Shim, D. J. Kim et al. 2011. Epigallocatechin-gallate suppresses tumorigenesis by directly targeting Pin1. *Cancer Prev Res* 4 (9):1366–77.

van Rees, B. P., K. Saukkonen, A. Ristimaki et al. 2002. Cyclooxygenase-2 expression during carcinogenesis in the human stomach. *J Pathol* 196 (2):171–9.

Weir, B., X. Zhao, and M. Meyerson. 2004. Somatic alterations in the human cancer genome. *Cancer Cell* 6 (5):433–8.

Widyarini, S., A. J. Husband, and V. E. Reeve. 2005. Protective effect of the isoflavonoid equol against hairless mouse skin carcinogenesis induced by UV radiation alone or with a chemical cocarcinogen. *Photochem Photobiol* 81 (1):32–7.

Williamson, M. P., T. G. McCormick, C. L. Nance, and W. T. Shearer. 2006. Epigallocatechin gallate, the main polyphenol in green tea, binds to the T-cell receptor, CD4: potential for HIV-1 therapy. *J Allergy Clin Immunol* 118 (6):1369–74.

Wolff, H., K. Saukkonen, S. Anttila et al. 1998. Expression of cyclooxygenase-2 in human lung carcinoma. *Cancer Res* 58 (22):4997–5001.

Wulf, G. M., A. Ryo, G. G. Wulf et al. 2001. Pin1 is overexpressed in breast cancer and cooperates with Ras signaling in increasing the transcriptional activity of c-Jun towards cyclin D1. *EMBO J* 20 (13):3459–72.

Wulf, G., G. Finn, F. Suizu, and K. P. Lu. 2005. Phosphorylation-specific prolyl isomerization: is there an underlying theme? *Nat Cell Biol* 7 (5):435–41.

Xiang, Z. 2006. Advances in homology protein structure modeling. *Curr Prot Pept Sci* 7 (3):217–27.

Yang, S., K. Irani, S. E. Heffron, F. Jurnak, and F. L. Meyskens, Jr. 2005. Alterations in the expression of the apurinic/apyrimidinic endonuclease-1/redox factor-1 (APE/Ref-1) in human melanoma and identification of the therapeutic potential of resveratrol as an APE/Ref-1 inhibitor. *Mol Cancer Ther* 4 (12):1923–35.

Yin, Z., E. C. Henry, and T. A. Gasiewicz. 2009. (-)-Epigallocatechin-3-gallate is a novel Hsp90 inhibitor. *Biochemistry* 48 (2):336–45.

Zykova, T. A., F. Zhu, X. Zhai et al. 2008. Resveratrol directly targets COX-2 to inhibit carcinogenesis. *Mol Carcinog* 47 (10):797–805.

6 Biomarkers for Diet in Cancer Prevention Studies

Zheng-Yuan Su, Limin Shu, and Ah-Ng Tony Kong

CONTENTS

6.1 INTRODUCTION

Tumorigenesis is the result of genetic alterations that drive the progressive transformation of normal cells into highly malignant derivatives. This process disrupts the normal functions of cells, tissues, and organs via the introduction of mutations, genome rearrangements, amplifications, deletions, and epigenetic modulation of gene expression (Hanahan and Weinberg 2000; Kelloff and Sigman 2012). DNA damage, oxidative stress, mitotic stress, proapoptotic stress, and metabolic stress have been identified as stress phenotypes of cancer (Luo et al. 2009). Molecules such as DNA, RNA, microRNA (miRNA), and proteins, and genetic and posttranslational modifications that participate in these stress responses in cells have been identified as cancer biomarkers and targets for preventive and therapeutic intervention (Bartsch et al. 2011; Kelloff and Sigman 2012). These biomarkers may be utilized for achieving an early diagnosis, prognosis, or classification of disease subtype; predicting the treatment response; and identifying potential targets for drug therapy (Leth-Larsen et al. 2010).

Dietary bioactive components in food that act as cancer preventive agents include essential nutrients (such as calcium; zinc; selenium; folate; and vitamins C, D, and E) and nonessential food components (such as carotenoids, flavonoids, indoles, allyl sulfur compounds, conjugated linoleic acid [CLA], and n-3 fatty acids) (Wiseman 2008). Bioactive food components simultaneously modify multiple events in cancer processes, including hormonal balance, carcinogen metabolism, cell-cycle control, apoptosis, cell signaling, and angiogenesis (Surh 2003). The target molecules

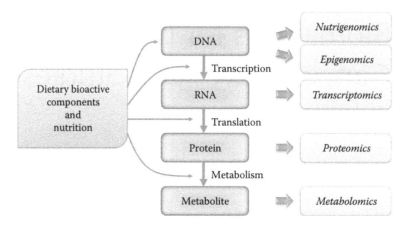

FIGURE 6.1 These "omics" approaches can be applied to understand the effects of dietary bioactive components and nutrition on biomarkers for cancer prevention.

of chemopreventive biomarkers, which play important roles in the development and behavior of cancer cells, have been classified into five "omics" systems: diet-associated gene polymorphisms (nutrigenomics); DNA methylation and chromatin alterations (epigenomics); gene expression (transcriptomics); synthesis and/or activation of proteins (proteomics); and the formation of cellular constituents with small molecular weights (metabolomics) (Figure 6.1).

In this review chapter, we will discuss and summarize the current progress related to studies of nutrigenomics, epigenomics, transcriptomics, proteomics, and metabolomics for the identification of cancer biomarkers for dietary chemoprevention. The well-known biomarkers of carcinogenesis for specific varieties of cancer will also be discussed regarding the chemopreventive effects of dietary bioactive components.

6.2 CANCER BIOMARKER APPROACHES FOR DIET

6.2.1 NUTRIGENOMICS

Single-nucleotide polymorphisms (SNPs) are genetic polymorphisms that represent the variations in single nucleotides between individuals, and more than 10 million SNPs in the human genome have been reported (Cargill et al. 1999; Thorisson and Stein 2003). Inherited SNPs are related to disease risk and nutrient metabolism (Potter 1999; Yan and Zhou 2004), and the interactions between individual genetic variability and diet can provide a greater understanding of the effects of bioactive food components on health and disease risk in humans (Fenech et al. 2011). Nutrigenomics is the science of the effect of nutrients and bioactive food compounds on gene expression, and correlations have been demonstrated between dietary and genetic variations (Trujillo et al. 2006; Kaput 2008; Ferguson 2009; Simopoulos 2010).

Increasing evidence from the field of nutrigenomics indicates that genetic and cultural differences, such as dietary habits, are related to the risk of cancer development. For example, the genetic polymorphism that replaces a valine with an alanine at the ninth position in the sequence of the enzyme manganese superoxide dismutase is associated with an increased risk of breast cancer in women who consume levels of fruits, vegetables, ascorbic acid, and α-tocopherol below the recommended median values (Ambrosone et al. 1999). Furthermore, the consumption of isothiocyanates from cruciferous vegetables lowers the risk for colorectal and gastric cancer in individuals with both the glutathione S-transferase (GST) M1- and T1-null genotypes (Seow et al. 2002; Moy et al. 2009). Inflammation and carcinogenesis of the prostate in individuals with the GSTM1 genotype were also shown to be reduced following the consumption of broccoli (Traka et al. 2008), whereas excessive red meat consumption was shown to increase the risk of colorectal cancer by interacting with allelic variant combinations of P450 polymorphisms (Kury et al. 2007).

6.2.2 EPIGENOMICS

Epigenetics refers to "the study of heritable changes in gene expression that occur without changes in the DNA sequence" (Wolffe and Matzke 1999). Carcinogenesis may be caused by epigenetic changes in oncogenes and tumor suppressor genes. Epigenetic events associated with cellular biological processes, including inflammation, carcinogenic metabolism, proliferation, apoptosis, cell-cycle control, and angiogenesis, may be altered by environmental and dietary factors, such as nutrients and bioactive food components. Epigenetic mechanisms consist of DNA methylation, posttranslational modifications of histones, and the regulation of noncoding RNAs (Baylin and Herman 2000; Ducasse and Brown 2006). Epigenetic alterations that cause transcriptional repression of suppressor genes can be reversible, which leads to the recovery of gene function (Issa 2002). Thus, dietary chemopreventive components or drugs may represent a novel approach for cancer prevention and therapy.

In mammalian cells, DNA methyltransferases (DNMTs), such as DNMT1, DNMT3a, and DNMT3b, catalyze DNA methylation by adding a methyl group to the 5' position of cytosine bases in CpG dinucleotides (Bird 2002; Esteller 2002). CpG islands are genomic regions consisting of a group of CpG dinucleotides, and these islands are not distributed evenly throughout the genome but are located at approximately 60% of human gene promoters (Bird 2002). Hypermethylation at CpG islands located in promoter regions results in silencing of the tumor suppressor genes p16^{ink4a} and breast cancer 1 (BRCA1) (Esteller 2005; Jones and Baylin 2002). DNA methylation of genes in most human cancers causes transcriptional silencing of tumor suppressor genes (Herman and Baylin 2003). For example, several cancer-related genes in different cellular pathways are inactivated by CpG island hypermethylation, including DNA repair–related human mutL homolog 1 (hMLH1) and methyl guanine methyl transferase (MGMT); cell-cycle–related p16^{INK4a}, p15^{INK4b}, and p14^{ARF}; apoptosis-related death-associated protein kinase 1 (DAPK); cell cadherin-related E-cadherin (CDH1) and CDH13; and detoxification-related glutathione S-transferase pi 1 (CSTP1) (Esteller 2002). The silencing of eight genes that are used as potential markers for the initiation and progression of lung cancer is induced via promoter hypermethylation, and supplements of leafy green vegetables and folate as well as multivitamins have been shown to reduce the incidence of lung cancer by reducing promoter methylation in the aerodigestive tracts of smokers (Stidley et al. 2010). In addition, methyl–CpG–binding domain proteins (MBDs) and methyl–CpG–binding protein 2 (MeCP2) interact with methylated DNA (Lewis et al. 1992; Hendrich and Bird 1998), and these binding proteins promote transcriptional repression by interacting with corepressor complexes such as histone deacetylases (HDACs) (Nan et al. 1998; Feng and Zhang 2001).

Chromatin is a densely packed macromolecular complex in eukaryotic cells that consists of DNA, histones, and nonhistone proteins. The structure of chromatin affects DNA replication and gene expression because DNA is packaged into a small volume for stability in the nucleus. The basic subunit of chromatin is the nucleosome, within which 146 bp of DNA is wrapped around a histone octamer containing an histone 3/histone 4 (H3/H4) tetramer and two histone 2A/histone 2B (H2A/H2B) dimers. Therefore, posttranslational modifications of histones play an important role in influencing chromatin structure and are therefore involved in gene expression (Berlowitz and Pallotta 1972; Luger et al. 1997; Tremethick 2007). Histone modifications also regulate gene expression associated with tumorigenesis (Esteller 2008; Ellis et al. 2009). For example, elevated expression of histone deacetylases(HDACs) has been observed in cases of gastric cancer (Weichert et al. 2008b), breast cancer (Krusche et al. 2005), renal cancer (Fritzsche et al. 2008), and ovarian endomethioid carcinoma (Weichert et al. 2008a). The lysine, arginine, and serine residues located at the N-terminal tails extending from the histone core can also be posttranscriptionally modified by acetylation, methylation, phosphorylation, sumoylation, or ubiquitination (Luger et al. 1997;

Berger 2007; Kouzarides 2007). For example, methylation at lysine 4 in the histone H3 tail results in active transcriptional chromatin, whereas methylation at lysine 9 in the same histone tail generates repressed transcriptional chromatin (Bannister et al. 2001; Jenuwein and Allis 2001; Nakayama et al. 2001). Histone modifications are reversible via the catalysis of specific enzymes such as histone deacetylases (HATs) and HDACs (Rodenhiser and Mann 2006; Ellis et al. 2009). Acetylation of histones is closely associated with DNA methylation, and the inhibitory potentials of HDAC inhibitors, such as trichostatin A and suberoylanilide hydroxamic acid (SAHA), have been investigated (Tamaru and Selker 2001; Jackson et al. 2002; Kim et al. 2010; Yu et al. 2010).

In addition, noncoding miRNAs can silence gene expression via antisense RNA–RNA interactions in various organisms (Lee et al. 1993; Pasquinelli et al. 2000). Reports of gene expression correlated with the expression of human miRNAs have increased in frequency (Griffiths-Jones et al. 2006; Zhang et al. 2007); miRNAs containing 17 to 25 nucleotides have been shown to inhibit translation and degrade target messenger RNAs (mRNAs), which results in various cellular biological responses, including cell proliferation, apoptosis, cell-cycle control, immunity, and tumorigenesis (Carleton et al. 2007; Negrini et al. 2007; Baltimore et al. 2008; Croce 2009). Recently, the effects of miRNAs on the regulation of epigenetics during carcinogenesis have been studied (Jones and Baylin 2002; Esteller 2007; Kai and Pasquinelli 2010; Krutovskikh and Herceg 2010), and studies identifying dietary phytochemicals that act as chemopreventive reagents by altering target miRNA expression in cancer cells are rapidly increasing in frequency (Sun et al. 2008; Izzotti et al. 2010; Li et al. 2010; Tsang and Kwok 2010).

6.2.3 Transcriptomics

Transcriptomic analyses evaluate global or a selected subset of gene expression profiles. High-throughput genomic technologies, such as DNA and mRNA microarrays, are important tools used to investigate changes in RNA expression patterns, which reflect the physiological status of the cell in response to external stimuli (Nambiar et al. 2005). Recent studies have reported that nutrition and bioactive food components, which have also been shown to reduce cancer risk, can influence gene transcription in cellular processes such as growth, differentiation, apoptosis, and energy restriction (Mariadason et al. 2000; Dong et al. 2002; Jiang et al. 2003). Therefore, transcriptomics studies related to cancer chemoprevention may serve to identify critical genes and pathways as molecular biomarkers that may be influenced by food components (Muller and Kersten 2003).

A low-fat/low-glycemic diet intervention was shown to significantly alter 23 of 5711 cDNAs in prostate tissue from men with newly diagnosed prostate cancer (Lin et al. 2007), and some of these genes were associated with cell migration and tissue remodeling, such as chemokine (C-X-C motif) receptor 4 (CXCR4), chemokine (C-X-C motif) ligand 2 (CXCL2), lumican, matrilysin, and secreted protein, acidic and rich in cysteine-like 1 (SPARCL1), or intracellular signal transduction, such as the immediate early response genes 2 and 3, dual specificity phosphatase 1, and the v-ets oncogene homologue. Furthermore, gene expression of the insulin-like growth factor-II receptor was upregulated, whereas the expression levels of antioxidant-protective peroxiredoxin 1 and prostate-specific membrane antigen were downregulated in these samples (Lin et al. 2007). Dietary energy restriction was also shown to be associated with the significant downregulation of genes involved in glycolytic and lipid synthesis pathways, such as stearoyl-CoA desaturase, fatty acid desaturase, and aldolase C in both breast tissues and epithelial cells, which may reduce the risk of spontaneous mammary cancers (Ong et al. 2009).

Selenium is known to modify the expression of cell growth–related genes in the intestines of C57B1/6J mice, including GADD153, cyclin A, cyclin-dependent kinase (CDK)1, CDK2, CDK4, CDC25, and E2Fs, as well as the activity of the mitogen-activated protein kinase (MAPK)/c-Jun NH_2-terminal kinase (JNK) and phosphoinositide 3-kinase pathways (Rao et al. 2001). Selenium was also shown to alter 2500 of 12,000 screened genes in 12 clusters of distinct kinetic patterns, including those related to the cell cycle, growth factors, apoptosis, angiogenesis, protein synthesis, tumor suppression, transcription factors, DNA repair, adhesion/invasion, signal transduction, and cytoskeletal function, in human prostate cancer cells (Dong et al. 2003). In addition, a pharmacogenomic study demonstrated that the combination of sulforaphane (SFN) and epigallocatechin gallate (EGCG) increased Nrf2-dependent gene expression pathways related to apoptosis/cell cycle, calcium ion binding, digestion, the extracellular space, the plasma membrane (PM), intracellular kinases, phosphatases, metal ion binding, transcription factors/interacting partners, transferases, and ubiquitination in the prostate (Nair et al. 2010). Thus, transcriptomics studies can be useful for comparing and contrasting gene expression profiles in response to the consumption of nutrients and food components.

6.2.4 PROTEOMICS

Polypeptides translated from a single gene may undergo different posttranslational modifications, such as alternative splicing, glycosylation, phosphorylation, oxidation, and reduction, which results in the generation of multiple proteins with various biological activities (Panisko et al. 2002; Tyers and Mann 2003). The rates of synthesis and degradation of a specific protein also lead to different cellular biological responses (Panisko et al. 2002), and protein function may also be affected by active dietary components via these posttranslational modifications. For instance, diallyl disulfide (DADS) has been shown to increase the phosphorylation of extracellular signal–regulated kinase (ERK) and lead to cell-cycle arrest in human colon tumor HCT-15 cells (Knowles and Milner 2003). In addition, EGCG was shown to suppress the activation of Ras and downstream ERK signaling following interactions with the Ras-GTPase–activating protein SH3 domain–binding protein 1 (G3BP1), which is one of the mechanisms by which EGCG is thought to interfere in lung tumorigenesis (Shim et al. 2010). The interaction between dietary SFN and the thiol groups in the cytoplasmic protein Keap1 was also shown to affect the binding of Keap1 to Nrf2, which activates GST and quinone reductase (Dinkova-Kostova et al. 2002).

Two-dimensional polyacrylamide gel electrophoresis (2D-PAGE) analysis combined with matrix-assisted laser desorption/ionization–time-of-flight (MALDI-TOF) mass spectrometry is generally performed to study proteomics (Gras et al. 1999; Nordhoff et al. 2001). In addition, other advanced techniques such as ProteinChip technology, protein microarrays, and targeted proteomic methods have also recently been introduced (Austin and Holway 2011; Hause et al. 2011; Woodbury et al. 2012). Using proteomic approaches, proteomic patterns have been established from serum samples of individuals with ovarian cancer in both high-risk and general populations (Petricoin et al. 2002), and human colorectal cancer has also been classified based on proteomic studies (Nambiar et al. 2010). Furthermore, breast cancers can be diagnosed early according to the detection of selected serum biomarkers, for which dietary habits have been shown to result in subtle changes in the levels of these markers (Li et al. 2002). Recently, additional proteomic techniques have been utilized to study the relationship between diet and cancer. For example, low levels of arsenite induced by benzo[a]pyrene (B[a]P)-treated lung cell transformation were found to be related to several uniquely identifiable proteins (He et al. 2003), and in a study of sodium butyrate–induced growth inhibition in human HT-29 colon cancer cells, proteomic results demonstrated that sodium butyrate affected the expression of proteins involved in control of the cell cycle, apoptosis, and differentiation (Tan et al. 2002).

6.2.5 METABOLOMICS

Metabolomics is the study of endogenous metabolites related to anabolism and catabolism in cells and tissues such as the blood, urine, and saliva (Bollard et al. 2005; German et al. 2005). Metabolic processes are influenced by various factors, such as the environment, diet, physiology, drugs, diseases, sex, genetic drift, and age (Bollard et al. 2005). In addition, other biological processes, such as absorption, distribution, and detoxification of natural and xenobiotic materials as well as energy utilization, also affect metabolomics (Claudino et al. 2007). The classes of metabolites include organic acids, amino acids, fatty acids, sugars, sugar alcohols, steroids, and nucleic acids (Chan et al. 2009).

Recently, biomarkers for various human cancers, including ovarian carcinoma (OC), prostate cancer, cervical cancer, and brain cancer, have been identified using a metabolomics approach (Mal et al. 2009). Higher glucose uptake, higher lactate conversion, and increased glycolysis have been identified within human colorectal cancer tissue as compared to normal colon tissue according to metabolomics analyses (Mal et al. 2009). In earlier studies, the use of nuclear magnetic resonance (NMR) spectra for metabolite analysis revealed different metabolome profiles in malignant and benign breast tumors, and histological grades of breast cancer have also been correctly distinguished using these techniques (Mountford et al. 2001; Lean et al. 2004).

Metabolomics has also been used for identifying and characterizing metabolites in cancer cells following exposure to active food ingredients. Regarding glucose metabolism, increases in glucose uptake and energy expenditure are hallmarks of tumor cell proliferation in comparison to normal cells (Amann et al. 2009; Yun et al. 2009). Moreover, dietary components such as green tea polyphenolics, cinnamon polyphenol extracts, fish n-3 fatty acids, and vegetable flavonoids have been shown to affect glucose uptake due to altered glucose transporter (GLUT1) expression (Pifferi et al. 2005; Strobel et al. 2005; Cao et al. 2007, 2008). In addition, tumor cells exhibit increased activity of fatty acid synthase, which is a critical enzyme to catalyze the production of fatty acids from acetyl CoA; however, active dietary components, such as luteolin in vegetables, catechin in tea, docosahexaenoic acid (DHA) in fish oil, resveratrol in red grapes, β-glucan in barley, and CLA in milk, have been shown to suppress this process by decreasing the expression and activity of fatty acid synthase (Brusselmans et al. 2005; Puig et al. 2008; Gotoh et al. 2009; Gnoni and Paglialonga 2009; Choi et al. 2010; Lau and Archer 2010).

6.3 REACTIVE OXYGEN AND NITROGEN SPECIES–RELATED BIOMARKERS

Reactive oxygen and nitrogen species participate in a wide variety of human diseases, and oxidative DNA damage is involved in chemical carcinogenesis and aging. Monocyclic chemicals induce mainly oxidative DNA damage, whereas polycyclic chemicals can induce oxidative DNA damage in addition to DNA adduct formation. Recently, chronic infection and inflammation have been recognized as important factors for carcinogenesis. As nitrative DNA damage as well as oxidative DNA damage are induced in inflammatory-related carcinogenesis, one study examined the formation of 8-nitroguanine, a nitrative DNA lesion, in humans and animals under inflammatory conditions, whereas an immunofluorescent labeling study demonstrated that significant levels of 8-nitroguanine were formed in gastric gland epithelial cells of gastritis patients with *Helicobacter pylori* infection, in hepatocytes of patients with hepatitis C, and in the oral epithelium of patients with oral lichen planus. 8-Nitroguanine was also detected in colonic epithelial cells in mouse models of inflammatory bowel diseases and patients with ulcerative colitis. Interestingly, 8-nitroguanine was formed at all sites of carcinogenesis, regardless of the etiology of the tumor. Therefore, 8-nitroguanine may be used as a potential biomarker to evaluate the risk of inflammatory-related carcinogenesis (Kawanishi and Hiraku 2006).

As previous results have suggested that oxidative and nitrative DNA damage occurs at sites of carcinogenesis, regardless of etiology, excessive amounts of reactive nitrogen species produced via inducible nitric oxide synthase (iNOS) during chronic inflammation may play a key role in carcinogenesis via the induction of DNA damage. Furthermore, we previously demonstrated that 8-nitroguanine is a promising biomarker for evaluating the potential risk of inflammation-mediated carcinogenesis (Kawanishi and Hiraku 2006).

Cytochrome P450 1B1 (CYP1B1), which catalyzes estrogen hydroxylation and the activation of potential carcinogenesis, is overexpressed in tumor cells and has been recognized as a biomarker of the tumor phenotype (McFadyen and Murray 2005). Immunohistochemical staining of endometrial carcinomas showed that CYP1B1 is upregulated in endometrial cancers, and CYP1B1 depletion in endometrial carcinoma cells had an extensive effect on cellular proliferation and cell-cycle arrest, whereby the expression levels of cyclin E1, S-phase kinase-associated protein 2 (SKP2), mini-chromosome maintenance complex component 4 (MCM4), RAD51, and p27 (Kip1) were specifically regulated (Saini et al. 2009).

6.4 INFLAMMATION-RELATED BIOMARKERS

Fifteen to twenty percent of cancer deaths are attributable to underlying infection or inflammation (Balkwill and Mantovani 2001). In the presence of chronic inflammation, cytokines, chemokines, reactive oxygen and nitrogen species, and the activation of some key transcription factors, such as nuclear factor kappaB (NF-κB), contribute to genetic instability and subsequent mutations in oncogenic and tumor suppressor pathways (Hussain and Harris 2007). Chronic inflammation also results in aberrant methylation patterns, which have been associated with cancer development (Valinluck and Sowers 2007).

Chronic inflammation is associated with various types of cancers (Aggarwal et al. 2006; Lu et al. 2006). C-reactive protein (CRP) is the classic "acute C-reactive protein" and can be used as a marker for immune system activation. During tissue injury and infection, CRP levels in the plasma increase over 10,000-fold (Danesh and Pepys 2000), and CRP is an inflammatory cell compound that has been associated with a wide range of diseases (Danesh et al. 2004). CRP has also been used for clinical studies to predict disease presence or recurrence, especially for a number of cancers (Coventry et al. 2009). High levels of CRP have been associated with an increased risk of cancer incidence, and the strongest association was demonstrated for lung cancer (Siemes et al. 2006). Although plasma CRP levels may not be able to predict an increased risk for developing colorectal cancer (Zhang et al. 2005), high levels (>3 mg/L) of CRP have been associated with an increased cancer incidence (hazard ratio, 1.4; 95% confidence interval [CI], 1.1 to 1.7). Decreased CRP levels in relation to SNPs were associated with an increased lung cancer risk of 2.6 (95% CI, 1.6 to 4.4) in homozygous carriers, suggesting that baseline CRP levels seem to represent a biomarker of chronic inflammation preceding the development of lung cancer (Siemes et al. 2006). However, these associations do not indicate that elevated CRP levels are responsible for cancer development; high circulating levels of CRP influenced by genetic polymorphisms may result from occult cancers that increase CRP levels or from confounding factors such as inflammation (Allin and Nordestgaard 2011). Furthermore, these associations may be cancer specific, as individuals with CRP levels in the highest quintile were shown to carry a 1.3-fold increased risk of any type of cancer but a 2-fold increased risk of lung cancer (Allin and Nordestgaard 2011; Singh and Newman 2011).

In addition to CRP, the inflammatory cytokine interleukin-6 (IL-6) is also associated with cancer development. One study revealed that IL-6, tumor necrosis factor alpha (TNFα), and CRP are strongly associated with cancer death, as these associations produced hazard ratios of 1.63, 1.82, and 1.64, respectively (Il'yasova et al. 2005), and were specific to the cancer type. For example, IL-5 and CRP levels were associated with colorectal cancer, CRP levels were associated with breast cancer, and neither level was associated with prostate cancer (Il'yasova et al. 2005). However, circulating levels of IL-6 have not been validated as predictors of cancer occurrence (Heikkila et al. 2008).

CD40–CD40L interactions are involved in inflammation and have greatly contributed to understanding the role of platelets in a variety of pathophysiological conditions, including atherothrombosis, immunoinflammatory diseases, and possibly cancer. Thus, CD40L is considered to be a biomarker in various human diseases that are characterized by underlying inflammation, such as atherothrombosis, cancer, and immunoinflammatory diseases (Ferroni et al. 2007).

The matrix metalloproteinase (MMP) family of proteins plays important roles in reproduction (Hulboy et al. 1997), embryogenesis (Vu and Werb 2000), angiogenesis (Roy et al. 2006), and tissue remodeling (Page-McCaw et al. 2007) by controlling the turnover and degradation of the extracellular matrix (ECM). Corresponding to ECM degradation, a number of signaling molecules, such as chemokines, cytokines, and growth factors, are released and subsequently activate numerous signaling molecules (Malemud 2006). The MMP family comprises 25 structurally and functionally related members, and 24 of these are found in mammals (Parks et al. 2004). MMP-8, also known as collagenase-2 or neutrophil collagenase, cleaves the triple-helix structure of native collagen, and the majority of MMP-8 is localized at the cell surface. MMP-8 is overexpressed in head and neck squamous carcinoma cells (Moilanen et al. 2002). In ovarian cancer patients, MMP-8 expression was shown to correlate with tumor stage and poor prognosis (Stadlmann et al. 2003), and in bladder cancer, MMP-8 genetic variations were shown to correlate with an increased bladder cancer risk in smokers (Kader et al. 2006). However, MMP-8 may also possess a tumor-suppressive role. MMP-8 was associated with a diminished risk of lymph node metastasis in breast cancer patients, and this factor was proposed to reduce cell invasion by modulating cell adhesion (Gutierrez-Fernandez et al. 2008). MMP expression was also associated with improved clinical outcome in squamous cell carcinoma patients. MMP-8 knockout (KO) mice showed an increased incidence of skin tumors (Balbin et al. 2003), and female MMP-8–deficient mice were shown to be more susceptible to tongue squamous cell carcinoma (Korpi et al. 2008). Furthermore, MMP-8 can be easily measured in oral fluids and serum, which suggests that it has strong potential to be used as a noninvasive, sensitive biomarker of disease progression. Moreover, MMP-8 levels may provide accurate point-of-care diagnoses and may be used to monitor inflammatory disorders and cancer progression, as these levels have been associated with the risk of lymph node metastasis (Dejonckheere et al. 2011).

Transforming growth factor beta (TGF-β) belongs to the transforming growth factor beta super-family, which includes activin, Nodal, and bone morphogenetic proteins (BMPs). The signaling pathways utilized by this superfamily are ubiquitous and essential regulators of a number of physi-ological processes, such as cell proliferation, differentiation, migration, and survival (Gordon and Blobe 2008). The serine and threonine kinase TGF-β receptors (TβRI and TβRII) form a hetero-complex after ligand binding, which activates TβRI and subsequently phosphorylates the R-Smad proteins (Massague and Chen 2000). The final Smad complex is formed when these Smad proteins complex with co-Smad and Smad 4, and it then translocates into the nucleus to regulate the tran-scription of downstream target genes with some cofactors (Chen and Xu 2011). In addition to TGF-β/Smad signaling, non-Smad pathways also participate in TGF-β signaling. For example, MAPKs, including ERK, p38 and JNK, phosphatidylinositol 3-kinase (PI3-K)/Akt, and small GTPases, can be activated by TGF-β (Moustakas and Heldin 2005; Huang and Chen 2012).

Epithelial-to-mesenchymal transition (EMT) enables polarized epithelial cells to adopt a mesen-chymal cell phenotype and an increased migratory and invasiveness capacity (Massague and Chen 2000). TGF-β signaling has been shown to be a major modulator of angiogenesis via the regulation of endothelial cell proliferation, EMT, and ECM metabolism. During the early stages of carcino-genesis, TGF-β inhibits angiogenesis and tumor cell growth, but in advanced tumors, TGF-β accel-erates disease progression. CD105 (endoglin) is a receptor for TGF-β1, and TGF-β3 is preferentially expressed in angiogenic vascular endothelial cells, especially the blood vessels of tumor tissues, which therefore makes it a promising vascular target for monitoring tumor growth and prognosis (Li et al. 2001; Duff et al. 2003). TGF-β1, CD105, and IL-6 have shown promise as biomarkers for the development of prostate cancer (Shariat et al. 2011).

Some phytochemical compounds and several nonsteroidal anti-inflammatory drugs (NSAIDs) have been associated with a lower cancer risk. Genistein, retinoids, and resveratrol were shown to inhibit prometastatic cell detachment, migration, and invasion, and TGF-β is one of the major mech-anisms that is targeted by these compounds (Li et al. 2000; Baek et al. 2005; Pavese et al. 2010).

Human macrophage–inhibitory cytokine-1 (MIC-1) belongs to the TGF-β superfamily and has also been designated as prostate-derived factor (PDF) or placental TGF-β (PTGF-β) (Mimeault and Batra 2010). MIC-1 regulates cellular stress; immune responses; and cell proliferation, dif-ferentiation, survival, migration, and invasion (Paralkar et al. 1998; Ding et al. 2009). In general, MIC-1 displays antitumorigenic activities in the early stages of cancer development (Bootcov et al. 1997; Hromas et al. 1997; Xu et al. 2006; Zimmers et al. 2006). In numerous cancers, such as brain cancer; melanoma; oral squamous cell carcinoma; and lung, thyroid, gastrointestinal, colorectal, pancreatic, prostate, breast, and cervical epithelial cancers, increased MIC-1 expression levels have been frequently observed, and these have also been associated with poor outcome and reduced patient survival (Karan et al. 2003; Lee et al. 2003; Nakamura et al. 2003; Brown et al. 2009; Koopmann et al. 2004; Rasiah et al. 2006; Chen et al. 2007; Shnaper et al. 2009; Zhang et al. 2009; Zhao et al. 2009; Cheung et al. 2004), which suggests that MIC-1 could be used as a biomarker for cancer progression. When combined with other biomarkers, such as allelic histidine 6-to-aspartate (H6D) polymorphic variations, MIC-1 was shown to independently predict the occurrence of cancer (Brown et al. 2003). Serum MIC-1 levels in combination with prostate-specific antigen (PSA) levels have also been shown to significantly improve diagnostic specificity (Brown et al. 2006). These results suggest that MIC-1 in combination with other cancer type-specific biomarkers may be beneficial for earlier and more accurate clinical cancer diagnoses (Mimeault and Batra 2010).

Decoy receptor 3 (DcR3), which is also known as tumor necrosis factor receptor (TNFR) superfamily member 6b (TNFRSF6B)/TR6/M68 (Pitti et al. 1998), is induced in the presence of inflammation (Fayad et al. 2006; Migone et al. 2002). In response to lipopolysaccharide (LPS) or TNF stimulation, NF-κB is activated, which is essential for the survival of intestinal epithelial cells and human pancreatic cancer cells (Funke et al. 2009). In addition, the activation of ERK1/2, JNK, Src-like protein tyrosine kinases, and PI3-K contributes to DcR3 release from human intestinal epithelial cell lines (Kim et al. 2005). Soluble DcR3 suppresses FasL-induced apoptosis and chemotaxis to evade cytotoxic attack via inhibition of the FasL–Fas interaction, which induces apoptosis (Roth et al. 2001; Green 1998). DcR3 is highly expressed in the lung and colon as well as many other malignant tissues (Macher-Goeppinger et al. 2008). In patients with oral cavity cancer, elevated serum DcR3 levels have been associated with nodal metastasis and a worse prognosis (Tu et al. 2011). Moreover, increased DcR3 copy numbers are common in recurrent oral tumors, glioblastoma, and gastric adenocarcinoma (Tu et al. 2011; Arakawa et al. 2005; Buffart et al. 2009), which suggests that DcR3 may serve as an important biomarker for staging differentiation, metastasis, and carcinoma (Lin and Hsieh 2011).

6.5 PM PROTEIN–ASSOCIATED BIOMARKERS

The PM is an organized biological system that serves as a structural barrier and communication interface with the extracellular environment (Harvey et al. 2001). The proteins associated with the PM mediate cell proliferation, adhesion, and migration, and alterations to the PM are associated with malignant transformation (Gschwind et al. 2004). For example, the increased expression of certain receptors, such as human epidermal growth factor receptor 2 (HER2), can contribute to tumor cell growth following activation by circulating or locally produced ligands or via the downregulation of certain adhesion molecules that enable the cells to detach from the primary tumor and spread (Swanton et al. 2006). These PM proteins may be subject to posttranslational modifications, such as altered phosphorylation or glycosylation (Leth-Larsen et al. 2010). While glycosylation is the most common form of posttranslational modification (occurring on 50% of all proteins), Asn (N)– and Thr/Ser (O)–linked glycans and proteoglycans (PGs) are the most frequently observed alterations in cancer cells (Apweiler et al. 1999). PGs are macromolecules that are located in basement membranes and composed of a specific core protein, which can be substituted with covalently linked glycosaminoglycan (GAG) chains termed chondroitin sulfate (CS), dermatan sulfate (DS), keratan sulfate, heparin, and heparan sulfate (HS). PGs can be divided into three main groups according to their cellular localization: extracellular, secreted molecules; cell surface molecules; and intracellular molecules (Iozzo 1998). Abnormal expression or deregulated function of these PGs can affect cancer progression and angiogenesis, and these steps are critical for the evolution of the tumor microenvironment (Iozzo et al. 2009). During carcinogenesis, the cell growth of malignant cells can be enhanced by secreted soluble growth factors. PG expression is markedly modified in the tumor microenvironment, which thereby affects the growth, survival, adhesion, migration, and angiogenesis of cancer cells. The type and organization of the structure of the GAG chains attached to PGs are markedly affected during malignant transformation as a result of the altered expression of GAG-synthesizing enzymes (Gschwind et al. 2004). Thus, proteomic analysis of these proteins would be useful in identifying biomarkers for early tumor detection, cancer prognosis, and prediction of the treatment response (Apweiler et al. 1999).

YKL-40 is a 40 kDa secreted human glycoprotein that was discovered over a decade ago (Johansen et al. 1992), and YKL-40 levels in the serum were shown to be significantly higher in some patients with various forms of inflammatory and degenerative joint disease (Johansen et al. 1993). YKL-40 is produced by cancer cells and tumor-associated macrophages, and its expression is associated with inflammation, cell proliferation, differentiation, protection against apoptosis, stimulation of angiogenesis, and regulation of the remodeling of the ECM surrounding the tumor (Kazakova and Sarafian 2009). Although there is insufficient evidence to support its value outside of clinical trials as a screening tool in the routine management of individual patients with cancer or diseases characterized by inflammation, elevated plasma YKL-40 levels have been shown to act as an independent prognostic biomarker of short survival (Johansen et al. 2009). YKL-40 has been shown to be a serum biomarker of prognosis in 13 different types of cancer and more than 2500 patients, and the highest serum levels of YKL-40 have been detected in patients with metastatic cancer and the shortest recurrence-free time intervals and shortest overall survival periods. YKL-40 measurements provide additional information in comparison to the use of other biomarkers, such as HER2, carcinoembryonic antigen, CA125, PSA, and lactate dehydrogenase, which supports its potential role as a cancer therapeutic target (Johansen et al. 2007).

The terminal laminin-like globular (LG3) domain of endorepellin is an antiangiogenesis factor. During tissue remodeling and cancer growth, endorepellin/LG3 is liberated via partial proteolysis by bone morphogenic protein-1 (BMP-1), which thereby represents an additional layer of control for angiogenesis (Iozzo et al. 2009). The plasma level of the endorepellin/LG3 fragment was found to be significantly lower in breast cancer patients as compared to healthy donors, which suggests that reduced titers of this molecule may serve as a useful biomarker of cancer progression and invasion (Chang et al. 2008; Theocharis et al. 2010).

6.6 CANCER BIOMARKERS IN VARIOUS TISSUES

6.6.1 Prostate Cancer Biomarkers

Based on case-control and cohort studies of prostate cancer patients, PSA is a common biomarker, and it is the most successful and widely used cancer serum marker to date (Linton and Hamdy 2003; van Leeuwen et al. 2010). The widespread use of PSA testing was demonstrated in a randomized, controlled trial, which found that PSA testing reduced prostate cancer (PCa) mortality (Schroder et al. 2009) due to earlier detection resulting in decreased prostate cancer mortality and a decline in metastatic disease (Albertsen 2002). However, PSA may not be a prostate cancer–specific biomarker because it has demonstrated unproven efficacy for affecting PCa outcomes. PSA levels above 10 ng/mL reflect a high probability of prostate cancer, while PSA levels between 4 and 10 ng/mL are considered to be in the diagnostic "gray zone" (Punglia et al. 2003). Furthermore, statins are known to reduce PSA levels, which can delay the decision for a prostate biopsy and subsequent PCa diagnosis. Consequently, patients who had been prescribed a statin were more likely to adhere to medical treatments and supervision and therefore underwent more frequent PSA testing and received more PCa diagnoses (Simons et al. 2011; Papadopoulos et al. 2011). Chromogranin A (CgA) is an acidic glycoprotein that is commonly expressed by neuroendocrine cells and constitutes one of the most profuse components of secretary granules. When a tumor develops in an endocrine tissue, it becomes the main source of circulating CgA. Thus, in patients with lower PSA levels, CgA could be a useful predictive marker (Khan and Ather 2011; Mikolajczyk et al. 2004).

6.6.2 Lung Cancer Biomarkers

Small cell lung carcinoma (SCLC) displays neuroendocrine differentiation and is a particularly malignant form of lung cancer with a poor prognosis (Ischia et al. 2009). Neuron-specific enolase (NSE) has long been the recommended tumor marker for SCLC (Issa et al. 2005). Gastrin-releasing peptide (GRP) and its receptor GRP-R are predominantly distributed throughout the central nervous system and gastrointestinal tract, and they play an important role in a multitude of physiological functions, including exocrine and endocrine secretions (Jensen et al. 2008). GRP is rarely detected in the serum of patients with lung cancer, whereas larger C-terminal proGRP fragments are more stable in the circulation, and proGRP has been detected in the serum and tumors of patients with lung cancer (Yamaguchi et al. 1983). Serum concentrations of proGRP are elevated in 68%–86% of patients with SCLC as compared to only 4%–30% of non-SCLC patients, 0%–7% of patients with benign lung disease, and 0% of healthy controls (Holst et al. 1989; Molina et al. 2005). Thus, proGRP has emerged as an alternative marker with greater sensitivity and specificity than either NSE or the other neuroendocrine marker, CgA (Shibayama et al. 2001).

6.6.3 Ovarian Cancer Biomarkers

BRCA1 protein inactivation in sporadic OC is common, and low BRCA1 expression is linked to platinum sensitivity. In an analysis of 251 patients, BRCA1 was shown to be a prognostic marker in sporadic OC patients with minimal residual disease (RD) (Weberpals et al. 2011).

Ovarian cancer is the most lethal of all gynecological cancers among women. Serum CA125 is the only biomarker that is used routinely for these patients, and there is a need for further complementary biomarkers both in terms of sensitivity and specificity. N-Glycosylation changes in ovarian cancer serum glycoproteins include decreases in the galactosylation of immunoglobulin G (IgG) and increases in sialyl Lewis X [SLe(x)] changes to the haptoglobin beta-chain, alpha1-acid glycoprotein, and alpha1-antichymotrypsin (Saldova et al. 2008).

6.6.4 Breast Cancer Biomarkers

Overexpression of HER2 in a subset of breast cancers (HER2+) is associated with a high histological grade and aggressive clinical course. Using immunohistochemistry staining to screen a tissue array cohort, protein arginine methyltransferases 2A (PRMT2A) was strongly associated with an outcome in HER2+ patients, which supports the use of PRMT2A as a biomarker of increased risk of recurrence in HER2+ breast cancer patients (Hicks et al. 2010). The folate receptor (FR) has also emerged as an attractive tumor biomarker with the potential to be exploited for therapeutic purposes, as the FR is believed to be a useful biological target for disease management (Leamon and Jackman 2008).

6.7 BIOMARKERS AND CANCER PREVENTION

In general, when a molecular target signifies a carcinogenic process, it will likely serve as an effective biomarker. Recently, many chemopreventive compounds have been investigated, and these studies have revealed extensive effects on alterations of important molecular targets involved in the regulation of antioxidant, anti-inflammatory, cell growth, and proliferation pathways (Kelloff et al. 2006). Thus, molecular biomarkers could be used for all aspects of chemoprevention, including the identification and optimization of new agents, the evaluation of cancer risk, and the prediction of the effects of mechanism-based interventions (Kelloff et al. 2006). Examples of the use of dietary bioactive compounds as cancer chemoprevention agents and their target biomarkers are listed in Table 6.1.

TABLE 6.1

Examples of Dietary Bioactive Compounds as Cancer Chemoprevention Agents and Their Target Biomarkers

Dietary Bioactive Components	Source	Cancer Biomarker
Agaricus bisporus polysaccharides	*Agaricus bisporus*	CYP1B1 (Jeong et al. 2012); NF-κB (Volman et al. 2010)
Apigenin	Chamomile, apples, celery, basil, parsley, onions, oranges, tea, wheat sprouts, endives, and cloves	IL-6 (Lamy et al. 2012); CD40L (Kawai et al. 2007); HER2 (Mafuvadze et al. 2012; Seo et al. 2012); NF-κB (Liao et al. 2012; Seo et al. 2012)
Astaxanthin	Microalgae, yeast, salmon, trout, shrimp, and other crustaceans	IL-6 (Yasui et al. 2011); NF-κB (Yasui et al. 2011; Nagendraprabhu et al. 2011)
Caffeic acid	Asparagus, cabbage, coffee, olives, olive oil, spinach, white grapes, and white wine	PSA (Zhao et al. 2001); NF-κB (Lin et al. 2012)
Caffeine	Tea leaves, coffee, cocoa beans, and kola nut	8-Nitroguanine (Castro et al. 2008); serum CA125 (Pauler et al. 2001); NF-κB (Ravi et al. 2008; Ahmed et al. 2009)
Catechin	Apple juice, black tea, cocoa, grapes, green tea, and wine	PSA (Zhao et al. 2001)
Carnosol	Rosemary	CYP1B1 (Johnson et al. 2010); NF-κB (Huang et al. 2005)
Chrysoeriol	Parsley	8-Nitroguanine (Takemura et al. 2010)
Conjugated linoleic acids	Eggs, meat and dairy products, safflower oil, and some mushrooms such as *Agaricus bisporus* and *Agaricus subrufescens*	CYP1B1 (Lee et al. 2006); HER2 (Flowers et al. 2009); NF-κB (Martinasso et al. 2010)
Curcumin	Turmeric (*Curcuma longa*)	MIC-1 (Prakobwong et al. 2011; Pinlaor et al. 2009); 8-nitroguanine (Walle et al. 2007); CYP1B1 (Kubota et al. 2012; Tu et al. 2012); CD40L (Belcaro et al. 2010); HER2 (Sun et al. 2012); NF-κB (Kim et al. 2012)
Delphinidin	Cranberries, grapes, and pomegranates	IL-6 (Lamy et al. 2012); HER2 (Ozbay et al. 2011); NF-κB (Bin Hafeez et al. 2008)
3,3′-Diindolylmethane (DIM)	Cruciferous vegetables such as broccoli, cabbage, brussels sprouts, and kale	NF-κB (Wang et al. 2012; Smith et al. 2008)
Dithiolethiones	Broccoli, brussels sprouts, cabbage, and cauliflower	8-Nitroguanine (Switzer et al. 2012); NF-κB (Switzer et al. 2012)
Ellagic acid	Grapes, peach, blackberries, cranberries, pomegranates, raspberries, strawberries, pecans, and walnuts	NF-κB (Umesalma et al. 2010); IL-6 (Vidya Priyadarsini et al. 2012; Anitha et al. 2011)
Epicatechin	Apple juice, black tea, cocoa, grapes, green tea, and wine	NF-κB (Zhao et al. 2001); CD40L (Oyama et al. 2010)
EGCG	Green tea	8-Nitroguanine (Baek et al. 2004); MIC-1 (Gasmi et al. 2010); PSA (Lamy et al. 2012); CD40L (Oyama et al. 2010); HER2 (Shimizu et al. 2008; Puig et al. 2008; Pan et al. 2007); NF-κB (Zhang et al. 2012)

(continued)

TABLE 6.1 (Continued)

Examples of Dietary Bioactive Compounds as Cancer Chemoprevention Agents and Their Target Biomarkers

Dietary Bioactive Components	Source	Cancer Biomarker
n-3 fatty acids	Fish and fish oil, eggs, meat, brown algae, and plant sources such as kiwifruit and flaxseed	PSA (Finocchiaro et al. 2012; van der Meij et al. 2010); CRP (Alfano et al. 2012; de Luis et al. 2008; Finocchiaro et al. 2012); CD40L (Alessandri et al. 2006; Aarsetoy et al. 2006); MMP8 (El-Sharkawy et al. 2010; Vardar-Sengul et al. 2008); BRCA1 (Jourdan et al. 2007); HER2 (Menendez et al. 2006); NF-κB (Cavazos et al. 2011)
Fisetin	Apples, grapes, strawberries, and onions	PSA (Khan et al. 2008); CD40L (Oyama et al. 2010); NF-κB (Liao et al. 2009)
Genistein	Soy, alfalfa sprouts, chickpeas, peanuts, and other legumes	8-Nitroguanine (Smith et al. 2008); MMP8 (Kim et al. 2002, 2001); BRCA1 (Fan et al. 2006); HER2 (Sakla et al. 2007; Mai et al. 2007); NF-κB (Pan et al. 2012)
Indole-3-carbinol (I3C)	Cruciferous vegetables such as broccoli, brussels sprouts, cabbage, and cauliflower	PSA (Wang et al. 2012); BRCA1 (Fan et al. 2006); NF-κB (Aronchik et al. 2010)
Kaempferol	Apples, grapes, grapefruit, strawberries, tomato, tea, beans, broccoli, brussels sprouts, cabbage, endive, and leek	IL-6 (Bobe et al. 2010); NF-κB (Yang et al. 2010)
Luteolin	Camomile tea, carrots, celery, green pepper, navel oranges, olive oil, peppermint, perilla, rosemary, and thyme	PSA (Lamy et al. 2012); CD40L (Hirano et al. 2006); HER2 (Chiang et al. 2007); NF-κB (Chen et al. 2012)
Lycopene	Papayas, red bell peppers, red carrots, tomatoes, and watermelons	IL-6 (Zhang, Wang et al. 2010; Vaishampayan et al. 2007); NF-κB (Palozza et al. 2010)
Nobiletin	Citrus peels such as in tangerine	8-Nitroguanine (Miyamoto et al. 2008); NF-κB (Lee et al. 2011)
Punicic acid	Pomegranate seed oil	CYP1B1 (Gasmi et al. 2010)
Quercetin	Apples, beans, buckwheat, cranberries, tea, wine, and red and yellow onions	PSA (Walle et al. 2007); CYP1B1 (Zhao et al. 2001); CD40L (Pignatelli et al. 2005); NF-κB (Priyadarsini et al. 2012)
Resveratrol	Red wine and grape juice, grape skins and seeds, nuts, and peanuts	NF-κB (Boddicker et al. 2011; Mbimba et al. 2012; Li et al. 2007); IL-6 (Kai et al. 2011; Wang et al. 2010); CD40L (Gocmen et al. 2011); YKL-40 (Zhang, Murao et al. 2010); CgA (Pinchot et al. 2011; Truong et al. 2011); BRCA1 (Papoutsis et al. 2010, 2012)
Sulforaphane	Cruciferous vegetables such as broccoli, brussels sprouts, and cabbages	IL-6 (Chan et al. 2008); NF-κB (Hamsa et al. 2011)

Cyclooxygenase 2 (COX2) is used as a biomarker of the inflammatory response to growth factors that are overexpressed in many cancers and precancers regulated by NF-κB (Anderson et al. 2002; Dannenberg and Subbaramaiah 2003; Subbaramaiah and Dannenberg 2003; Davis and Milner 2007). Inhibitors targeting COX2, such as aspirin and NSAIDs, have shown chemopreventive efficacy in both epidemiologic analyses and clinical studies (Kelloff 2000). In a colorectal cancer prevention trial, treatment with celecoxib, a selective COX2 inhibitor, was shown to significantly reduce the number of colorectal polyps (Steinbach et al. 2000).

The epidermal growth factor receptor (EGFR) is critical for prostate tumor growth; for example, when androgen is withdrawn, prostate tissue becomes more susceptible to the growth-promoting actions of epidermal growth factor (EGF)–family growth factors (Sherwood et al. 1998). Pretreatment of prostate cells with curcumin and beta-phenylethyl isothiocyanate (PEITC) dramatically suppressed EGFR phosphorylations (Y845 and Y1068), thereby inhibiting the downstream phosphorylation of IκBα and Akt (Ser473 and Thr308) and contributing to the anticancer effects of these compounds (Kim et al. 2006). The Selenium and Vitamin E Cancer Prevention Trial (SELECT) is a large-scale National Cancer Institute (NCI)-supported prostate cancer prevention trial that was conducted between July 2001 and June 2004 in the United States, and this trial provided a biorepository designed for future research (Lippman et al. 2005). In addition, inflammatory markers, such as iNOS, COX2, and prostaglandin E2 (PGE_2), have been associated with numerous pathological conditions including chronic inflammation and cancer (Rose et al. 2005). Moreover, combined treatment with SFN and PEITC or curcumin synergistically inhibited nitric oxide (NO) expression in LPS-stimulated RAW 264.7 cells as well as the expression levels of iNOS, TNFα, and IL-1 (Cheung et al. 2009).

For breast cancer, histological information concerning atypical ductal hyperplasia and carcinoma and BRCA1 or BRCA2 mutations provides targets for chemopreventive interventions, and BRCA1/2 testing has been shown to have a favorable effect on breast and ovarian cancer outcomes (Schwartz et al. 2012).

6.8   CONCLUSIONS AND PERSPECTIVES

Biomarkers that can differentiate between healthy and cancerous individuals can provide useful information for chemopreventive studies. Therefore, it is necessary to identify specific biomarkers that demonstrate predictive value in cancer prevention and treatment. Because the biological processes involved in carcinogenesis are complex and dietary bioactive components may affect more than one mechanism, integrated approaches such as nutrigenomics, epigenomics, transcriptomics, proteomics, and metabolomics will provide important clues about the specific target molecules or events that may be influenced by diet. In addition, interactions between different bioactive components in a food may result in numerous biological effects. For biomarkers identified on the basis of in vitro results, it is also important to verify the mechanisms of dietary active components in appropriate animal models and human samples.

REFERENCES

Aarsetoy, H., T. Brugger-Andersen, O. Hetland, H. Grundt, and D. W. Nilsen. 2006. Long term influence of regular intake of high dose n-3 fatty acids on CD40-ligand, pregnancy-associated plasma protein A and matrix metalloproteinase-9 following acute myocardial infarction. *Thromb Haemost* 95 (2):329–36.

Aggarwal, B. B., S. Shishodia, S. K. Sandur, M. K. Pandey, and G. Sethi. 2006. Inflammation and cancer: how hot is the link? *Biochem Pharmacol* 72 (11):1605–21.

Ahmed, K. M., D. Nantajit, M. Fan et al. 2009. Coactivation of ATM/ERK/NF-kappaB in the low-dose radiation-induced radioadaptive response in human skin keratinocytes. *Free Radic Biol Med* 46 (11):1543–50.

Albertsen, P. C. 2002. Prostate cancer mortality after introduction of prostate-specific antigen mass screening in the Federal State of Tyrol, Austria. *J Urol* 168 (2):880–1.

Alessandri, C., P. Pignatelli, L. Loffredo et al. 2006. Alpha-linolenic acid-rich wheat germ oil decreases oxidative stress and CD40 ligand in patients with mild hypercholesterolemia. *Arterioscler Thromb Vasc Biol* 26 (11):2577–8.

Alfano, C. M., I. Imayama, M. L. Neuhouser et al. 2012. Fatigue, inflammation, and omega-3 and omega-6 fatty acid intake among breast cancer survivors. *J Clin Oncol* 30 (12):1280–7.

Allin, K. H., and B. G. Nordestgaard. 2011. Elevated C-reactive protein in the diagnosis, prognosis, and cause of cancer. *Crit Rev Clin Lab Sci* 48 (4):155–70.

Amann, T., U. Maegdefrau, A. Hartmann et al. 2009. GLUT1 expression is increased in hepatocellular carcinoma and promotes tumorigenesis. *Am J Pathol* 174 (4):1544–52.

Ambrosone, C. B., J. L. Freudenheim, P. A. Thompson et al. 1999. Manganese superoxide dismutase (MnSOD) genetic polymorphisms, dietary antioxidants, and risk of breast cancer. *Cancer Res* 59 (3):602–6.

Anderson, W. F., A. Umar, J. L. Viner, and E. T. Hawk. 2002. The role of cyclooxygenase inhibitors in cancer prevention. *Curr Pharm Des* 8 (12):1035–62.

Anitha, P., R. V. Priyadarsini, K. Kavitha, P. Thiyagarajan, and S. Nagini. 2011. Ellagic acid coordinately attenuates Wnt/beta-catenin and NF-kappaB signaling pathways to induce intrinsic apoptosis in an animal model of oral oncogenesis. *Eur J Nutr* 52:75–84.

Apweiler, R., H. Hermjakob, and N. Sharon. 1999. On the frequency of protein glycosylation, as deduced from analysis of the SWISS-PROT database. *Biochim Biophys Acta* 1473 (1):4–8.

Aronchik, I., L. F. Bjeldanes, and G. L. Firestone. 2010. Direct inhibition of elastase activity by indole-3-carbinol triggers a CD40-TRAF regulatory cascade that disrupts NF-kappaB transcriptional activity in human breast cancer cells. *Cancer Research* 70 (12):4961–71.

Arakawa, Y., O. Tachibana, M. Hasegawa et al. 2005. Frequent gene amplification and overexpression of decoy receptor 3 in glioblastoma. *Acta Neuropathol* 109 (3):294–8.

Austin, J., and A. H. Holway. 2011. Contact printing of protein microarrays. *Methods Mol Biol* 785:379–94.

Baek, S. J., J. S. Kim, F. R. Jackson et al. 2004. Epicatechin gallate-induced expression of NAG-1 is associated with growth inhibition and apoptosis in colon cancer cells. *Carcinogenesis* 25 (12):2425–32.

Baek, S. J., J. S. Kim, S. M. Moore et al. 2005. Cyclooxygenase inhibitors induce the expression of the tumor suppressor gene EGR-1, which results in the up-regulation of NAG-1, an antitumorigenic protein. *Mol Pharmacol* 67 (2):356–64.

Balbin, M., A. Fueyo, A. M. Tester et al. 2003. Loss of collagenase-2 confers increased skin tumor susceptibility to male mice. *Nat Genet* 35 (3):252–7.

Balkwill, F., and A. Mantovani. 2001. Inflammation and cancer: back to Virchow? *Lancet* 357 (9255):539–45.

Baltimore, D., M. P. Boldin, R. M. O'Connell, D. S. Rao, and K. D. Taganov. 2008. MicroRNAs: new regulators of immune cell development and function. *Nat Immunol* 9 (8):839–45.

Bannister, A. J., P. Zegerman, J. F. Partridge et al. 2001. Selective recognition of methylated lysine 9 on histone H3 by the HP1 chromo domain. *Nature* 410 (6824):120–4.

Bartsch, H., K. Arab, and J. Nair. 2011. Biomarkers for hazard identification in humans. *Environ Health* 10 Suppl 1:S11.

Baylin, S. B., and J. G. Herman. 2000. DNA hypermethylation in tumorigenesis: epigenetics joins genetics. *Trends Genet* 16 (4):168–74.

Belcaro, G., M. R. Cesarone, M. Dugall et al. 2010. Efficacy and safety of Meriva(R), a curcumin-phosphatidylcholine complex, during extended administration in osteoarthritis patients. *Altern Med Rev* 15 (4):337–44.

Berger, S. L. 2007. The complex language of chromatin regulation during transcription. *Nature* 447 (7143): 407–12.

Berlowitz, L., and D. Pallotta. 1972. Acetylation of nuclear protein in the heterochromatin and euchromatin of mealy bugs. *Exp Cell Res* 71 (1):45–8.

Bin Hafeez, B., M. Asim, I. A. Siddiqui et al. 2008. Delphinidin, a dietary anthocyanidin in pigmented fruits and vegetables: a new weapon to blunt prostate cancer growth. *Cell Cycle* 7 (21):3320–6.

Bird, A. 2002. DNA methylation patterns and epigenetic memory. *Genes Dev* 16 (1):6–21.

Bobe, G., P. S. Albert, L. B. Sansbury et al. 2010. Interleukin-6 as a potential indicator for prevention of high-risk adenoma recurrence by dietary flavonols in the polyp prevention trial. *Cancer Prev Res (Phila)* 3 (6):764–75.

Boddicker, R. L., E. M. Whitley, J. E. Davis, D. F. Birt, and M. E. Spurlock. 2011. Low-dose dietary resveratrol has differential effects on colorectal tumorigenesis in adiponectin knockout and wild-type mice. *Nutr Cancer* 63 (8):1328–38.

Bollard, M. E., E. G. Stanley, J. C. Lindon, J. K. Nicholson, and E. Holmes. 2005. NMR-based metabonomic approaches for evaluating physiological influences on biofluid composition. *NMR Biomed* 18 (3):143–62.

Bootcov, M. R., A. R. Bauskin, S. M. Valenzuela et al. 1997. MIC-1, a novel macrophage inhibitory cytokine, is a divergent member of the TGF-beta superfamily. *Proc Natl Acad Sci U S A* 94 (21):11514–9.

Brown, D. A., F. Lindmark, P. Stattin et al. 2009. Macrophage inhibitory cytokine 1: a new prognostic marker in prostate cancer. *Clin Cancer Res* 15 (21):6658–64.

Brown, D. A., C. Stephan, R. L. Ward et al. 2006. Measurement of serum levels of macrophage inhibitory cytokine 1 combined with prostate-specific antigen improves prostate cancer diagnosis. *Clin Cancer Res* 12 (1):89–96.

Brown, D. A., R. L. Ward, P. Buckhaults et al. 2003. MIC-1 serum level and genotype: associations with progress and prognosis of colorectal carcinoma. *Clin Cancer Res* 9 (7):2642–50.

Brusselmans, K., R. Vrolix, G. Verhoeven, and J. V. Swinnen. 2005. Induction of cancer cell apoptosis by flavonoids is associated with their ability to inhibit fatty acid synthase activity. *J Biol Chem* 280 (7):5636–45.

Buffart, T. E., N. C. van Grieken, M. Tijssen et al. 2009. High resolution analysis of DNA copy-number aberrations of chromosomes 8, 13, and 20 in gastric cancers. *Virchows Arch* 455 (3):213–23.

Cao, H., J. F. Urban, Jr., and R. A. Anderson. 2008. Cinnamon polyphenol extract affects immune responses by regulating anti- and proinflammatory and glucose transporter gene expression in mouse macrophages. *J Nutr* 138 (5):833–40.

Cao, H., I. Hininger-Favier, M. A. Kelly et al. 2007. Green tea polyphenol extract regulates the expression of genes involved in glucose uptake and insulin signaling in rats fed a high fructose diet. *J Agric Food Chem* 55 (15):6372–8.

Cargill, M., D. Altshuler, J. Ireland et al. 1999. Characterization of single-nucleotide polymorphisms in coding regions of human genes. *Nat Genet* 22 (3):231–8.

Carleton, M., M. A. Cleary, and P. S. Linsley. 2007. MicroRNAs and cell cycle regulation. *Cell Cycle* 6 (17):2127–32.

Castro, D. J., Z. Yu, C. V. Lohr et al. 2008. Chemoprevention of dibenzo[a,l]pyrene transplacental carcinogenesis in mice born to mothers administered green tea: primary role of caffeine. *Carcinogenesis* 29 (8):1581–6.

Cavazos, D. A., R. S. Price, S. S. Apte, and L. A. deGraffenried. 2011. Docosahexaenoic acid selectively induces human prostate cancer cell sensitivity to oxidative stress through modulation of NF-kappaB. *Prostate* 71 (13):1420–8.

Chan, C., H. J. Lin, and J. Lin. 2008. Stress-associated hormone, norepinephrine, increases proliferation and IL-6 levels of human pancreatic duct epithelial cells and can be inhibited by the dietary agent, sulforaphane. *Int J Oncol* 33 (2):415–9.

Chan, E. C., P. K. Koh, M. Mal et al. 2009. Metabolic profiling of human colorectal cancer using high-resolution magic angle spinning nuclear magnetic resonance (HR-MAS NMR) spectroscopy and gas chromatography mass spectrometry (GC/MS). *J Proteome Res* 8 (1):352–61.

Chang, J. W., U. B. Kang, D. H. Kim et al. 2008. Identification of circulating endorepellin LG3 fragment: potential use as a serological biomarker for breast cancer. *Proteomics Clin Appl* 2 (1):23–32.

Chen, S. J., D. Karan, S. L. Johansson et al. 2007. Prostate-derived factor as a paracrine and autocrine factor for the proliferation of androgen receptor-positive human prostate cancer cells. *Prostate* 67 (5): 557–71.

Chen, S. S., A. Michael, and S. A. Butler-Manuel. 2012. Advances in the treatment of ovarian cancer: a potential role of antiinflammatory phytochemicals. *Discov Med* 13 (68):7–17.

Chen, X., and L. Xu. 2011. Mechanism and regulation of nucleocytoplasmic trafficking of smad. *Cell Biosci* 1 (1):40.

Cheung, K. L., T. O. Khor, and A. N. Kong. 2009. Synergistic effect of combination of phenethyl isothiocyanate and sulforaphane or curcumin and sulforaphane in the inhibition of inflammation. *Pharm Res* 26 (1):224–31.

Cheung, P. K., B. Woolcock, H. Adomat et al. 2004. Protein profiling of microdissected prostate tissue links growth differentiation factor 15 to prostate carcinogenesis. *Cancer Res* 64 (17):5929–33.

Chiang, C. T., T. D. Way, and J. K. Lin. 2007. Sensitizing HER2-overexpressing cancer cells to luteolin-induced apoptosis through suppressing p21(WAF1/CIP1) expression with rapamycin. *Mol Cancer Ther* 6 (7):2127–38.

Choi, J. S., H. Kim, M. H. Jung, S. Hong, and J. Song. 2010. Consumption of barley beta-glucan ameliorates fatty liver and insulin resistance in mice fed a high-fat diet. *Mol Nutr Food Res* 54 (7):1004–13.

Claudino, W. M., A. Quattrone, L. Biganzoli et al. 2007. Metabolomics: available results, current research projects in breast cancer, and future applications. *J Clin Oncol* 25 (19):2840–6.

Coventry, B. J., M. L. Ashdown, M. A. Quinn et al. 2009. CRP identifies homeostatic immune oscillations in cancer patients: a potential treatment targeting tool? *J Transl Med* 7:102.

Croce, C. M. 2009. Causes and consequences of microRNA dysregulation in cancer. *Nat Rev Genet* 10 (10):704–14.

Danesh, J., and M. B. Pepys. 2000. C-reactive protein in healthy and in sick populations. *Eur Heart J* 21 (19):1564–5.

Danesh, J., J. G. Wheeler, G. M. Hirschfield et al. 2004. C-reactive protein and other circulating markers of inflammation in the prediction of coronary heart disease. *N Engl J Med* 350 (14):1387–97.

Dannenberg, A. J., and K. Subbaramaiah. 2003. Targeting cyclooxygenase-2 in human neoplasia: rationale and promise. *Cancer Cell* 4 (6):431–6.

Davis, C. D., and J. A. Milner. 2007. Biomarkers for diet and cancer prevention research: potentials and challenges. *Acta Pharmacol Sin* 28 (9):1262–73.

de Luis, D. A., O. Izaola, R. Aller et al. 2008. Influence of a W3 fatty acids oral enhanced formula in clinical and biochemical parameters of head and neck cancer ambulatory patients. *An Med Interna* 25 (6):275–8.

Dejonckheere, E., R. E. Vandenbroucke, and C. Libert. 2011. Matrix metalloproteinase8 has a central role in inflammatory disorders and cancer progression. *Cytokine Growth Factor Rev* 22 (2):73–81.

Ding, Q., T. Mracek, P. Gonzalez-Muniesa et al. 2009. Identification of macrophage inhibitory cytokine-1 in adipose tissue and its secretion as an adipokine by human adipocytes. *Endocrinology* 150 (4):1688–96.

Dinkova-Kostova, A. T., W. D. Holtzclaw, R. N. Cole et al. 2002. Direct evidence that sulfhydryl groups of Keap1 are the sensors regulating induction of phase 2 enzymes that protect against carcinogens and oxidants. *Proc Natl Acad Sci U S A* 99 (18):11908–13.

Dong, Y., H. Zhang, L. Hawthorn, H. E. Ganther, and C. Ip. 2003. Delineation of the molecular basis for selenium-induced growth arrest in human prostate cancer cells by oligonucleotide array. *Cancer Res* 63 (1):52–9.

Dong, Y., H. E. Ganther, C. Stewart, and C. Ip. 2002. Identification of molecular targets associated with selenium-induced growth inhibition in human breast cells using cDNA microarrays. *Cancer Res* 62 (3):708–14.

Ducasse, M., and M. A. Brown. 2006. Epigenetic aberrations and cancer. *Molec Cancer* 5:60.

Duff, S. E., C. Li, J. M. Garland, and S. Kumar. 2003. CD105 is important for angiogenesis: evidence and potential applications. *FASEB J* 17 (9):984–92.

El-Sharkawy, H., N. Aboelsaad, M. Eliwa et al. 2010. Adjunctive treatment of chronic periodontitis with daily dietary supplementation with omega-3 Fatty acids and low-dose aspirin. *J Periodontol* 81 (11):1635–43.

Ellis, L., P. W. Atadja, and R. W. Johnstone. 2009. Epigenetics in cancer: targeting chromatin modifications. *Mol Cancer Ther* 8 (6):1409–20.

Esteller, M. 2008. Epigenetics in cancer. *N Engl J Med* 358 (11):1148–59.

Esteller, M. 2007. Epigenetic gene silencing in cancer: the DNA hypermethylome. *Hum Mol Genet* 16 Spec No 1:R50–9.

Esteller, M. 2005. Aberrant DNA methylation as a cancer-inducing mechanism. *Annu Rev Pharmacol Toxicol* 45:629–56.

Esteller, M. 2002. CpG island hypermethylation and tumor suppressor genes: a booming present, a brighter future. *Oncogene* 21 (35):5427–40.

Fan, S., Q. Meng, K. Auborn, T. Carter, and E. M. Rosen. 2006. BRCA1 and BRCA2 as molecular targets for phytochemicals indole-3-carbinol and genistein in breast and prostate cancer cells. *Br J Cancer* 94 (3):407–26.

Fayad, R., M. I. Brand, D. Stone, A. Keshavarzian, and L. Qiao. 2006. Apoptosis resistance in ulcerative colitis: high expression of decoy receptors by lamina propria T cells. *Eur J Immunol* 36 (8):2215–22.

Fenech, M., A. El-Sohemy, L. Cahill et al. 2011. Nutrigenetics and nutrigenomics: viewpoints on the current status and applications in nutrition research and practice. *J Nutrigenet Nutrigenomics* 4 (2):69–89.

Feng, Q., and Y. Zhang. 2001. The MeCP1 complex represses transcription through preferential binding, remodeling, and deacetylating methylated nucleosomes. *Genes Dev* 15 (7):827–32.

Ferguson, L. R. 2009. Nutrigenomics approaches to functional foods. *J Am Diet Assoc* 109 (3):452–8.

Ferroni, P., F. Santilli, F. Guadagni, S. Basili, and G. Davi. 2007. Contribution of platelet-derived CD40 ligand to inflammation, thrombosis and neoangiogenesis. *Curr Med Chem* 14 (20):2170–80.

Finocchiaro, C., O. Segre, M. Fadda et al. 2012. Effect of n-3 fatty acids on patients with advanced lung cancer: a double-blind, placebo-controlled study. *Br J Nutr* 108 (2):327–33.

Flowers, M., and P. A. Thompson. 2009. t10c12 conjugated linoleic acid suppresses HER2 protein and enhances apoptosis in SKBr3 breast cancer cells: possible role of COX2. *PLoS One* 4 (4):e5342.

Fritzsche, F. R., W. Weichert, A. Roske et al. 2008. Class I histone deacetylases 1, 2 and 3 are highly expressed in renal cell cancer. *BMC Cancer* 8:381.

Funke, B., F. Autschbach, S. Kim et al. 2009. Functional characterisation of decoy receptor 3 in Crohn's disease. *Gut* 58 (4):483–91.

Gasmi, J., and J. T. Sanderson. 2010. Growth inhibitory, antiandrogenic, and pro-apoptotic effects of punicic acid in LNCaP human prostate cancer cells. *J Agric Food Chem* 58:12149–56.

German, J. B., B. D. Hammock, and S. M. Watkins. 2005. Metabolomics: building on a century of biochemistry to guide human health. *Metabolomics* 1 (1):3–9.

Gnoni, G. V., and G. Paglialonga. 2009. Resveratrol inhibits fatty acid and triacylglycerol synthesis in rat hepatocytes. *Eur J Clin Invest* 39 (3):211–8.

Gocmen, A. Y., D. Burgucu, and S. Gumuslu. 2011. Effect of resveratrol on platelet activation in hypercholesterolemic rats: CD40-CD40L system as a potential target. *Appl Physiol Nutr Metab* 36 (3):323–30.

Gordon, K. J., and G. C. Blobe. 2008. Role of transforming growth factor-beta superfamily signaling pathways in human disease. *Biochim Biophys Acta* 1782 (4):197–228.

Gotoh, N., K. Nagao, S. Onoda et al. 2009. Effects of three different highly purified n-3 series highly unsaturated fatty acids on lipid metabolism in C57BL/KsJ-db/db mice. *J Agric Food Chem* 57 (22):11047–54.

Gras, R., M. Muller, E. Gasteiger et al. 1999. Improving protein identification from peptide mass fingerprinting through a parameterized multi-level scoring algorithm and an optimized peak detection. *Electrophoresis* 20 (18):3535–50.

Green, D. R. 1998. Apoptosis. Death deceiver. *Nature* 396 (6712):629–30.

Griffiths-Jones, S., R. J. Grocock, S. van Dongen, A. Bateman, and A. J. Enright. 2006. miRBase: microRNA sequences, targets and gene nomenclature. *Nucleic Acids Res* 34 (Database issue):D140–4.

Gschwind, A., O. M. Fischer, and A. Ullrich. 2004. The discovery of receptor tyrosine kinases: targets for cancer therapy. *Nat Rev Cancer* 4 (5):361–70.

Gutierrez-Fernandez, A., A. Fueyo, A. R. Folgueras et al. 2008. Matrix metalloproteinase-8 functions as a metastasis suppressor through modulation of tumor cell adhesion and invasion. *Cancer Res* 68 (8):2755–63.

Hamsa, T. P., P. Thejass, and G. Kuttan. 2011. Induction of apoptosis by sulforaphane in highly metastatic B16F-10 melanoma cells. *Drug Chem Toxicol* 34 (3):332–40.

Hanahan, D., and R. A. Weinberg. 2000. The hallmarks of cancer. *Cell* 100 (1):57–70.

Harvey, S., Y. Zhang, F. Landry, C. Miller, and J. W. Smith. 2001. Insights into a plasma membrane signature. *Physiol Genom* 5 (3):129–36.

Hause, R. J., H. D. Kim, K. K. Leung, and R. B. Jones. 2011. Targeted protein-omic methods are bridging the gap between proteomic and hypothesis-driven protein analysis approaches. *Expert Rev Proteomics* 8 (5):565–75.

He, Q. Y., T. T. Yip, M. Li, and J. F. Chiu. 2003. Proteomic analyses of arsenic-induced cell transformation with SELDI-TOF Protein Chip technology. *J Cell Biochem* 88 (1):1–8.

Heikkila, K., S. Ebrahim, and D. A. Lawlor. 2008. Systematic review of the association between circulating interleukin-6 (IL-6) and cancer. *Eur J Cancer* 44 (7):937–45.

Hendrich, B., and A. Bird. 1998. Identification and characterization of a family of mammalian methyl-CpG binding proteins. *Mol Cell Biol* 18 (11):6538–47.

Herman, J. G., and S. B. Baylin. 2003. Gene silencing in cancer in association with promoter hypermethylation. *N Engl J Med* 349 (21):2042–54.

Hicks, D. G., B. R. Janarthanan, R. Vardarajan et al. 2010. The expression of TRMT2A, a novel cell cycle regulated protein, identifies a subset of breast cancer patients with HER2 over-expression that are at an increased risk of recurrence. *BMC Cancer* 10:108.

Hirano, T., J. Arimitsu, S. Higa et al. 2006. Luteolin, a flavonoid, inhibits CD40 ligand expression by activated human basophils. *Int Arch Allergy Immunol* 140 (2):150–6.

Holst, J. J., M. Hansen, E. Bork, and T. W. Schwartz. 1989. Elevated plasma concentrations of C-flanking gastrin-releasing peptide in small-cell lung cancer. *J Clin Oncol* 7 (12):1831–8.

Hromas, R., M. Hufford, J. Sutton et al. 1997. PLAB, a novel placental bone morphogenetic protein. *Biochim Biophys Acta* 1354 (1):40–4.

Huang, F., and Y. G. Chen. 2012. Regulation of TGF-beta receptor activity. *Cell Biosci* 2:9.

Huang, S. C., C. T. Ho, S. Y. Lin-Shiau, and J. K. Lin. 2005. Carnosol inhibits the invasion of B16/F10 mouse melanoma cells by suppressing metalloproteinase-9 through down-regulating nuclear factor-kappa B and c-Jun. *Biochem Pharmacol* 69 (2):221–32.

Hulboy, D. L., L. A. Rudolph, and L. M. Matrisian. 1997. Matrix metalloproteinases as mediators of reproductive function. *Mol Hum Reprod* 3 (1):27–45.

Hussain, S. P., and C. C. Harris. 2007. Inflammation and cancer: an ancient link with novel potentials. *Int J Cancer* 121 (11):2373–80.

Il'yasova, D., L. H. Colbert, T. B. Harris et al. 2005. Circulating levels of inflammatory markers and cancer risk in the health aging and body composition cohort. *Cancer Epidemiol Biomarkers Prev* 14 (10):2413–8.

Iozzo, R. V. 1998. Matrix proteoglycans: from molecular design to cellular function. *Annu Rev Biochem* 67:609–52.

Iozzo, R. V., J. J. Zoeller, and A. Nystrom. 2009. Basement membrane proteoglycans: modulators Par Excellence of cancer growth and angiogenesis. *Mol Cells* 27 (5):503–13.

Ischia, J., O. Patel, A. Shulkes, and G. S. Baldwin. 2009. Gastrin-releasing peptide: different forms, different functions. *Biofactors* 35 (1):69–75.

Issa, J. P. 2002. Epigenetic variation and human disease. *J Nutr* 132 (8 Suppl):2388S–92S.

Issa, J. P., V. Gharibyan, J. Cortes et al. 2005. Phase II study of low-dose decitabine in patients with chronic myelogenous leukemia resistant to imatinib mesylate. *J Clin Oncol* 23 (17):3948–56.

Izzotti, A., G. A. Calin, V. E. Steele et al. 2010. Chemoprevention of cigarette smoke-induced alterations of MicroRNA expression in rat lungs. *Cancer Prev Res (Phila)* 3 (1):62–72.

Jackson, J. P., A. M. Lindroth, X. Cao, and S. E. Jacobsen. 2002. Control of CpNpG DNA methylation by the KRYPTONITE histone H3 methyltransferase. *Nature* 416 (6880):556–60.

Jensen, R. T., J. F. Battey, E. R. Spindel, and R. V. Benya. 2008. International Union of Pharmacology. LXVIII. Mammalian bombesin receptors: nomenclature, distribution, pharmacology, signaling, and functions in normal and disease states. *Pharmacol Rev* 60 (1):1–42.

Jenuwein, T., and C. D. Allis. 2001. Translating the histone code. *Science* 293 (5532):1074–80.

Jeong, S. C., S. R. Koyyalamudi, Y. T. Jeong, C. H. Song, and G. Pang. 2012. Macrophage immunomodulating and antitumor activities of polysaccharides isolated from Agaricus bisporus white button mushrooms. *J Med Food* 15 (1):58–65.

Jiang, W., Z. Zhu, and H. J. Thompson. 2003. Effect of energy restriction on cell cycle machinery in 1-methyl-1-nitrosourea-induced mammary carcinomas in rats. *Cancer Res* 63 (6):1228–34.

Johansen, J. S., N. A. Schultz, and B. V. Jensen. 2009. Plasma YKL-40: a potential new cancer biomarker? *Future Oncol* 5 (7):1065–82.

Johansen, J. S., B. V. Jensen, A. Roslind, and P. A. Price. 2007. Is YKL-40 a new therapeutic target in cancer? *Expert Opin Ther Targets* 11 (2):219–34.

Johansen, J. S., H. S. Jensen, and P. A. Price. 1993. A new biochemical marker for joint injury. Analysis of YKL-40 in serum and synovial fluid. *Br J Rheumatol* 32 (11):949–55.

Johansen, J. S., M. K. Williamson, J. S. Rice, and P. A. Price. 1992. Identification of proteins secreted by human osteoblastic cells in culture. *J Bone Miner Res* 7 (5):501–12.

Johnson, J. J., D. N. Syed, Y. Suh et al. 2010. Disruption of androgen and estrogen receptor activity in prostate cancer by a novel dietary diterpene carnosol: implications for chemoprevention. *Cancer Prev Res (Phila)* 3 (9):1112–23.

Jones, P. A., and S. B. Baylin. 2002. The fundamental role of epigenetic events in cancer. *Nat Rev Genet* 3 (6):415–28.

Jourdan, M. L., K. Maheo, A. Barascu et al. 2007. Increased BRCA1 protein in mammary tumours of rats fed marine omega-3 fatty acids. *Oncol Rep* 17 (4):713–9.

Kader, A. K., L. Shao, C. P. Dinney et al. 2006. Matrix metalloproteinase polymorphisms and bladder cancer risk. *Cancer Res* 66 (24):11644–8.

Kai, L., and A. S. Levenson. 2011. Combination of resveratrol and antiandrogen flutamide has synergistic effect on androgen receptor inhibition in prostate cancer cells. *Anticancer Res* 31 (10):3323–30.

Kai, Z. S., and A. E. Pasquinelli. 2010. MicroRNA assassins: factors that regulate the disappearance of miRNAs. *Nat Struct Mol Biol* 17 (1):5–10.

Kaput, J. 2008. Nutrigenomics research for personalized nutrition and medicine. *Curr Opin Biotechnol* 19 (2):110–20.

Karan, D., S. J. Chen, S. L. Johansson et al. 2003. Dysregulated expression of MIC-1/PDF in human prostate tumor cells. *Biochem Biophys Res Commun* 305 (3):598–604.

Kawai, M., T. Hirano, S. Higa et al. 2007. Flavonoids and related compounds as anti-allergic substances. *Allergol Int* 56 (2):113–23.

Kawanishi, S., and Y. Hiraku. 2006. Oxidative and nitrative DNA damage as biomarker for carcinogenesis with special reference to inflammation. *Antioxid Redox Signal* 8 (5–6):1047–58.

Kazakova, M. H., and V. S. Sarafian. 2009. YKL-40—a novel biomarker in clinical practice? *Folia Med (Plovdiv)* 51 (1):5–14.

Kelloff, G. J. 2000. Perspectives on cancer chemoprevention research and drug development. *Adv Cancer Res* 78:199–334.

Kelloff, G. J., and C. C. Sigman. 2012. Cancer biomarkers: selecting the right drug for the right patient. *Nat Rev Drug Discov* 11 (3):201–14.

Kelloff, G. J., S. M. Lippman, A. J. Dannenberg et al. 2006. Progress in chemoprevention drug development: the promise of molecular biomarkers for prevention of intraepithelial neoplasia and cancer—a plan to move forward. *Clin Cancer Res* 12 (12):3661–97.

Khan, M. O., and M. H. Ather. 2011. Chromogranin A—serum marker for prostate cancer. *J Pak Med Assoc* 61 (1):108–11.

Khan, N., M. Asim, F. Afaq, M. Abu Zaid, and H. Mukhtar. 2008. A novel dietary flavonoid fisetin inhibits androgen receptor signaling and tumor growth in athymic nude mice. *Cancer research* 68 (20):8555–63.

Kim, J. H., C. Xu, Y. S. Keum et al. 2006. Inhibition of EGFR signaling in human prostate cancer PC-3 cells by combination treatment with beta-phenylethyl isothiocyanate and curcumin. *Carcinogenesis* 27 (3):475–82.

Kim, J. M., E. M. Noh, K. B. Kwon et al. 2012. Curcumin suppresses the TPA-induced invasion through inhibition of PKCalpha-dependent MMP-expression in MCF-7 human breast cancer cells. *Phytomedicine* 19 (12):1085–92.

Kim, M. H., P. Albertsson, Y. Xue et al. 2001. Expression of neutrophil collagenase (MMP-8) in Jurkat T leukemia cells and its role in invasion. *Anticancer Res* 21 (1A):45–50.

Kim, M. H., A. M. Gutierrez, and R. H. Goldfarb. 2002. Different mechanisms of soy isoflavones in cell cycle regulation and inhibition of invasion. *Anticancer Res* 22 (6C):3811–7.

Kim, S., A. Fotiadu, and V. Kotoula. 2005. Increased expression of soluble decoy receptor 3 in acutely inflamed intestinal epithelia. *Clin Immunol* 115 (3):286–94.

Kim, S. H., H. J. Kang, H. Na, and M. O. Lee. 2010. Trichostatin A enhances acetylation as well as protein stability of ERalpha through induction of p300 protein. *Breast Cancer Res* 12 (2):R22.

Knowles, L. M., and J. A. Milner. 2003. Diallyl disulfide induces ERK phosphorylation and alters gene expression profiles in human colon tumor cells. *J Nutr* 133 (9):2901–6.

Koopmann, J., P. Buckhaults, D. A. Brown et al. 2004. Serum macrophage inhibitory cytokine 1 as a marker of pancreatic and other periampullary cancers. *Clin Cancer Res* 10 (7):2386–92.

Korpi, J. T., V. Kervinen, H. Maklin et al. 2008. Collagenase-2 (matrix metalloproteinase-8) plays a protective role in tongue cancer. *Br J Cancer* 98 (4):766–75.

Kouzarides, T. 2007. Chromatin modifications and their function. *Cell* 128 (4):693–705.

Krusche, C. A., P. Wulfing, C. Kersting et al. 2005. Histone deacetylase-1 and -3 protein expression in human breast cancer: a tissue microarray analysis. *Breast Cancer Res Treat* 90 (1):15–23.

Krutovskikh, V. A., and Z. Herceg. 2010. Oncogenic microRNAs (OncomiRs) as a new class of cancer biomarkers. *Bioessays* 32 (10):894–904.

Kubota, M., M. Shimizu, H. Sakai et al. 2012. Preventive effects of curcumin on the development of azoxymethane-induced colonic preneoplastic lesions in male C57BL/KsJ-db/db obese mice. *Nutr Cancer* 64 (1):72–9.

Kury, S., B. Buecher, S. Robiou-du-Pont et al. 2007. Combinations of cytochrome P450 gene polymorphisms enhancing the risk for sporadic colorectal cancer related to red meat consumption. *Cancer Epidemiol Biomarkers Prev* 16 (7):1460–7.

Lamy, S., N. Akla, A. Ouanouki, S. Lord-Dufour, and R. Beliveau. 2012. Diet-derived polyphenols inhibit angiogenesis by modulating the interleukin-6/STAT3 pathway. *Exp Cell Res* 318 (13):1586–96.

Lau, D. S., and M. C. Archer. 2010. The 10t,12c isomer of conjugated linoleic acid inhibits fatty acid synthase expression and enzyme activity in human breast, colon, and prostate cancer cells. *Nutr Cancer* 62 (1):116–21.

Leamon, C. P., and A. L. Jackman. 2008. Exploitation of the folate receptor in the management of cancer and inflammatory disease. *Vitam Horm* 79:203–33.

Lean, C., S. Doran, R. L. Somorjai et al. 2004. Determination of grade and receptor status from the primary breast lesion by magnetic resonance spectroscopy. *Technol Cancer Res Treat* 3 (6):551–6.

Lee, D. H., Y. Yang, S. J. Lee et al. 2003. Macrophage inhibitory cytokine-1 induces the invasiveness of gastric cancer cells by up-regulating the urokinase-type plasminogen activator system. *Cancer Res* 63 (15):4648–55.

Lee, R. C., R. L. Feinbaum, and V. Ambros. 1993. The C. elegans heterochronic gene lin-4 encodes small RNAs with antisense complementarity to lin-14. *Cell* 75 (5):843–54.

Lee, S. H., K. Yamaguchi, J. S. Kim et al. 2006. Conjugated linoleic acid stimulates an anti-tumorigenic protein NAG-1 in an isomer specific manner. *Carcinogenesis* 27 (5):972–81.

Lee, Y. C., T. H. Cheng, J. S. Lee et al. 2011. Nobiletin, a citrus flavonoid, suppresses invasion and migration involving FAK/PI3K/Akt and small GTPase signals in human gastric adenocarcinoma AGS cells. *Mol Cell Biochem* 347 (1–2):103–15.

Leth-Larsen, R., R. R. Lund, and H. J. Ditzel. 2010. Plasma membrane proteomics and its application in clinical cancer biomarker discovery. *Mol Cell Proteomics* 9 (7):1369–82.

Lewis, J. D., R. R. Meehan, W. J. Henzel et al. 1992. Purification, sequence, and cellular localization of a novel chromosomal protein that binds to methylated DNA. *Cell* 69 (6):905–14.

Li, C., B. Guo, C. Bernabeu, and S. Kumar. 2001. Angiogenesis in breast cancer: the role of transforming growth factor beta and CD105. *Microsc Res Tech* 52 (4):437–49.

Li, J., Z. Zhang, J. Rosenzweig, Y. Y. Wang, and D. W. Chan. 2002. Proteomics and bioinformatics approaches for identification of serum biomarkers to detect breast cancer. *Clin Chem* 48 (8):1296–304.

Li, P. X., J. Wong, A. Ayed et al. 2000. Placental transforming growth factor-beta is a downstream mediator of the growth arrest and apoptotic response of tumor cells to DNA damage and p53 overexpression. *J Biol Chem* 275 (26):20127–35.

Li, T., G. X. Fan, W. Wang, T. Li, and Y. K. Yuan. 2007. Resveratrol induces apoptosis, influences IL-6 and exerts immunomodulatory effect on mouse lymphocytic leukemia both in vitro and in vivo. *Int Immunopharmacol* 7 (9):1221–31.

Li, Y., T. G. Vandenboom, 2nd, Z. Wang et al. 2010. miR-146a suppresses invasion of pancreatic cancer cells. *Cancer Res* 70 (4):1486–95.

Liao, Y. C., Y. W. Shih, C. H. Chao, X. Y. Lee, and T. A. Chiang. 2009. Involvement of the ERK signaling pathway in fisetin reduces invasion and migration in the human lung cancer cell line A549. *J Agric Food Chem* 57 (19):8933–41.

Liao, Y. F., Y. K. Rao, and Y. M. Tzeng. 2012. Aqueous extract of Anisomeles indica and its purified compound exerts anti-metastatic activity through inhibition of NF-kappaB/AP-1-dependent MMP-9 activation in human breast cancer MCF-7 cells. *Food Chem Toxicol* 50 (8):2930–6.

Lin, D. W., M. L. Neuhouser, J. M. Schenk et al. 2007. Low-fat, low-glycemic load diet and gene expression in human prostate epithelium: a feasibility study of using cDNA microarrays to assess the response to dietary intervention in target tissues. *Cancer Epidemiol Biomarkers Prev* 16 (10):2150–4.

Lin, W. W., and S. L. Hsieh. 2011. Decoy receptor 3: a pleiotropic immunomodulator and biomarker for inflammatory diseases, autoimmune diseases and cancer. *Biochem Pharmacol* 81 (7):838–47.

Linton, K. D., and F. C. Hamdy. 2003. Early diagnosis and surgical management of prostate cancer. *Cancer Treat Rev* 29 (3):151–60.

Lippman, S. M., P. J. Goodman, E. A. Klein et al. 2005. Designing the Selenium and Vitamin E Cancer Prevention Trial (SELECT). *J Natl Cancer Inst* 97 (2):94–102.

Lu, H., W. Ouyang, and C. Huang. 2006. Inflammation, a key event in cancer development. *Mol Cancer Res* 4 (4):221–33.

Luger, K., A. W. Mader, R. K. Richmond, D. F. Sargent, and T. J. Richmond. 1997. Crystal structure of the nucleosome core particle at 2.8 A resolution. *Nature* 389 (6648):251–60.

Luo, J., N. L. Solimini, and S. J. Elledge. 2009. Principles of cancer therapy: oncogene and non-oncogene addiction. *Cell* 136 (5):823–37.

Macher-Goeppinger, S., S. Aulmann, N. Wagener et al. 2008. Decoy receptor 3 is a prognostic factor in renal cell cancer. *Neoplasia* 10 (10):1049–56.

Mafuvadze, B., Y. Liang, C. Besch-Williford, X. Zhang, and S. M. Hyder. 2012. Apigenin induces apoptosis and blocks growth of medroxyprogesterone acetate-dependent BT-474 xenograft tumors. *Horm Cancer* 3 (4):160–71.

Mai, Z., G. L. Blackburn, and J. R. Zhou. 2007. Genistein sensitizes inhibitory effect of tamoxifen on the growth of estrogen receptor-positive and HER2-overexpressing human breast cancer cells. *Mol Carcinog* 46 (7):534–42.

Mal, M., P. K. Koh, P. Y. Cheah, and E. C. Chan. 2009. Development and validation of a gas chromatography/mass spectrometry method for the metabolic profiling of human colon tissue. *Rapid Commun Mass Spectrom* 23 (4):487–94.

Malemud, C. J. 2006. Matrix metalloproteinases (MMPs) in health and disease: an overview. *Front Biosci* 11:1696–701.

Mariadason, J. M., G. A. Corner, and L. H. Augenlicht. 2000. Genetic reprogramming in pathways of colonic cell maturation induced by short chain fatty acids: comparison with trichostatin A, sulindac, and curcumin and implications for chemoprevention of colon cancer. *Cancer Res* 60 (16):4561–72.

Martinasso, G., S. Saracino, M. Maggiora et al. 2010. Conjugated linoleic acid prevents cell growth and cytokine production induced by TPA in human keratinocytes NCTC 2544. *Cancer Lett* 287 (1):62–6.

Massague, J., and Y. G. Chen. 2000. Controlling TGF-beta signaling. *Genes Dev* 14 (6):627–44.

Mbimba, T., P. Awale, D. Bhatia et al. 2012. Alteration of hepatic proinflammatory cytokines is involved in the resveratrol-mediated chemoprevention of chemically-induced hepatocarcinogenesis. *Curr Pharm Biotechnol* 13 (1):229–34.

McFadyen, M. C., and G. I. Murray. 2005. Cytochrome P450 1B1: a novel anticancer therapeutic target. *Future Oncol* 1 (2):259–63.

Menendez, J. A., A. Vazquez-Martin, S. Ropero, R. Colomer, and R. Lupu. 2006. HER2 (erbB-2)-targeted effects of the omega-3 polyunsaturated fatty acid, alpha-linolenic acid (ALA; 18:3n-3), in breast cancer cells: the "fat features" of the "Mediterranean diet" as an "anti-HER2 cocktail". *Clin Transl Oncol* 8 (11):812–20.

Migone, T. S., J. Zhang, X. Luo et al. 2002. TL1A is a TNF-like ligand for DR3 and TR6/DcR3 and functions as a T cell costimulator. *Immunity* 16 (3):479–92.

Mikolajczyk, S. D., Y. Song, J. R. Wong, R. S. Matson, and H. G. Rittenhouse. 2004. Are multiple markers the future of prostate cancer diagnostics? *Clin Biochem* 37 (7):519–28.

Mimeault, M., and S. K. Batra. 2010. Divergent molecular mechanisms underlying the pleiotropic functions of macrophage inhibitory cytokine-1 in cancer. *J Cell Physiol* 224 (3):626–35.

Miyamoto, S., Y. Yasui, T. Tanaka, H. Ohigashi, and A. Murakami. 2008. Suppressive effects of nobiletin on hyperleptinemia and colitis-related colon carcinogenesis in male ICR mice. *Carcinogenesis* 29 (5):1057–63.

Moilanen, M., E. Pirila, R. Grenman, T. Sorsa, and T. Salo. 2002. Expression and regulation of collagenase-2 (MMP-8) in head and neck squamous cell carcinomas. *J Pathol* 197 (1):72–81.

Molina, R., J. M. Auge, X. Filella et al. 2005. Pro-gastrin-releasing peptide (proGRP) in patients with benign and malignant diseases: comparison with CEA, SCC, CYFRA 21-1 and NSE in patients with lung cancer. *Anticancer Res* 25 (3A):1773–8.

Mountford, C. E., R. L. Somorjai, P. Malycha et al. 2001. Diagnosis and prognosis of breast cancer by magnetic resonance spectroscopy of fine-needle aspirates analysed using a statistical classification strategy. *Br J Surg* 88 (9):1234–40.

Moustakas, A., and C. H. Heldin. 2005. Non-Smad TGF-beta signals. *J Cell Sci* 118 (Pt 16):3573–84.

Moy, K. A., J. M. Yuan, F. L. Chung et al. 2009. Isothiocyanates, glutathione S-transferase M1 and T1 polymorphisms and gastric cancer risk: a prospective study of men in Shanghai, China. *Int J Cancer* 125 (11):2652–9.

Muller, M., and S. Kersten. 2003. Nutrigenomics: goals and strategies. *Nat Rev Genet* 4 (4):315–22.

Nair, S., A. Barve, T. O. Khor et al. 2010. Regulation of Nrf2- and AP-1-mediated gene expression by epigallocatechin-3-gallate and sulforaphane in prostate of Nrf2-knockout or C57BL/6J mice and PC-3 AP-1 human prostate cancer cells. *Acta Pharmacol Sin* 31 (9):1223–40.

Nagendraprabhu, P., and G. Sudhandiran. 2011. Astaxanthin inhibits tumor invasion by decreasing extracellular matrix production and induces apoptosis in experimental rat colon carcinogenesis by modulating the expressions of ERK-2, NFkB and COX-2. *Invest New Drugs* 29 (2):207–24.

Nakamura, T., A. Scorilas, C. Stephan et al. 2003. Quantitative analysis of macrophage inhibitory cytokine-1 (MIC-1) gene expression in human prostatic tissues. *Br J Cancer* 88 (7):1101–4.

Nakayama, J., J. C. Rice, B. D. Strahl, C. D. Allis, and S. I. Grewal. 2001. Role of histone H3 lysine 9 methylation in epigenetic control of heterochromatin assembly. *Science* 292 (5514):110–3.

Nambiar, P. R., R. R. Gupta, and V. Misra. 2010. An "Omics" based survey of human colon cancer. *Mutat Res* 693 (1–2):3–18.

Nambiar, P. R., S. R. Boutin, R. Raja, and D. W. Rosenberg. 2005. Global gene expression profiling: a complement to conventional histopathologic analysis of neoplasia. *Vet Pathol* 42 (6):735–52.

Nan, X., H. H. Ng, C. A. Johnson et al. 1998. Transcriptional repression by the methyl-CpG-binding protein MeCP2 involves a histone deacetylase complex. *Nature* 393 (6683):386–9.

Negrini, M., M. Ferracin, S. Sabbioni, and C. M. Croce. 2007. MicroRNAs in human cancer: from research to therapy. *J Cell Sci* 120 (Pt 11):1833–40.

Nordhoff, E., V. Egelhofer, P. Giavalisco et al. 2001. Large-gel two-dimensional electrophoresis-matrix assisted laser desorption/ionization-time of flight-mass spectrometry: an analytical challenge for studying complex protein mixtures. *Electrophoresis* 22 (14):2844–55.

Ong, K. R., A. H. Sims, M. Harvie et al. 2009. Biomarkers of dietary energy restriction in women at increased risk of breast cancer. *Cancer Prev Res (Phila)* 2 (8):720–31.

Oyama, J., T. Maeda, K. Kouzuma et al. 2010. Green tea catechins improve human forearm endothelial dysfunction and have antiatherosclerotic effects in smokers. *Circ J* 74 (3):578–88.

Ozbay, T., and R. Nahta. 2011. Delphinidin Inhibits HER2 and Erk1/2 Signaling and Suppresses Growth of HER2-Overexpressing and Triple Negative Breast Cancer Cell Lines. *Breast Cancer (Auckl)* 5:143–54.

Page-McCaw, A., A. J. Ewald, and Z. Werb. 2007. Matrix metalloproteinases and the regulation of tissue remodelling. *Nat Rev Mol Cell Biol* 8 (3):221–33.

Palozza, P., M. Colangelo, R. Simone et al. 2010. Lycopene induces cell growth inhibition by altering mevalonate pathway and Ras signaling in cancer cell lines. *Carcinogenesis* 31 (10):1813–21.

Pan, H., W. Zhou, W. He et al. 2012. Genistein inhibits MDA-MB-231 triple-negative breast cancer cell growth by inhibiting NF-kappaB activity via the Notch-1 pathway. *Int J Mol Med* 30 (2):337–43.

Pan, M. H., C. C. Lin, J. K. Lin, and W. J. Chen. 2007. Tea polyphenol (-)-epigallocatechin 3-gallate suppresses heregulin-beta1-induced fatty acid synthase expression in human breast cancer cells by inhibiting phosphatidylinositol 3-kinase/Akt and mitogen-activated protein kinase cascade signaling. *J Agric Food Chem* 55 (13):5030–7.

Panisko, E. A., T. P. Conrads, M. B. Goshe, and T. D. Veenstra. 2002. The postgenomic age: characterization of proteomes. *Exp Hematol* 30 (2):97–107.

Papadopoulos, G., D. Delakas, L. Nakopoulou, and T. Kassimatis. 2011. Statins and prostate cancer: molecular and clinical aspects. *Eur J Cancer* 47 (6):819–30.

Papoutsis, A. J., J. L. Borg, O. I. Selmin, and D. F. Romagnolo. 2012. BRCA-1 promoter hypermethylation and silencing induced by the aromatic hydrocarbon receptor-ligand TCDD are prevented by resveratrol in MCF-7 Cells. *J Nutr Biochem* 23 (10):1324–32.

Papoutsis, A. J., S. D. Lamore, G. T. Wondrak, O. I. Selmin, and D. F. Romagnolo. 2010. Resveratrol prevents epigenetic silencing of BRCA-1 by the aromatic hydrocarbon receptor in human breast cancer cells. *J Nutr* 140 (9):1607–14.

Paralkar, V. M., A. L. Vail, W. A. Grasser et al. 1998. Cloning and characterization of a novel member of the transforming growth factor-beta/bone morphogenetic protein family. *J Biol Chem* 273 (22):13760–7.

Parks, W. C., C. L. Wilson, and Y. S. Lopez-Boado. 2004. Matrix metalloproteinases as modulators of inflammation and innate immunity. *Nat Rev Immunol* 4 (8):617–29.

Pasquinelli, A. E., B. J. Reinhart, F. Slack et al. 2000. Conservation of the sequence and temporal expression of let-7 heterochronic regulatory RNA. *Nature* 408 (6808):86–9.

Pauler, D. K., U. Menon, M. McIntosh et al. 2001. Factors influencing serum CA125II levels in healthy postmenopausal women. *Cancer Epidemiol Biomarkers Prev* 10 (5):489–93.

Pavese, J. M., R. L. Farmer, and R. C. Bergan. 2010. Inhibition of cancer cell invasion and metastasis by genistein. *Cancer Metastasis Rev* 29 (3):465–82.

Petricoin, E. F., A. M. Ardekani, B. A. Hitt et al. 2002. Use of proteomic patterns in serum to identify ovarian cancer. *Lancet* 359 (9306):572–7.

Pifferi, F., F. Roux, B. Langelier et al. 2005. (n-3) polyunsaturated fatty acid deficiency reduces the expression of both isoforms of the brain glucose transporter GLUT1 in rats. *J Nutr* 135 (9):2241–6.

Pignatelli, P., S. Di Santo, R. Carnevale, and F. Violi. 2005. The polyphenols quercetin and catechin synergize in inhibiting platelet CD40L expression. *Thromb Haemost* 94 (4):888–9.

Pinchot, S. N., R. Jaskula-Sztul, L. Ning et al. 2011. Identification and validation of Notch pathway activating compounds through a novel high-throughput screening method. *Cancer* 117 (7):1386–98.

Pinlaor, S., P. Yongvanit, S. Prakobwong et al. 2009. Curcumin reduces oxidative and nitrative DNA damage through balancing of oxidant-antioxidant status in hamsters infected with Opisthorchis viverrini. *Mol Nutr Food Res* 53 (10):1316–28.

Pitti, R. M., S. A. Marsters, D. A. Lawrence et al. 1998. Genomic amplification of a decoy receptor for Fas ligand in lung and colon cancer. *Nature* 396 (6712):699–703.

Potter, J. D. 1999. Colorectal cancer: molecules and populations. *J Natl Cancer Inst* 91 (11):916–32.

Prakobwong, S., J. Khoontawad, P. Yongvanit et al. 2011. Curcumin decreases cholangiocarcinogenesis in hamsters by suppressing inflammation-mediated molecular events related to multistep carcinogenesis. *Int J Cancer* 129 (1):88–100.

Priyadarsini, R. V., and S. Nagini. 2012. Quercetin suppresses cytochrome P450 mediated ROS generation and NFkappaB activation to inhibit the development of 7,12-dimethylbenz[a]anthracene (DMBA) induced hamster buccal pouch carcinomas. *Free Radic Res* 46 (1):41–9.

Puig, T., J. Relat, P. F. Marrero et al. 2008. Green tea catechin inhibits fatty acid synthase without stimulating carnitine palmitoyltransferase-1 or inducing weight loss in experimental animals. *Anticancer Res* 28 (6A):3671–6.

Punglia, R. S., A. V. D'Amico, W. J. Catalona, K. A. Roehl, and K. M. Kuntz. 2003. Effect of verification bias on screening for prostate cancer by measurement of prostate-specific antigen. *N Engl J Med* 349 (4):335–42.

Rao, L., B. Puschner, and T. A. Prolla. 2001. Gene expression profiling of low selenium status in the mouse intestine: transcriptional activation of genes linked to DNA damage, cell cycle control and oxidative stress. *J Nutr* 131 (12):3175–81.

Rasiah, K. K., J. G. Kench, M. Gardiner-Garden et al. 2006. Aberrant neuropeptide Y and macrophage inhibitory cytokine-1 expression are early events in prostate cancer development and are associated with poor prognosis. *Cancer Epidemiol Biomarkers Prev* 15 (4):711–6.

Ravi, D., H. Muniyappa, and K. C. Das. 2008. Caffeine inhibits UV-mediated NF-kappaB activation in A2058 melanoma cells: an ATM-PKCdelta-p38 MAPK-dependent mechanism. *Mol Cell Biochem* 308 (1–2):193–200.

Rodenhiser, D., and M. Mann. 2006. Epigenetics and human disease: translating basic biology into clinical applications. *CMAJ* 174 (3):341–8.

Rose, P., Y. K. Won, C. N. Ong, and M. Whiteman. 2005. Beta-phenylethyl and 8-methylsulphinyloctyl isothiocyanates, constituents of watercress, suppress LPS induced production of nitric oxide and prostaglandin E2 in RAW 264.7 macrophages. *Nitric Oxide* 12 (4):237–43.

Roth, W., S. Isenmann, M. Nakamura et al. 2001. Soluble decoy receptor 3 is expressed by malignant gliomas and suppresses CD95 ligand-induced apoptosis and chemotaxis. *Cancer Res* 61 (6):2759–65.

Roy, R., B. Zhang, and M. A. Moses. 2006. Making the cut: protease-mediated regulation of angiogenesis. *Exp Cell Res* 312 (5):608–22.

Saini, S., H. Hirata, S. Majid, and R. Dahiya. 2009. Functional significance of cytochrome P450 1B1 in endometrial carcinogenesis. *Cancer Res* 69 (17):7038–45.

Sakla, M. S., N. S. Shenouda, P. J. Ansell, R. S. Macdonald, and D. B. Lubahn. 2007. Genistein affects HER2 protein concentration, activation, and promoter regulation in BT-474 human breast cancer cells. *Endocrine* 32 (1):69–78.

Saldova, R., M. R. Wormald, R. A. Dwek, and P. M. Rudd. 2008. Glycosylation changes on serum glycoproteins in ovarian cancer may contribute to disease pathogenesis. *Dis Markers* 25 (4–5):219–32.

Schroder, F. H., J. Hugosson, M. J. Roobol et al. 2009. Screening and prostate-cancer mortality in a randomized European study. *N Engl J Med* 360 (13):1320–8.

Schwartz, M. D., C. Isaacs, K. D. Graves et al. 2012. Long-term outcomes of BRCA1/BRCA2 testing: risk reduction and surveillance. *Cancer* 118 (2):510–7.

Seo, H. S., H. S. Choi, S. R. Kim et al. 2012. Apigenin induces apoptosis via extrinsic pathway, inducing p53 and inhibiting STAT3 and NFkappaB signaling in HER2-overexpressing breast cancer cells. *Mol Cell Biochem* 366 (1–2):319–34.

Seow, A., J. M. Yuan, C. L. Sun et al. 2002. Dietary isothiocyanates, glutathione S-transferase polymorphisms and colorectal cancer risk in the Singapore Chinese Health Study. *Carcinogenesis* 23 (12):2055–61.

Shariat, S. F., D. S. Scherr, A. Gupta et al. 2011. Emerging biomarkers for prostate cancer diagnosis, staging, and prognosis. *Arch Esp Urol* 64 (8):681–94.

Sherwood, E. R., J. L. Van Dongen, C. G. Wood et al. 1998. Epidermal growth factor receptor activation in androgen-independent but not androgen-stimulated growth of human prostatic carcinoma cells. *Br J Cancer* 77 (6):855–61.

Shibayama, T., H. Ueoka, K. Nishii et al. 2001. Complementary roles of pro-gastrin-releasing peptide (ProGRP) and neuron specific enolase (NSE) in diagnosis and prognosis of small-cell lung cancer (SCLC). *Lung Cancer* 32 (1):61–9.

Shim, J. H., Z. Y. Su, J. I. Chae et al. 2010. Epigallocatechin gallate suppresses lung cancer cell growth through Ras-GTPase-activating protein SH3 domain-binding protein 1. *Cancer Prev Res (Phila)* 3 (5):670–9.

Shimizu, M., Y. Shirakami, and H. Moriwaki. 2008. Targeting receptor tyrosine kinases for chemoprevention by green tea catechin, EGCG. *Int J Mol Sci* 9 (6):1034–49.

Shnaper, S., I. Desbaillets, D. A. Brown et al. 2009. Elevated levels of MIC-1/GDF15 in the cerebrospinal fluid of patients are associated with glioblastoma and worse outcome. *Int J Cancer* 125 (11):2624–30.

Siemes, C., L. E. Visser, J. W. Coebergh et al. 2006. C-reactive protein levels, variation in the C-reactive protein gene, and cancer risk: the Rotterdam Study. *J Clin Oncol* 24 (33):5216–22.

Simons, L. A., M. Ortiz, and G. Calcino. 2011. Long term persistence with statin therapy—experience in Australia 2006–2010. *Aust Fam Phys* 40 (5):319–22.

Simopoulos, A. P. 2010. Nutrigenetics/nutrigenomics. *Annu Rev Public Health* 31:53–68.

Singh, T., and A. B. Newman. 2011. Inflammatory markers in population studies of aging. *Ageing Res Rev* 10 (3):319–29.

Smith, S., D. Sepkovic, H. L. Bradlow, and K. J. Auborn. 2008. 3,3'-Diindolylmethane and genistein decrease the adverse effects of estrogen in LNCaP and PC-3 prostate cancer cells. *J Nutr* 138 (12):2379–85.

Stadlmann, S., J. Pollheimer, P. L. Moser et al. 2003. Cytokine-regulated expression of collagenase-2 (MMP-8) is involved in the progression of ovarian cancer. *Eur J Cancer* 39 (17):2499–505.

Steinbach, G., P. M. Lynch, R. K. Phillips et al. 2000. The effect of celecoxib, a cyclooxygenase-2 inhibitor, in familial adenomatous polyposis. *N Engl J Med* 342 (26):1946–52.

Stidley, C. A., M. A. Picchi, S. Leng et al. 2010. Multivitamins, folate, and green vegetables protect against gene promoter methylation in the aerodigestive tract of smokers. *Cancer Res* 70 (2):568–74.

Strobel, P., C. Allard, T. Perez-Acle et al. 2005. Myricetin, quercetin and catechin-gallate inhibit glucose uptake in isolated rat adipocytes. *Biochem J* 386 (Pt 3):471–8.

Subbaramaiah, K., and A. J. Dannenberg. 2003. Cyclooxygenase 2: a molecular target for cancer prevention and treatment. *Trends Pharmacol Sci* 24 (2):96–102.

Sun, M., Z. Estrov, Y. Ji et al. 2008. Curcumin (diferuloylmethane) alters the expression profiles of microRNAs in human pancreatic cancer cells. *Mol Cancer Ther* 7 (3):464–73.

Sun, S. H., H. C. Huang, C. Huang, and J. K. Lin. 2012. Cycle arrest and apoptosis in MDA-MB-231/Her2 cells induced by curcumin. *Eur J Pharmacol* 690 (1–3):22–30.

Surh, Y. J. 2003. Cancer chemoprevention with dietary phytochemicals. *Nat Rev Cancer* 3 (10):768–80.

Swanton, C., A. Futreal, and T. Eisen. 2006. Her2-targeted therapies in non-small cell lung cancer. *Clin Cancer Res* 12 (14 Pt 2):4377s–4383s.

Switzer, C. H., R. Y. Cheng, L. A. Ridnour et al. 2012. Dithiolethiones inhibit NF-kappaB activity via covalent modification in human estrogen receptor-negative breast cancer. *Cancer Research* 72 (9):2394–404.

Takemura, H., H. Nagayoshi, T. Matsuda et al. 2010. Inhibitory effects of chrysoeriol on DNA adduct formation with benzo[a]pyrene in MCF-7 breast cancer cells. *Toxicology* 274 (1–3):42–8.

Tamaru, H., and E. U. Selker. 2001. A histone H3 methyltransferase controls DNA methylation in *Neurospora crassa*. *Nature* 414 (6861):277–83.

Tan, S., T. K. Seow, R. C. Liang et al. 2002. Proteome analysis of butyrate-treated human colon cancer cells (HT-29). *Int J Cancer* 98 (4):523–31.

Theocharis, A. D., S. S. Skandalis, G. N. Tzanakakis, and N. K. Karamanos. 2010. Proteoglycans in health and disease: novel roles for proteoglycans in malignancy and their pharmacological targeting. *FEBS J* 277 (19):3904–23.

Thorisson, G. A., and L. D. Stein. 2003. The SNP Consortium website: past, present and future. *Nucleic Acids Res* 31 (1):124–7.

Traka, M., A. V. Gasper, A. Melchini et al. 2008. Broccoli consumption interacts with GSTM1 to perturb oncogenic signalling pathways in the prostate. *PLoS One* 3 (7):e2568.

Tremethick, D. J. 2007. Higher-order structures of chromatin: the elusive 30 nm fiber. *Cell* 128 (4):651–4.

Trujillo, E., C. Davis, and J. Milner. 2006. Nutrigenomics, proteomics, metabolomics, and the practice of dietetics. *J Am Diet Assoc* 106 (3):403–13.

Truong, M., M. R. Cook, S. N. Pinchot, M. Kunnimalaiyaan, and H. Chen. 2011. Resveratrol induces Notch2-mediated apoptosis and suppression of neuroendocrine markers in medullary thyroid cancer. *Ann Surg Oncol* 18 (5):1506–11.

Tsang, W. P., and T. T. Kwok. 2010. Epigallocatechin gallate up-regulation of miR-16 and induction of apoptosis in human cancer cells. *J Nutr Biochem* 21 (2):140–6.

Tu, H. F., C. J. Liu, S. Y. Liu et al. 2011. Serum decoy receptor 3 level: a predictive marker for nodal metastasis and survival among oral cavity cancer patients. *Head Neck* 33 (3):396–402.

Tu, S. P., H. Jin, J. D. Shi et al. 2012. Curcumin induces the differentiation of myeloid-derived suppressor cells and inhibits their interaction with cancer cells and related tumor growth. *Cancer Prev Res (Phila)* 5 (2):205–15.

Tyers, M., and M. Mann. 2003. From genomics to proteomics. *Nature* 422 (6928):193–7.

Umesalma, S., and G. Sudhandiran. 2010. Differential inhibitory effects of the polyphenol ellagic acid on inflammatory mediators NF-kappaB, iNOS, COX-2, TNF-alpha, and IL-6 in 1,2-dimethylhydrazine-induced rat colon carcinogenesis. *Basic Clin Pharmacol Toxicol* 107 (2):650–5.

Vaishampayan, U., M. Hussain, M. Banerjee et al. 2007. Lycopene and soy isoflavones in the treatment of prostate cancer. *Nutr Cancer* 59 (1):1–7.

Valinluck, V., and L. C. Sowers. 2007. Inflammation-mediated cytosine damage: a mechanistic link between inflammation and the epigenetic alterations in human cancers. *Cancer Res* 67 (12):5583–6.

van der Meij, B. S., J. A. Langius, E. F. Smit et al. 2010. Oral nutritional supplements containing (n-3) polyunsaturated fatty acids affect the nutritional status of patients with stage III non-small cell lung cancer during multimodality treatment. *J Nutr* 140 (10):1774–80.

van Leeuwen, P. J., D. Connolly, A. Gavin et al. 2010. Prostate cancer mortality in screen and clinically detected prostate cancer: estimating the screening benefit. *Eur J Cancer* 46 (2):377–83.

Vardar-Sengul, S., E. Buduneli, O. Turkoglu et al. 2008. The effects of selective COX-2 inhibitor/celecoxib and omega-3 fatty acid on matrix metalloproteinases, TIMP-1, and laminin-5gamma2-chain immunolocalization in experimental periodontitis. *J Periodontol* 79 (10):1934–41.

Vidya Priyadarsini, R., N. Kumar, I. Khan et al. 2012. Gene expression signature of DMBA-induced hamster buccal pouch carcinomas: modulation by chlorophyllin and ellagic acid. *PLoS One* 7 (4):e34628.

Volman, J. J., J. P. Helsper, S. Wei et al. 2010. Effects of mushroom-derived beta-glucan-rich polysaccharide extracts on nitric oxide production by bone marrow-derived macrophages and nuclear factor-kappaB transactivation in Caco-2 reporter cells: can effects be explained by structure? *Mol Nutr Food Res* 54 (2):268–76.

Vu, T. H., and Z. Werb. 2000. Matrix metalloproteinases: effectors of development and normal physiology. *Genes Dev* 14 (17):2123–33.

Walle, T., and U. K. Walle. 2007. Novel methoxylated flavone inhibitors of cytochrome P450 1B1 in SCC-9 human oral cancer cells. *J Pharm Pharmacol* 59 (6):857–62.

Wang, T. T., N. W. Schoene, J. A. Milner, and Y. S. Kim. 2012. Broccoli-derived phytochemicals indole-3-carbinol and 3,3'-diindolylmethane exerts concentration-dependent pleiotropic effects on prostate cancer cells: comparison with other cancer preventive phytochemicals. *Mol Carcinog* 51 (3):244–56.

Weberpals, J. I., D. Tu, J. A. Squire et al. 2011. Breast cancer 1 (BRCA1) protein expression as a prognostic marker in sporadic epithelial ovarian carcinoma: an NCIC CTG OV.16 correlative study. *Ann Oncol* 22 (11):2403–10.

Weichert, W., C. Denkert, A. Noske et al. 2008a. Expression of class I histone deacetylases indicates poor prognosis in endometrioid subtypes of ovarian and endometrial carcinomas. *Neoplasia* 10 (9):1021–7.

Weichert, W., A. Roske, V. Gekeler et al. 2008b. Association of patterns of class I histone deacetylase expression with patient prognosis in gastric cancer: a retrospective analysis. *Lancet Oncol* 9 (2):139–48.

Wiseman, M. 2008. The second World Cancer Research Fund/American Institute for Cancer Research expert report. Food, nutrition, physical activity, and the prevention of cancer: a global perspective. *Proc Nutr Soc* 67 (3):253–6.

Wolffe, A. P., and M. A. Matzke. 1999. Epigenetics: regulation through repression. *Science* 286 (5439):481–6.

Woodbury, R. L., D. L. McCarthy, and A. L. Bulman. 2012. Profiling of urine using ProteinChip(R) technology. *Methods Mol Biol* 818:97–107.

Xu, J., T. R. Kimball, J. N. Lorenz et al. 2006. GDF15/MIC-1 functions as a protective and antihypertrophic factor released from the myocardium in association with SMAD protein activation. *Circ Res* 98 (3):342–50.

Yamaguchi, K., K. Abe, T. Kameya et al. 1983. Production and molecular size heterogeneity of immunoreactive gastrin-releasing peptide in fetal and adult lungs and primary lung tumors. *Cancer Res* 43 (8):3932–9.

Yan, H., and W. Zhou. 2004. Allelic variations in gene expression. *Curr Opin Oncol* 16 (1):39–43.

Yang, J. H., T. P. Kondratyuk, L. E. Marler et al. 2010. Isolation and evaluation of kaempferol glycosides from the fern Neocheiropteris palmatopedata. *Phytochemistry* 71 (5–6):641–7.

Yasui, Y., M. Hosokawa, N. Mikami, K. Miyashita, and T. Tanaka. 2011. Dietary astaxanthin inhibits colitis and colitis-associated colon carcinogenesis in mice via modulation of the inflammatory cytokines. *Chem Biol Interact* 193 (1):79–87.

Yu, S. W., T. O. Khor, K. L. Cheung et al. 2010. Nrf2 Expression is regulated by epigenetic mechanisms in prostate cancer of TRAMP mice. *PLoS One* 5 (1).

Yun, J., C. Rago, I. Cheong et al. 2009. Glucose deprivation contributes to the development of KRAS pathway mutations in tumor cells. *Science* 325 (5947):1555–9.

Zhang, B., X. Pan, G. P. Cobb, and T. A. Anderson. 2007. microRNAs as oncogenes and tumor suppressors. *Dev Biol* 302 (1):1–12.

Zhang, L., X. Yang, H. Y. Pan et al. 2009. Expression of growth differentiation factor 15 is positively correlated with histopathological malignant grade and in vitro cell proliferation in oral squamous cell carcinoma. *Oral Oncol* 45 (7):627–32.

Zhang, S. M., J. E. Buring, I. M. Lee, N. R. Cook, and P. M. Ridker. 2005. C-reactive protein levels are not associated with increased risk for colorectal cancer in women. *Ann Intern Med* 142 (6):425–32.

Zhao, K., M. Whiteman, J. P. Spencer, and B. Halliwell. 2001. DNA damage by nitrite and peroxynitrite: protection by dietary phenols. *Methods Enzymol* 335:296–307.

Zhao, L., B. Y. Lee, D. A. Brown et al. 2009. Identification of candidate biomarkers of therapeutic response to docetaxel by proteomic profiling. *Cancer Res* 69 (19):7696–703.

Zimmers, T. A., X. Jin, E. C. Hsiao et al. 2006. Growth differentiation factor-15: induction in liver injury through p53 and tumor necrosis factor-independent mechanisms. *J Surg Res* 130 (1):45–51.

Section III

In Vivo Absorption and Pharmacokinetics of Nutritional Phytochemicals

7 Metabolism and Transport of Anticancer and Anti-Inflammatory Phytochemicals across the Gastrointestinal Tract

Yong Ma and Ming Hu

CONTENTS

7.1   INTRODUCTION

For thousands of years, humans have continued to undertake strenuous exploration on how to utilize natural resources better. Even in early civilization, humans realized that ingestion of certain foods or herbals could make their body better by being free from diseases or recovering from diseases faster. This practice lasted for thousands of years, although the specific phytochemical ingredients responsible for the observed beneficial effects were largely unknown. The advent of modern chemistry, biology, and medicine made it possible to identify some of the chemical ingredients responsible for the beneficial effects. Today, natural compounds and their derivatives represent a large section of approved drugs. We are experiencing an increasing beneficial effect from using these health-promoting and disease-preventing phytochemicals (Chin et al. 2006).

Extensive studies have successfully demonstrated that phytochemicals have diverse pharmacological properties, including antioxidant, anti-inflammation, and antiproliferation, and a significant number of these chemicals also induce apoptosis and suppress metastasis in cell lines or animal models (Shu et al. 2010; Murakami and Ohigashi 2007). However, these results could not be extrapolated directly to illustrate their beneficial effects in human beings, because these studies were often conducted at a very high concentration (or dose), which is not achievable in vivo for humans. Low bioavailability often prevents phytochemicals from exerting their activities due to the low plasma and/or low local concentrations at target tissues or organs.

The human gastrointestinal tract often represents the first barrier to the absorption of these phytochemicals, exerting a very important influence on their bioavailability. Thus, a thorough comprehension of the disposition behaviors of phytochemicals along the gastrointestinal tract is not only very important for researchers to understand the gap between in vitro and in vivo data but also critical in designing new approaches to increase their bioavailability in vivo.

Phytochemicals are classified according to their backbone structures and functional groups. According to Harborne (1999), phytochemicals can be categorized in three main biogenetic classes:

terpenoids, alkaloids and other nitrogen-containing metabolites, and phenolics. Under each class, there are several subclasses that are distinguished from each other based on more detailed classification rules (Harborne 1999). Due to their distinct molecular structures, phytochemicals usually display different properties during their absorption by the gastrointestinal tract. In this chapter, we will review disposition behaviors of representative phytochemicals in each class that is reported to possess anti-inflammation and anticancer activities. Factors that influence their absorption along the gastrointestinal tract will be discussed in detail.

The barriers to absorption of intact phytochemicals include solubility, permeation, metabolism, and excretion (Hu 2007). Solubility is important because phytochemicals have to be soluble to be available for absorption. Permeation is the obvious necessary step for getting the phytochemicals into the blood, whereas metabolisms in the intestine and liver are the first-pass metabolic barriers to the absorbed phytochemicals, since they have to overcome these barriers to get into the systemic circulation. Excretion may occur at the intestinal apical membrane, which is an antiabsorption mechanism that prevents absorption. Excretion may also occur at the liver and kidney, where it eliminates the absorbed phytochemicals. Both types of excretion will decrease the exposure of the biologically active phytochemicals in vivo, but antiabsorption mechanisms at the apical membrane of the intestine are often called *efflux* because they prevent the absorption of phytochemicals.

7.2 SOLUBILITY AND GASTROINTESTINAL ABSORPTION

Solubility is the physicochemical property of a solute (a solid, liquid, or gaseous substance) that measures its tendency to dissolve in a solvent and form a homogeneous solution. For nutrients and drug molecules, solubility is a very important factor that determines the oral bioavailability since substances must be dissolved first before they can move cross the gastrointestinal epithelium via major absorption mechanisms such as passive diffusion and transporter-mediated translocation across the intestinal epithelium. Together with another two parameters, intestinal permeability and dissolution rate, solubility can be used to predict intestinal drug absorption, according to the Biopharmaceutics Classification System (BCS) (Amidon et al. 1995). BCS can separate drugs into four classes: high solubility and high permeability (BCS class I), low solubility and high permeability (BCS class II), high solubility and low permeability (BCS class III), and low solubility and low permeability (BCS class IV). Pade and Stavchansky (1998) determined effective permeability coefficients of a series of model drugs in the Caco-2 cell line and their saturated solubility. By linking these data with the extent of absorption in vivo, they arrived at a conclusion that drugs in BCS class I are completely absorbed; however, for other drugs, low permeability or low solubility may be the rate-limiting factor in determining their absorption (Pade and Stavchansky 1998).

7.2.1 Solubility of Terpenoids

Due to the structural diversity of terpenoids, solubility for compounds in this class varies greatly. For example, terpenes displayed low solubilities (0.037–0.22 mmol/L), whereas oxygenated monoterpenes exhibited solubilities that are 20 orders of magnitude higher, in the range of 2–20 mmol/L at 25°C (Fichan et al. 1998). Thus, solubility of different terpenoids will be discussed separately.

7.2.1.1 Solubility of Carotenoids

Carotenoids are naturally occurring tetraterpenoids that are present in fruits and vegetables as organic pigments. As antioxidants or anticancer agents, carotenoids have been extensively studied. For example, lycopene (Figure 7.1, 1) and β-carotene (Figure 7.1, 2) have been shown to have an inhibitory effect on metastatic lung cancer (Heber 2000). Featuring a long polyunsaturated fatty acid chain, carotenoids, especially carotenes, are nearly insoluble in water, unless some water-soluble components such as a carbonyl group or hydroxyl group are included in the structure to form xanthophylls (or yellow pigments). Even for these compounds, aqueous solubilities are only

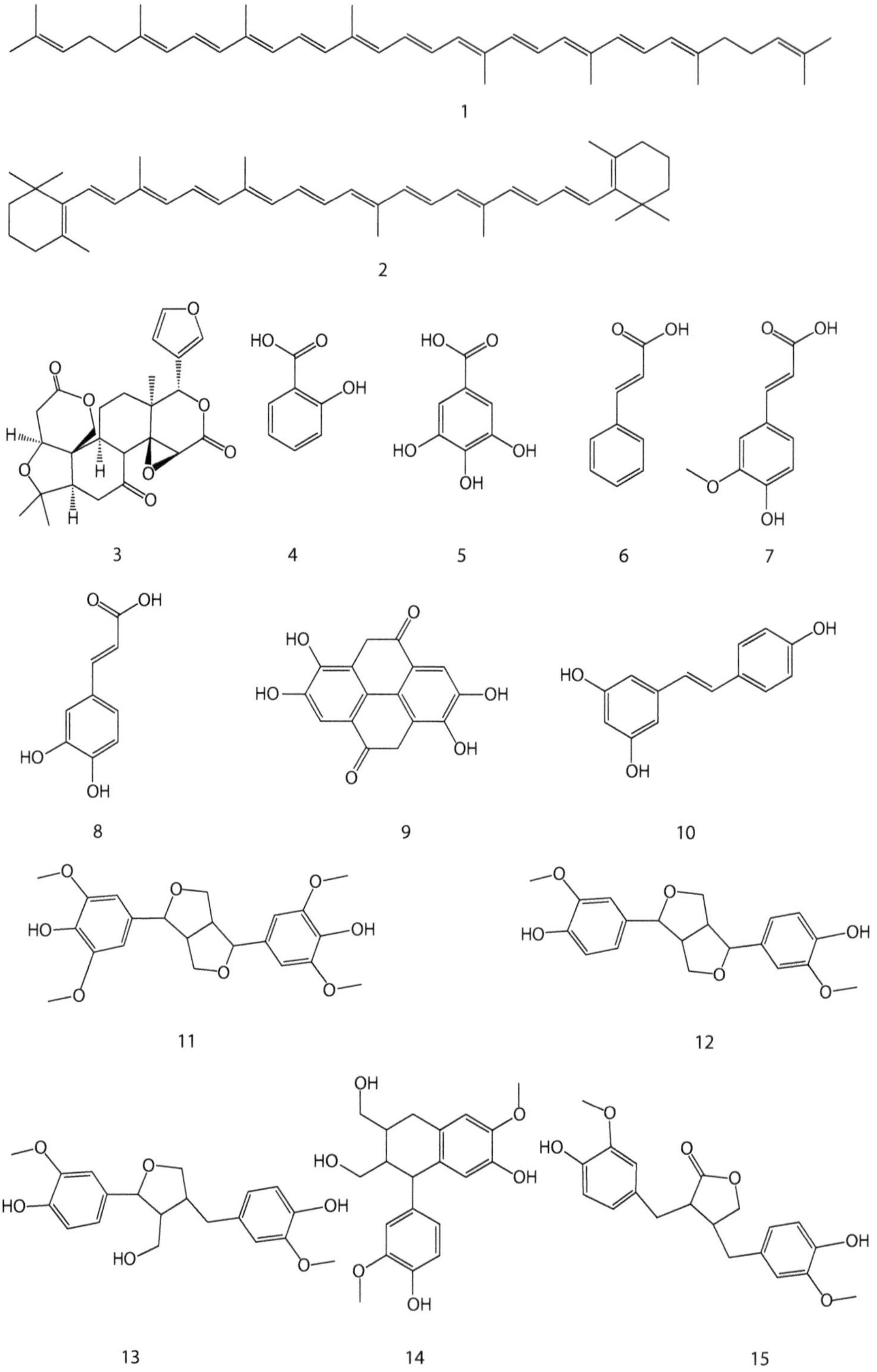

FIGURE 7.1 Structures of phytochemicals.

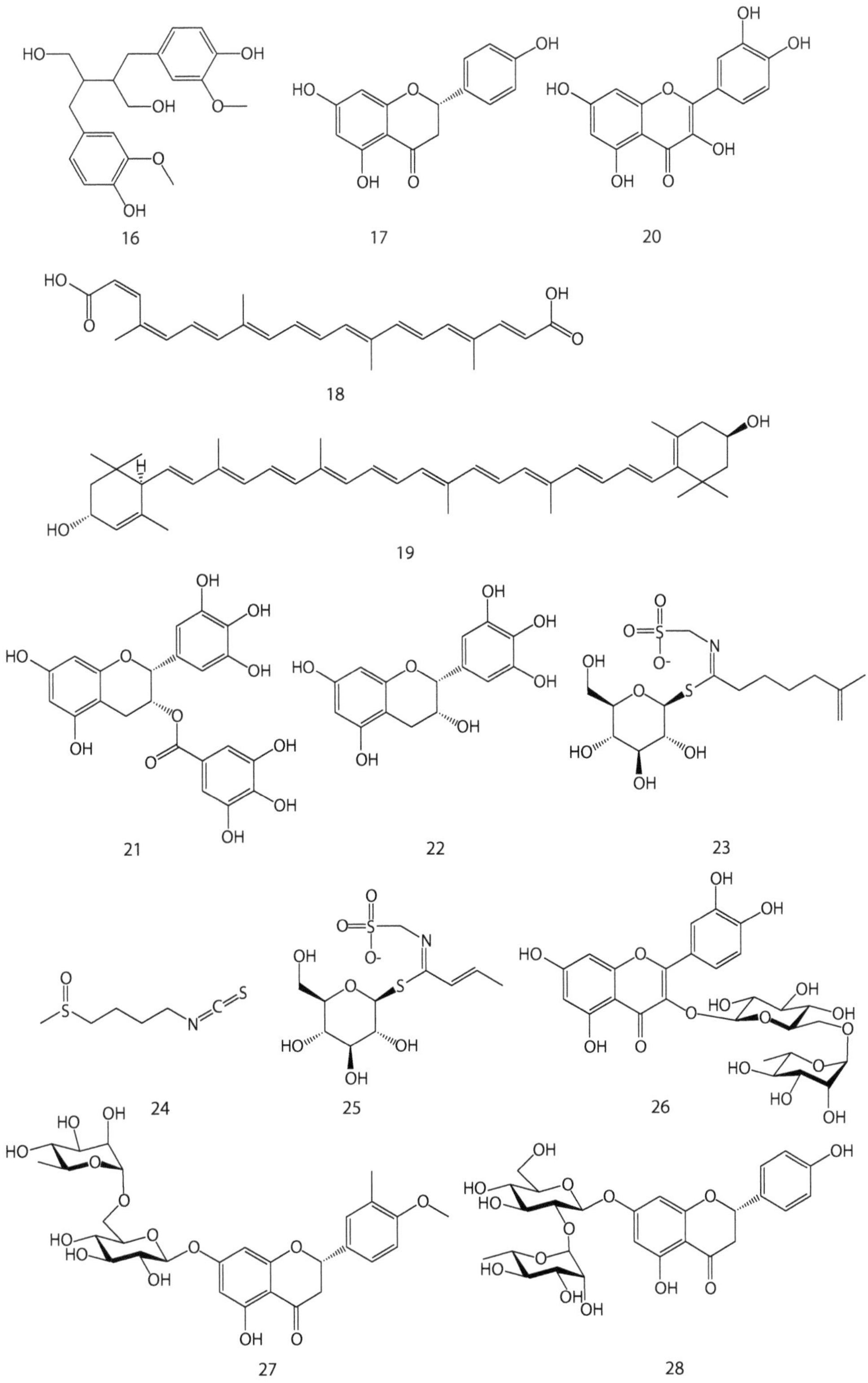

FIGURE 7.1 (Continued) Structures of phytochemicals.

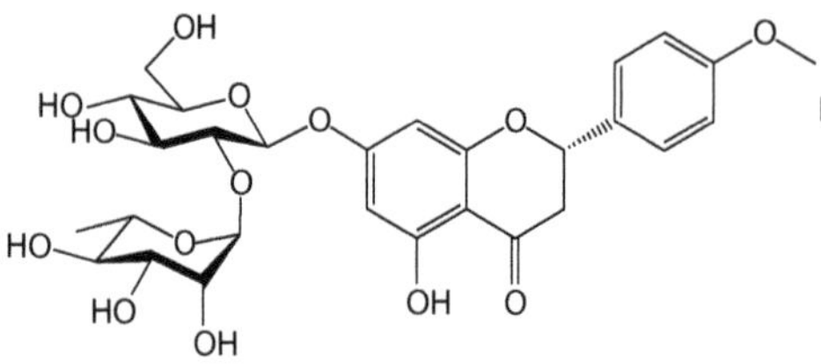

FIGURE 7.1 (Continued) Structures of phytochemicals.

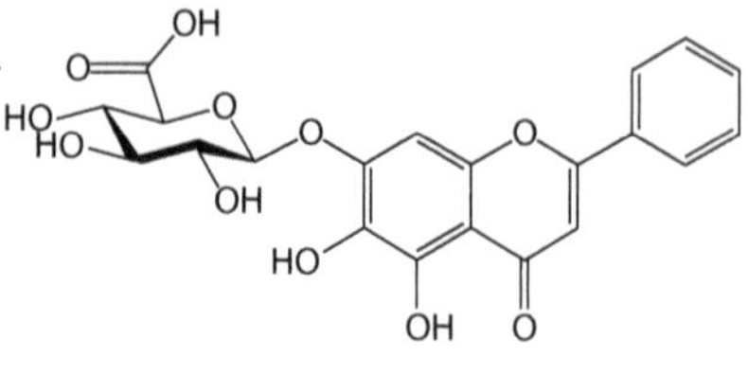

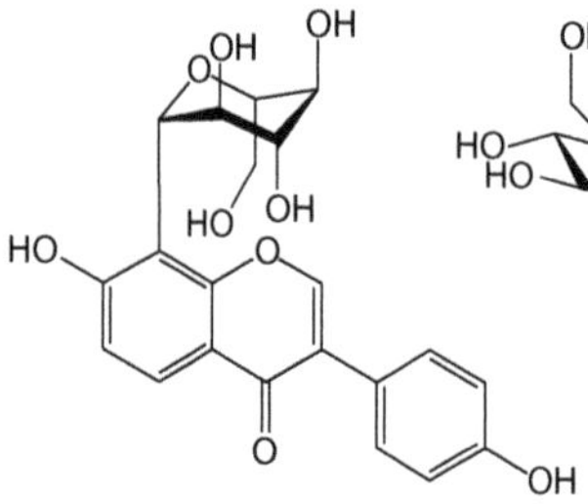

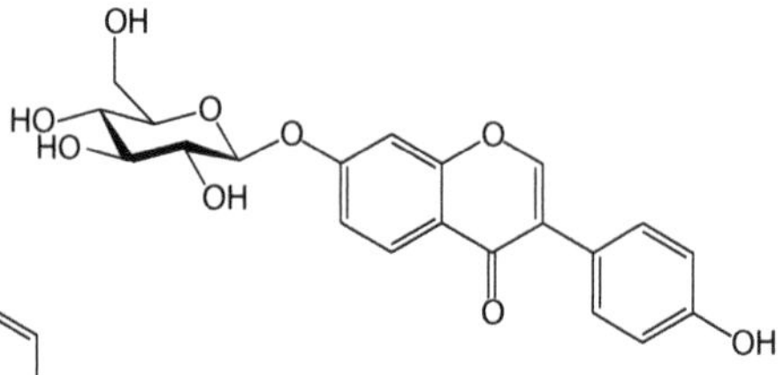

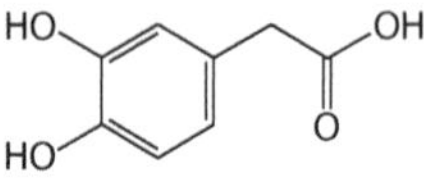

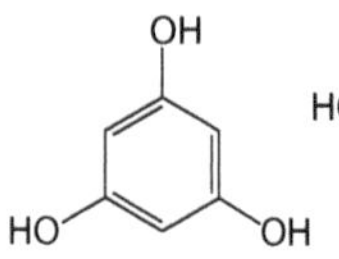

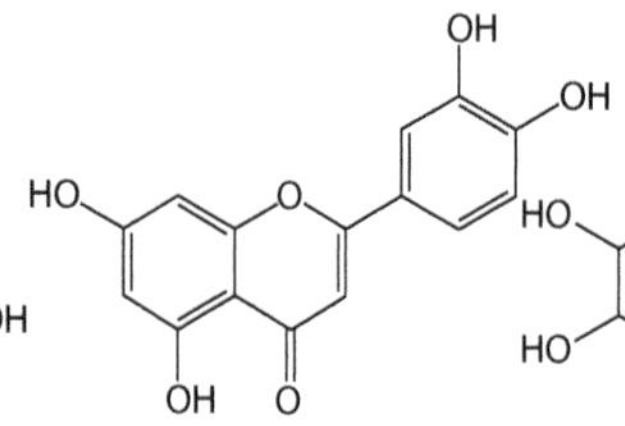

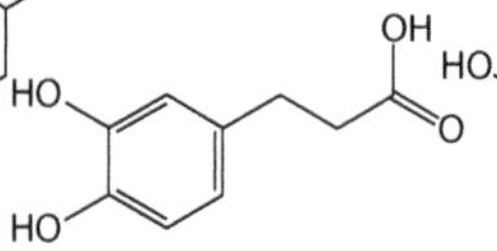

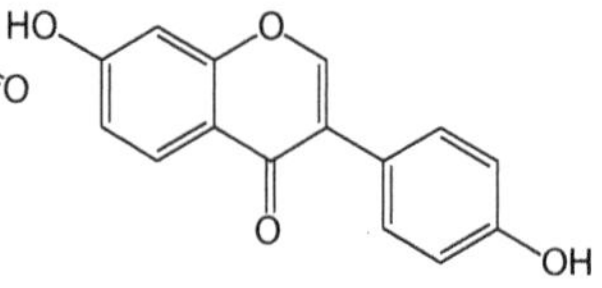

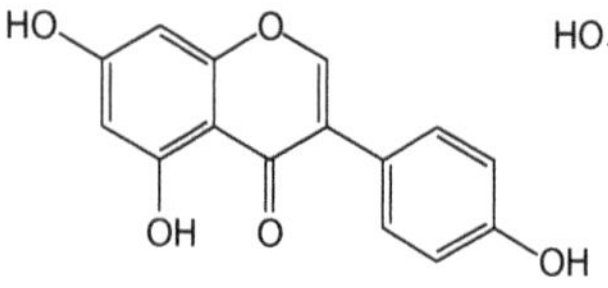

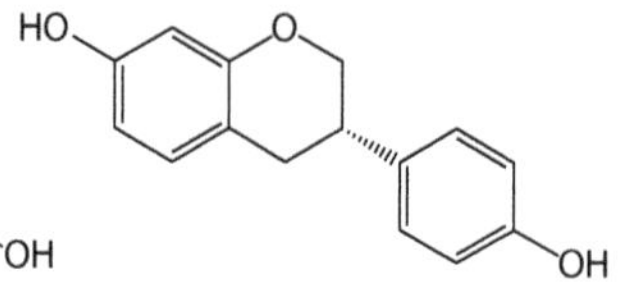

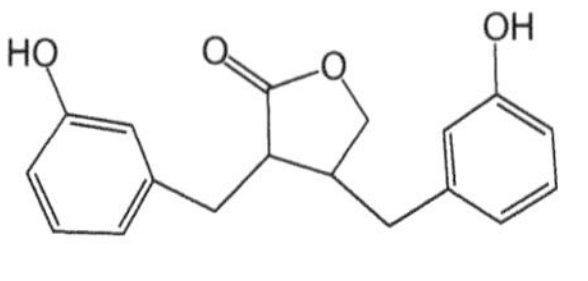

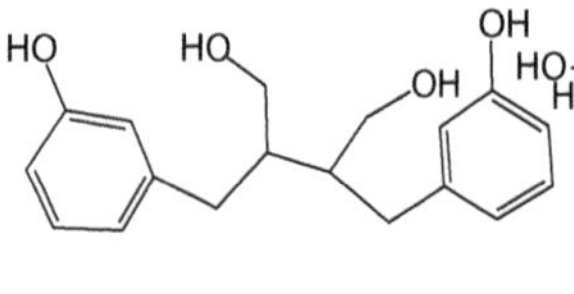

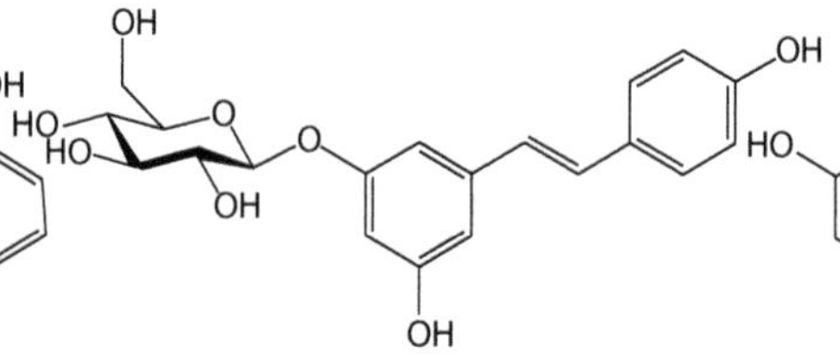

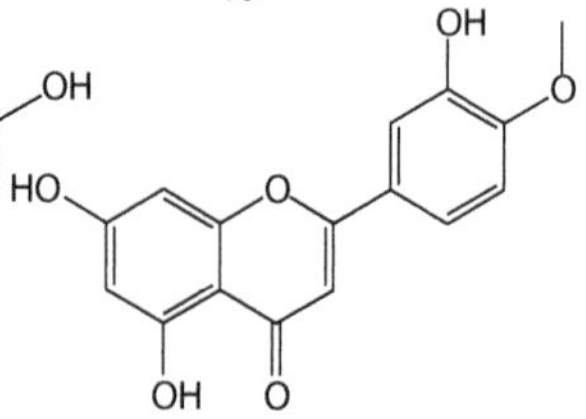

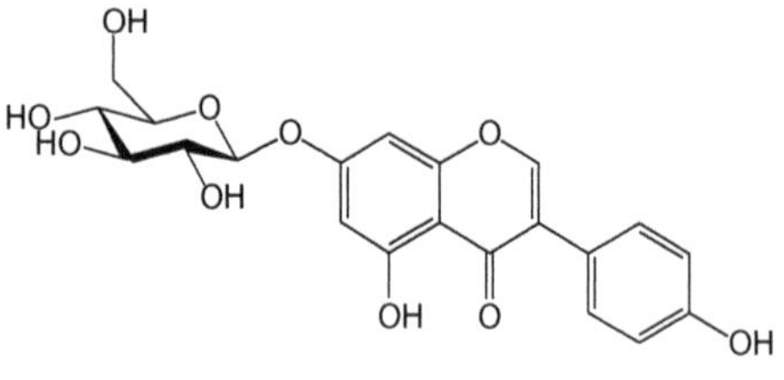

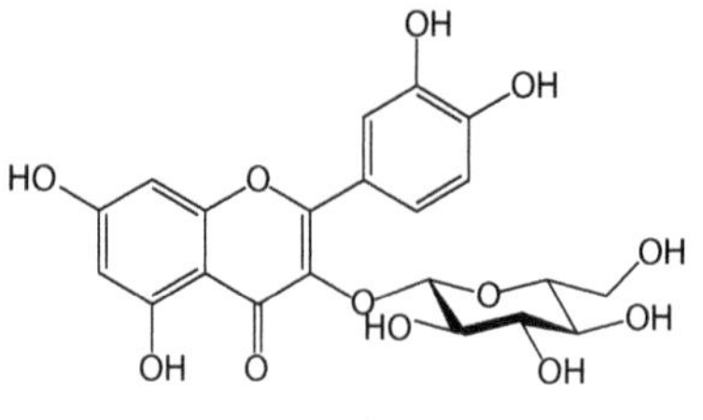

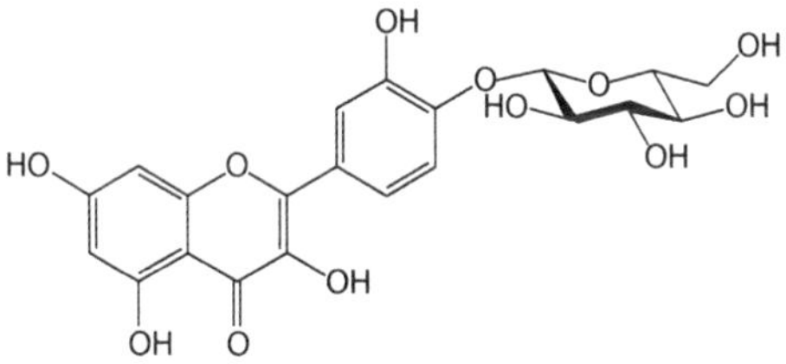

46

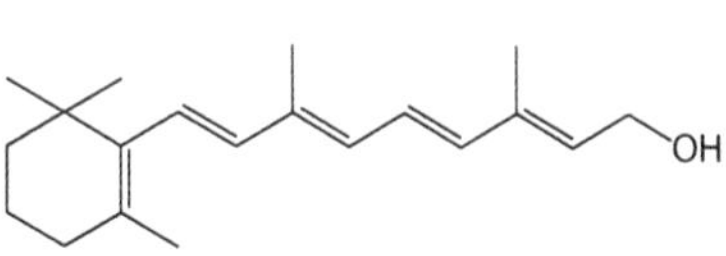

47

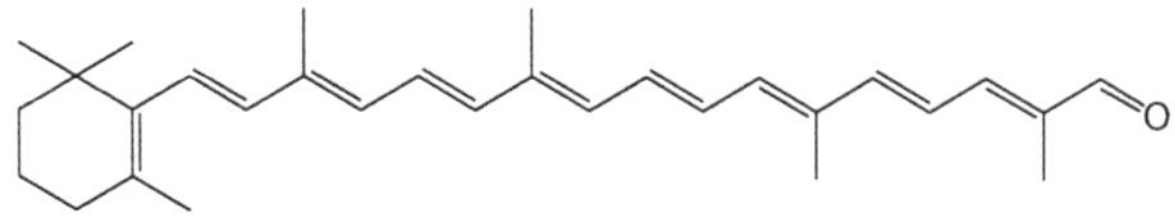

48

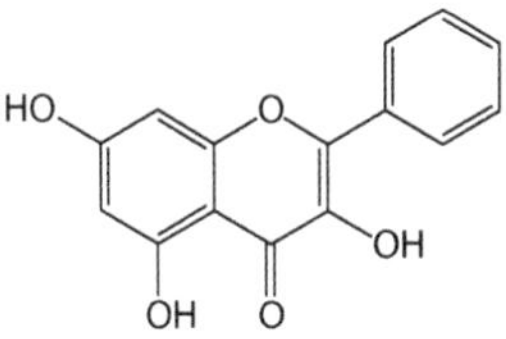

49

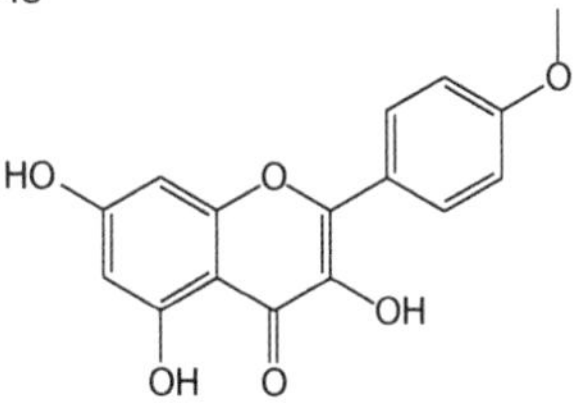

50

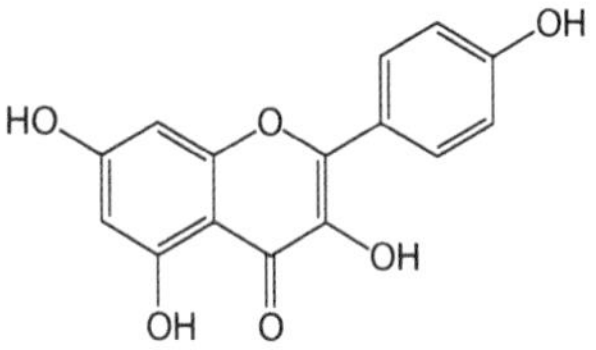

51

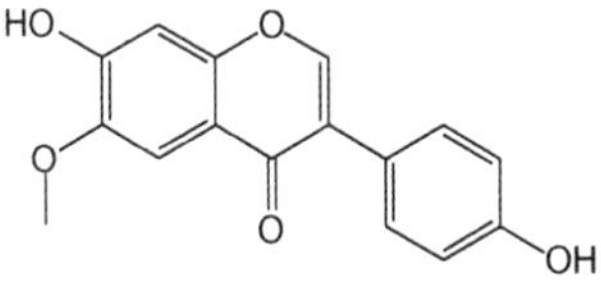

52

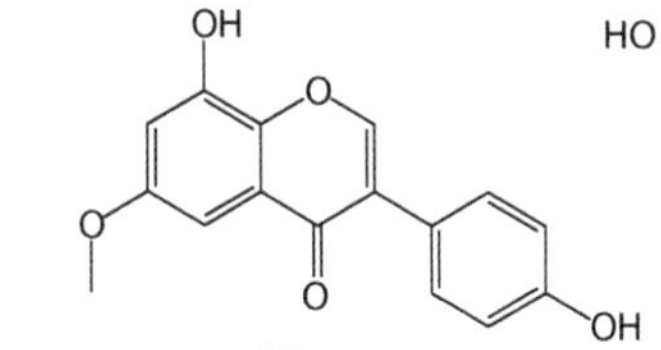

53

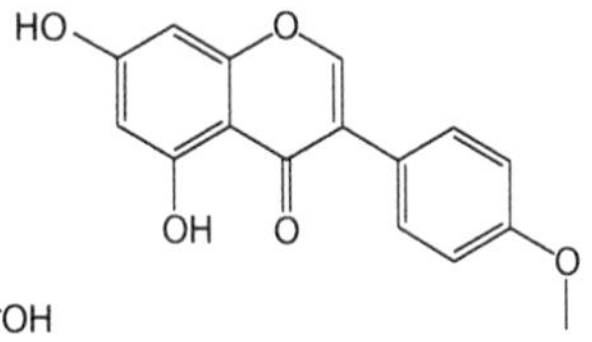

54

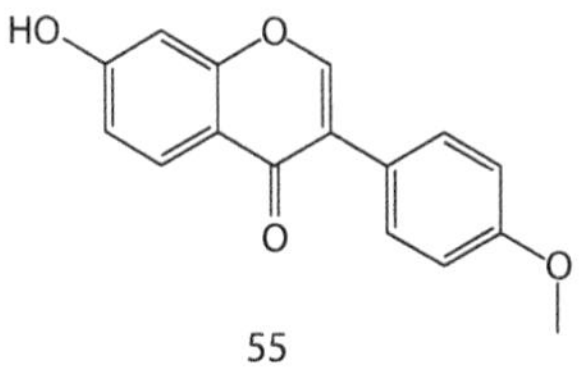

55

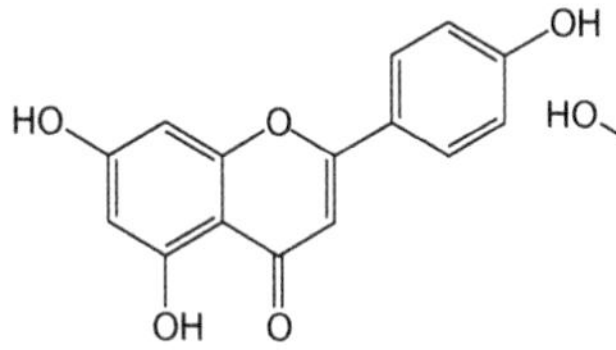

56

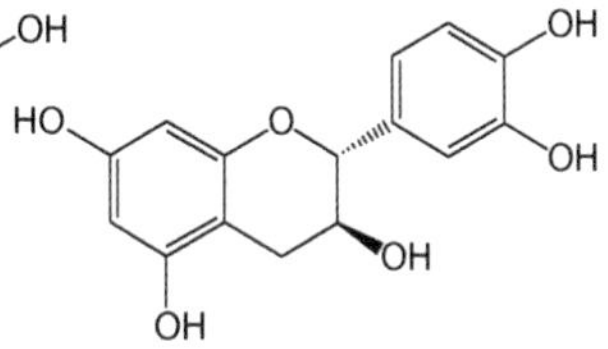

57

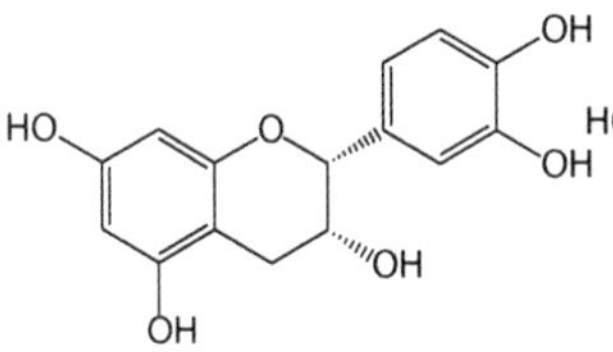

58

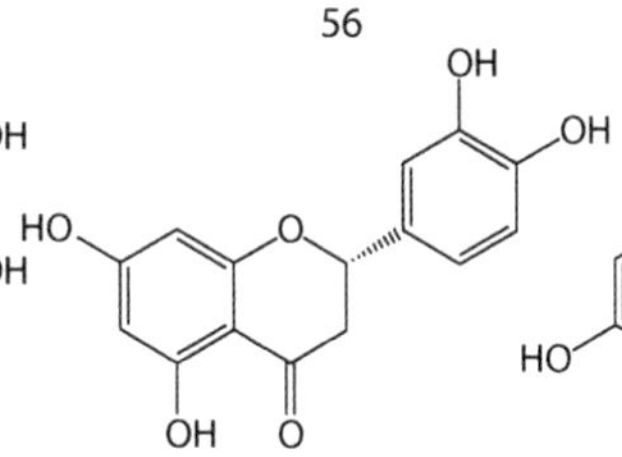

59

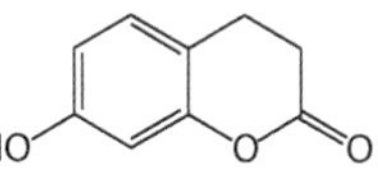

60

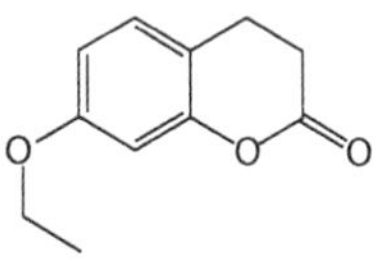

61

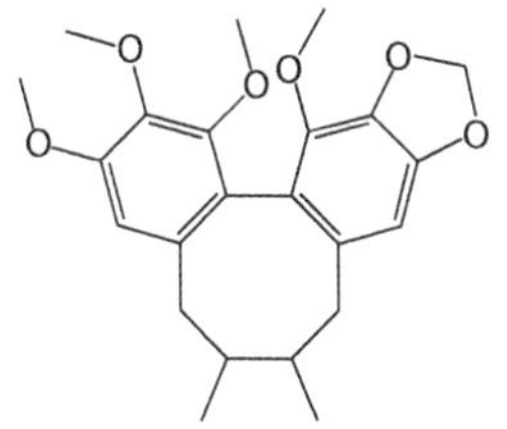

62

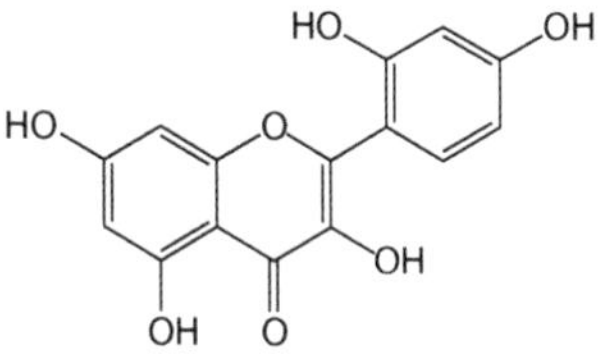

63

FIGURE 7.1 (Continued) Structures of phytochemicals.

slightly improved. And as such, only about 5% of the total carotenoids in raw vegetables are absorbed by the intestine directly, whereas 50% or more are absorbed from micellar solutions (formed by the action of surface-active bile acids) (Olson et al. 1994). Thus, two initial and also crucial steps in the in vivo intestinal absorption of carotenoids are released from the food matrix and solubilization into the mixed lipid micelles in the lumen (Borel 2003). The micellar structure has a disklike shape with an approximate diameter of 4–60 nm, consisting of an outer shell of bile salts surrounding a core formed by more hydrophobic lipids. The detergent action of bile salts plays an essential role in the absorption of carotenoids (Yonekura and Nagao 2007).

7.2.1.2 Solubility of Limonoids

Limonoids are highly oxidized triterpenes present in all citrus fruits. Several citrus limonoid aglycones or glycosides have been found to possess substantial anticancer activity in laboratory screening using animal models and human cancer cell lines (Poulose et al. 2006; Ejaz et al. 2006). Concentration of limonoid glycosides, mainly glucosides, can be as high as 900 ppm in orange juice and in excess of 2 g/L in certain byproducts of citrus processing (Schoch et al. 2001; Ozaki et al. 1995). Limonoids are water soluble, tasteless, and abundant in nature and may prove to be ideal functional food additives for cancer prevention (Hasegawa et al. 2000a). Limonoid aglycones that occur at low levels in citrus juice are water insoluble and bitter, similar to limonin (Figure 7.1, 3). However, water solubility of limonoid aglycones can be improved through their conversion from lactone to carboxylic form in aqueous solution by adjusting the pH to a value higher than 6.5, making both aglycone and glycoside soluble so they can be available for absorption by the enterocytes (Hasegawa et al. 2000b).

7.2.2 Solubility of Phenolics

Among the dietary phytochemicals used in cancer chemoprevention, phenolic compounds have perhaps been the most attractive ones. Cai et al. (2004) characterized antioxidant activity in 112 species of traditional plants with anticancer activities and found that phenolic compounds were the dominant antioxidant components. The phenolics include phenolic acids, flavonoids, tannins, coumarins, lignans, stilbenes, and curcuminoids. The chemistry, bioavailability, and beneficial effects of phenolics have been reviewed extensively (Crozier et al. 2009; Dai and Mumper 2010; Soobrattee et al. 2006). Their solubilities are summarized below, separated by various subclasses.

7.2.2.1 Solubility of Phenolic Acids

Mota et al. (2008) determined aqueous solubility of several natural phenolic acids at 30°C and found them to be relatively soluble with salicylic acid at 2.18 g/L (Figure 7.1, 4), gallic acid at 18.86 g/L (Figure 7.1, 5), *trans*-cinnamic acid at 0.31 g/L (Figure 7.1, 6), ferulic acid at 0.92 g/L (Figure 7.1, 7), and caffeic acid at 1.23 g/L (Figure 7.1, 8). Another phenolic acid, ellagic acid (Figure 7.1, 9), which was a promising anticancer and antiproliferation agent, was reported to have a relatively low aqueous solubility (9.7 μg/mL in water, 33.1 μg/mL in pH 7.4 phosphate buffer, 37°C). The poor absorption of ellagic acid after oral administration could be partially due to its low solubility (Bala et al. 2006). However, in a food matrix, most phenolic acids mainly occur as soluble or insoluble (or bound) esters, depending on the ester and structures of the phenolic acids. Chlorogenic acid, a soluble ester of caffeic acid, was found to be absorbed in their intact form from the stomach of rats (Lafay et al. 2006a). For insoluble esters, hydrolysis is required to release free phenolic acids for absorption. Phenolic acids are significantly better absorbed than their esters, indicating the importance of aqueous solubility in determining their bioavailability (Adam et al. 2002; Azuma et al. 2000; Lafay et al. 2006b).

7.2.2.2 Solubility of Stilbenoids

Stilbenoids are hydroxylated derivatives of stilbene. Recently, natural and synthetic stilbenoids have been actively and extensively investigated to reveal their potentials in cancer therapy and prevention (Kimura et al. 2008; Rimando and Suh 2008). Resveratrol (Figure 7.1, 10), a phytoalexin found in grapes and wines, has been a "superstar" phytochemical due to its well-acknowledged biological beneficial effects such as cancer prevention and life extension (Howitz et al. 2003; Jang et al. 1997). However, oral bioavailability of resveratrol in humans is very low, which may impede its pharmacological activities in vivo (Delmas et al. 2006). Although resveratrol is a lipophilic molecule with log $P > 3.1$ and solubility of 0.03 g/L, the direct role of aqueous solubility on oral bioavailability of resveratrol was not actively examined until recently. Das et al. (2008) found that although cyclodextrin could increase resveratrol solubility substantially, no significant improvement in bioavailability was observed when resveratrol formulated in cyclodextrin solution was administrated to rats, indicating that poor availability of resveratrol was not due to poor solubility, provided that resveratrol did not actually bind too tightly to cyclodextrin.

7.2.2.3 Solubility of Lignans

Lignans are one of the major classes of phytochemicals widely distributed in cereals, fruits, vegetables, and beverages, especially in flaxseed (0.4% dried mass) (Milder et al. 2005). The major lignans in natural products are syringiresinol (Figure 7.1, 11), pinoresinol (Figure 7.1, 12), lariciresinol (Figure 7.1, 13), isolariciresinol (Figure 7.1, 14), matairesinol (MAT) (Figure 7.1, 15), and secoisolariciresinol (SECO) (Figure 7.1, 16), which are usually found in nature as glucosides and/or diglucosides (Bowey et al. 2003). As phytoestrogens, lignans have been well studied with respect to their potential in treatment or prevention of diseases such as breast cancer, prostate cancer, and several hormone-related disorders (Ward and Kuhnle 2010; Virk-Baker et al. 2010). Some of the most extensively studied lignans are MAT and SECO, as well as their diglucosides (secoisolariciresinol diglucoside [SDG]). When studying the oral bioavailability of lignans, researchers usually pay more attention to microflora transformation than their solubilities. However, it is generally believed that lignan glycosides are water soluble, while their aglycones are less soluble (Kim et al. 2006). As estimated by Hu et al. (2003), after oral administration, colon epithelial cells may be exposed to SECO at concentrations as high as 100 µM, which was enabled by colonic microflora-mediated SDG hydrolysis. This level of solubility was also reported by Kulling et al. (1998), who incubated 100 µM SECO Chinese hamster with Chinese hamster V79 cells (Kitts et al. 1999). Thus, it appears that oral absorption of SDG and SECO is not limited by their solubilities.

7.2.2.4 Solubility of Flavonoids

In the human daily diet, a large percentage of phenolics are consumed as flavonoids. Their protective effects as antioxidant, anticancer, and anti-inflammatory agents have been demonstrated both in vitro and in vivo (Ramos 2007; Kale et al. 2008; González et al. 2011). Dietary flavonoid glycosides could not rapidly diffuse across the intestinal membrane during ingestion because of their hydrophilic property (Liu and Hu 2002). However, for highly permeable flavonoid aglycones, oral bioavailability is not high, either, at least partially due to their poor solubility, which is often less than 20 µg/mL in water (Hu 2007). The low solubility can limit dissolution rates, which could lead to a slow absorption. No systematic studies have been performed to determine the relationship between aglycone solubilities and their diverse molecular structures, featuring different substitutions on the carbon backbone. Several researchers have shown that flavonoid solubility and dissolution rate could be improved by complexation with pharmaceutical excipients like β-cyclodextrin or by being formulated as a solid dispersion (Rezende et al. 2009; Lee et al. 2007; Tommasini et al. 2004; Kanaze et al. 2006). Shulman et al. (2011) found that after complexation with hydroxylpropyl-β-cyclodextrin, naringenin (Figure 7.1, 17) solubility in water and permeability in a Caco-2 cell model increased by over 400-fold and 11-fold, respectively. More attractively, when fed to rats, both area under the curve (AUC) and C_{max} values increased by 7.4-fold and 14.6-fold, respectively (Shulman et al. 2011).

7.3 STABILITY AND GUT MICROFLORA BIOTRANSFORMATION

Usually, the whole process of human digestion takes more than 24 h, indicating that certain bioactive constituents in food may be subject to fast degradation or biotransformation before absorption. For

TABLE 7.1

Digestive Degradation of Selected Phytochemicals

Class	Phytochemicals	Factors or Mechanisms that Influence Digestive Stability	Reference
Anthocyanidins and anthocyanins	Anthocyanidins	pH	(Yonekura-Sakakibara et al. 2009)
	Procyanidin oglimers	Acidic hydrolysis	(Spencer et al. 2000)
Glucosinolate	Glucosinolates from broccoli	Acidic decomposition	(Vallejo et al. 2003)
	Allyl isothiocyanate	Nucleophilic addition reactions with amino acid or small peptides	(Cejpek et al. 2000)
Flavonoids	Flavonoids from broccoli	pH	(Vallejo et al. 2003)
	Flavonoids from *Ginkgo biloba*	pH	(Goh and Barlow 2004)
	EGCG and EGC	Dimerization	(Neilson et al. 2007)
	EGCG	Epimerization	(Wang et al. 2008)
	Quercetin	Oxidative degradation	(Boulton et al. 1999)
Carotenoids	Xanthophylls/carotenes	Containing oxygen or not	(Blanquet-Diot et al. 2009)
	Lycopene	Isomeric conformation	(Blanquet-Diot et al. 2009)
	β-Carotene	Isomeric conformation	(Ferruzzi et al. 2006)

example, some phytochemicals, which work as excellent antioxidant agents, may be very easily oxidized. Recently, a booming metabonomics analysis has revealed a very important role of large bowel microflora in shaping the metabolic profiles of xenobiotics or nutrients (Wikoff et al. 2009). Here, chemical stability and gut microflora biotransformation are included in our discussion of oral bioavailability of phytochemicals. Selective presentation of the information related to the digestive degradation of selected phytochemicals was briefly summarized and can be found in Table 7.1.

7.3.1 Chemical Stability of Selected Phytochemicals

7.3.1.1 Chemical Stability of Carotenoids

For carotenoids such as lutein (Figure 7.1, 18), β-carotene, and lycopene, their stability is a major concern during food storage (Lin and Chen 2005). Recently Boon et al. thoroughly reviewed research on the chemical stability of carotenoids in foods (Boon et al. 2010). Degradation of carotenoids during food storage involves reaction with singlet oxygen, acid, metal ions, and free radicals, via multiple mechanisms such as autoxidation, thermal degradation, and photodegradation (Henry et al. 2000; Perez-Galvez et al. 2005; Konovalova et al. 2001; Edge et al. 1997; Konovalov and Kispert 1999; Gao et al. 2006). Polar-Cabrera et al. (2010) investigated the stability of norbixin (Figure 7.1, 19), an abundant 24-carbon carotenoid in annatto, during digestion, and they found that norbixin added in milk was highly stable during simulated gastric and small intestinal digestion. By employing a dynamic in vitro gastrointestinal system, Blanquet-Diot et al. (2009) assessed and compared digestive stability of different subclasses of carotenoids. Xanthophylls, or oxygenated carotenoids, showed a decent digestive stability throughout the artificial digestion process, whereas unoxygenated carotenoids, or carotenes, were partially degraded during this process (Blanquet-Diot et al. 2009). The isomeric conformation of a compound also influences the stability of different carotenoid isomers during digestion (Blanquet-Diot et al. 2009; Ferruzzi et al. 2006). The impact of the stability of carotenoids on their absorption in the human gastrointestinal tract and their oral bioavailabilities is unclear and merits further investigations.

7.3.1.2 Chemical Stability of Glucosinolate

More than 100 different glucosinolates are known to occur as secondary metabolites in cruciferous vegetables like broccoli and cauliflower (Bednarek et al. 2009; Halkier and Gershenzon 2006).

Derived from glucose and amino acid, this class of compounds contains sulfur and nitrogen and exhibits toxicity at high doses in both humans and animals (Nugon-Baudon et al. 1990; Donkin 1995). However, at exposure below the toxic level, hydrolytic and metabolic products of glucosinolates can act as liver detoxification enzyme activators and provide protection against mutagenesis, carcinogenesis, and oxidative damages (Hayes et al. 2008; Steinkellner et al. 2001).

Bioavailability of glucosinolates from *Brassica* vegetables was influenced by storage, processing, and cooking procedures (Song and Thornalley 2007). Vallejo et al. (2003) demonstrated a major loss (up to 69%) in glucosinolates during in vitro gastric digestion of broccoli, revealing that digestive stability of glucosinolates could be a critical factor in determining their oral bioavailability. Besides biotransformation pathways, nonenzymic degradation also contributes to the conversion of glucosinolates to their health-promoting metabolic products. Recently, Bones and Rossiter (2006) published a comprehensive review on both enzymatic and chemically induced decomposition of glucosinolates. Generally, chemical stability of glucosinolates depends on pH, temperature, and other factors such as concentrations of metal ions in the solution (Bones and Rossiter 2006; MacLeod and Rossiter 1986). In particular, acid decomposition of glucosinolates generates corresponding carboxylic acids and hydroxylammonium ions, which may be responsible for the losses of glucosinolates during gastric digestion (Ettlinger and Lundeen 1956). Moreover, certain electrophilic derivatives of glucosinolates such as allyl or benzyl isothiocyanate can react with small peptides and amino acids to generate new products in a pH-dependent manner (Cejpek et al. 2000; Kroll and Rawel 1996). Enzyme-mediated metabolic pathways will be discussed elsewhere in this chapter.

7.3.1.3 Chemical Stability of Anthocyanidins and Anthocyanins

Anthocyanidins and their sugar-containing (glycosidic) counterparts, anthocyanins, are common pigments in plants. Health benefits of these pigments have attracted a lot of attention because of their potential curative or preventive effects against cancer, inflammation, diabetes, aging, and cardiovascular diseases (Wang and Stoner 2008; Zafra-Stone et al. 2007). Anthocyanidins are inherently unstable, and their stability is largely dependent on pH (Yonekura-Sakakibara et al. 2009). Spencer et al. (2000) found that in an acidic environment like the gastric milieu, procyanidin oglimers (trimers to hexamer) would be hydrolyzed to a mixture of epicatechin monomer and dimer, resulting in enhanced potential for absorption in the small intestine.

Anthocyanins are products of anthocyanidin glycosylation, usually present as 3-*O*-glucoside. Although stability of anthocyanins is largely improved compared to their aglycones, these pigments are still subject to significant physiochemical degradation. After oral consumption, low pH in the stomach renders anthocyanins to stay in their most stable form as the flavylium cation (Talavéra et al. 2003). However, in the intestine with a neutral or alkaline pH, anthocyanins exist in multiple other forms, which are less stable (Seeram et al. 2001). Dai et al. (2009) reported that total anthocyanins extracted from blackberries degraded rapidly when incubated in biologically relevant buffers such as pH 7.4 phosphate buffered saline (PBS) with 10% fetal bovine serum (FBS) or Roswell Park Memorial Institute (RPMI) 1640 cell culture medium with 10% FBS at 37°C, with a half-life of 5.0 and 6.2 h, respectively. It has also been demonstrated that the degradation of anthocyanins to their phenolic acid and aldehyde residues involves B-ring hydroxylation (Woodward et al. 2009). Thus, after oral consumption, ingested anthocyanins are likely to degrade in the intestinal tract before absorption, which may contribute to their low bioavailability and low plasma concentration.

7.3.1.4 Chemical Stability of Flavonoids

Digestive stability of flavonoids has been investigated in several studies by an in vitro digestion model that simulates in vivo gastrointestinal digestion with respect to pH, temperature, enzymes, and chemicals (Goh and Barlow 2004; Walsh et al. 2003). In general, flavonoids showed high stability at low pH, while they were vulnerable at neutral or higher pH values (Xing et al. 2005; Zhu et al. 2002). For example, Vallejo et al. (2003) conducted simulated gastrointestinal digestion of flavonoids from broccoli, and their results showed almost no losses of flavonoids in gastric digestion, in contrast to up to 80% losses of total flavonoids after intestinal digestion. Boulton et al. (1999) examined the elimination of quercetin (Figure 7.1, 20), which was incubated in Hank's balanced salt solution (HBSS) buffer or cell culture medium together with human cell lines. Besides cellular metabolism, oxidative degradation also contributed significantly to the complete depletion of quercetin in 8 h, resulting in C-ring opening and carboxylic acid formation (Boulton et al. 1999).

For flavan-3-ols, which are also known as catechins, degradation occurs simultaneously via several pathways. For example, (-)-epigallocatechin gallate (EGCG) (Figure 7.1, 21) and (-)-epigallocatechin (EGC) (Figure 7.1, 22) degrade in a simulated digestion model with concurrent formation of homocatechin and heterocatechin dimers (Neilson et al. 2007). Meanwhile, for EGCG, both degradation and epimerization occur at the same time in a temperature-dependent manner, and degradation is more profound than epimerization at the physiological temperature (Wang et al. 2008).

7.3.2 BIOTRANSFORMATION OF PHYTOCHEMICALS BY GUT MICROFLORA

The human gut is populated by diverse bacterial species that are prominently involved in the digestion, biotransformation, and absorption of nutrition constituents along the intestinal tract, exerting various effects on the health status of the host. Reciprocal influences and complicated interactions have been described between gut microflora and dietary components, including not only nutrients but also bioactive phytochemicals. For example, phytochemicals may inhibit pathogenic bacteria growth directly or change gut microflora composition and their metabolic profiles, bringing beneficial efforts to human health (Laparra and Sanz 2010). For phytochemicals, their bioavailability and pharmacological behavior would be affected, at least partially, by gut microflora-mediated biotransformation, via either activation or degradation/inactivation. Here we will discuss the roles of gut microflora in determining the fate of several anticancer or anti-inflammation phytochemicals after oral consumption. A brief summary on the degradation and biotransformation of selected phytochemicals by gut microflora is provided in Table 7.2.

TABLE 7.2
Biotransformation of Selected Phytochemicals by the Microflora in the Human Gastrointestinal Tract

Class	Phytochemical	Biotransformation	Products	Reference
Glucosinolates	Glucoraphanin	Hydrolysis	Sulforaphane	(Lai et al. 2010)
Flavonoids	Flavonoid glycosides	Hydrolysis	Flavonoid aglycones	(Kim et al. 1998)
	Flavonoid aglycones	Ring fission	Phenolic acids	(Braune et al. 2001)
		Reduction	Dihydroflavonoids	(Yuan et al. 2007)
Lignans	SDG	Hydrolysis	SECO	(Roncaglia et al. 2011)
	SECO	Oxidation/	Enterolactone and/or	(Borriello et al. 1985)
	MAT	reduction	enterodiol	
Stilbenes	Piceid	Hydrolysis	*Trans*-resveratrol	(Wang et al. 2011)
	Resveratrol	Hydrogenation	5-(4-hydroxyphenethyl) benzene-1,3-diol	(Walle et al. 2004)
Anthocyanins	Anthocyanin glucosides	Hydrolysis	Anthocyanin aglycones	(Keppler and Humpf 2005)
	Anthocyanin aglycones	Ring fission	Phenolic acids	(Keppler and Humpf 2005)

7.3.2.1 Microflora and Carotenoids in Food

By employing an in vitro digestion and colonic (microflora) fermentation method, Laparra et al. found that both enzymatic digestion and colonic (microflora) fermentation facilitated the release of carotenoids, such as β-carotene and lutein, from the food matrix (Laparra and Sanz 2010). In another study, Goñi et al. (2006) investigated the large intestinal accessibility of carotenoids in the food matrix, and they arrived at a similar conclusion that colonic fermentation was important for carotenoid oral bioavailability. However, Grolier et al. (1998) reported that when rats were fed with a diet supplemented with carotenoids, a reduction in the intestinal microflora resulted in the accumulation of carotenoids and their derivatives in the liver. They also found that bacteria in rat or human feces neither contributed to the degradation of β-carotene during in vitro incubation nor had a direct impact on its bioavailability (Grolier et al. 1998). These divergent facts indicate that further exploration is needed for researchers to establish an explicit association between gut microflora and the bioavailability of carotenoids in food.

7.3.2.2 Microflora and Glucosinolates

Cruciferous vegetables and certain bacterial species resident in the human and rat intestine are able to produce an enzyme called myrosinase. Functioning synergistically, myrosinases from different origins may cleave off the glucose group from a glucosinolate and convert it to a corresponding isothiocyanate (ITC) during digestion of raw cruciferous vegetables (Rouzaud et al. 2003, 2004).

Recently, it has been found that after oral consumption of cooked broccoli, where plant or dietary myrosinase was deactivated, glucoraphanin (Figure 7.1, 23), a major glucosinolate in broccoli, remained intact during passage through the rat gastrointestinal tract until it reached the cecum, where it was hydrolyzed by bacterial myrosinases and absorbed by the bowel epithelium. The absorption resulted in the appearance of an ITC known as sulforaphane (Figure 7.1, 24), in the mesenteric plasma (Lai et al. 2010). By simulating the digestion of cooked brussels sprouts in a dynamic large intestinal model in vitro, Krul et al. (2002) also demonstrated the local release of ITCs from 2-propenyl glucosinolate (sinigrin) (Figure 7.1, 25) in the colon by human intestinal microflora.

7.3.2.3 Microflora and Flavonoids

Microflora-mediated metabolism of flavonoids has been extensively studied, and three areas of research are highlighted here.

7.3.2.3.1 Hydrolysis

Flavonoids are commonly present in food as glycosides with decent water solubility but poor permeability across the gut epithelial membrane (Slimestad et al. 2007). Bacterial glycoside hydrolases in the animal intestinal tract catalyze the hydrolysis of the glycosidic linkage and transform glycosides to their aglycones with lower water solubility but high permeability, thus enhancing their overall absorption (Bowey et al. 2003; Selma et al. 2009). As reported by Kim et al. (1998), rutin (Figure 7.1, 26), hesperidin (Figure 7.1, 27), naringin (Figure 7.1, 28), and poncirin (Figure 7.1, 29) were hydrolyzed by the bacteria producing α-rhamnosidase and β-glucosidase or endo-β-glucosidase, while baicalin (Figure 7.1, 30), puerarin (Figure 7.1, 31), and daidzin (Figure 7.1, 32) were hydrolyzed by the bacteria producing β-glucuronidase, c-glycosidase, and β-glycosidase, forming aglycones that are much more rapidly absorbed.

7.3.2.3.2 Ring Fission

Intestinal microflora-mediated ring fission has been known as a degradation pathway for isoflavones, flavonols, flavones, and flavan-3-ols for more than 50 years (Selma et al. 2009; Booth et al. 1956). In this pathway, the C ring breaks from certain particular positions, followed by an internal split between the A and B rings and generation of simpler phenolic compounds (Winter et al. 1989). For example, by an anaerobe named *Eubacertium ramulus* found in human intestinal tract, quercetin was converted to 3,4-dihydroxyphenylacetic acid (Figure 7.1, 33) and phloroglucinol (Figure 7.1, 34), while luteolin (Figure 7.1, 35) was converted to 3-(3,4-dihydroxyphenyl)-propionic acid (Figure 7.1, 36) and phloroglucinol (Braune et al. 2001). A similar degradation pathway is responsible for the ring fission of multiple flavonoids, including daidzein (Figure 7.1, 37), genistein (Figure 7.1, 38), rutin, and naringin (Hur et al. 2002; Schoefer et al. 2002; Cheng et al. 1969, 1971; Krishnamurty et al. 1970). After oral administration of flavonoids, several phenolic acids are detected in the urine of normal animals but not in animals without normal intestinal microflora, validating a microfloral origin of these metabolic products (Griffiths 1972).

7.3.2.3.3 Reduction

Reduction is also a metabolic pathway of flavonoids mediated by intestinal microflora. In fact, for daidzein, genistein, quercetin, and luteolin, the C-ring fission process is usually initiated after the hydrogenation (i.e., reduction) of the C2–C3 double bond to form dihydroflavonoids (Braune et al. 2001; Aura 2008; Yuan et al. 2007). Among these dihydroflavonoids, dihydrolyzed daidzein is the most extensively investigated one because it is subject to further reduction, generating a more potent estrogenic metabolite, equol (Figure 7.1, 39), a compound whose exposure is associated with lower cancer risk in humans (Yuan et al. 2007; Lampe 2010).

7.3.2.4 Microflora and Lignan

The lignans are wildly distributed natural products, usually present as glucosides and diglucosides. After losing sugar moieties by acidic or bacterial hydrolase-mediated hydrolysis, the aglycones undergo extensive metabolism by intestinal microflora (Bowey et al. 2003). For example, a major dietary lignan, SDG, undergoes hydrolysis to form SECO, which is also further transformed to become biologically active (Roncaglia et al. 2011). By conducting in vitro incubation of lignans with human fecal materials, Borriello et al. (1985) found that enterolactone (Figure 7.1, 40) was produced from MAT and enterodiol (Figure 7.1, 41) was produced from SECO by bacteria present in stools. Enterodiol can be further oxidized to enterolactone by bacteria. Both enterodiol and enterolactone were sometimes referenced as "mammalian lignans." Wang (2000) isolated seven metabolites including enterodiol and enterolactone from anaerobic incubation of SDG with a human fecal suspension, and they also identified two bacterial strains that were responsible for their biotransformation. Heinonen et al. (2001) quantitatively analyzed human fecal microflora-mediated biotransformation of eight major lignan species in food to enterodiol and enterolactone and depicted their overall conversion schemes.

7.3.2.5 Microflora and Stilbenes

5,4′-Dihydroxystilbene-3-*O*-β-D-glucopyranoside, also known as piceid (Figure 7.1, 42), is the 3-β-glucoside of resveratrol. It is probably the most abundant form of resveratrol in nature (Regev-Shoshani et al. 2003). When exposed to intestinal microflora, cleavage of sugar moieties by bacterial hydrolases occurs to release resveratrol for absorption (Wang et al. 2011).

After oral administration of [^{3}H]*trans*-resveratrol in rats, El-Mohsen et al. (2006) studied its distribution. Unlike flavonoids, urinary excretion of simple phenolic acids as colonic bacterial degradation products was not observed after gavage of resveratrol in rats, leading to a conclusion that resveratrol aglycone is not degraded by colonic microflora (El-Mohsen et al. 2006). However in another study by Walle et al. (2004), oral ingestion, bioavailability, and metabolism of [^{14}C] *trans*-resveratrol in humans was examined, and the hydrogenation of the aliphatic double bond was identified as a new and interesting metabolic pathway. The researchers claimed that this pathway might be mediated by the intestinal microflora.

7.3.2.6 Microflora and Anthocyanins

Different from the absorption of flavonoids, intact anthocyanin glycosides can be absorbed without hydrolysis and that the intact glycosides can be detected in plasma and even in urine, as animal studies have demonstrated (Matsumoto et al. 2001; Passamonti et al. 2005; Felgines et al. 2002; He et al. 2006).

However, when exposed to intestinal microflora, anthocyanin molecules are likely to be extensively modified or degraded, particularly in the colon. Keppler and Humpf (2005) investigated the fate of anthocyanins after exposure to microflora isolated from pig cecum in an in vitro model. They reported that after rapid deglycosylation, the corresponding aglycones of anthocyanins were unstable at neutral pH and suffered from further phenolic degradation involving demethylation, finally generating phenolic acids with better chemical and microbial stability than their precursors (Keppler and Humpf 2005). Several other studies employing bacterial population isolated from human feces have also shown that anthocyanins, which did not undergo gastric and small intestinal absorption, are subject to substantial biotransformation by colonic microflora, which may decrease bioavailability of the aglycone but may generate metabolites with new biological activities (Aura et al. 2005; Fleschhut et al. 2006).

7.4 UPTAKE MECHANISMS

Permeation of molecules across the intestinal epithelium may involve both uptake and efflux. Uptake is a process that a cell uses to take up an endogenous compound or a xenobiotic. Uptake or efflux may employ the same or different transport mechanisms, including, for example, transcellular and/or paracellular passive diffusion, facilitated and/or active transport mediated by transporters, or sometimes a combination of both. In this section, uptake of phytochemicals by enterocytes will be discussed in detail, while efflux will be discussed later.

7.4.1 Intestinal Epithelium as a Biological Barrier to Oral Absorption

The intestinal tract is the main site where digestion of drugs and foods takes place. The intestinal epithelium is where nutrient and xenobiotic absorption occurs; however, it is also the first biological barrier to their bioavailability since absorption could be selective. A comprehension of the anatomic structure of the intestinal epithelium may be helpful to understanding its function in the absorption process. The finger-shaped projections protruding from the intestinal epithelium are named villi, and the cellular membrane protrusions of epithelial cells are named microvilli. Villi and microvilli tremendously increase the absorptive surface area and facilitate contact between the epithelial surface and the fluid in the lumen. Uptake transporters (e.g., peptide transporters [PEPTs], organic anion-transporting polypeptides [OATPs], organic anion transporters [OATs], glucose transporters [GLUTs]) and efflux transporters (e.g., breast cancer resistance protein [BCRPs], multidrug-resistant proteins [MRPs], P-glycoprotein [P-gp]) are distributed on the membrane of intestinal epithelial cells. These cells are tightly joined together by junctional proteins, forming an impermeable barrier (Lee 2000; Murakami and Takano 2008). The cellular structure of the human intestinal epithelium is delineated in Figure 7.2.

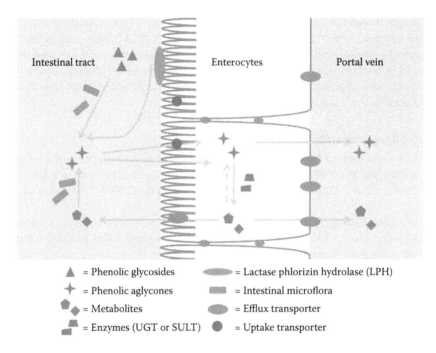

▲ = Phenolic glycosides   ⬭ = Lactase phlorizin hydrolase (LPH)

✦ = Phenolic aglycones   ▭ = Intestinal microflora

⬟◆ = Metabolites   ⬯ = Efflux transporter

▬◼ = Enzymes (UGT or SULT)   ● = Uptake transporter

FIGURE 7.2 Schematic depiction of absorption, metabolism, and efflux of phenolics in the human intestinal tract.

7.4.2 Uptake of Phytochemicals and Their Derivatives by Intestinal Epithelium

Permeability is often used to describe the ability of a molecule to traverse a membrane barrier. It may be the dominant factor to determine the intestinal absorption of certain compounds.

Generally, passive permeability of lipophilic compounds in the cell membrane is much higher than that of hydrophilic compounds; neutral molecules or uncharged molecular species are more permeable than charged molecules or species; molecules with a molecular weight (MW) < 500 usually have a better permeability than those with a larger size (Gao 2010). In vitro assays such as the parallel artificial membrane permeability assay (PAMPA) and human intestinal epithelial cell line Caco-2 assay are commonly used to predict the passive permeability of drug candidates (Reis et al. 2010). The majority of phytochemicals were found to be lipophilic, indicating that they might cross the epithelial membrane by passive diffusion. However, other types of transport mechanisms, for example, facilitated or active transport by transporters, have also been reported in the transport of certain phytochemicals or their derivatives.

7.4.2.1 Uptake of Carotenoids

Carotenoids belong to the class of highly lipophilic food microconstituents (HLFMs). Solubilization of carotenoids into mixed lipid micelles in the lumen may be needed for cellular uptake of carotenoids by intestinal mucosal cells (Harrison 2009). It has long been assumed that intestinal absorption of carotenoids depends on passive diffusion of micelles, based on an original study, which performed recirculating perfusion of micelles containing β-carotene through jejunal and ileal intestinal loops (Hollander and Ruble 1978). However, some experimental facts could not be explained by passive diffusion of carotenoids. For example, different isomers of β-carotene are selectively absorbed, there are interactions between absorption of different carotenoids in Caco-2 cells, and β-carotene absorption in the distal part of the intestine can be saturated in an intestinal perfusion model (Hollander and Ruble 1978; During et al. 2002). These observations indicate the likely existence of a protein-mediated transport mechanism, which, at the functional level, is important and may be complementary to the passive diffusion. Currently, several functional proteins on the membrane of epithelial cells have been identified as possible candidate proteins, and they include scavenger receptor class B type I (SR-BI), cluster determinant 36 (CD36), and Niemann-Pick C1-like 1 (NPC1L1) (During et al. 2005; Lobo et al. 2001). In a recent review on proteins involved in the transport of carotenoids, Reboul and Borel (2011) made a comment that protein-mediated transport works efficiently at dietary concentrations of carotenoids, while passive diffusion plays a more important role in carotenoid transport at pharmacological doses.

7.4.2.2   Uptake of ITC as Derivatives of Glucosinolates

Intact glucosinolates are hydrophilic and have a low permeability in the cell membrane, and thus, they are not expected to permeate the intestinal epithelium efficiently. However, after their hydrolysis (catalyzed by myrosinases), the metabolic products ITCs are found to be rapidly absorbed. Several studies showed that consuming foods rich in myrosinase would substantially improve the bioavailability of sulforaphane, an ITC derived from glucoraphanin, and accelerate its appearance in the plasma (Cramer and Jeffery 2011; Vermeulen et al. 2008). These facts confirm the differences that existed between the uptake of glucosinolates and that of ITCs. In in situ jejunum perfusion, the average effective jejunal permeability (P_{eff}) and percentage absorbed for sulforaphane were $18.7 \pm 12.6 \times 10^4$ cm/s and $74 \pm 29\%$, respectively, indicating a rapid absorption, possibly via passive transcellular diffusion (Petri et al. 2003).

7.4.2.3   Uptake of Flavonoids

Flavonoids are usually present in plants as glycosides with higher molecular weights and lower lipophilicity than their aglycones. The glycosides are usually too polar to be permeable in the lipid bilayer and thus cannot be absorbed rapidly from the small intestine. However, the absorption could be significantly improved upon the cleavage of the glycoside moieties by either lactase–phlorizin hydrolase (LPH) on the brush border of small intestine epithelial cells or hydrolases from colonic microflora. Once released, aglycones will passively diffuse across the membrane due to their smaller size and better lipophilicity. Serra et al. (2008) characterized the permeability of three flavonoid aglycones (diosmetin [Figure 7.1, 43], hesperitin, and naringenin) as well as their glycosides in a Caco-2 cell model and PAMPA. It was concluded that the permeability of these glycosides was extremely low when compared to their aglycones (Serra et al. 2008). For humans consuming soy or unfermented soy foods, isoflavone glycosides were not well absorbed until they were converted to aglycones by gut microflora (Xu et al. 1995). In vitro data also indicated that genistein (Figure 7.1, 44) and daidzin were hardly absorbed across the Caco-2 cell monolayer, while their aglycones were rapidly absorbed (Steensma et al. 1999). However, there is an alternative route for absorption of flavonoid glucosides other than hydrolysis and passive perfusion. The glucose moiety may enable transport of glucosides into epithelial cells by an apically located sodium-dependent glucose transporter 1 (SGLT1) (Gee et al. 2000). After uptake, these glucosides are hydrolyzed by an endogenous cytosolic β-glucosidase (CBG) inside enterocytes (Day et al. 1998). Glucoside conjugation position may decide the route by which flavonoids will be absorbed. As suggested by Day et al. (2003), quercetin-3-*O*-glucoside (Figure 7.1, 45) appears to be hydrolyzed by LPH first and then diffuses passively into enterocytes, whereas absorption of quercetin-4′-*O*-glucoside (Figure 7.1, 46) involves both active transport mediated by SGLT1 and luminal hydrolysis by LPH (Day et al. 2003).

7.4.2.4   Uptake of Stilbenes

Uptake of resveratrol and its 3-β-glucoside piceid across the intestinal apical membrane is quite similar to that of flavonoids and their glucosides. Resveratrol aglycones are quite lipophilic and display a decent permeability across the cell membrane. Piceid is proposed to be hydrolyzed into aglycone by the microfloral hydrolases or intestinal LPH before absorption.

For the glucoside, an alternative route of active transport is also present in the intestine. In Caco-2 cell lines, Henry et al. (2005) found that resveratrol accumulated faster than its glucoside and that transport of the aglycone depended on passive diffusion, while transport of the glucoside was likely active. They also identified the transporter involved as SGLT1 by using specific inhibitors of SGLT1 (Henry et al. 2005).

7.4.2.5 Uptake of Anthocyanins

As glucosides or diglucosides of anthocyanidins, anthocyanins possess a peculiar molecular structure derived from a flavylium cation. Water-soluble and charged properties substantially decrease permeability of anthocyanins in membrane. Thus, these molecules could not be transported into intestinal epithelial cells efficiently if passive diffusion was the only absorption pathway. However, intact anthocyanins are demonstrated to be absorbed in the stomach and small intestine in vivo, before hydrolysis by intestinal LPH or colonic microflora (McGhie and Walton 2007; Talavéra et al. 2003). Passamonti et al. (2003) demonstrated the involvement of the stomach in the absorption of grape anthocyanins in rats, providing a possible explanation for the fast appearance of anthocyanins in plasma. In another study, they identified anthocyanins as a new class of substrates for an organic anion carrier called bilitranslocase, located on the membrane of epithelial cells of the gastric mucosa (Passamonti et al. 2002).

In situ perfusion has demonstrated that intact anthocyanins were efficiently absorbed in the jejunum and ileum of rats and reached the systemic circulation rapidly (Talavéra et al. 2004). Active transport of anthocyanins is observed in the jejunum, which may interfere with glucose or quercetin glycoside uptake (McGhie and Walton 2007; Walton et al. 2006). However, no transporters have been unequivocally demonstrated to be responsible for the active transport of anthocyanins in intestine. On the other hand, sugar transporters such as SGLT1 or facilitative GLUT2 appeared to be putatively involved (Bitsch et al. 2004; McGhie and Walton 2007; Tian et al. 2009).

7.5 METABOLISM IN ENTEROCYTES

The gastrointestinal epithelium is a metabolic barrier against absorption of xenobiotics including most drugs and phytochemicals, including those with significant health-promoting effects. Inside enterocytes, these compounds would possibly be substrates for different enzymes. Together with the liver, the gastrointestinal tract is considered as an important site for "first-pass" metabolism, which impedes the appearance of xenobiotics in peripheral circulation and decreases their bioavailability in systemic circulation.

7.5.1 PHASE I AND PHASE II METABOLISM

The metabolism of xenobiotics is generally divided into phase I and phase II metabolism. These two major metabolic pathways may arise independently or be sequentially connected. Phase I metabolism could be considered as a functionalization phase, while phase II metabolism as a conjugation phase. Lipophilicity is required for most substrates to diffuse into enterocytes, and phase I metabolism often generates more hydrophilic metabolites with functional groups such as -OH, -NH₂, -SH, or -COOH. These new functional groups may render the molecular structures of metabolites ready for conjugative reactions by phase II enzymes (Gibson and Fil 2001).

7.5.1.1 Cytochrome P450s

Mediated by cytochrome P450s (CYPs) or other functional enzymes, phase I reactions include oxidation, reduction, hydrolysis, hydration, and isomerization, as well as other unusual or miscellaneous reaction types (Gibson and Fil 2001). The CYP enzyme superfamily currently has more than

2000 members, and many of them have been identified to be in charge of the metabolism of both xenobiotics and endogenous compounds (Rendic 2002; Rendic and Di Carlo 1997). In mammals, P450s from CYP1, CYP2, and CYP3 families play a major role for phase I metabolism of xenobiotics, and they mediate over 90% of all drug metabolism in humans (Lewis 2003). Although the liver is usually regarded as the most important organ for metabolism, intestinal CYP450s also contribute significantly to the first-pass metabolism, especially those from the CYP3A and CYP2C subfamilies, which account for approximately 80% and 18% of total intestinal CYP contents, respectively (Thelen and Dressman 2009).

Phase II reactions are usually a conjugation of sugar moiety, sulfonate, glutathione (GSH), or amino acid to substrates by transferases that require endogenous cofactors, producing metabolites with increased molecular weight and water solubility (Coleman 2010). Major reactions in phase II metabolism include glucuronidation, sulfation, GSH conjugation, methylation, and acetylation, but glucuronidation and sulfation are mainly responsible for the conjugation of compounds presented in this review except for ITCs, which are metabolized mainly by GSH transferases.

7.5.1.2 Uridine 5′-diphospho-glucuronosyltransferases

Glucuronidation is catalyzed by uridine 5′-diphospho-glucuronosyltransferases (UGTs). UGTs are a superfamily of membrane-bound enzymes embedded in the endoplasmic reticulum inside the cell. UGT isoforms involved in glucuronidation of phenolics and other relevant compounds discussed here usually belong to the UGT1A or UGT2B family. Although a broad distribution in humans has been described, the most abundant expression of UGTs is found in the liver and intestine, with significant expression in the kidney as well (Nakamura et al. 2008). The expression profiles of UGTs revealed that the intestine expresses not only UGT 1A1, 1A3, 1A4, 1A6, 2B15, and 2B4 but also 1A7, 1A8, and 1A10, with the latter three not present in the liver (Zhang et al. 2007b; Harbourt et al. 2011). Regardless of their distinctive distribution pattern, many UGT isoforms have broad overlaps in substrate specificities. Hence, a compound could be metabolized in an equally efficient manner by two different isoforms present in two different organs. Because the intestine would be the site where the absorbed substrates first encounter extensive metabolism, the intestinal glucuronidation contributes significantly to the role of limiting the oral bioavailability of many compounds.

7.5.1.3 Sulfotransferases

Sulfation or sulfonation, catalyzed by cytosolic sulfotransferases (SULTs), is another important phase II metabolism pathway for compounds discussed in this review. Recently, human SULTs and their roles in chemical metabolism have been reviewed by Gamage et al. (2006). At least 13 distinct SULT isoforms have been identified in humans, represented by three subfamilies: SULT1, SULT2, and SULT4. SULT1A1 is the main isoform in the liver and also widely distributed in other organs including the intestine, brain, and kidney, while SULT1A3 is highly expressed in the small intestine but is barely detectable in the adult liver (Honma et al. 2001; Meinl et al. 2008). Another important isoform significantly expressed in the small intestine is SULT1B1, while only marginal expression of SULT2A1 and 1E1 was found in the small intestine (Teubner et al. 2007; Riches et al. 2009).

7.5.1.4 Modulation of Metabolic Enzymes

Certain dietary phytochemicals such as flavonoids could modulate expression and activity of drug-metabolizing enzymes and transporters to promote detoxification and efflux of exogenous carcinogens (Satsu et al. 2008; Křížková 2009; Wilkinson 1997). Thus, the gastrointestinal epithelium may be used for evaluating both pharmacological and pharmaceutical profiles of these phytochemicals. Complicated interactions may occur because biotransformation of phytochemicals leads to gain or loss of activities, while these activities may be linked with their pharmacologic effects on metabolizing enzymes.

7.5.2 Intestinal Metabolism of Selected Phytochemicals

7.5.2.1 Intestinal Metabolism of Carotenoids

In humans, vitamin A (Figure 7.1, 47), or retinol, cannot be synthesized de novo, and thus, a supply of exogenous vitamin A or carotenoids as precursors must be available in the diet or other food sources (Tanumihardjo 2011). The carotenoids are precursors of vitamin A and are also known as provitamin A. An abundant provitamin A in dietary plants, β-carotene, is often considered as the most potent one. Although more β-carotene is converted in the human liver, the intestine is also a major site for its metabolism (During et al. 2001).

Once absorbed into the enterocytes, the carotenoids may undergo different patterns of cleavage and be converted to different products with a shorter polyene chain (Harrison 2012). β-Carotene is cleaved by a cytosolic enzyme called β-carotene 15,15′-monooxygenase, which cuts the central 15,15′ double bond, generating a retinal, a direct precursor of retinol (Leuenberger et al. 2001). Besides central cleavage, another cleavage pattern for β-carotene is called eccentric cleavage (Wolf 1995; van Vliet et al. 1996). Eccentric cleavage occurs at other positions, like the 13′,14′, 11′,12′, or 9′,10′ double bond of the polyene chain, producing apocarotenals (e.g., *trans*-β-apo-8′-carotenal [Figure 7.1, 48]) with different lengths in an asymmetric way (Wang et al. 1991). Apocarotenals may be oxidized to apocartenoic acids and then further transformed to retinoic acid, an active form of vitamin A (Wolf 1995). Kiefer et al. (2001) have identified another enzyme called β-carotene-9′,10′-monooxygenase, which cleaves β-carotene at the 9′,10′ double bond and produces β-apo-10′-carotenal and β-ionone asymmetrically. Inside the enterocytes, most retinol derived from carotenoids would be complexed with cellular retinol-binding protein type 2 (CRBP2) and then esterified by the enzyme lecithin:retinol acyltransferase (LRAT) before subsequent transport to other tissues (During and Harrison 2004).

7.5.2.2 Intestinal Metabolism of ITCs

ITCs, as hydrolysis products of corresponding glucosinolates, are rapidly absorbed by enterocytes both in rodents and in humans (Mennicke et al. 1983, 1988). The major route of metabolism for ITCs in the enterocytes is GSH conjugation either via a nonenzymatic pathway or with the help of GSH S-transferases (GSTs), followed by hepatic metabolism via the mercapturic acid pathway (Zhang et al. 1995; Jösch et al. 1998). In this pathway, glutamate and glycine residues in GSH conjugates of ITCs are hydrolyzed by multiple enzymes (Shapiro et al. 1998). The derived ITC–cysteine conjugates are further *N*-acetylated by *N*-acetyltransferase and eventually excreted as *N*-acetylcysteine–ITC in the urine.

Although mainly metabolized in the liver, ITC metabolism is initiated in enterocytes by GSTs, which are abundantly expressed in humans in both the liver and the intestinal tract (de Waziers et al. 1990). Petri et al. (2003) conducted an in vivo jejunal perfusion in volunteers with an extract of broccoli, and an analysis of perfusate revealed the presence of a sulforaphane–GSH conjugate but not cysteine or *N*-acetylcysteine conjugates (Petri et al. 2003). In several cultured cell lines, ITCs were observed to accumulate at very high concentrations, and the accumulated product was predominantly identified as the GSH conjugates, as well as compounds that are possibly cysteinylglycine conjugates (Zhang 2000; Callaway et al. 2004).

7.5.2.3 Intestinal Metabolism of Flavonoids

Due to the presence of hydroxyl groups in their structures, flavonoids are already decent substrates for phase II metabolism, and the majority of the terminal metabolites are conjugates (Gao 2010). However, recombinant CYPs and liver microsomes from human or Aroclor 1254–induced rats have demonstrated oxidative metabolism of several flavonoids mediated by CYPs (Breinholt et al. 2002; Duarte Silva et al. 1997; Nielsen et al. 1998; Otake and Walle 2002). For example, both galangin (Figure 7.1, 49) and kaempferide (Figure 7.1, 50) can be transformed to kaempferol (Figure 7.1, 51) through ring hydroxylation or *O*-demethylation (Otake and Walle 2002). Quantitative exploration revealed that the same human microsomes exhibited an intrinsic conjugation clearance (V_{max}/K_m) value nearly 50-fold higher than that of CYP-mediated oxidation (Otake et al. 2002). Thus, the phase I metabolic pathway is usually a minor contributor to flavonoid disposition and has never been shown to be important in vivo or in primary cultured cells (Thomas 2004).

Glucuronidation and sulfation in phase II metabolism have been recognized as the two main routes for the metabolism of phenolics, including flavonoids. Conjugation with glucuronic acid or sulfonic acid to free hydroxyl groups will increase polarity and aqueous solubility of these flavonoids, which facilitates their ultimate elimination from the body. Combined with excretion, phase II conjugation works as a barrier against dietary carcinogens by detoxifying them or reducing exposure to them, and it also limits plasma concentration and oral bioavailability of flavonoids (Malfatti et al. 2006).

Certain flavonoids could be a substrate for multiple UGTs' isoforms with different binding affinities and reaction kinetics (Otake et al. 2002; Boersma et al. 2002; Zhang et al. 2007a). Tang et al. (2009) reported that soy isoflavones such as genistein, daidzein, glycitein (Figure 7.1, 52), prunetin (Figure 7.1, 53), biochanin A (Figure 7.1, 54), and formononetin (Figure 7.1, 55) were metabolized most rapidly by one of the following four UGT isoforms: 1A1, 1A8, 1A9, and 1A10. Flavonoid glucuronidation by different UGT isoforms has been reviewed and summarized (Zhang et al. 2007b). Meanwhile, regioselectivity is observed in the glucuronidation of flavonoids with multiple hydroxyl groups. During incubation with human small intestine S9 fractions, quercetin could be conjugated with glucuronic acid at the 3-, 7-, 3′- or 4′-positions, respectively (van der Woude et al. 2004). In another study on a Caco-2 cell model, the 7-hydroxy group of soy isoflavones was the main site for glucuronidation, although hydroxyl groups in other positions were also available (Chen et al. 2005). Flavonoid diglucuronides have also been detected and identified from the intestine after oral administration of quercetin in rats; however, they are sparsely reported to be present in humans in vivo (Graf et al. 2006; Mullen et al. 2008).

For several flavonoids, monosulfates of formononetin, prunetin and apigenin (Figure 7.1, 56), were also found to be their major metabolites in the Caco-2 cell model, rat intestinal perfusion, or intestinal cytosol fraction incubation (Chen et al. 2005; Jeong et al. 2005; Hu et al. 2003). Besides glucuronides, incubation of quercetin with human small intestinal S9 fractions also produced comparable amounts of sulfates with a relative composition of 12% 7-O-sulfate and 88% 3′-O-sulfate, showing a regioselectivity (van der Woude et al. 2004). Huang et al. (2009) investigated sulfation of four dietary flavonoids—catechin (Figure 7.1, 57), epicatechin (Figure 7.1, 58), eriodictyol (Figure 7.1, 59), and hesperetin—by recombinant human SULT1A1 and SULT1A3, and they found that these substrates could be potent inhibitors for both enzymes at a high concentration.

Methylation of flavonoids, which is usually mediated by the enzyme catechol-O-methyltransferase (COMT) and the cofactor S-adenosylmethionine, has also been demonstrated in isolated or in situ rat small intestine perfusion, although with a smaller amount than glucuronidation and sulfation (Donovan et al. 2001; Kuhnle et al. 2000b). Moreover, methylation often occurs in combination with glucuronidation or sulfation to those substrates with multiple hydroxyl groups, especially catechols or phenolics with two neighboring hydroxyl groups, resulting in mixed conjugates. For example, methylated quercetin and their glucuronides or sulfates were detected when quercetin was incubated with rat small intestinal S9 fractions but were not detected when it was incubated with human small intestinal S9 fractions (van der Woude et al. 2004).

7.5.2.4 Intestinal Metabolism of Stilbenes

Intact piceid can be absorbed actively via the action of SGLT1 and then rapidly converted to its aglycones, after encountering hydrolysis by CBG inside epithelial cells (Henry-Vitrac et al. 2006). Phase II metabolism of resveratrol aglycone is responsible for its limited oral bioavailability.

Kuhnle et al. (2000a) studied the absorption and metabolism of resveratrol in an isolated rat small intestinal model, and they found that only small amounts of resveratrol remained intact when crossing enterocytes, while the major metabolites detected on the serosal side were the glucuronides.

However, Kaldas et al. (2003) reported that in Caco-2 cells, the main metabolites of resveratrol tended to be sulfates, with a smaller amount of glucuronide. Phase II metabolism in the small intestine and the liver can almost prevent the appearance of resveratrol aglycone in plasma, leaving sulfate and glucuronide conjugates instead (Meng et al. 2004; Goldberg et al. 2003). In vitro glucuronidation of *trans*-resveratrol by human liver and intestinal microsomes demonstrated that compared with human liver microsomes, human intestinal microsomes exhibited a 3- to 10-fold higher glucuronidation efficiency for resveratrol, producing a higher level of 4'-*O*-glucuronide than 3-*O*-glucuronide (Brill et al. 2006).

7.5.2.5 Intestinal Metabolism of Coumarins

Pathways of coumarin metabolism may be very complicated in vivo, where monohydroxylation or multihydroxylation at six different positions (carbon atoms 3 to 8) could occur along with lactone ring fission (Lake 1999). In humans, the majority of coumarin is metabolized to 7-hydroxylcoumarin (7-HC) (Figure 7.1, 60) and the responsible CYP isoform here is mainly CYP2A6. When 7-HC is generated, it is extensively metabolized by phase II enzymes and excreted in urine (Lake 1999). Because CYP2A6 is primarily expressed in the liver and not detected in the small intestine, the contribution of the small intestine to coumarin phase I metabolism after oral administration is supposed to be relatively small, compared with the liver (Ding and Kaminsky 2003). Hence, more metabolic studies are focused on the liver instead of the small intestine (Mäenpää et al. 1993; Wang et al. 2005). The *O*-deethylation rate of 7-ethoxycoumarin (Figure 7.1, 61) was adopted as an index for comparing the drug metabolizing ability of the rat intestine and liver by Shirkey et al. (1979), and their results showed that liver microsomes were 20-fold more potent than intestinal microsomes in the metabolism of coumarin.

7.6 ENTERIC EXCRETION

Membrane-bound transporters may be involved in both apical and basolateral efflux of their substrates with decent hydrophilicity, or when the substrates are transported against a concentration gradient. The most pharmacologically relevant transporters expressed on the apical side of enterocytes include P-gp (ATP-binding cassette transporter B1 [ABCB1]), MRP2 (ABCC2), MRP4 (ABCC4), and BCRP (ABCG2), while MRP1 (ABCC1), MRP3 (ABCC3), and MRP5 (ABCC5) are localized on the basolateral side (Oostendorp et al. 2009).

7.6.1 Excretion of Chemicals from Enterocytes

The human intestine is an important site for absorption and metabolism of phytochemicals, but in most cases, it is far from the terminus of their journey inside the human body. For some phytochemicals, the intestinal tract also serves as a target organ where they can modulate the activities of their disposition machinery such as conjugation enzymes and efflux transporters (Sergent et al. 2008). However, the systemic beneficial effects require a broader distribution of these phytochemicals in various tissues and organs. Therefore, it is necessary for these compounds to be transported from the basolateral side of enterocytes into the portal vein or lymph duct, from which they can then be distributed throughout the body. Unfortunately, some phytochemicals and their metabolites are excreted from the apical side back into the intestinal lumen (also called apical efflux), which limits their exposure in vivo.

7.6.2 Enteric Excretion of Selected Phytochemicals

7.6.2.1 Excretion of Carotenoids

After absorption by enterocytes, carotenoids and their esterified metabolites are transported or secreted to the basolateral side and then delivered to the systemic circulation. Before their inward transport, these hydrophobic compounds are incorporated into relevant lipoprotein particles called chylomicron, which consists of dietary lipids (mainly triglyceride, phospholipids, and cholesterol) and apoproteins (mainly apoprotein B-48) (Hussain 2000; Hussain et al. 2003). The chylomicrons carrying carotenoids and retinyl esters are secreted by enterocytes into the mesenteric lymph and finally enter blood circulation through the thoracic duct (During and Harrison 2004). For unesterified retinol inside enterocytes, facilitated efflux to the portal vein can serve as an alternative transport route, with the help of ABCA1 transporters that are located on the basolateral side of enterocytes (During et al. 2005).

7.6.2.2 Efflux of GSH-Conjugated ITCs

ITCs are derived from dietary glucosinolates. For sulforaphane, a representative ITC, the major phase II metabolism product in enterocytes has been demonstrated to be GSH conjugates (Petri et al. 2003). In addition to basolateral excretion into the portal vein and further metabolism in the liver, GSH conjugates of sulforaphane are also excreted back to the lumen. Due to the hydrophilicity and ionizability, excretion of GSH conjugates of sulforaphane is probably dependent on facilitated transport by membrane transporters rather than the passive diffusion. According to Callaway et al., P-gp and MRP1 transporters were involved in the rapid export of GSH conjugates of several ITCs in human prostate carcinoma or leukemia cell lines (Callaway et al. 2004; Zhang and Callaway 2002). Thus, in a schematic mechanism proposed by Petri et al. (2003), apical efflux of sulforaphane–GSH is mediated by P-gp, while basolateral efflux is mediated by MRP1, partially due to their locations on the cell membrane of enterocytes (Petri et al. 2003; Beedholm-Ebsen et al. 2010). However, no direct evidence has been provided for the further identification and characterization of transporters responsible for the enteric efflux of GSH conjugates of sulforaphane.

7.6.2.3 Excretion of Phenolics: Flavonoids, Coumarins, Stilbenes

Enteric excretion is also very important in determining the oral absorption of phenolics and their phase II metabolites. The bioavailability of these substances will be affected by either the apical or the basolateral efflux (Suzuki and Sugiyama 2000).

Interaction between substrates and efflux transporters can be identified by incubation of substrates with or without transporter-specific inhibitors in different models. Vaidyanathan and Walle (2003) reported that in the presence of an MRP2 inhibitor, MK-571, uptake of epicatechin-3-gallate was increased in Caco-2 cells or Madin-Darby canine kidney epithelial (MDCK) cells transfected with MRP2, suggesting the involvement of this transporter in its efflux. Similarly, Henry et al. (2005) reported that *trans*-resveratrol was effluxed by MRP2 in Caco-2 cells. Efflux of gomisin N (Figure 7.1, 62), a lignan extracted from *Schisandra chinensis*, was inhibited by MK-571 and verapamil, indicating that both MRP2 and P-gp might be involved in its efflux (Madgula et al. 2008).

Phase II metabolites of phenolics, mainly glucuronides or sulfates, are usually good substrates for transporters, and their excretion out of epithelial cells is sometimes termed as phase III metabolism (Toshihisa 1992). According to Brand et al. (2008), hesperetin was conjugated to glucuronides and sulfates in Caco-2 cells and then excreted to the apical side mainly by BCRP, since the presence of BCRP inhibitor Ko143 could significantly reduce the efflux of metabolites to the apical side. In a rat intestinal perfusion model, perfusion of naringenin with either MK-571 or dipyridamole (inhibitor of BCPR) did not change excretion of naringenin glucuronides in the perfusate; however, when employed together, they significantly decreased excretion, suggesting a possible compensating effect of the two transporters on excretion of flavonoid glucuronides (Xu et al. 2009).

Compared to the efflux transporters on the apical membrane of enterocytes, the ones on the basolateral side are less thoroughly studied. 4-Methylumbelliferone glucuronide was used as an MRP3 substrate (Hirohashi et al. 1999; Bock-Hennig et al. 2002). Preliminary data on the function of MRP3 have indicated that several nonconjugated organic anions and glucuronide conjugates are good substrates of MRP3, while GSH conjugates are poor substrates (Hirohashi et al. 1999; Kool et al. 1999). Further investigation is necessary to define the functional details of MRP3. As for MRP1,

Nguyen et al. (2003) reported that several dietary flavonoids such as morin (Figure 7.1, 63), genistein, and quercetin could inhibit MRP1-mediated drug transport in a human pancreatic adenocarcinoma cell line, Panc-1. However, detailed mechanisms delineating the interactions between MRP1 and phytochemicals or their metabolites in the enterocytes remain largely unexplored.

Among transporters with overlapping substrate specificities, the relative contribution of a single transporter to the total transport of a substrate is perhaps best determined by the relative expression levels of these transporters in enterocytes, as well as affinity between the substrate and each transporter. For example, in Caco-2 cells, chrysin glucuronide was mostly excreted to the apical side (Walle et al. 1999). For resveratrol, at low concentrations, its main metabolites in Caco-2 cells are found to be excreted to the apical side, presumably by MRP2, while at high concentrations, a shift toward the excretion from the basolateral side, possibly involving MRP3, can be observed, probably due to the saturation of apical efflux transporter(s) (Kaldas et al. 2003). A schematic depiction of absorption, metabolism, and efflux of phenolics along the human intestinal tract is given in Figure 7.2.

7.6.3 ENTEROHEPATIC RECYCLING AND ENTERIC RECYCLING

Enterohepatic recycling is a very important concept for the in vivo disposition of relevant endogenous or exogenous substances, including phenolics (Roberts et al. 2002). Dietary phenolics and their enteric metabolites that are delivered to the liver by the portal vein undergo hepatic metabolism. Sometimes, a considerable percentage of these compounds in their intact form or, more often, as sulfates and glucuronides are excreted to the sinusoidal side of hepatocytes, which will then reach the intestinal tract again via biliary excretion. Conjugated metabolites such as glucuronides and sulfates can be converted back to aglycones by microfloral hydrolases in the colon, where novel metabolic products from ring fission or reduction reactions are also formed. The resulting aglycone is then available for reabsorption in the intestinal tract, completing a circulation (Yang et al. 2001).

As a coherent process involving biotransformation and transport at different sites in vivo, enterohepatic recycling is very important for assessing the bioavailability of dietary phenolics. For example, lignans and their metabolites could be detected in the intestinal tract for up to 48 h after oral administration in rats, perhaps due to the enterohepatic recycling that prolonged its systemic exposure (Rickard and Thompson 1998).

Chen et al. (2003) proposed that enteric recycling involving reconversion of conjugates excreted by the intestine is another component of flavonoids' disposition process in vivo, which is at least as important as the enterohepatic recycling in the first-pass metabolism process of flavonoids. Compared to the enterohepatic recycling, the enteric recycling may provide more constant systemic exposure to dietary flavonoids, because the gallbladder (holding the bile) empties only with a meal. Combing these two recycling processes, the reason for poor systemic bioavailability but reasonably long half-lives of flavonoids may be relatively clear (Chen et al. 2003).

7.7 CONCLUSION

Anti-inflammatory or anticancer effects of health-promoting phytochemicals have been demonstrated at the cellular and molecular levels. However, the issues concerning their bioavailability are beginning to attract more attention because there is a clear gap between in vitro IC50 concentrations and in vivo exposure levels.

As the main site for phytochemical absorption and metabolism, the gastrointestinal tract is also a barrier that may limit the bioavailability of various anti-inflammatory compounds. As discussed throughout the text, solubility, permeability, metabolism by bacteria or enterocytes, and enteric efflux are included as important barriers to their oral bioavailability. Further exploration on the behaviors of these phytochemicals along the gastrointestinal tract is necessary for a better understanding of how to amplify their beneficial effects in humans. For developing anti-inflammatory and anticancer drugs from phytochemicals or their derivatives, new approaches may be required to overcome various barriers to absorption in order to elevate their bioavailability.

ACKNOWLEDGMENT

This work is supported by a grant from the National Institutes of Health (GM070737).

REFERENCES

Adam, A., V. Crespy, M.-A. Levrat-Verny, F. Leenhardt, M. Leuillet, C. Demigné, and C. Rémésy. "The Bioavailability of Ferulic Acid Is Governed Primarily by the Food Matrix Rather Than Its Metabolism in Intestine and Liver in Rats." *The Journal of Nutrition* 132, no. 7 (2002): 1962–8.

Amidon, G. L., H. Lennernäs, V. P. Shah, and J. R. Crison. "A Theoretical Basis for a Biopharmaceutic Drug Classification: The Correlation of *in Vitro* Drug Product Dissolution and *in Vivo* Bioavailability." *Pharmaceutical Research* 12, no. 3 (1995): 413–20.

Aura, A.-M. "Microbial Metabolism of Dietary Phenolic Compounds in the Colon." *Phytochemistry Reviews* 7, no. 3 (2008): 407–29.

Aura, A. M., P. Martin-Lopez, K. A. O'Leary, G. Williamson, K. M. Oksman-Caldentey, K. Poutanen, and C. Santos-Buelga. "In Vitro Metabolism of Anthocyanins by Human Gut Microflora." *European Journal of Nutrition* 44, no. 3 (2005): 133–42.

Azuma, K., K. Ippoushi, M. Nakayama, H. Ito, H. Higashio, and J. Terao. "Absorption of Chlorogenic Acid and Caffeic Acid in Rats after Oral Administration." *Journal of Agricultural and Food Chemistry* 48, no. 11 (2000): 5496–500.

Bala, I., V. Bhardwaj, S. Hariharan, and M. N. V. Ravi Kumar. "Analytical Methods for Assay of Ellagic Acid and Its Solubility Studies." *Journal of Pharmaceutical and Biomedical Analysis* 40, no. 1 (2006): 206–10.

Bednarek, P., M. Piślewska-Bednarek, A. Svatoš, B. Schneider, J. Doubský, M. Mansurova, M. Humphry, C. Consonni, R. Panstruga, A. Sanchez-Vallet, A. Molina, and P. Schulze-Lefert. "A Glucosinolate Metabolism Pathway in Living Plant Cells Mediates Broad-Spectrum Antifungal Defense." *Science* 323, no. 5910 (2009): 101–6.

Beedholm-Ebsen, R., K. van de Wetering, T. Hardlei, E. Nexø, P. Borst, and S. K. Moestrup. "Identification of Multidrug Resistance Protein 1 (Mrp1/Abcc1) as a Molecular Gate for Cellular Export of Cobalamin." *Blood* 115, no. 8 (2010): 1632–9.

Bitsch, R., M. Netzel, T. Frank, G. Strass, and I. Bitsch. "Bioavailability and Biokinetics of Anthocyanins from Red Grape Juice and Red Wine." *Journal of Biomedicine and Biotechnology* 2004, no. 5 (2004): 293–8.

Blanquet-Diot, S., M. Soufi, M. Rambeau, E. Rock, and M. Alric. "Digestive Stability of Xanthophylls Exceeds That of Carotenes as Studied in a Dynamic in vitro Gastrointestinal System." *The Journal of Nutrition* 139, no. 5 (2009): 876–83.

Bock-Hennig, B. S., C. Köhle, K. Nill, and K. W. Bock. "Influence of T-Butylhydroquinone and β-Naphthofla-vone on Formation and Transport of 4-Methylumbelliferone Glucuronide in Caco-2/Tc-7 Cell Monolayers." *Biochemical Pharmacology* 63, no. 2 (2002): 123–8.

Boersma, M. G., H. van der Woude, J. Bogaards, S. Boeren, J. Vervoort, N. H. P. Cnubben, M. L. P. S. van Iersel, P. J. van Bladeren, and I. M. C. M. Rietjens. "Regioselectivity of Phase II Metabolism of Luteolin and Quercetin by Udp-Glucuronosyl Transferases." *Chemical Research in Toxicology* 15, no. 5 (2002): 662–70.

Bones, A. M., and J. T. Rossiter. "The Enzymic and Chemically Induced Decomposition of Glucosinolates." *Phytochemistry* 67, no. 11 (2006): 1053–67.

Boon, C. S., D. J. McClements, J. Weiss, and E. A. Decker. "Factors Influencing the Chemical Stability of Carotenoids in Foods." *Critical Reviews in Food Science and Nutrition* 50, no. 6 (2010): 515–32.

Booth, A. N., C. W. Murray, F. T. Jones, and F. DeEds. "The Metabolic Fate of Rutin and Quercetin in the Animal Body." *Journal of Biological Chemistry* 223, no. 1 (1956): 251–7.

Borel, P. "Factors Affecting Intestinal Absorption of Highly Lipophilic Food Microconstituents (Fat-Soluble Vitamins, Carotenoids and Phytosterols)." *Clinical Chemistry and Laboratory Medicine* 41, no. 8 (2003): 979–94.

Borriello, S. P., K. D. R. Setchell, M. Axelson, and A. M. Lawson. "Production and Metabolism of Lignans by the Human Faecal Flora." *Journal of Applied Microbiology* 58, no. 1 (1985): 37–43.

Boulton, D. W., U. K. Walle, and T. Walle. "Fate of the Flavonoid Quercetin in Human Cell Lines: Chemical Instability and Metabolism." *Journal of Pharmacy and Pharmacology* 51, no. 3 (1999): 353–9.

Bowey, E., H. Adlercreutz, and I. Rowland. "Metabolism of Isoflavones and Lignans by the Gut Microflora: A Study in Germ-Free and Human Flora Associated Rats." *Food and Chemical Toxicology* 41, no. 5 (2003): 631–6.

Brand, W., P. A. I. van der Wel, M. J. Rein, D. Barron, G. Williamson, P. J. van Bladeren, and I. M. C. M. Rietjens. "Metabolism and Transport of the Citrus Flavonoid Hesperetin in Caco-2 Cell Monolayers." *Drug Metabolism and Disposition* 36, no. 9 (2008): 1794–802.

Braune, A., M. Gutschow, W. Engst, and M. Blaut. "Degradation of Quercetin and Luteolin by Eubacterium Ramulus." *Applied and Environmental Microbiology* 67, no. 12 (2001): 5558–67.

Breinholt, V. M., E. A. Offord, C. Brouwer, S. E. Nielsen, K. Brøsen, and T. Friedberg. "In Vitro Investigation of Cytochrome P450-Mediated Metabolism of Dietary Flavonoids." *Food and Chemical Toxicology* 40, no. 5 (2002): 609–16.

Brill, S. S., A. M. Furimsky, M. N. Ho, M. J. Furniss, Y. Li, A. G. Green, C. E. Green, L. V. Iyer, W. W. Bradford, and I. M. Kapetanovic. "Glucuronidation of Trans-Resveratrol by Human Liver and Intestinal Microsomes and Ugt Isoforms." *Journal of Pharmacy and Pharmacology* 58, no. 4 (2006): 469–79.

Cai, Y., Q. Luo, M. Sun, and H. Corke. *Antioxidant Activity and Phenolic Compounds of 112 Traditional Chinese Medicinal Plants Associated with Anticancer*. Vol. 74. Kidlington, Royaume-Uni: Elsevier, 2004.

Callaway, E. C., Y. Zhang, W. Chew, and H. H. S. Chow. "Cellular Accumulation of Dietary Anticarcinogenic Isothiocyanates Is Followed by Transporter-Mediated Export as Dithiocarbamates." *Cancer Letters* 204, no. 1 (2004): 23–31.

Cejpek, K., J. Valusek, and J. Velisek. "Reactions of Allyl Isothiocyanate with Alanine, Glycine, and Several Peptides in Model Systems." *Journal of Agricultural and Food Chemistry* 48, no. 8 (2000): 3560–5.

Chen, J., H. Lin, and M. Hu. "Absorption and Metabolism of Genistein and Its Five Isoflavone Analogs in the Human Intestinal Caco-2 Model." *Cancer Chemotherapy and Pharmacology* 55, no. 2 (2005): 159–69.

Chen, J., H. Lin, and M. Hu. "Metabolism of Flavonoids Via Enteric Recycling: Role of Intestinal Disposition." *Journal of Pharmacology and Experimental Therapeutics* 304, no. 3 (2003): 1228–35.

Cheng, K. J., H. G. Krishnamurty, G. A. Jones, and F. J. Simpson. "Identification of Products Produced by the Anaerobic Degradation of Naringin by Butyrivibrio Sp. C3." *Canadian Journal of Microbiology* 17, no. 1 (1971): 129–31.

Cheng, K. J., G. A. Jones, F. J. Simpson, and M. P. Bryant. "Isolation and Identification of Rumen Bacteria Capable of Anaerobic Rutin Degradation." *Canadian Journal of Microbiology* 15, no. 12 (1969): 1365–71.

Chin, Y.-W., M. Balunas, H. Chai, and A. Kinghorn. "Drug Discovery from Natural Sources." *The AAPS Journal* 8, no. 2 (2006): E239–53.

Coleman, M. D. "Conjugation and Transport Processes." In *Human Drug Metabolism*, 125–57. Chichester: John Wiley & Sons, Ltd, 2010.

Cramer, J. M., and E. H. Jeffery. "Sulforaphane Absorption and Excretion Following Ingestion of a Semi-Purified Broccoli Powder Rich in Glucoraphanin and Broccoli Sprouts in Healthy Men." *Nutrition and Cancer* 63, no. 2 (2011): 196–201.

Crozier, A., I. B. Jaganath, and M. N. Clifford. "Dietary Phenolics: Chemistry, Bioavailability and Effects on Health." *Natural Product Reports* 26, no. 8 (2009): 1001–43.

Dai, J., and R. J. Mumper. "Plant Phenolics: Extraction, Analysis and Their Antioxidant and Anticancer Properties." *Molecules* 15, no. 10 (2010): 7313–52.

Dai, J., A. Gupte, L. Gates, and R. J. Mumper. "A Comprehensive Study of Anthocyanin-Containing Extracts from Selected Blackberry Cultivars: Extraction Methods, Stability, Anticancer Properties and Mechanisms." *Food and Chemical Toxicology* 47, no. 4 (2009): 837–47.

Das, S., H.-S. Lin, P. Ho, and K.-Y. Ng. "The Impact of Aqueous Solubility and Dose on the Pharmacokinetic Profiles of Resveratrol." *Pharmaceutical Research* 25, no. 11 (2008): 2593–600.

Day, A. J., J. M. Gee, M. S. DuPont, I. T. Johnson, and G. Williamson. "Absorption of Quercetin-3-Glucoside and Quercetin-4′-Glucoside in the Rat Small Intestine: The Role of Lactase Phlorizin Hydrolase and the Sodium-Dependent Glucose Transporter." *Biochemical Pharmacology* 65, no. 7 (2003): 1199–206.

Day, A. J., M. S. DuPont, S. Ridley, M. Rhodes, M. J. C. Rhodes, M. R. A. Morgan, and G. Williamson. "Deglycosylation of Flavonoid and Isoflavonoid Glycosides by Human Small Intestine and Liver β-Glucosidase Activity." *FEBS Letters* 436, no. 1 (1998): 71–5.

de Waziers, I., P. H. Cugnenc, C. S. Yang, J. P. Leroux, and P. H. Beaune. "Cytochrome P 450 Isoenzymes, Epoxide Hydrolase and Glutathione Transferases in Rat and Human Hepatic and Extrahepatic Tissues." *Journal of Pharmacology and Experimental Therapeutics* 253, no. 1 (1990): 387–94.

Delmas, D., A. Lançon, D. Colin, B. Jannin, and N. Latruffe. "Resveratrol as a Chemopreventive Agent: A Promising Molecule for Fighting Cancer." *Current Drug Targets* 7, no. 4 (2006): 423–42.

Ding, X., and L. S. Kaminsky. "Human Extrahepatic Cytochromes P450: Function in Xenobiotic Metabolism and Tissue-Selective Chemical Toxicity in the Respiratory and Gastrointestinal Tracts*." *Annual Review of Pharmacology and Toxicology* 43, no. 1 (2003): 149–73.

Donkin, S. G. "Toxicity of Glucosinolates and Their Enzymatic Decomposition Products to *Caenorhabditis elegans*." *Journal of Nematology* 27, no. 3 (1995): 258–62.

Donovan, J. L., V. Crespy, C. Manach, C. Morand, C. Besson, A. Scalbert, and C. Rémésy. "Catechin Is Metabolized by Both the Small Intestine and Liver of Rats." *The Journal of Nutrition* 131, no. 6 (2001): 1753–7.

Duarte Silva, I., A. S. Rodrigues, J. Gaspar, A. Laires, and J. Rueff. "Metabolism of Galangin by Rat Cytochromes P450: Relevance to the Genotoxicity of Galangin." *Mutation Research/Genetic Toxicology and Environmental Mutagenesis* 393, no. 3 (1997): 247–57.

During, A., and E. H. Harrison. "Intestinal Absorption and Metabolism of Carotenoids: Insights from Cell Culture." *Archives of Biochemistry and Biophysics* 430, no. 1 (2004): 77–88.

During, A., H. D. Dawson, and E. H. Harrison. "Carotenoid Transport Is Decreased and Expression of the Lipid Transporters Sr-Bi, Npc1l1, and Abca1 Is Downregulated in Caco-2 Cells Treated with Ezetimibe." *The Journal of Nutrition* 135, no. 10 (2005): 2305–12.

During, A., M. M. Hussain, D. W. Morel, and E. H. Harrison. "Carotenoid Uptake and Secretion by Caco-2 Cells." *Journal of Lipid Research* 43, no. 7 (2002): 1086–95.

During, A., M. K. Smith, J. B. Piper, and J. C. Smith. "β-Carotene 15,15′-Dioxygenase Activity in Human Tissues and Cells: Evidence of an Iron Dependency." *The Journal of Nutritional Biochemistry* 12, no. 11 (2001): 640–7.

Edge, R., D. J. McGarvey, and T. G. Truscott. "The Carotenoids as Anti-Oxidants—A Review." *Journal of Photochemistry and Photobiology B: Biology* 41, no. 3 (1997): 189–200.

Ejaz, S., A. Ejaz, K. Matsuda, and C. W. Lim. "Limonoids as Cancer Chemopreventive Agents." *Journal of the Science of Food and Agriculture* 86, no. 3 (2006): 339–45.

El-Mohsen, M. A., H. Bayele, G. Kuhnle, G. Gibson, E. Debnam, S. K. Srai, C. Rice-Evans, and J. P. E. Spencer. "Distribution of [3h] Trans-Resveratrol in Rat Tissues Following Oral Administration." *British Journal of Nutrition* 96, no. 01 (2006): 62–70.

Ettlinger, M. G., and A. J. Lundeen. "The Structures of Sinigrin and Sinalbin; an Enzymatic Rearrangement." *Journal of the American Chemical Society* 78, no. 16 (1956): 4172–3.

Felgines, C., O. Texier, C. Besson, D. Fraisse, J.-L. Lamaison, and C. Rémésy. "Blackberry Anthocyanins Are Slightly Bioavailable in Rats." *The Journal of Nutrition* 132, no. 6 (2002): 1249–53.

Ferruzzi, M. G., J. L. Lumpkin, S. J. Schwartz, and M. Failla. "Digestive Stability, Micellarization, and Uptake of β-Carotene Isomers by Caco-2 Human Intestinal Cells." *Journal of Agricultural and Food Chemistry* 54, no. 7 (2006): 2780–5.

Fichan, I., C. Larroche, and J. B. Gros. "Water Solubility, Vapor Pressure, and Activity Coefficients of Terpenes and Terpenoids." *Journal of Chemical & Engineering Data* 44, no. 1 (1998): 56–62.

Fleschhut, J., F. Kratzer, G. Rechkemmer, and S. Kulling. "Stability and Biotransformation of Various Dietary Anthocyanins *in Vitro*" *European Journal of Nutrition* 45, no. 1 (2006): 7–18.

Gamage, N., A. Barnett, N. Hempel, R. G. Duggleby, K. F. Windmill, J. L. Martin, and M. E. McManus. "Human Sulfotransferases and Their Role in Chemical Metabolism." *Toxicological Sciences* 90, no. 1 (2006): 5–22.

Gao, S. "Bioavailability Challenges Associated with Development of Anti-Cancer Phenolics." *Mini Reviews in Medicinal Chemistry* 10, no. 6 (2010): 550–67.

Gao, Y., A. L. Focsan, L. D. Kispert, and D. A. Dixon. "Density Functional Theory Study of the β-Carotene Radical Cation and Deprotonated Radicals." *The Journal of Physical Chemistry B* 110, no. 48 (2006): 24750–6.

Gee, J. M., M. S. DuPont, A. J. Day, G. W. Plumb, G. Williamson, and I. T. Johnson. "Intestinal Transport of Quercetin Glycosides in Rats Involves Both Deglycosylation and Interaction with the Hexose Transport Pathway." *The Journal of Nutrition* 130, no. 11 (2000): 2765–71.

Gibson, G. G., and P. S. Fil. "Pathways of Drug Metabolism." In *Introduction to Drug Metabolism*, 1–13. Cheltenham, UK: Nelson Thornes Publishers, 2001.

Goh, L. M. L., and P. J. Barlow. "Flavonoid Recovery and Stability from Ginkgo Biloba Subjected to a Simulated Digestion Process." *Food Chemistry* 86, no. 2 (2004): 195–202.

Goldberg, D. M., J. Yan, and G. J. Soleas. "Absorption of Three Wine-Related Polyphenols in Three Different Matrices by Healthy Subjects." *Clinical Biochemistry* 36, no. 1 (2003): 79–87.

Goñi, I., J. Serrano, and F. Saura-Calixto. "Bioaccessibility of β-Carotene, Lutein, and Lycopene from Fruits and Vegetables." *Journal of Agricultural and Food Chemistry* 54, no. 15 (2006): 5382–7.

González, R., I. Ballester, R. López-Posadas, M. D. Suárez, A. Zarzuelo, O. Martínez-Augustin, and F. Sánchez De Medina. "Effects of Flavonoids and Other Polyphenols on Inflammation." *Critical Reviews in Food Science and Nutrition* 51, no. 4 (2011): 331–62.

Graf, B. A., C. Ameho, G. G. Dolnikowski, P. E. Milbury, C.-Y. Chen, and J. B. Blumberg. "Rat Gastrointestinal Tissues Metabolize Quercetin." *The Journal of Nutrition* 136, no. 1 (2006): 39–44.

Griffiths, L. A. "Metabolism of Flavonoid Compounds in Germ-Free Rats." *Biochemical Journal* 130, no. 4 (1972): 1161–2.

Grolier, P., P. Borel, C. Duszka, S. Lory, M. C. Alexandre-Gouabau, V. Azais-Braesco, and L. Nugon-Baudon. "The Bioavailability of A- and β-Carotene Is Affected by Gut Microflora in the Rat." *British Journal of Nutrition* 80, no. 02 (1998): 199–204.

Halkier, B. A., and J. Gershenzon. "Biology and Biochemistry of Glucosinolates." *Annual Review of Plant Biology* 57, no. 1 (2006): 303–33.

Harborne, J. B. "Classes and Functions of Secondary Products from Plants." In *Chemicals from Plants: Perspectives on Plant Secondary Products*, edited by Nicholas J. Walton and Diane E. Brown, 1–26. London: Imperial College Press, 1999.

Harbourt, D. E., J. K. Fallon, S. Ito, T. Baba, J. K. Ritter, G. L. Glish, and P. C. Smith. "Quantification of Human Uridine-Diphosphate Glucuronosyl Transferase (Ugt) 1a Isoforms in Liver, Intestine and Kidney Using Nanolc-Ms/Ms." *Analytical Chemistry* 84, no. 1 (2011): 98–105.

Harrison, E. H. "Mechanisms Involved in the Intestinal Absorption of Dietary Vitamin a and Provitamin a Carotenoids." *Biochimica et Biophysica Acta (BBA)—Molecular and Cell Biology of Lipids* 1821, no. 1 (2012): 70–7.

Harrison, E. "Mechanisms of Intestinal Absorption of Carotenoids." In *Carotenoids*, 367–79. Boca Raton, FL: CRC Press, 2009.

Hasegawa, S., L. K. T. Lam, and E. G. Miller. "Citrus Limonoids: Biochemistry and Possible Importance to Human Nutrition." In *Phytochemicals and Phytopharmaceuticals*, edited by F. Shahidi and C.-T. Ho, 79–94. Champaign, IL: AOCS Press, 2000a.

Hasegawa, S., M. A. Berhow, and G. D. Manners. "Citrus Limonoid Research: An Overview." In *Citrus Limonoids*, 1–8. Washington, DC: American Chemical Society, 2000b.

Hayes, J., M. Kelleher, and I. Eggleston. "The Cancer Chemopreventive Actions of Phytochemicals Derived from Glucosinolates." *European Journal of Nutrition* 47, (2008): 73–88.

He, J., B. A. Magnuson, G. Lala, Q. Tian, S. J. Schwartz, and M. M. Giusti. "Intact Anthocyanins and Metabolites in Rat Urine and Plasma after 3 Months of Anthocyanin Supplementation." *Nutrition and Cancer* 54, no. 1 (2006): 3–12.

Heber, D. "Colorful Cancer Prevention: A-Carotene, Lycopene, and Lung Cancer." *The American Journal of Clinical Nutrition* 72, no. 4 (2000): 901–2.

Heinonen, S., T. Nurmi, K. Liukkonen, K. Poutanen, K. Wähälä, T. Deyama, S. Nishibe, and H. Adlercreutz. "In Vitro Metabolism of Plant Lignans: New Precursors of Mammalian Lignans Enterolactone and Enterodiol." *Journal of Agricultural and Food Chemistry* 49, no. 7 (2001): 3178–86.

Henry, C., X. Vitrac, A. Decendit, R. Ennamany, S. Krisa, and J.-M. Merillon. "Cellular Uptake and Efflux of Trans-Piceid and Its Aglycone Trans-Resveratrol on the Apical Membrane of Human Intestinal Caco-2 Cells." *Journal of Agricultural and Food Chemistry* 53, no. 3 (2005): 798–803.

Henry, L. K., N. L. Puspitasari-Nienaber, M. Jaren-Galan, R. B. van Breemen, G. L. Catignani, and S. J. Schwartz. "Effects of Ozone and Oxygen on the Degradation of Carotenoids in an Aqueous Model System." *Journal of Agricultural and Food Chemistry* 48, no. 10 (2000): 5008–13.

Henry-Vitrac, C., A. Desmoulière, D. Girard, J.-M. Mérillon, and S. Krisa. "Transport, Deglycosylation, and Metabolism of *Trans*-Piceid by Small Intestinal Epithelial Cells." *European Journal of Nutrition* 45, no. 7 (2006): 376–82.

Hirohashi, T., H. Suzuki, and Y. Sugiyama. "Characterization of the Transport Properties of Cloned Rat Multidrug Resistance-Associated Protein 3 (Mrp3)." *Journal of Biological Chemistry* 274, no. 21 (1999): 15181–5.

Hollander, D., and P. E. Ruble. "Beta-Carotene Intestinal Absorption: Bile, Fatty Acid, Ph, and Flow Rate Effects on Transport." *American Journal of Physiology—Endocrinology And Metabolism* 235, no. 6 (1978): E686–91.

Honma, W., Y. Kamiyama, K. Yoshinari, H. Sasano, M. Shimada, K. Nagata, and Y. Yamazoe. "Enzymatic Characterization and Interspecies Difference of Phenol Sulfotransferases, St1a Forms." *Drug Metabolism and Disposition* 29, no. 3 (2001): 274–81.

Howitz, K. T., K. J. Bitterman, H. Y. Cohen, D. W. Lamming, S. Lavu, J. G. Wood, R. E. Zipkin, P. Chung, A. Kisielewski, L.-L. Zhang, B. Scherer, and D. A. Sinclair. "Small Molecule Activators of Sirtuins Extend *Saccharomyces cerevisiae* Lifespan." *Nature* 425, no. 6954 (2003): 191–6.

Hu, M. "Commentary: Bioavailability of Flavonoids and Polyphenols: Call to Arms." *Molecular Pharmaceutics* 4, no. 6 (2007): 803–6.

Hu, M., J. Chen, and H. Lin. "Metabolism of Flavonoids Via Enteric Recycling: Mechanistic Studies of Disposition of Apigenin in the Caco-2 Cell Culture Model." *Journal of Pharmacology and Experimental Therapeutics* 307, no. 1 (2003): 314–21.

Huang, C., Y. Chen, T. Zhou, and G. Chen. "Sulfation of Dietary Flavonoids by Human Sulfotransferases." *Xenobiotica* 39, no. 4 (2009): 312–22.

Hur, H.-G., R. Beger, T. Heinze, J. Lay, J. Freeman, J. Dore, and F. Rafii. "Isolation of an Anaerobic Intestinal Bacterium Capable of Cleaving the C-Ring of the Isoflavonoid Daidzein." *Archives of Microbiology* 178, no. 1 (2002): 8–12.

Hussain, M. M. "A Proposed Model for the Assembly of Chylomicrons." *Atherosclerosis* 148, no. 1 (2000): 1–15.

Hussain, M. M., J. Shi, and P. Dreizen. "Microsomal Triglyceride Transfer Protein and Its Role in Apob-Lipoprotein Assembly." *Journal of Lipid Research* 44, no. 1 (2003): 22–32.

Jang, M., L. Cai, G. O. Udeani, K. V. Slowing, C. F. Thomas, C. W. W. Beecher, H. H. S. Fong, N. R. Farnsworth, A. D. Kinghorn, R. G. Mehta, R. C. Moon, and J. M. Pezzuto. "Cancer Chemopreventive Activity of Resveratrol, a Natural Product Derived from Grapes." *Science* 275, no. 5297 (1997): 218–20.

Jeong, E. J., X. Jia, and M. Hu. "Disposition of Formononetin Via Enteric Recycling: Metabolism and Excretion in Mouse Intestinal Perfusion and Caco-2 Cell Models." *Molecular Pharmaceutics* 2, no. 4 (2005): 319–28.

Jösch, C., H. Sies, and T. P. M. Akerboom. "Hepatic Mercapturic Acid Formation: Involvement of Cytosolic Cysteinylglycine S-Conjugate Dipeptidase Activity." *Biochemical Pharmacology* 56, no. 6 (1998): 763–71.

Kaldas, M. I., U. K. Walle, and T. Walle. "Resveratrol Transport and Metabolism by Human Intestinal Caco-2 Cells." *Journal of Pharmacy and Pharmacology* 55, no. 3 (2003): 307–12.

Kale, A., S. Gawande, and S. Kotwal. "Cancer Phytotherapeutics: Role for Flavonoids at the Cellular Level." *Phytotherapy Research* 22, no. 5 (2008): 567–77.

Kanaze, F. I., E. Kokkalou, I. Niopas, M. Georgarakis, A. Stergiou, and D. Bikiaris. "Dissolution Enhancement of Flavonoids by Solid Dispersion in Pvp and Peg Matrixes: A Comparative Study." *Journal of Applied Polymer Science* 102, no. 1 (2006): 460–71.

Keppler, K., and H.-U. Humpf. "Metabolism of Anthocyanins and Their Phenolic Degradation Products by the Intestinal Microflora." *Bioorganic and Medicinal Chemistry* 13, no. 17 (2005): 5195–205.

Kiefer, C., S. Hessel, J. M. Lampert, K. Vogt, M. O. Lederer, D. E. Breithaupt, and J. von Lintig. "Identification and Characterization of a Mammalian Enzyme Catalyzing the Asymmetric Oxidative Cleavage of Provitamin A." *Journal of Biological Chemistry* 276, no. 17 (2001): 14110–16.

Kim, D.-H., E.-A. Jung, I.-S. Sohng, J.-A. Han, T.-H. Kim, and M. Han. "Intestinal Bacterial Metabolism of Flavonoids and Its Relation to Some Biological Activities." *Archives of Pharmacal Research* 21, no. 1 (1998): 17–23.

Kim, K. S., S. H. Park, and M. G. Choung. "Nondestructive Determination of Lignans and Lignan Glycosides in Sesame Seeds by near Infrared Reflectance Spectroscopy." *Journal of Agricultural and Food Chemistry* 54, no. 13 (2006): 4544–50.

Kimura, Y., M. Sumiyoshi, and K. Baba. "Antitumor Activities of Synthetic and Natural Stilbenes through Antiangiogenic Action." *Cancer Science* 99, no. 10 (2008): 2083–96.

Kitts, D. D., Y. V. Yuan, A. N. Wijewickreme, and L. U. Thompson. "Antioxidant Activity of the Flaxseed Lignan Secoisolariciresinol Diglycoside and Its Mammalian Lignan Metabolites Enterodiol and Enterolactone." *Molecular and Cellular Biochemistry* 202, no. 1 (1999): 91–100.

Konovalov, V. V., and L. D. Kispert. "Am1, Indo/S and Optical Studies of Carbocations of Carotenoid Molecules. Acid Induced Isomerization." *Journal of the Chemical Society, Perkin Transactions* 2, no. 4 (1999): 901–10.

Konovalova, T. A., Y. Gao, R. Schad, L. D. Kispert, C. A. Saylor, and L.-C. Brunel. "Photooxidation of Carotenoids in Mesoporous Mcm-41, Ni-Mcm-41 and Al-Mcm-41 Molecular Sieves." *The Journal of Physical Chemistry B* 105, no. 31 (2001): 7459–64.

Kool, M., M. van der Linden, M. de Haas, G. L. Scheffer, J. M. L. de Vree, A. J. Smith, G. Jansen, G. J. Peters, N. Ponne, R. J. Scheper, R. P. J. Oude Elferink, F. Baas, and P. Borst. "Mrp3, an Organic Anion Transporter Able to Transport Anti-Cancer Drugs." *Proceedings of the National Academy of Sciences* 96, no. 12 (1999): 6914–9.

Krishnamurty, H. G., K. J. Cheng, G. A. Jones, F. J. Simpson, and J. E. Watkin. "Identification of Products Produced by the Anaerobic Degradation of Rutin and Related Flavonoids by Butyrivibrio Sp. C3." *Canadian Journal of Microbiology* 16, no. 8 (1970): 759–67.

Křížková, J. "The Effects of Selected Flavonoids on Cytochromes P450 in Rat Liver and Small Intestine." *Interdisciplinary Toxicology* 2, no. 3 (2009): 201–4.

Kroll, J, and H. Rawel. "Chemical Reactions of Benzyl Isothiocyanate with Myoglobin." *Journal of the Science of Food and Agriculture* 72, no. 3 (1996): 376–84.

Krul, C., C. Humblot, C. Philippe, M. Vermeulen, M. van Nuenen, R. Havenaar, and S. Rabot. "Metabolism of Sinigrin (2-Propenyl Glucosinolate) by the Human Colonic Microflora in a Dynamic in vitro Large-Intestinal Model." *Carcinogenesis* 23, no. 6 (2002): 1009–16.

Kuhnle, G., J. P. E. Spencer, G. Chowrimootoo, H. Schroeter, E. S. Debnam, S. K. S. Srai, C. Rice-Evans, and U. Hahn. "Resveratrol Is Absorbed in the Small Intestine as Resveratrol Glucuronide." *Biochemical and Biophysical Research Communications* 272, no. 1 (2000a): 212–17.

Kuhnle, G., J. P. E. Spencer, H. Schroeter, B. Shenoy, E. S. Debnam, S. K. S. Srai, C. Rice-Evans, and U. Hahn. "Epicatechin and Catechin Are O-Methylated and Glucuronidated in the Small Intestine." *Biochemical and Biophysical Research Communications* 277, no. 2 (2000b): 507–12.

Kulling, S. E., E. Jacobs, E. Pfeiffer, and M. Metzler. "Studies on the Genotoxicity of the Mammalian Lignans Enterolactone and Enterodiol and Their Metabolic Precursors at Various Endpoints in Vitro." *Mutation Research/Genetic Toxicology and Environmental Mutagenesis* 416, nos. 1–2 (1998): 115–24.

Lafay, S., A. Gil-Izquierdo, C. Manach, C. Morand, C. Besson, and A. Scalbert. "Chlorogenic Acid Is Absorbed in Its Intact Form in the Stomach of Rats." *The Journal of Nutrition* 136, no. 5 (2006a): 1192–7.

Lafay, S., C. Morand, C. Manach, C. Besson, and A. Scalbert. "Absorption and Metabolism of Caffeic Acid and Chlorogenic Acid in the Small Intestine of Rats." *British Journal of Nutrition* 96, no. 01 (2006b): 39–46.

Lai, R.-H., M. J. Miller, and E. Jeffery. "Glucoraphanin Hydrolysis by Microbiota in the Rat Cecum Results in Sulforaphane Absorption." *Food & Function* 1, no. 2 (2010): 161–66.

Lake, B. G. "Coumarin Metabolism, Toxicity and Carcinogenicity: Relevance for Human Risk Assessment." *Food and Chemical Toxicology* 37, no. 4 (1999): 423–53.

Lampe, J. W. "Emerging Research on Equol and Cancer." *The Journal of Nutrition* 140, no. 7 (2010): 1369S–72S.

Laparra, J. M., and Y. Sanz. "Interactions of Gut Microbiota with Functional Food Components and Nutraceuticals." *Pharmacological Research* 61, no. 3 (2010): 219–25.

Lee, S.-H., Y. H. Kim, H.-J. Yu, N.-S. Cho, T.-H. Kim, D.-C. Kim, C.-B. Chung, Y.-I. Hwang, and K. H. Kim. "Enhanced Bioavailability of Soy Isoflavones by Complexation with β-Cyclodextrin in Rats." *Bioscience, Biotechnology, and Biochemistry* 71, no. 12 (2007): 2927–33.

Lee, V. H. L. "Membrane Transporters." *European Journal of Pharmaceutical Sciences* 11, Supplement 2, (2000): S41–50.

Leuenberger, M. G., C. Engeloch-Jarret, and W.-D. Woggon. "The Reaction Mechanism of the Enzyme-Catalyzed Central Cleavage of β-Carotene to Retinal." *Angewandte Chemie International Edition* 40, no. 14 (2001): 2613–7.

Lewis, D. F. V. "Human Cytochromes P450 Associated with the Phase 1 Metabolism of Drugs and Other Xenobiotics: A Compilation of Substrates and Inhibitors of the Cyp1, Cyp2 and Cyp3 Families." *Current Medicinal Chemistry* 10, no. 19 (2003): 1955.

Lin, C. H., and B. H. Chen. "Stability of Carotenoids in Tomato Juice During Storage." *Food Chemistry* 90, no. 4 (2005): 837–46.

Liu, Y., and M. Hu. "Absorption and Metabolism of Flavonoids in the Caco-2 Cell Culture Model and a Perused Rat Intestinal Model." *Drug Metabolism and Disposition* 30, no. 4 (2002): 370–7.

Lobo, M. V. T., L. Huerta, N. Ruiz-Velasco, E. Teixeiro, P. de la Cueva, A. Celdrán, A. Martín-Hidalgo, M. A. Vega, and R. Bragado. "Localization of the Lipid Receptors Cd36 and Cla-1/Sr-Bi in the Human Gastrointestinal Tract: Towards the Identification of Receptors Mediating the Intestinal Absorption of Dietary Lipids." *Journal of Histochemistry & Cytochemistry* 49, no. 10 (2001): 1253–60.

M. Reis, J., B. Sinko, and C. H. R. Serra. "Parallel Artificial Membrane Permeability Assay (Pampa)—Is It Better Than Caco-2 for Human Passive Permeability Prediction?" *Mini Reviews in Medicinal Chemistry* 10, no. 11 (2010): 1071–6.

MacLeod, A. J., and J. T. Rossiter. "Non-Enzymic Degradation of 2-Hydroxybut-3-Enylglucosinolate (Progoitrin)." *Phytochemistry* 25, no. 4 (1986): 855–8.

Madgula, V. L. M., B. Avula, Y. W. Choi, S. V. Pullela, I. A. Khan, L. A. Walker, and S. I. Khan. "Transport of Schisandra Chinensis Extract and Its Biologically-Active Constituents across Caco-2 Cell Monolayers—An In-Vitro Model of Intestinal Transport." *Journal of Pharmacy and Pharmacology* 60, no. 3 (2008): 363–70.

Mäenpää, J., H. Sigusch, H. Raunio, T. Syngelmä, P. Vuorela, H. Vuorela, and O. Pelkonen. "Differential Inhibition of Coumarin 7-Hydroxylase Activity in Mouse and Human Liver Microsomes." *Biochemical Pharmacology* 45, no. 5 (1993): 1035–42.

Malfatti, M. A., K. H. Dingley, S. Nowell-Kadlubar, E. A. Ubick, N. Mulakken, D. Nelson, N. P. Lang, J. S. Felton, and K. W. Turteltaub. "The Urinary Metabolite Profile of the Dietary Carcinogen 2-Amino-1-Methyl-6-Phenylimidazo[4,5-B]Pyridine Is Predictive of Colon DNA Adducts after a Low-Dose Exposure in Humans." *Cancer Research* 66, no. 21 (2006): 10541–7.

Matsumoto, H., H. Inaba, M. Kishi, S. Tominaga, M. Hirayama, and T. Tsuda. "Orally Administered Delphinidin 3-Rutinoside and Cyanidin 3-Rutinoside Are Directly Absorbed in Rats and Humans and Appear in the Blood as the Intact Forms." *Journal of Agricultural and Food Chemistry* 49, no. 3 (2001): 1546–51.

McGhie, T. K., and M. C. Walton. "The Bioavailability and Absorption of Anthocyanins: Towards a Better Understanding." *Molecular Nutrition & Food Research* 51, no. 6 (2007): 702–13.

Meinl, W., B. Ebert, H. Glatt, and A. Lampen. "Sulfotransferase Forms Expressed in Human Intestinal Caco-2 and Tc7 Cells at Varying Stages of Differentiation and Role in Benzo[a]Pyrene Metabolism." *Drug Metabolism and Disposition* 36, no. 2 (2008): 276–83.

Meng, X., P. Maliakal, H. Lu, M.-J. Lee, and C. S. Yang. "Urinary and Plasma Levels of Resveratrol and Quercetin in Humans, Mice, and Rats after Ingestion of Pure Compounds and Grape Juice." *Journal of Agricultural and Food Chemistry* 52, no. 4 (2004): 935–42.

Mennicke, W. H., K. Görler, G. Krumbiegel, D. Lorenz, and N. Rittmann. "Studies on the Metabolism and Excretion of Benzyl Isothiocyanate in Man." *Xenobiotica* 18, no. 4 (1988): 441–7.

Mennicke, W. H., K. Görler, and G. Krumbiegel. "Metabolism of Some Naturally Occurring Isothiocyanates in the Rat." *Xenobiotica* 13, no. 4 (1983): 203–7.

Milder, I. E. J., I. C. W. Arts, B. van de Putte, D. P. Venema, and P. C. H. Hollman. "Lignan Contents of Dutch Plant Foods: A Database Including Lariciresinol, Pinoresinol, Secoisolariciresinol and Matairesinol." *British Journal of Nutrition* 93, no. 03 (2005): 393–402.

Mota, F. L., A. J. Queimada, S. P. Pinho, and E. A. Macedo. "Aqueous Solubility of Some Natural Phenolic Compounds." *Industrial & Engineering Chemistry Research* 47, no. 15 (2008): 5182–9.

Mullen, W., J.-M. Rouanet, C. Auger, P.-L. Teissèdre, S. T. Caldwell, R. C. Hartley, M. E. J. Lean, C. A. Edwards, and A. Crozier. "Bioavailability of [2-14c]Quercetin-4′-Glucoside in Rats." *Journal of Agricultural and Food Chemistry* 56, no. 24 (2008): 12127–37.

Murakami, A., and H. Ohigashi. "Targeting Nox, Inos and Cox-2 in Inflammatory Cells: Chemoprevention Using Food Phytochemicals." *International Journal of Cancer* 121, no. 11 (2007): 2357–63.

Murakami, T., and M. Takano. "Intestinal Efflux Transporters and Drug Absorption." *Expert Opinion on Drug Metabolism & Toxicology* 4, no. 7 (2008): 923–39.

Nakamura, A., M. Nakajima, H. Yamanaka, R. Fujiwara, and T. Yokoi. "Expression of Ugt1a and Ugt2b Mrna in Human Normal Tissues and Various Cell Lines." *Drug Metabolism and Disposition* 36, no. 8 (2008): 1461–4.

Neilson, A. P., A. S. Hopf, B. R. Cooper, M. A. Pereira, J. A. Bomser, and M. G. Ferruzzi. "Catechin Degradation with Concurrent Formation of Homo- and Heterocatechin Dimers During in vitro Digestion." *Journal of Agricultural and Food Chemistry* 55, no. 22 (2007): 8941–9.

Nguyen, H., S. Zhang, and M. E. Morris. "Effect of Flavonoids on Mrp1-Mediated Transport in Panc-1 Cells." *Journal of Pharmaceutical Sciences* 92, no. 2 (2003): 250–7.

Nielsen, S. E., V. Breinholt, U. Justesen, C. Cornett, and L.O. Dragsted. "In Vitro Biotransformation of Flavonoids by Rat Liver Microsomes." *Xenobiotica* 28, no. 4 (1998): 389–401.

Nugon-Baudon, L., S. Rabot, O. Szylit, and P. Raibaud. "Glucosinolates Toxicity in Growing Rats: Interactions with the Hepatic Detoxification System." *Xenobiotica* 20, no. 2 (1990): 223–30.

Olson, J. A. "Absorption, Transport, and Metabolism of Carotenoids in Humans." *Pure and Applied Chemistry* 66, no. 5(1994): 1011–16

Oostendorp, R. L., J. H. Beijnen, and J. H. M. Schellens. "The Role of Transporters at the Intestinal Barrier." In *Abc Transporters and Multidrug Resistance*, edited by Ahcène Boumendjel, Jean Boutonnat and Jacques Robert, 386–401. Hoboken: Wiley, 2009.

Otake, Y., and T. Walle. "Oxidation of the Flavonoids Galangin and Kaempferide by Human Liver Microsomes and Cyp1a1, Cyp1a2, and Cyp2c9." *Drug Metabolism and Disposition* 30, no. 2 (2002): 103–5.

Otake, Y., F. Hsieh, and T. Walle. "Glucuronidation Versus Oxidation of the Flavonoid Galangin by Human Liver Microsomes and Hepatocytes." *Drug Metabolism and Disposition* 30, no. 5 (2002): 576–81.

Ozaki, Y., S. Ayano, N. Inaba, M. Miyake, M. A. Berhow, and S. Hasegawa. "Limonoid Glucosides in Fruit, Juice and Processing by-Products of Satsuma Mandarin (Chus Unshiu Marcov.)." *Journal of Food Science* 60, no. 1 (1995): 186–9.

Pade, V., and S. Stavchansky. "Link between Drug Absorption Solubility and Permeability Measurements in Caco-2 Cells." *Journal of Pharmaceutical Sciences* 87, no. 12 (1998): 1604–7.

Passamonti, S., A. Vanzo, U. Vrhovsek, M. Terdoslavich, A. Cocolo, G. Decorti, and F. Mattivi. "Hepatic Uptake of Grape Anthocyanins and the Role of Bilitranslocase." *Food Research International* 38, nos. 8–9 (2005): 953–60.

Passamonti, S., U. Vrhovsek, A. Vanzo, and F. Mattivi. "The Stomach as a Site for Anthocyanins Absorption from Food." *FEBS Letters* 544, nos. 1–3 (2003): 210–3.

Passamonti, S., U. Vrhovsek, and F. Mattivi. "The Interaction of Anthocyanins with Bilitranslocase." *Biochemical and Biophysical Research Communications* 296, no. 3 (2002): 631–6.

Perez-Galvez, A., J. J. Rios, and M. I. Minguez-Mosquera. "Thermal Degradation Products Formed from Carotenoids During a Heat-Induced Degradation Process of Paprika Oleoresins (Capsicum Annuum L.)." *Journal of Agricultural and Food Chemistry* 53, no. 12 (2005): 4820–6.

Petri, N., C. Tannergren, B. Holst, F. A. Mellon, Y. Bao, G. W. Plumb, J. Bacon, K. A. O'Leary, P. A. Kroon, L. Knutson, P. Forsell, T. Eriksson, H. Lennernas, and G. Williamson. "Absorption/Metabolism of Sulforaphane and Quercetin, and Regulation of Phase II Enzymes, in Human Jejunum in Vivo." *Drug Metabolism and Disposition* 31, no. 6 (2003): 805–13.

Polar-Cabrera, K., T. Huo, S. J. Schwartz, and M. L. Failla. "Digestive Stability and Transport of Norbixin, a 24-Carbon Carotenoid, across Monolayers of Caco-2 Cells." *Journal of Agricultural and Food Chemistry* 58, no. 9 (2010): 5789–94.

Poulose, S. M., E. D. Harris, and B. S. Patil. "Antiproliferative Effects of Citrus Limonoids against Human Neuroblastoma and Colonic Adenocarcinoma Cells." *Nutrition and Cancer* 56, no. 1 (2006): 103–12.

Ramos, S. "Effects of Dietary Flavonoids on Apoptotic Pathways Related to Cancer Chemoprevention." *The Journal of Nutritional Biochemistry* 18, no. 7 (2007): 427–42.

Reboul, E., and P. Borel. "Proteins Involved in Uptake, Intracellular Transport and Basolateral Secretion of Fat-Soluble Vitamins and Carotenoids by Mammalian Enterocytes." *Progress in Lipid Research* 50, no. 4 (2011): 388–402.

Regev-Shoshani, G., O. Shoseyov, I. Bilkis, and Z. Kerem. "Glycosylation of Resveratrol Protects It from Enzymic Oxidation." *Biochemical Journal* 374, no. 1 (2003): 157–63.

Rendic, S. "Summary of Information on Human Cyp Enzymes: Human P450 Metabolism Data." *Drug Metabolism Reviews* 34, no. 1/2 (2002): 83.

Rendic, S., and F. J. Di Carlo. "Human Cytochrome P450 Enzymes: A Status Report Summarizing Their Reactions, Substrates, Inducers, and Inhibitors." *Drug Metabolism Reviews* 29, nos. 1–2 (1997): 413–580.

Rezende, B. A., S. F. Cortes, F. B. De Sousa, I. S. Lula, M. Schmitt, R. D. Sinisterra, and V. S. Lemos. "Complexation with β-Cyclodextrin Confers Oral Activity on the Flavonoid Dioclein." *International Journal of Pharmaceutics* 367, nos. 1–2 (2009): 133–9.

Riches, Z., E. L. Stanley, J. C. Bloomer, and M. W. H. Coughtrie. "Quantitative Evaluation of the Expression and Activity of Five Major Sulfotransferases (Sults) in Human Tissues: The Sult "Pie"." *Drug Metabolism and Disposition* 37, no. 11 (2009): 2255–61.

Rickard, S. E., and L. U. Thompson. "Chronic Exposure to Secoisolariciresinol Diglycoside Alters Lignan Disposition in Rats." *The Journal of Nutrition* 128, no. 3 (1998): 615–23.

Rimando, A. M., and N. Suh. "Biological/Chemopreventive Activity of Stilbenes and Their Effect on Colon Cancer." *Planta Med* 74, 2008 Oct; 74(13):1635–43.

Roberts, M. S., B. M. Magnusson, F. J. Burczynski, and M. Weiss. "Enterohepatic Circulation: Physiological, Pharmacokinetic and Clinical Implications." *Clinical Pharmacokinetics* 41, no. 10 (2002): 751–90.

Roncaglia, L., A. Amaretti, S. Raimondi, A. Leonardi, and M. Rossi. "Role of Bifidobacteria in the Activation of the Lignan Secoisolariciresinol Diglucoside." *Applied Microbiology and Biotechnology* 92, no. 1 (2011): 159–68.

Rouzaud, G., S. A. Young, and A. J. Duncan. "Hydrolysis of Glucosinolates to Isothiocyanates after Ingestion of Raw or Microwaved Cabbage by Human Volunteers." *Cancer Epidemiology Biomarkers & Prevention* 13, no. 1 (2004): 125–31.

Rouzaud, G., S. Rabot, B. Ratcliffe, and A. J. Duncan. "Influence of Plant and Bacterial Myrosinase Activity on the Metabolic Fate of Glucosinolates in Gnotobiotic Rats." *British Journal of Nutrition* 90, no. 02 (2003): 395–404.

Satsu, H., Y. Hiura, K. Mochizuki, M. Hamada, and M. Shimizu. "Activation of Pregnane X Receptor and Induction of Mdr1 by Dietary Phytochemicals." *Journal of Agricultural and Food Chemistry* 56, no. 13 (2008): 5366–73.

Schoch, T. K., G. D. Manners, and S. Hasegawa. "Analysis of Limonoid Glucosides from Citrus by Electrospray Ionization Liquid Chromatography–Mass Spectrometry." *Journal of Agricultural and Food Chemistry* 49, no. 3 (2001): 1102–08.

Schoefer, L., R. Mohan, A. Braune, M. Birringer, and M. Blaut. "Anaerobic C-Ring Cleavage of Genistein and Daidzein by Eubacterium Ramulus." *FEMS Microbiology Letters* 208, no. 2 (2002): 197–202.

Seeram, N. P., L. D. Bourquin, and M. G. Nair. "Degradation Products of Cyanidin Glycosides from Tart Cherries and Their Bioactivities." *Journal of Agricultural and Food Chemistry* 49, no. 10 (2001): 4924–9.

Selma, M. V., J. C. Espín, and F. A. Tomás-Barberán. "Interaction between Phenolics and Gut Microbiota: Role in Human Health." *Journal of Agricultural and Food Chemistry* 57, no. 15 (2009): 6485–501.

Sergent, T., L. Ribonnet, A. Kolosova, S. Garsou, A. Schaut, S. De Saeger, C. Van Peteghem, Y. Larondelle, L. Pussemier, and Y.-J. Schneider. "Molecular and Cellular Effects of Food Contaminants and Secondary Plant Components and Their Plausible Interactions at the Intestinal Level." *Food and Chemical Toxicology* 46, no. 3 (2008): 813–41.

Serra, H., T. Mendes, M. R. Bronze, and A. L. Simplício. "Prediction of Intestinal Absorption and Metabolism of Pharmacologically Active Flavones and Flavanones." *Bioorganic & Medicinal Chemistry* 16, no. 7 (2008): 4009–18.

Shapiro, T. A., J. W. Fahey, K. L. Wade, K. K. Stephenson, and P. Talalay. "Human Metabolism and Excretion of Cancer Chemoprotective Glucosinolates and Isothiocyanates of Cruciferous Vegetables." *Cancer Epidemiology Biomarkers & Prevention* 7, no. 12 (1998): 1091–100.

Shirkey, R. S., J. Chakraborty, and J. W. Bridges. "Comparison of the Drug Metabolising Ability of Rat Intestinal Mucosal Microsomes with That of Liver." *Biochemical Pharmacology* 28, no. 18 (1979): 2835–39.

Shu, L., K.-L. Cheung, T. Khor, C. Chen, and A.-N. Kong. "Phytochemicals: Cancer Chemoprevention and Suppression of Tumor Onset and Metastasis." *Cancer and Metastasis Reviews* 29, no. 3 (2010): 483–502.

Shulman, M., M. Cohen, A. Soto-Gutierrez, H. Yagi, H. Wang, J. Goldwasser, C. W. Lee-Parsons, O. Benny-Ratsaby, M. L. Yarmush, and Y. Nahmias. "Enhancement of Naringenin Bioavailability by Complexation with Hydroxypropoyl-β-Cyclodextrin." *PLoS ONE* 6, no. 4 (2011): e18033.

Slimestad, R., T. Fossen, and I. Molund Vågen. "Onions: A Source of Unique Dietary Flavonoids." *Journal of Agricultural and Food Chemistry* 55, no. 25 (2007): 10067–80.

Song, L., and P. J. Thornalley. "Effect of Storage, Processing and Cooking on Glucosinolate Content of Brassica Vegetables." *Food and Chemical Toxicology* 45, no. 2 (2007): 216–24.

Soobrattee, M. A., T. Bahorun, and O. I. Aruoma. "Chemopreventive Actions of Polyphenolic Compounds in Cancer." *BioFactors* 27, nos. 1–4 (2006): 19–35.

Spencer, J. P. E., F. Chaudry, A. S. Pannala, S. K. Srai, E. Debnam, and C. Rice-Evans. "Decomposition of Cocoa Procyanidins in the Gastric Milieu." *Biochemical and Biophysical Research Communications* 272, no. 1 (2000): 236–41.

Steensma, A., H. P. J. M. Noteborn, R. C. M. van der Jagt, T. H. G. Polman, M. J. B. Mengelers, and H. A. Kuiper. "Bioavailability of Genistein, Daidzein, and Their Glycosides in Intestinal Epithelial Caco-2 Cells." *Environmental Toxicology and Pharmacology* 7, no. 3 (1999): 209–12.

Steinkellner, H., S. Rabot, C. Freywald, E. Nobis, G. Scharf, M. Chabicovsky, S. Knasmüller, and F. Kassie. "Effects of Cruciferous Vegetables and Their Constituents on Drug Metabolizing Enzymes Involved in the Bioactivation of DNA-Reactive Dietary Carcinogens." *Mutation Research/Fundamental and Molecular Mechanisms of Mutagenesis* 480–481, (2001): 285–97.

Suzuki, H., and Y. Sugiyama. "Role of Metabolic Enzymes and Efflux Transporters in the Absorption of Drugs from the Small Intestine." *European Journal of Pharmaceutical Sciences* 12, no. 1 (2000): 3–12.

Talavéra, S., C. Felgines, O. Texier, C. Besson, C. Manach, Jean-Louis Lamaison, and Christian Rémésy. "Anthocyanins Are Efficiently Absorbed from the Small Intestine in Rats." *The Journal of Nutrition* 134, no. 9 (2004): 2275–9.

Talavéra, S., C. Felgines, O. Texier, C. Besson, J.-L. Lamaison, and C. Rémésy. "Anthocyanins Are Efficiently Absorbed from the Stomach in Anesthetized Rats." *The Journal of Nutrition* 133, no. 12 (2003): 4178–82.

Tang, L., R. Singh, Z. Liu, and M. Hu. "Structure and Concentration Changes Affect Characterization of Ugt Isoform-Specific Metabolism of Isoflavones." *Molecular Pharmaceutics* 6, no. 5 (2009): 1466–82.

Tanumihardjo, S. A. "Vitamin A: Biomarkers of Nutrition for Development." *The American Journal of Clinical Nutrition* 94, no. 2 (2011): 658S–65S.

Teubner, W., W. Meinl, S. Florian, Michael Kretzschmar, and Hansruedi Glatt. "Identification and Localization of Soluble Sulfotransferases in the Human Gastrointestinal Tract." *The Biochemical Journal* 404, no. 2 (2007): 207–15.

Thelen, K., and J. B. Dressman. "Cytochrome P450-Mediated Metabolism in the Human Gut Wall." *Journal of Pharmacy and Pharmacology* 61, no. 5 (2009): 541–58.

Thomas, W. "Absorption and Metabolism of Flavonoids." *Free Radical Biology and Medicine* 36, no. 7 (2004): 829–37.

Tian, X.-J., X.-W. Yang, X. Yang, and K. Wang. "Studies of Intestinal Permeability of 36 Flavonoids Using Caco-2 Cell Monolayer Model." *International Journal of Pharmaceutics* 367, nos. 1–2 (2009): 58–64.

Tommasini, S., D. Raneri, R. Ficarra, M. L. Calabrò, R. Stancanelli, and P. Ficarra. "Improvement in Solubility and Dissolution Rate of Flavonoids by Complexation with β-Cyclodextrin." *Journal of Pharmaceutical and Biomedical Analysis* 35, no. 2 (2004): 379–87.

Toshihisa, I. "The Atp-Dependent Glutathione S-Conjugate Export Pump." *Trends in Biochemical Sciences* 17, no. 11 (1992): 463–8.

Vaidyanathan, J. B., and T. Walle. "Cellular Uptake and Efflux of the Tea Flavonoid (-)Epicatechin-3-Gallate in the Human Intestinal Cell Line Caco-2." *Journal of Pharmacology and Experimental Therapeutics* 307, no. 2 (2003): 745–52.

Vallejo, F., A. Gil-Izquierdo, A. Pérez-Vicente, and C. García-Viguera. "In Vitro Gastrointestinal Digestion Study of Broccoli Inflorescence Phenolic Compounds, Glucosinolates, and Vitamin C." *Journal of Agricultural and Food Chemistry* 52, no. 1 (2003): 135–8.

van der Woude, H., M. G. Boersma, J. Vervoort, and I. M. C. M. Rietjens. "Identification of 14 Quercetin Phase Ii Mono- and Mixed Conjugates and Their Formation by Rat and Human Phase II in vitro Model Systems." *Chemical Research in Toxicology* 17, no. 11 (2004): 1520–30.

van Vliet, T., M. F. van Vlissingen, F. van Schaik, and H. van den Berg. "β-Carotene Absorption and Cleavage in Rats Is Affected by the Vitamin a Concentration of the Diet." *The Journal of Nutrition* 126, no. 2 (1996): 499–508.

Vermeulen, M., I. W. A. A. Klöpping-Ketelaars, R. van den Berg, and W. H. J. Vaes. "Bioavailability and Kinetics of Sulforaphane in Humans after Consumption of Cooked Versus Raw Broccoli." *Journal of Agricultural and Food Chemistry* 56, no. 22 (2008): 10505–9.

Virk-Baker, M. K., T. R. Nagy, and S. Barnes. "Role of Phytoestrogens in Cancer Therapy." *Planta Med* 76, no. EFirst (2010): 1132,42.

Walle, T., F. Hsieh, M. H. DeLegge, J. E. Oatis, and U. K. Walle. "High Absorption but Very Low Bioavailability of Oral Resveratrol in Humans." *Drug Metabolism and Disposition* 32, no. 12 (2004): 1377–82.

Walle, U. K., A. Galijatovic, and T. Walle. "Transport of the Flavonoid Chrysin and Its Conjugated Metabolites by the Human Intestinal Cell Line Caco-2." *Biochemical Pharmacology* 58, no. 3 (1999): 431–8.

Walsh, K. R., Y. C. Zhang, Y. Vodovotz, S. J. Schwartz, and M. L. Failla. "Stability and Bioaccessibility of Isoflavones from Soy Bread During in vitro Digestion." *Journal of Agricultural and Food Chemistry* 51, no. 16 (2003): 4603–9.

Walton, M. C., T. K. McGhie, G. W. Reynolds, and W. H. Hendriks. "The Flavonol Quercetin-3-Glucoside Inhibits Cyanidin-3-Glucoside Absorption in Vitro." *Journal of Agricultural and Food Chemistry* 54, no. 13 (2006): 4913–20.

Wang, D., Z. Zhang, J. Ju, X. Wang, and W. Qiu. "Investigation of Piceid Metabolites in Rat by Liquid Chromatography Tandem Mass Spectrometry." *Journal of Chromatography B* 879, no. 1 (2011): 69–74.

Wang, L. Q. "Human Intestinal Bacteria Capable of Transforming Secoisolariciresinol Diglucoside to Mammalian Lignans, Enterodiol and Enterolactone." *Chemical & Pharmaceutical Bulletin* 48, no. 11 (2000): 1606–10.

Wang, L.-S., and G. D. Stoner. "Anthocyanins and Their Role in Cancer Prevention." *Cancer Letters* 269, no. 2 (2008): 281–90.

Wang, Q., R. Jia, C. Ye, M. Garcia, J. Li, and I. Hidalgo. "Glucuronidation and Sulfation of 7-Hydroxycoumarin in Liver Matrices from Human, Dog, Monkey, Rat, and Mouse." *In Vitro Cellular & Developmental Biology—Animal* 41, no. 3 (2005): 97–103.

Wang, R., W. Zhou, and X. Jiang. "Reaction Kinetics of Degradation and Epimerization of Epigallocatechin Gallate (Egcg) in Aqueous System over a Wide Temperature Range." *Journal of Agricultural and Food Chemistry* 56, no. 8 (2008): 2694–701.

Wang, X.-D., G.-W. Tang, J. G. Fox, N. I. Krinsky, and R. M. Russell. "Enzymatic Conversion of β-Carotene into β-Apo-Carotenals and Retinoids by Human, Monkey, Ferret, and Rat Tissues." *Archives of Biochemistry and Biophysics* 285, no. 1 (1991): 8–16.

Ward, H. A., and G. G. C. Kuhnle. "Phytoestrogen Consumption and Association with Breast, Prostate and Colorectal Cancer in Epic Norfolk." *Archives of Biochemistry and Biophysics* 501, no. 1 (2010): 170–5.

Wikoff, W. R., A. T. Anfora, J. Liu, P. G. Schultz, S. A. Lesley, E. C. Peters, and G. Siuzdak. "Metabolomics Analysis Reveals Large Effects of Gut Microflora on Mammalian Blood Metabolites." *Proceedings of the National Academy of Sciences* 106, no. 10 (2009): 3698–703.

Wilkinson, G. R. "The Effects of Diet, Aging and Disease-States on Presystemic Elimination and Oral Drug Bioavailability in Humans." *Advanced Drug Delivery Reviews* 27, nos. 2–3 (1997): 129–59.

Winter, J., L. H. Moore, V. R. Dowell, and V. D. Bokkenheuser. "C-Ring Cleavage of Flavonoids by Human Intestinal Bacteria." *Applied and Environmental Microbiology* 55, no. 5 (1989): 1203–8.

Wolf, G. "The Enzymatic Cleavage of β-Carotene: Still Controversial." *Nutrition Reviews* 53, no. 5 (1995): 134–7.

Woodward, G., P. Kroon, A. Cassidy, and C. Kay. "Anthocyanin Stability and Recovery: Implications for the Analysis of Clinical and Experimental Samples." *Journal of Agricultural and Food Chemistry* 57, no. 12 (2009): 5271–8.

Xing, J., X. Chen, and D. Zhong. "Stability of Baicalin in Biological Fluids in Vitro." *Journal of Pharmaceutical and Biomedical Analysis* 39, nos. 3–4 (2005): 593–600.

Xu, H., K. H. Kulkarni, R. Singh, Z. Yang, S. W. J. Wang, V. H. Tam, and M. Hu. "Disposition of Naringenin Via Glucuronidation Pathway Is Affected by Compensating Efflux Transporters of Hydrophilic Glucuronides." *Molecular Pharmaceutics* 6, no. 6 (2009): 1703–15.

Xu, X., K. S. Harris, H.-J. Wang, P. A. Murphy, and S. Hendrich. "Bioavailability of Soybean Isoflavones Depends Upon Gut Microflora in Women." *The Journal of Nutrition* 125, no. 9 (1995): 2307–15.

Yang, C. S., J. M. Landau, M.-T. Huang, and H. L. Newmark. "Inhibition of Carcinogenesis by Dietary Polyphenolic Compounds." *Annual Review of Nutrition* 21, no. 1 (2001): 381–406.

Yonekura-Sakakibara, K., T. Nakayama, M. Yamazaki, and K. Saito. "Modification and Stabilization of Anthocyanins." In *Anthocyanins: Biosynthesis, Functions, and Applications*, edited by Kevin Gould, Kevin Davies and Chris Winefield, 169–90. New York: Springer 2009.

Yonekura, L., and A. Nagao. "Intestinal Absorption of Dietary Carotenoids." *Molecular Nutrition & Food Research* 51, no. 1 (2007): 107–15.

Yuan, J.-P., J.-H. Wang, and X. Liu. "Metabolism of Dietary Soy Isoflavones to Equol by Human Intestinal Microflora—Implications for Health." *Molecular Nutrition & Food Research* 51, no. 7 (2007): 765–81.

Zafra-Stone, S., T. Yasmin, M. Bagchi, A. Chatterjee, J. A. Vinson, and D. Bagchi. "Berry Anthocyanins as Novel Antioxidants in Human Health and Disease Prevention." *Molecular Nutrition & Food Research* 51, no. 6 (2007): 675–83.

Zhang, L., G. Lin, and Z. Zuo. "Involvement of Udp-Glucuronosyltransferases in the Extensive Liver and Intestinal First-Pass Metabolism of Flavonoid Baicalein." *Pharmaceutical Research* 24, no. 1 (2007a): 81–9.

Zhang, L., Z. Zuo, and G. Lin. "Intestinal and Hepatic Glucuronidation of Flavonoids." *Molecular Pharmaceutics* 4, no. 6 (2007b): 833–45.

Zhang, Y. S., R. H. Kolm, B. Mannervik, and P. Talalay. "Reversible Conjugation of Isothiocyanates with Glutathione Catalyzed by Human Glutathione Transferases." *Biochemical and Biophysical Research Communications* 206, no. 2 (1995): 748–55.

Zhang, Y.. "Role of Glutathione in the Accumulation of Anticarcinogenic Isothiocyanates and Their Glutathione Conjugates by Murine Hepatoma Cells." *Carcinogenesis* 21, no. 6 (2000): 1175–82.

Zhang, Y., and E. C. Callaway. "High Cellular Accumulation of Sulphoraphane, a Dietary Anticarcinogen, Is Followed by Rapid Transporter-Mediated Export as a Glutathione Conjugate." *The Biochemical Journal* 364, no. 1 (2002): 301–7.

Zhu, Q. Y., J. F. Hammerstone, S. A. Lazarus, H. H. Schmitz, and C. L. Keen. "Stabilizing Effect of Ascorbic Acid on Flavan-3-Ols and Dimeric Procyanidins from Cocoa." *Journal of Agricultural and Food Chemistry* 51, no. 3 (2002): 828–33.

8 Pharmacokinetics of Dietary Isothiocyanates and Flavonoids

Yoshihiko Ito, Shizuo Yamada, and Marilyn E. Morris

CONTENTS

8.1   INTRODUCTION

This review will focus on the bioavailability and pharmacokinetics (PK) of two classes of dietary compounds, namely, isothiocyanates (ITCs) and flavonoids. Isothiocyanates form a class of dietary compounds that are present in *Brassica* and other vegetables of the family Cruciferae (e.g., broccoli, brussels sprouts, cauliflower, kale, watercress) and the genus *Raphanus* (radishes and daikons). Organic isothiocyanates (R-N = C = S) (Figure 8.1) occur in plants as thioglycoside conjugates known as glucosinolates. Flavonoids comprise the most common type of plant polyphenols and provide much of the flavor and color to fruits and vegetables (Ross and Kasum 2002). Some major subclasses of flavonoids include the flavanones (e.g., hesperetin, naringenin); flavonols (e.g., quercetin, myricetin); flavan-3-ols (e.g., catechins); isoflavones (e.g., genistein, biochanin A, daidzein); and flavones (e.g., apigenin, chrysin, luteolin) (Figure 8.2). Flavonoids are present in fruits, vegetables, and plant-derived beverages, as well as in a multitude of dietary supplements, either as a single flavonoid or as simple or complex mixtures.

8.2   ISOTHIOCYANATES

Organic isothiocyanates are not only ubiquitous in the diet as their glucosinolate precursors, but because they have anticancer activities, they are also available as dried vegetable extracts in dietary supplements. As a result of isothiocyanates' wide availability, human exposure to them can be significant. The pharmacokinetic properties of several isothiocyanates have been investigated in rats and humans (see review by Lamy et al. 2011). Isothiocyanates have high oral bioavailability and do not exhibit adverse reactions at the doses consumed (Ji et al. 2005). Isothiocyanates undergo metabolism mediated by glutathione-S-transferases and are substrates for ATP-dependent binding cassette (ABC) transporters (Tseng et al. 2002; Ji and Morris 2004, 2005b; Ji et al. 2005); these dietary compounds exhibit nonlinear elimination profiles, which could be a result of enzyme or

Name	Structure
Sulforaphane	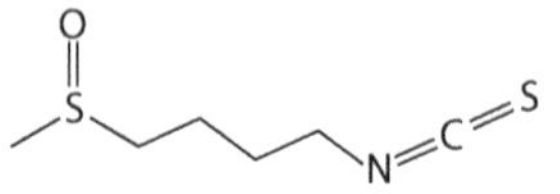
Phenethyl isothiocyanate	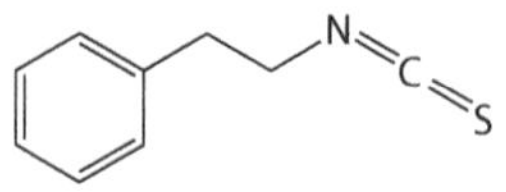
Napthyl isothiocyanate	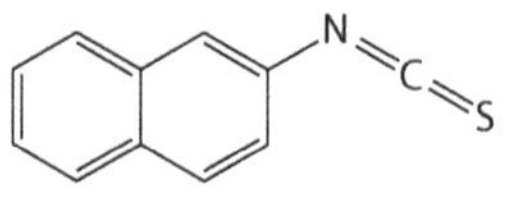

FIGURE 8.1   Chemical structures of dietary organic isothiocyanates.

transporter saturation or both (Ji et al. 2005). Some pharmacokinetic studies have used nonspecific methods where total dithiocarbamates, consisting of the isothiocyanate of interest, its metabolites, and other thionyl compounds, are determined, and findings from these studies will not be reported.

Phenylethyl isothiocyanate (PEITC) has rapid absorption, high oral bioavailability, and low clearance (11.6 mL/min/kg at the lowest dose of 2 μmol/kg) in rats (Ji et al. 2005). Nonlinear elimination and distribution are evident at high doses. Ji et al. (2005) evaluated the clearance and bioavailability of PEITC after the administration of varying oral and intravenous (IV) doses in rats, demonstrating nonlinearity at higher doses. In humans, following the ingestion of watercress at a 100 g dose, the half-life was 4.9 h, and the mean C_{max} value was 928 nM (Figure 8.3). The average oral clearance [clearance/availability (CL/F)] was 490 mL/min (Ji and Morris 2003). α-Naphthyl isothiocyanate (NITC) also exhibits nonlinear pharmacokinetics with a plasma half-life of 6.1 h at a high dose of 75 mg/kg (Hu and Morris 2005). A high dose of sulforaphane (50 μmol) in rats produces high concentrations in plasma after oral administration, with a C_{max} of 20 μM and a half-life of about 2.2 h; a second study examined the PK of sulforaphane 25 mg/kg (100 μmol/kg) and reported a clearance of 48 mL/min/kg and a half-life of 3.2 h (Hu et al. 2004; Cornblatt et al. 2007). Oral bioavailability of ITCs in human studies following the administration of fresh watercress, garden cress, broccoli, cabbage, or mustard, based on ITC metabolite recovery in the urine, ranges from 14% to 85% (Lamy et al. 2011). The bioavailability of sulforaphane from broccoli sprouts is dependent on the availability of the enzyme myrosinase (β-thioglucoside glucohydrolase) (Cramer and Jeffery 2011).

Isothiocyanates are widely distributed into tissues, leading to the suggestion that isothiocyanates may affect transporter-mediated distribution of coadministered drug substrates. Both PEITC and phenhexyl isothiocyanate (PHITC), following their administration to F344 rats, were detected as ^{14}C in all 13 tissues examined, although concentrations of ^{14}C-PHITC were higher than ^{14}C-PEITC in tissues (Conaway et al. 1999). ITCs covalently bind to proteins by reacting with sulfhydryl groups, leading to extensive protein binding in plasma and tissues. The apparent volume of distribution at steady state (Vss) of PEITC following a 400 μmol/kg dose is much greater than at lower doses, suggesting saturation of efflux transporters or saturation of tissue metabolism.

The metabolism of isothiocyanates has mainly been studied in humans. The conjugation and excretion of isothiocyanates is predominantly catalyzed by glutathione S-transferase M1 (GSTM1) and GSTT1 (Ketterer 1998), although a variety of other GSTs, including A1, P1, M2, and M4, are also involved to a minor extent. GSTM1 and GSTT1 exhibit genetic polymorphisms, and a GSTM1-null phenotype results in no activity in 52% of European Americans and 28% of African Americans. Thus, human exposure and metabolism of ITCs may be highly dependent on the genetic variability of GSTs. Lin et al. (1998) reported that the colon cancer chemoprotective effect of broccoli was

	Structure	Members of the Subgroup	Representative Food Sources
Flavone	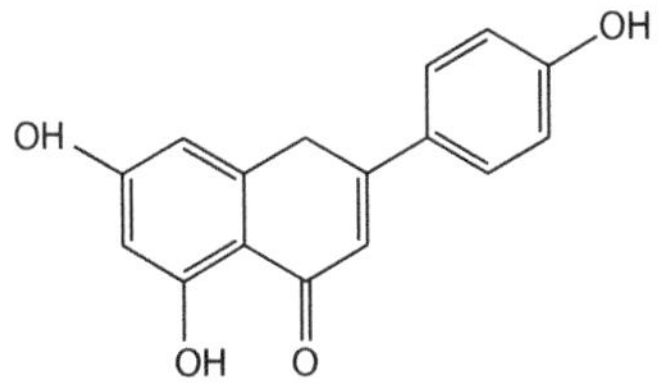 Apigenin	Apigenin Baicalein Chrysin Diosmetin Luteolin Tangeretin	Parsley, thyme, celery, sweet red peppers, honey
Flavonol	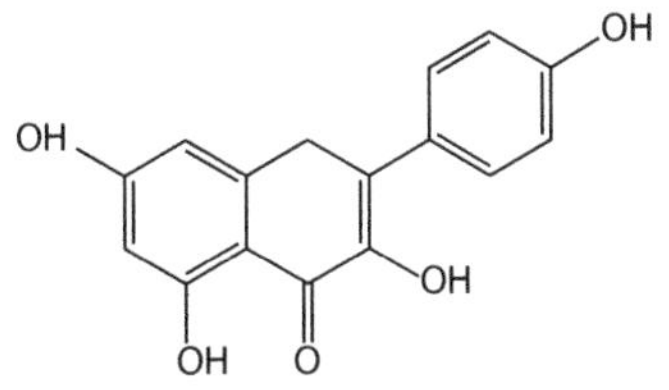 Kaempferol	Galangin Kaempferol Morin Myricetin Quercetin	Onions, kale, broccoli, tomato, beans, apples, cherries, berries, tea, red wine
Flavanone	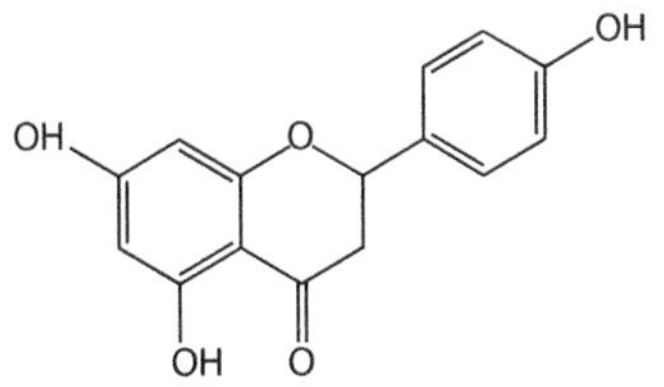 Naringenin	Eriodictyol Hesperetin Naringenin	Citrus
Flavan-3-ols	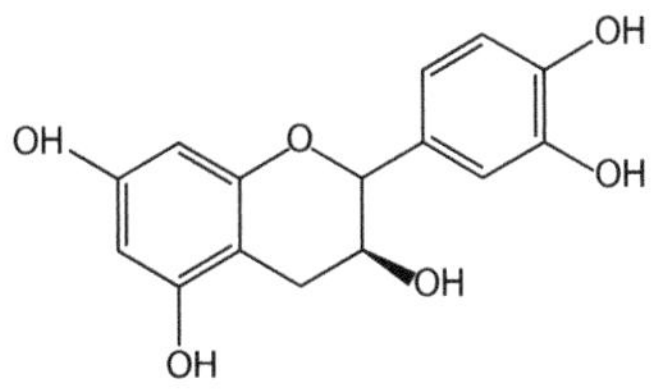 Epicatechin	Catechin Epicatechin Epigallocatechin gallate	Cocoa, green tea, chocolate, red wine, hawthorn, bilberry
Isoflavone	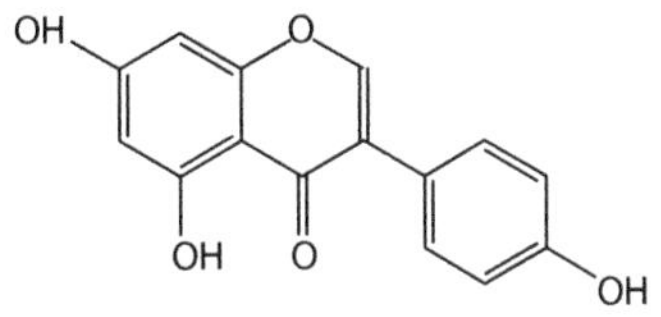 Genistein	Biochanin A Daidzein Equol Genistein	Red clover, legumes, soybeans, soy milk, tofu

FIGURE 8.2 Chemical structures and major food sources of the major flavonoid subgroups. (From Ross, J.A., and Kasum, C.M., *Annu. Rev. Nutr.*, 22, 19–34, 2002; Moon, Y.J. et al., *Toxicol. In Vitro*, 20, 187–210, 2006b.)

observed only in subjects with a GSTM1-null phenotype, who would be expected to exhibit higher concentrations of isothiocyanates.

The glutathione conjugates of ITCs are effluxed from cells by the family of ABCC transporters. As well, glutathione conjugation of ITCs is likely responsible for the intracellular glutathione depletion observed in vitro (Dietrich et al. 2001). The nonlinear pharmacokinetics of ITCs observed in

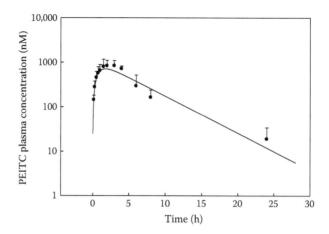

FIGURE 8.3 Plasma concentrations of PEITC in humans after the administration of 100 g watercress. Data are expressed as mean ± SD, $n = 4$. The line represents the fitted line, determined by nonlinear regression analysis (WinNonlin 2.1). (Reprinted from *Anal. Biochem.*, 323, Ji, Y., and Morris, M.E., Determination of phenethyl isothiocyanate in human plasma and urine by ammonia derivatization and liquid chromatography-tandem mass spectrometry, 39–47. Copyright 2003, with permission from Elsevier.)

vivo might be a result of saturation of this efflux, or the decreased metabolism of the parent itself, with glutathione depletion contributing to this nonlinearity. Isothiocyanate–glutathione conjugates (ITC-SG), present intracellularly, may be further metabolized or hydrolyzed back to the parent ITC, and the formed ITC-SG conjugate may be effluxed out of the cell by members of the ABCC family (Zhang 2001; Ji and Morris 2005b). Isothiocyanates are present in the urine as glutathione, cysteine, and mercapturic acid conjugates in both rats and humans, and conjugates may also undergo biliary excretion and enterohepatic cycling (Ji et al. 2005).

Certain dietary ITCs can inhibit ABCB1- (P-glycoprotein), ABCC1-, and ABCG2-mediated transport in multidrug-resistant cancer cells (Tseng et al. 2002; Ji and Morris 2004; Telang et al. 2009) either as unchanged ITC or as a glutathione conjugate. Studies using membrane vesicle preparations have demonstrated that ITCs are inhibitors of ABCG2 ATPase activity and PEITC itself is a substrate for ABCG2 (Ji and Morris 2005a). In vivo studies in rats have demonstrated that benzyl ITC can significantly increase the systemic exposure and decrease the elimination of the ABCG2 substrates, topotecan, and nitrofurantoin, in a dose-dependent manner (Telang et al. 2009).

8.3 FLAVONOIDS

Flavonoids are polyphenolic compounds, widely present in fruits, vegetables, and plant-derived beverages, and in many dietary supplements, either alone or combined with other flavonoids. Flavonoids are present in the diet in glycosylated forms, and generally, research indicates that glycosides are hydrolyzed to the aglycones by intestinal enzymes including lactase–phlorizin hydrolase and β-glucosidases or by colonic microflora before absorption (D'Archivio et al. 2007). However, quercetin glucosides may exhibit greater absorption than quercetin aglycone, and it has been suggested that transport of flavonoid glucosides may be facilitated through interactions with the sodium-dependent glucose transporters. On the other hand, increased stability of flavonoids in the intestine when present as glycosides might contribute to decreased conjugative metabolism in the intestine and increased bioavailability (Prasain and Barnes 2007; D'Archivio et al. 2007). The pharmacokinetics of flavonoids is characterized by extensive conjugative metabolism in the intestine and liver, resulting in poor bioavailability and high clearance (Prasain and Barnes 2007). The major circulating forms are conjugated (sulfate, glucuronide, and methyl) metabolites, which are cleared by both urinary and biliary excretion, with glucuronide conjugates subject to enterohepatic cycling. Flavonoids are inhibitors and substrates for a number of classes of both influx and efflux transporters, both in unchanged form and as their conjugated metabolites, and these represent important determinants of their bioavailability, clearance, and tissue distribution. Interactions of flavonoids with various transporters have been previously summarized (Morris and Zhang 2006; An and Morris 2009) but involve a range of transporters, including ABCB1 (P-glycoprotein), ABCC2 (multidrug resistance protein 2 [MRP2]), ABCG2 (breast cancer resistance protein [BCRP]), organic anion transporting polypeptide 1B1 (OATP1B1), and monocarboxylate transporters (MCTs). Based on chemical structure, flavonoids have been divided into different chemical classes (Figure 8.2). The following discussion will focus on the different classes of flavonoids and the PK of selected members of each class.

8.3.1 FLAVONOLS

Quercetin (3,3′,4′,5,7-pentahydroxyflavone), a flavonol with a wide range of biological activities, is an ingredient in a large number of dietary supplements and multivitamin preparations. Quercetin represents a major dietary flavonoid, with the richest sources of quercetin being onions, apples, tea, and red wine. It mainly occurs in plants as glycosides such as rutin (quercetin rutinoside) (Murota and Terao 2003). Despite the widespread use of flavonoids and the fact that many studies suggest beneficial pharmacological activity, little is known about the pharmacokinetics of quercetin aglycone. Due to the lack of sensitivity of many published assays, most of the clinical studies have measured total quercetin (unchanged quercetin plus conjugated quercetin metabolites following enzymatic hydrolysis) (Hollman et al. 1996, 1997; Olthof et al. 2000; Graefe et al. 2001). To our knowledge, there are only a few clinical studies that have reported the plasma concentration–time profile of unchanged quercetin following the administration of quercetin.

In humans, quercetin is extensively conjugated to sulfate and glucuronide conjugates, which are the major metabolites present in plasma (Walle et al. 2000). In rats, part of the quercetin dose absorbed in the small intestine is conjugated and excreted back into the intestinal lumen through biliary secretion (Crespy et al. 1999). Quercetin (23.0%–81.1% of doses) is recovered as $^{14}CO_2$ in the expired air from volunteers after both oral and IV ^{14}C-quercetin administration, indicating extensive metabolism (Walle et al. 2001). Bioavailability of quercetin is poor to moderate, and the bioavailability of quercetin glycosides is dependent on the type and position of the sugar moieties (Hollman et al. 1999).

We reported plasma quercetin aglycone concentration–time profiles, following the ingestion of quercetin 500 mg three times daily (Moon et al. 2008). The mean C_{max} values for the quercetin aglycone and quercetin conjugated metabolites were 15.4 and 448 ng/mL, respectively. When the plasma samples were treated with the glucuronidase and sulfatase enzymes, the plasma concentrations of quercetin increased ~30-fold. The average oral clearance (CL/F) was high (3.5×10^4 L/h), with an average terminal half-life of 3.5 h for quercetin. Plasma reentry peaks for quercetin were observed, suggesting enterohepatic cycling. A one-compartment model that included enterohepatic recirculation best described the plasma data (Moon et al. 2008).

Another common flavonoid in the diet, kaempferol, also exhibits cancer chemopreventative properties. Similarly to quercetin, kaempferol exhibits high clearance and low bioavailability. After IV doses of 10 and 25 mg/kg in rats, the clearance of kaempferol was about 55 mL/min/kg, and its half-life was ~4 h; bioavailability of oral doses of 100 and 250 mg/kg was less than 3%, likely due to extensive first-pass metabolism (Wang et al. 2011).

8.3.2 FLAVAN-3-OLS

Green tea is extensively ingested in many Eastern countries, with increasing popularity in the West. It is a rich source of several flavan-3-ol monomers, including (-)-epigallocatechin-3-O-gallate (EGCG), (-)-epigallocatechin, and (-)-epicatechin (Del Rio et al. 2004). Green tea delivers these bioactive compounds in a water-soluble form, which contains various amounts of caffeine, depending on the brewing method, and is reported to reduce the risk of cardiovascular diseases and certain cancers (Arab and Liebeskind 2010; Mineharu et al. 2011; Williamson et al. 2011).

Chen et al. (1997) compared the plasma pharmacokinetics of EGCG in rats after IV (10 mg/kg) and oral (75 mg/kg) administration and reported an oral bioavailability of 1.6%. Lambert et al. (2003) determined the pharmacokinetics of EGCG in mice after oral and IV dosing, reporting an oral bioavailability of 15.8%. Cai et al. (2002) reported that the plasma concentration–time curve of EGCG was similar in rats following IV and intraportal administration, suggesting that this tea catechin does not undergo significant first-pass hepatic metabolism. EGCG, administered at a dose of 100 mg/kg to rats by intraperitoneal injection, results in higher dose-normalized plasma concentrations compared with that observed after oral administration, suggesting the possibility of presystemic loss/metabolism within the gastrointestinal tract (Kao et al. 2000). Therefore, gastrointestinal first-pass extraction may contribute more significantly than hepatic first-pass extraction to the low oral bioavailability of green tea catechins.

Chen et al. (1997) administered green tea containing 73, 68, and 27 mg/g of EGCG, (-)-epigallocatechin, and (-)-epicatechin, respectively, to rats via IV and oral routes. The oral bioavailability was found to be 0.1%, 13.7%, and 31.2% for EGCG, (-)-epigallocatechin, and (-)-epicatechin, respectively. Epigallocatechin and epicatechin exhibited higher C_{max} and bioavailability values compared with EGCG (Chen et al. 1997).

In a recent clinical study, 10 healthy human subjects, who had been on a low-flavonoid-content diet for 2 days, consumed 500 mL of green tea containing 648 µmol of flavan-3-ols, after which plasma and urine were collected over a 24-h period and analyzed by liquid chromatography-tandem mass spectrometry (LC/MS/MS) (Stalmach et al. 2009). Plasma contained a total of 12 metabolites, in the form of O-methyl, sulfate, and glucuronide conjugates of epicatechin and epigallocatechin along with EGCG and (-)-epicatechin-O-gallate. The main metabolites were epigallocatechin-O-glucuronide with a C_{max} of 29 nmol/L and a T_{max} of 2.2 h and epicatechin-O-glucuronide, probably the 3′-O-conjugate, with a C_{max} of 29 nmol/L and a T_{max} of 1.7 h. The unmetabolized flavan-3-ols, EGCG and (-)-epicatechin-3-O-gallate, had C_{max} values of 55 and 25 nmol/L. The T_{max} values ranged from 1.6 to 2.3 h, and all the flavan-3-ols and their metabolites were present only in trace quantities after 8 h and were not detected in the 24-h plasma samples. This indicates low intestinal absorption, a fact confirmed when a similar flavan-3-ol metabolite plasma profile was obtained after the ingestion of green tea by human subjects with an ileostomy (Stalmach et al. 2010). Stalmach et al. (2010) reported that after subjects with ileostomies drank green tea containing 634 µmol of flavan-3-ols, 69% of the intake was recovered in 0- to 24-h ileal fluid as a mixture of unchanged compounds and metabolites.

8.3.3 FLAVANONES

The flavanones hesperetin and naringenin are abundant in citrus fruits and constitute a major part of the total flavonoids intake in many European countries (Justesen et al. 1997; Knekt et al. 2002; Bredsdorff et al. 2010). Hesperetin and naringenin are naturally present in citrus fruits as their respective 7-O-rutinosides, hesperidin and narirutin (Bredsdorff et al. 2010). By enzymatic treatment with α-rhamnosidase, the rutinoside moiety can be hydrolyzed to yield hesperetin-7-O-glucoside and narigenin-7-O-glucoside, respectively (Nielsen et al. 2006). The sugar moiety is a major determinant of the absorption site and bioavailability of the flavonoid since flavonoid monoglucoside bioavailability is several fold higher than that of flavonoid rutinoside (Hollman et al. 1999; Manach et al. 2003; Nielsen et al. 2006). Flavonoid monoglucosides are absorbed in the small intestine after hydrolysis by lactase-phlorizin hydrolase (Day et al. 2000; Sesink et al. 2003) or cytosolic β-glucosidases (Day et al. 1998; Nemeth et al. 2003), whereas flavonoids rutinosides must reach the microflora in the colon before they can be hydrolyzed and absorbed. Both small intestinal and colonic epithelium can metabolize flavonoids via glucuronidation or sulfation reactions (Brand et al. 2008).

In a recent study, Mullen et al. (2008) evaluated the human bioavailability and metabolism of orange juice flavanones. They collected human plasma and urine over a 24-h period after the consumption of 250 mL of orange juice containing a total of 168 μM of hesperetin-7-O-rutinoside and 17 μM of naringenin-7-O-rutinoside. They reported extensive conjugation of orange juice flavonoids in the gastrointestinal tract, particularly in the large intestine and colon. The excretion of hesperetin metabolites in the urine corresponded to 6.3% of intake, whereas urinary naringenin metabolites were equivalent to about 17.7% of the amount ingested, suggesting higher bioavailability of naringenin. This may represent a dose-dependent effect on bioavailability or suggest differences in the permeability and/or gastrointestinal metabolism of these two orange juice flavonoids.

8.3.4 Isoflavones

The interest in soy isoflavones, especially genistein and daidzein, has increased owing to scientific data showing a wide range of biological activities by these phytoestrogens, including beneficial effects of soy on a range of hormone-dependent conditions, including breast cancer, osteoporosis, postmenopausal symptoms, and hypercholesterolemia (Setchell and Cassidy 1999; Messina and Loprinzi 2001; Burke et al. 2003; Setchell and Lydeking-Olsen 2003; Nielsen and Williamson 2007).

Genistein and daidzein are present as glucosides in soy and in many unfermented foods (Day et al. 2000). There is some absorption in the small intestine, as shown by the appearance of a small plasma peak present approximately 1 h after ingestion (Day et al. 2000; King and Bursill 1998). A larger peak appears after 5–8 h, which is due to enterohepatic recycling of conjugates, first-time absorption in the colon, or a combination of both. Most of the absorbed genistein and daidzein are conjugated in plasma, although a proportion is present in plasma as aglycone (Piskula 2000). In approximately 40% of the population, specific colon microfloras (Setchell et al. 2002) are present and can convert daidzein to equol (Lampe et al. 1998). The ability to produce equol in these subjects may improve the outcome in studies involving measuring health benefits from isoflavones (Setchell et al. 2002).

In a clinical study (Rufer et al. 2008), seven male volunteers ingested either pure daidzein or pure daidzein-7-O-glucoside, both at a dose of 3.9 μmol/kg body weight. The bioavailability of daidzein following glucoside ingestion was three to six times greater than that following consumption of the aglycone. The bioavailability reported in this study contrasts markedly with the results obtained when tablets containing a crude preparation of soy saponins and either daidzein and genistein aglycone or their mixed glycosides were ingested by eight volunteers at doses of 0.11 and 1.7 mmol (Izumi et al. 2000). The isoflavone aglycone mixture (1.7 mmol) produced plasma C_{max} concentrations up to five times higher than the preparation containing the daidzein and genistein glycosides. The T_{max} in this study was 4 h, which is much earlier than the 8–9 h previously reported (Rufer et al. 2008). These differences are not easily explained, but a possible role for the influence of the type of glycoside present, as well as the influence of isoflavones and other dietary constituents on each other's metabolism and transport, is suggested (Crozier et al. 2010).

A number of studies in rats have characterized the pharmacokinetics of the isoflavone biochanin A at different doses and examined effects of multiple flavonoids on its transport and metabolism (Moon and Morris 2007; Zhang and Morris 2003; Zhang et al. 2005; Moon et al. 2006a). Biochanin A is present in the diet in legumes and red clover and in many dietary supplements, again due to suggested beneficial health effects. Biochanin A was present in plasma samples mainly as its conjugated metabolites and as conjugated metabolites of its demethylated metabolite genistein. Both biochanin A and genistein exhibited low bioavailability after oral administration of the aglycones (<4%), high clearance, and large volumes of distribution (Moon et al. 2006a). Biochanin A and genistein conjugates are eliminated in the bile, and the plasma concentration–time profiles of biochanin A and genistein are characterized by reentry peaks, suggesting enterohepatic cycling. A two-compartment model that included both linear and nonlinear clearance terms and enterohepatic recirculation best described the plasma data (Moon et al. 2006a; Figure 8.4). Biochanin A was administered to rats

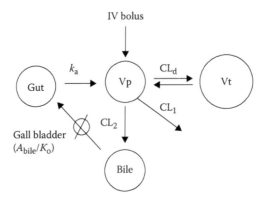

FIGURE 8.4 PK model to describe the disposition and enterohepatic cycling of the isoflavone biochanin A in rats. CL_1 and CL_2 represent linear and nonlinear clearances. Vp, CL_d, Vt, and k_a are the volume of the central compartment, the intercompartmental diffusion, the volume of the peripheral compartment, and the first-order absorption rate constant, respectively. A_{bile}/K_o is the zero-order release rate of drug from the bile compartment. A lag time (t_{lag}) was added to better describe the data. The assumptions of this model are that (1) biochanin A undergoes nonlinear metabolism, (2) biochanin A glucuronide and sulfate conjugates are the major metabolites and are combined in the modeling, (3) there is no elimination from the bile compartment, and (4) rates of absorption and reabsorption are equal. (With kind permission from Springer Science+Business Media: Pharmacokinetics and bioavailability of the isoflavone biochanin A in rats, *AAPS J*, 8, 2006, E433–E442, Moon YJ, Sagawa K, Frederick K, Zhang S and Morris ME.)

intravenously (5 mg/kg) or orally (16.67 or 50 mg/kg) with or without concomitant EGCG and quercetin (Moon and Morris 2007). The administration of multiple flavonoids increased the area under the plasma concentration–time curve (AUC) of biochanin A after both IV and oral administration. The increases in biochanin A AUC reflected predominantly increased bioavailability; this was true even after IV administration due to an apparent increase in the enterohepatic cycling of biochanin A. The mechanism was investigated in in vitro studies, which indicated decreased intestinal and hepatic conjugation of biochanin A in the presence of EGCG and quercetin. Inhibition of the intestinal efflux of flavonoids or their conjugated metabolites may also represent important interaction mechanisms resulting in higher bioavailability (An and Morris 2011).

8.3.5 FLAVONES

Dietary flavones include compounds such as apigenin, chrysin, and 7,8-benzoflavone. The dose-dependent pharmacokinetics and bioavailability of 7,8-benzoflavone have been studied in rats. 7,8-Benzoflavone exhibited a large volume of distribution (Vss ~1.5 L/kg) and rapid absorption after oral administration (Walle et al. 2007; Wang and Morris 2008). The clearance was dose dependent, decreasing at higher doses, and bioavailability was low and variable (0.61%–13.2%). Walle et al. (2007) reported that the methylated flavone, 5,7-dimethoxyflavone, was detectable in plasma with a peak concentration of 2.5 μM, whereas chrysin, the demethylated analog of 5,7-dimethoxyflavone, was not. These authors suggest that methylated flavones may exhibit better bioavailability due to decreased metabolism in the gastrointestinal tract.

8.4 CONCLUSIONS AND PERSPECTIVES

The pharmacokinetics and bioavailability of two groups of dietary compounds, isothiocyanates and flavonoids, have been briefly reviewed here. Most of the studies on isothiocyanates have focused on sulforaphane and PEITC due to interest in their cancer chemopreventive and other pharmacological effects. PEITC aglycone exhibits good bioavailability, high protein binding and metabolism due to glutathione conjugation, with nonlinear clearance reported in rat studies at high doses (Ji et al. 2005). Human oral bioavailability of isothiocyanates from food is estimated to be 14%–85% (D'Archivio et al. 2007). Flavonoids, as a group, exhibit low bioavailability due to first-pass extraction resulting from conjugative metabolism forming methyl, glucuronide, and sulfate conjugates. Both groups of dietary compounds can be substrates for membrane transport proteins and can inhibit the transport of other drug substrates. Interestingly, the administration of multiple flavonoids together, as present in food or dietary supplements, can influence the pharmacokinetics and bioavailability of one another due to competition for enzymes and/or transporters (An and Morris 2011). Additionally, methylated flavonoids have been reported to exhibit better bioavailability due to decreased intestinal metabolism (Walle et al. 2007). A number of formulation approaches have also been investigated to increase bioavailability. For example, the use of nanosized nobiletin resulted in a 13-fold increase in bioavailability in rats (Onoue et al. 2011), and the use of an oil-based nanocarrier for silymarin increased its oral bioavailability in animal studies (Parveen et al. 2011). Due to the important health benefits of dietary flavonoids, including their chemopreventive effects, further investigations characterizing the reasons for the poor bioavailability of flavonoids and evaluating methods to increase bioavailability are needed.

ACKNOWLEDGMENT

This work is supported in part by the Susan G. Komen Foundation for MEM.

REFERENCES

An G and Morris ME (2011). The sulfated conjugate of biochanin A is a substrate of breast cancer resistant protein (ABCG2). *Biopharm Drug Dispos* 32:446–457.

An G and Morris ME (2009). Herbal supplement-based drug interactions, in: *Enzymatic- and Transporter-mediated Drug Drug Interactions: Progress and Future Challenges* (Pang KS, Rodrigues AD and Peter R eds), pp 555–584, Springer, New York.

Arab L and Liebeskind DS (2010). Tea, flavonoids and stroke in man and mouse. *Arch Biochem Biophys* 501:31–36.

Brand W, van der Wel PA, Rein MJ, Barron D, Williamson G, van Bladeren PJ and Rietjens IM (2008). Metabolism and transport of the citrus flavonoid hesperetin in Caco-2 cell monolayers. *Drug Metab Dispos* 36:1794–1802.

Bredsdorff L, Nielsen IL, Rasmussen SE, Cornett C, Barron D, Bouisset F, Offord E and Williamson G (2010). Absorption, conjugation and excretion of the flavanones, naringenin and hesperetin from alpha-rhamnosidase-treated orange juice in human subjects. *Br J Nutr* 103:1602–1609.

Burke GL, Legault C, Anthony M, Bland DR, Morgan TM, Naughton MJ, Leggett K, Washburn SA and Vitolins MZ (2003). Soy protein and isoflavone effects on vasomotor symptoms in peri- and postmenopausal women: the Soy Estrogen Alternative Study. *Menopause* 10:147–153.

Cai Y, Anavy ND and Chow HH (2002). Contribution of presystemic hepatic extraction to the low oral bioavailability of green tea catechins in rats. *Drug Metab Dispos* 30:1246–1249.

Chen L, Lee MJ, Li H and Yang CS (1997). Absorption, distribution, elimination of tea polyphenols in rats. *Drug Metab Dispos* 25:1045–1050.

Conaway CC, Jiao D, Kohri T, Liebes L and Chung FL (1999). Disposition and pharmacokinetics of phenethyl isothiocyanate and 6-phenylhexyl isothiocyanate in F344 rats. *Drug Metab Dispos* 27:13–20.

Cornblatt BS, Ye L, Dinkova-Kostova AT, Erb M, Fahey JW, Singh NK, Chen MS, Stierer T, Garrett-Mayer E, Argani P, Davidson NE, Talalay P, Kensler TW and Visvanathan K (2007). Preclinical and clinical evaluation of sulforaphane for chemoprevention in the breast. *Carcinogenesis* 28:1485–1490.

Cramer JM and Jeffery EH (2011). Sulforaphane absorption and excretion following ingestion of a semi-purified broccoli powder rich in glucoraphanin and broccoli sprouts in healthy men. *Nutr Cancer* 63:196–201.

Crespy V, Morand C, Manach C, Besson C, Demigne C and Remesy C (1999). Part of quercetin absorbed in the small intestine is conjugated and further secreted in the intestinal lumen. *Am J Physiol* 277:G120–G126.

Crozier A, Del Rio D and Clifford MN (2010). Bioavailability of dietary flavonoids and phenolic compounds. *Mol Aspects Med* 31:446–467.

D'Archivio M, Filesi C, Di Benedetto R, Gargiulo R, Giovannini C and Masella R (2007). Polyphenols, dietary sources and bioavailability. *Ann Ist Super Sanita* 43:348–361.

Day AJ, Canada FJ, Diaz JC, Kroon PA, McLauchlan R, Faulds CB, Plumb GW, Morgan MR and Williamson G (2000). Dietary flavonoid and isoflavone glycosides are hydrolysed by the lactase site of lactase phlorrhizin hydrolase. *FEBS Lett* 468:166–170.

Day AJ, DuPont MS, Ridley S, Rhodes M, Rhodes MJ, Morgan MR and Williamson G (1998). Deglycosylation of flavonoid and isoflavonoid glycosides by human small intestine and liver beta-glucosidase activity. *FEBS Lett* 436:71–75.

Del Rio D, Stewart AJ, Mullen W, Burns J, Lean ME, Brighenti F and Crozier A (2004). HPLC-MSn analysis of phenolic compounds and purine alkaloids in green and black tea. *J Agric Food Chem* 52:2807–2815.

Dietrich CG, Ottenhoff R, de Waart DR and Oude Elferink RP (2001). Role of MRP2 and GSH in intrahepatic cycling of toxins. *Toxicology* 167:73–81.

Graefe EU, Wittig J, Mueller S, Riethling AK, Uehleke B, Drewelow B, Pforte H, Jacobasch G, Derendorf H and Veit M (2001). Pharmacokinetics and bioavailability of quercetin glycosides in humans. *J Clin Pharmacol* 41:492–499.

Hollman PC, Bijsman MN, van Gameren Y, Cnossen EP, de Vries JH and Katan MB (1999). The sugar moiety is a major determinant of the absorption of dietary flavonoid glycosides in man. *Free Radic Res* 31:569–573.

Hollman PC, van Trijp JM, Buysman MN, van der Gaag MS, Mengelers MJ, de Vries JH and Katan MB (1997). Relative bioavailability of the antioxidant flavonoid quercetin from various foods in man. *FEBS Lett* 418:152–156.

Hollman PC, vd Gaag M, Mengelers MJ, van Trijp JM, de Vries JH and Katan MB (1996). Absorption and disposition kinetics of the dietary antioxidant quercetin in man. *Free Radic Biol Med* 21:703–707.

Hu K and Morris ME (2005). Pharmacokinetics of alpha-naphthyl isothiocyanate in rats. *J Pharm Sci* 94:2441–2451.

Hu R, Hebbar V, Kim BR, Chen C, Winnik B, Buckley B, Soteropoulos P, Tolias P, Hart RP and Kong AN (2004). In vivo pharmacokinetics and regulation of gene expression profiles by isothiocyanate sulforaphane in the rat. *J Pharmacol Exp Ther* 310:263–271.

Izumi T, Piskula MK, Osawa S, Obata A, Tobe K, Saito M, Kataoka S, Kubota Y and Kikuchi M (2000). Soy isoflavone aglycones are absorbed faster and in higher amounts than their glucosides in humans. *J Nutr* 130:1695–1699.

Ji Y and Morris ME (2005a). Membrane transport of dietary phenethyl isothiocyanate by ABCG2 (breast cancer resistance protein). *Mol Pharm* 2:414–419.

Ji Y and Morris ME (2005b). Transport of dietary phenethyl isothiocyanate is mediated by multidrug resistance protein 2 but not P-glycoprotein. *Biochem Pharmacol* 70:640–647.

Ji Y and Morris ME (2004). Effect of organic isothiocyanates on breast cancer resistance protein (ABCG2)-mediated transport. *Pharm Res* 21:2261–2269.

Ji Y and Morris ME (2003). Determination of phenethyl isothiocyanate in human plasma and urine by ammonia derivatization and liquid chromatography-tandem mass spectrometry. *Anal Biochem* 323:39–47.

Ji Y, Kuo Y and Morris M (2005). Pharmacokinetics of dietary phenethyl isothiocyanate in rats. *Pharm Res* 22:1658–1666.

Justesen U, Knuthsen P and Leth T (1997). Determination of plant polyphenols in Danish foodstuffs by HPLC-UV and LC-MS detection. *Cancer Lett* 114:165–167.

Kao YH, Hiipakka RA and Liao S (2000). Modulation of endocrine systems and food intake by green tea epigallocatechin gallate. *Endocrinology* 141:980–987.

Ketterer B (1998). Dietary isothiocyanates as confounding factors in the molecular epidemiology of colon cancer. *Cancer Epidemiol Biomarkers Prev* 7:645–646.

King RA and Bursill DB (1998). Plasma and urinary kinetics of the isoflavones daidzein and genistein after a single soy meal in humans. *Am J Clin Nutr* 67:867–872.

Knekt P, Kumpulainen J, Jarvinen R, Rissanen H, Heliovaara M, Reunanen A, Hakulinen T and Aromaa A (2002). Flavonoid intake and risk of chronic diseases. *Am J Clin Nutr* 76:560–568.

Lambert JD, Lee MJ, Lu H, Meng X, Hong JJ, Seril DN, Sturgill MG and Yang CS (2003). Epigallocatechin-3-gallate is absorbed but extensively glucuronidated following oral administration to mice. *J Nutr* 133:4172–4177.

Lampe JW, Karr SC, Hutchins AM and Slavin JL (1998). Urinary equol excretion with a soy challenge: influence of habitual diet. *Proc Soc Exp Biol Med* 217:335–339.

Lamy E, Scholtes C, Herz C and Mersch-Sundermann V (2011). Pharmacokinetics and pharmacodynamics of isothiocyanates. *Drug Metab Rev* 43:387–407.

Lin HJ, Probst-Hensch NM, Louie AD, Kau IH, Witte JS, Ingles SA, Frankl HD, Lee ER and Haile RW (1998). Glutathione transferase null genotype, broccoli, and lower prevalence of colorectal adenomas. *Cancer Epidemiol Biomarkers Prev* 7:647–652.

Manach C, Morand C, Gil-Izquierdo A, Bouteloup-Demange C and Remesy C (2003). Bioavailability in humans of the flavanones hesperidin and narirutin after the ingestion of two doses of orange juice. *Eur J Clin Nutr* 57:235–242.

Messina MJ and Loprinzi CL (2001). Soy for breast cancer survivors: a critical review of the literature. *J Nutr* 131:3095S–3108S.

Mineharu Y, Koizumi A, Wada Y, Iso H, Watanabe Y, Date C, Yamamoto A, Kikuchi S, Inaba Y, Toyoshima H, Kondo T and Tamakoshi A (2011). Coffee, green tea, black tea and oolong tea consumption and risk of mortality from cardiovascular disease in Japanese men and women. *J Epidemiol Community Health* 65:230–240.

Moon YJ and Morris ME (2007). Pharmacokinetics and bioavailability of the bioflavonoid biochanin A: effects of quercetin and EGCG on biochanin A disposition in rats. *Mol Pharm* 4:865–872.

Moon YJ, Sagawa K, Frederick K, Zhang S and Morris ME (2006). Pharmacokinetics and bioavailability of the isoflavone biochanin A in rats. *AAPS J* 8:E433–E442.

Moon YJ, Wang X and Morris ME (2006b). Dietary flavonoids: effects on xenobiotic and carcinogen metabolism. *Toxicol In Vitro* 20:187–210.

Moon YJ, Wang L, DiCenzo R and Morris ME (2008). Quercetin pharmacokinetics in humans. *Biopharm Drug Dispos* 29:205–217.

Morris ME and Zhang S (2006). Flavonoid-drug interactions: effects of flavonoids on ABC transporters. *Life Sci* 78:2116–2130.

Mullen W, Archeveque MA, Edwards CA, Matsumoto H and Crozier A (2008). Bioavailability and metabolism of orange juice flavanones in humans: impact of a full-fat yogurt. *J Agric Food Chem* 56:11157–11164.

Murota K and Terao J (2003). Antioxidative flavonoid quercetin: implication of its intestinal absorption and metabolism. *Arch Biochem Biophys* 417:12–17.

Nemeth K, Plumb GW, Berrin JG, Juge N, Jacob R, Naim HY, Williamson G, Swallow DM and Kroon PA (2003). Deglycosylation by small intestinal epithelial cell beta-glucosidases is a critical step in the absorption and metabolism of dietary flavonoid glycosides in humans. *Eur J Nutr* 42:29–42.

Nielsen IL and Williamson G (2007). Review of the factors affecting bioavailability of soy isoflavones in humans. *Nutr Cancer* 57:1–10.

Nielsen IL, Chee WS, Poulsen L, Offord-Cavin E, Rasmussen SE, Frederiksen H, Enslen M, Barron D, Horcajada MN and Williamson G (2006). Bioavailability is improved by enzymatic modification of the citrus flavonoid hesperidin in humans: a randomized, double-blind, crossover trial. *J Nutr* 136:404–408.

Olthof MR, Hollman PC, Vree TB and Katan MB (2000). Bioavailabilities of quercetin-3-glucoside and quercetin-4′-glucoside do not differ in humans. *J Nutr* 130:1200–1203.

Onoue S, Uchida A, Takahashi H, Seto Y, Kawabata Y, Ogawa K, Yuminoki K, Hashimoto N and Yamada S (2011). Development of high-energy amorphous solid dispersion of nanosized nobiletin, a citrus polymethoxylated flavone, with improved oral bioavailability. *J Pharm Sci* 100:3793–3801.

Parveen R, Baboota S, Ali J, Ahuja A, Vasudev SS and Ahmad S (2011). Oil based nanocarrier for improved oral delivery of silymarin: in vitro and in vivo studies. *Int J Pharm* 413:245–253.

Piskula MK (2000). Soy isoflavone conjugation differs in fed and food-deprived rats. *J Nutr* 130:1766–1771.

Prasain JK and Barnes S (2007). Metabolism and bioavailability of flavonoids in chemoprevention: current analytical strategies and future prospectus. *Mol Pharm* 4:846–864.

Ross JA and Kasum CM (2002). Dietary flavonoids: bioavailability, metabolic effects, and safety. *Annu Rev Nutr* 22:19–34.

Rufer CE, Bub A, Moseneder J, Winterhalter P, Sturtz M and Kulling SE (2008). Pharmacokinetics of the soybean isoflavone daidzein in its aglycone and glucoside form: a randomized, double-blind, crossover study. *Am J Clin Nutr* 87:1314–1323.

Sesink AL, Arts IC, Faassen-Peters M and Hollman PC (2003). Intestinal uptake of quercetin-3-glucoside in rats involves hydrolysis by lactase phlorizin hydrolase. *J Nutr* 133:773–776.

Setchell KD and Lydeking-Olsen E (2003). Dietary phytoestrogens and their effect on bone: evidence from in vitro and in vivo, human observational, and dietary intervention studies. *Am J Clin Nutr* 78:593S–609S.

Setchell KD and Cassidy A (1999). Dietary isoflavones: biological effects and relevance to human health. *J Nutr* 129:758S–767S.

Setchell KD, Brown NM and Lydeking-Olsen E (2002). The clinical importance of the metabolite equol—a clue to the effectiveness of soy and its isoflavones. *J Nutr* 132:3577–3584.

Stalmach A, Mullen W, Steiling H, Williamson G, Lean ME and Crozier A (2010). Absorption, metabolism, and excretion of green tea flavan-3-ols in humans with an ileostomy. *Mol Nutr Food Res* 54:323–334.

Stalmach A, Troufflard S, Serafini M and Crozier A (2009). Absorption, metabolism and excretion of Choladi green tea flavan-3-ols by humans. *Mol Nutr Food Res* 53 Suppl 1:S44–S53.

Telang U, Ji Y and Morris ME (2009). ABC transporters and isothiocyanates: potential for pharmacokinetic diet-drug interactions. *Biopharm Drug Dispos* 30:335–344.

Tseng E, Kamath A and Morris ME (2002). Effect of organic isothiocyanates on the P-glycoprotein- and MRP1-mediated transport of daunomycin and vinblastine. *Pharm Res* 19:1509–1515.

Walle T, Ta N, Kawamori T, Wen X, Tsuji PA and Walle UK (2007). Cancer chemopreventive properties of orally bioavailable flavonoids—methylated versus unmethylated flavones. *Biochem Pharmacol* 73:1288–1296.

Walle T, Walle UK and Halushka PV (2001). Carbon dioxide is the major metabolite of quercetin in humans. *J Nutr* 131:2648–2652.

Walle T, Otake Y, Walle UK and Wilson FA (2000). Quercetin glucosides are completely hydrolyzed in ileostomy patients before absorption. *J Nutr* 130:2658–2661.

Wang H, Lin W, Shen G, Khor TO, Nomeir AA and Kong AN (2011). Development and validation of an LC-MS-MS method for the simultaneous determination of sulforaphane and its metabolites in rat plasma and its application in pharmacokinetic studies. *J Chromatogr Sci* 49:801–806.

Wang X and Morris ME (2008). Pharmacokinetics and bioavailability of the flavonoid 7,8-benzoflavone in rats. *J Pharm Sci* 97:4546–4556.

Williamson G, Dionisi F and Renouf M (2011). Flavanols from green tea and phenolic acids from coffee: critical quantitative evaluation of the pharmacokinetic data in humans after consumption of single doses of beverages. *Mol Nutr Food Res* 55:864–873.

Zhang S and Morris ME (2003). Effects of the flavonoids biochanin A, morin, phloretin, and silymarin on P-glycoprotein-mediated transport. *J Pharmacol Exp Ther* 304:1258–1267.

Zhang S, Yang X, Coburn RA and Morris ME (2005). Structure activity relationships and quantitative structure activity relationships for the flavonoid-mediated inhibition of breast cancer resistance protein. *Biochem Pharmacol* 70:627–639.

Zhang Y (2001). Molecular mechanism of rapid cellular accumulation of anticarcinogenic isothiocyanates. *Carcinogenesis* 22:425–431.

Section IV

Vitamins A, D, and E Cancer Prevention and Clinical Perspective

9 Retinoic Acid Signaling in Hematopoiesis and Immune Functions, and Options for Chemoprevention

Rodica P. Bunaciu and Andrew Yen

CONTENTS

9.1 INTRODUCTION

Retinoic acid, through its signaling and downstream transcriptional targets, regulates the development and activity of hematopoietic cells and their myeloid and lymphocytic progenitors. The hematopoietic sites and the circulatory system (including both blood and lymph) have important multifaceted roles in the relationship between inflammation and cancer. Their components are responsible for the homeostasis in the entire organism. They are involved in many processes, including delivering nutrients and removing waste; removing the preneoplastic/neoplastic cells or infectious agents like viruses, which could promote cancer, or in contrast, promoting angiogenesis and sustained inflammation, which promotes solid tumor growth and metastasis; or becoming malignant themselves, as in the case of leukemias and lymphomas. Retinoic acid (RA), a metabolite of vitamin A, is an important regulator of differentiation, development, and functions of the hematopoietic and immune systems. This chapter tries to highlight some of the signaling events elicited by RA in the blood and immune cells.

9.2 VITAMIN A

Vitamin A is a class of lipid-soluble essential micronutrients for all vertebrates (Zempleni et al. 2007). According to the International Union of Pure and Applied Chemistry and International Union of Biochemistry and Molecular Biology, "vitamin A" is a generic term covering all the retinoids with the biological activity of all-*trans*-retinol (Liebecq 1997). There are three parent compounds: retinol, retinal, and RA (tretinoin). RA is, biologically, a metabolite of vitamin A, not a form of vitamin A, since it cannot be transformed to retinol. There are two main forms of dietary vitamin A: vitamin A (retinyl esters and retinol) and provitamin A carotenoids (β-carotene, α-carotene, and β-cryptoxanthin). Dietary precursors serve as substrates for the biosynthesis of two metabolites of vitamin A: 11-*cis*-retinal, essential for vision, and all-*trans*-RA (ATRA), essential for cell differentiation, cell survival, and the regulation of gene transcription. Retinol, by oxidation, generates retinal. The reaction is reversible and catalyzed by alcohol dehydrogenase (ADH). Retinal, by oxidation, generates RA. The reaction is irreversible and catalyzed by aldehyde dehydrogenase. All-*trans*-retinal is also the immediate product of the central cleavage of β-carotene. Retinol, retinal, and RA forms may be further metabolically modified, generating a myriad of products with biological activity still to be elucidated. Besides the natural forms of vitamin A, structural analogs have been synthesized. A full description of the nomenclature of retinoids, carotenoids, and their derivatives is available online (http://www.chem.qmul.ac.uk/iubmb/index.html) (Liebecq 1997). Numerous retinoids are used as chemopreventive and/or therapeutic agents, especially in the treatment of dermatological diseases and certain cancers, since the discovery of inducing almost complete remission in acute promyelocytic leukemia (APL).

RA and its metabolites, including its isomerization product, 9-*cis*-RA, and many synthetic retinoids are ligands for two classes of ligand-activated transcription factors, retinoic acid receptors (RARs) and retinoid X receptors (RXRs) (Mangelsdorf et al. 1990, 1992). RARs and RXRs each have three subtypes, α, β, and gamma, encoded by different genes (Germain et al. 2006). RARs and RXRs are members of the superfamily of steroid thyroid hormone receptors. They can form homodimers and heterodimers. They bind DNA at hexad consensus sequences, AGGTCA, that occur in repeated (direct repeat [DR]) or palindromic configurations separated by several nucleotides (Germain et al. 2006; Mangelsdorf and Evans 1995), although exceptions are known (Wang and Yen 2004). 9-*cis*-RA is capable of binding to the nuclear receptors and may be a principal ligand of the RXR. 13-*cis*-RA is effectively used as a therapeutic agent for dermatological diseases, is present in human plasma, and does not have high affinity for RAR or RXR but localizes predominantly to the nuclei (Ruhl et al. 2001). Although ATRA binds both RAR and RXR classes of receptors, it presents higher concentrations in the cytosol than in the nuclei (Ruhl et al. 2001). Its modalities of eliciting biological response are not limited to the interaction with RARs or RXRs, and some of those processes are highlighted in this review.

Vitamin A is indispensable for vision, reproduction, cell differentiation, organogenesis, and immune function. Excluding vision (where retinal is the active form) and spermatogenesis, all the other activities of vitamin A are generally attributed to ATRA. ATRA restores growth and tissue differentiation and prevents mortality when fed to vitamin A–deficient animals. This suggests that RA or its metabolites are responsible for those functions of vitamin A.

9.3 ALL-*TRANS*-RA (ATRA)

ATRA is an important developmental morphogen with pleiotropic actions. One of the most studied effects is the specification of the anterior–posterior axis. The mammalian embryo has two signaling centers: one in the anterior visceral endoderm (AVE) and one in the node (Foley, Skromne, and Stern 2000; Gilbert 2010). AVE originates from the visceral endoderm that migrates forward while secreting Lefty-1 and Cerberus. Those two proteins are antagonists of Nodal. Lefty-1 expression is regulated by both RA and sonic hedgehog protein (Shh) (Tsukui et al. 1999). Nodal contains an

RA-responsive element in the first intron (Uehara et al. 2009). If at the time of migration, RA concentrations are higher than normal, AVE precursors cannot migrate. The consequence is a double body axis, leading to conjoined twins (Liao and Collins 2008). There is a negative gradient of Nodal, bone morphogenetic proteins (BMPs), Wnt3a, FGF8 proteins, and RA, from the posterior region of the axis toward the anterior region where Nodal is totally absent and RA is very low (Chen and Solursh 1992; Gilbert 2010). The RA gradient is controlled by the expression of RA-synthesizing (retinol dehydrogenase and aldehyde dehydrogenase) and -degrading enzymes (Cyp26) (Uehara et al. 2009; Sandell et al. 2007; Sakai et al. 2001; Oosterveen, Meijlink, and Deschamps 2004). The Cyp26 promoter contains an RA-responsive element. Cyp26 is responsible for removing the maternal RA (Uehara et al. 2009). If on day 8, RA concentrations are higher than normal, a cervical vertebra develops with thoracic vertebra morphology as RA drives homeobox B8 (HOXB8). If the RA concentration is lower than normal, a thoracic vertebra develops as a cervical vertebra (Charite, de Graaff, and Deschamps 1995; Gilbert 2010). RA controls those processes, at least at two levels: Cdx proteins and HOX proteins (Gilbert 2010). The anterior–posterior patterning signals of RA, Wnt3a, and FGF8 converge at the transcriptional regulation of caudate-type homeobox gene Cdx1 (Lohnes 2003; Houle, Sylvestre, and Lohnes 2003; Gilbert 2010). Cdx1 activates HOX genes. HOX genes also have RA response elements (RAREs) in their promoters or enhancers (Boncinelli et al. 1991; Tabin 1995; Dupe et al. 1997; Oosterveen et al. 2003b; Lohnes 2003; Houle, Sylvestre, and Lohnes 2003; Conlon and Rossant 1992; Sakai et al. 2001; Kessel 1992). RA is also essential for the left–right patterning (Gilbert 2010). RA and Shh are contained in the membrane-bound nodal vesicular parcels (NVPs). The ciliary movement directs NVPs to the left side of the body. The nodal is predominantly expressed on the left side of the embryo. RA is involved also in the organ-specific level of left–right regulation, as was demonstrated in ocular, craniofacial, and cardiac development (Gilbert 2010).

HOX genes are involved in hematopoiesis (Thorsteinsdottir, Sauvageau, and Humphries 1997). Methylation of CpG islands at the promoter region of the HOXA gene cluster is increased in leukemia patients and leukemia cell lines, especially in T-cell leukemia and B-cell leukemia. In normal cells, the same region is unmethylated. In acute myelogenous leukemia (AML), acute lymphocytic leukemia (ALL), and chronic myelogenous leukemia (CML) patients in complete remission and in RA-treated HL-60 and K562 cells, the methylation levels are downregulated (Fang et al. 2009). Specifically during granulocytic differentiation, HOX antisense intergenic RNA myeloid 1 gene (HOTAIRM1) is upregulated under the control of RA-ligated RAR (Zhang et al. 2009). The Hoxa1–Pbx1/2–Meis2 protein complex is also involved in ALDH1a2 gene expression (Vitobello et al. 2011). HOXB genes are RA regulated in a context-dependent manner (Oosterveen, Meijlink, and Deschamps 2004; Oosterveen et al. 2003a). HOXB7 is important in myelomonocytic differentiation. Upon 1,25-dihydroxy vitamin D_3–induced monocytic differentiation in HL-60, the expression of HOXB7 messenger RNA (mRNA) was upregulated (Lill et al. 1995). Constitutive overexpression of HOXB7 in the same cell line inhibited the RA-induced granulocytic differentiation but did not hinder the monocytic differentiation induced by vitamin D_3. There are two lines of evidence suggesting that the expression of HOXB7 occurs only during the differentiation process. Firstly, human bone marrow (BM) cells express HOXB7 in response to granulocyte-macrophage colony-stimulating factor (GM-CSF), and antisense oligonucleotides directed against HOX B7 inhibited the formation of colonies derived from GM-CSF–stimulated BM. Secondly, normal human monocytes do not constitutively express HOXB7, nor are they able to be induced to do so (Lill et al. 1995). Likewise, HOXB8 promotes monopoiesis and inhibits granulopoiesis, at least in part by upregulating the transcription factor Egr-1 (Krishnaraju, Hoffman, and Liebermann 1997). During the T-cell activation with PHA and RA, the expression of HOXB cluster genes is markedly upregulated. Antisense oligonucleotides directed toward HOXB2 or HOXB4 mRNA cause a drastic inhibition of T-cell proliferation and a decreased expression of T-cell activation markers (Care et al. 1994). Cdx4 is known to regulate HOX genes, and defects in this cascade generate acute myeloid leukemia (Bansal et al. 2006).

POU-family transcription factors are known to be important regulators of cardiovascular system development (Farooqui-Kabir et al. 2008), thymic organogenesis (Yukawa et al. 1993), hematopoietic cell development, lymphoid gene expression (Sivaraja et al. 1994; Messier et al. 1993; Kang et al. 1992; Clerc et al. 1988; Wu et al. 1997; de Grazia et al. 1994), and myeloid series cell differentiation (Seta and Kuwana 2010). Octamer-binding transcription factor 4 (Oct4) is a homeodomain transcription factor that is a member of the POU family and important in maintenance of stem cell characteristics. It is known that the Oct4 promoter contains RAREs responsible for Oct4 repression (Pikarsky et al. 1994). Moreover, recently it has been shown that RA downregulates Oct4 also in an indirect way by upregulating aryl hydrocarbon receptor, which in turn diminishes Oct4 levels (Bunaciu and Yen 2011). It was long known that aryl hydrocarbon–inducible cytochrome P450 genes are upregulated in myeloid blasts during RA-induced differentiation (Liu et al. 2000). Another Oct family member, Oct2, is important in the maintenance of the B-cell compartment (Schubart et al. 2001) and is transcriptionally negatively regulated by RA bound to RAR-α (de Grazia et al. 1994).

Thus, it is clear that RA is a fundamental regulator of cell differentiation and proliferation especially in the context of development and stem cell fate.

9.4   RA IN EARLY HEMATOPOIESIS

During the first 2 months of embryonic development, hematopoiesis consists almost exclusively of erythropoiesis and takes place in the blood islands of the yolk sac. RA is an important developmental regulator of early hematopoiesis, signaling downstream of Cdx4 and upstream of scl (de Jong et al. 2010). In the vitamin A–deficient (VAD) quail embryo, there is a significant reduction in erythroid cells. The GATA2 gene fails to be expressed normally in VAD embryos, due to diminished expression of its regulator, BMP4. Moreover, the cell clusters of primitive blood islands undergo apoptosis in the VAD embryo, which can explain the deficit in differentiated primitive blood cells (Ghatpande et al. 2002).

9.5   RA IN ADULT HEMATOPOIESIS; REGULATION OF BM HEMATOPOIETIC PROGENITOR CELL LINEAGE-SPECIFIC DIFFERENTIATION

Vitamin A and RA are regulators of hematopoiesis. Early studies showed that vitamin A–deficient children and animals present with anemia (Mejia, Hodges, and Rucker 1979), T-cell dysfunctions (Cantorna, Nashold, and Hayes 1994), and decreased ability to combat infections. An excess of vitamin A has toxic effects on the cellular compartment of the BM by upregulating p21(Cip1) and p27(Kip1) (Perrotta et al. 2002). 13-cis-RA enhanced myeloid progenitor cell growth in culture (Bleiberg et al. 1988). BM CD34-committed and -proliferating precursors express CD38, a molecule under RAR-α regulation due to the presence of a RARE in its first intron (Malavasi et al. 2008). Within the BM cellular compartment, RA promotes granulocytic development to the detriment of the erythroid (Gratas et al. 1993) and myeloid dendritic cell (DC) differentiation (Hengesbach and Hoag 2004).

9.5.1   ERYTHROID SERIES

RA is a positive regulator of yolk sac erythropoiesis and a negative regulator of erythrocyte differentiation in the adult, involving scl and probably regulating GATA1 (de Jong et al. 2010). Erythropoietin is under RA (RAR/RXR) transcriptional control during yolk sac hematopoiesis and under hypoxia-inducible factor-1 (HIF-1; hypoxia)/HNF4 control during adult hematopoiesis. Moreover, RA inhibits the BFU-E response to erythropoietin (Rusten et al. 1996). However, the regulation is far from being well elucidated. For example, hypervitaminose A, as expected, leads to anemia (Perrotta et al. 2002), but vitamin A deficiency also leads to anemia (Mejia, Hodges, and Rucker 1979), possibly due to the interdependence of vitamin A and iron metabolism.

9.5.2 NEUTROPHIL SERIES

Probably the most notable effect of RA on hematopoiesis is in the neutrophil series, both in normal granulopoiesis and, especially, in APL treatment. RA induces remission in almost all of APL PML/RAR-α+ patients (Nilsson 1984); however, the remission is not long lasting, and the relapsed cases are resistant to the retinoid treatment. RA regulation of the myeloid compartment is very complex. For example, not only do retinoids induce differentiation to neutrophils but also vitamin A–deficient mice present expansion of both precursor and mature myeloid cells due to a downregulation of RXR α and β; the numbers of myeloid cells are restored by RA supplementation in the diet (Kuwata et al. 2000). The complexity of the role of RA in granulopoiesis is reflected by the large variety and number of papers on this topic. In vitro model systems have been potent tools used to study the molecular events governed by RA in myeloid series cells. Because RA has been used chemotherapeutically against myelogenous leukemia, there are probably more details mechanistically known about RA-regulated myeloid differentiation than other cells. Bipotent human AML HL-60 cells have a high proliferative rate in culture and do not bear the t(15,17) translocation that characterizes clinical response for APL, yet they are ATRA responsive. RA causes G0 arrest and myeloid differentiation characterized by the upregulated expression of CD38, CD11b, and inducible oxidative metabolism. Onset of G0 arrest and terminal differentiation is slow, requiring approximately 48 h of treatment, during which the cells undergo approximately two division cycles (Yen, Brown, and Fishbaugh 1987; Yen, Reece, and Albright 1984; Yen et al. 1987; Yen and Forbes 1990). During the first cycle, cells undergo early differentiation events common to both myeloid and monocytic differentiation, and the determination of lineage specifically occurs in the second cycle as a function of the inducer, for example, RA or vitamin D_3, present in that second cycle (Yen, Brown, and Fishbaugh 1987; Yen et al. 1987). This differentiation is driven by numerous cascades of events. Some are nuclear, and some involve membrane receptor signal transduction. There are numerous protein tyrosine phosphorylation events, a prolonged mitogen-activated protein kinase (MAPK) activation cascade, and expression of specific neutrophil functions. Although there is a significant body of information, the integration of all those events is not fully elucidated yet.

RA and its derivatives act as ligands for the RAR and RXR ligand-activated nuclear receptors that regulate transcription. Studies with RAR and RXR selective retinoids showed that both RAR and RXR activation are needed to elicit differentiation (Battle et al. 2001; Brooks et al. 1996, 1997). C/EBP epsilon transcription factor is critical for granulopoiesis (Yamanaka et al. 1997) and has RARE in its promoter (Park et al. 1999). Two of the earliest cell surface markers of differentiation upon HL-60 RA treatment are BLR1/CXCR5 and CD38, proteins that have a significant role in propelling the differentiation process. The BLR1 (CXCR5) promoter contains a novel 17 bp GT box that is a noncanonical RARE (Wang and Yen 2004). CD38 is highly expressed in granulocytes (Malavasi et al. 2008). CD38 contains a RARE in the first intron, and transcription is regulated by RAR-α (Mehta et al. 1997; Kishimoto et al. 1998). CD38 is a 46 kD type II transmembrane glycoprotein associated with lipid rafts (Zubiaur et al. 2002). This receptor has a long cysteine-rich C-terminal extracellular domain and a short N-terminal cytoplasmic domain. The C-terminal domain (CTD) contains the 273–285 sequence (with Cys275) responsible for NADase ectoenzymatic activity (Kontani et al. 1997). Myeloid precursors ectopically overexpressing CD38 show an enhanced rate of differentiation indicated by increased inducible oxidative metabolism by 48 h and G1/0 arrest by 72 h (Lamkin et al. 2006), and RNA interference (RNAi) directed toward CD38 hinders RA-induced differentiation (Munshi, Graeff, and Lee 2002). The CD38 cytoplasmic domain is associated with multiple proteins, one of which is the adaptor c-Cbl (Shen and Yen 2008). If the CD38 protein of myeloid precursors is stimulated by a certain anti-CD38 monoclonal antibody, the RA-induced differentiation is enhanced (Kontani et al. 1996). There are also other cases of other anti-CD38 antibodies (IB4) that increase the rate of cell division in AML patient samples and cell lines, including HL-60 (Konopleva et al. 1998). The differential effect is probably due to eliciting different signaling pathways through different epitopes of CD38 or different cellular contexts (Funaro et al. 1993). In the case where the cells arrest, multiple tyrosine phosphorylation events are occurring as part of the signal transmembrane transduction. The epitope on the CD38 molecule responsible for transmembrane signal transduction reported in the initial studies is also located in the 273–285 sequence (Kontani et al. 1997). One of those tyrosine phosphorylation events is the phosphorylation of E3 ubiquitin ligase and adaptor c-Cbl (Kontani et al. 1996). Moreover, overexpression of c-Cbl augmented CD38 basal level and propelled RA-induced differentiation and MAPK activation, whereas c-Cbl knockdown transfectants blunted them (Shen and Yen 2008). A c-Cbl tyrosine kinase–binding domain mutant (G306E) is unable to complex with CD38 and to drive MAPK signaling and differentiation (Shen and Yen 2009). Another protein that is tyrosine phosphorylated is CrkL (Alsayed et al. 2000). CrkL is a member of the Crk family, SH2 and SH3 domain–containing adaptor proteins (the other two members are CR II, containing the domain SH2–SH3–SH3, and Crk I, containing a shorter form, SH2–SH3). CrkL was initially cloned from chronic myelogenous leukemia (ten Hoeve et al. 1993). Consequent to RA-induced differentiation in HL-60 cells, c-Cbl directly binds the SH2 domain of CrkL (Alsayed et al. 2000) and IRF-1 (Shen et al. 2011), two molecules at the intersection of retinoic and interferon pathways. IRF-1 association with c-Cbl during RA-induced differentiation is accompanied by enhanced MAPK signaling (Shen et al. 2011).

The Src-family protein tyrosine kinases (SFKs) Lyn and Fgr are progressively activated by tyrosine phosphorylation after RA treatment of HL-60 cells and reach a maximum 48 h posttreatment (Katagiri et al. 1996). Their different localizations in membrane domains suggest participation in distinct signaling cascades (Welch and Maridonneau-Parini 1997). Recently, a possible feedback loop involving KSR1-scaffolded c-Raf and extracellular signal–regulated kinase (ERK) complexed with Lyn and CK2 was suggested to be a mechanistic basis for augmenting RA-induced differentiation with SFK inhibitors (PP2 and dasatinib). PP2 and dasatinib increase ATRA-induced expression of Lyn, total c-Raf, and c-RafpS259 and their association as revealed by coimmunoprecipitation. The Lyn-associated serine/threonine kinase CK2 also complexed with c-Raf and c-RafpS259, and the KSR1 scaffold protein bound c-Raf, Lyn, and ERK. c-Raf/ERK association was increased by the inhibitors and was associated with c-Raf CTD phosphorylation. Lyn knockdown decreased c-Raf CTD and S259 phosphorylation (Congleton, MacDonald, and Yen 2012).

Fes/Fps is a protein tyrosine kinase characteristic of the myeloid lineage (Ferrari et al. 1985; Yu, Smithgall, and Glazer 1989). Its expression is enhanced during RA-induced differentiation of HL-60 cells and APL blasts (Ferrari et al. 1994) and protects against apoptosis (Ferrari et al. 1990). During RA-induced differentiation, Fes was shown to form oligomers and exhibit nuclear localization (Tagliafico et al. 2003). Fes tyrosine phosphorylates signal transducer and activator of transcription 3 (STAT3) and increases its DNA binding activity (Nelson et al. 1998).

The guanine nucleotide exchange factor Vav1 has both cytoplasmic and nuclear localization. After RA treatment of HL-60 cells, Vav is tyrosine phosphorylated and associates (via its SH2 domain) with c-Cbl in the cytosol and SLP-76, with tyrosine kinase Syk (which can phosphorylate Vav) in the nuclei, as well as with p85 of PI3-K (Bertagnolo et al. 2001). A consequence of Vav phosphorylation and interactions is the nuclear cytoskeleton reorganization specific to granulocytic differentiation. Vav has been implicated as an important regulator of myeloid series cell differentiation in vivo as well as in vitro, and the mechanism involves CD38 receptor (Bertagnolo et al. 2005; Shen and Yen 2009).

Another later event in the same differentiation process is the association of FcgammaRIIα (CD32) to lipid rafts. Although in neutrophils, Lyn is constitutively associated with the cytosolic tail of FcgammaRIIα, this pool of Lyn is not active (phosphorylated) until immunoglobulin G (IgG) binds the FcR and the ligated receptor undergoes cross-linking–dependent association to lipid rafts. Lyn activation leads to subsequent events necessary for mounting respiratory burst activity (Katsumata et al. 2001). Less clear is the consequence of FcgammaRIIα and FcR-associated c-Cbl phosphorylation in this process. Nevertheless, it is clear that all those molecular events are important for neutrophil function.

A prolonged MAPK activation is a characteristic of RA-induced myeloid differentiation in HL-60. During the priming period of the induced differentiation process, RA slowly elicits the MEK-dependent activations of the Raf kinase and also ERK1/2 activation (Yen et al. 1998; Hong, Varvayanis, and Yen 2001; Yen and Varvayanis 2000). c-Raf seems to be the most important part in the Raf/MEK/ERK axis during RA-induced differentiation of HL-60. If Raf is inhibited, then ERK fails to activate, and the cells do not arrest or differentiate in response to RA. While inhibiting Raf blocks ERK activation and RA-induced differentiation, indicating a necessary role for Raf in induced differentiation, ectopic expression of activated Raf accelerates RA-induced differentiation. During the early priming process, Raf activation in response to RA thus appears to be both a necessary and rate-limiting process for RA-induced differentiation. Raf also presents nuclear localization after Ra treatment (Smith et al. 2009).

RA-inducible gene-I (RIG-I) is expressed in response to RA during RA-induced differentiation of HL-60 and NB4 myelogenous leukemia cells and is expressed at high levels in mature neutrophils (Zhang et al. 2008; Liu et al. 2000). As shown using knockout mice, RIG-I is important in inducing growth arrest of granulocytic precursors and commitment toward differentiation; after 9 months of age, the knockout mice develop chronic myeloid leukemia (Zhang et al. 2008). In part, the commitment to differentiation is the result of RIG-I–dependent induction of interferon consensus sequence binding protein (ICSBP) (Zhang et al. 2008) and of the Gα(i2) subunit of heterotrimeric G proteins (Wang et al. 2007b). Moreover, neutrophil Gα(i2) is necessary for chemokine-induced neutrophil recruitment to sites of acute inflammation (Zarbock et al. 2007). RIG-I, through its antiviral activity, has a role against oncogenic viruses.

mi-R15a is a tumor suppressor upregulated by RA in HL-60, NB4, and U937 (Gao et al. 2011). It has high levels in AML patients in remission and low levels in relapsed AML (Ofir, Hacohen, and Ginsberg 2011) and in chronic lymphocytic leukemia (CLL) patients (Cimmino et al. 2005). mi-R15 is regulated by E2F1, a transcription factor regulated by retinoblastoma, targets cyclin E and inhibits proliferation (Ofir, Hacohen, and Ginsberg 2011) and targets BCL2 and induces apoptosis (Cimmino et al. 2005) (Table 9.1).

9.5.3 MONOCYTES

Monocytes and granulocytes emerge from the same hematopoietic precursor cell. It is plausible that some agents enhancing the differentiation process toward one lineage would inhibit the other. RA is an inducer of granulopoiesis as shown above, and although the precommitment stage (the first 24 hours after the treatment with the differentiating agent) is induced equally well by RA and vitamin D_3, the later stages of monopoiesis are inhibited by RA (Yen, Reece, and Albright 1984; Yen et al. 1987). Thus, 9-*cis*-RA or SR11237 (agonists of RXR) inhibit PMA-induced THP-1 cell monopoiesis (Zhou et al. 2010). However, RA does regulate aspects of monocytic differentiation. Osteoclasts are specialized macrophages in the bone. The proliferation of human osteoclast progenitors is increased by RA. At the same time, the osteoclast differentiation is suppressed in a RAR-dependent process, as shown by using a RAR pan-antagonist (Hu et al. 2010). RA activates RARs, and in turn, those activated receptors (1) inhibit the expression of the receptor activator of nuclear factor kappaB (NF-κB) (RANK); (2) suppress the expression of the transcription factor nuclear factor of activated T cells, cytoplasmic 1 (NFATc1); and (3) increase the expression of interferon regulatory factor 8 (IRF-8) (Hu et al. 2010). RANK and NFATc1 are positive regulators, whereas IRF-8 is a negative regulator of osteoclastogenesis. IRF-1 is also RA regulated, and the interferon and RA pathways are known to overlap in various myelomonocytic cells (Nakamura et al. 1986; Rhodes and Stokes 1982). During ATRA-induced differentiation of monoblastic U937 cells toward monocytes, there is a transcriptional upregulation of Wnt13B and Wnt13C that correlates with transcriptional upregulation of MAFB transcription factors (Bunaciu, Tang, and Mao 2008). MAFB deletion is frequently encountered in myeloid malignancies (Wang et al. 1998, 1999). The MAFB transcription factor was shown to set the M-CSF sensitivity thresholds in the hematopoietic stem

TABLE 9.1

Summary of RA-Elicited Molecular Events Leading to Differentiation in HL-60 Bipotent Human AML Cells

Transcription Factors		
RAR and RXR	Activation brings forth differentiation	Brooks et al. 1996, 1997; Battle et al. 2001
C/EBP epsilon	Critical for granulopoiesis	Yamanaka et al. 1997
	Has RARE in its promoter	Park et al. 1999
IRF-1	Upregulated	Shen et al. 2011
AhR	Upregulated	Bunaciu and Yen 2011

Stem Cell Markers		
Oct4	Transcription factor downregulated	Bunaciu and Yen 2011
ALDH1	Activity downregulated	Bunaciu and Yen 2011

Earliest Cell Surface Proteins Upregulated after RA Induced Differentiation and Propelled the Differentiation Process		
BLR1/CXCR5	Promoter contains a novel 17 bp GT box that is a noncanonical RARE	Wang and Yen 2004
CD38	Highly expressed in granulocytes	Malavasi et al. 2008
	Contains an RARE in the first intron; transcription is regulated by RAR-α	Mehta et al. 1997; Kishimoto et al. 1998

Phosphorylation Events		
Prolonged MAPK activation	During the priming period: MEK-dependent activations of the Raf kinase and of ERK1/2. c-Raf: the most important part in the Raf/MEK/ERK axis during RA-induced differentiation of HL-60	Yen et al. 1998; Yen and Varvayanis 2000; Hong et al. 2001
	Raf nuclear localization	Smith et al. 2009
c-Cbl	Phosphorylation of E3 ubiquitin ligase and adaptor c-Cbl	Kontani et al. 1996
	c-Cbl tyrosine kinase binding domain is necessary for c-Cbl and CD38 complex formation and to drive MAPK signaling and differentiation	Shen and Yen 2009
SFKs Lyn and Fgr	Progressively activated by tyrosine phosphorylation	Katagiri et al. 1996
	Lyn activation necessary for mounting respiratory burst activity	Katsumata et al. 2001
Fes/Fps	A protein tyrosine kinase characteristic to myeloid lineage; expression is enhanced during RA-induced differentiation of HL-60 cells and APL blasts	Ferrari et al. 1985; Yu et al. 1989; Ferrari et al. 1994
	Fes tyrosine phosphorylates STAT3 and increases its DNA binding activity	Nelson et al. 1998
Vav	Tyrosine phosphorylated and associates with c-Cbl, SLP-76, Syk, and p85 of PI3-K	Bertagnolo et al. 2001

cells, specifically to restrict the ability of those cells to become myeloid committed (Sarrazin et al. 2009). Moreover, a correlation between RA signaling pathways and MAFB functions is suggested by cleft lip/palate pathologies, both in MAFB dysfunctions (Pan et al. 2011) and RA teratogenic effects (Mitchell et al. 2003). MAFB, and the other large MAFs, share the response elements they bind to (antioxidant response element [ARE]) with other bZIP transcription factors, such as Nrfs, small MAFs, and Jun (Jaiswal 2004). The small MAF proteins are known to heterodimerize with

Nrf2 and stabilize Nrf2 signaling (Li et al. 2008). Known risk factors for neoplastic transformation, such as hepatitis C virus, are able to disrupt the interaction between small MAF proteins and Nrf2 (Carvajal-Yepes et al. 2011). Low concentrations of RA are able to inhibit Nrf2, whereas therapeutic doses of RA activated Nrf2 (Tan et al. 2008). However, those effects are context (cell type and microenvironment) specific, as high doses of RA are also reported to inhibit Nrf2 through RAR-α (Wang et al. 2007a).

Generally, RA inhibits excessive monocyte/macrophage activity. For example, tissue factor (TF) is a membrane-bound glycoprotein that is expressed in many cell types and that initiates the blood coagulation cascade. RA inhibits the expression of lipopolysaccharide (LPS)-induced TF in monocytes (Oeth et al. 1998). This is especially significant for the management of APL, since many patients have severe coagulopathy before starting ATRA-induced differentiation therapy for APL (Chang et al. 2012). The excessive bleeding in APL patients is due mainly to excessive expression of TF in the blasts. The PML/RAR-α fusion protein transactivates the TF promoter through an indirect interaction with a GAGC element (Yan et al. 2010). However, it is of significant clinical advantage that the same agent, RA, is effective in differentiation therapy and downregulation of TF in the blasts as well as downregulation of the TF in the circulating monocytes.

Monocytes also appear to be regulated by RA through CD38. CD38, the expression of which is RA regulated, is expressed in circulating monocytes but not in the resident macrophages. It is highly expressed in circulating osteoclast and osteoblast precursors (specialized monocytes). During the inflammatory process, monocytes lose CD38 and CD14 and acquire CD1a, transitioning to becoming immature DCs (iDCs). Lipopolysaccharide induces iDCs to reexpress CD30 and become mature DCs (Malavasi et al. 2008).

9.5.4 MYELOID DCs

DCs are important determinants of T-cell immunity, both in terms of the type of T-cell immunity and in terms of homing. Blood DCs are able to migrate to both gut and skin. Tissue-specific DCs exhibit tissue-specific homing and induce tissue-specific T cells. When DCs are exposed to the colonic environment, they acquire gut-specific DC phenotype with the result of inducing gut-specific T cells. This process is dependent on RA and transforming growth factor β (TGF-β) (Mann et al. 2012). Those DCs express CD103 and become part of the mucosa-associated lymphoid tissue (MALT), also known as gut-associated lymphoid tissue (GALT). The GALT consists of Peyer's patches and mesenteric lymph nodes linked by intestinal lymphatics. GALT contains precursors of T cells and IgA-secreting plasma cells. Their role is very important as they confer both tolerance toward dietary antigens and immunocompetence against infectious agents in the gut. The mechanism of this distinction is not understood, but a central role likely lies with CD103 DCs, which instruct the lymphoid cells (thymus independent). RIG-I knockout mice have decreased DCs in GALT (Wang et al. 2007b). Intraepithelial lymphocytes are the first line of defense against intestinal neoplasms but are also the players in GALT lymphomas. CD103 DCs are able to synthesize RA from retinaldehyde, as these cells express ALDH1A2, and to elicit expression of CCR9 on CD8+ T cells (Svensson et al. 2008). Their ability to instruct lymphocytes depends on the RA concentrations. As it was already shown that exogenous RA is effective as a vaccine adjuvant to protect against viral infections (Tan et al. 2011), it might be plausible that RA could be an adjuvant in antitumor vaccination. DCs can take up and deliver exogenous ATRA to T cells during antigen presentation (Saurer, McCullough, and Summerfield 2007).

9.5.5 EOSINOPHIL AND BASOPHIL SERIES

RA seems to be important in maintaining the eosinophil population and thereby in controlling acute inflammation. One aspect is the inhibition of differentiation of BM aspirates and cord blood CD34+ cells toward eosinophil and basophil lineages. The mechanism involves downregulation of interleukin 5 (IL-5) receptor α, the most critical cytokine for eosinophils (Upham et al. 2002). RA is also important for maintaining normal eosinophil counts, by ligand activation of RAR and RXR and inhibition of apoptosis (Ueki et al. 2008). In a further potential regulatory loop, when activated by IL-3, eosinophils activate PI3-K and NF-κB and, as consequence, express aldehyde dehydrogenase and release RA (Spiegl et al. 2008). RA is important for T-cell instruction inducing the expression of CD38 receptor and α4/β7 integrins and Th2 activation (Spiegl et al. 2008). Moreover, in an autocrine loop, RA induces IL-3, CD25 (positive feedback), and granzyme B (negative feedback) (Spiegl et al. 2008).

9.5.6 Lymphocytes—T Cells

RA can influence T-cell immunity both directly, by effects on T-cell activation, and indirectly, by effects on DC maturation and function, as DCs are important regulators of T cells. CD4+ T-cell–mediated immunity is triggered by RA signaling, which correlates, spatially and temporarily, with inflammation. If the RA signal is perturbed, CD4+ T cells present impaired effector functions, migration, and polarity (Pino-Lagos et al. 2011). Double-positive thymocytes, CD4+/CD45RA+ naive T, a subset of regulatory CD4+/CD25+ T cells, and CD8+ T cells during chronic infection express CD38, a molecule induced by RA (Malavasi et al. 2008). Moreover, CD45+/CD4+/CD3– lymphoid tissue inducer cells express CXCR5 (Kim 2005), another membrane receptor under RA transcriptional control (Wang and Yen 2004). CD4+ and CD8+ T cells during primed in vitro in the presence of ATRA or DCs isolated from intestinal sites express high levels of the integrin α4β7 and the chemokine receptor CCR9. The CCR9 promoter has a RARE (Ohoka et al. 2011; Takeuchi et al. 2011). CCR9, upon binding to MAdCAM-1 and CCL25, mediates the migration of T cells to gut mucosa (Iwata et al. 2004; Johansson-Lindbom et al. 2003; Stenstad et al. 2006). ATRA modulates the balance between Th1 and Th2 cells. RA and vitamin A favor the development and function of Th2 to the detriment of Th1 (Iwata, Eshima, and Kagechika 2003; Stephensen et al. 2002). In both cases, the retinoid receptors are involved. Conversely, vitamin A deficiency favors Th1 responses (Cantorna, Nashold, and Hayes 1994, 1995), which means a chronic inflammatory phenotype (Assenmacher et al. 1998). Resting T cells enter the cell cycle and proliferate as a response to antigen stimulation. The binding of the antigen to TCR/CD3 prompts the synthesis of cyclins and cyclin-dependent kinases and, consequently, transition from G0 to G1. However, just the antigen cannot blunt the levels of p27Kip1 (Mohapatra, Agrawal, and Pledger 2001). This is achieved under IL-2 binding to TL-2R in those antigen-stimulated T cells (Firpo et al. 1994). RA bound to RAR enhances this process of T-cell proliferation by increasing IL-2R expression and both the phosphorylation of retinoblastoma protein and the expression of cyclin D3 (Engedal et al. 2006). The effect on cyclin D3 expression was dependent on the intact signaling pathway originating from IL-2R and Janus kinase (JAK), without altering the phosphorylation level of STAT3 or STAT5 (Engedal et al. 2006).

An important aspect of maintaining the balance between tolerance to food antigens and protection against toxins and pathogens present in the gastrointestinal tract is the upregulation of the expression of gut-homing receptors (CCR9 and α4β7) on T cells (Iwata et al. 2004). This process is RAR dependent and leads to T cells homing to the small intestine (Iwata et al. 2004). Studies done with knockout mice showed that CCR9 is essential for CD8+ T-cell localization to the small intestinal epithelium (Johansson-Lindbom et al. 2003).

In the past 10 years, over 5000 papers were published on the differentiation and function of CD4+ T cells expressing the forkhead-winged helix transcription factor Foxp3 (scurfin). Foxp3-defective individuals present an autoimmune and inflammatory syndrome (Hori, Nomura, and Sakaguchi 2003). CD4+/Foxp3+ T cells are regulatory T cells responsible for suppressing self-reactive lymphocytes and therefore are a therapeutic target for ameliorating exacerbated inflammation or graft tolerance conditions (Wang et al. 2010). Although in naive CD4+ T-cells RA inhibits the production of the immunosuppressive IL-10, in regulatory CD4+/Foxp3+ T cells, it has an opposite overall effect (Maynard et al. 2009). Through its forkhead domain, Foxp3 acts as a repressor of transcription (Schubert et al. 2001). As a consequence, Foxp3 inhibits activation-induced cytokine production by CD4+ T cells (Schubert et al. 2001) and suppresses B-cell Ig response (Lim et al. 2005). CD4+/Foxp3+ T cells express Cyp26b1, which provides a feedback inhibition to RA-induced CCR9 expression (Takeuchi et al. 2011). Moreover, RA promotes TGF-β–induced regulatory T cells by directly upregulating Foxp3 expression (Lu et al. 2011) in a RAR-α–dependent manner (Elias et al. 2008). The mechanism also involves upregulation and phosphorylation of Smad3 (Xiao et al. 2008). In contrast to the immunosuppressive T regulatory cells, the Th17 cells are proinflammatory, able to cause autoimmunity and inflammation. The same growth factor, TGF-β, is a positive inducer of naive T-cell differentiation both to regulatory T cells and to T helper cells secreting IL-17 (Th17). The key regulator of TGF-β responses in naive T cells is RA: it inhibits the differentiation to Th17 and promotes Foxp3+ regulatory T cells (Mucida et al. 2007). In the case of autoimmune inflammation, although the effect of RA is efficient both on suppressing Th17 and promoting Foxp3+ regulatory cells, the former is predominant (Xiao et al. 2008). The IL-17+/Foxp3+/CD4+ T cells present complex and largely unexplored biology and might link chronic inflammation to carcinogenesis (Kryczek et al. 2011).

9.5.7 LYMPHOCYTES—B CELLS

Oct2 is an important transcriptional factor required for the proliferation of pre–B cells as response to polyclonal mitogens and differentiation to newly formed antibody-secreting cells (Corcoran and Karvelas 1994). Oct2 knockout mice present no CD5+ B cells. Oct2 is negatively regulated by RA and positively regulates BLR1 (CXCR5) and CD36 (Konig et al. 1995). BLR1 is important for the homing of newly formed B cells to the lymphoid follicle. Memory B cells require NFATc1 transcriptional activity for differentiation and antibody production. NFATc1 is under transcriptional regulation of RA (Maruya et al. 2011). CD38 is downregulated in resting B cells and is upregulated in terminally differentiated plasma cells and chronic lymphocytic leukemia (Malavasi et al. 2008). IgA and IgM production depends largely on adequate local concentrations of vitamin A. Vitamin A–deficient rats are not able to produce sufficient amounts of IgA upon bacterial infection (Puengtomwatanakul and Sirisinha 1986). IgE production presents a biphasic modulation by RA: it is inhibited at high concentrations and augmented at moderate doses (Scheffel et al. 2005; Matheu et al. 2009).

9.5.8 NATURAL KILLER CELLS

Interferon gamma (IFN-gamma) is primarily produced by natural killer cells (NKs). RA inhibits IFN-gamma transcription (Cantorna, Nashold, and Hayes 1995). CD38 is highly expressed in NKs (Malavasi et al. 2008) and has an important role in NK-specific signal transduction by association with CD16 (Deaglio et al. 2002).

9.5.9 MEGAKARYOCYTES

Although this lineage is not as strongly related to inflammation, RA also regulates the megakaryocytic series cells. For example, an excess of vitamin A causes thrombocytopenia (Perrotta et al. 2002).

9.6 INFLAMMATION, VITAMIN A, AND CANCER

There are more than 100 pathologies described in the World Health Organization's *Classification of Tumours of Haematopoietic and Lymphoid Tissues*. Each is postulated to derive from a different single cell type and be characterized by a molecular fingerprint. It is estimated that with the advancement of laboratory techniques, those pathologies will be classified in even more detail. The classification not only is useful for the hematological pathologies but also serves as a starting point for the diagnosis of cutaneous lymphomas (Khamaysi et al. 2008; Slater 2005). One theory of carcinogenesis is that of cancer stem cells. AML fusion proteins induce genes responsible for the stemness of the cell. For example, ectopic expression of fusion proteins constitutively activates pathways, leading to increased stem cell renewal (such as the Jagged1/Notch pathway) (Alcalay et al. 2003). Notch4 overexpression in HL-60 myeloid leukemia cells hindered RA-induced differentiation (Ye et al. 2004). NB4, an APL PML/RAR-α–positive cell line, undergoes neutrophilic differentiation and apoptosis following RA treatment. When cells were treated with RA plus Delta-1 (a Notch ligand), the neutrophilic differentiation was hindered and apoptosis suppressed, and part of the cell population presented monocytic characteristics (Murata-Ohsawa et al. 2005). There is an increasing recognition of the role of persistent inflammation in stem cell biology (Zhou et al. 2012; Ye and Gimble 2011).

However, long ago, the German physician Rudolph Virchow (1821–1902) pointed out the association between inflammation (white blood cells infiltration) and cancer. He also coined the terms "leukemia" and "cancerous lymphoid glands" (Lindkvist 1999). Chronic inflammation is accompanied by reactive oxygen species, cytokines, and growth factors, which are all able to induce or promote carcinogenesis (Morrison 2012). In contrast, a healthy immune response facilitates the removal of preneoplastic cells. As previously shown, vitamin A, and especially RA, has multiple regulatory effects on the immune system. To summarize, RA regulates differentiation and function of diverse immune cells. Vitamin A deficiency causes immune dysfunctions such as the following: mucosal barrier defects; perturbation in the balance between regulatory T cells and Th17; blunted antibody production; decreased maturation of neutrophils and macrophages; and decreased functional capacities for CD103 DCs and eosinophils. Hypervitaminosis A is equally deleterious for the immune system. As shown in this chapter, the entire cellular component of the blood and lymphatic system is influenced by RA. The signaling elicited is complex, with intracellular and intercellular components, and only starting to be understood. Here we have sketched RA control of molecular regulation of the hematopoietic cells involved in inflammatory response.

We regret that because of the limitations in space, it was not possible to cite all of the important work that has been reported in this broad and active field, and we apologize for any omissions.

ACKNOWLEDGMENTS

We gratefully acknowledge partial support from the National Institutes of Health (NIH) grants CA033505 (Yen), CA152870 (Yen), and 1U54 CA143876 (Shuler), and from New York State Stem Cell Science (NYSTEM) (Yen). The flow cytometry core laboratory acknowledges support by the Empire State Stem Cell Fund through New York State Department of Health Contract #C026718.

REFERENCES

Alcalay, M., N. Meani, V. Gelmetti, A. Fantozzi, M. Fagioli, A. Orleth, D. Riganelli, C. Sebastiani, E. Cappelli, C. Casciari, M. T. Sciurpi, A. R. Mariano, S. P. Minardi, L. Luzi, H. Muller, P. P. Di Fiore, G. Frosina, and P. G. Pelicci. 2003. Acute myeloid leukemia fusion proteins deregulate genes involved in stem cell maintenance and DNA repair. *J Clin Invest* 112 (11):1751–61.

Alsayed, Y., S. Modi, S. Uddin, N. Mahmud, B. J. Druker, E. N. Fish, R. Hoffman, and L. C. Platanias. 2000. All-trans-retinoic acid induces tyrosine phosphorylation of the CrkL adapter in acute promyelocytic leukemia cells. *Exp Hematol* 28 (7):826–32.

Assenmacher, M., M. Lohning, A. Scheffold, A. Richter, S. Miltenyi, J. Schmitz, and A. Radbruch. 1998. Commitment of individual Th1-like lymphocytes to expression of IFN-gamma versus IL-4 and IL-10: selective induction of IL-10 by sequential stimulation of naive Th cells with IL-12 and IL-4. *J Immunol* 161 (6):2825–32.

Bansal, D., C. Scholl, S. Frohling, E. McDowell, B. H. Lee, K. Dohner, P. Ernst, A. J. Davidson, G. Q. Daley, L. I. Zon, D. G. Gilliland, and B. J. Huntly. 2006. Cdx4 dysregulates Hox gene expression and generates acute myeloid leukemia alone and in cooperation with Meis1a in a murine model. *Proc Natl Acad Sci U S A* 103 (45):16924–9.

Battle, T. E., M. S. Roberson, T. Zhang, S. Varvayanis, and A. Yen. 2001. Retinoic acid-induced blr1 expression requires RARα, RXR, and MAPK activation and uses ERK2 but not JNK/SAPK to accelerate cell differentiation. *Eur J Cell Biol* 80 (1):59–67.

Bertagnolo, V., F. Brugnoli, C. Mischiati, A. Sereni, A. Bavelloni, C. Carini, and S. Capitani. 2005. Vav promotes differentiation of human tumoral myeloid precursors. *Exp Cell Res* 306 (1):56–63.

Bertagnolo, V., M. Marchisio, F. Brugnoli, A. Bavelloni, L. Boccafogli, M. L. Colamussi, and S. Capitani. 2001. Requirement of tyrosine-phosphorylated Vav for morphological differentiation of all-trans-retinoic acid-treated HL-60 cells. *Cell Growth Differ* 12 (4):193–200.

Bleiberg, I., I. Fabian, S. Kantor, and Y. Kletter. 1988. The effect of 13-cis retinoic acid on hematopoiesis in human long-term bone marrow culture. *Leuk Res* 12 (7):545–50.

Boncinelli, E., A. Simeone, D. Acampora, and F. Mavilio. 1991. HOX gene activation by retinoic acid. *Trends Genet* 7 (10):329–34.

Brooks, S. C., 3rd, R. Sturgill, J. Choi, and A. Yen. 1997. An RXR-selective analog attenuates the RAR α-selective analog-induced differentiation and non-G1-restricted growth arrest of NB4 cells. *Exp Cell Res* 234 (2):259–69.

Brooks, S. C., 3rd, S. Kazmer, A. A. Levin, and A. Yen. 1996. Myeloid differentiation and retinoblastoma phosphorylation changes in HL-60 cells induced by retinoic acid receptor- and retinoid X receptor-selective retinoic acid analogs. *Blood* 87 (1):227–37.

Bunaciu, R. P., and A. Yen. 2011. Activation of the aryl hydrocarbon receptor AhR Promotes retinoic acid-induced differentiation of myeloblastic leukemia cells by restricting expression of the stem cell transcription factor Oct4. *Cancer Res* 71 (6):2371–80.

Bunaciu, R. P., T. Tang, and C. D. Mao. 2008. Differential expression of Wnt13 isoforms during leukemic cell differentiation. *Oncol Rep* 20 (1):195–201.

Cantorna, M. T., F. E. Nashold, and C. E. Hayes. 1994. In vitamin A deficiency multiple mechanisms establish a regulatory T helper cell imbalance with excess Th1 and insufficient Th2 function. *J Immunol* 152 (4):1515–22.

Cantorna, M. T., F. E. Nashold, and C. E. Hayes. 1995. Vitamin A deficiency results in a priming environment conducive for Th1 cell development. *Eur J Immunol* 25 (6):1673–9.

Care, A., U. Testa, A. Bassani, E. Tritarelli, E. Montesoro, P. Samoggia, L. Cianetti, and C. Peschle. 1994. Coordinate expression and proliferative role of HOXB genes in activated adult T lymphocytes. *Mol Cell Biol* 14 (7):4872–7.

Carvajal-Yepes, M., K. Himmelsbach, S. Schaedler, D. Ploen, J. Krause, L. Ludwig, T. Weiss, K. Klingel, and E. Hildt. 2011. Hepatitis C virus impairs the induction of cytoprotective Nrf2 target genes by delocalization of small Maf proteins. *J Biol Chem* 286 (11):8941–51.

Chang, H., M. C. Kuo, L. Y. Shih, P. Dunn, P. N. Wang, J. H. Wu, T. L. Lin, Y. S. Hung, and T. C. Tang. 2012. Clinical bleeding events and laboratory coagulation profiles in acute promyelocytic leukemia. *Eur J Haematol* 88 (4):321–8.

Charite, J., W. de Graaff, and J. Deschamps. 1995. Specification of multiple vertebral identities by ectopically expressed Hoxb-8. *Dev Dyn* 204 (1):13–21.

Chen, Y., and M. Solursh. 1992. Comparison of Hensen's node and retinoic acid in secondary axis induction in the early chick embryo. *Dev Dyn* 195 (2):142–51.

Cimmino, A., G. A. Calin, M. Fabbri, M. V. Iorio, M. Ferracin, M. Shimizu, S. E. Wojcik, R. I. Aqeilan, S. Zupo, M. Dono, L. Rassenti, H. Alder, S. Volinia, C. G. Liu, T. J. Kipps, M. Negrini, and C. M. Croce. 2005. miR-15 and miR-16 induce apoptosis by targeting BCL2. *Proc Natl Acad Sci U S A* 102 (39):13944–9.

Clerc, R. G., L. M. Corcoran, J. H. LeBowitz, D. Baltimore, and P. A. Sharp. 1988. The B-cell-specific Oct-2 protein contains POU box- and homeo box-type domains. *Genes Dev* 2 (12A):1570–81.

Congleton, J., R. MacDonald, and A. Yen. 2012. Src inhibitors, PP2 and dasatinib, increase retinoic acid-induced association of Lyn and c-Raf (S259) and enhance MAPK dependent differentiation of myeloid leukemia cells. *Leukemia* 26 (6):1180–8.

Conlon, R. A., and J. Rossant. 1992. Exogenous retinoic acid rapidly induces anterior ectopic expression of murine Hox-2 genes in vivo. *Development* 116 (2):357–68.

Corcoran, L. M., and M. Karvelas. 1994. Oct-2 is required early in T cell-independent B cell activation for G1 progression and for proliferation. *Immunity* 1 (8):635–45.

de Grazia, U., M. P. Felli, A. Vacca, A. R. Farina, M. Maroder, L. Cappabianca, D. Meco, M. Farina, I. Screpanti, L. Frati, and A. Gulino. 1994. Positive and negative regulation of the composite octamer motif of the interleukin 2 enhancer by AP-1, Oct-2, and retinoic acid receptor. *J Exp Med* 180 (4):1485–97.

de Jong, J. L., A. J. Davidson, Y. Wang, J. Palis, P. Opara, E. Pugach, G. Q. Daley, and L. I. Zon. 2010. Interaction of retinoic acid and scl controls primitive blood development. *Blood* 116 (2):201–9.

Deaglio, S., M. Zubiaur, A. Gregorini, F. Bottarel, C. M. Ausiello, U. Dianzani, J. Sancho, and F. Malavasi. 2002. Human CD38 and CD16 are functionally dependent and physically associated in natural killer cells. *Blood* 99 (7):2490–8.

Dupe, V., M. Davenne, J. Brocard, P. Dolle, M. Mark, A. Dierich, P. Chambon, and F. M. Rijli. 1997. In vivo functional analysis of the Hoxa-1 3′ retinoic acid response element (3′RARE). *Development* 124 (2):399–410.

Elias, K. M., A. Laurence, T. S. Davidson, G. Stephens, Y. Kanno, E. M. Shevach, and J. J. O'Shea. 2008. Retinoic acid inhibits Th17 polarization and enhances FoxP3 expression through a Stat-3/Stat-5 independent signaling pathway. *Blood* 111 (3):1013–20.

Engedal, N., T. Gjevik, R. Blomhoff, and H. K. Blomhoff. 2006. All-trans retinoic acid stimulates IL-2-mediated proliferation of human T lymphocytes: early induction of cyclin D3. *J Immunol* 177 (5):2851–61.

Fang, M. H., W. L. Liu, F. K. Meng, and H. Y. Sun. 2009. [Aberrant methylation at promoter region of HOX A gene cluster in leukemia cells]. *Zhonghua Xue Ye Xue Za Zhi* 30 (7):468–72.

Farooqui-Kabir, S. R., J. K. Diss, D. Henderson, M. S. Marber, D. S. Latchman, V. Budhram-Mahadeo, and R. J. Heads. 2008. Cardiac expression of Brn-3a and Brn-3b POU transcription factors and regulation of Hsp27 gene expression. *Cell Stress Chaperones* 13 (3):297–312.

Ferrari, S., R. Manfredini, E. Tagliafico, A. Grande, D. Barbieri, R. Balestri, M. Pizzanelli, P. Zucchini, G. Citro, G. Zupi et al. 1994. Antiapoptotic effect of c-fes protooncogene during granulocytic differentiation. *Leukemia* 8 Suppl 1:S91–4.

Ferrari, S., A. Donelli, R. Manfredini, M. Sarti, R. Roncaglia, E. Tagliafico, E. Rossi, G. Torelli, and U. Torelli. 1990. Differential effects of c-myb and c-fes antisense oligodeoxynucleotides on granulocytic differentiation of human myeloid leukemia HL60 cells. *Cell Growth Differ* 1 (11):543–8.

Ferrari, S., U. Torelli, L. Selleri, A. Donelli, D. Venturelli, L. Moretti, and G. Torelli. 1985. Expression of human c-fes onc-gene occurs at detectable levels in myeloid but not in lymphoid cell populations. *Br J Haematol* 59 (1):21–5.

Firpo, E. J., A. Koff, M. J. Solomon, and J. M. Roberts. 1994. Inactivation of a Cdk2 inhibitor during interleukin 2-induced proliferation of human T lymphocytes. *Mol Cell Biol* 14 (7):4889–901.

Foley, A. C., I. Skromne, and C. D. Stern. 2000. Reconciling different models of forebrain induction and patterning: a dual role for the hypoblast. *Development* 127 (17):3839–54.

Funaro, A., L. B. De Monte, U. Dianzani, M. Forni, and F. Malavasi. 1993. Human CD38 is associated to distinct molecules which mediate transmembrane signaling in different lineages. *Eur J Immunol* 23 (10):2407–11.

Gao, S. M., J. Yang, C. Chen, S. Zhang, C. Y. Xing, H. Li, J. Wu, and L. Jiang. 2011. miR-15a/16-1 enhances retinoic acid-mediated differentiation of leukemic cells and is up-regulated by retinoic acid. *Leuk Lymphoma* 52 (12):2365–71.

Germain, P., P. Chambon, G. Eichele, R. M. Evans, M. A. Lazar, M. Leid, A. R. De Lera, R. Lotan, D. J. Mangelsdorf, and H. Gronemeyer. 2006. International Union of Pharmacology. LX. Retinoic acid receptors. *Pharmacol Rev* 58 (4):712–25.

Ghatpande, S., A. Ghatpande, J. Sher, M. H. Zile, and T. Evans. 2002. Retinoid signaling regulates primitive (yolk sac) hematopoiesis. *Blood* 99 (7):2379–86.

Gilbert, S. F. 2010. *Developmental Biology*, 9th Ed. Sunderland, MA Sinauer Associates, Inc.

Gratas, C., M. L. Menot, C. Dresch, and C. Chomienne. 1993. Retinoid acid supports granulocytic but not erythroid differentiation of myeloid progenitors in normal bone marrow cells. *Leukemia* 7 (8):1156–62.

Hengesbach, L. M., and K. A. Hoag. 2004. Physiological concentrations of retinoic acid favor myeloid dendritic cell development over granulocyte development in cultures of bone marrow cells from mice. *J Nutr* 134 (10):2653–9.

Hong, H. Y., S. Varvayanis, and A. Yen. 2001. Retinoic acid causes MEK-dependent RAF phosphorylation through RARα plus RXR activation in HL-60 cells. *Differentiation* 68 (1):55–66.

Hori, S., T. Nomura, and S. Sakaguchi. 2003. Control of regulatory T cell development by the transcription factor Foxp3. *Science* 299 (5609):1057–61.

Houle, M., J. R. Sylvestre, and D. Lohnes. 2003. Retinoic acid regulates a subset of Cdx1 function in vivo. *Development* 130 (26):6555–67.

Hu, L., T. Lind, A. Sundqvist, A. Jacobson, and H. Melhus. 2010. Retinoic acid increases proliferation of human osteoclast progenitors and inhibits RANKL-stimulated osteoclast differentiation by suppressing RANK. *PLoS One* 5 (10):e13305.

Iwata, M., A. Hirakiyama, Y. Eshima, H. Kagechika, C. Kato, and S. Y. Song. 2004. Retinoic acid imprints gut-homing specificity on T cells. *Immunity* 21 (4):527–38.

Iwata, M., Y. Eshima, and H. Kagechika. 2003. Retinoic acids exert direct effects on T cells to suppress Th1 development and enhance Th2 development via retinoic acid receptors. *Int Immunol* 15 (8):1017–25.

Jaiswal, A. K. 2004. Nrf2 signaling in coordinated activation of antioxidant gene expression. *Free Radic Biol Med* 36 (10):1199–207.

Johansson-Lindbom, B., M. Svensson, M. A. Wurbel, B. Malissen, G. Marquez, and W. Agace. 2003. Selective generation of gut tropic T cells in gut-associated lymphoid tissue (GALT): requirement for GALT dendritic cells and adjuvant. *J Exp Med* 198 (6):963–9.

Kang, S. M., W. Tsang, S. Doll, P. Scherle, H. S. Ko, A. C. Tran, M. J. Lenardo, and L. M. Staudt. 1992. Induction of the POU domain transcription factor Oct-2 during T-cell activation by cognate antigen. *Mol Cell Biol* 12 (7):3149–54.

Katagiri, K., K. K. Yokoyama, T. Yamamoto, S. Omura, S. Irie, and T. Katagiri. 1996. Lyn and Fgr protein-tyrosine kinases prevent apoptosis during retinoic acid-induced granulocytic differentiation of HL-60 cells. *J Biol Chem* 271 (19):11557–62.

Katsumata, O., M. Hara-Yokoyama, C. Sautes-Fridman, Y. Nagatsuka, T. Katada, Y. Hirabayashi, K. Shimizu, J. Fujita-Yoshigaki, H. Sugiya, and S. Furuyama. 2001. Association of FcgammaRII with low-density detergent-resistant membranes is important for cross-linking-dependent initiation of the tyrosine phosphorylation pathway and superoxide generation. *J Immunol* 167 (10):5814–23.

Kessel, M. 1992. Respecification of vertebral identities by retinoic acid. *Development* 115 (2):487–501.

Khamaysi, Z., Y. Ben-Arieh, O. B. Izhak, R. Epelbaum, E. J. Dann, and R. Bergman. 2008. The applicability of the new WHO-EORTC classification of primary cutaneous lymphomas to a single referral center. *Am J Dermatopathol* 30 (1):37–44.

Kim, C. H. 2005. The greater chemotactic network for lymphocyte trafficking: chemokines and beyond. *Curr Opin Hematol* 12 (4):298–304.

Kishimoto, H., S. Hoshino, M. Ohori, K. Kontani, H. Nishina, M. Suzawa, S. Kato, and T. Katada. 1998. Molecular mechanism of human CD38 gene expression by retinoic acid. Identification of retinoic acid response element in the first intron. *J Biol Chem* 273 (25):15429–34.

Konig, H., P. Pfisterer, L. M. Corcoran, and T. Wirth. 1995. Identification of CD36 as the first gene dependent on the B-cell differentiation factor Oct-2. *Genes Dev* 9 (13):1598–607.

Konopleva, M., Z. Estrov, S. Zhao, M. Andreeff, and K. Mehta. 1998. Ligation of cell surface CD38 protein with agonistic monoclonal antibody induces a cell growth signal in myeloid leukemia cells. *J Immunol* 161 (9):4702–8.

Kontani, K., I. Kukimoto, Y. Kanda, S. Inoue, H. Kishimoto, S. Hoshino, H. Nishina, K. Takahashi, O. Hazeki, and T. Katada. 1997. Signal transduction via the CD38/NAD+ glycohydrolase. *Adv Exp Med Biol* 419:421–30.

Kontani, K., I. Kukimoto, H. Nishina, S. Hoshino, O. Hazeki, Y. Kanaho, and T. Katada. 1996. Tyrosine phosphorylation of the c-cbl proto-oncogene product mediated by cell surface antigen CD38 in HL-60 cells. *J Biol Chem* 271 (3):1534–7.

Krishnaraju, K., B. Hoffman, and D. A. Liebermann. 1997. Lineage-specific regulation of hematopoiesis by HOX-B8 (HOX-2.4): inhibition of granulocytic differentiation and potentiation of monocytic differentiation. *Blood* 90 (5):1840–9.

Kryczek, I., K. Wu, E. Zhao, S. Wei, L. Vatan, W. Szeliga, E. Huang, J. Greenson, A. Chang, J. Rolinski, P. Radwan, J. Fang, G. Wang, and W. Zou. 2011. IL-17+ regulatory T cells in the microenvironments of chronic inflammation and cancer. *J Immunol* 186 (7):4388–95.

Kuwata, T., I. M. Wang, T. Tamura, R. M. Ponnamperuma, R. Levine, K. L. Holmes, H. C. Morse, L. M. De Luca, and K. Ozato. 2000. Vitamin A deficiency in mice causes a systemic expansion of myeloid cells. *Blood* 95 (11):3349–56.

Lamkin, T. J., V. Chin, S. Varvayanis, J. L. Smith, R. M. Sramkoski, J. W. Jacobberger, and A. Yen. 2006. Retinoic acid-induced CD38 expression in HL-60 myeloblastic leukemia cells regulates cell differentiation or viability depending on expression levels. *J Cell Biochem* 97 (6):1328–38.

Li, W., S. Yu, T. Liu, J. H. Kim, V. Blank, H. Li, and A. N. Kong. 2008. Heterodimerization with small Maf proteins enhances nuclear retention of Nrf2 via masking the NESzip motif. *Biochim Biophys Acta* 1783 (10):1847–56.

Liao, X., and M. D. Collins. 2008. All-trans retinoic acid-induced ectopic limb and caudal structures: murine strain sensitivities and pathogenesis. *Dev Dyn* 237 (6):1553–64.

Liebecq, C. 1997. IUPAC-IUBMB Joint Commission on Biochemical Nomenclature (JCBN) and Nomenclature Committee of IUBMB (NC-IUBMB). Newsletter 1996. *Eur J Biochem* 247 (2):733–9.

Lill, M. C., J. F. Fuller, R. Herzig, G. M. Crooks, and J. C. Gasson. 1995. The role of the homeobox gene, HOX B7, in human myelomonocytic differentiation. *Blood* 85 (3):692–7.

Lim, H. W., P. Hillsamer, A. H. Banham, and C. H. Kim. 2005. Cutting edge: direct suppression of B cells by CD4+ CD25+ regulatory T cells. *J Immunol* 175 (7):4180–3.

Lindkvist, L. 1999. [Rudolf Virchow 1821–1902. Physician, politician, historian and anthropologist]. *Sven Med Tidskr* 3 (1):57–82.

Liu, T. X., J. W. Zhang, J. Tao, R. B. Zhang, Q. H. Zhang, C. J. Zhao, J. H. Tong, M. Lanotte, S. Waxman, S. J. Chen, M. Mao, G. X. Hu, L. Zhu, and Z. Chen. 2000. Gene expression networks underlying retinoic acid-induced differentiation of acute promyelocytic leukemia cells. *Blood* 96 (4):1496–504.

Lohnes, D. 2003. The Cdx1 homeodomain protein: an integrator of posterior signaling in the mouse. *Bioessays* 25 (10):971–80.

Lu, L., J. Ma, Z. Li, Q. Lan, M. Chen, Y. Liu, Z. Xia, J. Wang, Y. Han, W. Shi, V. Quesniaux, B. Ryffel, D. Brand, B. Li, Z. Liu, and S. G. Zheng. 2011. All-trans retinoic acid promotes TGF-β-induced Tregs via histone modification but not DNA demethylation on Foxp3 gene locus. *PLoS One* 6 (9):e24590.

Malavasi, F., S. Deaglio, A. Funaro, E. Ferrero, A. L. Horenstein, T. Ortolan, T. Vaisitti, and S. Aydin. 2008. Evolution and function of the ADP ribosyl cyclase/CD38 gene family in physiology and pathology. *Physiol Rev* 88 (3):841–86.

Mangelsdorf, D. J., and R. M. Evans. 1995. The RXR heterodimers and orphan receptors. *Cell* 83 (6):841–50.

Mangelsdorf, D. J., U. Borgmeyer, R. A. Heyman, J. Y. Zhou, E. S. Ong, A. E. Oro, A. Kakizuka, and R. M. Evans. 1992. Characterization of three RXR genes that mediate the action of 9-cis retinoic acid. *Genes Dev* 6 (3):329–44.

Mangelsdorf, D. J., E. S. Ong, J. A. Dyck, and R. M. Evans. 1990. Nuclear receptor that identifies a novel retinoic acid response pathway. *Nature* 345 (6272):224–9.

Mann, E. R., D. Bernardo, H. O. Al-Hassi, N. R. English, S. K. Clark, N. E. McCarthy, A. N. Milestone, S. A. Cochrane, A. L. Hart, A. J. Stagg, and S. C. Knight. 2012. Human gut-specific homeostatic dendritic cells are generated from blood precursors by the gut microenvironment. *Inflamm Bowel Dis* 18 (7):1275–86.

Maruya, M., K. Suzuki, H. Fujimoto, M. Miyajima, O. Kanagawa, T. Wakayama, and S. Fagarasan. 2011. Vitamin A-dependent transcriptional activation of the nuclear factor of activated T cells c1 (NFATc1) is critical for the development and survival of B1 cells. *Proc Natl Acad Sci U S A* 108 (2):722–7.

Matheu, V., K. Berggard, Y. Barrios, Y. Barrios, M. R. Arnau, J. M. Zubeldia, M. L. Baeza, O. Back, and S. Issazadeh-Navikas. 2009. Impact on allergic immune response after treatment with vitamin A. *Nutr Metab (Lond)* 6:44.

Maynard, C. L., R. D. Hatton, W. S. Helms, J. R. Oliver, C. B. Stephensen, and C. T. Weaver. 2009. Contrasting roles for all-trans retinoic acid in TGF-β-mediated induction of Foxp3 and Il10 genes in developing regulatory T cells. *J Exp Med* 206 (2):343–57.

Mehta, K., T. McQueen, T. Manshouri, M. Andreeff, S. Collins, and M. Albitar. 1997. Involvement of retinoic acid receptor-α-mediated signaling pathway in induction of CD38 cell-surface antigen. *Blood* 89 (10):3607–14.

Mejia, L. A., R. E. Hodges, and R. B. Rucker. 1979. Clinical signs of anemia in vitamin A-deficient rats. *Am J Clin Nutr* 32 (7):1439–44.

Messier, H., H. Brickner, J. Gaikwad, and A. Fotedar. 1993. A novel POU domain protein which binds to the T-cell receptor β enhancer. *Mol Cell Biol* 13 (9):5450–60.

Mitchell, L. E., J. C. Murray, S. O'Brien, and K. Christensen. 2003. Retinoic acid receptor α gene variants, multivitamin use, and liver intake as risk factors for oral clefts: a population-based case-control study in Denmark, 1991–1994. *Am J Epidemiol* 158 (1):69–76.

Mohapatra, S., D. Agrawal, and W. J. Pledger. 2001. p27Kip1 regulates T cell proliferation. *J Biol Chem* 276 (24):21976–83.

Morrison, W. B. 2012. Inflammation and cancer: a comparative view. *J Vet Intern Med* 26 (1):18–31.

Mucida, D., Y. Park, G. Kim, O. Turovskaya, I. Scott, M. Kronenberg, and H. Cheroutre. 2007. Reciprocal TH17 and regulatory T cell differentiation mediated by retinoic acid. *Science* 317 (5835):256–60.

Munshi, C. B., R. Graeff, and H. C. Lee. 2002. Evidence for a causal role of CD38 expression in granulocytic differentiation of human HL-60 cells. *J Biol Chem* 277 (51):49453–8.

Murata-Ohsawa, M., S. Tohda, H. Kogoshi, S. Sakano, and N. Nara. 2005. The Notch ligand, Delta-1, alters retinoic acid (RA)-induced neutrophilic differentiation into monocytic and reduces RA-induced apoptosis in NB4 cells. *Leuk Res* 29 (2):197–203.

Nakamura, T., H. Hemmi, H. Aso, and N. Ishida. 1986. Variants of a human monocytic leukemia cell line (THP-1): induction of differentiation by retinoic acid, interferon-gamma, and T-lymphocyte-derived differentiation-inducing activity. *J Natl Cancer Inst* 77 (1):21–7.

Nelson, K. L., J. A. Rogers, T. L. Bowman, R. Jove, and T. E. Smithgall. 1998. Activation of STAT3 by the c-Fes protein-tyrosine kinase. *J Biol Chem* 273 (12):7072–7.

Nilsson, B. 1984. Probable in vivo induction of differentiation by retinoic acid of promyelocytes in acute promyelocytic leukaemia. *Br J Haematol* 57 (3):365–71.

Oeth, P., J. Yao, S. T. Fan, and N. Mackman. 1998. Retinoic acid selectively inhibits lipopolysaccharide induction of tissue factor gene expression in human monocytes. *Blood* 91 (8):2857–65.

Ofir, M., D. Hacohen, and D. Ginsberg. 2011. MiR-15 and miR-16 are direct transcriptional targets of E2F1 that limit E2F-induced proliferation by targeting cyclin E. *Mol Cancer Res* 9 (4):440–7.

Ohoka, Y., A. Yokota, H. Takeuchi, N. Maeda, and M. Iwata. 2011. Retinoic acid-induced CCR9 expression requires transient TCR stimulation and cooperativity between NFATc2 and the retinoic acid receptor/retinoid X receptor complex. *J Immunol* 186 (2):733–44.

Oosterveen, T., F. Meijlink, and J. Deschamps. 2004. Expression of retinaldehyde dehydrogenase II and sequential activation of 5′ Hoxb genes in the mouse caudal hindbrain. *Gene Expr Patterns* 4 (3):243–7.

Oosterveen, T., K. Niederreither, P. Dolle, P. Chambon, F. Meijlink, and J. Deschamps. 2003a. Retinoids regulate the anterior expression boundaries of 5′ Hoxb genes in posterior hindbrain. *EMBO J* 22 (2):262–9.

Oosterveen, T., P. van Vliet, J. Deschamps, and F. Meijlink. 2003b. The direct context of a hox retinoic acid response element is crucial for its activity. *J Biol Chem* 278 (26):24103–7.

Pan, Y., W. Zhang, Y. Du, N. Tong, Y. Han, H. Zhang, M. Wang, J. Ma, L. Wan, and L. Wang. 2011. Different roles of two novel susceptibility loci for nonsyndromic orofacial clefts in a Chinese Han population. *Am J Med Genet A* 155A (9):2180–5.

Park, D. J., A. M. Chumakov, P. T. Vuong, D. Y. Chih, A. F. Gombart, W. H. Miller, Jr., and H. P. Koeffler. 1999. CCAAT/enhancer binding protein epsilon is a potential retinoid target gene in acute promyelocytic leukemia treatment. *J Clin Invest* 103 (10):1399–408.

Perrotta, S., B. Nobili, F. Rossi, M. Criscuolo, A. Iolascon, D. Di Pinto, I. Passaro, L. Cennamo, A. Oliva, and F. Della Ragione. 2002. Infant hypervitaminosis A causes severe anemia and thrombocytopenia: evidence of a retinol-dependent bone marrow cell growth inhibition. *Blood* 99 (6):2017–22.

Pikarsky, E., H. Sharir, E. Ben-Shushan, and Y. Bergman. 1994. Retinoic acid represses Oct-3/4 gene expression through several retinoic acid-responsive elements located in the promoter-enhancer region. *Mol Cell Biol* 14 (2):1026–38.

Pino-Lagos, K., Y. Guo, C. Brown, M. P. Alexander, R. Elgueta, K. A. Bennett, V. De Vries, E. Nowak, R. Blomhoff, S. Sockanathan, R. A. Chandraratna, E. Dmitrovsky, and R. J. Noelle. 2011. A retinoic acid-dependent checkpoint in the development of CD4+ T cell-mediated immunity. *J Exp Med* 208 (9):1767–75.

Puengtomwatanakul, S., and S. Sirisinha. 1986. Impaired biliary secretion of immunoglobulin A in vitamin A-deficient rats. *Proc Soc Exp Biol Med* 182 (4):437–42.

Rhodes, J., and P. Stokes. 1982. Interferon-induced changes in the monocyte membrane: inhibition by retinol and retinoic acid. *Immunology* 45 (3):531–6.

Ruhl, R., C. Plum, M. M. Elmazar, and H. Nau. 2001. Embryonic subcellular distribution of 13-cis- and all-trans-retinoic acid indicates differential cytosolic/nuclear localization. *Toxicol Sci* 63 (1):82–9.

Rusten, L. S., I. Dybedal, H. K. Blomhoff, R. Blomhoff, E. B. Smeland, and S. E. Jacobsen. 1996. The RAR-RXR as well as the RXR-RXR pathway is involved in signaling growth inhibition of human CD34+ erythroid progenitor cells. *Blood* 87 (5):1728–36.

Sakai, Y., C. Meno, H. Fujii, J. Nishino, H. Shiratori, Y. Saijoh, J. Rossant, and H. Hamada. 2001. The retinoic acid-inactivating enzyme CYP26 is essential for establishing an uneven distribution of retinoic acid along the anterio-posterior axis within the mouse embryo. *Genes Dev* 15 (2):213–25.

Sandell, L. L., B. W. Sanderson, G. Moiseyev, T. Johnson, A. Mushegian, K. Young, J. P. Rey, J. X. Ma, K. Staehling-Hampton, and P. A. Trainor. 2007. RDH10 is essential for synthesis of embryonic retinoic acid and is required for limb, craniofacial, and organ development. *Genes Dev* 21 (9):1113–24.

Sarrazin, S., N. Mossadegh-Keller, T. Fukao, A. Aziz, F. Mourcin, L. Vanhille, L. Kelly Modis, P. Kastner, S. Chan, E. Duprez, C. Otto, and M. H. Sieweke. 2009. MafB restricts M-CSF-dependent myeloid commitment divisions of hematopoietic stem cells. *Cell* 138 (2):300–13.

Saurer, L., K. C. McCullough, and A. Summerfield. 2007. In vitro induction of mucosa-type dendritic cells by all-trans retinoic acid. *J Immunol* 179 (6):3504–14.

Scheffel, F., G. Heine, B. M. Henz, and M. Worm. 2005. Retinoic acid inhibits CD40 plus IL-4 mediated IgE production through alterations of sCD23, sCD54 and IL-6 production. *Inflamm Res* 54 (3):113–8.

Schubart, K., S. Massa, D. Schubart, L. M. Corcoran, A. G. Rolink, and P. Matthias. 2001. B cell development and immunoglobulin gene transcription in the absence of Oct-2 and OBF-1. *Nat Immunol* 2 (1):69–74.

Schubert, L. A., E. Jeffery, Y. Zhang, F. Ramsdell, and S. F. Ziegler. 2001. Scurfin (FOXP3) acts as a repressor of transcription and regulates T cell activation. *J Biol Chem* 276 (40):37672–9.

Seta, N., and M. Kuwana. 2010. Derivation of multipotent progenitors from human circulating CD14+ monocytes. *Exp Hematol* 38 (7):557–63.

Shen, M., and A. Yen. 2009. c-Cbl tyrosine kinase-binding domain mutant G306E abolishes the interaction of c-Cbl with CD38 and fails to promote retinoic acid-induced cell differentiation and G0 arrest. *J Biol Chem* 284 (38):25664–77.

Shen, M., and A. Yen. 2008. c-Cbl interacts with CD38 and promotes retinoic acid-induced differentiation and G0 arrest of human myeloblastic leukemia cells. *Cancer Res* 68 (21):8761–9.

Shen, M., R. P. Bunaciu, J. Congleton, H. A. Jensen, L. G. Sayam, J. D. Varner, and A. Yen. 2011. Interferon regulatory factor-1 binds c-Cbl, enhances mitogen activated protein kinase signaling and promotes retinoic acid-induced differentiation of HL-60 human myelo-monoblastic leukemia cells. *Leuk Lymphoma* 52 (12):2372–9.

Sivaraja, M., M. C. Botfield, M. Mueller, A. Jancso, and M. A. Weiss. 1994. Solution structure of a POU-specific homeodomain: 3D-NMR studies of human B-cell transcription factor Oct-2. *Biochemistry* 33 (33):9845–55.

Slater, D. N. 2005. The new World Health Organization-European Organization for Research and Treatment of Cancer classification for cutaneous lymphomas: a practical marriage of two giants. *Br J Dermatol* 153 (5):874–80.

Smith, J., R. P. Bunaciu, G. Reiterer, D. Coder, T. George, M. Asaly, and A. Yen. 2009. Retinoic acid induces nuclear accumulation of Raf1 during differentiation of HL-60 cells. *Exp Cell Res* 315 (13):2241–8.

Spiegl, N., S. Didichenko, P. McCaffery, H. Langen, and C. A. Dahinden. 2008. Human basophils activated by mast cell-derived IL-3 express retinaldehyde dehydrogenase-II and produce the immunoregulatory mediator retinoic acid. *Blood* 112 (9):3762–71.

Stenstad, H., A. Ericsson, B. Johansson-Lindbom, M. Svensson, J. Marsal, M. Mack, D. Picarella, D. Soler, G. Marquez, M. Briskin, and W. W. Agace. 2006. Gut-associated lymphoid tissue-primed CD4+ T cells display CCR9-dependent and -independent homing to the small intestine. *Blood* 107 (9):3447–54.

Stephensen, C. B., R. Rasooly, X. Jiang, M. A. Ceddia, C. T. Weaver, R. A. Chandraratna, and R. P. Bucy. 2002. Vitamin A enhances in vitro Th2 development via retinoid X receptor pathway. *J Immunol* 168 (9):4495–503.

Svensson, M., B. Johansson-Lindbom, F. Zapata, E. Jaensson, L. M. Austenaa, R. Blomhoff, and W. W. Agace. 2008. Retinoic acid receptor signaling levels and antigen dose regulate gut homing receptor expression on CD8+ T cells. *Mucosal Immunol* 1 (1):38–48.

Tabin, C. 1995. The initiation of the limb bud: growth factors, Hox genes, and retinoids. *Cell* 80 (5):671–4.

Tagliafico, E., M. Siena, T. Zanocco-Marani, R. Manfredini, E. Tenedini, M. Montanari, A. Grande, and S. Ferrari. 2003. Requirement of the coiled-coil domains of p92(c-Fes) for nuclear localization in myeloid cells upon induction of differentiation. *Oncogene* 22 (11):1712–23.

Takeuchi, H., A. Yokota, Y. Ohoka, and M. Iwata. 2011. Cyp26b1 regulates retinoic acid-dependent signals in T cells and its expression is inhibited by transforming growth factor-β. *PLoS One* 6 (1):e16089.

Tan, K. P., K. Kosuge, M. Yang, and S. Ito. 2008. NRF2 as a determinant of cellular resistance in retinoic acid cytotoxicity. *Free Radic Biol Med* 45 (12):1663–73.

Tan, X., J. L. Sande, J. S. Pufnock, J. N. Blattman, and P. D. Greenberg. 2011. Retinoic acid as a vaccine adjuvant enhances CD8+ T cell response and mucosal protection from viral challenge. *J Virol* 85 (16):8316–27.

ten Hoeve, J., C. Morris, N. Heisterkamp, and J. Groffen. 1993. Isolation and chromosomal localization of CRKL, a human crk-like gene. *Oncogene* 8 (9):2469–74.

Thorsteinsdottir, U., G. Sauvageau, and R. K. Humphries. 1997. Hox homeobox genes as regulators of normal and leukemic hematopoiesis. *Hematol Oncol Clin North Am* 11 (6):1221–37.

Tsukui, T., J. Capdevila, K. Tamura, P. Ruiz-Lozano, C. Rodriguez-Esteban, S. Yonei-Tamura, J. Magallon, R. A. Chandraratna, K. Chien, B. Blumberg, R. M. Evans, and J. C. Belmonte. 1999. Multiple left-right asymmetry defects in Shh(−/−) mutant mice unveil a convergence of the shh and retinoic acid pathways in the control of Lefty-1. *Proc Natl Acad Sci U S A* 96 (20):11376–81.

Uehara, M., K. Yashiro, K. Takaoka, M. Yamamoto, and H. Hamada. 2009. Removal of maternal retinoic acid by embryonic CYP26 is required for correct Nodal expression during early embryonic patterning. *Genes Dev* 23 (14):1689–98.

Ueki, S., G. Mahemuti, H. Oyamada, H. Kato, J. Kihara, M. Tanabe, W. Ito, T. Chiba, M. Takeda, H. Kayaba, and J. Chihara. 2008. Retinoic acids are potent inhibitors of spontaneous human eosinophil apoptosis. *J Immunol* 181 (11):7689–98.

Upham, J. W., R. Sehmi, L. M. Hayes, K. Howie, J. Lundahl, and J. A. Denburg. 2002. Retinoic acid modulates IL-5 receptor expression and selectively inhibits eosinophil-basophil differentiation of hemopoietic progenitor cells. *J Allergy Clin Immunol* 109 (2):307–13.

Vitobello, A., E. Ferretti, X. Lampe, N. Vilain, S. Ducret, M. Ori, J. F. Spetz, L. Selleri, and F. M. Rijli. 2011. Hox and Pbx factors control retinoic acid synthesis during hindbrain segmentation. *Dev Cell* 20 (4):469–82.

Wang, G., A. Zhong, S. Wang, N. Dong, Z. Sun, and J. Xia. 2010. Retinoic acid attenuates acute heart rejection by increasing regulatory T cell and repressing differentiation of Th17 cell in the presence of TGF-β. *Transpl Int* 23 (10):986–97.

Wang, J., and A. Yen. 2004. A novel retinoic acid-responsive element regulates retinoic acid-induced BLR1 expression. *Mol Cell Biol* 24 (6):2423–43.

Wang, P. W., J. D. Eisenbart, S. P. Cordes, G. S. Barsh, M. Stoffel, and M. M. Le Beau. 1999. Human KRML (MAFB): cDNA cloning, genomic structure, and evaluation as a candidate tumor suppressor gene in myeloid leukemias. *Genomics* 59 (3):275–81.

Wang, P. W., K. Iannantuoni, E. M. Davis, R. Espinosa, 3rd, M. Stoffel, and M. M. Le Beau. 1998. Refinement of the commonly deleted segment in myeloid leukemias with a del(20q). *Genes Chromosomes Cancer* 21 (2):75–81.

Wang, X. J., J. D. Hayes, C. J. Henderson, and C. R. Wolf. 2007a. Identification of retinoic acid as an inhibitor of transcription factor Nrf2 through activation of retinoic acid receptor α. *Proc Natl Acad Sci U S A* 104 (49):19589–94.

Wang, Y., H. X. Zhang, Y. P. Sun, Z. X. Liu, X. S. Liu, L. Wang, S. Y. Lu, H. Kong, Q. L. Liu, X. H. Li, Z. Y. Lu, S. J. Chen, Z. Chen, S. S. Bao, W. Dai, and Z. G. Wang. 2007b. Rig-I–/– mice develop colitis associated with downregulation of G α i2. *Cell Res* 17 (10):858–68.

Welch, H., and I. Maridonneau-Parini. 1997. Lyn and Fgr are activated in distinct membrane fractions of human granulocytic cells. *Oncogene* 15 (17):2021–9.

Wu, G. D., E. J. Lai, N. Huang, and X. Wen. 1997. Oct-1 and CCAAT/enhancer-binding protein (C/EBP) bind to overlapping elements within the interleukin-8 promoter. The role of Oct-1 as a transcriptional repressor. *J Biol Chem* 272 (4):2396–403.

Xiao, S., H. Jin, T. Korn, S. M. Liu, M. Oukka, B. Lim, and V. K. Kuchroo. 2008. Retinoic acid increases Foxp3+ regulatory T cells and inhibits development of Th17 cells by enhancing TGF-β-driven Smad3 signaling and inhibiting IL-6 and IL-23 receptor expression. *J Immunol* 181 (4):2277–84.

Yamanaka, R., C. Barlow, J. Lekstrom-Himes, L. H. Castilla, P. P. Liu, M. Eckhaus, T. Decker, A. Wynshaw-Boris, and K. G. Xanthopoulos. 1997. Impaired granulopoiesis, myelodysplasia, and early lethality in CCAAT/enhancer binding protein epsilon-deficient mice. *Proc Natl Acad Sci U S A* 94 (24):13187–92.

Yan, J., K. Wang, L. Dong, H. Liu, W. Chen, W. Xi, Q. Ding, N. Kieffer, J. P. Caen, S. Chen, Z. Chen, and X. Xi. 2010. PML/RARα fusion protein transactivates the tissue factor promoter through a GAGC-containing element without direct DNA association. *Proc Natl Acad Sci U S A* 107 (8):3716–21.

Ye, J., and J. M. Gimble. 2011. Regulation of stem cell differentiation in adipose tissue by chronic inflammation. *Clin Exp Pharmacol Physiol* 38 (12):872–8.

Ye, Q., J. H. Shieh, G. Morrone, and M. A. Moore. 2004. Expression of constitutively active Notch4 (Int-3) modulates myeloid proliferation and differentiation and promotes expansion of hematopoietic progenitors. *Leukemia* 18 (4):777–87.

Yen, A., and M. E. Forbes. 1990. c-myc down regulation and precommitment in HL-60 cells due to bromodeoxyuridine. *Cancer Res* 50 (5):1411–20.

Yen, A., and S. Varvayanis. 2000. Retinoic acid increases amount of phosphorylated RAF; ectopic expression of cFMS reveals that retinoic acid-induced differentiation is more strongly dependent on ERK2 signaling than induced GO arrest is. *In Vitro Cell Dev Biol Anim* 36 (4):249–55.

Yen, A., M. S. Roberson, S. Varvayanis, and A. T. Lee. 1998. Retinoic acid induced mitogen-activated protein (MAP)/extracellular signal-regulated kinase (ERK) kinase-dependent MAP kinase activation needed to elicit HL-60 cell differentiation and growth arrest. *Cancer Res* 58 (14):3163–72.

Yen, A., D. Brown, and J. Fishbaugh. 1987. Precommitment states induced during HL-60 myeloid differentiation: possible similarities of retinoic acid- and DMSO-induced early events. *Exp Cell Res* 173 (1):80–4.

Yen, A., M. Forbes, G. DeGala, and J. Fishbaugh. 1987. Control of HL-60 cell differentiation lineage specificity, a late event occurring after precommitment. *Cancer Res* 47 (1):129–34.

Yen, A., S. L. Reece, and K. L. Albright. 1984. Dependence of HL-60 myeloid cell differentiation on continuous and split retinoic acid exposures: precommitment memory associated with altered nuclear structure. *J Cell Physiol* 118 (3):277–86.

Yu, G., T. E. Smithgall, and R. I. Glazer. 1989. K562 leukemia cells transfected with the human c-fes gene acquire the ability to undergo myeloid differentiation. *J Biol Chem* 264 (17):10276–81.

Yukawa, K., T. Yasui, A. Yamamoto, H. Shiku, T. Kishimoto, and H. Kikutani. 1993. Epoc-1: a POU-domain gene expressed in murine epidermal basal cells and thymic stromal cells. *Gene* 133 (2):163–9.

Zarbock, A., T. L. Deem, T. L. Burcin, and K. Ley. 2007. Gαi2 is required for chemokine-induced neutrophil arrest. *Blood* 110 (10):3773–9.

Zempleni, J., R. B. Rucker, J. W. Suttie, and D. B. McCormick. 2007. *Handbook of Vitamins*, 4th ed. Edited by R. B. R. Janos Zempleni, John W. Suttie, Donald B. McCormick. Boca Raton, FL: CRC Press.

Zhang, N. N., S. H. Shen, L. J. Jiang, W. Zhang, H. X. Zhang, Y. P. Sun, X. Y. Li, Q. H. Huang, B. X. Ge, S. J. Chen, Z. G. Wang, Z. Chen, and J. Zhu. 2008. RIG-I plays a critical role in negatively regulating granulocytic proliferation. *Proc Natl Acad Sci U S A* 105 (30):10553–8.

Zhang, X., Z. Lian, C. Padden, M. B. Gerstein, J. Rozowsky, M. Snyder, T. R. Gingeras, P. Kapranov, S. M. Weissman, and P. E. Newburger. 2009. A myelopoiesis-associated regulatory intergenic noncoding RNA transcript within the human HOXA cluster. *Blood* 113 (11):2526–34.

Zhou, L., L. H. Shen, L. H. Hu, H. Ge, J. Pu, D. J. Chai, Q. Shao, L. Wang, J. Z. Zeng, and B. He. 2010. Retinoid X receptor agonists inhibit phorbol-12-myristate-13-acetate (PMA)-induced differentiation of monocytic THP-1 cells into macrophages. *Mol Cell Biochem* 335 (1–2):283–9.

Zhou, Y., X. Jiang, P. Gu, W. Chen, X. Zeng, and X. Gao. 2012. Gsdma3 Mutation Causes Bulge Stem Cell Depletion and Alopecia Mediated by Skin Inflammation. *Am J Pathol* 180 (2):763–74.

Zubiaur, M., O. Fernandez, E. Ferrero, J. Salmeron, B. Malissen, F. Malavasi, and J. Sancho. 2002. CD38 is associated with lipid rafts and upon receptor stimulation leads to Akt/protein kinase B and Erk activation in the absence of the CD3-zeta immune receptor tyrosine-based activation motifs. *J Biol Chem* 277 (1):13–22.

10 Vitamin D and Inflammation in Cancer
Emerging Concepts

Katrina M. Simmons, Wei-Lin W. Wang,
Martin P. R. Tenniswood, and JoEllen Welsh

CONTENTS

10.1 INTRODUCTION

Epidemiologic and laboratory data suggest that vitamin D protects against inflammation and reduces the incidence and severity of many types of cancer. The vitamin D receptor (VDR) is highly expressed in epithelial cells at risk for carcinogenesis (including those resident in the skin, breast, prostate, and colon) and in immune cells that infiltrate the tumor microenvironment and participate in tumor surveillance. In epithelial cells, activation of VDR by its ligand, 1,25-dihydroxyvitamin D (1,25D), triggers genomic changes that contribute to maintenance of differentiation via regulation of the cell cycle and apoptosis. Vitamin D also regulates inflammatory pathways and modulates cross talk between epithelial cells and immune cells in the context of cancer. Both epithelial and immune cells express the vitamin D metabolizing enzyme cytochrome P450 27B1 (CYP27B1), which enables autocrine generation of 1,25D from the circulating vitamin D metabolite 25-hydroxyvitamin D (25D), critically linking overall vitamin D status with antitumor and anti-inflammatory actions. In animal models, dietary vitamin D supplementation, chronic treatment with VDR agonists, and/or VDR deletion alters both inflammation and tumorigenesis in the skin, colon, prostate, and breast. Because VDR expression is retained in many human tumors, control of inflammatory signaling by vitamin D likely contributes to its ability to reduce cancer development or progression, but clinical data in this area are scarce. Collectively, these observations reinforce the need to further define the anti-inflammatory actions of vitamin D in both the epithelial cells at risk for cancer and in immune cell populations that populate the tumor microenvironment.

10.2   VITAMIN D BIOLOGY

There are two forms of vitamin D: vitamin D_2 (ergocalciferol, synthesized from ergosterol in yeast and fungi) and vitamin D_3 (cholecalciferol, synthesized from 7-dehydrocholesterol in the animal epidermis). Vitamins D_2 and D_3 are obtained from natural foods, fortified products, and supplements, and significant amounts of vitamin D_3 are synthesized in skin exposed to ultraviolet B (UVB) radiation. In animal systems, metabolic activation by cytochrome P450 enzymes is required for biological activity of both vitamin D_2 and D_3. Because the metabolism and activity of both forms of vitamin D are similar, the generic term "vitamin D" will be used for either D_2 or D_3 in this review. Hepatic hydroxylation of vitamin D by CYP2R1 and CYP27A1 (25-hydroxylases) generates 25-hydroxyvitamin D (25D), which is the most abundant circulating metabolite and accurately reflects an individual's overall vitamin D status. Although not itself biologically active, 25D serves as the precursor to 1,25D, the active metabolite. 1,25D is generated by CYP27B1 (1α-hydroxylase), a mitochondrial enzyme first characterized in renal proximal tubules but now known to function in many extrarenal tissues as well. During hypocalcemia, renal CYP27B1 is activated, resulting in elevated serum 1,25D, which acts as an endocrine factor to enhance calcium absorption and retention. Sustained increases in serum 1,25D are prevented through classical negative feedback mechanisms involving CYP24A1 (24-hydroxylase). Once normocalcemia is restored, renal CYP27B1 activity is suppressed, and CYP24A1 is activated, resulting in 25D conversion to 24,25-dihydroxyvitamin D (24,25D), a biologically inactive metabolite that is ultimately converted to calcitroic acid and excreted. In contrast to the renal enzyme, activity of the extrarenal CYP27B1 and CYP24A1 enzymes is regulated not by calcium status but by tissue-specific signals such as growth factors, cytokines, and disease states. 1,25D produced in extrarenal tissues acts as a paracrine or autocrine factor to regulate differentiation, proliferation, and immune functions.

1,25D exerts both genomic and nongenomic actions through the VDR (Haussler et al. 2011). The best characterized mechanism of action for the 1,25D–VDR complex involves heterodimerization with retinoid X receptor (RXR) and binding to vitamin D response elements (VDREs) in target genes to regulate transcription. 1,25D also mediates rapid, nongenomic actions on signaling pathways via membrane-localized VDRs concentrated at caveolae. VDR is highly expressed in virtually every cell type including epithelial cells (including skin, breast, prostate, and colon, which are at risk for carcinogenesis) and immune cells (such as macrophages and dendritic cells).

Extensive studies support the concept that 1,25D acts on epithelial cells to maintain the quiescent, differentiated phenotype and protect the epithelium against endogenous and exogenous stresses—actions that translate to reduced risk for carcinogenic conversion. More recently, the concept that the antitumor effects of vitamin D may also involve effects on accessory cells in tumors (i.e., immune cells, stromal cells, endothelial cells) has gained credence. This review will focus on the effects of vitamin D on cellular effectors and soluble mediators of inflammation in the context of tumorigenesis in colon, breast, prostate, and skin tissue.

10.3   VITAMIN D AND CANCER OVERVIEW

Epidemiologic and laboratory research indicates that the alterations associated with cancer development result from complex interactions between individuals' genetic makeup and their exposure to environmental risk factors. Based on data suggesting that environmental factors contribute substantially to overall cancer risk, attention has focused on exploiting specific lifestyle and dietary factors in cancer prevention strategies. Among dietary factors, vitamin D has been linked to cancer prevention in epidemiological, laboratory, animal, and clinical studies (Woloszynska-Read, Johnson, and Trump 2011). Although the epidemiologic evidence for cancer prevention by vitamin D is not entirely consistent, the strongest correlations have been observed for the common age-related solid cancers (i.e., skin, colon, breast, and prostate tissue). However, large-scale intervention trials to define the circulating 25D levels associated with the lowest cancer risk in humans have yet to be completed. Epidemiological studies indicate that maintenance of serum 25D levels above 40 ng/mL (100 nmol/L) correlates with reduced risk of breast, colon, and rectal cancer (Giovannucci 2011). Depending on an individual's sun exposure, age, sex, body weight, and baseline vitamin D status, supplements in the range of 2000–4000 IU daily may be necessary to maintain serum 25D above 100 nmol/L. Due to considerable individual variability, monitoring vitamin D status by serum 25D analysis is the most accurate way to determine the appropriate level and route of supplementation.

In human cell lines derived from normal epithelial tissues and cancers (including skin, colon, breast, and prostate), 1,25D and other VDR agonists induce cell cycle arrest, differentiation, apoptosis, and/or autophagy depending on the particular cell type, microenvironment, and activity of other signaling pathways (Matthews et al. 2010; Hoyer-Hansen et al. 2005; Kemmis et al. 2006; Pendas-Franco et al. 2007). Data from transformed mammary cells isolated from VDR-null mice indicate that the growth-inhibitory effects of 1,25D are mediated by the VDR (Zinser, McEleney, and Welsh 2003). However, the concentrations of 1,25D (10–100 nmol/L) required to mediate these anticancer effects are well above the physiological range and are associated with undesirable side effects in vivo. Based on these considerations, it is unlikely that 1,25D acts at the systemic level to regulate epithelial cell growth in vivo. Instead, the identification of CYP27B1 in skin, colon, breast, and prostate epithelium supports the concept that locally generated 1,25D acts in an autocrine or paracrine manner to protect cells against transformation and/or slow cancer progression. In support of this concept, low circulating levels of the CYP27B1 substrate 25D are positively correlated with biomarkers and/or risk for prostate, colon, and breast cancer (Chen et al. 2010; Yin et al. 2010). Moreover, extrarenal expression of CYP27B1 appears to be of biological significance since locally generated 1,25D inhibited growth and induced differentiation of transformed keratinocytes in a xenograft model (Huang et al. 2002). In addition, loss of CYP27B1 in prostate cancer cells correlated with reduced sensitivity to 25D (Hsu et al. 2001).

10.4 IMPACT OF VITAMIN D ON IMMUNE CELLS

The effects of vitamin D on immune cells, including macrophages, dendritic cells, and T cells, have been well documented, but relatively few studies have focused on these actions in the context of cancer-associated inflammatory processes. VDR and CYP27B1 are expressed in monocytes, macrophages, dendritic cells, and activated B and T cells (Chen et al. 2007; Sigmundsdottir et al. 2007; Bikle 2011), and vitamin D treatment elicits cell type–specific effects as described below.

The maturation, proliferation, differentiation, and survival of dendritic cells are inhibited by 1,25D (Mora, Iwata, and von Andrian 2008; Guillot et al. 2010). In these cells, 1,25D also reduces the expression of human leukocyte antigen-DR (HLA), CD40, CD80, and CD86, which reduces their ability to present antigen and activate T cells (Fritsche et al. 2003). 1,25D also reduces the secretion of interleukin 12 (IL-12) and the proinflammatory cytokines (IL-1 and tumor necrosis factor α [TNFα]) and increases the secretion of IL-10 (Penna and Adorini 2000; D'Ambrosio et al. 1998; Guillot et al. 2010).

In contrast to dendritic cells, the differentiation and function of cells of the monocytic lineage are predominantly stimulated by 1,25D. 1,25D promotes the differentiation of monocytes to macrophages (as demonstrated by increased expression of macrophage markers such as CD14) and promotes phagocytosis (Helming et al. 2005). In mature macrophages, 1,25D decreases the secretion of proinflammatory cytokines (IL-1, IL-6, and TNFα) and the toll-like receptors (TLR2, TLR4, and TLR9) while increasing the production of the bactericidal peptide cathelicidin and the immunosuppressor prostaglandin E2 (Guillot et al. 2010). Mechanistically, 1,25D blocks monocyte/macrophage proinflammatory cytokine production via increasing signaling through mitogen-activated protein kinase (MAPK) phosphatase-1, which prevents lipopolysaccharide (LPS)-induced p38 activation (Zhang et al. 2012). 1,25D also inhibits the antigen-presenting properties of macrophages via reduction of major histocompatibility complex, class II (MHC-II) expression, which affects the activation of adaptive immune cells (Sadeghi et al. 2006; Dickie et al. 2010; Liu et al. 2006).

The activation and function of adaptive immune cells are, for the most part, inhibited by 1,25D—either directly or indirectly through antigen-presenting cells. 1,25D inhibits T-cell proliferation, recruitment, and function (Mora, Iwata, and von Andrian 2008). The VDR–RXR complex binds to the promoter regions of IL-2 and interferon gamma (IFNγ) to inhibit transcription, resulting in reduced cytokine expression (Alroy, Towers, and Freedman 1995; Rigby, Stacy, and Fanger 1984; Bhalla, Amento, and Krane 1986; Lemire et al. 1985; Reichel et al. 1987). The reduced production of IL-2 and IFNγ by T cells reduces their proliferation (function of IL-2) and recruitment (function of IFNγ). T helper (TH1) cell proliferation is decreased, while the production of TH2 cells is stimulated. TH2 cells secrete IL-4, IL-5, and IL-10, which further skews TH2-mediated immunity relative to TH1-mediated immunity. CD4+/CD25+ T regulatory cells (TREGs) are also promoted by 1,25D since 1,25D induces FoxP3 expression and IL-10 production (Penna et al. 2005; Daniel et al. 2008). TH17 production is also inhibited by 1,25D due to the reduction of IL-6 and IL-23 secretion from macrophages (Gregori et al. 2001). Lastly B cell proliferation, immunoglobulin production, and differentiation to plasma cells are also inhibited by 1,25D (Chen et al. 2007).

Given the well-documented and comprehensive effects of vitamin D on specific immune cells, it is highly likely that the complex interactions that occur between immune cells and tumor cells during carcinogenesis are modulated by 1,25D. However, the extent and significance of vitamin D signaling in the context of tumor inflammatory processes have been examined only in a few models, and mechanistic details are lacking.

10.5   INTRODUCTION TO INFLAMMATION AND CANCER

As originally defined by Hanahan and Weinberg, the "hallmarks of cancer" comprise six biological properties required for tumor development and progression. These properties include acquisition of autocrine proliferative signaling, immortality, angiogenesis, and invasion/metastasis coupled with resistance to negative growth regulators and cell death. Emerging data suggest that inflammation and evasion of immune destruction constitute additional hallmarks that accelerate the cancer process (Hanahan and Weinberg 2011). Cellular regulators and soluble mediators represent important contributors to inflammation in the tumor microenvironment, which enhances proliferation and survival of malignant cells, promotes angiogenesis and metastasis, and impairs adaptive immunity. Immune cells commonly found in the tumor microenvironment include T cells, dendritic cells, and tumor-associated macrophages (TAMs). TAMs primarily exert protumorigenic effects and are generally correlated with poor prognosis (Giovannucci 2011). Regardless of their cellular sources, specific cytokines and chemokines can either promote or inhibit tumor development and progression (Sun et al. 2011). Through activation of various downstream effectors, in particular, nuclear factor kappaB (NF-κB) and signal transducer and activator of transcription (STAT) transcription factors, proinflammatory cytokines have direct effects on cancer cell growth and survival and modify the tumor microenvironment to favor tumor progression (i.e., via promotion of invasion, angiogenesis, and metastasis).

10.6   TISSUE-SPECIFIC LINKS BETWEEN VITAMIN D,
INFLAMMATION, AND CANCER

The effects of vitamin D supplementation and VDR ablation have been extensively studied in relation to spontaneous and induced cancers of the skin, breast, prostate, and colon. As detailed below for specific tumor types, it is clear that dietary supplementation with vitamin D or administration of synthetic VDR agonists reduces tumor burden and/or tumor growth rates (Lamprecht and Lipkin 2001; Hussain et al. 2003; Murillo et al. 2007). Furthermore, VDR ablation in mice influences tissue proliferation and apoptosis (Zinser and Welsh 2004), enhances oxidative DNA damage, is associated with chronic inflammation, and enhances sensitivity to carcinogenesis triggered by chemical carcinogens or genetic mutations (Welsh et al. 2011; Kallay et al. 2001). Even though the effects of VDR deficiency are tissue specific, some common mechanistic links have emerged from these studies, including control of inflammation.

10.6.1 VITAMIN D AND INFLAMMATION IN COLITIS AND COLON CANCER

10.6.1.1 In Vitro Studies

The antiproliferative and prodifferentiating effects of 1,25D in colon cancer cells were recognized more than 20 years ago (Brehier and Thomasset 1988), and recent molecular studies have uncovered effects of vitamin D on the Wnt pathway and inflammatory signaling in the gut epithelium (Byers et al. 2011). The liganded VDR directly interacts with β-catenin to suppress its transcriptional activity, leading to inhibition of Wnt target genes, such as dickoff homolog (DKK)-4, in Caco-2 cells (Shah et al. 2006; Egan et al. 2010). In addition to direct effects of VDR on Wnt signaling in epithelial cells, 1,25D modulates heterotypic signaling between tumor cells and TAMs. Soluble factors released from TAMs activate Wnt signaling in cocultures of HCT116 colon cancer cells and THP-1 macrophages. IL-1β was identified as a macrophage-derived cytokine that stimulated Wnt activity and induced resistance to TNF related apoptosis inducing ligand (TRAIL)-mediated apoptosis in colon cancer cells (McCombie, Mason, and Damian 2009; Dixon et al. 2005). Activation of VDR by 1,25D in macrophages blocked the production of IL-1β and abrogated both Wnt activation and TRAIL resistance in the cocultured HCT116 cells. The inhibition of macrophage IL-1β secretion by 1,25D was VDR dependent and involved inhibition of STAT1 signaling. These studies demonstrated a unique mechanism whereby 1,25D exerts antitumor activity by interrupting cross talk between tumor epithelial cells and macrophages in the tumor microenvironment.

Factors that disrupt the integrity of 1,25D/VDR signaling at the level of the gut mucosa would be anticipated to increase the risk for gut inflammation and development or progression of colorectal cancer. Clinical data indicate that VDR is highly expressed in early-stage colon cancer but not in aggressive late-stage colon cancer (Palmer et al. 2004). The reduction in VDR expression during colon cancer progression has been linked to the upregulation of transcriptional repressors such as SNAIL, which directly bind and repress the VDR promoter (Larriba et al. 2009). In addition, changes in the vitamin D metabolizing enzymes CYP27B1 and CYP24A1 in advanced colon cancer favor catabolism of both 25D and 1,25D, limiting their effectiveness in growth control. In particular, aberrant expression and the occurrence of splice variants of CYP24A1 correlate with high proliferative rate in advanced colon cancers (Horvath, Khabir et al. 2010; Horvath, Lakatos et al. 2010). These tumor-associated changes in VDR signaling would be predicted to significantly impair the ability of vitamin D to control inflammation during the progression of both colitis and colon cancer.

10.6.1.2 In Vivo Studies

The effect of vitamin D on colon carcinogenesis in vivo has been studied in spontaneous, chemically induced, and genetic models (Raman et al. 2011; Byers et al. 2011). As early as 1992, it was reported that administration of 1,25D to mice prior to challenge with the colon carcinogen 1,2-dimethylhydrazine dihydrochloride reduced the development of colon adenocarcinomas by 50% (Belleli et al. 1992). Consistent with an antitumor effect of dietary vitamin D, chronic feeding of a vitamin D–deficient diet containing adequate calcium significantly enhanced the growth of MC-26 murine colon cancer xenografts (Tangpricha et al. 2005). In a more clinically relevant model, mice chronically fed with a Western-style diet containing low levels of both calcium and vitamin D spontaneously developed benign and malignant colonic tumors, which were inhibited by supplementation with dietary calcium and vitamin D (Newmark et al. 2009). Furthermore, mice fed with the Western-style diet exhibited increased circulating IL-1β, monocyte chemotactic protein (MCP-1), and regulated on activation, normal T cell expressed and secreted (RANTES), as well as tissue inflammation, which were largely prevented by supplementing the diet with calcium and vitamin D (Dissanayake, Greenoak, and Mason 1993).

Chronic inflammation in the gut promotes tumorigenesis in mice and is a risk factor for colon cancer in humans; thus, protection against intestinal tumorigenesis by vitamin D may involve anti-inflammatory mechanisms. In support of this concept, VDR-null mice were highly susceptible to intestinal inflammation induced by chemical irritants such as dextran sulfate sodium (DSS) (Kong et al. 2008; Froicu and Cantorna 2007) and developed severe chronic gut inflammation when crossed to IL-10–null mice, a model of inflammatory bowel disease (Froicu et al. 2003). VDR ablation also enhanced tumorigenesis in a genetic model of colon cancer driven by loss of the tumor suppressor adenomatous polyposis coli (APC), a negative regulator of Wnt signaling (Zheng et al. 2011; Larriba et al. 2011). A recent intriguing study demonstrated that inhibition of chemically induced inflammation, dysplasia, and carcinoma in the colon of rats by a probiotic agent was associated with upregulation of VDR expression (Appleyard et al. 2011). Collectively, these data link VDR to prevention of inflammation and carcinoma in colonic epithelium.

Multiple studies have examined the effects of VDR ligands on colon tumorigenesis in rodent models. Although mice are relatively resistant to the chemical carcinogen azoxymethane (AOM), development of preneoplastic lesions and carcinomas is enhanced if mice are pretreated with DSS to induce inflammation. In this AOM/DSS model, vitamin D analogs inhibited colitis, proliferation, and the development of preneoplastic aberrant crypt foci (Fichera et al. 2007; Wali et al. 2002). Mechanistically, vitamin D analogs such as Ro26-2198 inhibited the AOM/DSS-stimulated increases in c-MYC, COX2, and phospho-extracellular regulated kinase (pERK). More recently, the effect of dietary supplementation with vitamin D_3 or the circulating metabolite 25D has been studied in mice treated with AOM/DSS (Murillo et al. 2010). Both vitamin D_3 and 25D reduced the incidence of colon tumors by approximately 50% without adverse effects such as weight loss. Collectively, these data suggest a model whereby vitamin D and the VDR influence risk for carcinogen-induced colon cancer via effects on the development of inflammation in the gut; however, the involvement and responses of specific cell types remain to be determined. As discussed above, in vitro studies demonstrated that 1,25D acts on macrophages to block the release of IL-1β, which drives proliferation and survival of colon cancer cells (Dixon et al. 2005), yet this cross talk has not been explored in vivo.

The most commonly studied genetic model of colon tumorigenesis is the APC[+/−] mouse, which spontaneously develops intestinal tumors driven by loss of APC function and subsequent activation of the Wnt pathway. Interestingly, Western-style diets low in calcium and vitamin D (discussed above) accelerated the tumor phenotype of APC[+/−] mice, indicating that dietary and genetic modulation of intestinal tumorigenesis involves at least partially distinct and interactive effects (Yang et al. 2008). The first study to specifically examine the efficacy of vitamin D in this model where mice were fed with a standard rodent diet containing vitamin D found that chronic administration of 1,25D reduced total tumor load by approximately 50% but had no effect on the number of tumors (Huerta et al. 2002). A similar study using mice fed with a vitamin D–deficient diet found that 1,25D administration significantly reduced both the size and number of aberrant crypt foci and polyps (Xu et al. 2010). Although these data provide proof of principle that vitamin D signaling through VDR inhibits colon tumorigenesis driven by aberrant Wnt signaling, the intervention studies utilized 1,25D administered via injection rather than orally. No studies thus far have tested the impact of manipulating dietary vitamin D per se on tumorigenesis in APC[+/−] mice or the interactions between vitamin D signaling and inflammation in this model.

A small clinical trial recently examined the effects of calcium and vitamin D on biomarkers of inflammation in 92 colorectal adenoma patients (Mason, Chinn, and Crews 1987). The randomized, double-blinded trial compared plasma inflammatory markers in patients receiving 800 IU/day vitamin D_3 supplementation (with or without 2 g/day calcium) or placebo. After 6 months of intervention, vitamin D_3 supplementation was associated with decreases in plasma C-reactive protein (CRP), TNFα, IL-6, IL-1β, and IL-8 relative to placebo. There was no evidence of synergy between calcium and vitamin D_3 in regulation of inflammatory biomarkers. Vitamin D_3 supplementation reduced the combined inflammatory markers' z-score by 77% relative to placebo. These results are consistent with the laboratory and animal model data indicating that vitamin D reduces inflammation in colon cancer, but additional clinical trials are needed to confirm these findings.

10.6.2 Vitamin D and Inflammation in Breast Cancer

In primary cultures of normal human mammary epithelial (HME) cells, vitamin D signaling mediates growth arrest and induction of differentiation markers (such as E-cadherin), but apoptosis has not been observed (Kemmis et al. 2006). Our lab has recently conducted genomic profiling of HME cells and identified a number of 1,25D-responsive genes involved in immune responses, including CD14, cathelicidin, beta-defensin-1, macrophage colony stimulating factor (M-CSF), and IL-1 receptor-like 1. Using protein arrays and enzyme linked immunosorbent assay (ELISAs), we identified a series of cytokines whose secretion from HME cells was altered by 1,25D (CD14, IL-6, IL-15, IL-16, insulin like growth factor binding protein 4 [IGFBP4]). Interestingly, in the presence of 1,25D, LPS synergistically enhanced the secretion of some cytokines (IL-1β, IL-1α, chemokine X3 motif ligand 1 [CX3CL1]) while antagonizing the secretion of others (IGFBP4). These studies demonstrate that 1,25D controls the expression of immune regulatory genes and induces the secretion of numerous cytokines from normal mammary epithelial cells, indicating that it may influence inflammatory signaling in the tissue microenvironment both directly (on immune cells) and indirectly (through mammary epithelial cells). In support of the concept that vitamin D exerts anti-inflammatory signaling in the breast, we found that VDR-null mice developed chronic inflammation in the mammary gland (Welsh et al. 2011). Further studies are required to clarify the possible contribution of these immunoregulatory actions of vitamin D in normal mammary cells to chemoprevention of breast cancer.

Like normal mammary cells, most established breast cancer cell lines express functional VDR and undergo growth inhibition in response to 1,25D (Matthews et al. 2010). VDR agonists inhibit growth and induce regression of established human breast cancer xenografts in animal models (James et al. 1998; VanWeelden et al. 1998). Tumor cells derived from VDR-null mice were used to demonstrate that the VDR is necessary and sufficient for the antiproliferative effects of 1,25D (Zinser, McEleney, and Welsh 2003). Studies on xenografts derived from wild type (WT)- and VDR-null cells indicate that expression of functional VDR in tumor epithelial cells (rather than in accessory cells such as immune, stromal, or endothelial cells) is necessary for the antitumor effects of the vitamin D analog EB1089 and UV-generated vitamin D in vivo (Valrance et al. 2007). These data suggest a model whereby VDR agonists primarily mediate effects on the tumor microenvironment through actions on epithelial tumor cells.

In support of this model, systems biology approaches in breast cancer cells exposed to VDR agonists have identified a broad range of downstream targets (Swami et al. 2003; Lee et al. 2006; Byrne and Welsh 2007) involved in the cell cycle (cyclins, cyclin-dependent kinases, and their inhibitors), apoptosis/autophagy (BCL-2 family, caspases, cathepsins), and inflammation (NF-κB and COX2). While most research has focused on the antiproliferative and apoptotic effects of vitamin D signaling in breast cancer, a few studies have mechanistically examined the role of inflammatory processes, specifically, the role of prostaglandins and NF-κB. In MCF-7 breast cancer cells, 1,25D suppresses the expression of the prostaglandin-endoperoxide synthase 2 (PTGS2) that encodes the inducible isoform of cyclooxygenase, COX2, which is the rate-limiting enzyme in prostaglandin synthesis and a known target for cancer therapy. 1,25D also increases the expression of the 15-hydroxy prostaglandin dehydrogenase (15-PGDH) gene (15-PGDH), which degrades and inactivates prostaglandins. Thus, the net effect of 1,25D is inhibition of prostaglandin actions, which reduces inflammation and also disrupts estrogen synthesis since prostaglandins are major stimulators of aromatase gene expression.

Numerous studies have identified NF-κB as a target of vitamin D signaling in breast cancer. The RelB subunit of NF-κB regulates growth of mammary epithelium during pregnancy and is highly expressed in a subset of breast cancers, where it promotes survival via induction of antiapoptotic genes. In breast cancer cells with high RelB expression, 1,25D decreased the expression of RelB and its pro-survival targets (baculoviral IAP repeat containing 5 [BIRC-5], superoxide dismutase 2 [SOD2], and B-cell CLL/lymphoma 2 [BCL2]) while enhancing cellular sensitivity to gamma irradiation (Mineva et al. 2009). In MCF-7 breast cancer cells, 1,25D suppressed TNFα-mediated gene expression via inhibition of the transactivation potential of the RelA subunit of NF-κB (Tse et al. 2010). These and other data show that vitamin D consistently inhibits NF-κB signaling in breast cancer cells regardless of the specific subunits being expressed in different cells. The impact of vitamin D–mediated changes in prostaglandin and NF-κB signaling with respect to inflammation in the tissue microenvironment and disease progression in women living with breast cancer remains to be determined. However, a recent study demonstrated that serum 25D was inversely related to serum TNFα concentration in healthy women, supporting a connection between vitamin D status and inflammatory biomarkers.

10.6.3 VITAMIN D AND INFLAMMATION IN PROSTATE CANCER

Primary cultures derived from normal human prostate and many established prostate cancer cell lines express VDR and undergo growth inhibition in response to 1,25D. In primary cultures of human prostate cells, 1,25D inhibited TNFα-stimulated IL-6 production, suggesting anti-inflammatory actions (Nonn et al. 2006). Consistent with these data, recent genomic profiling of the temporal changes induced by 1,25D in immortalized but nontumorigenic prostate epithelial cells revealed rapid suppression of NF-kB signaling and sustained reductions in proinflammatory media-tors (Kovalenko et al. 2010). In contrast, 1,25D treatment of progenitor/stem cells (PrP/SCs) isolated from murine prostate was associated with induction of the proinflammatory cytokine IL-1α, which was functionally linked to the antiproliferative effects and luminal differentiation induced by 25D and 1,25D in these cells. These divergent effects of vitamin D signaling in prostate cells from different lineages at specific stages of differentiation have yet to be fully explored mechanistically.

Specific anti-inflammatory effects of 1,25D that have been characterized in established prostate cancer cell lines include inhibition of prostaglandin synthesis and action through suppression of COX2, upregulation of 15-PGDH, and downregulation of prostaglandin receptors (Krishnan and Feldman 2011). 1,25D also downregulates the proinflammatory cytokine IL-8 secondary to inhibition of signaling through p38 stress kinase and NF-κB in prostate cancer cells. Growth of prostate cancer cells treated with 1,25D and nonsteroidal anti-inflammatory drugs is synergistically inhibited, indicating a functional link between regulation of inflammatory pathways and growth in these cells.

Emerging studies also indicate that vitamin D signaling interacts significantly with androgen signaling in both normal and cancerous prostate cells. Using genomic profiling of LNCaP prostate cancer cells treated with 1,25D ± testosterone, we identified over 250 genes that are synergistically modulated by the combination of the two steroids (Wang et al. 2011). A subset of these genes lack obvious androgen receptor (AR) or VDR binding sites in their promoter regions and appear to be regulated by 1,25D and testosterone indirectly through changes in microRNA (miRNA) abundance. David pathway analysis (Huang, Sherman, and Lempicki 2009) indicated synergistic actions of 1,25D and testosterone on genes associated with inflammatory responses, including chemokines and their receptors (chemokine (C-X-C motif) ligand 11 [CXCL11], chemokine (C-C motif) ligand 8 [CCL8], chemokine (C-X-C motif) receptor 4 [CXCR4]); cytokines (TNFα, IL-8); TLR path-way genes (TLR3, lymphocyte antigen 96 [LY96], CD14); transcription factors (FBJ murine osteo-sarcoma viral oncogene homolog [FOS], E74-like factor 3 [ELF3], interferon regulatory factor-7 [IRF-7]); downstream mediators (serum amyloid A [SAA2], SAA1); metabolic enzymes (NADPH oxidase 1 [NOX1], hemo oxygenase 1 [HMOX1], 15-PGDH); and acute-phase proteins (orosomu-coid [ORM1], ORM2, serpin peptidase inhibitor A3 [SERPINA3]). Synergistic upregulation of 15-PGDH in response to 1,25D and testosterone was confirmed by quantitative polymerase chain reaction (qPCR) in these studies (Wang et al. 2011). These data indicate that 1,25D regulates multiple facets of the inflammatory response in prostate cancer cells and that testosterone significantly influences both the growth-inhibitory and -immunoregulatory effects of 1,25D.

The capacity of VDR agonists to treat benign prostatic hyperplasia (BPH), a complex syndrome characterized by tissue overgrowth that includes an inflammatory component, has also been investigated (Adorini et al. 2007). Preclinical data demonstrate that VDR agonists not only reduce the growth component of BPH by inhibiting the activity of intraprostatic growth factors but also inhibit production of proinflammatory cytokines and chemokines by human BPH cells. The anti-inflammatory effects of VDR agonists have been demonstrated in murine models of autoimmune prostatitis. Although these studies offer proof of principle that VDR agonists reduce tissue inflammation when administered systemically, BPH is not considered a precursor lesion to prostate cancer. It is known that VDR deletion alters cell turnover and hormonal responsiveness in normal murine prostate tissue and increases susceptibility to prostate intraepithelial neoplasia (PIN) and tumorigenesis (Mordan-McCombs et al. 2010; Kovalenko et al. 2011); however, the possibility that inflammation contributes to or synergizes with these effects of VDR ablation in vivo has not been experimentally addressed.

10.6.4 Vitamin D and Inflammation in Skin Cancer

A recent unbiased systems biology approach to map genetic loci that underlie susceptibility to skin cancer linked the VDR to coordinated control of epidermal barrier function, inflammation, and tumor susceptibility (Quigley et al. 2009). Consistent with these findings, the skin of VDR-null mice exhibits abnormal barrier function, decreased differentiation markers, and impaired innate immunity. VDR-null mice are also highly sensitive to skin tumorigenesis triggered by chemical carcinogens or UV radiation (Zinser, Sundberg, and Welsh 2002; Ellison et al. 2008; Oda et al. 2009). In VDR-null animals, hyperplastic epidermis and carcinogen-induced tumors exhibit hyperactivity of the hedgehog pathway, which plays a critical role in epidermal stem cell fate determination (Teichert et al. 2011). Several additional mechanisms have been shown to contribute to the protective effects of vitamin D against UV-induced carcinogenesis. In Skh:hr1 mice exposed to UV radiation, administration of 1,25D reduces the accumulation of mutagenic cyclobutane pyrimidine dimers (CPDs), which are strongly associated with tumorigenesis, suggesting a role for vitamin D in optimizing DNA repair (Dixon et al. 2011). Chronic administration of 1,25D also inhibits the development of papillomas and squamous cell carcinomas in this model.

In addition to a role for VDR in regulation of keratinocyte differentiation and DNA repair, both VDR and 1,25D modulate inflammatory responses triggered by chronic UV exposure (Dixon et al. 2011; Ellison et al. 2008). 1,25D treatment was shown to minimize expression of the proinflammatory cytokine IL-6 and increase the anti-inflammatory cytokine IL-10 in epidermis exposed to UV. Interestingly, regulation of these cytokines by 1,25D in the skin is mediated in different cell types. 1,25D directly inhibits IL-6 expression in keratinocytes but stimulates synthesis and secretion of IL-10 by mast cells (Biggs et al. 2010). Furthermore, transplantation studies indicate that VDR in mast cells is required for 1,25D stimulation of IL-10 following UV exposure. VDR in mast cells was also required for optimal mast cell–dependent suppression of inflammation, local production of proinflammatory cytokines, epidermal hyperplasia, and epidermal ulceration associated with chronic UVB irradiation of the skin. Collectively, these data point to a complex role for VDR in the regulation of epidermal proliferation, inflammation, and tumorigenesis that involves several cell types and multiple mechanisms. Clarification of the underlying mechanisms of action, especially the role of inflammatory signaling, will likely provide insight into new strategies for prevention of human skin cancer, which, some data suggest, is inversely related to vitamin D status (Tang and Epstein 2011).

10.7 CONCLUSIONS

In summary, the VDR and CYP27B1 are highly expressed in epithelial cells and infiltrating immune cells of skin, colon, breast, and prostate tumors. Using distinct animal models, vitamin D signaling has been shown to inhibit the development and progression of spontaneous, induced, and genetically engineered forms of these common cancers. For several tissues, predictable changes in cancer incidence are induced during states of vitamin D deficiency and excess as well as with VDR deletion. Even under normal conditions, vitamin D signaling alters tissue homeostasis via effects on conserved pathways that regulate cell proliferation, differentiation, and/or survival. In addition, emerging data support the concept that vitamin D modulates the expression of proinflammatory mediators in epithelial cells and regulates the functions of immune cells such as macrophages within the tumor microenvironment. Importantly, the effects of vitamin D on tissue homeostasis are VDR dependent, and VDR agonists mimic the effects of natural vitamin D metabolites. A caveat to these findings is that sensitivity to vitamin D often becomes reduced as cancer progresses due to abrogated expression or activity of VDR and CYP27B1 in the epithelial compartment. Therefore, it appears that optimization of vitamin D status will most often be beneficial prior to cancer development or during the earliest disease stages rather than in advanced disease.

REFERENCES

Adorini, L., G. Penna, S. Amuchastegui, C. Cossetti, F. Aquilano, R. Mariani, B. Fibbi, A. Morelli, M. Uskokovic, E. Colli, and M. Maggi. 2007. "Inhibition of prostate growth and inflammation by the vitamin D receptor agonist BXL-628 (elocalcitol)." *J Steroid Biochem Mol Biol* no. 103 (3–5):689–93. doi: 10.1016/j.jsbmb.2006.12.065.

Alroy, I., T. L. Towers, and L. P. Freedman. 1995. "Transcriptional repression of the interleukin-2 gene by vitamin D3: direct inhibition of NFATp/AP-1 complex formation by a nuclear hormone receptor." *Molec Cell Biol* no. 15 (10):5789–99.

Appleyard, C. B., M. L. Cruz, A. A. Isidro, J. C. Arthur, C. Jobin, and C. De Simone. 2011. "Pretreatment with the probiotic VSL#3 delays transition from inflammation to dysplasia in a rat model of colitis-associated cancer." *Am J Physiol Gastrointest Liver Physiol.* no. 301 (6):G1004–13. doi:10.1152/ajpgi.00167.2011.

Belleli, A., S. Shany, J. Levy, R. Guberman, and S. A. Lamprecht. 1992. "A protective role of 1,25-dihydroxyvitamin D3 in chemically induced rat colon carcinogenesis." *Carcinogenesis* no. 13 (12):2293–8.

Bhalla, A. K., E. P. Amento, and S. M. Krane. 1986. "Differential effects of 1,25-dihydroxyvitamin D3 on human lymphocytes and monocyte/macrophages: inhibition of interleukin-2 and augmentation of interleukin-1 production." *Cell Immunol* no. 98 (2):311–22.

Biggs, L., C. Yu, B. Fedoric, A. F. Lopez, S. J. Galli, and M. A. Grimbaldeston. 2010. "Evidence that vitamin D(3) promotes mast cell-dependent reduction of chronic UVB-induced skin pathology in mice." *J Exp Med* no. 207 (3):455–63. doi: jem.20091725 [pii]; 10.1084/jem.20091725.

Bikle, D. D. 2011. "Vitamin D regulation of immune function." *Vitam Horm Adv Res Appl* no. 86:1–21. doi: B978-0-12-386960-9.00001-0 [pii]; 10.1016/B978-0-12-386960-9.00001-0.

Brehier, A., and M. Thomasset. 1988. "Human colon cell line HT-29: characterisation of 1,25-dihydroxyvitamin D3 receptor and induction of differentiation by the hormone." *J Steroid Biochem* no. 29 (2):265–70.

Byers, S. W., T. Rowlands, M. Beildeck, and Y. S. Bong. 2011. "Mechanism of action of vitamin D and the vitamin D receptor in colorectal cancer prevention and treatment." *Rev Endocr Metab Disord.* doi: 10.1007/s11154-011-9196-y.

Byrne, B., and J. Welsh. 2007. "Identification of novel mediators of Vitamin D signaling and 1,25(OH)2D3 resistance in mammary cells." *J Steroid Biochem Molec Biol* no. 103 (3–5):703–7. doi: S0960-0760(06)00440-7 [pii]; 10.1016/j.jsbmb.2006.12.061.

Chen, P., P. Hy, D. Xie, Y. Qin, F. Wang, and H. Wang. 2010. "Meta-analysis of vitamin D, calcium and the prevention of breast cancer." *Breast Cancer Res Treatment* no. 121:469–77.

Chen, S., G. P. Sims, X. X. Chen, Y. Y. Gu, S. Chen, and P. E. Lipsky. 2007. "Modulatory effects of 1,25-dihydroxyvitamin D3 on human B cell differentiation." *J Immunol* no. 179 (3):1634–47.

D'Ambrosio, D., M. Cippitelli, M. G. Cocciolo, D. Mazzeo, P. Di Lucia, R. Lang, F. Sinigaglia, and P. Panina-Bordignon. 1998. "Inhibition of IL-12 production by 1,25-dihydroxyvitamin D3. Involvement of NF-kappaB downregulation in transcriptional repression of the p40 gene." *J Clin Invest* no. 101 (1):252–62. doi: 10.1172/JCI1050.

Daniel, C., N. A. Sartory, N. Zahn, H. H. Radeke, and J. M. Stein. 2008. "Immune modulatory treatment of trinitrobenzene sulfonic acid colitis with calcitriol is associated with a change of a T helper (Th) 1/Th17 to a Th2 and regulatory T cell profile." *J Pharmacol Exp Ther* no. 324 (1):23–33. doi: 10.1124/jpet.107.127209.

Dickie, L. J., L. D. Church, L. R. Coulthard, R. J. Mathews, P. Emery, and M. F. McDermott. 2010. "Vitamin D3 down-regulates intracellular Toll-like receptor 9 expression and Toll-like receptor 9-induced IL-6 production in human monocytes." *Rheumatology (Oxford)* no. 49 (8):1466–71. doi: 10.1093/rheumatology/keq124.

Dissanayake, N. S., G. E. Greenoak, and R. S. Mason. 1993. "Effects of ultraviolet irradiation on human skin-derived epidermal cells in vitro." *J Cell Physiol* no. 157 (1):119–27. doi: 10.1002/jcp.1041570116.

Dixon, K. M., S. S. Deo, G. Wong, M. Slater, A. W. Norman, J. E. Bishop, G. H. Posner, S. Ishizuka, G. M. Halliday, V. E. Reeve, and R. S. Mason. 2005. "Skin cancer prevention: a possible role of 1,25dihydroxyvitamin D3 and its analogs." *J Steroid Biochem Molec Biol* no. 97 (1–2):137–43. doi: S0960-0760(05)00231-1 [pii]; 10.1016/j.jsbmb.2005.06.006.

Dixon, K. M., A. W. Norman, V. B. Sequeira, R. Mohan, M. S. Rybchyn, V. E. Reeve, G. M. Halliday, and R. S. Mason. 2011. "1{alpha},25(OH)2-vitamin D and a non-genomic vitamin D analog inhibit ultraviolet radiation-induced skin carcinogenesis." *Cancer Prev Res (Phila)*. doi: 1940-6207.CAPR-11-0165 [pii]; 10.1158/1940-6207.CAPR-11-0165.

Egan, J. B., P. A. Thompson, M. V. Vitanov, L. Bartik, E. T. Jacobs, M. R. Haussler, E. W. Gerner, and P. W. Jurutka. 2010. "Vitamin D receptor ligands, adenomatous polyposis coli, and the vitamin D receptor FokI polymorphism collectively modulate beta-catenin activity in colon cancer cells." *Molec Carcinog* no. 49 (4):337–52. doi: 10.1002/mc.20603.

Ellison, T. I., M. K. Smith, A. C. Gilliam, and P. N. MacDonald. 2008. "Inactivation of the vitamin D receptor enhances susceptibility of murine skin to UV-induced tumorigenesis." *J Invest Dermatol* no. 128 (10):2508–17. doi: jid2008131 [pii]; 10.1038/jid.2008.131.

Fichera, A., N. Little, U. Dougherty, R. Mustafi, S. Cerda, Y. C. Li, J. Delgado, A. Arora, L. K. Campbell, L. Joseph, J. Hart, A. Noffsinger, and M. Bissonnette. 2007. "A vitamin D analogue inhibits colonic carcinogenesis in the AOM/DSS model." *J Surg Res* no. 142 (2):239-45. doi: S0022-4804(07)00118-7 [pii]; 10.1016/j.jss.2007.02.038.

Fritsche, J., K. Mondal, A. Ehrnsperger, R. Andreesen, and M. Kreutz. 2003. "Regulation of 25-hydroxyvitamin D3-1 alpha-hydroxylase and production of 1 alpha,25-dihydroxyvitamin D3 by human dendritic cells." *Blood* no. 102 (9):3314–6. doi: 10.1182/blood-2002-11-3521.

Froicu, M., and M. T. Cantorna. 2007. "Vitamin D and the vitamin D receptor are critical for control of the innate immune response to colonic injury." *BMC Immunol* no. 8:5. doi: 1471-2172-8-5 [pii]; 10.1186/1471-2172-8-5.

Froicu, M., V. Weaver, T. A. Wynn, M. A. McDowell, J. E. Welsh, and M. T. Cantorna. 2003. "A crucial role for the vitamin D receptor in experimental inflammatory bowel diseases." *Molec Endocrinol (Baltimore, Md.)* no. 17 (12):2386–92. doi: 10.1210/me.2003-0281; me.2003-0281 [pii].

Giovannucci, E. 2011. "The epidemiology of vitamin D and cancer risk." In *Vitamin D*, edited by D. Feldman, J.S. Adams and J.W. Pike. Academic Press, London.

Gregori, S., M. Casorati, S. Amuchastegui, S. Smiroldo, A. M. Davalli, and L. Adorini. 2001. "Regulatory T cells induced by 1 alpha,25-dihydroxyvitamin D3 and mycophenolate mofetil treatment mediate transplantation tolerance." *J Immunol* no. 167 (4):1945–53.

Guillot, X., L. Semerano, N. Saidenberg-Kermanac'h, G. Falgarone, and M. C. Boissier. 2010. "Vitamin D and inflammation." *Joint Bone Spine* no. 77 (6):552–7. doi: 10.1016/j.jbspin.2010.09.018.

Hahn, E. W., P. Peschke, R. P. Mason, E. E. Babcock, and P. P. Antich. 1993. "Isolated tumor growth in a surgically formed skin pedicle in the rat: a new tumor model for NMR studies." *Magn Reson Imaging* no. 11 (7):1007–17. doi: 0730-725X(93)90219-4 [pii].

Hanahan, D., and R. A. Weinberg. 2011. "Hallmarks of cancer: the next generation." *Cell* no. 144 (5):646–74. doi: 10.1016/j.cell.2011.02.013.

Haussler, M. R., P. W. Jurutka, M. Mizwicki, and A. W. Norman. 2011. "Vitamin D receptor (VDR)-mediated actions of 1alpha,25(OH)vitamin D: genomic and non-genomic mechanisms." *Best Pract Res Clin Endocrinol Metab* no. 25 (4):543–59. doi: 10.1016/j.beem.2011.05.010.

Helming, L., J. Bose, J. Ehrchen, S. Schiebe, T. Frahm, R. Geffers, M. Probst-Kepper, R. Balling, and A. Lengeling. 2005. "1alpha,25-Dihydroxyvitamin D3 is a potent suppressor of interferon gamma-mediated macrophage activation." *Blood* no. 106 (13):4351–8. doi: 10.1182/blood-2005-03-1029.

Horvath, H. C., Z. Khabir, T. Nittke, S. Gruber, G. Speer, T. Manhardt, E. Bonner, and E. Kallay. 2010. "CYP24A1 splice variants—implications for the antitumorigenic actions of 1,25-(OH)2D3 in colorectal cancer." *J Steroid Biochem Molec Biol* no. 121 (1–2):76–9. doi: S0960-0760(10)00179-2 [pii]; 10.1016/j.jsbmb.2010.03.080.

Horvath, H. C., P. Lakatos, J. P. Kosa, K. Bacsi, K. Borka, G. Bises, T. Nittke, P. A. Hershberger, G. Speer, and E. Kallay. 2010. "The candidate oncogene CYP24A1: a potential biomarker for colorectal tumorigenesis." *J Histochem Cytochem* no. 58 (3):277–85. doi: jhc.2009.954339 [pii]; 10.1369/jhc.2009.954339.

Hoyer-Hansen, M., L. Bastholm, I. S. Mathiasen, F. Elling, and M. Jaattela. 2005. "Vitamin D analog EB1089 triggers dramatic lysosomal changes and Beclin 1-mediated autophagic cell death." *Cell Death Different* no. 12 (10):1297–309. doi: 4401651 [pii]; 10.1038/sj.cdd.4401651.

Hsu, J. Y., D. Feldman, J. E. McNeal, and D. M. Peehl. 2001. "Reduced 1alpha-hydroxylase activity in human prostate cancer cells correlates with decreased susceptibility to 25-hydroxyvitamin D3-induced growth inhibition." *Cancer Res* no. 61 (7):2852–6.

Huang, D. C., V. Papavasiliou, J. S. Rhim, R. L. Horst, and R. Kremer. 2002. "Targeted disruption of the 25-hydroxyvitamin D3 1alpha-hydroxylase gene in ras-transformed keratinocytes demonstrates that locally produced 1alpha,25-dihydroxyvitamin D3 suppresses growth and induces differentiation in an autocrine fashion." *Mol Cancer Res* no. 1 (1):56–67.

Huang, D. W., B. T. Sherman, and R. A. Lempicki. 2009. "Bioinformatics enrichment tools: paths toward the comprehensive functional analysis of large gene lists." *Nucleic Acids Res* no. 37 (1):1–13. doi: 10.1093/nar/gkn923.

Huerta, S., R. W. Irwin, D. Heber, V. L. Go, H. P. Koeffler, M. R. Uskokovic, and D. M. Harris. 2002. "1alpha,25-(OH)(2)-D(3) and its synthetic analogue decrease tumor load in the Apc(min) Mouse." *Cancer Res* no. 62 (3):741–6.

Hussain, E. A., R. R. Mehta, R. Ray, T. K. Das Gupta, and R. G. Mehta. 2003. "Efficacy and mechanism of action of 1alpha-hydroxy-24-ethyl-cholecalciferol (1alpha[OH]D5) in breast cancer prevention and therapy." *Recent Results Cancer Res Fortschritte Der Krebsforschung. Progres Dans Les Recherches Sur Le Cancer* no. 164:393–411.

James, S.Y., E. Mercer, M. Brady, L. Binderup, and K. W. Colston. 1998. "EB1089, a synthetic analogue of vitamin D, induces apoptosis in breast cancer cells in vivo and in vitro." *Br J Pharmacol* no. 125 (5):953–62.

Kallay, E., P. Pietschmann, S. Toyokuni, E. Bajna, P. Hahn, K. Mazzucco, C. Bieglmayer, S. Kato, and H.S. Cross. 2001. "Characterization of a vitamin D receptor knockout mouse as a model of colorectal hyperproliferation and DNA damage." *Carcinogenesis* no. 22 (9):1429–35.

Kemmis, C. M., S. M. Salvador, K. M. Smith, and J. Welsh. 2006. "Human mammary epithelial cells express CYP27B1 and are growth inhibited by 25-hydroxyvitamin D-3, the major circulating form of vitamin D-3." *J Nutr* no. 136 (4):887–92. doi: 136/4/887 [pii].

Kong, J., Z. Zhang, M. W. Musch, G. Ning, J. Sun, J. Hart, M. Bissonnette, and Y. C. Li. 2008. "Novel role of the vitamin D receptor in maintaining the integrity of the intestinal mucosal barrier." *Am J Physiol Gastrointest Liver Physiol* no. 294 (1):G208–16. doi: 00398.2007 [pii]; 10.1152/ajpgi.00398.2007.

Kovalenko, P. L., Z. Zhang, J. G. Yu, Y. Li, S. K. Clinton, and J. C. Fleet. 2011. "Dietary vitamin D and vitamin D receptor level modulate epithelial cell proliferation and apoptosis in the prostate." *Cancer Prev Res (Phila)* 1617–25. doi: 1940-6207.CAPR-11-0035 [pii]; 10.1158/1940-6207.CAPR-11-0035.

Kovalenko, P. L., Z. Zhang, M. Cui, S. K. Clinton, and J. C. Fleet. 2010. "1,25 dihydroxyvitamin D-mediated orchestration of anticancer, transcript-level effects in the immortalized, non-transformed prostate epithelial cell line, RWPE1." *BMC Genom* no. 11:26. doi: 1471-2164-11-26 [pii]; 10.1186/1471-2164-11-26.

Krishnan, A. V., and D. Feldman. 2011. "Mechanisms of the anti-cancer and anti-inflammatory actions of vitamin D." *Annu Rev Pharmacol Toxicol* no. 51:311–36. doi: 10.1146/annurev-pharmtox-010510-100611.

Lamprecht, S. A., and M. Lipkin. 2001. "Cellular mechanisms of calcium and vitamin D in the inhibition of colorectal carcinogenesis." *Ann N Y Acad Sci* no. 952:73–87.

Larriba, M. J., P. Ordonez-Moran, I. Chicote, G. Martin-Fernandez, I. Puig, A. Munoz, and H. G. Palmer. 2011. "Vitamin D receptor deficiency enhances Wnt/beta-catenin signaling and tumor burden in colon cancer." *PLoS One* no. 6 (8):e23524. doi: 10.1371/journal.pone.0023524; PONE-D-11-05092 [pii].

Larriba, M. J., E. Martin-Villar, J. M. Garcia, F. Pereira, C. Pena, A. G. de Herreros, F. Bonilla, and A. Munoz. 2009. "Snail2 cooperates with Snail1 in the repression of vitamin D receptor in colon cancer." *Carcinogenesis* no. 30 (8):1459–68. doi: bgp140 [pii]; 10.1093/carcin/bgp140.

Lee, H. J., H. Liu, C. Goodman, Y. Ji, H. Maehr, M. Uskokovic, D. Notterman, M. Reiss, and N. Suh. 2006. "Gene expression profiling changes induced by a novel Gemini Vitamin D derivative during the progression of breast cancer." *Biochemical Pharmacology* no. 72 (3):332–43. doi: S0006-2952(06)00264-4 [pii]; 10.1016/j.bcp.2006.04.030.

Lemire, J. M., J. S. Adams, V. Kermani-Arab, A. C. Bakke, R. Sakai, and S. C. Jordan. 1985. "1,25-Dihydroxyvitamin D3 suppresses human T helper/inducer lymphocyte activity in vitro." *J Immunol* no. 134 (5):3032–5.

Liu, P. T., S. Stenger, H. Li, L. Wenzel, B. H. Tan, S. R. Krutzik, M. T. Ochoa, J. Schauber, K. Wu, C. Meinken, D. L. Kamen, M. Wagner, R. Bals, A. Steinmeyer, U. Zugel, R. L. Gallo, D. Eisenberg, M. Hewison, B. W. Hollis, J. S. Adams, B. R. Bloom, and R. L. Modlin. 2006. "Toll-like receptor triggering of a vitamin D-mediated human antimicrobial response." *Science* no. 311 (5768):1770–3. doi: 10.1126/science.1123933.

Mason, R. T., J. W. Chinn, and D. Crews. 1987. "Sex and seasonal differences in the skin lipids of garter snakes." *Comp Biochem Physiol B* no. 87 (4):999–1003.

Matthews, D., E. LaPorta, G. M. Zinser, C. J. Narvaez, and J. Welsh. 2010. "Genomic vitamin D signaling in breast cancer: insights from animal models and human cells." *J Steroid Biochem Molec Biol* no. 121 (1–2):362–7. doi: S0960-0760(10)00160-3 [pii]; 10.1016/j.jsbmb.2010.03.061.

McCombie, A. M., R. S. Mason, and D. L. Damian. 2009. "Vitamin D deficiency in Sydney skin cancer patients." *Med J Aust* no. 190 (2):102. doi: letters_190109_fm-7 [pii].

Mineva, N. D., X. Wang, S. Yang, H. Ying, Z. X. Xiao, M. F. Holick, and G. E. Sonenshein. 2009. "Inhibition of RelB by 1,25-dihydroxyvitamin D3 promotes sensitivity of breast cancer cells to radiation." *J Cell Physiol* no. 220 (3):593–9. doi: 10.1002/jcp.21765.

Mora, J. R., M. Iwata, and U. H. von Andrian. 2008. "Vitamin effects on the immune system: vitamins A and D take centre stage." *Nat Rev Immunol* no. 8 (9):685–98. doi: 10.1038/nri2378.

Mordan-McCombs, S., T. Brown, W. L. Wang, A. C. Gaupel, J. Welsh, and M. Tenniswood. 2010. "Tumor progression in the LPB-Tag transgenic model of prostate cancer is altered by vitamin D receptor and serum testosterone status." *J Steroid Biochem Molec Biol* no. 121 (1–2):368–71. doi: S0960-0760(10)00161-5 [pii]; 10.1016/j.jsbmb.2010.03.062.

Murillo, G., V. Nagpal, N. Tiwari, R. V. Benya, and R. G. Mehta. 2010. "Actions of vitamin D are mediated by the TLR4 pathway in inflammation-induced colon cancer." *J Steroid Biochem Molec Biol* no. 121 (1–2):403–7. doi: S0960-0760(10)00098-1 [pii]; 10.1016/j.jsbmb.2010.03.009.

Murillo, G., D. Matusiak, R. V. Benya, and R. G. Mehta. 2007. "Chemopreventive efficacy of 25-hydroxyvitamin D3 in colon cancer." *J Steroid Biochem Molec Biol* no. 103 (3–5):763–7. doi: S0960-0760(06)00418-3 [pii]; 10.1016/j.jsbmb.2006.12.074.

Newmark, H. L., K. Yang, N. Kurihara, K. Fan, L. H. Augenlicht, and M. Lipkin. 2009. "Western-style diet-induced colonic tumors and their modulation by calcium and vitamin D in C57Bl/6 mice: a preclinical model for human sporadic colon cancer." *Carcinogenesis* no. 30 (1):88–92. doi: bgn229 [pii]; 10.1093/carcin/bgn229.

Nonn, L., L. Peng, D. Feldman, and D. M. Peehl. 2006. "Inhibition of p38 by vitamin D reduces interleukin-6 production in normal prostate cells via mitogen-activated protein kinase phosphatase 5: implications for prostate cancer prevention by vitamin D." *Cancer Res* no. 66 (8):4516–24. doi: 10.1158/0008-5472.CAN-05-3796.

Oda, Y., Y. Uchida, S. Moradian, D. Crumrine, P. M. Elias, and D. D. Bikle. 2009. "Vitamin D receptor and coactivators SRC2 and 3 regulate epidermis-specific sphingolipid production and permeability barrier formation." *J Invest Dermatol* no. 129 (6):1367–78. doi: jid2008380 [pii]; 10.1038/jid.2008.380.

Palmer, H. G., M. J. Larriba, J. M. Garcia, P. Ordonez-Moran, C. Pena, S. Peiro, I. Puig, R. Rodriguez, R. de la Fuente, A. Bernad, M. Pollan, F. Bonilla, C. Gamallo, A. G. de Herreros, and A. Munoz. 2004. "The transcription factor SNAIL represses vitamin D receptor expression and responsiveness in human colon cancer." *Nat Med* no. 10 (9):917–9. doi: 10.1038/nm1095; nm1095 [pii].

Pendas-Franco, N., J. M. Gonzalez-Sancho, Y. Suarez, O. Aguilera, A. Steinmeyer, C. Gamallo, M. T. Berciano, M. Lafarga, and A. Munoz. 2007. "Vitamin D regulates the phenotype of human breast cancer cells." *Differentiation* no. 75 (3):193–207. doi: S0301-4681(09)60115-8 [pii]; 10.1111/j.1432-0436.2006.00131.x.

Penna, G., and L. Adorini. 2000. "1 Alpha,25-dihydroxyvitamin D3 inhibits differentiation, maturation, activation, and survival of dendritic cells leading to impaired alloreactive T cell activation." *J Immunol* no. 164 (5):2405–11.

Penna, G., A. Roncari, S. Amuchastegui, K. C. Daniel, E. Berti, M. Colonna, and L. Adorini. 2005. "Expression of the inhibitory receptor ILT3 on dendritic cells is dispensable for induction of CD4+Foxp3+ regulatory T cells by 1,25-dihydroxyvitamin D3." *Blood* no. 106 (10):3490–7. doi: 10.1182/blood-2005-05-2044.

Quigley, D. A., M. D. To, J. Perez-Losada, F. G. Pelorosso, J. H. Mao, H. Nagase, D. G. Ginzinger, and A. Balmain. 2009. "Genetic architecture of mouse skin inflammation and tumour susceptibility." *Nature* no. 458 (7237):505–8. doi: nature07683 [pii]; 10.1038/nature07683.

Raman, M., A. N. Milestone, J. R. Walters, A. L. Hart, and S. Ghosh. 2011. "Vitamin D and gastrointestinal diseases: inflammatory bowel disease and colorectal cancer." *Therap Adv Gastroenterol* no. 4 (1):49–62. doi: 10.1177/1756283X10377820.

Reichel, H., H. P. Koeffler, A. Tobler, and A. W. Norman. 1987. "1 alpha,25-Dihydroxyvitamin D3 inhibits gamma-interferon synthesis by normal human peripheral blood lymphocytes." *Proc Natl Acad Sci U S A* no. 84 (10):3385–9.

Rigby, W. F., T. Stacy, and M. W. Fanger. 1984. "Inhibition of T lymphocyte mitogenesis by 1,25-dihydroxyvitamin D3 (calcitriol)." *J Clin Invest* no. 74 (4):1451–5. doi: 10.1172/JCI111557.

Sadeghi, K., B. Wessner, U. Laggner, M. Ploder, D. Tamandl, J. Friedl, U. Zugel, A. Steinmeyer, A. Pollak, E. Roth, G. Boltz-Nitulescu, and A. Spittler. 2006. "Vitamin D3 down-regulates monocyte TLR expression and triggers hyporesponsiveness to pathogen-associated molecular patterns." *Eur J Immunol* no. 36 (2):361–70. doi: 10.1002/eji.200425995.

Shah, S., M. N. Islam, S. Dakshanamurthy, I. Rizvi, M. Rao, R. Herrell, G. Zinser, M. Valrance, A. Aranda, D. Moras, A. Norman, J. Welsh, and S. W. Byers. 2006. "The molecular basis of vitamin D receptor and beta-catenin crossregulation." *Mol Cell* no. 21 (6):799–809.

Sigmundsdottir, H., J. Pan, G. F. Debes, C. Alt, A. Habtezion, D. Soler, and E. C. Butcher. 2007. "DCs metabolize sunlight-induced vitamin D3 to 'program' T cell attraction to the epidermal chemokine CCL27." *Nat Immunol* no. 8 (3):285–93. doi: 10.1038/ni1433.

Sun, Y., C. Kojima, C. Chignell, R. Mason, and M. P. Waalkes. 2011. "Arsenic transformation predisposes human skin keratinocytes to UV-induced DNA damage yet enhances their survival apparently by diminishing oxidant response." *Toxicol Appl Pharmacol* no. 255 (3):242–50. doi: S0041-008X(11)00266-3 [pii]; 10.1016/j.taap.2011.07.006.

Swami, S., N. Raghavachari, U. R. Muller, Y. P. Bao, and D. Feldman. 2003. "Vitamin D growth inhibition of breast cancer cells: gene expression patterns assessed by cDNA microarray." *Breast Cancer Res Treat* no. 80 (1):49–62.

Tang, J. Y., and E. H. Epstein. 2011. Vitamin D and skin cancer. In *Vitamin D*, 3rd ed., edited by D. Feldman, J. W. Pike and J. S. Adams. Elsevier. 1751–62.

Tangpricha, V., C. Spina, M. Yao, T. C. Chen, M. M. Wolfe, and M. F. Holick. 2005. "Vitamin D deficiency enhances the growth of MC-26 colon cancer xenografts in Balb/c mice." *J Nutr* no. 135 (10):2350–4. doi: 135/10/2350 [pii].

Teichert, A. E., H. Elalieh, P. M. Elias, J. Welsh, and D. D. Bikle. 2011. "Overexpression of hedgehog signaling is associated with epidermal tumor formation in vitamin D receptor-null mice." *J Invest Dermatol* 2289–97. doi: jid2011196 [pii]; 10.1038/jid.2011.196.

Tse, A. K., G. Y. Zhu, C. K. Wan, X. L. Shen, Z. L. Yu, and W. F. Fong. 2010. "1alpha,25-Dihydroxyvitamin D3 inhibits transcriptional potential of nuclear factor kappa B in breast cancer cells." *Mol Immunol* no. 47 (9):1728–38. doi: 10.1016/j.molimm.2010.03.004.

Valrance, M. E., A. H. Brunet, A. Acosta, and J. Welsh. 2007. "Dissociation of growth arrest and CYP24 induction by VDR ligands in mammary tumor cells." *J Cell Biochem* 101 (6):1505–19.

VanWeelden, K., L. Flanagan, L. Binderup, M. Tenniswood, and J. Welsh. 1998. "Apoptotic regression of MCF-7 xenografts in nude mice treated with the vitamin D3 analog, EB1089." *Endocrinology* no. 139 (4):2102–10.

Wali, R. K., S. Khare, M. Tretiakova, G. Cohen, L. Nguyen, J. Hart, J. Wang, M. Wen, A. Ramaswamy, L. Joseph, M. Sitrin, T. Brasitus, and M. Bissonnette. 2002. "Ursodeoxycholic acid and F(6)-D(3) inhibit aberrant crypt proliferation in the rat azoxymethane model of colon cancer: roles of cyclin D1 and E-cadherin." *Cancer Epidemiol Biomarkers Prev* no. 11 (12):1653–62.

Wang, W. L., N. Chatterjee, S. V. Chittur, J. Welsh, and M. P. Tenniswood. 2011. "Effects of 1alpha,25 dihydroxyvitamin D3 and testosterone on miRNA and mRNA expression in LNCaP cells." *Mol Cancer* no. 10:58. doi: 1476-4598-10-58 [pii]; 10.1186/1476-4598-10-58.

Welsh, J., L. N. Zinser, L. Mianecki-Morton, J. Martin, S. E. Waltz, H. James, and G. M. Zinser. 2011. "Age-related changes in the epithelial and stromal compartments of the mammary gland in normocalcemic mice lacking the vitamin D3 receptor." *PLoS One* no. 6 (1):e16479. doi: 10.1371/journal.pone.0016479.

Woloszynska-Read, A., C. S. Johnson, and D. L. Trump. 2011. "Vitamin D and cancer: clinical aspects." *Best Pract Res Clin Endocrinol Metab* no. 25 (4):605–15. doi: S1521-690X(11)00070-4 [pii]; 10.1016/j.beem.2011.06.006.

Xu, H., G. H. Posner, M. Stevenson, and F. C. Campbell. 2010. "Apc(MIN) modulation of vitamin D secosteroid growth control." *Carcinogenesis* no. 31 (8):1434–41. doi: bgq098 [pii]; 10.1093/carcin/bgq098.

Yang, K., S. A. Lamprecht, H. Shinozaki, K. Fan, W. Yang, H. L. Newmark, L. Kopelovich, W. Edelmann, B. Jin, C. Gravaghi, L. Augenlicht, R. Kucherlapati, and M. Lipkin. 2008. "Dietary calcium and cholecalciferol modulate cyclin D1 expression, apoptosis, and tumorigenesis in intestine of adenomatous polyposis coli1638N/+ mice." *J Nutr* no. 138 (9):1658–63. doi: 138/9/1658 [pii].

Yin, L., N. Grandi, E. Rawm, U. Haug, V. Arndt, and H. Brenner. 2010. "Meta-analysis: serum vitamin D and breast cancer risk." *Eur J Cancer (Oxford, England : 1990)* no. 46:2196–205.

Zhang, Y., D. Y. Leung, B. N. Richers, Y. Liu, L. K. Remigio, D. W. Riches, and E. Goleva. 2012. "Vitamin D inhibits monocyte/macrophage proinflammatory cytokine production by targeting MAPK phosphatase-1." *J Immunol* no. 188 (5):2127–35. doi: 10.4049/jimmunol.1102412.

Zheng, W., K. E. Wong, Z. Zhang, U. Dougherty, R. Mustafi, J. Kong, D. K. Deb, H. Zheng, M. Bissonnette, and Y. C. Li. 2011. "Inactivation of the vitamin D receptor in APC(min/+) mice reveals a critical role for the vitamin D receptor in intestinal tumor growth." *Int J Cancer* doi: 10.1002/ijc.25992.

Zinser, G. M., and J. Welsh. 2004. "Effect of Vitamin D3 receptor ablation on murine mammary gland development and tumorigenesis." *J Steroid Biochem Molec Biol* no. 89–90 (1–5):433–6. doi: 10.1016/j.jsbmb.2004.03.012; S0960076004000585 [pii].

Zinser, G. M., K. McEleney, and J. Welsh. 2003. "Characterization of mammary tumor cell lines from wild type and vitamin D(3) receptor knockout mice." *Molec Cell Endocrinol* no. 200 (1–2):67–80.

Zinser, G. M., J. P. Sundberg, and J. Welsh. 2002. "Vitamin D(3) receptor ablation sensitizes skin to chemically induced tumorigenesis." *Carcinogenesis* no. 23 (12):2103–9.

11 Vitamin E Family of Compounds and Cancer Prevention

*Kimberly Kline, Weiping Yu, Richa Tiwary,
and Bob G. Sanders*

CONTENTS

11.1 INTRODUCTION: BASIC INFORMATION ABOUT THE VITAMIN E FAMILY OF COMPOUNDS

Many excellent reviews have been published recently addressing present trends in vitamin E research and the possible roles of vitamin E in preventing cancer and inflammation (Dietrich et al. 2006; Sen et al. 2007; Constantinou et al. 2008; Brigelius-Flohe 2009; Aggarwal et al. 2010; Ju et al. 2010; Galli and Azzi 2010; Smolarek 2010; Mamede et al. 2011; Nesaretnam and Meganathan 2011; Traber and Stevens 2011; Kannappan et al. 2012).

Vitamin E is a fat-soluble vitamin that is naturally present in some foods, added by the food industry to others, and available in dietary supplements. It is a general term used indiscriminately to refer to a group of chemically related yet distinct, small bioactive lipids originally recognized and characterized by the essential role they played in rat reproduction (Evans and Bishop 1922). Eight different vitamin E compounds are synthesized by plants in various combinations and amounts, namely, alpha-, beta-, gamma-, and delta-tocopherol and alpha-, beta-, gamma-and delta-tocotrienol (Figure 11.1). In addition to these eight natural-source forms, α-tocopheryl phosphate, a phosphoric acid ester of RRR-α-tocopherol (RRR-α-T), has been found in foods, plants, and animal tissues (reviewed by Zingg et al. 2010). Synthetic vitamin E (*all-rac[emic]*-α-tocopherol, also referred to as DL-α-tocopherol) is made commercially for use in multivitamin/ mineral supplements and as a food additive. Synthetic vitamin E (*all-rac*-α-tocopherol) is a mixture of eight stereoisomers, only one of which (namely, RRR-α-T) is equivalent to a natural-source form (Figure 11.1).

At variance with past definitions and recommendations for vitamin E, the most recent committee for establishing Dietary Reference Intakes (DRIs) for vitamin E limited the definition of vitamin E to RRR-α-T and the 2*R* stereoisomeric forms (Institute of Medicine 2000). Thus, to achieve the Recommended Dietary Allowance (RDA) of 15 mg of α-tocopherol/day, individuals can consume 15 mg RRR-α-T/day or 30 mg of *all-rac*-α-tocopherol/day. It is important to note that the concept of α-tocopherol equivalence and conversion factors for the other tocopherol and tocotrienol forms of vitamin E in calculating α-tocopherol equivalence is no longer used. The Tolerable Upper Intake Level (UL) for vitamin E, which is set at 1000 mg α-tocopherol (1500 IU RRR-α-T)/ day for adults (males and females 19 years of age or older), includes any form of supplemental α-tocopherol (Institute of Medicine 2000). Commercially available acetate and succinate esters of either RRR-α-T or *all-rac*-α-tocopherol are manufactured to protect the labile hydroxyl (OH) group on the chromanol head of vitamin E, preventing its destruction (oxidation) and extending shelf life. These ester-linked acetate and succinic acid additions are removed readily by cellular esterases in the digestive tract, resulting in the release of the parent compounds for absorption. Genetic variance in esterase levels and activity among individuals may lead to varying levels of vitamin E among individuals taking the acetate or succinate derivatives. Additionally, a number of novel vitamin E derivatives and tocopherol or tocotrienol combinations have been produced and tested for anticancer properties in preclinical studies (reviewed by Neuzil et al. 2004; Tomic-Vatic et al. 2005; Wang et al. 2006; Zingg 2007; Constantinou et al. 2008; Ju et al. 2010). Thus, the vitamin E family of compounds and mixtures is quite varied, presenting a number of challenges to researchers interested in its anticancer properties, not the least of which is accurate citation of the precise form of vitamin E being tested. For example, both RRR-α-T and *all-rac*-α-tocopherol are frequently referred to simply as α-tocopherol without differentiating between these two markedly different chemical entities.

Despite the fact that vitamin E was discovered over 80 years ago, important fundamental basic information regarding the roles of the various vitamin Es in biology remains unknown (Brigelius-Flohe 2009). Although many theories have been proposed to explain the function of RRR-α-T, the form of vitamin E with the highest tissue bioavailability and greatest vitamin E activity, as defined using a rat fertility restoration assay (referred to as a rat resorption–gestation test), the most widely accepted explanation is that it acts in concert with other antioxidants in cells to prevent damage from oxygen radicals (Brigelius-Flohe 2009). Yet strongly held differing viewpoints persist, best summarized in the point/counterpoint articles by Traber and Adkinson (2007), suggesting vitamin E is an antioxidant and only an antioxidant, and the companion article by Azzi (2007b), suggesting functions that appear to be independent of antioxidant properties and based on regulation of various signal transduction events and gene regulation.

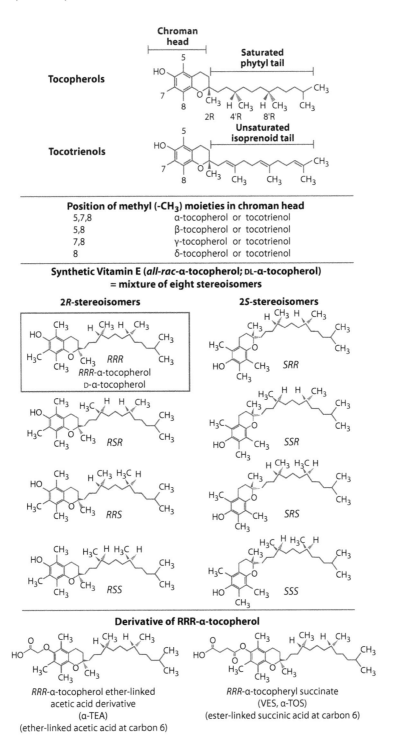

FIGURE 11.1 Vitamin E is a generic term used to refer collectively to structurally distinct yet similar small bioactive lipids. Chemical structures are given for natural-source vitamin E compounds (tocopherols and tocotrienols), commercially produced synthetic vitamin E, and two analogs of vitamin E: α-TEA (RRR-α-T–ether–acetic acid analog), also referred to as α-tocopheryloxyacetic acid in the literature, and RRR-α-T succinate (also referred to as VES [vitamin E succinate]). (Modified from Kline, K. et al., *Vitam. Horm.*, 76, 435–461, 2007.)

11.2 HUMAN INTERVENTION TRIALS ABOUT VITAMIN E'S ROLE IN CANCER HAVE LED TO NECK-SNAPPING NEWS: SOMETIMES PROTECTIVE, SOMETIMES NO SIGNIFICANT IMPACT, SOMETIMES DANGEROUS

Without a doubt, vitamin E meets the descriptor of an agent that produces "neck-snapping news." Multiple mixed outcomes from numerous epidemiological studies investigating the possibility of using vitamin E as a cancer chemoprevention agent have been reported in the literature (reviewed by Ju et al. 2010). For example, the Alpha-Tocopherol, Beta-Carotene Lung Cancer Prevention Study (ATBC), a randomized, controlled human intervention trial, asked the question of whether daily oral doses of vitamin E (50 mg DL-α-tocopherol acetate) or beta-carotene (20 mg), singly or in combination, would reduce rates of lung cancer in male smokers (The Alpha-Tocopherol, Beta-Carotene Cancer Prevention Study Group 1994). They observed an 18% increase in incidence and 8% increase in deaths from lung cancer in the beta-carotene group, a 34% decrease in incidence and 41% decrease in death from prostate cancer in the vitamin E group, and a small but statistically insignificant decrease in colorectal cancer in the vitamin E group (Virtamo et al. 2003). Results from the ATBC trial were a key consideration in the initiation and conduct of another randomized, controlled human intervention trial known as SELECT (selenium [200 µg/day of L-selenomethionine] and vitamin E [400 IU/day of *all-rac-*α-tocopheryl acetate] cancer prevention trial) involving supplementation of 35,533 relatively healthy men for more than 5 years (Klein et al. 2003). This study came to the conclusion that neither selenium nor vitamin E, alone or in combination, at the doses and formulations used, prevented prostate cancer (Lippman et al. 2009). In fact, the study was halted early, in part because the supplements were associated with a slight increase in the risk of prostate cancer and diabetes, coupled with the fact that no reduction in the incidence of prostate cancer had been observed. Recently, a longer follow-up study reported that compared with the placebo, the healthy men receiving the vitamin E supplementation had a significantly increased risk of developing prostate cancer (Klein et al. 2012). These mixed results showing success in heavy smokers but null or increased risk of synthetic *all-rac-*α-tocopherol acetate supplementation in healthy men have led to further confusion about the possible role of synthetic vitamin E in human health and certainly highlight the great gaps in our knowledge about synthetic vitamin E and mechanisms of action. A paper addressing the post-SELECT status of selenium and vitamin E for preventing prostate cancer points out that perhaps the most effective doses and formulations of these agents have yet to be tested and that improved understanding of selenium and vitamin E biology is needed in order to achieve this goal (Ledesma et al. 2011).

11.3 IMPACT OF VITAMIN E COMPOUNDS ON GENES THAT PROMOTE INFLAMMATION

Vitamin E compounds, especially the tocotrienols, have been shown to inhibit a variety of proinflammatory genes and mediators (reviewed by Aggarwal et al. 2010). One major regulator of proinflammatory responses that is inhibited by tocotrienols is nuclear factor kappaB (NF-κB). NF-κB is a transcription factor that promotes tumor development via increases in proinflammatory enzymes cyclooxygenase (Cox2) and inducible nitric oxide synthase (iNOS) as well as increases in proinflammatory cytokines interleukin 1 (IL-1), IL-2, IL-6, and tumor necrosis factor α (TNFα) (Gupta et al. 2011). Vitamin E compounds have been reported to inhibit both basal as well as stimulated levels of NF-κB activity in a variety of cell types (reviewed by Aggarwal et al. 2010). Vitamin E compounds have also been shown to suppress protein levels of Cox2 and iNOS and, subsequently, their products, prostaglandin E2 and nitric oxide (NO) (Table 11.1). Additionally, vitamin E compounds have been shown to reduce levels of inflammatory mediators IL-4, IL-6, and IL-8, as well as TNFα (Table 11.1).

Another key proinflammatory promoting factor that has been shown to be downregulated by tocotrienols is signal transducer and activator of transcription 3 (Stat3). Stat3, an acute-phase

TABLE 11.1
Mechanisms of Anticancer Actions by Vitamin E Compounds

Cellular Targets		Vitamin E Compounds	Cell Types/In Vivo Model	References
		Induction of Apoptosis		
Extrinsic Death Receptor Mediated Proapoptotic Pathway Mediators				
Fas (CD95) cell surface expression	↑	VES, α-TEA, δ-T3	Leukemia, breast, gastric ovarian prostate	*
Fas ligand expression	↑	VES, α-TEA	Breast, prostate	*
Fas ligand secretion	↑	VES	Prostate	*
Death receptor 4/5 (DR4/5)	↑	VES, γ-T, γ-T3, α-TEA	Mesothelioma, breast, colon	Yu et al. 2008a, 2010, Park et al. 2010, Tiwary et al. 2010, Kannappan et al. 2010a
TRAIL	↑	α-TEA	Breast	Yu et al. 2010
FADD associated with Fas	↑	VES, α-TEA	Gastric, prostate	*
Daxx associated Fas	↑	α-TEA	Prostate	*
Caspase-8 activation	↑	VES, γ-T, γ-T3, α-TEA	Gastric, breast, ovarian, prostate	* Yu et al. 2008a, 2010, Park et al. 2010, Yap et al. 2008, Tiwary et al. 2010
Intrinsic Mitochondrial-Mediated Proapoptotic Pathway Mediators				
Mitochondrial complex II	↓	VES	Leukemia	Dong et al. 2008, 2011
Mitochondria permeability transition	↑	γ-T, VES, α-TEA, γ-T3	Breast, gastric, leukemia, neuroblastoma	* Yu et al. 2008a, 2010, Zhao et al. 2010, Prochazka et al. 2010
Cytochrome c release	↑	γ-T, VES, α-TEA	Breast, ovarian, prostate, leukemia	* Yu et al. 2008, 2010
Bid activation (cleavage)	↑	γ-T, α-TEA, VES	Breast, ovarian, prostate, gastric	* Yu et al. 2008a, 2010, Zhao et al. 2010
Bax conformation change	↑	VES, γ-T, α-TEA	Breast, ovarian, prostate, lung	* Yu et al. 2008a, 2010, Prochazka et al. 2010
Bax translocation to mitochondria	↑	VES	Breast, leukemia, prostate	*
Bak conformation change	↑	VES	Breast, leukemia, lung	Prochazka et al. 2010
Bak translocation to mitochondria	↑	VES	Breast, lung, leukemia	*Prochazka et al. 2010
Bak binding with Bcl-2/Bcl-Xl	↓	VES	Prostate	*
Bak channel	↑	VES	Breast, lung, leukemia	Prochazka et al. 2010
B-cell lymphoma 2 (Bcl-2) protein	↓	γ-T, γ-T3, α-TEA	Breast, pancreatic, prostate	*Gopalan et al. 2012, Tiwary et al. 2010, Kunnumakkara et al. 2010, Yap et al. 2008

(*continued*)

TABLE 11.1 (Continued)

Mechanisms of Anticancer Actions by Vitamin E Compounds

Cellular Targets		Vitamin E Compounds	Cell Types/In Vivo Model	References
Bcl-xL	↓	γ-T3	MM, myeloid, gastric, hepatocellular	Kannappan et al. 2010b, Ahn et al. 2007, Manu et al. 2012, Rajendran et al. 2011
Mcl-1	↓	γ-T3	MM, hepatocellular	Kannappan et al. 2010b, Rajendran et al. 2011
Phospho-Bcl-2 (ser-70)	↑	VES	Prostate	*
NOXA	↑	α-TEA, VES	Breast, lung, leukemia	Wang et al. 2008, Prochazka et al. 2010
NOXA binding with MCl-1	↑	VES	Lung	Prochazka et al. 2010
Phospho-Bim EL	↑	VES	Prostate	*
Phospho-Bad	↓	α-TEA	Breast	Tiwary et al. 2011a
Phospho-caspase-9	↓	α-TEA	Breast	Tiwary et al. 2011a
Caspase-9 activation	↑	γ-T, γ-T3, VES, α-TEA TRF	Breast, ovarian, prostate, gastric nueroblastoma, colon, leukemia	* Tiwary et al. 2010, Park et al. 2010, Yu et al. 2008, 2010, Yap et al. 2008
Apoptotic Execution Phase Mediators				
Caspase-3 protein	↑	VES	Prostate	*
Caspase-3 activation	↑	γ-T, γ-T3, VES, α-TEA, TRF	Breast, colon, Leukemia ovarian, prostate, neuroblastoma	* Yap et al. 2008
Caspase-7	↑	γ-T, γ-T3	Colon, prostate	* Yap et al. 2008
Lysosomal Instability in Apoptosis				
Disability of lysosomal membranes	↑	VES	Leukemia	*
Cathepsin D	↑	VES	Leukemia	*
Reactive Oxygen Species (ROS) Mediated Apoptosis				
ROS generation/ Accumulation	↑	VES, α-TEA, γ-T3	Leukemia, neuroblastoma, endothelial, colon	* Dong et al. 2007, Kannappan et al. 2010a
Endoplasmic Reticulum (ER) Stress Mediated Apoptosis				
CHOP protein	↑	γ-T3, α-TEA, γ-T, VES	Breast, gastric	Park et al. 2010, Tiwary et al. 2010, Huang et al. 2010, Gopalan et al. 2012
Phospho-JNK	↑	γ-T3, α-TEA, γ-T, VES	Breast, gastric	Sook et al. 2010, Tiwary et al. 2010, Huang et al. 2010, Gopalan et al. 2012
ATF3	↑	γ-T3	Breast	Patacsil et al. 2012

(continued)

TABLE 11.1 (Continued)
Mechanisms of Anticancer Actions by Vitamin E Compounds

Cellular Targets		Vitamin E Compounds	Cell Types/In Vivo Model	References
Caspase-4 activation	↑	VES	Prostate, gastric	Malafa et al. 2006, Huang et al. 2010
Cytosolic Ca (2+)	↑	VES	Gastric	Huang et al. 2010
Phospho-p38	↑	α-TEA	Breast	Park et al. 2010
Ceramide Pathway Mediated Apoptosis				
Acid sphingomyelinase activation	↑	α-TEA, VES	Breast, leukemia	Li, J. et al. 2010
Increase in membrane ceramide	↑	α-TEA	Breast	Li, J. et al. 2010
Increase in de novo ceramide	↑	γ-T, γ-T3	Breast	Gopalan et al. 2012
Dihydrosphingosine/ dihydroceramide	↑	γ-T, γ-T3	Prostate	*Jiang et al. 2012
Blockage of Prosurvival Pathways and Antiapoptotic Mediators				
EGFR	↓	α-TEA, γ-T3	Breast, ovarian, prostate	Tiwary et al. 2011a, Shun et al. 2010, Yap et al. 2008
Her-2	↓	TE, α-TEA, VES, γ-T3, δ-T3	Breast, ovarian, pancreatic	*Tiwary et al. 2011a, 2011c, Shin-Kang et al. 2011, Shun et al. 2010
IGFR	↓	α-TEA	Breast	Tiwary et al. 2011a
Estrogen receptor-α/β	↓	α-TEA, *all-rac*-T, MT	Breast	*Tiwary et al. 2011c, Lee et al. 2009
Androgen receptor	↓	VES	Prostate	*
Phospho-Akt	↓	TE, α-TEA, γ-T3, δ-T3, VES, MT	Breast, ovarian, prostate, pancreatic, mammary tumor	*Jia et al. 2008, Tiwary et al. 2011a, 2011c, Shun et al. 2010, Shin-Kang et al. 2011, Lee et al. 2009
Phospho-ERK1/2	↓↑	VES, α-TEA, γ-T3, δ-T3	Gastric, breast, ovarian, pancreatic, colon	*Shin-Kang et al. 2011, Tiwary et al. 2011a, 2011c, Kannappan et al. 2010a, Bi et al. 2010
Phospho-mTOR	↓	α-TEA	Breast	Tiwary et al. 2011a
c-FLIP-L	↓	γ-T, α-TEA	Breast, prostate, ovarian	Tiwary et al. 2010, 2011c, Yu et al. 2008b, Shun et al. 2010, Jia et al. 2008
Survivin	↓	γ-T, γ-T3, α-TEA	Breast, ovarian, prostate, MM pancreatic, myeloid, hepatocellular	Jia et al. 2008, Shun et al. 2010, Yu et al. 2009, Tiwary et al. 2010, Gopalan et al. 2012, Kunnumakkara et al. 2010, Kannappan et al. 2010b, Ahn et al. 2007
IAP-1/IAP-2	↓	γ-T3	Pancreatic, myeloid	Kunnumakkara et al. 2010, Ahn et al. 2007
K-Ras	↓	VES	Breast, colon	*

(*continued*)

TABLE 11.1 (Continued)
Mechanisms of Anticancer Actions by Vitamin E Compounds

Cellular Targets		Vitamin E Compounds	Cell Types/In Vivo Model	References
XIAP	↓	γ-T3	Myeloid, gastric, hepatocellular	Ahn et al. 2007, Manu et al. 2012, Rajendran et al. 2011
TRAF-1	↓	γ-T3	Myeloid	Ahn et al. 2007
BFI-1/A1	↓	γ-T3	Myeloid	Ahn et al. 2007
Transcription Factor Mediated Apoptosis				
c-Jun	↑	VES, α-TEA, δ-T3, γ-T3	Breast, gastric, leukemia, prostate	* Yap et al. 2008
c-Fos	↑	VES	Breast	*
ATF-2	↑	VES, γ-T3	Breast, prostate	* Yap et al. 2008
AP-1 activation	↑	VES	Breast	*
Phospho-FOXO1	↑	α-TEA	Prostate	*
Nuclear translocation of Foxo3	↑	γ-T3, δ-T3	Pancreatic	Shin-Kang et al. 2011
p53	↑	VES, γ-T3	Mesothelioma, colon	* Kannappan et al. 2010a
p73	↑	α-TEA	Breast	Wang et al. 2008
Other Factors Associated with Apoptosis Outcomes				
Lipid raft disruption	↑	α-TEA	Breast	Tiwary et al. 2011c
TGF-β receptor	↑	α-TEA, δ-T3, VES	Breast	*
Protein kinase Cα	↓↑	VES, γ-T, δ-T3	Breast, leukemia, colon	*
Protein phosphatase 2A activity	↑	VES	Leukemia, colon	*
Phospho-Ask-1	↑	VES	Prostate	*
Phospho-MKK4/JNK	↑	γ-T3	Prostate	* Yap et al. 2008
GADD45β	↑	VES	Prostate	*
Autophagy	↑	γ-T3, γ-T	Prostate	Jiang et al. 2012
Inhibition of Cellular Proliferation/DNA Synthesis and Blockage of Cell Cycle				
DNA synthesis arrest	↑	α-T, β-T, γ-T, VES,	Breast, prostate, colon	*
p21	↑	VES, MT	Breast, colon, TRAMP mice mammary tumor	* Lee et al. 2009, Barve et al. 2010
p27	↑	VES, MT	Prostate, mammary tumor, TRAMP mice	* Lee et al. 2009, Barve et al. 2010
TGF-β	↑	VES, γ-T3	Breast, gastric, prostate	*Campbell et al. 2011
TGF-β receptor	↑	VES, α-TEA, δ-T3	Breast	*
E2F-1	↓	VES	Breast, mesothelioma	*
FGF-R2	↓	VES	Mesothelioma	*
FGF2	↓	VES	Mesothelioma	*
Oxidative stress	↑	VES	Mesothelioma	*
Erg1	↓	VES	Mesothelioma	*
PPAR-γ	↑	γ-T3, γ-T, MT	Colon, prostate, mammary tumor	*Campbell et al. 2009, 2011, Lee et al. 2009, Smolarek and Suh 2011

(continued)

TABLE 11.1 (Continued)

Mechanisms of Anticancer Actions by Vitamin E Compounds

Cellular Targets		Vitamin E Compounds	Cell Types/In Vivo Model	References
PPAR-γ activity	↑	γ-T, δ-T, MT	Breast	Lee et al. 2009
15-hydroxyeicosatetraenoic acid	↑	γ-T	Prostate	Campbell et al. 2009
Cyclin D1	↓	α-T, γ-T, VES, γ-T3	Prostate, breast, pancreatic, MM myeloid, gastric, hepatocellular	* Kunnumakkara et al. 2010, Kannappan et al. 2010b, Ahn et al. 2007, Manu et al. 2012, Hsieh et al. 2010b, Rajendran et al. 2011
c-Myc	↓	VES, γ-T3	Breast, pancreatic, myeloid	* Kunnumakkara et al. 2010, Ahn et al. 2007
Cyclin E	↓	α-T, γ-T, VES, MT	Prostate, TRAMP mice	* Barve et al. 2010
Cdk2/cdk4	↓	VES	Prostate	*
Cdk2/cyclin A complex	↓	VES	Breast	*
Phospho-Rb	↓	VES	Prostate, leukemia, breast	* Hsieh et al. 2010b
Induction of Differentiation				
c-Jun	↑	VES	Breast	*
ERK	↑	VES	Breast, leukemia	*
p21	↑	VES	Breast, leukemia	*
Id1	↓	γ-T3	Prostate	Yap et al. 2008, 2010a
Id3	↓	γ-T3	Prostate	Yap et al. 2008
Inhibition of Metastasis				
MMP-2	↓	γ-T3	Gastric	Liu et al. 2010
MMP-9	↓	VES, γ-T3	Gastric, prostate, pancreatic, myeloid	* Liu et al. 2010, Kunnumakkara et al. 2010, Ahn et al. 2007, Manu et al. 2012
TIMP-1, TIMP-2	↓	γ-T3	Gastric	Liu et al. 2010
E-Cadherin	↑	γ-T3	Prostate	Yap et al. 2008
γ-Cadherin	↑	γ-T3	Prostate	Yap et al. 2008
Snail	↓	γ-T3	Prostate	Yap et al. 2008
αSMA	↓	γ-T3	Prostate	Yap et al. 2008
Vimentin	↓	γ-T3	Prostate	Yap et al. 2008
Twist	↓	γ-T3	Prostate	Yap et al. 2008
ICAM-1	↓	γ-T3, δ-T3	Pancreatic, MM, macrophages, gastric	Kunnumakkara et al. 2010, Ahn et al. 2007, Manu et al. 2012, Qureshi et al. 2011b
VCAM-1	↓	γ-T3, δ-T3	Endothelial, macrophages	Theriault et al. 2002, Qureshi et al. 2011b
E-selectin	↓	γ-T3	Endothelial	Theriault et al. 2002

(continued)

TABLE 11.1 (Continued)
Mechanisms of Anticancer Actions by Vitamin E Compounds

Cellular Targets		Vitamin E Compounds	Cell Types/In Vivo Model	References
Inhibition of Angiogenesis				
HIF-1α	↓	δ-T3, γ-T3	Colon, gastric	Shibata et al. 2008a, Bi et al. 2010
Phospho-VEGFR	↓	γ-T3, δ-T3	Endothelial	Li et al. 2011, Shibata et al. 2009, Miyazawa et al. 2009
Phospho-Akt	↓	δ-T3	Endothelial	Miyazawa et al. 2009, Shibata et al. 2008b
Phospho-ERK	↓	δ-T3	Endothelial	Miyazawa et al. 2009, Bi et al. 2010
Phospho-p38	↓	δ-T3	Endothelial	Miyazawa et al. 2009
β-catenin	↓	γ-T3	Endothelial	Li et al. 2011
VEGF expression	↓	γ-T3, δ-T3	Pancreatic, colon, breast, MM myeloid, gastric, hepatocellular	*Kunnumakkara et al. 2010, Shibata et al. 2008a, Kannappan et al. 2010b, Ahn et al. 2007, Manu et al. 2012, Rajendran et al. 2011
VEGF release	↓	VES	Breast, glioma, gastric	* Bi et al. 2010
ROS	↑	α-TEA, VES	Endothelial, mesothelioma	Dong et al. 2007, Neuzil et al. 2007, Shibata et al. 2008b
MMP-9	↓	γ-T3	Endothelial	Li et al. 2011
Cyclin D1	↓	γ-T3	Endothelial, gastric	Li et al. 2011
EGF2	↓	VES	mesothelioma	Neuzil et al. 2007
Elimination of Tumor Initiating Cells				
	↓	γ-T3	Prostate	Luk et al. 2011
Anti-Inflammation				
5-lipoxygenase	↓	γ-T, δ-T, γ-T3	Neutrophils, leukemia	Jiang et al. 2011
Prostaglandin E2	↓	γ-T, δ-T, α-T3, δ-T3, TRF, MT	Macrophage, epithelial, monocytic, colon, mice, mammary hyperplasia	* Jiang et al. 2000, 2008, Jiang and Ames 2003 Mun-Li et al. 2009, Wu et al. 2008, Yang et al. 2010, Smolarek and Suh 2011
Leukotriene B4	↓	MT, γ-T, TRF	Colon, mice, rat	Yang, C.S. et al. 2010, Jiang and Ames 2003, Ju et al. 2009
Nitrotyrosine	↓	MT, TRF	Colon	Yang, C.S. et al. 2010, Ju et al. 2009
Cox-2 expression	↓	γ-T3, TRF, δ-T3, α-T3, MT	Pancreatic, monocytic, colon, myeloid Macrophages, hepatoma, mammary hyperplasia, gastric	Wu et al. 2008, Kunnumakkara et al. 2010, Shibata et al. 2008a,b, Mun-Li et al. 2009, Lee et al. 2009, Smolarek and Suh 2011, Manu et al. 2012, Qureshi et al. 2011b, Ahn et al. 2007

(continued)

TABLE 11.1 (Continued)

Mechanisms of Anticancer Actions by Vitamin E Compounds

Cellular Targets		Vitamin E Compounds	Cell Types/In Vivo Model	References
Cox-2 activity	↓	γ-T, δ-T	Macrophages, epithelial, lung	*Jiang et al. 2008
RNS	↓	γ-T	Human plasma, rat	Christen et al. 1997, Jiang et al. 2000, Jiang and Ames 2003
Peroxynitrite	↓	γ-T	Human plasma	Christen et al. 1997
iNOS	↓	TRF, δ-T3	Monocytic, macrophages	Wu et al. 2008, Qureshi et al. 2011a,b
NO	↓	γ-T3, TRF, δ-T3, α-T3	Macrophages	Mun-Li et al. 2009, Qureshi et al. 2011a,b
IL-1α/β	↓	δ-T3	Macrophages	Qureshi et al. 2011b
IL-6	↓	γ-T3, TRF, δ-T3, α-T3	Macrophages	Mun-Li et al. 2009, Qureshi et al. 2011b
IL-4	↓	TRF	Monocytic	Wu et al. 2008
IL-8	↓	TRF	Monocytic	Wu et al. 2008
TNF-α	↓	γ-T, TRF, δ-T3	Monocytic, macrophages, rat	Wu et al. 2008, Qureshi et al. 2011a,b, Jiang and Ames 2003b
Phospho-Stat-3 (Tyr-705)	↓	γ-T3	MM, prostate, pancreatic, hepatocellular	Kannappan et al. 2010b, Rajendran et al. 2011
Phospho-JAK1/JAK2	↓	γ-T3	Multiple myeloma, hepatocellular	Kannappan et al. 2010b, Rajendran et al. 2011
Phospho-Src	↓	γ-T3	Multiple myeloma, hepatocellular	Kannappan et al. 2010b, Rajendran et al. 2011
SHP-1	↑	γ-T3	Multiple myeloma, prostate, pancreatic, hepatocellular	Kannappan et al. 2010b, Rajendran et al. 2011
NF-kB	↓	VES, γ-T3, TRF, δ-T3, α-T3	Breast, leukemia, monocytic, gastric pancreatic, prostate, macrophage, lung hepatocellular	*Husain et al. 2011, Wu et al. 2008, Ahn et al. 2007, Qureshi et al. 2011a,b, Yap et al. 2008, Kunnumakkara et al. 2010, Mun-Li et al. 2009, Manu et al. 2012, Rajendran et al. 2011
TRAF1	↓	δ-T3	Macrophages	Qureshi et al. 2011b
KEAP1	↓	α-T3, γ-T3, δ-T3	Breast	Hsieh et al. 2010a
NRF2	↑	α-T3, γ-T3, δ-T3, MT, α-T	Breast, TRAMP mice, ACI rats, retinal	Hsieh et al. 2010a, Feng et al. 2010, Smolarek and Suh 2011

(*continued*)

TABLE 11.1 (Continued)

Mechanisms of Anticancer Actions by Vitamin E Compounds

Cellular Targets		Vitamin E Compounds	Cell Types/In Vivo Model	References
Immune Functions				
Dendritic cell vaccines	↑	α-TEA, VES, TRF	Mammary cancer cell line in mice	Ramanathapuram et al. 2005, 2006, Hafid et al. 2010
IFN-γ	↑	VES + TRAIL + dendritic, α-T, γ-T3, α-TEA, TRF + tumor lysate + dendritic	T lymphocytes, rat, splenocytes in mice Mammary cancer cell line in mice	Tomasetti and Neuzil 2007, Gu et al. 1999, Hafid et al. 2010, Hahn et al. 2011a
IL-12	↑	TRF + tumor lysate + dendritic	Splenocytes in mice	Hafid et al. 2010
Lymphocytes	↑	TRF + tumor lysate + dendritic TRF, α-T3, γ-T3, δ-T3	Splenocytes in mice	Hafid et al. 2010, Ren et al. 2010
IL-2	↑	α-T	CD4+ T cells from aged humans or mice	Molano and Meydani 2012
Sensitization of Tumor Cells to Killing by Other Anticancer Agents and Drugs				
Fas	↑	VES, α-TEA, α-T	Breast, ovarian, prostate	*
TRAIL	↑	VES, γ-T3, γ-T	Breast, leukemia, mesothelioma, colon	*Yu et al. 2008, Kannappan et al. 2010
Celecoxib	↑	α-TEA	Breast	*
Etoposide	↑	α-T	Prostate	*
Cisplatin	↑	α-TEA, γ-T3	Ovarian, hepatocellular	* Rajendran et al. 2011
5-Fluorouracil	↑	VES	Colon	*
Doxorubicin	↑	TE, VES, α-TEA, γ-T3	Gastric, breast, hepatocellular	*Tiwary et al. 2011b, Zhang et al. 2011, Rajendran et al. 2011
Trastuzumab (monoclonal to Her-2)	↑	α-TEA	Breast	Hahn et al. 2011b
Vitamin K3 + ascorbate	↑	VES	Prostate	Tomasetti et al. 2010
Gemcitabine	↑	γ-T3, δ-T3	Pancreatic	Kunnumakkara et al. 2010, Husain et al. 2011
Thalidomide	↑	γ-T3	Multiple myeloma	Kannappan et al. 2010
Paclitaxel	↑	VES	Lung, bladder cancer	Kanai et al. 2010, Lim et al. 2009
Atorvastatin	↑	γ-T3	Colon	Yang, Z. et al. 2010
Docetaxel	↑	γ-T3	Prostate	Yap et al. 2008, 2010b

(continued)

TABLE 11.1 (Continued)
Mechanisms of Anticancer Actions by Vitamin E Compounds

Cellular Targets		Vitamin E Compounds	Cell Types/In Vivo Model	References
Rapamycin	↑	α-TEA	Breast	Tiwary et al. 2011a
Tamoxifen	↑	α-TEA	Breast	Tiwary et al. 2011c
Capecitabine	↑	γ-T3	Gastric	Manu et al. 2012

Note: ↑ enhance; ↓ suppress; MT: mixed tocotrienol; TRF: tocotrienol-rich fraction from palm oil; α-T: RRR-α-tocopherol; γ-T: gamma-tocopherol; δ-T: delta-tocopherol; α-T3: α-tocotrienol; γ-T3: gamma-tocotrienol; δ-T3: delta-tocotrienol; TE: α-tocopheryloxybutyric acid; VES: vitamin E succinate or RRR-α-tocopheryl succinate; α-TEA: RRR-α-tocopherol acetic acid derivative; MM: multiple myeloma.

* This symbol denotes references that can be found in our earlier review paper (Kline et al. 2007).

response factor, plays important roles in promoting inflammation (Kunnumakkara et al. 2010). The active form of Stat3 (phospho-Stat3 at Tyr 705) is suppressed by gamma-tocotrienol (γ-T3) in several cell types (Kannappan et al. 2010b; Rajendran et al. 2011). The activity of Stat3 upstream activators Janus kinase 1 (JAK1), JAK2, and Src-1 is also suppressed by γ-T3, suggesting that γ-T3 suppresses Stat3 via inhibition of IL-6/JAK signaling (Kannappan et al. 2010b; Rajendran et al. 2011). Furthermore, data show that γ-T3 upregulates SH2 domain-containing inositol 5′-phosphatase-1 (SHIP-1), a tyrosine kinase phosphatase. Downregulation of SHIP-1 blocks the ability of γ-T3 to suppress Stat3, indicating that SHIP-1 plays a critical role in γ-T3's regulation of Stat3-mediated inflammation (Kannappan et al. 2010b; Rajendran et al. 2011).

In addition to inhibiting NF-κB and Stat3 signaling, tocotrienols have been reported to impact several other proinflammatory mediators. Hypoxia-inducible factor (HIF), a key transcription factor for hypoxia adaptation, plays an important role in proinflammatory responses via upregulation of Cox2 and acts cooperatively with NF-κB (Imtiyaz and Simon 2010; Koeppen et al. 2011). HIF-α levels are suppressed by γ-T3 and δ-T3 in colon and gastric cancer cells (Shibata et al. 2008a; Bi et al. 2010). Furthermore, γ-tocopherol has been demonstrated to enhance peroxisome proliferator–activated receptor-gamma (PPAR-γ) protein levels and activity via the formation of 15-S-hydroxyeicosatetraenoic acid, an endogenous PPAR-γ ligand (Campbell et al. 2009). Since ligand-activated PPAR-γ inhibits proinflammatory mediators Cox2, NF-κB, iNOS, IL-1β, IL-6, and TNFα, this is another mechanism whereby tocotrienols may inhibit inflammation (Kapadia et al. 2008). Vitamin E compounds that enhance PPAR-γ protein levels and activity are listed in Table 11.1. Taken together, accumulating data show that tocotrienols are potent anti-inflammation agents and that they exert their effects via multiple signaling events. Emerging data support an important role for the tumor microenvironment in tumorigenesis and how oxidative stress and inflammation contribute, and how vitamin E compounds, especially tocotrienols, can block these tumor-promoting events is clearly an area in need of additional experimentation.

11.4   VITAMIN E's AND THE VALUABLE INSIGHTS THEY HAVE GIVEN US INTO ABERRANT CANCER CELL SIGNALING PATHWAYS AND CANCER CELL DRUG RESISTANCE

Cancer development is a multistep process leading to a heterogeneous population of cells with disrupted survival and death signaling pathways that have been selected for enhanced survival and enhanced cellular proliferation under adverse conditions (Hanahan and Weinberg 2011). Cancers of different origins share characteristics of self-sufficiency in growth factors, insensitivity to growth-inhibitory signals, evasion of programmed cell death, limitless replication potential, sustained angiogenesis, tissue invasion and metastasis, ability to acquire stemness (tumor initiation and self-renewal), and ability to evade elimination by innate and adaptive immune systems (Hanahan and Weinberg 2011; Chaffer and Weinberg 2011). Thus, cancers provide a multitude of challenges to the discovery and development of dietary agents for prevention and treatment without causing adverse outcomes in normal cells and tissues. An even greater challenge is the discovery of dietary agents for treatment of aggressive relapsed cancers that have poor outcomes due to resistance to chemotherapeutics and the capacity to spread to distant sites (metastatic capability).

The discovery that certain members of the vitamin E group exhibit potent anticancer actions in a wide range of cancer types in preclinical studies conducted with both cancer cells in culture as well as animal models of cancer has led to investigations into vitamin E's anticancer mechanisms of action. As illustrated in Figure 11.2, various vitamin E forms have been shown to have a multitude of promising anticancer effects.

As summarized in Table 11.1, a number of different forms of vitamin E and cancer models have been used to better understand mechanisms of action. (Please note that this is not a complete listing of important studies. Those conducted prior to 2006 are not included since they were cataloged in an earlier review [Kline et al. 2007].) Unfortunately, like other dietary agents that elicit a multitude of intracellular outcomes, there is no clear understanding of the fundamental biological basis for this multitude of effects and no understanding of if or where the apical event occurs.

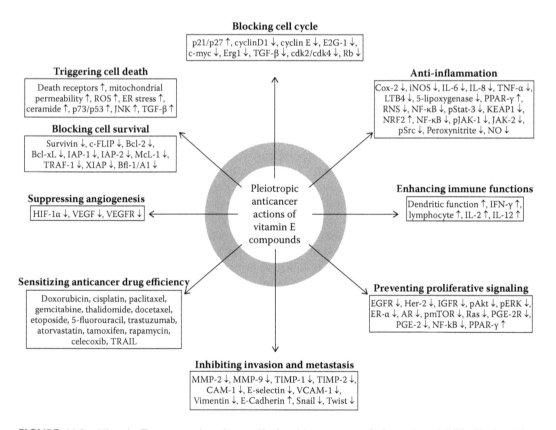

FIGURE 11.2 Vitamin E compounds enhance (depicted by arrows pointing up) or inhibit (depicted by arrows pointing down) a multitude of genes and proteins that are involved in cancer.

11.5 DUAL-ACTING VITAMIN E COMPOUNDS THAT SIMULTANEOUSLY TRIGGER PRODEATH SIGNALING AND BLOCK PROSURVIVAL/ ANTIDEATH FACTORS ARE POTENT ANTICANCER AGENTS

It is becoming increasingly clear that the efficacy of anticancer agents that target a single factor, for example, a single prosurvival signaling pathway mediator, is transient, with the development of treatment resistance often being the ultimate outcome. Failure of single-target agents is due, in part, to the genetic heterogeneity that exists within each tumor leading to enhanced expression of prosurvival mediators (e.g., growth factor signaling pathways and prosurvival/antiapoptotic mediators) and suppression of prodeath signaling (intrinsically and extrinsically mediated apoptotic signaling pathways). Agents that target only one arm of the dysfunctional signaling pathways are insufficient. Dietary anticancer agents, including anticancer-acting forms of vitamin E, that simultaneously suppress proliferation/prosurvival/antiapoptotic pathways and enhance prodeath signaling pathways show promise in the prevention and treatment of cancer (Tiwary et al. 2011c).

Emerging concepts in cancer are the following: (1) Tumors are composed of a small number of tumor-initiating cells (TICs), also referred to as cancer stem cells (CSCs), with the bulk of tumor cells being non-TICs. (2) TICs are resistant to killing by chemotherapeutics. (3) Bioactive dietary agents, including curcumin plus piperine (breast), sulforaphane (breast), and γ-T3 (prostate), show promise in the elimination of TICs (Kakarala et al. 2010; Li, Y. et al. 2010; Luk et al. 2011). An important question that often comes up is how do you think dietary agents can eliminate TICs when highly toxic chemotherapeutics do not? This is an important question that is actively being studied. One possible answer is that some dietary anticancer agents are dual acting, that is, they activate prodeath and inactivate prosurvival/antiapoptotic mediators—a one-two punch that is necessary for eliminating TICs. Investigation of the impact of vitamin E compounds on eliminating TICs is predicted to be a promising field of study.

11.6 CONTROVERSIES AND THINGS THAT CONTINUE TO PUZZLE RESEARCHERS AND THE PUBLIC

Here we will address a few of the controversies and questions that exist in the vitamin E field and offer our perspective.

11.6.1 CAN RRR-α-T AND THE TWO 2R STEREOISOMERS OF ALL-RAC-α- TOCOPHEROL BE BAD ACTORS IN CANCER PREVENTION?

As covered earlier in this review, supplementation of humans with *all-rac*-α-tocopheryl acetate (composed of four 2R stereoisomers and four 2S stereoisomers of α-tocopheryl acetate) gave conflicting results in two large randomized, controlled clinical trials, ATBC and SELECT (ATBC Study Group 1994; Klein et al. 2012). A daily dose of 50 mg *all-rac*-α-tocopheryl acetate in the ATBC trial protected against prostate cancer in male heavy smokers, whereas a daily dose of 400 IU increased the incidence of prostate cancer in healthy males in SELECT. One of several possible explanations proposed for the differences is the possibility that γ-tocopherol is displaced by large doses of α-tocopherol (Giovannucci 2000; reviewed by Dunn et al. 2010). Supplementation of diets with α-tocopherol is known to reduce serum concentrations of γ- and δ-tocopherol in humans (Handelman et al. 1985; reviewed by Devaraj et al. 2008). Since it has been estimated that approximately 70% of the vitamin E intake in the United States from unsupplemented diet is in the form of γ-tocopherol due to its abundance in corn, soybean, and canola oils (i.e., comprising 50% or more of total tocopherol forms found in these oils) (reviewed by Dietrich et al. 2006) and since γ-tocopherol has been shown to exhibit potent anticancer properties (reviewed by Ju et al. 2010), the possibility that 2R forms of α-tocopherol might reduce the bioavailability of γ-tocopherol (γ-T), especially in tissues, is clearly a gap in our knowledge that needs addressing. To further illustrate the possibility that RRR-α-T might be a bad actor in cancer, we have preclinical data in a human breast cancer xenograft nude mouse model that shows that the anticancer properties of γ-tocopherol are blocked by concurrent administration of RRR-α-T (Yu et al. 2009). γ-T levels in serum were significantly decreased in mice supplemented with RRR-α-T + γ-T in comparison to mice supplemented with only γ-T.

11.6.2 Does RRR-α-T Really Function as an Antioxidant In Vivo?

Although the conventional view is that vitamin Es function solely as lipophilic antioxidants that protect polyunsaturated lipids in membranes from peroxidation, a study by Roberts II and colleagues showed, in a dose-ranging study in humans using 0, 100, 200, 400, 800, 1600, or 3200 IU/day of RRR-α-T for 16 weeks, that the maximum suppression of a biomarker of systemic oxidative stress (plasma F2-isoprostane concentration) did not occur until 16 weeks of supplementation, and only the two highest doses, 1600 and 3200 IU/day, both of which exceed the current UL, showed a significant reduction in the stress biomarker (Roberts II et al. 2007). This study highlights the limitations of our current understanding of systemic oxidative stress and the role vitamin E plays in the antioxidant defenses (reviewed by Azzi 2007b).

Oxidation–reduction reactions occur rapidly and most likely within tightly conscripted locations within cells. Furthermore, it is known that in addition to the well-documented harmful outcomes reactive oxygen and nitrogen species play in biology, they also play critical beneficial cell-specific and cell-context–specific roles in signal transduction. These limitations in basic knowledge combined with technical limitations in accurately measuring biologically meaningful outcomes leave a critical gap in our understanding of the role various vitamin E compounds may play as lipid-soluble antioxidants (reviewed by Azzi 2007b).

11.6.3 How Bioavailable Are the Various Vitamin E Forms?

While γ-tocopherol, which is found in corn, soybean, canola, and sesame oils, walnuts, peanuts, and pecans, is the most common form of vitamin E in the US diet, it is typically found in plasma at 10 times lower concentrations than RRR-α-T (Giovannucci 2000; reviewed by Dunn et al. 2010). Although all dietary-source tocopherols and tocotrienols are reported to be equally absorbed from the gastrointestinal tract in chylomicrons, due to the presence of the RRR-α-T transfer protein (α-TTP) found in the liver, endogenous fat transport greatly favors RRR-α-T (Traber 2007). How various vitamin E forms are taken up and selectively retained by various tissues and cancer cells is unknown.

11.6.4 What about the Tocotrienols? Are They the Answer to Beneficial Anticancer Outcomes?

A recent extensive review of tocotrienols by Aggarwal et al. (2010) examined in detail the molecular targets of tocotrienols and their roles in cancer, bone resorption, diabetes, and cardiovascular and neurological diseases at the preclinical and clinical levels. Tocotrienols are found in the seed endosperm of monocots such as wheat, rice, barley, oats, and rye and are especially abundant in palm oil and annatto beans (Aggarwal et al. 2010; Nesaretnam and Meganathan 2011). Preclinical studies show that the anticancer effects of tocotrienols include inhibiting cell proliferation and inducing apoptosis (Sen et al. 2007). A tocotrienol-rich fraction (TRF) extracted from palm oil as well as individual tocotrienol forms have exhibited anticancer efficacy in human breast cancer, colorectal cancer, gastric adenocarcinoma, liver cancer, lung carcinoma, pancreatic cancer, and prostate cancers (reviewed by Park 2010). Dual mechanisms of tocotrienol anticancer actions include suppression of prosurvival/antiapoptotic mediators (i.e., phosphatidylinositol 3-kinase [PI3-K]/Akt and NF-κB signaling pathways) and activation of prodeath signaling mediators (i.e., transforming growth factor beta receptor II [TGF-βRII], Fas/cluster determinant (CD)95-, and c-Jun N-terminal kinase [JNK] signaling pathways) as well as induction of endoplasmic reticulum stress and upregulation of the extrinsic death receptor (DR)5 (reviewed by Aggarwal et al. 2010; Park 2010). Further studies on the anticancer potential of tocotrienols are clearly warranted.

11.7 WHAT ABOUT THE POSSIBILITY OF VITAMIN E DERIVATIVES AS POTENT ANTICANCER AGENTS? (SUBTITLE: CAN YOU IMPROVE ON MOTHER NATURE?)

Clearly, there is an unmet need for new strategies for prevention of primary cancers and prevention of cancer recurrence and metastases in survivors. The development and investigation of the anticancer efficacy of novel vitamin E–based derivatives is an ongoing endeavor by several labs (Neuzil et al. 2002, 2004; Lawson et al. 2003, 2004; Birringer 2003; Tomic-Vatic et al. 2005; Wang et al. 2006; Elnagar et al. 2010; reviewed by Kline et al. 2007; mini review by Constantinou et al. 2008; review by Zhao 2009). Here, we will review briefly the anticancer properties of two RRR-α-T derivatives, vitamin E succinate (VES) and α-TEA (please see Figure 11.1), and α- and γ-tocotrienol derivatives produced by attaching an ether-linked acetic acid at carbon 6 to α-tocotrienol (α-T3EA) and γ-tocotrienol (γ-T3EA) (Park 2010).

11.7.1 VES AND α-TEA DERIVATIVES

Both VES and α-TEA exhibit potent anticancer efficacy in several preclinical cell and animal models, whereas the parent RRR-α-T form from which they are synthesized is ineffective as an anticancer agent. VES has been shown to inhibit human breast cancer, colon cancer, and mesothelioma, and mouse melanoma, lung cancer, and mammary cancer in animal models when administered intraperitoneally (reviewed by Wang et al. 2006). Importantly, the anticancer efficacy of VES depends on the intact molecule. Thus, esterases, which hydrolyze the ester linkage to the C6 position of RRR-α-T (Figure 11.1), yield succinic acid and RRR-α-T, neither of which has been shown to possess anticancer efficacy (Anderson et al. 2004). In an effort to develop a clinically relevant RRR-α-T–based anticancer agent that can be administered orally, a nonhydrolyzable ether derivative, α-TEA, was developed (Figure 11.1) (Lawson et al. 2003; reviewed by Kline et al. 2007). α-TEA, when fed orally, has been shown to be effective at reducing tumor burden and metastasis in xenograft models of transplanted human breast and prostate cancer cells and in the syngeneic 66cl-4 and 4T1 syngenic murine mammary cancer models, as well as in mouse mammary tumor virus (MMTV)-polyomavirus middle T antigen (PyMT) transgenic mice and in ultraviolet (UV)-induced skin cancer mouse model (Lawson et al. 2003, 2004; Hahn et al. 2006, 2009; Wang et al. 2007; Jia et al. 2008b; Riedel et al. 2008). α-TEA has also been shown to enhance outcomes when combined with cisplatin in the treatment of cisplatin-resistant ovarian cancer cells both in vitro and in a xenograft model (Anderson et al. 2004), and in combination with antibodies to human epidermal growth factor receptor-2 in the 4T1 mouse mammary cancer model as well as in an MMTV-PyMT transgenic mouse model (Hahn et al. 2006, 2011a,b).

Importantly, α-TEA does not induce apoptosis in normal human prostate epithelial cells (PrECs) or normal human mammary epithelial cells (HMECs) and does not produce toxic side effects in animal models of cancer, making it an excellent prospect as a preventive and therapeutic agent (Anderson et al. 2004; Latimer et al. 2009; Hahn and Akporiaye 2011). Furthermore, limited toxicity assessments in normal mice show no signs of any major toxicity (Latimer et al. 2009; Hahn and Akporiaye 2011), and no genotoxic activity was reported when α-TEA was evaluated for bacterial mutagenesis in the *Salmonella–Escherichia coli* assay, for mammalian mutagenesis in mouse lymphoma cells, for chromosome aberrations in Chinese hamster ovary (CHO) cells, and for micronucleus induction in bone marrow (Doppalapudi et al. 2007). Our current understanding of α-TEA's mechanisms of action is that it is a potent inducer of apoptosis in cancer but not normal cells. This ability to induce apoptosis is the result of α-TEA triggering and amplifying both extrinsic and intrinsic prodeath pathways while simultaneously downregulating several key prosurvival factors. More specifically, α-TEA induces endoplasmic reticulum stress, activates prodeath mediators Fas/CD95 and DR5, and triggers mito-chondrial-dependent apoptosis by increasing Bax and decreasing Bcl-2 (Wang et al. 2008; Jia et al. 2008a; Tiwary et al. 2010). Additionally, α-TEA inhibits the expression of numerous prosurvival signaling pathway mediators including phosphorylated (active) Akt, HER-1, HER-2, and HER-3 as well as FADD-[Fas-associated protein with death domain] like IL-I beta [interleukin-1 beta]-converting enzyme (FLICE)-like inhibitory protein (FLIP) and survivin protein levels (Shun et al. 2010; Tiwary et al. 2011a). α-TEA acts cooperatively with both chemotherapeutic agents and signal transduction inhibitors (e.g., tamoxifen, rapamycin, PI3-K inhibitor [wortmannin], mitogen-activated protein kinase (MAPK)/extracellular signal-regulated kinase (ERK) kinase (MEK) inhibi-tor [U01260], fatty acid synthase inhibitor [C75], and lipid raft disruptor methyl-β-cyclodextrin [MβCD]) to induce apoptosis in cancer cells (Tiwary et al. 2011a,b). Recently, Hahn et al. (2011a) showed that α-TEA enhances the antitumor immune responses by enhancing levels of CD8 cytotoxic T cells. We credit the success of α-TEA's anticancer actions with the strength and duration of its simultaneous impact on prodeath and antisurvival mediators.

11.7.2 α-T3EA and γ-T3EA Derivatives

α-T3EA and γ-T3EA induce apoptosis in both a mouse mammary cancer cell line as well as human breast cancer cell lines (Park et al. 2010). Moreover, studies using human vascular endothelial cells in culture showed that the tocotrienol derivatives exhibited strong antiangiogenic activities, which were markedly improved over those of the parent compounds (Park 2010). When the tocotrienol derivatives were delivered in the diet, they significantly suppressed mammary tumor growth in a syngeneic mouse model (Park 2010). In conclusion, vitamin E derivatives (VES, α-TEA, α-T3EA, and γ-T3EA) have con-sistently demonstrated potent anticancer activities in a variety of human and murine cancer cell lines and animal models and appear to mediate their anticancer effects by similar mechanisms of action.

Our data support the hypothesis that anticancer forms of natural-source vitamin Es and derivatives are acting, at least in part, at the membrane level to inhibit cholesterol-enriched procellular division signal transductors and inhibit prosurvival mediators while simultaneously enhancing ceramide-enriched prodeath signaling. The exact nature of this dual "membrane effect" remains an enigma.

11.8 CONCLUSIONS

Many things about vitamin E remain puzzling. As concluded by the Institute of Medicine in 2000, when they were setting the DRI for vitamin E, there are no conclusive data supporting a preventive role for vitamin E in cancer (Institute of Medicine 2000). The question "To E or Not to E?" as posed by Friedrich (2004) remains a question, as does the question "If you E, what forms of E should you use, and how much and how often should you use it?" It is our sincere hope that current and future research into the biological actions of this interesting group of bioactive lipids leads to increased scientific knowledge and health benefits for humans in the near future.

ACKNOWLEDGMENTS

We would like to take this opportunity to acknowledge Kedar N. Prasad, Lawrence J. Machlin, Adrianne Bendich, Anita Roberts, Tom J. Slaga, L. H. Hurley, Dudley Dobie, and Lena Powers for their kindness and influence on our research over the years. Although too numerous to name, we gratefully acknowledge the contributions of all our undergraduate and graduate students, postdoc-toral fellows, research assistants and associates, visiting scientists, collaborators, and researchers who shared valuable reagents and cell lines. Finally, we would like to thank the American Institute for Cancer Research (AICR), Clayton Foundation for Research, US Government (the National Institutes of Health and the Department of Defense), and the University of Texas at Austin for their generous support of our research.

ABBREVIATIONS

pAkt: a three letter name (not an abbreviation); "p" stands for phosphorylated (active) form
AR: androgen receptor
Bcl-2: B cell leukemia oncogene that inhibits apoptosis
Bcl-xL: Bcl family member that inhibits apoptosis
Bfl-1/A1: B cell lymphoma-1-related gene expressed in fetal liver-1/A1
CAM-1: cell adhesion molecule-1
CD: cluster determinant
Cdk2/cdk4: cyclin dependent kinases 2 and 4
c-myc: transcription factor, oncogene
c-FLIP: cellular (caspase 8)-like inhibitory protein
Cox-2: cyclooxygenase-2
DR5: death receptor 5
E2F-1: transcription factor family including E2F and Dp-like subunits
EGFR: epidermal growth factor receptor
pERK: phosphorylated (active) extracellular signal-regulated kinase
ER stress: endoplasmic reticulum stress
ER-α: estrogen receptor-alpha
Erg1: ETS-related gene 1, transcription factor in the ETS family
FLICE: FADD-[Fas-associated protein with death domain] like IL-I beta [interleukin-1 beta]-converting enzyme (FLICE)
HER-2: human epidermal growth factor receptor
HIF-1α: hypoxia inducible factor-1 alpha
IAP-1, -2: inhibitor of apoptosis proteins
IFN-γ: interferon-gamma
IGFR: insulin-like growth factor receptor
IL-2, -6, -8, -12: interleukins
pJAK-1, -2: phosphorylated Janus-family tyrosine kinase-1 or 2
pJNK: phosphorylated (active) c-Jun N-terminal kinase
KEAP1: Kelch like-ECH-associated protein 1
LTB4: leukotriene B4
MCL-1: myeloid cell leukemia sequence, Bcl-2 family member
MEK: mitogen-activated protein kinase (MAPK)/extracellular signal-regulated kinase (ERK) kinase
MMP-2, -9: matrix metalloproteinases
MMTV: mouse mammary tumor virus
NF-κB: nuclear factor-kappa B
NO: nitric oxide
iNOS: inducible nitric oxygen synthase
Nrf2: transcription factor: nuclear factor (erythroid-derived 2)-like 2
PGE-2: prostaglandin E2
PGE-2R: prostaglandin E2 receptor
pmTOR: phosphorylated mammalian target of rapamycin
PPAR-γ: proxisomal proliferator activator receptor-gamma
PyMT: polyomavirus middle T antigen
Ras: small GTPase; abbreviation of rat sarcoma
Rb: retinoblastoma protein, a tumor suppressor

ROS: reactive oxygen species
RNS: reactive nitrogen species
SHIP-1: SH2 domain-containing inositol 5'-phosphatase-1
pSrc: tyrosine kinase (abbreviation is short for sarcoma)
pStat-3: phosphorylated (active) signal transducer and activator of transcription-3
γ-T: gamma tocopherol
α-TEA: RRR-alpha-tocopherol ether-linked acetic acid derivative
TGF-β: transforming growth factor-beta
TRIAL: TNF-related apoptosis-inducing ligand
TIMP-1, -2: tissue inhibitor of metalloproteinases
TNF-α: tumor necrosis factor-alpha
TRAF-1: TNF receptor-associated factor 1
VCAM-1: vascular cell adhesion molecule
VEGF: vascular endothelial growth factor
VEGFR: vascular endothelial growth factor receptor
VES: vitamin E succinate
XIAP: X-linked inhibitor of apoptosis protein

REFERENCES

Aggarwal, B.B., A.B. Kunnumakkara, K.B. Harikumar et al. 2009. Signal transducer and activator of transcription-3, inflammation, and cancer: how intimate is the relationship? *Ann N Y Acad Sci* 1171:59–76.

Aggarwal, B.B., C. Sundaram, S. Prasad, and R. Kannappan. 2010. Tocotrienols, the vitamin E of the 21st century: Its potential against cancer and other chronic diseases. *Biochem Pharm* 80:1613–31.

Ahn, K.S., G. Sethi, K. Krishnan, and B.B. Aggarwal. 2007. Gamma-tocotrienol inhibits nuclear factor-kappaB signaling pathway through inhibition of receptor-interacting protein and TAK1 leading to suppression of antiapoptotic gene products and potentiation of apoptosis. *J Biol Chem* 282:809–20.

Anderson, K., K.A. Lawson, M. Simmons-Menchaca, L.-Z. Sun, B.G. Sanders, and K. Kline. 2004. Alpha-TEA plus cisplatin reduces human cisplatin-resistant ovarian cancer cell tumor burden and metastasis. *Exp Biol Med* 229(11):1169–76.

Azzi, A. 2007a. Molecular mechanism of alpha-tocopherol action. *Free Radic Biol Med* 43:16–21.

Azzi, A. 2007b. Oxidative stress: A dead end or a laboratory hypothesis? *Biochem Biophy Res Commun* 362:230–2.

Barve, A., T.O. Khor, K. Reuhl, B. Reddy, H. Newmark, and A.N. Kong. 2010. Mixed tocotrienols inhibit prostate carcinogenesis in TRAMP mice. *Nutr Cancer* 62(6):789–94.

Bi, S., J.R. Liu, Y. Li et al. 2010. Gamma-tocotrienol modulates the paracrine secretion of VEGF induced by cobalt(II) chloride via ERK signaling pathway in gastric adenocarcinoma SGC-7901 cell line. *Toxicology* 274(1–3):27–33.

Birringer, M., J.H. Eytina, B.A. Salvatore, and J. Neuzil. 2003. Vitamin E analogues as inducers of apoptosis: structure-function relation. *Br J Cancer* 88(12):1948–55.

Brigelius-Flohe, R. and M.G. Traber. 1999. Vitamin E: function and metabolism. *FASEB J* 13:1145–55.

Brigelius-Flohe, R. 2009. Vitamin E. The shrew waiting to be tamed. *Free Radic Biol Med* 46:543–54.

Campbell, S.E., P.R. Musich, S.G. Whaley et al. 2009. Gamma tocopherol upregulates the expression of 15-S-HETE and induces growth arrest through a PPAR gamma-dependent mechanism in PC-3 human prostate cancer cells. *Nutr Cancer* 61(5):649–62.

Campbell, S.E., B. Rudder, R.B. Phillips et al. 2011. γ-Tocotrienol induces growth arrest through a novel pathway with TGFβ2 in prostate cancer. *Free Radic Biol Med* 50(10):1344–54.

Chaffer, C.L. and R.A. Weinberg. 2011. A perspective on cancer cell metastasis. *Science* 331:1559–64.

Christen, S., A.A. Woodall, M.K. Shigenaga, P.T. Southwell-Keely, M.W. Duncan, and B.N. Ames. 1997. Gamma-tocopherol traps mutagenic electrophiles such as NO (X) and complements alpha-tocopherol: physiological implications. *Proc Natl Acad Sci* 94(7):3217–22.

Constantinou, C., A. Papas, and A.I. Constantinou. 2008. Vitamin E and cancer: An insight into the anticancer activities of vitamin E isomers and analogs. *Int J Cancer* 123:739–52.

Devaraj, S., S. Lenard, M.G. Traber, and I. Jialal. 2008. Gamma-tocopherol supplementation alone and in combination with alpha-tocopherol alters biomarkers of oxidative stress and inflammation in subjects with metabolic syndrome. *Free Rad Biol Med* 44:1203–8.

Dietrich, M., M.G. Traber, P.F. Jacques, C.E. Cross, Y. Hu, and G. Block. 2006. Does γ-tocopherol play a role in the primary prevention of heart disease and cancer? *J Am Coll Nutr* 25(4):292–9.

Dong, L.F., E. Swettenham, J. Eliasson et al. 2007. Vitamin E analogues inhibit angiogenesis by selective induction of apoptosis in proliferating endothelial cells: the role of oxidative stress. *Cancer Res* 67(24):11906–13.

Dong, L.F., P. Low, J.C. Dyason et al. 2008. Alpha-tocopheryl succinate induces apoptosis by targeting ubiquinone-binding sites in mitochondrial respiratory complex II. *Oncogene* 27(31):4324–35.

Dong, L.F., V.J. Jameson, D. Tilly et al. 2011. Mitochondrial targeting of vitamin E succinate enhances its proapoptotic and anti-cancer activity via mitochondrial complex II. *J Biol Chem* 286(5):3717–28.

Doppalapudi, R.S., E.S. Riccio, L.L. Rausch et al. 2007. Evaluation of chemopreventive agents for genotoxic activity. *Mutat Res* 18;629(2):148–60.

Dunn, B.K., E.S. Richmond, L.M. Minasian, A.M. Ryan, and L.G. Ford. 2010. A nutrient approach to prostate cancer prevention: The selenium and vitamin E cancer prevention trial (SELECT). *Nutr Cancer* 62(7):896–918.

Elnagar, A.Y., V.B. Wali, P.W. Sylvester, and K.A. El Sayed. 2010. Design and preliminary structure-activity relationship of redox-silent semisynthetic tocotrienol analogues as inhibitors for breast cancer proliferation and invasion. *Bioorg Med Chem* 18(2):755–68.

Evans, H.M. and K.S. Bishop. 1922. On the existence of a hitherto unrecognized dietary factor essential for reproduction. *Science* 56:650–1.

Feng Z., Z. Liu. X. Li et al. 2010. alpha-Tocopherol is an effective Phase II enzyme inducer: Protective effects on acrolein-induced oxidative stress and mitochondrial dysfunction in human retinal pigment epithelial cells. *J Nutr Biochem* 21:1222–31.

Friedrich, M.J. 2004. To "E" or not to "E", vitamin E's role in health and disease is the question. *JAMA* 292:671–3.

Galli, F. and A. Azzi. 2010. Present trends in vitamin E research. *Int Union Biochem Mol Biol* 36(1):33–42.

Giovannucci, E. 2000. γ-tocopherol: A new player in prostate cancer prevention. *J Natl Cancer Inst* 92 (24):1966–7.

Gopalan, A., W. Yu, Q. Jiang et al. 2012. Involvement of de novo ceramide synthesis in gamma-tocopherol and gamma-tocotrienol—induced apoptosis in human breast cancer cells. *Mol Nutr Food Res* 56(12):1803–11.

Gu, J.Y., Y. Wakizono, Y. Sunada et al. 1999. Dietary effect of tocopherols and tocotrienols on the immune function of spleen and mesenteric lymph node lymphocytes in Brown Norway rats. *Biosci Biotechnol Biochem* 63:1697–702.

Gupta, S.C., J.H. Kim, R. Kannappan, S. Reuter, P.M. Dougherty, and B.B. Aggarwal. 2011. Role of nuclear factor κB-mediated inflammatory pathways in cancer-related symptoms and their regulation by nutritional agents. *Exp Biol Med* 236(6):658–71.

Hahn, T. and E.T. Akporiaye. 2011. Repeat dose study of the novel proapoptotic chemotherapeutic agent alpha-tocopheryloxy acetic acid in mice. *Anticancer Drugs* 23(4):455–64.

Hahn, T., L. Szabo, M. Gold, L. Ramanathapuram, L.H. Hurley, and E.T. Akporiaye. 2006. Dietary administration of the proapoptotic vitamin E analogue alpha-tocopheryloxyacetic acid inhibits metastatic murine breast cancer. *Cancer Res* 66(19):9374–8.

Hahn, T., K. Fried, L.H. Hurley, and E.T. Akporiaye. 2009. Orally active alpha-tocopheryloxyacetic acid suppresses tumor growth and multiplicity of spontaneous murine breast cancer. *Mol Cancer Ther* 8(6):1570–8.

Hahn, T., B. Jagadish, E.A. Mash, K. Garrison, and E.T. Akporiaye. 2011a. α-Tocopheryloxyacetic acid: a novel chemotherapeutic that stimulates the antitumor immune response. *Breast Cancer Res* 13(1):R4.

Hahn, T., D.J. Bradley-Dunlop, L.H. Hurley et al. 2011b. The vitamin E analog, alpha-tocopheryloxyacetic acid enhances the anti-tumor activity of trastuzumab against HER2/neu-expressing breast cancer. *BMC Cancer* 11:471.

Handelman, G.J., L.J. Machlin, K. Fitch, J.J. Weiter, and E.A. Dratz. 1985. Oral alpha-tocopherol supplements decrease plasma gamma-tocopherol levels in humans. *J Nutr* 115:807–13.

Hafid, S.R., A.K. Radhakrishnan, and K. Nesaretnam. 2010. Tocotrienols are good adjuvants for developing cancer vaccines. *BMC Cancer* 10:5.

Hanahan, D. and R.A. Weinberg. 2011. Hallmarks of cancer: The next generation. *Cell* 144:646–74.

Hsieh, T.C., S. Elangovan, and J.M. Wu. 2010a. Differential suppression of proliferation in MCF-7 and MDA-MB-231 breast cancer cells exposed to alpha-, gamma- and delta-tocotrienols is accompanied by altered expression of oxidative stress modulatory enzymes. *Anticancer Res* 30(10):4169–76.

Hsieh, T.C., S. Elangovan, and J.M. Wu. 2010b. Gamma-tocotrienol controls proliferation, modulates expression of cell cycle regulatory proteins and up-regulates quinone reductase NQO2 in MCF-7 breast cancer cells. *Anticancer Res* 30(7):2869–74.

Huang, X., Z. Zhang, L. Jia, Y. Zhao, X. Zhang, and K. Wu. 2010. Endoplasmic reticulum stress contributes to vitamin E succinate-induced apoptosis in human gastric cancer SGC-7901 cells. *Cancer Lett* 296(1):123–31.

Husain, K., R.A. Francois, T. Yamauchi, M. Perez, S.M. Sebti, and M.P. Malafa. 2011. Vitamin E δ-tocotrienol augments the antitumor activity of gemcitabine and suppresses constitutive NF-κB activation in pancreatic cancer. *Mol Cancer Ther* 10(12):2363–72.

Imtiyaz, H.Z. and M.C. Simon. 2010. Hypoxia-inducible factors as essential regulators of inflammation. *Curr Top Microbiol Immunol* 345:105–20.

Institute of Medicine. Food and Nutrition Board Panel on Dietary Antioxidants and Related Compounds. 2000. *Dietary Reference Intakes for Vitamin C, Vitamin E, Selenium, and Carotenoids*, 1–486. Washington, DC: National Academy Press.

Jia, L., W. Yu, P. Wang, J. Li, B.G. Sanders, and K. Kline. 2008a. Critical roles for JNK, c-Jun, and Fas/FasL-Signaling in vitamin E analog-induced apoptosis in human prostate cancer cells. *Prostate* 68(4):427–41.

Jia, L., W. Yu, P. Wang, B.G. Sanders, and K. Kline. 2008b. In vivo and in vitro studies of anticancer actions of alpha-TEA for human prostate cancer cells. *Prostate* 68(8):849–60.

Jiang, Q. and B.N. Ames. 2003. Gamma-tocopherol, but not alpha-tocopherol, decreases proinflammatory eicosanoids and inflammation damage in rats. *FASEB J* 17(8):816–22.

Jiang, Q., I. Elson-Schwab, C. Courtemanche, and B.N. Ames. 2000. Gamma-tocopherol and its major metabolite, in contrast to alpha-tocopherol, inhibit cyclooxygenase activity in macrophages and epithelial cells. *Proc Natl Acad Sci* 97(21):11494–9.

Jiang, Q., X. Yin, M.A. Lill, M.L. Danielson, H. Freiser, and J. Huang. 2008. Long-chain carboxychromanols, metabolites of vitamin E, are potent inhibitors of cyclooxygenases. *Proc Natl Acad Sci* 105(51):20464–9.

Jiang, Q., X. Rao, C.Y. Kim et al. 2012. Gamma-tocotrienol induces apoptosis and autophagy in prostate cancer cells by increasing intracellular dihydrosphingosine and dihydroceramide. *Int J Cancer* 130(3):685–93.

Jiang, Z., X. Yin, and Q. Jiang. 2011. Natural forms of vitamin E and 13′-carboxychromanol, a long-chain vitamin E metabolite, inhibit leukotriene generation from stimulated neutrophils by blocking calcium influx and suppressing 5-lipoxygenase activity, respectively. *J Immunol* 186(2):1173–9.

Ju, J., X. Hao, M.J. Lee et al. 2009. A gamma-tocopherol-rich mixture of tocopherols inhibits colon inflammation and carcinogenesis in azoxymethane and dextran sulfate sodium-treated mice. *Cancer Prev Res* 2(2):143–52.

Ju, J., S.C. Picinich, Y. Zhihong et al. 2010. Cancer preventive activities of tocopherols and tocotrienols. *Carcinogenesis* 31(4):533–42.

Kakarala, M., D.E. Brenner, H. Korkaya et al. 2010. Targeting breast stem cells with the cancer preventive compounds curcumin and piperine. *Breast Cancer Res Treat* 122(3):777–85.

Kanai, K., E. Kikuchi, S. Mikami et al. 2010. Vitamin E succinate induced apoptosis and enhanced chemosensitivity to paclitaxel in human bladder cancer cells in vitro and in vivo. *Cancer Sci* 101(1):216–23.

Kannappan, R., J. Ravindran, S. Prasad et al. 2010a. Gamma-tocotrienol promotes TRAIL-induced apoptosis through reactive oxygen species/extracellular signal-regulated kinase/p53-mediated upregulation of death receptors. *Mol Cancer Ther* 9:2196–07.

Kannappan, R., V.R. Yadav, and B.B. Aggarwal. 2010b. γ-Tocotrienol but not γ-tocopherol blocks STAT3 cell signaling pathway through induction of protein-tyrosine phosphatase SHP-1 and sensitizes tumor cells to chemotherapeutic agents. *J Biol Chem* 285(43):33520–8.

Kannappan, R., S.C. Gupta, J.H. Kim, and B.B. Aggarwal. 2012. Tocotrienols fight cancer by targeting multiple cell signaling pathways. *Genes Nutr* 7(1):43–52.

Kapadia, R., J.H. Yi, and R. Vemuganti. 2008. Mechanisms of anti-inflammatory and neuroprotective actions of PPAR-gamma agonists. *Front Biosci* 1(13):1813–26.

Klein, E.A., S.M. Lippman, I.M. Thompson et al. 2003. The selenium and vitamin E cancer prevention trial. *World J Urol* 21:21–7.

Klein, E.A., I.M. Thompson, C.M. Tangen et al. 2012. Vitamin E and the risk of prostate cancer: The selenium and vitamin E cancer prevention trial (SELECT). *JAMA* 306(14):1549–56.

Kline, K., K.A. Lawson, W. Yu, and B.G. Sanders. 2007. Vitamin E and cancer. *Vitam Horm* 76:435–61.

Koeppen, M., T. Eckle, and H.K. Eltzschig. 2011. The hypoxia-inflammation link and potential drug targets. *Curr Opin Anaesthesiol* 24(4):363–9.

Kunnumakkara, A.B., B. Sung, J. Ravindran et al. 2010. Gamma-tocotrienol inhibits pancreatic tumors and sensitizes them to gemcitabine treatment by modulating the inflammatory microenvironment. *Cancer Res* 70(21):8695–705.

Latimer, P., M. Menchaca, R.M. Snyder et al. 2009. Aerosol delivery of liposomal formulated paclitaxel and vitamin E analog reduces murine mammary tumor burden and metastases. *Exp Biol Med* 234:1244–52.

Lawson, K.A., K. Anderson, M. Menchaca et al. 2003. Novel vitamin E analogue decreases syngeneic mouse mammary tumor burden and reduces lung metastasis. *Mol Cancer Ther* 2(5):437–44.

Lawson, K.A., K. Anderson, and M. Simmons-Menchaca. 2004. Comparison of vitamin E derivatives alpha-TEA and VES in reduction of mouse mammary tumor burden and metastasis. *Exp Biol Med* 229(9):954–63.

Ledesma, M.C., B. Jung-Hynes, T.L. Schmit, R. Kumar, H. Mukhtar, and N. Ahmad. 2011. Selenium and vitamin E for prostate cancer: Post-SELECT (Selenium and Vitamin E Cancer Prevention Trial) status. *Mol Med* 17(1–2):134–43.

Lee, H.J., J. Ju, S. Paul et al. 2009. Mixed tocopherols prevent mammary tumorigenesis by inhibiting estrogen action and activating PPAR-gamma. *Clin Cancer Res* 15(12):4242–9.

Li, J., W. Yu, R. Tiwary et al. 2010. α-TEA-induced death receptor dependent apoptosis involves activation of acid sphingomyelinase and elevated ceramide-enriched cell surface membranes. *Cancer Cell Int* 10:40.

Li, Y., T. Zhang, H. Korkaya et al. 2010. Sulforaphane, a dietary component of broccoli/broccoli sprouts, inhibits breast cancer stem cells. *Clin Cancer Res* 16(9):2580–90.

Li, Y., W.G. Sun, H.K. Liu et al. 2011. γ-Tocotrienol inhibits angiogenesis of human umbilical vein endothelial cell induced by cancer cell. *J Nutr Biochem* 22(12):1127–36.

Lim, S.J., M.K. Choi, M.J. Kim, and J.K. Kim. 2009. Alpha-tocopheryl succinate potentiates the paclitaxel-induced apoptosis through enforced caspase 8 activation in human H460 lung cancer cells. *Exp Mol Med* 41(10):737–45.

Lippman, S.M., E.A. Klein, P.J. Goodman et al. 2009. Effect of selenium and vitamin E on risk of prostate cancer and other cancers: the Selenium and Vitamin E Cancer Prevention Trial (SELECT). *JAMA* 301(1):39–51.

Liu, H.K., Q. Wang, Y. Li et al. 2010. Inhibitory effects of gamma-tocotrienol on invasion and metastasis of human gastric adenocarcinoma SGC-7901 cells. *J Nutr Biochem* 21(3):206–13.

Luk, S.U., W.N. Yap, Y.T. Chiu et al. 2011. Gamma-tocotrienol as an effective agent in targeting prostate cancer stem cell-like population. *Int J Cancer* 128(9):2182–91.

Malafa, M.P., F.D. Fokum, J. Andoh et al. 2006. Vitamin E succinate suppresses prostate tumor growth by inducing apoptosis. *Int J Cancer* 118(10):2441–7.

Mamede, A.C., S.D. Tavares, A.M. Abrantes, J. Trindale, J.M. Maia, and M.F. Botelho. 2011. The role of vitamins in cancer: *Nutr Cancer* 63(4):479–94.

Manu, K.A., M.K. Shanmugam, L. Ramachandran et al. 2012. First evidence that γ-tocotrienol inhibits the growth of human gastric cancer and chemosensitizes it to capecitabine in a xenograft mouse model through the modulation of NF-KB pathway. *Clin Cancer Res* 18(8):2220–9.

Miyazawa, T., A. Shibata, P. Sookwong et al. 2009. Antiangiogenic and anticancer potential of unsaturated vitamin E (tocotrienol). *J Nutr Biochem* 20:79–86.

Molano, A. and S.N. Meydani. 2012. Vitamin E, signalosomes and gene expression in T cells. *Mol Aspects Med* 33(1):55–62.

Mun-Li, Y., S.R. Hafid, C. Hwee-Ming, and K. Nesaretnam. 2009. Tocotrienols suppress proinflammatory markers and cyclooxygenase-2 expression in RAW264.7 macrophages. *Lipids* 44:787–97.

Nesaretnam, K. and P. Meganathan. 2011. Tocotrienols: inflammation and cancer. *Ann NY Acad Sci* 1229:18–22.

Neuzil, J., K. Kågedal, L. Andera, C. Weber, and U.T. Brunk. 2002. Vitamin E analogs: a new class of multiple action agents with anti-neoplastic and anti-atherogenic activity. *Apoptosis* 7(2):179–87.

Neuzil, J.M., A.S. Tomasetti, R. Mellick, B.A. Alleva, S.M. Birringer, and M.W. Fariss. 2004. Vitamin E analogues: A new class of inducers of apoptosis with selective anti-cancer effects. *Curr Cancer Drug Targets* 4:355–72.

Neuzil, J., E. Swettenham, X.F. Wang, L.F. Dong, and M. Stapelberg. 2007. alpha-Tocopheryl succinate inhibits angiogenesis by disrupting paracrine FGF2 signalling. *FEBS Lett* 581(24):4611–5.

Park, S.K. 2010. Studies of natural vitamin E forms and their synthetic derivatives for potential anticancer application in human breast cancer cell lines and mouse tumor models. PhD diss., (University of Texas at Austin).

Park, S.K., B.G. Sanders, and K. Kline. 2010. Tocotrienols induce apoptosis in breast cancer cell lines via an endoplasmic reticulum stress-dependent increase in extrinsic death receptor signaling. *Breast Cancer Res Treat* 124(2):361–75.

Patacsil, D., A.T. Tran, Y.S. Cho et al. 2012. Gamma-tocotrienol induced apoptosis is associated with unfolded protein response in human breast cancer cells. *J Nutr Biochem* 23(1):93–100.

Prochazka, L., L.F. Dong, K. Valis et al. 2010. alpha-Tocopheryl succinate causes mitochondrial permeabilization by preferential formation of Bak channels. *Apoptosis* 15(7):782–94.

Qureshi, A.A., X. Tan, J.C. Reis et al. 2011a. Suppression of nitric oxide induction and pro-inflammatory cytokines by novel proteasome inhibitors in various experimental models. *Lipids Health Dis* 10:177.

Qureshi, A.A., X. Tan, J.C. Reis et al. 2011b. Inhibition of nitric oxide in LPS-stimulated macrophages of young and senescent mice by δ-tocotrienol and quercetin. *Lipids Health Dis* 10:239.

Ramanathapuram, L.V., T. Hahn, S.M. Dial, and E.T. Akporiaye. 2005. Chemo-immunotherapy of breast cancer using vesiculated alpha-tocopheryl succinate in combination with dendritic cell vaccination. *Nutr Cancer* 53(2):177–93.

Ramanathapuram, L.V., T. Hahn, M.W. Graner, E. Katsanis, and E.T. Akporiaye. 2006. Vesiculated alpha-tocopheryl succinate enhances the anti-tumor effect of dendritic cell vaccines. *Cancer Immunol Immunother* 55(2):166–77.

Rajendran, P., F. Li, K.A. Manu et al. 2011. γ-Tocotrienol is a novel inhibitor of constitutive and inducible STAT3 signalling pathway in human hepatocellular carcinoma: potential role as an antiproliferative, proapoptotic and chemosensitizing agent. *Br J Pharmacol* 163(2):283–98.

Ren, Z., M. Pae, M.C. Dao, D. Smith, S.N. Meydani, and D. Wu 2010. Dietary supplementation with tocotrienols enhances immune function in C57BL/6 mice. *J Nutr* 140(7):1335–41.

Riedel, S.B., S.M. Fischer, B.G. Sanders, and K. Kline. 2008. Vitamin E analog, alpha-tocopherol ether-linked acetic acid analog, alone and in combination with celecoxib, reduces multiplicity of ultraviolet-induced skin cancers in mice. *Anticancer Drugs* 19(2):175–81.

Roberts II, L.J., J.A. Oates, M.F. Linton et al. 2007. The relationship between dose in vitamin E and suppression of oxidative stress in humans. *Free Radic Biol Med* 43:1388–93.

Sen, C.K., S.K. Khanna, and S. Roy. 2007. Tocotrienols in health and disease: the other half of the natural vitamin E family. *Mol Aspects Med* 28: 692–728.

Shibata, A., K. Nakagawa, P. Sookwong et al. 2008a. Tocotrienol inhibits secretion of angiogenic factors from human colorectal adenocarcinoma cells by suppressing hypoxia-inducible factor-1alpha. *J Nutr* 138: 2136–42.

Shibata, A., K. Nakagawa, P. Sookwong et al. 2008b. Tumor antiangiogenic effect and mechanism of action of delta-tocotrienol. *Biochem Pharmacol* 76:330–9.

Shibata, A., K. Nakagawa, P. Sookwong et al. 2009. Delta-tocotrienol suppresses VEGF induced angiogenesis whereas alpha-tocopherol does not. *J Agric Food Chem* 57:8696–704.

Shin-Kang, S., V.P. Ramsauer, J. Lightner et al. 2011. Tocotrienols inhibit AKT and ERK activation and suppress pancreatic cancer cell proliferation by suppressing the ErbB2 pathway. *Free Radic Biol Med* 51(6):1164–74.

Shun, M.C., W. Yu, S.K. Park, B.G. Sanders, and K. Kline. 2010. Downregulation of epidermal growth factor receptor expression contributes to alpha-TEA's proapoptotic effects in human ovarian cancer cell lines. *J Oncol* 2010:824571.

Smolarek, A.K. and N. Suh. 2011. Chemopreventive activity of vitamin E in breast cancer: a focus on γ- and δ-tocopherol. *Nutrients* 3(11):962–86.

The Alpha-Tocopherol, Beta-Carotene Lung Cancer Prevention Study Group. 1994. The effect of vitamin E and beta carotene on the incidence of lung cancer and other cancers in male smokers. *N Engl J Med* 330:1029–35.

Theriault, A., J.T. Chao, and A. Gapor. 2002. Tocotrienol is the most effective vitamin E for reducing endothelial expression of adhesion molecules and adhesion to monocytes. *Atherosclerosis* 160(1):21–30.

Tiwary, R., W. Yu, J. Li, S.K. Park, B.G. Sanders, and K. Kline. 2010. Role of endoplasmic reticulum stress in alpha-TEA mediated TRAIL/DR5 death receptor dependent apoptosis. *PLoS One* 5(7):e11865.

Tiwary, R., W. Yu, B.G. Sanders, and K. Kline. 2011a. α-TEA cooperates with MEK or mTOR inhibitors to induce apoptosis via targeting IRS/PI3K pathways. *Br J Cancer* 104(1):101–9.

Tiwary, R., W. Yu, B.G. Sanders, and K. Kline. 2011b. α-TEA cooperates with chemotherapeutic agents to induce apoptosis of p53 mutant, triple-negative human breast cancer cells via activating p73. *Breast Cancer Res* 13(1):R1

Tiwary, R., W. Yu, L.A. deGraffenried, B.G. Sanders, and K. Kline. 2011c. Targeting cholesterol-rich microdomains to circumvent tamoxifen-resistant breast cancer. *Breast Cancer Res* 13(6):R120.

Tomasetti, M. and J. Neuzil. 2007. Vitamin E analogues and immune response in cancer treatment. *Vitam Horm* 76:463–91.

Tomasetti, M., E. Strafella, S. Staffolani, L. Santarelli, J. Neuzil, and R. Guerrieri. 2010. Alpha-tocopheryl succinate promotes selective cell death induced by vitamin K3 in combination with ascorbate. *Br J Cancer* 102(8):1224–34.

Tomic-Vatic, A.J., E. Chapman, J. Neuzil, and B.A. Salvatore. 2005. Vitamin E amindes, a new class of vitamin E analogues with enhanced proapoptotic activity. *Int J Cancer* 117:188–93.

Traber, M.G. 2007. Vitamin E regulatory mechanisms. *Annu Rev Nutr* 27:347–62.

Traber, M.G. and J. Atkinson. 2007. Vitamin E, antioxidant and nothing more. *Free Radic Biol Med* 43:4–15.

Traber, M.G. and J.F. Stevens. 2011. Vitamins C and E: Beneficial effects from a mechanistic perspective. *Free Rad Biol Med* 51:1000–13.

Virtamo, J., P. Pietinen, J.K. Huttunen et al. (ATBC Study Group). 2003. Incidence of cancer and mortality following alpha-tocopherol and beta-carotene supplementation: a post intervention follow-up. *JAMA* 290(4):476–85.

Wang, P., L. Jia, B.G. Sanders, and K. Kline. 2007. Liposomal or nanoparticle alpha-TEA reduced 66cl-4 murine mammary cancer burden and metastasis. *Drug Deliv* 14(8):497–505.

Wang, P., W. Yu, Z. Hu et al. 2008. Involvement of JNK/p73/NOXA in vitamin E analog-induced apoptosis of human breast cancer cells. *Mol Carcinog* 47(6):436–45.

Wang, X.F., L. Dong, Y. Zhao, M. Tomasetti, K. We, and J. Neuzil. 2006. Vitamin E analogues as anticancer agents: Lessons from studies with α-tocopheryl succinate. *Mol Nutr Food Res* 50:675–85.

Weng-Yew, W., K.R. Selvaduray, C.H. Ming, and K. Nesaretnam. 2009. Suppression of tumor growth by palm tocotrienols via the attenuation of angiogenesis. *Nutr Cancer* 61(3):367–73.

Wu, S.J., P.L. Liu, and L.T. Ng. 2008. Tocotrienol-rich fraction of palm oil exhibits anti-inflammatory property by suppressing the expression of inflammatory mediators in human monocytic cells. *Mol Nutr Food Res* 52:921–9.

Yang, C.S., G. Lu, J. Ju, and G.X. Li. 2010. Inhibition of inflammation and carcinogenesis in the lung and colon by tocopherols. *Ann N Y Acad Sci* 1203:29–34.

Yang, Z., H. Xiao, H. Jin, P.T. Koo, D.J. Tsang, and C.S. Yang. 2010. Synergistic actions of atorvastatin with gamma-tocotrienol and celecoxib against human colon cancer HT29 and HCT116 cells. *Int J Cancer* 126(4):852–63.

Yang, Z., M.J. Lee, Y. Zhao, and C.S. Yang. 2011. Metabolism of tocotrienols in animals and synergistic inhibitory actions of tocotrienols with atorvastatin in cancer cells. *Genes Nutr* 7(1):11–8.

Yap, W.N., P.N. Chang, H.Y. Han et al. 2008. Gamma-tocotrienol suppresses prostate cancer cell proliferation and invasion through multiple-signalling pathways. *Br J Cancer* 99:1832–41.

Yap, W.N., N. Zaiden, Y.L. Tan et al. 2010a. Id1, inhibitor of differentiation, is a key protein mediating antitumor responses responses of gamma-tocotrienol in breast cancer cells. *Cancer Lett* 291:187–99.

Yap, W.N., N. Zaiden, S.Y. Luk et al. 2010b. In vivo evidence of gamma-tocotrienol as a chemosensitizer in the treatment of hormone-refractory prostate cancer. *Pharmacology* 85(4):248–58.

Yu, W., S.K. Park, L. Jia et al. 2008a. RRR-gamma-tocopherol induces human breast cancer cells to undergo apoptosis via death receptor 5 (DR5)-mediated apoptotic signaling. *Cancer Lett* 259(2):165–76.

Yu, W., L. Jia, P. Wang et al. 2008b. In vitro and in vivo evaluation of anticancer actions of natural and synthetic vitamin E forms. *Mol Nutr Food Res* 52(4):447-56.

Yu, W., L. Jia, S.K. Park et al. 2009. Anticancer actions of natural and synthetic vitamin E forms: RRR-alpha-tocopherol blocks the anticancer actions of gamma-tocopherol. *Mol Nutr Food Res* 53(12):1573–81.

Yu, W., R. Tiwary, J. Li et al. 2010. α-TEA induces apoptosis of human breast cancer cells via activation of TRAIL/DR5 death receptor pathway. *Mol Carcinog* 49(11):964–73.

Zhang, X., X. Peng, W. Yu et al. 2011. Alpha-tocopheryl succinate enhances doxorubicin-induced apoptosis in human gastric cancer cells via promotion of doxorubicin influx and suppression of doxorubicin efflux. *Cancer Lett* 307(2):174–81.

Zhao, Y., J. Neuzil, and K. Wu. 2009. Vitamin E analogues as mitochondria-targeting compounds: from the bench to the bedside? *Mol Nutr Food Res* 53:129–39.

Zhao, Y., R. Li, W. Xia et al. 2010. Bid integrates intrinsic and extrinsic signaling in apoptosis induced by alpha-tocopheryl succinate in human gastric carcinoma cells. *Cancer Lett* 288(1):42–9.

Zingg, J.M. 2007. Molecular and cellular activities of vitamin E analogues. *Med Chem* 7:545–60.

Zingg, J.M., M. Meydani, and A. Azzi. 2010. Alpha-tocopheryl phosphate-An active lipid mediator? *Mol Nutr Food Res* 54: 679–92.

12 The Protective Role of Vitamin E in Inflammation and Cancer

Amanda K. Smolarek and Nanjoo Suh

CONTENTS

12.1 INTRODUCTION

Chronic inflammation plays a role in developing certain diseases such as cancer, cardiovascular disease (CVD), type 2 diabetes, Alzheimer's disease (AD), and renal disease. Cancer and CVD account for nearly one out of two deaths in the United States (Heron 2011). Prevention and treatment with diet, pharmacological agents, and nutrition factors may be more effective in the reduction of premature mortality arising from these diseases. Dietary micronutrients may control intracellular events such as antioxidant activity, anti-inflammatory activity, and induction of apoptosis (Surh 2003). One such dietary micronutrient is vitamin E. Vitamin E is recognized as a lipid-soluble antioxidant that has been suggested to reduce cancer risk (Taylor et al. 2003). Besides cancers, vitamin E has been investigated in preventing numerous human diseases such as CVD, neurodegenerative conditions such as AD and Parkinson's disease, and immune response, which may be linked to chronic inflammation (Galli and Azzi 2010). In this chapter, we will focus on the chemoprevention activities and anti-inflammatory actions by vitamin E.

12.1.1 DISCOVERY AND STRUCTURES OF VITAMIN E

Vitamin E was first discovered in 1922, when it was noted to restore fertility function (Evans and Bishop 1922; Wolf 2005). In 1936, vitamin E was aptly named "tocopherol," from the Greek, *tocos*, which means "childbirth," and *phero*, which means "to bring" (Wolf 2005). Tocotrienols were not discovered until 1964 (Pennock et al. 1964), and since then, vitamin E has consisted of eight structurally related compounds, four tocopherols and four tocotrienols. Both tocopherols and tocotrienols have the same denotation for the number and position of methyl groups on the chromanol ring, designated as α, β, γ, and δ (Constantinou et al. 2008). α-Tocopherol is trimethylated at the 5-, 7-, and 8-positions; β-tocopherol is dimethylated at the 5- and 8-positions; γ-tocopherol is dimethylated at the 7- and 8-positions; and δ-tocopherol is monomethylated at the 8-position on the chromanol ring. Tocopherols have a saturated 16-carbon side chain, while tocotrienols have an unsaturated 16-carbon side chain with double bonds at 3′, 7′, and 11′ positions (Traber 2007; Constantinou et al. 2008).

12.1.2 Vitamin E in the Human Diet

The most significant sources of vitamin E are plant oils and fats. α-Tocopherol is most commonly found in wheat germ, almond, and sunflower oil (McLaughlin and Weihrauch 1979). However, γ-tocopherol is more prominent than α-tocopherol in the American diet and is found in vegetable oils such as soybean, corn, and cottonseed (Traber 2007). δ-Tocopherol is primarily found in soybean and castor oils and, to a lesser extent, in wheat germ oil (Aggarwal et al. 2010). A γ-tocopherol–enriched mixture (γ-TmT) containing 58% γ-tocopherol, 24% δ-tocopherol, 13% α-tocopherol, and 0.5% β-tocopherol can be easily available as a by-product of refining vegetable oil (Lee et al. 2009; Ju et al. 2009). Tocotrienols are found primarily in palm and annatto oils and more readily consumed in East South Asian diets (Sen et al. 2007).

12.1.3 Transport and Metabolism of Vitamin E

Vitamin E is taken up by intestinal cells and released into circulation in chylomicrons, where they reach the liver. In the liver, the α-tocopherol transfer protein, a 30–35 kDa protein (Murphy and Mavis 1981), preferentially transfers α-tocopherol from the liver to the blood (Sontag and Parker 2002). The relative affinities of α-tocopherol transfer protein for the variants of vitamin E as determined in vitro were 100% for α-tocopherol, 38% for β-tocopherol, 9% for γ-tocopherol, 2% for δ-tocopherol, and 12% for α-tocotrienol (Hosomi et al. 1997). Thus, α-tocopherol is the most abundant form found in human tissues and serum.

Another protein involved with vitamin E is tocopherol-associated protein, which is a cytosolic lipid-binding and transfer protein. Tocopherol-associated protein is a 46 kDa protein and has the highest levels in the liver > prostate > whole brain > spinal cord > kidney > mammary gland > stomach (Zimmer et al. 2000). Tocopherol-binding protein is a 15 kDa cystolic protein initially found in the rat liver and heart (Dutta-Roy et al. 1993) and later found in the human placenta (Gordon et al. 1996). Tocopherol-binding protein is involved in intracellular transport and metabolism for α-tocopherol (Gordon et al. 1995). The first nonantioxidant function of vitamin E determined that α-tocopherol inhibited the activity of smooth muscle proliferation and protein kinase C (PKC) (Boscoboinik, Szewczyk, and Azzi 1991; Boscoboinik, Szewczyk, Hensey et al. 1991).

Vitamin E is metabolized in the liver by cytochrome P450 4F2 (CYP4F2). CYP4F2 catalyzes the initial step in the vitamin E–ω-hydroxylase pathway, followed by β-oxidation, which removes two carbons from the side chain in each cycle, ending in the short-chain metabolite, carboxyethyl hydroxychromans (CEHCs) (Sontag and Parker 2002; Birringer et al. 2002). Since α-tocopherol is preferentially transferred to the blood by α-tocopherol transfer protein, γ-tocopherol and δ-tocopherol are more readily metabolized in the liver (Sontag and Parker 2002). Due to the abundance in the serum and tissue, α-tocopherol has been termed the "classic" vitamin E and been the primary variant used in dietary supplements and in studies over the years (Brigelius-Flohe and Traber 1999).

12.2 POSSIBLE MECHANISMS OF CANCER PREVENTION BY VITAMIN E

The mechanisms of the anticancer activity of vitamin E have been investigated for many years (Kline et al. 2003, 2007; Stone et al. 2004) and include the induction of apoptosis, modulation of nuclear receptors, inhibition of cell growth, and antioxidative and anti-inflammatory activities (Stone et al. 2004; Kline et al. 2003; Jiang et al. 2000; Chamras et al. 2005; Barve et al. 2009; Guthrie et al. 1997; Comitato et al. 2009). More specifically, vitamin E has been shown to interact with PKC, Akt/PKB, the mitogen-activated protein kinase (MAPK) family, cell cycle–related kinases, and activation of nuclear factor kappaB (NF-κB) (Shah and Sylvester 2005; Jiang et al. 2008; Munteanu et al. 2004; Zingg 2007; Betti et al. 2006).

12.2.1 REGULATION OF APOPTOSIS AND CELL PROLIFERATION BY VITAMIN E

Apoptosis is defined as programmed cell death and is characterized by cell shrinkage, chromatin condensation, internucleosomal DNA fragmentation, and apoptotic bodies (Kerr 2002; Kerr et al. 1972; Hacker 2000). Apoptotic bodies are formed, and the tightly packed organelles leave the cell through "budding" (Elmore 2007). Dietary compounds that induce apoptosis are highly beneficial since apoptosis has the ability to remove cells with neoplastic transformation when upstream cellular defenses have failed. The caspases cascade is important for both the extrinsic and intrinsic pathways (Igney and Krammer 2002). The proteolytic activity of procaspases leads to the activation and cleavage of downstream caspases. There are 10 major caspases with 3 main subgroups: initiators (-2, -8, -9, and -10), effectors (-3, -6, and -7), and inflammatory (-1, -4, and -5) (Cohen 1997; Rai et al. 2005). Caspase 3 is of particular interest since it has the ability to cleave over a hundred different substrates that lead to apoptosis (Tan et al. 2011).

In breast, colon, and prostate cancer cells, apoptosis was induced by γ-tocopherol (Jiang, Wong, and Ames 2004; Yu et al. 1999, 2008; Campbell et al. 2006; Jiang, Wong, Fyrst et al. 2004). More specifically, γ-tocopherol, but not α-tocopherol, induced cleaved caspase 8 and 9 in MDA-MB-435 human breast cancer cells (Yu et al. 2008). nu/nu mice injected MDA-MB-231 cells reduced tumor burden and increased apoptosis when administered with γ-tocopherol (Yu et al. 2009). In a lung xenograft model, both δ- and γ-tocopherol inhibited tumor growth, while α-tocopherol did not (Li et al. 2011). γ-Tocotrienol induced apoptosis and inhibited cell proliferation in HT-29 colon cancer cells (Xu et al. 2009) and induced apoptosis in human gastric cancer SGC-7901 cells (Sun et al. 2008).

In breast, colon, lung, and prostate cancer cell lines, γ-tocopherol was shown to be more effective at inhibiting cell growth than α-tocopherol (Campbell et al. 2006; Gysin et al. 2002; Jiang, Wong, Fyrst et al. 2004; Lee et al. 2009). Treatment with γ-TmT and γ- and δ-tocopherol inhibited cell proliferation in MCF-7 breast cancer cells in a dose-dependent manner, while treatment with α-tocopherol did not (Lee et al. 2009). In addition, a colony growth inhibition assay utilizing MDA-MB-435 breast cancer cells showed that γ- and δ-tocopherol showed potential to inhibit colony formation, whereas α-tocopherol was not active (Kline et al. 2003). Tocotrienols differ in their inhibition of proliferation, with relative potencies in the order of δ-tocotrienol > γ-tocotrienol > α-tocotrienol (McIntyre et al. 2000; Kamal-Eldin and Appelqvist 1996; Inokuchi et al. 2003).

Mammary tumor growth and burden were decreased by administration of a γ-TmT diet in Sprague-Dawley rats induced with a synthetic carcinogen N-methyl-N-nitrosourea (NMU) (Suh et al. 2007; Lee et al. 2009). Proliferating cell nuclear antigen (PCNA) was decreased in mammary hyperplasia (Smolarek, So, Thomas et al. 2012) and in mammary tumors when administered with γ-TmT (Suh et al. 2007). Administration of γ-TmT increased the levels of cleaved caspase 3 in mammary hyperplasia (Smolarek, So, Thomas et al. 2012) and in mammary tumors (Lee et al. 2009). Furthermore, γ-TmT and individual tocopherols were administered to Sprague-Dawley rats, which were induced with a carcinogen, NMU; treatment with γ-TmT and γ- and δ-tocopherol decreased PCNA levels while increasing the levels of cleaved caspase 3 in mammary tumors, whereas α-tocopherol was not active (Smolarek, So, Kong et al. 2012).

12.2.2 DIRECT AND INDIRECT ANTIOXIDATIVE ACTIVITIES OF VITAMIN E

Vitamin E is an important dietary antioxidant, which prevents the propagation of free radical reactions (Traber 2007; Burton and Traber 1990). The antioxidant properties are mostly due to the phenolic hydrogens in the chromanol ring that are donated to lipid free radicals (Burton and Ingold 1989). Due to the structural differences on the chromanol ring, α-tocopherol with two *ortho*-methyl groups is expected to be a more potent hydrogen donor than either γ-tocopherol (one *ortho*-methyl group) or δ-tocopherol (zero *ortho*-methyl group) (Kamal-Eldin and Appelqvist 1996). The antioxidant activity of α-tocopherol is similar to that of α-tocotrienol and superior to that of γ- and δ-tocopherol (Suarna et al. 1993). However, γ-tocopherol is more effective in trapping reactive nitrogen species (RNS) than α-tocopherol (Jiang et al. 2000, 2001, 2002; Jiang and Ames 2003; Christen et al. 1997; Cooney et al. 1993). The tocopherols with a free 5^- position on the chromanol ring, such as γ- and δ-tocopherol, are expected to react with nitrogen species, forming C-nitroso derivatives at this position (Cooney et al. 1993). α-Tocopherol is trimethylated, and consequently, the nitrosating agent has the possibility to add only to the *para*- position on the chromanol ring of α-tocopherol, forming a highly unstable compound, and may form toxic *N*-nitroso derivatives from amines (Cooney et al. 1993). The high hydrogen donation ability of α-tocopherol may cause undesirable side effects, such as prooxidant and toxic nitro derivatives (Cillard and Cillard 1980).

There are differences in the efficacy of tocopherols and tocotrienols. The structural difference in the side chain may allow tocotrienols to be more uniformly distributed throughout the lipid bilayer. In addition, tocotrienols may have a higher recycling efficiency (Serbinova and Packer 1994) as well as a 70-times-higher cellular uptake than tocopherols (Saito et al. 2004).

Vitamin E may also be an indirect antioxidant by activating nuclear factor (erythroid-derived 2)–like 2 (Nrf2) enzymes. Nrf2 is a transcription factor that is a key regulator of cellular antioxidant and detoxification enzymes (Saw et al. 2010). Kelch-like ECH-associated protein 1 (KEAP1) inhibits Nrf2 in the cytoplasm, and thus, Nrf2 is marked for degradation through the proteasomal pathway (Saw et al. 2010). Chemopreventive agents or oxidative stress may modify the cysteine bonds on KEAP1, which allows the release and the consequential activation of Nrf2 (Saw et al. 2010; Surh 2003; Frohlich et al. 2008). Nrf2 translocates into the nucleus, dimerizes with small Maf proteins, and binds to the antioxidant-responsive element (ARE) to stimulate gene expression of antioxidant enzymes (thioredoxin, superoxide dismutase [SOD], catalase, glutathione peroxidase, and heme oxygenase 1 [HO-1]) and phase II detoxification enzymes (glutathione s-transferases [GSTs], UDP-glucuronosyltransferases, sulfotransferases, and NAD(P)H dehydrogenase, quinone 1 [NQO1]) (Kwak and Kensler 2010; Surh 2003; Saw et al. 2010; Barve et al. 2009; Frohlich et al. 2008). The stimulated detoxifying and antioxidant enzymes are able to protect the cells from neoplastic transformation by maintaining oxidative stress homeostasis (Khor et al. 2008; Barve et al. 2009). In Nrf2-knockout mice, the induction of cyclooxygenase 2 (COX2), 5-lipoxygenase, prostaglandin E_2 (PGE$_2$), and leukotriene B_4 was significantly higher when compared to that of the wild-type mice (Li et al. 2008). Thus, the loss of Nrf2 may play an important role in the protection against inflammation and lead to a decrease in cellular defense against oxidative stress, which may result in tumorigenesis (Chen and Kong 2005).

Pretreatment with α-tocopherol inhibits reactive oxygen species (ROS) generation, increases Nrf2 expression, and induces phase II enzymes (glutamate cysteine ligase, NQO1, HO-1, GST, and SOD) in human retinal pigment epithelial cells (Feng et al. 2010). In prostate tumors, the expression of Nrf2 was suppressed (Yu et al. 2010), and treatment with γ-TmT upregulated the expression of Nrf2 and detoxifying enzymes and inhibited tumor development in TRAMP (transgenic adenocarcinoma of mouse prostate) mice (Barve et al. 2009; Yu et al. 2010). In mammary hyperplasia, administration of γ-TmT increased the protein expression level of Nrf2 (Smolarek, So, Thomas et al. 2012). Both δ- and γ-tocotrienol increased Nrf2 expression in MDA-MB-231 breast cancer cells but not in MCF-7 estrogen receptor (ER)–positive breast cancer cells (Hsieh et al. 2010a). In addition, δ- and γ-tocotrienol were found to upregulate downstream targets of Nrf2 such as glutathione peroxidase, thioredoxin, and catalase (Hsieh et al. 2010a). In MCF-7 breast cancer cells, γ-tocotrienol was found to upregulate NQO2 (Hsieh et al. 2010b).

12.2.3 REGULATION OF ERs BY VITAMIN E

ER is a nuclear receptor that consists of two different subtypes (α and β) and stimulates cell growth and proliferation (Mense et al. 2008). Upon ligand activation, ER dimerizes, enters the nucleus, and binds to the estrogen response element sequence. The DNA binding domains of ERα and ERβ are highly homologous, while the ligand binding domain is 60% homologous (Rice and Whitehead 2008). ERα and ERβ are both present in breast tissue; however, the ratio of ERα to ERβ is increased in breast tumors (Rice and Whitehead 2008). Some studies have shown that activation of ERβ in breast cancer cell lines inhibits cell growth and that the dimerization of ERβ with ERα silences the growth-promoting effects of ERα (Rice and Whitehead 2008; Comitato et al. 2009).

In ER-positive breast cancer cell lines MCF-7 and T47D, vitamin E has been shown to inhibit proliferation and work as antagonists of estrogen signaling (Chamras et al. 2005). MCF-7 cells were treated with γ-TmT, and the expression of ERα was downregulated (Lee et al. 2009). In mammary tumors, ERα messenger RNA (mRNA) and protein levels were downregulated by treatment with γ-TmT (Lee et al. 2009). Treatment with γ-TmT reduced ERα mRNA and protein levels in hyperplastic mammary tissues in estrogen-treated August Copenhagen Irish (ACI) rats, while mRNA levels of ERβ were increased (Smolarek, So, Thomas et al. 2012). The circulating levels of E_2 in the serum were decreased when γ-TmT was administered, suggesting that γ-TmT may modify the response to estrogen (Smolarek, So, Thomas et al. 2012). Tocotrienols have also been shown to alter ER expression. Both γ- and δ-tocotrienol increased ERβ in MDA-MB-231 breast cancer cells (Comitato et al. 2009), and a tocotrienol-rich fraction from palm oil increased ERβ and decreased ERα protein levels in MCF-7 breast cancer cells (Comitato et al. 2010).

12.2.4 ACTIVATION OF PEROXISOME PROLIFERATOR-ACTIVATED RECEPTOR γ BY VITAMIN E

Another nuclear receptor of importance in cancers is peroxisome proliferator–activated receptor (PPAR). This nuclear hormone receptor superfamily comprises three subtypes (α, γ, and δ), which are ligand-regulated transcription factors (Desvergne and Wahli 1999). PPAR-γ forms a heterodimer with the retinoid X receptor after ligand activation (Michalik et al. 2004). One known PPAR-γ ligand is troglitazone (Campbell et al. 2003), and the chromanol ring of vitamin E is structurally similar. However, vitamin E is not a direct ligand of PPAR-γ, but rather γ-tocopherol was shown to induce the formation of 15-S-hydroxyeicosatetraenoic acid, an endogenous PPAR-γ ligand (Campbell et al. 2009). PPAR-γ is known to be involved in fatty acid uptake and transport and acts to control inflammation by inducing apoptosis and inhibiting cell proliferation and cell survival (Michalik et al. 2004; Mansure et al. 2009). PPAR-γ signaling is connected to the inhibition of inflammatory markers (COX2, cytokines, and inducible nitric oxide synthase [iNOS]), the phosphoinositide 3-kinase (PI3-K)/Akt pathway, and angiogenesis while inducing cyclin dependent kinase (CDK) inhibitors, differentiation, and apoptosis markers in cancers (Mansure et al. 2009).

γ-Tocopherol displayed the strongest activity in inducing the mRNA and protein levels of PPAR-γ in SW480 colon cancer cells (Campbell et al. 2003) and transcriptional activity in the NCTC 2544 keratinocyte cell line (De Pascale et al. 2006). In MCF-7 and T47D breast cancer cells, γ-TmT, γ-tocopherol, and more strongly, δ-tocopherol enhance the transactivation of PPAR-γ (Lee et al. 2009). In an NMU-induced breast cancer model in Sprague-Dawley rats, γ-TmT increased PPAR-γ mRNA and protein levels (Lee et al. 2009). There are limited data with tocotrienols and PPAR-γ, but one study showed that γ-tocopherol induced PPAR-γ in PC-3 prostate cancer cells (Campbell et al. 2011).

12.3 ANTI-INFLAMMATORY ACTIVITIES OF VITAMIN E

Inflammation is a response to heal tissue afflicted with injury. Under normal conditions, chemotactic factors such as transforming growth factor beta (TGF-β) and platelet-derived growth factor remodel the extracellular matrix (Coussens and Werb 2002). Once the wound is healed, the signaling subsides. However, under chronic inflammation, growth factors and cytokines such as tumor necrosis factor α (TNFα) are deregulated, leading to abnormalities and neoplastic progression. Inflammation may play a critical role in tumorigenesis at both the initiation and progression stages. During the tumor initiation stage, where a normal cell acquires the first mutation, the inflammatory microenvironment may increase mutation rates by generating ROS and RNS that cause DNA damage to nearby cells or by producing growth factors and cytokines (Grivennikov et al. 2010). In addition, the tumor microenvironment may recruit leukocytes and cytokines and help the cancer cells survive by recruiting more inflammatory cells (Grivennikov et al. 2010). For tumor promotion, tumor growth comes from a single initiated cell. Both cell proliferation and reduced cell death are stimulated by inflammation-driven mechanisms. Immune cells such as macrophages are able to produce cytokines, which are able to activate key transcription factors such as NF-κB or signal transducer and activator of transcription 3 (STAT3). In addition, NF-κB and STAT3 are able to produce chemokines that attract more inflammatory cells to increase a positive feed-forward loop. As a result, the stimulated malignant cells are able to induce survival, proliferation, growth, angiogenesis, and invasion (Grivennikov et al. 2010).

12.3.1 INHIBITION OF COX2 BY VITAMIN E

There are two major types of COX, constitutive (COX1) and inducible (COX2). COX1 is a "housekeeping protein" in most tissues and does not change in response to stimuli (O'Leary et al. 2004). COX2 is an inducible prostaglandin synthase, which is upregulated by growth factors, tumor promoters, and cytokines (Herschman 1996) and is responsive to several oncogenes, such as human epidermal growth factor receptor 2 (HER2) (Howe et al. 2001; Ristimaki et al. 2002). Prostaglandin synthesis is increased in inflamed and neoplastic tissues (Howe et al. 2001). High levels of COX2 are associated with about 40% of aggressive human breast cancers and correlate with large tumor sizes, high proliferation rates, and metastases (Ristimaki et al. 2002). When a COX2 inhibitor, celecoxib, was administered to HER2/neu transgenic mice, mammary tumor onset was delayed, and there was a 50% reduction in mammary tumor PGE_2 levels (Howe et al. 2002). When stimulated with cytokines, PGE_2 and COX2 production was accompanied by an increase in nitric oxide (NO) and corresponding iNOS enzyme in the A549 human lung adenocarcinoma cell line (Banerjee et al. 2002).

In various model systems, vitamin E supplementation can inhibit COX2 activity (Wu et al. 1998, 2000; Jiang et al. 2000). Tocopherols are known anti-inflammatory agents, and γ-tocopherol is more effective in inhibiting the activity of COX2 than α-tocopherol (Jiang et al. 2000, 2001). In addition, γ-tocopherol was shown to reduce PGE_2 synthesis in macrophages and human epithelial cells (Jiang et al. 2000), and the inhibitory effect was due to the decrease in COX2 activity (Jiang et al. 2000, 2008). Serum levels of PGE_2 and 8-isoprostane, a marker of oxidative stress, were reduced when estrogen-induced ACI rats were treated with γ-TmT, and COX2 levels decreased in the mammary gland when treated with dietary γ-TmT (Smolarek, So, Thomas et al. 2012).

12.3.2 SUPPRESSION OF NF-κB BY VITAMIN E

NF-κB is a transcription factor that is closely linked to inflammation. Under normal conditions, NF-κB is located in the cytoplasm and bound to inhibitor IκB proteins. Once activated, IκB proteins are degraded, which leads to the activation and translocation of NF-κB into the nucleus (Aggarwal and Gehlot 2009). Activation of NF-κB can be a response to environmental stimuli, inflammatory cytokines, and stress and is responsible for regulating the activity of proinflammatory genes such as TNFα, interleukin 1 (IL-1), IL-6, IL-8, matrix metalloproteinase 9 (MMP-9), vascular endothelial growth factor (VEGF), and 5-lipoxygenase (Aggarwal and Gehlot 2009). Constitutive activation of NF-κB may be found in breast, colon, prostate, ovary, liver, pancreas, leukemia, and lymphoma cancers and correlates with recurrence, poor survival, aggressiveness, and tumor progression (Nesaretnam and Meganathan 2011).

In lipopolysaccharide (LPS)-activated RAW 264.7 macrophages, apigenin blocked LPS-induced NF-κB activation and also suppressed the promoter activity of COX2 (Liang et al. 1999), which thus shows that another potential mechanism that inhibits COX2 gene expression is by the alteration of the NF-κB pathway. Furthermore, it has recently been shown that NF-κB could repress Nrf2 by competing for the transcription coactivator CREB-binding protein and by recruiting histone deacetylase 3 to cause local hypoacetylation to hamper Nrf2 signaling (Liu et al. 2008). Further studies are needed to understand the relationship between NF-κB, COX2, and Nrf2.

TNFα was used to stimulate the A549 human type II alveolar epithelial cell line, and treatment with α-tocopherol resulted in decreased levels of intracellular adhesion molecule 1 (ICAM-1), vascular adhesion molecule-1, IL-8, NF-κB, phospho-Erk (p-Erk), and p38 (Ekstrand-Hammarstrom et al. 2007). A vitamin E analog, α-tocopheryl succinate, was shown to inhibit NF-κB translocation and phospho-AKT (p-Akt) in MDA-MB-453 and MCF-7 breast cancer cell lines (Wang et al. 2010). NF-κB was inhibited by α-tocopheryl succinate in KU-19-19 and 5637 bladder cancer cell lines as well as KU-19-19 preestablished tumors (Kanai et al. 2010). In androgen-independent PC-3, DU-145, and CA-HPV prostate cancer cells, α-tocopheryl succinate inhibits NF-κB; reduces the expression of IL-6, IL-8, and VEGF; suppresses cell adhesion molecule ICAM-1; and augments activator protein 1 (AP-1) (Crispen et al. 2007).

Treatment with γ-tocotrienol suppressed constitutive activation of NF-κB as well as NF-κB activation induced by TNFα, phorbol myristate acetate (PMA), okadaic acid, cigarette smoke, LPS, IL-1β, and epidermal growth factor (Ahn et al. 2007). In addition, the anti-inflammatory effect of γ-tocotrienol on the suppression of NF-κB was found in human lung adenocarcinoma H1299, human embryonic kidney A293, human breast cancer MCF-7, multiple myeloma U266, and human squamous cell carcinoma SCC-4 cell lines (Ahn et al. 2007). Tocotrienol-rich fraction from palm oil was able to reduce PGE_2, TNFα, IL-4, IL-8, iNOS, COX2, and NF-κB in LPS-induced human monocytic leukemia cells (Wu et al. 2008).

12.3.3 PROTECTIVE EFFECTS OF VITAMIN E IN CARDIOVASCULAR AND NEURODEGENERATIVE DISEASES

CVD is a leading cause of morbidity and mortality in the United States, and several studies have indicated that biomarkers of inflammation predict an increased risk for CVD (Jialal et al. 2004; Libby 2002). One marker of inflammation is C-reactive protein (CRP), a member of the pentraxin family, and it is active in atherosclerosis (Jialal et al. 2004; Verma et al. 2006). Atherosclerosis is a chronic inflammatory disease where there is an accumulation of lipids, cells (macrophages, T lymphocytes, and smooth muscle cells [SMCs]), and extracellular matrix in the arterial wall. Monocytes and macrophages produce biologically active proinflammatory mediators and cytokines such as IL-1β, TNFα, and IL-6 (Singh and Devaraj 2007). Both IL-1β and TNFα stimulate adhesion molecules, and atherosclerosis is associated with impaired endothelial dysfunction such as changes induced by adhesion and migration of monocytes (Jialal et al. 2004; Singh and Devaraj 2007). Furthermore, apolipoprotein E knockout (ApoE KO) mice are deficient in IL-1β and demonstrate a decrease in severity of atherosclerosis, which put forth the evidence that IL-1 signaling promotes inflammation in the vascular wall (Kirii et al. 2003; Jialal et al. 2004). In the ApoE KO mice, vitamin E deficiency caused by disruption of the α-tocopherol transport protein (α-TTP) gene increased the severity of atherosclerotic lesions in the proximal aorta (Terasawa et al. 2000). Vitamin E is a potent lipid-soluble antioxidant in plasma and low density lipoprotein (LDL) and has demonstrated anti-inflammatory activity in atherosclerosis.

In an additional study, Apo E KO and Apo E/α-TTP KO mice were fed with a high-fat diet with or without α-tocopherol (Suarna et al. 2006). The study concluded that an α-tocopherol supplement ameliorated atherosclerosis in hyperlipidemic mice with severe vitamin E deficiency (Suarna et al. 2006). In Sprague-Dawley rats, α-tocopherol and, to a greater extent, γ-tocopherol supplementation decreased platelet aggregation, delayed intraarterial thrombus formation, and increased super oxide dismutase activity (Saldeen et al. 1999). An atherogenic diet supplemented with palm tocotrienols (33% α-tocopherol, 32.2% γ-tocotrienol, 16.1% α-tocotrienol, 16.1% δ-tocopherol, and 2.3% β-tocotrienol) fed to ApoE$^{+/-}$ mice reduced atherosclerotic lesions, while α-tocopherol supplementation did not (Black et al. 2000). α-Tocopherol has been shown to reduce oxidative stress on cells that participate in atherogenesis; however, clinical trials have failed to demonstrate a benefit of antioxidant supplementation in the prevention of CVD (Singh and Devaraj 2007).

AD is a neurodegenerative disease characterized by the development of senile plaques and neurofibrillary tangles in the brain (Usoro and Mousa 2010). The neuroinflammation that occurs in AD is thought to originate from amyloid accumulation in the senile plaques, which undergoes autocrine cycling that is able to regulate cytokine expression, glial activation, and oxidative and nitrosative production (Williamson et al. 2002). Oxidative stress may play a major role in the pathophysiology of neurodegenerative diseases since the central nervous system has a high oxygen consumption rate, abundant lipid content, and deficient antioxidant systems (Halliwell 1999). For instance, ROS may produce normal and abnormal cellular reactions and cause cell damage by way of lipid peroxidation, protein oxidation, and DNA oxidation (Coyle and Puttfarcken 1993). Vitamin E is a lipid-soluble, chain-breaking antioxidant in the biological membrane and may be able to protect against AD.

Williamson et al. (2002) examined brain tissue from individuals afflicted with AD and found that there was an increase in the lipid nitration product nitro-γ-tocopherol. Further investigation determined that there was a difference between α- and γ-tocopherol treatment in rat brain mitochondria after exposure to a peroxynitrite-generating compound, 3-morpholinosydnonimine (SIN-1). They revealed that oxidation-sensitive α-ketoglutarate dehydrogenase was inactivated by SIN-1 and was attenuated by γ-tocopherol but not α-tocopherol (Williamson et al. 2002). Thus, their findings suggest that nitrogen species contribute to the oxidative stress in the AD brain and that γ-tocopherol, but not α-tocopherol, may be protective (Williamson et al. 2002). In one population study, 8-iso-prostaglandin F2α, a lipid-peroxidation product and oxidative stress marker, was examined in AD patients before and after vitamin E treatment of 400 mg/day for 6 months; the study revealed that there was a 28% decrease in 8-iso-PGF2α levels after vitamin E treatment (Guan et al. 2012).

12.4 CONCLUSION

Inflammation is linked to cancer and CVD, which are leading causes of mortality in the United States. Although a very complex process, inflammation may be prevented by decreasing ROS and RNS as well as cytokine pathways. Once cells become exhausted in the ability to eliminate ROS, dietary sources of antioxidants are needed to help alleviate the stress. Vitamin E is a widely used dietary antioxidant. Both tocopherols and tocotrienols exhibit anti-inflammatory and cancer-preventive effects. Tables 12.1 and 12.2 summarize the protective effects of the different tocopherols and tocotrienols in vitro and in vivo, respectively. The in vitro and in vivo data show that γ/δ-tocopherol and γ/δ-tocotrienol, but not α-tocopherol, may inhibit inflammation, oxidative stress, and cell proliferation while inducing apoptosis. There is a need to further investigate the activities of individual forms of vitamin E to determine their differential efficacy against inflammation, cancer, and CVD.

TABLE 12.1

Molecular Events and Targets Modulated by Vitamin E in Vitro

Vitamin E	Cell Type/Cancer Model	Result	References
Apoptosis and Cell Proliferation			
γ-Tocopherol	Prostate cancer cells (LNCaP and PC-3) and lung cancer cells (A549)	↓Proliferation, ↑apoptosis	(Jiang, Wong, and Ames 2004)
Combination of tocopherols, γ-tocopherol, δ-tocopherol	Prostate cancer cells (LNCaP)	↓Proliferation, ↑apoptosis	(Jiang, Wong, Fyrst et al. 2004)
γ-Tocopherol	Colon cancer cells (SW480, HCT-15, HCT-116, HT-29)	↓Proliferation, ↑apoptosis	(Campbell et al. 2006)
γ-Tocopherol	Prostate cancer cells (DU-145 and LNCaP)	↓Proliferation, ↓cyclin D1, ↓cyclin E	(Gysin et al. 2002)
γ-Tocopherol	Prostate cancer cells (LNCaP)	↓Proliferation, ↑apoptosis	(Jiang, Wong, and Ames 2004)
δ-Tocopherol	Breast cancer cells (MCF-7 and MDA-MB-435)	↑Apoptosis	(Yu et al. 1999)
γ-Tocopherol	Breast cancer cells (MCF-7 and MDA-MB-435) and murine 66cl-4	↓Proliferation, ↑apoptosis	(Yu et al. 2008)
γ-Tocopherol, δ-tocopherol, γ-tocotrienol, δ-tocotrienol	Prostate cancer cells (PC-3 and LNCaP)	↓Proliferation	(Campbell et al. 2011)
γ-Tocotrienol	Prostate cancer cells (PC-3)	↑Apoptosis	(Campbell et al. 2011)
α-Tocotrienol, γ-tocotrienol, δ-tocotrienol	Breast cancer cells (MCF-7 and MDA-MB-231)	↓Proliferation	(Guthrie et al. 1997)
γ-Tocotrienol, δ-tocotrienol	Breast cancer cells (MCF-7 and MDA-MB-231)	↓Proliferation	(Hsieh et al. 2010a)
γ-Tocotrienol	Breast cancer cells (MCF-7)	↓Proliferation	(Hsieh et al. 2010b)
γ-Tocotrienol	Colon cancer cells (HT-29)	↓Proliferation, ↑apoptosis	(Xu et al. 2009)
γ-Tocotrienol	Gastric cancer cells (SGC-7901)	↑Apoptosis	(Sun et al. 2008)
Direct and Indirect Antioxidant Activities			
γ-Tocopherol	Human plasma	↓RNS, ↓peroxynitrite	(Christen et al. 1997)
Tocotrienol-rich fraction from palm oil	Human monocytic cells (THP-1) induced by LPS	↓NO	(Wu et al. 2008)
α-Tocopherol	Human retinal pigment epithelial cells (ARPE-19)	↑Nrf2 protein levels, ↑glutamate cysteine ligase, ↑NQO1, ↑HO-1, ↑GST, ↑SOD	(Feng et al. 2010)
γ-Tocotrienol, δ-tocotrienol	Breast cancer cells (MDA-MB-231)	↓KEAP1 levels, ↑Nrf2 protein levels, ↑catalase, ↑glutathione peroxidase, ↑quinone reductase 2	(Hsieh et al. 2010a)
γ-Tocotrienol	Breast cancer cells (MCF-7)	↑NQO2	(Hsieh et al. 2010b)
γ-Tocopheryl quinone	Neuronal cells (PC-12)	↑Activating transcription factor 4, ↑glutathione	(Ogawa et al. 2008)

(continued)

TABLE 12.1 (Continued)
Molecular Events and Targets Modulated by Vitamin E in Vitro

Vitamin E	Cell Type/Cancer Model	Result	References
Nuclear Receptors			
γ-TmT	Breast cancer cells (MCF-7)	↓ERα protein level	(Lee et al. 2009)
γ-Tocotrienol, δ-tocotrienol	Breast cancer cells (MDA-MB-231)	↑ERβ, ↑*MIC-1*, ↑*EGR-1*, ↑*cathepsin D*	(Comitato et al. 2009)
Tocotrienol-rich fraction from palm oil	Breast cancer cells (MCF-7)	↓ERα mRNA and protein levels, ↑ERβ protein levels, ↑*MIC-1*, ↑*EGR-1*, ↑*cathepsin D*	(Comitato et al. 2010)
γ-Tocopherol	Colon cancer cells (SW480)	↑PPAR-γ mRNA and protein level	(Campbell et al. 2003)
γ-Tocopherol	Keratinocytes cells (NCTC 2544)	↑PPAR-γ mRNA levels	(De Pascale et al. 2006)
γ-TmT, γ-tocopherol, δ-tocopherol	Breast cancer cells (MCF-7 and T47D)	↑PPAR-γ transactivation	(Lee et al. 2009)
γ-Tocotrienol	Prostate cancer cells (PC-3)	↑PPAR-γ	(Campbell et al. 2011)
Anti-Inflammation			
γ-Tocopherol	Macrophages (RAW 264.7) and human epithelial cells (A549)	↓COX2, ↓PGE$_2$	(Jiang et al. 2000)
γ-Tocopherol, δ-tocopherol	Human epithelial cells (A549)	↓COX2	(Jiang et al. 2008)
α-Tocopherol	Human epithelial cells (A549)	↓NF-κB, ↓ICAM-1, ↓IL-8, ↓p-Erk, ↓p38	(Ekstrand-Hammarstrom et al. 2007)
α-Tocopheryl succinate	Breast cancer cells (MDA-MB-453 and MCF-7)	↓NF-κB, ↓p-Akt	(Wang et al. 2010)
α-Tocopheryl succinate	Bladder cancer cells (KU-19-19 and 5637)	↓NF-κB	(Kanai et al. 2010)
α-Tocopheryl succinate	Prostate cancer cells (PC-3, DU-145, CA-HPV)	↓NF-κB, ↓IL-6, ↓IL-8, ↓VEGF, ↓ICAM-1, ↑AP-1	(Crispen et al. 2007)
γ-Tocotrienol	Prostate cancer cells (PC-3)	↓NF-κB, ↓p38, ↓TGF-β2, ↓MKK3/6	(Campbell et al. 2011)
γ-Tocotrienol	Human myeloid cells (KBM-5), lung cells (H1299), embryonic kidney cells (A293), breast cancer cells (MCF-7), multiple myeloma cells (U266), squamous cell carcinoma (SCC-4)	↓Inducible and constitutive NF-κB activation, ↓p-p65, ↓p-Akt	(Ahn et al. 2007)
Tocotrienol-rich fraction from palm oil	Prostate cancer cells (PCa)	↓NF-κB	(Yap et al. 2008)
γ-Tocotrienol	Melanoma cells (C32)	↓NF-κB	(Chang et al. 2009)
Tocotrienol-rich fraction from palm oil	Human acute monocytic leukemia cells (THP-1) induced by LPS	↓PGE$_2$, ↓TNFα, ↓IL-4, ↓IL-8, ↓iNOS, ↓COX2, ↓NF-κB	(Wu et al. 2008)

Note: EGR-1, early growth response-1; MIC-1, human macrophage–inhibitory cytokine-1, MKK3/6, MAPK kinase.

TABLE 12.2

Molecular Events and Targets Modulated by Vitamin E in Vivo

Vitamin E	Cell Type/Cancer Model	Result	References
Apoptosis and Cell Proliferation			
γ-Tocopherol	Breast cancer MDA-MB-231 xenograft in nu/nu mice	↑Apoptosis	(Yu et al. 2009)
γ-TmT	NNK-induced A/J mice and lung cancer xenograft in nu/nu mice (H1299)	↑Apoptosis	(Lu et al. 2010)
γ-Tocopherol, δ-tocopherol	Lung cancer H1299 xenograft in nu/nu mice	↑Apoptosis	(Li et al. 2011)
γ-TmT	NMU-induced mammary tumors in female Sprague-Dawley rats	↓Proliferation	(Suh et al. 2007)
γ-TmT	NMU-induced mammary tumors in female Sprague-Dawley rats	↑Apoptosis	(Lee et al. 2009)
γ-Tocopherol, δ-tocopherol, γ-TmT	NMU-induced mammary tumors in female Sprague-Dawley rats	↑Apoptosis	(Smolarek, So, Kong et al. 2012)
γ-TmT	Estrogen-induced mammary hyperplasia in female ACI rats	↓Proliferation, ↑apoptosis	(Smolarek, So, Thomas et al. 2012)
γ-TmT	Colon cancer in AOM/DSS-treated mice	↑Apoptosis	(Ju et al. 2009)
Mixed tocotrienols	TRAMP mice	↑Apoptosis, ↑CDK inhibitors, ↓cyclins	(Barve et al. 2010)
Direct and Indirect Antioxidant Activities			
γ-Tocopherol	Zymosan-induced acute peritonitis in male Fischer 344 rats	↓RNS	(Jiang et al. 2002)
γ-Tocopherol	Carrageenan-induced inflammation in Wistar male rats	↓RNS	(Jiang et al. 2003)
γ-TmT	NNK-induced A/J mice and lung cancer xenograft in nu/nu mice (H1299)	↓8-OHdG, ↓γ-H2AX, ↓nitrotyrosine	(Lu et al. 2010)
γ-Tocopherol, δ-tocopherol, γ-TmT	Lung cancer xenograft in nu/nu mice (H1299)	↓8-OHdG, ↓γ-H2AX, ↓nitrotyrosine	(Li et al. 2011)
γ-TmT	Colon cancer in AOM/DSS-treated mice	↓Nitrotyrosine	(Ju et al. 2009)
γ-TmT	Prostate carcinogenesis in TRAMP male mice	↑Nrf2 protein levels, ↑GSTm1, UGT1A1, SOD, HO-1, catalase, glutathione peroxidase	(Barve et al. 2009)
γ-TmT	Estrogen-induced mammary hyperplasia in female ACI rats	↑Nrf2 protein levels	(Smolarek, So, Thomas et al. 2012)
Nuclear Receptors			
γ-TmT	NMU-induced mammary tumors in female Sprague-Dawley rats	↓ERα mRNA and protein level	(Lee et al. 2009)
γ-TmT	Estrogen-induced mammary hyperplasia in female ACI rats	↓ERα mRNA and protein level, ↑ERβ mRNA level, ↓E_2 in the serum	(Smolarek, So, Thomas et al. 2012)
γ-TmT	NMU-induced mammary tumors in female Sprague-Dawley rats	↑PPAR-γ mRNA and protein level	(Lee et al. 2009)
γ-TmT	Estrogen-induced mammary hyperplasia in female ACI rats	↑PPAR-γ mRNA and protein level	(Smolarek, So, Thomas et al. 2012)

(continued)

TABLE 12.2 (Continued)
Molecular Events and Targets Modulated by Vitamin E in Vivo

Vitamin E	Cell Type/Cancer Model	Result	References
	Anti-Inflammation		
γ-Tocopherol	Carrageenan-induced inflammation in Wistar male rats	↓PGE$_2$, ↓LTB$_4$, ↓TNFα	(Jiang et al. 2003)
γ-TmT	NNK-induced A/J mice and lung cancer xenograft in nu/nu mice (H1299)	↓PGE$_2$, ↓LTB$_4$	(Lu et al. 2010)
γ-TmT	Colon cancer in AOM/DSS-treated mice	↓PGE$_2$, ↓LTB$_4$	(Ju et al. 2009)
γ-TmT	Estrogen-induced mammary hyperplasia in female ACI rats	↓COX2, ↓PGE$_2$, ↓8-isoprostane	(Smolarek, So, Thomas et al. 2012)

Note: AOM/DSS, azoxymethane/dextran sulfate sodium; LTB$_4$, leukotriene B$_4$; NNK, 4-(methylnitrosamino)-1-(3-pyridyl)-1-butanone; 8-OHdG, hydroxy-2'-deoxyguanosine; UGT1A1, UDP-glucuronosyltransferase.

ACKNOWLEDGMENTS

This work was supported in part by NIH R03 CA141756, NIEHS Center Grant P30 ES005022, and the Trustees Research Fellowship Program at Rutgers, the State University of New Jersey.

REFERENCES

Aggarwal, B. B., and P. Gehlot. 2009. Inflammation and cancer: how friendly is the relationship for cancer patients? *Curr Opin Pharmacol* 9 (4):351–69.

Aggarwal, B. B., C. Sundaram, S. Prasad, and R. Kannappan. 2010. Tocotrienols, the vitamin E of the 21st century: its potential against cancer and other chronic diseases. *Biochem Pharmacol* 80 (11):1613–31.

Ahn, K. S., G. Sethi, K. Krishnan, and B. B. Aggarwal. 2007. Gamma-tocotrienol inhibits nuclear factor-kappaB signaling pathway through inhibition of receptor-interacting protein and TAK1 leading to suppression of antiapoptotic gene products and potentiation of apoptosis. *J Biol Chem* 282 (1):809–20.

Banerjee, T., A. Van der Vliet, and V. A. Ziboh. 2002. Downregulation of COX-2 and iNOS by amentoflavone and quercetin in A549 human lung adenocarcinoma cell line. *Prostaglandins Leukot Essent Fatty Acids* 66 (5–6):485–92.

Barve, A., T. O. Khor, S. Nair et al. 2009. Gamma-tocopherol-enriched mixed tocopherol diet inhibits prostate carcinogenesis in TRAMP mice. *Int J Cancer* 124 (7):1693–9.

Barve, A., T. O. Khor, K. Reuhl et al. 2010. Mixed tocotrienols inhibit prostate carcinogenesis in TRAMP mice. *Nutr Cancer* 62 (6):789–94.

Betti, M., A. Minelli, B. Canonico et al. 2006. Antiproliferative effects of tocopherols (vitamin E) on murine glioma C6 cells: homologue-specific control of PKC/ERK and cyclin signaling. *Free Radic Biol Med* 41 (3):464–72.

Birringer, M., P. Pfluger, D. Kluth, N. Landes, and R. Brigelius-Flohe. 2002. Identities and differences in the metabolism of tocotrienols and tocopherols in HepG2 cells. *J Nutr* 132 (10):3113–8.

Black, T. M., P. Wang, N. Maeda, and R. A. Coleman. 2000. Palm tocotrienols protect ApoE +/– mice from diet-induced atheroma formation. *J Nutr* 130 (10):2420–6.

Boscoboinik, D., A. Szewczyk, and A. Azzi. 1991. Alpha-tocopherol (vitamin E) regulates vascular smooth muscle cell proliferation and protein kinase C activity. *Arch Biochem Biophys* 286 (1):264–9.

Boscoboinik, D., A. Szewczyk, C. Hensey, and A. Azzi. 1991. Inhibition of cell proliferation by alpha-tocopherol. Role of protein kinase C. *J Biol Chem* 266 (10):6188–94.

Brigelius-Flohe, R., and M. G. Traber. 1999. Vitamin E: function and metabolism. *FASEB J* 13 (10):1145–55.

Burton, G. W., and K. U. Ingold. 1989. Vitamin E as an in vitro and in vivo antioxidant. *Ann N Y Acad Sci* 570:7–22.

Burton, G. W., and M. G. Traber. 1990. Vitamin E: antioxidant activity, biokinetics, and bioavailability. *Annu Rev Nutr* 10:357–82.

Campbell, S. E., B. Rudder, R. B. Phillips et al. 2011. gamma-Tocotrienol induces growth arrest through a novel pathway with TGFbeta2 in prostate cancer. *Free Radic Biol Med* 50 (10):1344–54.

Campbell, S. E., P. R. Musich, S. G. Whaley et al. 2009. Gamma tocopherol upregulates the expression of 15-S-HETE and induces growth arrest through a PPAR gamma-dependent mechanism in PC-3 human prostate cancer cells. *Nutr Cancer* 61 (5):649–62.

Campbell, S. E., W. L. Stone, S. Lee et al. 2006. Comparative effects of RRR-alpha- and RRR-gamma-tocopherol on proliferation and apoptosis in human colon cancer cell lines. *BMC Cancer* 6:13.

Campbell, S. E., W. L. Stone, S. G. Whaley, M. Qui, and K. Krishnan. 2003. Gamma (gamma) tocopherol upregulates peroxisome proliferator activated receptor (PPAR) gamma (gamma) expression in SW 480 human colon cancer cell lines. *BMC Cancer* 3:25.

Chamras, H., S. H. Barsky, A. Ardashian et al. 2005. Novel interactions of vitamin E and estrogen in breast cancer. *Nutr Cancer* 52 (1):43–8.

Chang, P. N., W. N. Yap, D. T. Lee et al. 2009. Evidence of gamma-tocotrienol as an apoptosis-inducing, invasion-suppressing, and chemotherapy drug-sensitizing agent in human melanoma cells. *Nutr Cancer* 61 (3):357–66.

Chen, C., and A. N. Kong. 2005. Dietary cancer-chemopreventive compounds: from signaling and gene expression to pharmacological effects. *Trends Pharmacol Sci* 26 (6):318–26.

Christen, S., A. A. Woodall, M. K. Shigenaga et al. 1997. Gamma-tocopherol traps mutagenic electrophiles such as NO(X) and complements alpha-tocopherol: physiological implications. *Proc Natl Acad Sci U S A* 94 (7):3217–22.

Cillard, J., and P. Cillard. 1980. [Prooxidant effect of alpha-tocopherol on essential fatty acids in aqueous media]. *Ann Nutr Aliment* 34 (3):579–91.

Cohen, G. M. 1997. Caspases: the executioners of apoptosis. *Biochem J* 326 (Pt 1):1–16.

Comitato, R., G. Leoni, R. Canali et al. 2010. Tocotrienols activity in MCF-7 breast cancer cells: involvement of ERbeta signal transduction. *Mol Nutr Food Res* 54 (5):669–78.

Comitato, R., K. Nesaretnam, G. Leoni et al. 2009. A novel mechanism of natural vitamin E tocotrienol activity: involvement of ERbeta signal transduction. *Am J Physiol Endocrinol Metab* 297 (2):E427–37.

Constantinou, C., A. Papas, and A. I. Constantinou. 2008. Vitamin E and cancer: an insight into the anticancer activities of vitamin E isomers and analogs. *Int J Cancer* 123 (4):739–52.

Cooney, R. V., A. A. Franke, P. J. Harwood et al. 1993. Gamma-tocopherol detoxification of nitrogen dioxide: superiority to alpha-tocopherol. *Proc Natl Acad Sci U S A* 90 (5):1771–5.

Coussens, L. M., and Z. Werb. 2002. Inflammation and cancer. *Nature* 420 (6917):860–7.

Coyle, J. T., and P. Puttfarcken. 1993. Oxidative stress, glutamate, and neurodegenerative disorders. *Science* 262 (5134):689–95.

Crispen, P. L., R. G. Uzzo, K. Golovine et al. 2007. Vitamin E succinate inhibits NF-kappaB and prevents the development of a metastatic phenotype in prostate cancer cells: implications for chemoprevention. *Prostate* 67 (6):582–90.

De Pascale, M. C., A. M. Bassi, V. Patrone et al. 2006. Increased expression of transglutaminase-1 and PPARgamma after vitamin E treatment in human keratinocytes. *Arch Biochem Biophys* 447 (2):97–106.

Desvergne, B., and W. Wahli. 1999. Peroxisome proliferator-activated receptors: nuclear control of metabolism. *Endocr Rev* 20 (5):649–88.

Dutta-Roy, A. K., M. J. Gordon, D. J. Leishman et al. 1993. Purification and partial characterisation of an alpha-tocopherol-binding protein from rabbit heart cytosol. *Mol Cell Biochem* 123 (1–2):139–44.

Ekstrand-Hammarstrom, B., C. Osterlund, B. Lilliehook, and A. Bucht. 2007. Vitamin E down-modulates mitogen-activated protein kinases, nuclear factor-kappaB and inflammatory responses in lung epithelial cells. *Clin Exp Immunol* 147 (2):359–69.

Elmore, S. 2007. Apoptosis: a review of programmed cell death. *Toxicol Pathol* 35 (4):495–516.

Evans, H. M., and K. S. Bishop. 1922. On the existence of a hitherto unrecognized dietary factor essential for reproduction. *Science* 56 (1458):650–1.

Feng, Z., Z. Liu, X. Li et al. 2010. alpha-Tocopherol is an effective Phase II enzyme inducer: protective effects on acrolein-induced oxidative stress and mitochondrial dysfunction in human retinal pigment epithelial cells. *J Nutr Biochem* 21 (12):1222–31.

Frohlich, D. A., M. T. McCabe, R. S. Arnold, and M. L. Day. 2008. The role of Nrf2 in increased reactive oxygen species and DNA damage in prostate tumorigenesis. *Oncogene* 27 (31):4353–62.

Galli, F., and A. Azzi. 2010. Present trends in vitamin E research. *Biofactors* 36 (1):33–42.

Gordon, M. J., F. M. Campbell, and A. K. Dutta-Roy. 1996. alpha-Tocopherol-binding protein in the cytosol of the human placenta. *Biochem Soc Trans* 24 (2):202S.

Gordon, M. J., F. M. Campbell, G. G. Duthie, and A. K. Dutta-Roy. 1995. Characterization of a novel alpha-tocopherol-binding protein from bovine heart cytosol. *Arch Biochem Biophys* 318 (1):140–6.

Grivennikov, S. I., F. R. Greten, and M. Karin. 2010. Immunity, inflammation, and cancer. *Cell* 140 (6):883–99.

Guan, J. Z., W. P. Guan, T. Maeda, and N. Makino. 2012. Effect of vitamin E administration on the elevated oxygen stress and the telomeric and subtelomeric status in Alzheimer's disease. *Gerontology* 58 (1):62–9.

Guthrie, N., A. Gapor, A. F. Chambers, and K. K. Carroll. 1997. Inhibition of proliferation of estrogen receptor-negative MDA-MB-435 and -positive MCF-7 human breast cancer cells by palm oil tocotrienols and tamoxifen, alone and in combination. *J Nutr* 127 (3):544S–548S.

Gysin, R., A. Azzi, and T. Visarius. 2002. Gamma-tocopherol inhibits human cancer cell cycle progression and cell proliferation by down-regulation of cyclins. *FASEB J* 16 (14):1952–4.

Hacker, G. 2000. The morphology of apoptosis. *Cell Tissue Res* 301 (1):5–17.

Halliwell, B. 1999. Antioxidant defence mechanisms: from the beginning to the end (of the beginning). *Free Radic Res* 31 (4):261–72.

Heron, M. 2011. Deaths: leading causes for 2007. *Natl Vital Stat Rep* 59 (8):1–95.

Herschman, H. R. 1996. Prostaglandin synthase 2. *Biochim Biophys Acta* 1299 (1):125–40.

Hosomi, A., M. Arita, Y. Sato et al. 1997. Affinity for alpha-tocopherol transfer protein as a determinant of the biological activities of vitamin E analogs. *FEBS Lett* 409 (1):105–8.

Howe, L. R., K. Subbaramaiah, A. M. Brown, and A. J. Dannenberg. 2001. Cyclooxygenase-2: a target for the prevention and treatment of breast cancer. *Endocr Relat Cancer* 8 (2):97–114.

Howe, L. R., K. Subbaramaiah, J. Patel et al. 2002. Celecoxib, a selective cyclooxygenase 2 inhibitor, protects against human epidermal growth factor receptor 2 (HER-2)/neu-induced breast cancer. *Cancer Res* 62 (19):5405–7.

Hsieh, T. C., S. Elangovan, and J. M. Wu. 2010a. Differential suppression of proliferation in MCF-7 and MDA-MB-231 breast cancer cells exposed to alpha-, gamma- and delta-tocotrienols is accompanied by altered expression of oxidative stress modulatory enzymes. *Anticancer Res* 30 (10):4169–76.

Hsieh, T. C., S. Elangovan, and J. M. Wu. 2010b. gamma-Tocotrienol controls proliferation, modulates expression of cell cycle regulatory proteins and up-regulates quinone reductase NQO2 in MCF-7 breast cancer cells. *Anticancer Res* 30 (7):2869–74.

Igney, F. H., and P. H. Krammer. 2002. Death and anti-death: tumour resistance to apoptosis. *Nat Rev Cancer* 2 (4):277–88.

Inokuchi, H., H. Hirokane, T. Tsuzuki et al. 2003. Anti-angiogenic activity of tocotrienol. *Biosci Biotechnol Biochem* 67 (7):1623–7.

Jialal, I., S. Devaraj, and S. K. Venugopal. 2004. C-reactive protein: risk marker or mediator in atherothrombosis? *Hypertension* 44 (1):6–11.

Jiang, Q., and B. N. Ames. 2003. Gamma-tocopherol, but not alpha-tocopherol, decreases proinflammatory eicosanoids and inflammation damage in rats. *FASEB J* 17 (8):816–22.

Jiang, Q., X. Yin, M. A. Lill et al. 2008. Long-chain carboxychromanols, metabolites of vitamin E, are potent inhibitors of cyclooxygenases. *Proc Natl Acad Sci U S A* 105 (51):20464–9.

Jiang, Q., J. Wong, and B. N. Ames. 2004. Gamma-tocopherol induces apoptosis in androgen-responsive LNCaP prostate cancer cells via caspase-dependent and independent mechanisms. *Ann N Y Acad Sci* 1031:399–400.

Jiang, Q., J. Wong, H. Fyrst, J. D. Saba, and B. N. Ames. 2004. gamma-Tocopherol or combinations of vitamin E forms induce cell death in human prostate cancer cells by interrupting sphingolipid synthesis. *Proc Natl Acad Sci U S A* 101 (51):17825–30.

Jiang, Q., J. Lykkesfeldt, M. K. Shigenaga et al. 2002. Gamma-tocopherol supplementation inhibits protein nitration and ascorbate oxidation in rats with inflammation. *Free Radic Biol Med* 33 (11):1534–42.

Jiang, Q., S. Christen, M. K. Shigenaga, and B. N. Ames. 2001. Gamma-tocopherol, the major form of vitamin E in the US diet, deserves more attention. *Am J Clin Nutr* 74 (6):714–22.

Jiang, Q., I. Elson-Schwab, C. Courtemanche, and B. N. Ames. 2000. Gamma-tocopherol and its major metabolite, in contrast to alpha-tocopherol, inhibit cyclooxygenase activity in macrophages and epithelial cells. *Proc Natl Acad Sci U S A* 97 (21):11494–9.

Ju, J., X. Hao, M. J. Lee et al. 2009. A gamma-tocopherol-rich mixture of tocopherols inhibits colon inflammation and carcinogenesis in azoxymethane and dextran sulfate sodium-treated mice. *Cancer Prev Res (Phila Pa)* 2 (2):143–52.

Kamal-Eldin, A., and L. A. Appelqvist. 1996. The chemistry and antioxidant properties of tocopherols and tocotrienols. *Lipids* 31 (7):671–701.

Kanai, K., E. Kikuchi, S. Mikami et al. 2010. Vitamin E succinate induced apoptosis and enhanced chemosensitivity to paclitaxel in human bladder cancer cells in vitro and in vivo. *Cancer Sci* 101 (1):216–23.

Kerr, J. F. 2002. History of the events leading to the formulation of the apoptosis concept. *Toxicology* 181–182:471–4.

Kerr, J. F., A. H. Wyllie, and A. R. Currie. 1972. Apoptosis: a basic biological phenomenon with wide-ranging implications in tissue kinetics. *Br J Cancer* 26 (4):239–57.

Khor, T. O., S. Yu, and A. N. Kong. 2008. Dietary cancer chemopreventive agents—targeting inflammation and Nrf2 signaling pathway. *Planta Med* 74 (13):1540–7.

Kirii, H., T. Niwa, Y. Yamada et al. 2003. Lack of interleukin-1beta decreases the severity of atherosclerosis in ApoE-deficient mice. *Arterioscler Thromb Vasc Biol* 23 (4):656–60.

Kline, K., K. A. Lawson, W. Yu, and B. G. Sanders. 2007. Vitamin E and cancer. *Vitam Horm* 76:435–61.

Kline, K., K. A. Lawson, W. Yu, and B. G. Sanders. 2003. Vitamin E and breast cancer prevention: current status and future potential. *J Mammary Gland Biol Neoplasia* 8 (1):91–102.

Kwak, M. K., and T. W. Kensler. 2010. Targeting NRF2 signaling for cancer chemoprevention. *Toxicol Appl Pharmacol* 244 (1):66–76.

Lee, H. J., J. Ju, S. Paul et al. 2009. Mixed tocopherols prevent mammary tumorigenesis by inhibiting estrogen action and activating PPAR-gamma. *Clin Cancer Res* 15 (12):4242–9.

Li, G. X., M. J. Lee, A. B. Liu et al. 2011. Delta-tocopherol is more active than alpha- or gamma-tocopherol in inhibiting lung tumorigenesis in vivo. *Cancer Prev Res (Phila)* 4 (3):404–13.

Li, W., T. O. Khor, C. Xu et al. 2008. Activation of Nrf2-antioxidant signaling attenuates NFkappaB-inflammatory response and elicits apoptosis. *Biochem Pharmacol* 76 (11):1485–9.

Liang, Y. C., Y. T. Huang, S. H. Tsai et al. 1999. Suppression of inducible cyclooxygenase and inducible nitric oxide synthase by apigenin and related flavonoids in mouse macrophages. *Carcinogenesis* 20 (10):1945–52.

Libby, P. 2002. Inflammation in atherosclerosis. *Nature* 420 (6917):868–74.

Liu, G. H., J. Qu, and X. Shen. 2008. NF-kappaB/p65 antagonizes Nrf2-ARE pathway by depriving CBP from Nrf2 and facilitating recruitment of HDAC3 to MafK. *Biochim Biophys Acta* 1783 (5):713–27.

Lu, G., H. Xiao, G. X. Li et al. 2010. A gamma-tocopherol-rich mixture of tocopherols inhibits chemically induced lung tumorigenesis in A/J mice and xenograft tumor growth. *Carcinogenesis* 31 (4):687–94.

Mansure, J. J., R. Nassim, and W. Kassouf. 2009. Peroxisome proliferator-activated receptor gamma in bladder cancer: a promising therapeutic target. *Cancer Biol Ther* 8 (7):6–15.

McIntyre, B. S., K. P. Briski, A. Gapor, and P. W. Sylvester. 2000. Antiproliferative and apoptotic effects of tocopherols and tocotrienols on preneoplastic and neoplastic mouse mammary epithelial cells. *Proc Soc Exp Biol Med* 224 (4):292–301.

McLaughlin, P. J., and J. L. Weihrauch. 1979. Vitamin E content of foods. *J Am Diet Assoc* 75 (6):647–65.

Mense, S. M., F. Remotti, A. Bhan et al. 2008. Estrogen-induced breast cancer: alterations in breast morphology and oxidative stress as a function of estrogen exposure. *Toxicol Appl Pharmacol* 232 (1):78–85.

Michalik, L., B. Desvergne, and W. Wahli. 2004. Peroxisome-proliferator-activated receptors and cancers: complex stories. *Nat Rev Cancer* 4 (1):61–70.

Munteanu, A., J. M. Zingg, and A. Azzi. 2004. Anti-atherosclerotic effects of vitamin E—myth or reality? *J Cell Mol Med* 8 (1):59–76.

Murphy, D. J., and R. D. Mavis. 1981. Membrane transfer of alpha-tocopherol. Influence of soluble alpha-tocopherol-binding factors from the liver, lung, heart, and brain of the rat. *J Biol Chem* 256 (20):10464–8.

Nesaretnam, K., and P. Meganathan. 2011. Tocotrienols: inflammation and cancer. *Ann N Y Acad Sci* 1229: 18–22.

O'Leary, K. A., S. de Pascual-Tereasa, P. W. Needs et al. 2004. Effect of flavonoids and vitamin E on cyclooxygenase-2 (COX-2) transcription. *Mutat Res* 551 (1–2):245–54.

Ogawa, Y., Y. Saito, K. Nishio et al. 2008. Gamma-tocopheryl quinone, not alpha-tocopheryl quinone, induces adaptive response through up-regulation of cellular glutathione and cysteine availability via activation of ATF4. *Free Radic Res* 42 (7):674–87.

Pennock, J. F., F. W. Hemming, and J. D. Kerr. 1964. A reassessment of tocopherol in chemistry. *Biochem Biophys Res Commun* 17 (5):542–8.

Rai, N. K., K. Tripathi, D. Sharma, and V. K. Shukla. 2005. Apoptosis: a basic physiologic process in wound healing. *Int J Low Extrem Wounds* 4 (3):138–44.

Rice, S., and S. A. Whitehead. 2008. Phytoestrogens oestrogen synthesis and breast cancer. *J Steroid Biochem Mol Biol* 108 (3–5):186–95.

Ristimaki, A., A. Sivula, J. Lundin et al. 2002. Prognostic significance of elevated cyclooxygenase-2 expression in breast cancer. *Cancer Res* 62 (3):632–5.

Saito, Y., Y. Yoshida, K. Nishio, M. Hayakawa, and E. Niki. 2004. Characterization of cellular uptake and distribution of vitamin E. *Ann N Y Acad Sci* 1031:368–75.

Saldeen, T., D. Li, and J. L. Mehta. 1999. Differential effects of alpha- and gamma-tocopherol on low-density lipoprotein oxidation, superoxide activity, platelet aggregation and arterial thrombogenesis. *J Am Coll Cardiol* 34 (4):1208–15.

Saw, C. L., Q. Wu, and A. N. Kong. 2010. Anti-cancer and potential chemopreventive actions of ginseng by activating Nrf2 (NFE2L2) anti-oxidative stress/anti-inflammatory pathways. *Chin Med* 5:37.

Sen, C. K., S. Khanna, and S. Roy. 2007. Tocotrienols in health and disease: the other half of the natural vitamin E family. *Mol Aspects Med* 28 (5–6):692–728.

Serbinova, E. A., and L. Packer. 1994. Antioxidant properties of alpha-tocopherol and alpha-tocotrienol. *Methods Enzymol* 234:354–66.

Shah, S. J., and P. W. Sylvester. 2005. Gamma-tocotrienol inhibits neoplastic mammary epithelial cell proliferation by decreasing Akt and nuclear factor kappaB activity. *Exp Biol Med (Maywood)* 230 (4):235–41.

Singh, U., and S. Devaraj. 2007. Vitamin E: inflammation and atherosclerosis. *Vitam Horm* 76:519–49.

Smolarek, A. K., J. Y. So, A. N. Kong et al. 2012. Dietary administration of gamma- and delta-tocopherol inhibits mammary carcinogenesis. In *Proceedings of Society of Toxicology's 51st Annual Meeting & ToxExpo*, 363, San Francisco, CA, USA, Abstract.

Smolarek, A. K., J. Y. So, P. E. Thomas et al. 2012. Dietary tocopherols inhibit cell proliferation, regulate expression of ERalpha, PPARgamma, and Nrf2, and decrease serum inflammatory markers during the development of mammary hyperplasia. *Mol Carcinog* 52(7):514–25.

Sontag, T. J., and R. S. Parker. 2002. Cytochrome P450 omega-hydroxylase pathway of tocopherol catabolism. Novel mechanism of regulation of vitamin E status. *J Biol Chem* 277 (28):25290–6.

Stone, W. L., K. Krishnan, S. E. Campbell et al. 2004. Tocopherols and the treatment of colon cancer. *Ann N Y Acad Sci* 1031:223–33.

Suarna, C., R. L. Hood, R. T. Dean, and R. Stocker. 1993. Comparative antioxidant activity of tocotrienols and other natural lipid-soluble antioxidants in a homogeneous system, and in rat and human lipoproteins. *Biochim Biophys Acta* 1166 (2–3):163–70.

Suarna, C., B. J. Wu, K. Choy et al. 2006. Protective effect of vitamin E supplements on experimental atherosclerosis is modest and depends on preexisting vitamin E deficiency. *Free Radic Biol Med* 41 (5):722–30.

Suh, N., S. Paul, H. J. Lee et al. 2007. Mixed tocopherols inhibit N-methyl-N-nitrosourea-induced mammary tumor growth in rats. *Nutr Cancer* 59 (1):76–81.

Sun, W., Q. Wang, B. Chen et al. 2008. Gamma-tocotrienol-induced apoptosis in human gastric cancer SGC-7901 cells is associated with a suppression in mitogen-activated protein kinase signalling. *Br J Nutr* 99 (6):1247–54.

Surh, Y. J. 2003. Cancer chemoprevention with dietary phytochemicals. *Nat Rev Cancer* 3 (10):768–80.

Tan, A. C., I. Konczak, D. M. Sze, and I. Ramzan. 2011. Molecular pathways for cancer chemoprevention by dietary phytochemicals. *Nutr Cancer* 63 (4):495–505.

Taylor, P. R., Y. L. Qiao, C. C. Abnet et al. 2003. Prospective study of serum vitamin E levels and esophageal and gastric cancers. *J Natl Cancer Inst* 95 (18):1414–6.

Terasawa, Y., Z. Ladha, S. W. Leonard et al. 2000. Increased atherosclerosis in hyperlipidemic mice deficient in alpha-tocopherol transfer protein and vitamin E. *Proc Natl Acad Sci U S A* 97 (25):13830–4.

Traber, M. G. 2007. Vitamin E regulatory mechanisms. *Annu Rev Nutr* 27:347–62.

Usoro, O. B., and S. A. Mousa. 2010. Vitamin E forms in Alzheimer's disease: a review of controversial and clinical experiences. *Crit Rev Food Sci Nutr* 50 (5):414–9.

Verma, S., S. Devaraj, and I. Jialal. 2006. Is C-reactive protein an innocent bystander or proatherogenic culprit? C-reactive protein promotes atherothrombosis. *Circulation* 113 (17):2135–50; discussion 2150.

Wang, X. F., Y. Xie, H. G. Wang et al. 2010. alpha-Tocopheryl succinate induces apoptosis in erbB2-expressing breast cancer cell via NF-kappaB pathway. *Acta Pharmacol Sin* 31 (12):1604–10.

Williamson, K. S., S. P. Gabbita, S. Mou et al. 2002. The nitration product 5-nitro-gamma-tocopherol is increased in the Alzheimer brain. *Nitric Oxide* 6 (2):221–7.

Wolf, G. 2005. The discovery of the antioxidant function of vitamin E: the contribution of Henry A. Mattill. *J Nutr* 135 (3):363–6.

Wu, D., M. Meydani, A. A. Beharka et al. 2000. In vitro supplementation with different tocopherol homologues can affect the function of immune cells in old mice. *Free Radic Biol Med* 28 (4):643–51.

Wu, D., C. Mura, A. A. Beharka et al. 1998. Age-associated increase in PGE2 synthesis and COX activity in murine macrophages is reversed by vitamin E. *Am J Physiol* 275 (3 Pt 1):C661–8.

Wu, S. J., P. L. Liu, and L. T. Ng. 2008. Tocotrienol-rich fraction of palm oil exhibits anti-inflammatory property by suppressing the expression of inflammatory mediators in human monocytic cells. *Mol Nutr Food Res* 52 (8):921–9.

Xu, W. L., J. R. Liu, H. K. Liu et al. 2009. Inhibition of proliferation and induction of apoptosis by gamma-tocotrienol in human colon carcinoma HT-29 cells. *Nutrition* 25 (5):555–66.

Yap, W. N., P. N. Chang, H. Y. Han et al. 2008. Gamma-tocotrienol suppresses prostate cancer cell proliferation and invasion through multiple-signalling pathways. *Br J Cancer* 99 (11):1832–41.

Yu, S., T. O. Khor, K. L. Cheung et al. 2010. Nrf2 expression is regulated by epigenetic mechanisms in prostate cancer of TRAMP mice. *PLoS One* 5 (1):e8579.

Yu, W., L. Jia, S. K. Park et al. 2009. Anticancer actions of natural and synthetic vitamin E forms: RRR-alpha-tocopherol blocks the anticancer actions of gamma-tocopherol. *Mol Nutr Food Res* 53 (12):1573–81.

Yu, W., L. Jia, P. Wang et al. 2008. In vitro and in vivo evaluation of anticancer actions of natural and synthetic vitamin E forms. *Mol Nutr Food Res* 52 (4):447–56.

Yu, W., M. Simmons-Menchaca, A. Gapor, B. G. Sanders, and K. Kline. 1999. Induction of apoptosis in human breast cancer cells by tocopherols and tocotrienols. *Nutr Cancer* 33 (1):26–32.

Zimmer, S., A. Stocker, M. N. Sarbolouki et al. 2000. A novel human tocopherol-associated protein: cloning, in vitro expression, and characterization. *J Biol Chem* 275 (33):25672–80.

Zingg, J. M. 2007. Modulation of signal transduction by vitamin E. *Mol Aspects Med* 28 (5–6):481–506.

13 Vitamin D and Cancer
Research Update and Clinical Recommendations

Kathleen M. Wesa and Barrie R. Cassileth

CONTENTS

13.1 VITAMIN D BACKGROUND

13.1.1 VITAMIN D SYNTHESIS AND FORMS

Vitamin D has long been known as the major regulator of calcium homeostasis, and adequate serum vitamin D levels are required for bone mineralization. Vitamin D maintains calcium balance through actions in the intestines, bones, kidneys, and parathyroid glands (Feldman et al. 2007). The extraskeletal beneficial effects of vitamin D are increasingly recognized. The vitamin D receptor (VDR) has been demonstrated in nearly all tissues throughout the body. VDR binding results in local tissue-specific calcitriol synthesis, including many cancers. Calcitriol is the active

265

form of vitamin D and has a short half-life of 8–12 h. The local tissue-specific calcitriol stores act independently of the systemic calcitriol-calcium homeostasis modulation and may be responsible for the anti-inflammatory and anticancer effects of vitamin D (Ma Yingyu, Trump, and Johnson 2010).

Technically, vitamin D is not a vitamin, but rather it is a secosteroid hormone. Although some vitamin D is obtained through diet, the primary source of vitamin D in humans is from either sunlight ultraviolet B (UVB) exposure or dietary supplements. There are two forms of vitamin D: D_2 and D_3, both of which are vitamin D precursors that undergo multiple chemical conversions to ultimately form calcitriol. Cholecalciferol (D_3) comes from animal sources and is what humans synthesize in response to skin exposure to UVB rays 290–310 nm. Once the UVB rays contact the skin, vitamin D is synthesized from the precursor 7-dehydrocholesterol, which is then converted into the secosteroid vitamin D_3. Sunscreen use filters out the UVB rays, effectively preventing cutaneous vitamin D synthesis. Ergocalciferol (D_2) originates in plants and is also synthesized by mushrooms in response to UVB exposure. For the purpose of this discussion, unless D_2, D_3, or calcitriol is specified, "vitamin D" or "D" refers to serum 25-hydroxy vitamin D (calcidiol).

D_3 and D_2 are converted through hydroxylation in the liver into 25-hydroxy vitamin D (calcidiol). Calcidiol then undergoes a second hydroxylation step in the kidneys by the enzyme 1α-hydroxylase to form the secosteroid hormone calcitriol (1α,25-dihydroxyvitamin D_3). Calcitriol binds to the VDR and, through this VDR binding, exerts its distant effects (Ma Yingyu, Trump, and Johnson 2010).

Calcitriol is also synthesized locally in most tissues. This local tissue conversion is not as tightly regulated by the 1α-hydroxylase as the conversion of D_3 into calcitriol in the kidney (Krishnan and Feldman 2011). The tissue-specific calcidiol concentration acts as a substrate and regulates the rate of local tissue calcidiol conversion into calcitriol, which then acts locally in a paracrine manner (Hewison 2007). It is the local tissue-specific calcitriol synthesis and local calcitriol concentrations that may be responsible for the extraskeletal beneficial effects (Krishnan et al. 2010; Krishnan and Feldman 2011). Malignant tissues such as breast cancer and more highly differentiated colorectal cancers (CRCs) contain high levels of 1α-hydroxylase. Enhancing serum vitamin D levels in these clinical situations may provide chemoprotective effects through facilitating increased calcitriol synthesis (Ma et al. 2011).

13.1.2 Vitamin D Degradation

The initial step in vitamin D degradation into less active metabolites is catalyzed through the enzyme 24-hydroxylase (cytochrome P450 24 [CYP24]) (Henry 2011). The presence of calcitriol induces the expression of 24-hydroxylase; however, not all cells or tissues contain the same concentration of 24-hydroxylase (Miller 1995). In malignant cells, the CYP24 concentration determines the rate of calcitriol and 25-hydroxy D degradation. Prostate cancer cells often contain higher concentrations of the 24-hydroxylase, and coadministration of CYP24 inhibitors such as liarozole, ketoconazole, or genistein, a soy isoflavone that directly inhibits 24-hydroxylase enzyme activity, renders the cells more responsive to calcitriol (Swami et al. 2005).

13.1.3 Increased Vitamin D Supplement Sales and Volume of Testing

The volume of vitamin D supplement sales has increased steadily (Bailey et al. 2011), and vitamin D is among the top 5 of all supplements sold to consumers (Supplement Business Report 2010). The number of laboratory tests ordered to measure D levels also has increased exponentially. At the Memorial Sloan–Cancer Center in New York, 396 vitamin D tests were ordered in 2003, 846 in 2006, and 1711 in 2007, and in 2011, 3000 tests were ordered each month. Most tests were ordered for patients with breast cancer (57%) and CRC (14%) and for patients from the leukemia/lymphoma survivorship clinic (14%) (Wesa et al. 2011).

13.1.4 Vitamin D Mechanisms of Action

Vitamin D has multiple antiproliferative, proapoptotic, and prodifferentiating actions on malignant cells. It decreases tumor growth in animal models of cancer and was implicated in the regulation and transcription of over 200 different genes (Nagpal, Na, and Rathnachalam 2005). Vitamin D increases anti-inflammatory activity via inhibition of both cyclooxygenase 2 (COX2) and interleukin 6 (IL-6) production, increases prostaglandin degradation, decreases angiogenesis, downregulates estrogen receptor (ER) activity, increases aromatase inhibition activity, enhances insulin sensitivity, inhibits nuclear factor kappaB activity, and decreases hypoxia-inducing factor synthesis through decreasing vascular endothelial growth factor (VEGF) and IL-8 synthesis (Krishnan and Feldman 2011). There is also evidence that vitamin D acts synergistically with platinum-based chemotherapy (Hershberger 2002; Moffatt 1999; Saunders 1993) and with paclitaxel (Hershberger 2001) to increase apoptosis in multiple cell lines and in animal models.

13.1.5 Serum Vitamin D Measurement and Sufficiency

The accepted marker for D status is the serum 25-hydroxyvitamin D level. Values are reported as ng/mL in the United States and as nmol/L in Canada and Europe. To convert nmol/L to ng/mL, divide by a factor of 2.5. The term "sufficient" refers to levels of at least 30 ng/mL (75 nmol/L). "Insufficient" describes 20–30 ng/mL, and "deficient" is defined as <20 ng/mL. Most clinical laboratories will provide a reference range for the practitioner to interpret the serum values; typical reference ranges include 30–80 or 30–100 ng/mL. These values are in reference to skeletal health and are the subject of ongoing debate.

No clinical trials have yet defined optimal vitamin D levels for cancer patients. The US 2010 Institute of Medicine (IOM) report defining the new dietary reference intakes indicates that serum levels >20 ng/mL are sufficient for skeletal health (Ross et al. 2011), although the scientific community continues to debate the issue of optimal levels (Heaney and Holick 2011; Giovannucci 2011; Holick et al. 2011; Hollis 2009). The IOM report also concluded that there was insufficient evidence to support benefits aside from skeletal health (Ross et al. 2011). This conclusion was based on the lack of large-scale randomized clinical trial (RCT) evidence with the specific outcome of interest, including cancer incidence as the primary end point.

Vitamin D deficiency induces secondary hyperparathyroidism and increased serum parathyroid hormone (PTH) levels in an effort to maintain calcium homeostasis. Maximal PTH suppression is then considered the gold standard for defining skeletal vitamin D sufficiency. A recent cross-sectional analysis of the National Health and Nutrition Examination Survey (NHANES), 2003–2006, involving 14,681 participants concluded that maximal PTH suppression does not occur until the serum D level is ≥40 ng/mL (Ginde 2011).

13.1.6 D₂ versus D₃ Supplementation

The prescription form of vitamin D is D_2 (Drisdol) at 50,000 international units (units). D_3 is widely available over the counter and is also available at the 50,000-unit dose without a prescription. When doses of 1000 units of D_2 or D_3 are administered daily, the two forms have similar pharmacokinetics and pharmacodynamics (Holick et al. 2008). When the high-dose 50,000 units are used, D_2 is not as efficient as D_3 for either increasing or maintaining stable serum D levels (Armas, Hollis, and Heaney 2004; Chel et al. 2008; Pepper et al. 2009). D_2 has a much shorter serum half-life, with rapid return to baseline levels after 5–7 days (Armas, Hollis, and Heaney 2004). There is also evidence that high-dose D_2 administration induces calcidiol degradation, with resultant serum D levels lower than baseline following a single 50,000-unit dose of D_2 (Heaney et al. 2011). Since the local tissue calcitriol synthesis is dependent on calcidiol concentration (Hewison 2007), using D_2 for vitamin D repletion and maintenance may provide undesirable roller coaster serum D levels and suboptimal local tissue calcidiol levels.

After the initial 2- to 3-day rapid serum peak following a single oral dose of 50,000 units of D_3, pharmacokinetic curves demonstrate steady serum levels for an additional 10–14 days following D_3 administration with a very gradual decrease (Armas, Hollis, and Heaney 2004). D_3 relative potency is 56%–87% more efficient at raising serum D levels than D_2 and produces a 2- to 3-fold greater adipose tissue storage of calcidiol compared with D_2 (Heaney et al. 2011).

13.2   VITAMIN D CLINICAL STUDIES

13.2.1   Epidemiologic Studies of Vitamin D and Cancer Incidence

Multiple epidemiologic studies have examined the relationship between vitamin D and cancer incidence. The strongest and most consistent evidence for a protective effect was shown for CRC (Jenab et al. 2009; Giovannucci 2010; Wactawaski-Wende 2006; Ding 2008; Jenab et al. 2010; Wactawski-Wende 2006) and breast cancer (Goodwin et al. 2009; Grant 2009; Garland et al. 2007; Rejnmark et al. 2009; Bertone-Johnson et al. 2005; Abbas et al. 2008; Lappe et al. 2007), with the strongest association in women who never used hormonal therapy (Ding et al. 2008). Prostate cancer data are inconsistent on whether vitamin D is protective (Giovannucci 2005, 2009; Hanchette and Schwartz 1992; Schwartz and Hanchette 2006; Li et al. 2007). Studies on non–small-cell lung cancer patients (Zhou et al. 2007; Heist et al. 2008) and those with ovarian (Yin et al. 2011; Bakhru et al. 2010), endometrial (Mohr et al. 2007), and pancreatic (Bao et al. 2010; Pubudu, Kostas, and Muhammad 2010) cancer and non-Hodgkin's lymphoma (Drake et al. 2010; Negri 2010) produced conflicting results (Helzlsouer 2010; Eliassen et al. 2011; Stolzenberg-Solomon et al. 2010).

The European Prospective Investigation into Cancer (EPIC) study was a large cohort involving 519,978 participants 35–70 years of age from 10 countries including Denmark, France, Germany, Greece, Italy, the Netherlands, Norway, Spain, Sweden, and the United Kingdom (Jenab et al. 2010). The objective was to examine the association between prediagnostic circulating vitamin D levels, dietary intake of vitamin D and calcium, and the risk of CRC. Results were reported as a nested case control with 1248 cases matched with 12,478 controls. Serum D levels showed a strong inverse correlation and a linear dose–response association with risk of CRC. Compared with the predefined serum D level of 50–75 nmol/L, levels <25 nmol/L had an increased CRC incidence rate of 1.32, levels 25–49.9 had an increased rate of 1.28, and serum levels >75–99.9 nmol/L had a decreased risk rate of 0.88. Those with serum levels >100 nmol/L (corresponding to >40 ng/mL) had a decreased risk rate of 0.77, with $P < .001$ for highest versus lowest quartile of serum D levels.

The Vitamin D Pooling Project of Rarer Cancers (VDPP) involved 10 large international cohorts to conduct a prospective study of the association of serum vitamin D levels with the incidence of seven of the rarer forms of cancer including endometrial, esophageal, gastric, kidney, and non-Hodgkin lymphoma, and ovarian and pancreatic cancers. (Helzlsouer 2010). This was a nested case-control study, with the vast majority of serum samples analyzed specifically for this project. Most of the evaluations did not show any association between serum vitamin D levels >75 nmol/L and cancer incidence. There was a suggestion from the VDPP that serum vitamin D levels >100 nmol/L may be associated with increased pancreatic cancer incidence, with an odds ratio of 2.12 for cancer incidence (Stolzenberg-Solomon et al. 2010). However, 313 of the 952 pancreatic cancer cases were from the Finnish alpha-tocopherol, beta-carotene study, which consisted entirely of male cigarette smokers (Stolzenberg-Solomon et al. 2010), introducing significant confounding. Other published reports show improved clinical outcome and decreased pancreatic cancer incidence with serum D levels >30 ng/mL (75 nmol/L) (Pubudu, Kostas, and Muhammad 2010; Bao et al. 2010).

13.2.2   Women's Health Initiative

The Women's Health Initiative (WHI) was one of the largest US RCTs examining the use of estrogen and progesterone in 68,132 postmenopausal women. A separate WHI arm evaluated the clinical effects of calcium and vitamin D (CaD) supplementation on hip fracture prevention (Jackson et al. 2006). There were 36,282 WHI participants randomized to receive calcium 1000 mg plus vitamin D 400 units daily (administered as 500 mg calcium + 200 units vitamin D_3 twice daily) or double placebo for approximately 7 years. The hypothesis was that calcium plus vitamin D would reduce the risk of hip fracture as the primary end point and decrease the incidence of CRC and breast cancer as secondary end points. Study participants were postmenopausal women ages 50–79 with life expectancy >3 years, no previous history of breast or colon cancer, and no other cancer within 10 years of study entry. Exclusion criteria included hypercalcemia, kidney stones, and current corticosteroid or calcitriol use.

Participants in both study arms were initially allowed to take additional daily vitamin D up to 600 units, which was liberalized to an additional 1000 units of vitamin D daily. At study randomization, 57% of the women were taking nonprotocol CaD supplements. Study medication adherence was poor, and there was considerable cross-contamination between groups (Chlebowski et al. 2008). At study end, 68% were taking calcium or vitamin D, with 60% taking both, 6% taking calcium alone, and 2% taking only D. Of those who were taking supplements at randomization, 84% had continued throughout the study. The active arm "drop-in" rate was 47% for women not taking supplements at entry who were taking supplements at last questionnaire (Bolland 2011). The mean vitamin D intake in both groups was <1000 units daily and substantially overlapped in all quintiles of vitamin D intake, with only 238 units/day separating the highest versus lowest quintiles (Chlebowski et al. 2008). A separate WHI arm evaluated the clinical effects fo calcium and vitamin D (CaD) supplementation of hip fracture prevention (Jackson 2006).

13.2.2.1 Breast Cancer Incidence in WHI

There were 1067 incident cases of breast cancer in the WHI CaD portion, with 528 cases in the CaD group and 546 cases in the placebo group. The Kaplan–Meier breast cancer incidence curves were essentially superimposed between the two groups, with a hazard ratio (HR) of 0.96 (95% confidence interval, 0.85–1.09) (Chlebowski et al. 2008). The mean baseline serum D level was 50 ± 21.0 nmol/L in participants subsequently diagnosed with breast cancer compared with 52.0 ± 21.2 nmol/L among the control subjects.

Recent reanalysis of a limited-access data set (Bolland 2011) showed significant interaction between CaD use at entry and breast cancer incidence. The women not taking supplements at entry randomized to active CaD had decreased incidence of invasive breast cancer, with an HR of 0.82, $P = .021$, P interaction $= .012$, and decreased risk of in situ breast cancer, with an HR of 0.80, $P = .015$, P interaction $= .005$ compared with placebo. Those taking CaD at entry had no change in breast cancer incidence compared with placebo. The authors did not stratify by estrogen group assignment.

13.2.2.2 CRC Incidence in WHI

There were 168 CRC cases in the CaD arm and 154 in the placebo arm. Baseline serum levels between the two groups and CRC incidence showed no significant interaction based on treatment assignment ($P = .54$), and the Kaplan–Meier curves were largely superimposed. However, when the groups were assessed based on baseline quintiles of serum vitamin D levels, the groups in the lowest quintile of baseline serum D levels (31.0 nmol/L or 12.4 ng/mL) compared with the highest quintile (58.4 nmol/L or 23.3 ng/mL) had significantly increased risk of CRC, with an odds ratio of 2.53, $P = .02$ (Wactawaski-Wende 2006). A recent reanalysis of the WHI data (Ding et al. 2008) has demonstrated a significant interaction with estrogen and CRC incidence. The group receiving placebo estrogen/progesterone (EP) had significantly reduced risk of CRC, with an HR of 0.71, compared with the group receiving active EP, with an HR of 1.5, with $P = .018$ for the interaction.

13.2.2.3 Skin Cancer Incidence in WHI

A recent post hoc analysis of WHI data on the risk of skin cancer demonstrated that, in women at high risk for melanoma, calcium plus vitamin D supplementation decreased their risk of developing melanoma (Tang et al. 2011). Whether vitamin D alone would decrease risk is unknown, although retrospective data show improved survival with higher baseline D levels at melanoma diagnosis (Field 2011; Newton Bishop 2009).

13.2.3 BREAST CANCER PREVENTION: POOLED ANALYSIS

In 2007, a pooled review estimating the serum vitamin D level required to prevent breast cancer was undertaken by Garland et al. (2007). A search of all studies reporting breast cancer risk by quintiles of vitamin D levels was performed. Two studies were identified, with a total of 1760 individuals. One study was from England, containing 179 cases and 179 controls, and the other study was part of the Harvard Nurses' Health Study (NHS) cohort, which included prediagnostic vitamin D levels taken between 1989 and 1990 in 701 breast cancer cases and 724 matched controls.

Data were pooled to assess the dose–response association between serum D levels and risk of breast cancer. The pooled quintiles of serum D levels were 6, 18, 29, 37, and 48 ng/mL. Pooled odds ratios for breast cancer, from lowest to highest quintile, were 1.00, 0.90, 0.70, 0.70, and 0.50 (P trend < .001). From the pooled analysis, those with a serum D level >52 ng/mL had 50% decreased risk of breast cancer compared with those with a serum level <13 ng/mL. The raw data from London showed 50% decreased risk with a serum level of 48 ng/mL and, from the NHS, 30% decreased risk with a serum level of 42 ng/mL. They estimated that healthy individuals would require approximately 4000 units of D_3 daily to achieve serum levels in the 52 ng/mL range.

13.2.4 PROGNOSTIC EFFECTS OF VITAMIN D LEVELS IN BREAST CANCER

Three recent studies of baseline serum D levels in women with breast cancer found improved prognosis with higher D levels (Peppone et al. 2012; Yao et al. 2011; Goodwin et al. 2009). Goodwin et al. (2009) showed a significant predictive effect of baseline vitamin D on distant disease-free and overall survival. Women with serum D levels <50 nmol/L had an HR for recurrence of 1.94 and an HR for death of 1.73. Five-year distant disease-free survival rates for women with deficient, insufficient, and sufficient levels were 82%, 85%, and 88%, respectively. Corresponding 10-year distant disease-free survival rates were 69%, 79%, and 83%. It was suggested that serum levels between 80 and 110 nmol/L may be optimal for overall survival, but the wide confidence intervals limited the accuracy of this prediction (Goodwin et al. 2009).

A prospective study compared 192 women undergoing breast cancer surgical resection with matched cancer-free controls. A significant association between D deficiency and poor prognostic indicators was found, including ER-negative, triple negative, and high-risk tumor subtypes. Breast cancer patients deficient in D were more likely to have aggressive tumor profiles and unfavorable prognostic markers than women with normal levels of D (Rickels et al. 2011).

In a recent case-control and case-series analysis, serum D levels were determined in relation to breast cancer prognostic characteristics, including histologic grade; ER; and molecular subtypes defined by ER, progesterone receptor (PR), and human epidermal growth factor receptor 2 (HER2) status. A total of 579 breast cancer patients and 574 controls were matched on age and time of blood draw. Breast cancer cases had significantly lower serum D concentrations than controls, with an adjusted mean of 22.8 ng/mL in cases versus 26.2 ng/mL in control patients (P = .001). Women with triple negative tumor markers had the lowest mean baseline D levels, 17.5 ng/mL (Yao et al. 2011).

13.2.5 NON–SMALL-CELL LUNG CANCER

An observational study examining serum D levels in 447 non–small-cell lung cancer patients evaluated between 1992 and 2002 demonstrated improved survival for those with early disease, stage

IB–IIB, in the highest (>21 ng/mL) versus lowest quartile (<10 mg/mL), with an HR of 0.45 (Zhou et al. 2007). A similar analysis was performed for more advanced disease, and there was no difference in survival (Heist et al. 2008). It is to be noted, however, that even the highest quartile of D levels for these patients was still very low, at 21 ng/mL, so it remains to be determined whether serum levels that are >30 or even >40 ng/mL would provide improved clinical outcomes.

13.2.6 CALCITRIOL IN PROSTATE CANCER

As prostate cancer cells become increasingly malignant, it is suggested that they lose their VDR and are less responsive to the effects of D_3 but still may retain their responsiveness to calcitriol (Giovannucci 2009; Holt et al. 2010). Not all studies show consistent effects of various VDR gene expressions on cancer risk and progression (Holt et al. 2009; McCulough, Bostick, and Mayo 2009). Clinical trials using calcitriol in advanced hormone-resistant prostate cancer also show mixed results. A phase II trial showed minimal toxicity using calcitriol 30 μg three times per week, plus monthly zoledronate 4 mg (Morris et al. 2004), and suggested clinical benefit with the calcitriol. The Androgen-Independent Prostate Cancer Study of Calcitriol Enhancing Taxotere (ASCENT) trial used high-dose calcitriol with docetaxel and weekly dexamethasone for 3 of every 4 weeks or prednisone with docetaxel every 3 weeks. Interim analysis showed more deaths in the ASCENT arm than among controls, and the trial was halted (Scher et al. 2011).

13.2.7 COLORECTAL CANCER

A meta-analysis of 5 large RCTs determined that a baseline serum level of at least 34 ng/mL decreased the incidence of CRC by 50% (Gorham et al. 2005). Ng et al. (2011) evaluated CRC incidence in the NHS, involving 32,826 women, and in the Health Professionals Follow-up Study, involving 18,018 physicians. A total of 304 participants developed CRC from 1991 to 2002. Those who were D deficient had increased CRC incidence and higher mortality. A baseline D level of 40 versus 16.5 ng/mL showed an HR of 0.52 for overall mortality (Ng et al. 2008). In addition, survival was longer for stage III and IV CRC patients with higher serum vitamin D levels. A similar association was not found for serum D levels and survival in earlier-stage CRC patients.

Recently, Ng et al. (2011) evaluated a subgroup of 515 stage IV CRC patients from 1379 patients in an intergroup trial and found no association between vitamin D and survival or time to progression. Conversely, others found better survival in stage IV CRC patients with higher D levels. In 250 newly diagnosed stage IV CRC patients, multivariate analysis showed that those with D levels >30 ng/mL lived, on average, 1.5 times longer compared with those who had D levels <30 ng/mL. The median survival time was 35 months for patients with D ≥30 compared to 25 months for patients with vitamin D <30. The median serum D level was 21.5 ng/mL, and 83% of patients had a serum D level <30 ng/mL (Wesa et al. 2010).

13.3 OPTIMAL VITAMIN D LEVELS AND CLINICAL RECOMMENDATIONS

13.3.1 OPTIMAL VITAMIN D LEVELS

Different serum levels are likely required for various disease end points and symptom management. Some epidemiologic studies suggest that a serum D level of at least 30 ng/mL may protect against breast cancer (Bertone-Johnson et al. 2005; Garland and Garland 1980), while other studies conclude that at least 52 ng/mL is required to decrease the risk of breast cancer by 50% (Garland et al. 2007). Serum levels of at least 33 ng/mL are reported from meta-analyses to be similarly protective against CRC (Gorham et al. 2005, 2007). Still other trials demonstrate that women with breast cancer require serum D levels of at least 68 ng/mL to decrease the risk of aromatase inhibitor (AI)–associated arthralgias (Khan et al. 2010; Rastelli et al. 2011).

13.3.2 Vitamin D Supplementation Recommendations

For adult patients with or at risk for fractures, falls, cardiovascular or autoimmune diseases, and cancer, a target serum D level of at least 30 to 50 ng/mL is recommended (Dawson Hughes et al. 2010; Holick et al. 2011; Michael et al. 2010; Holick 2008; Souberbielle et al. 2010; Pietras et al. 2009). It is estimated that healthy women require a daily D_3 supplement of 1000–2000 units to achieve and maintain serum levels of approximately 30 ng/mL (Chlebowski et al. 2008). To maintain serum levels in the 52 ng/mL range, healthy individuals require approximately 4000 units of D_3 daily. It takes approximately 1000 units to increase serum levels by 10 ng/mL, starting at 10 ng/mL (Heaney et al. 2003). Repletion regimens containing at least 600,000 units administered over a mean 3-month period were successful in achieving D levels >30 ng/mL without toxicity in 64% of patients (Pepper et al. 2009). D_3 is preferable to D_2 for both repletion and maintenance supplementation. Because response to treatment varies by environmental factors and baseline D levels, testing may be warranted 3 months after initiation of supplementation (Stalgis Bilinski et al. 2011).

13.3.3 Cautions

Rapid increases in vitamin D may exacerbate hypercalcemia or precipitate symptomatic renal stone disease (Pierides 1981; Whiting and Calvo 2010). Therefore, care must be taken when repleting patients at risk for hypercalcemia or those with nephrolithiasis or autoimmune diseases such as sarcoid. Medications such as corticosteroids, Dilantin, and cholesterol resin binders often decrease serum D levels and increase repletion/maintenance dose requirements (Pierides 1981). Statins and thiazide diuretics increase serum D levels (Pierides 1981).

The upper limit of 4000 units daily recommended by the US IOM may be conservative. Based on guidelines and clinical trials including elderly patients, doses up to 8000 units daily can be given safely over extended periods of time if serum levels are monitored (Holick 2011; Garland 2011; Bacon 2009; Ross 2011). The International Osteoporosis Foundation (IOF) recommendations include maintaining levels between 35 and 50 ng/mL, which they state is possible without any untoward toxicity (Pietras et al. 2009).

Although unprotected UV sunlight exposure is the primary natural source of vitamin D, obtaining adequate levels through UV exposure is difficult in many parts of the world. Further, the risks of high unprotected UV exposure, including melanoma and other skin cancers, must be considered against the potential benefits of natural D synthesis. The amount of D obtained through UV exposure varies greatly by geography, sunlight, air quality, and host factors such as body mass index (BMI), age, and skin melanin content (Stalgis Bilinski et al. 2011). Oral vitamin D supplementation may be required to ensure adequate D status for most people.

ACKNOWLEDGMENT

The authors wish to acknowledge Jyothi Gubili for her editorial assistance.

AUTHORS' DISCLOSURES OF POTENTIAL CONFLICTS OF INTEREST

The authors indicated no potential conflicts of interest.

REFERENCES

Abbas, Sascha, Jakob Linseisen, Tracy Slanger, Silke Kropp, Elke Mutschelknauss, Dieter Flesch-Janys, and Jenny Chang-Claude. 2008. Serum 25-hydroxyvitamin D and risk of post-menopausal breast cancer—results of a large case-control study. *Carcinogenesis* 29 (1):93–99.

Armas, Laura A. G., Bruce Hollis, and Robert Heaney. 2004. Vitamin D2 is much less effective than vitamin D3 in humans. *The Journal of Clinical Endocrinology and Metabolism* 89 (11):5387–5391.

Bacon, C. J., G. D. Gamble, A. M. Horne, and M. A. Scott. High-dose oral vitamin D3 supplementation in the elderly. *Osteoporosis International* 20 (8):1407–1415.

Bailey, Regan, Jaime Gahche, Cindy Lentino, Johanna Dwyer, Jody Engel, Paul Thomas, Joseph Betz, Christopher Sempos, and Mary Frances Picciano. 2011. Dietary supplement use in the United States, 2003–2006. *Journal of Nutrition* 141 (2):261–266.

Bakhru, Arvind, Julie Mallinger, Ronald Buckanovich, and Jennifer Griggs. 2010. Casting light on 25-hydroxy-vitamin D deficiency in ovarian cancer: a study from the NHANES. *Gynecologic Oncology* 119 (2):314–318.

Bao, Y., Kimmie Ng, B. M. Wolpin, D. S. Michaud, Edward Giovannucci, and Charles Fuchs. 2010. Predicted vitamin D status and pancreatic cancer risk in two prospective cohort studies. *British Journal of Cancer* 102 (9):1422–1427.

Bertone-Johnson, Elizabeth, Wendy Chen, Michael Holick, Bruce Hollis, Graham Colditz, Walter Willett, and Susan Hankinson. 2005. Plasma 25-hydroxyvitamin D and 1,25-dihydroxyvitamin D and risk of breast cancer. *Cancer Epidemiology, Biomarkers & Prevention* 14 (8):1991–1997.

Bolland Mark, Andrew Grey, Greg Gamble, and Ian Reid. 2011. Calcium and vitamin D supplements and health outcomes: a reanalysis of the Women's Health Initiative (WHI) limited-access data set. *American Journal of Clinical Nutrition* 94 (4):1144–1149.

Bulathsinghala Pubudu, Syrigos Kostas, and Maif Muhammad. 2010. Role of vitamin D in the prevention of pancreatic cancer. *Journal of Nutrition and Metabolism*.

Chel, V., H. A. H. Wijnhoven, J. H. Smit, M. Ooms, and P. Lips. 2008. Efficacy of different doses and time intervals of oral vitamin D supplementation with or without calcium in elderly nursing home residents. *Osteoporosis International* 19 (5):663–671.

Chlebowski, Rowan, Karen Johnson, Charles Kooperberg, Mary Pettinger, Jean Wactawski-Wende, Tom Rohan, Jacques Rossouw, Dorothy Lane, Mary O'Sullivan, Shagufta Yasmeen, Robert Hiatt, James Shikany, Mara Vitolins, Janu Khandekar, and F. Allan Hubbell. 2008. Calcium plus vitamin D supplementation and the risk of breast cancer. *Journal of the National Cancer Institute* 100 (22):1581–1591.

Dawson Hughes, B., A. Mithal, J. P. Bonjour, S. Boonen, P. Burckhardt, G. E. H. Fuleihan, R. G. Josse, P. Lips, J. Morales Torres, and N. Yoshimura. 2010. IOF position statement: vitamin D recommendations for older adults. *Osteoporosis International* 21 (7):1151–1154.

Ding, Eric, Saurabh Mehta, Wafaie Fawzi, and Edward Giovannucci. 2008. Interaction of estrogen therapy with calcium and vitamin D supplementation on colorectal cancer risk: reanalysis of Women's Health Initiative randomized trial. *International Journal of Cancer* 122 (8):1690–1694.

Drake, Matthew, Matthew Maurer, Brian Link, Thomas Habermann, Stephen Ansell, Ivana Micallef, Jennifer Kelly, William Macon, Grzegorz Nowakowski, David Inwards, Patrick Johnston, Ravinder Singh, Cristine Allmer, Susan Slager, George Weiner, Thomas Witzig, and James Cerhan. 2010. Vitamin D insufficiency and prognosis in non-Hodgkin's lymphoma. *Journal of Clinical Oncology* 28 (27):4191–4198.

Eliassen, A. Heather, Donna Spiegelman, Bruce Hollis, Ronald Horst, Walter Willett, and Susan Hankinson. 2011. Plasma 25-hydroxyvitamin D and risk of breast cancer in the Nurses' Health Study II. *Breast Cancer Research* 13 (3):R50–R50.

Feldman, David, P. J. Malloy, Aruna Krishnan et al. 2007. *Vitamin D: Biology, Action and Clinical Implications.* Edited by Marcus, R., Feldman, David, Nelson, D. A. et al. 3rd edition, Vol. 1, *Osteoporosis.* San Diego: Academic Press.

Field, Sinead, and Julia Newton-Bishop. 2011. Melanoma and vitamin D. *Molecular Oncology* 5 (2):197–214.

Garland, Cedric, and Frank Garland. 1980. Do sunlight and vitamin D reduce the likelihood of colon cancer? *International Journal of Epidemiology* 9 (3):227–231.

Garland, Cedric, Edward Gorham, Sharif Mohr, William Grant, Edward Giovannucci, Martin Lipkin, Harold Newmark, Michael Holick, and Frank Garland. 2007. Vitamin D and prevention of breast cancer: pooled analysis. *The Journal of Steroid Biochemistry and Molecular Biology* 103 (3–5):708–711.

Garland, Cedric, Christine French, Leo Baggerly, and Robert Heaney. 2011. Vitamin D supplement doses and serum 25-hydroxyvitamin D in the range associated with cancer prevention. *Anticancer Research* 31 (2):L607–611.

Ginde A. A., P. Wolfe, C. A. Camargo Jr., and R. S. Schwartz. 2011. Defining vitamin D status by secondary hyperparathyroidism in the U.S. population. *Journal of Endocrinological Investigation* 35 (1):42–48.

Giovannucci, Edward. 2005. The epidemiology of vitamin D and cancer incidence and mortality: a review (United States). *Cancer Causes & Control* 16 (2):83–95.

Giovannucci, Edward. 2009. Vitamin D and cancer incidence in the Harvard cohorts. *Annals of Epidemiology* 19 (2):84–88.

Giovannucci, Edward. 2010. Epidemiology of vitamin D and colorectal cancer: casual or causal link? *The Journal of Steroid Biochemistry and Molecular Biology* 121 (1–2):349–354.

Giovannucci, Edward. 2011. Vitamin D, how much is enough and how much is too much? *Public Health Nutrition* 14 (4):740–741.

Goodwin, Pamela, Marguerite Ennis, Kathleen Pritchard, Jarley Koo, and Nicky Hood. 2009. Prognostic effects of 25-hydroxyvitamin D levels in early breast cancer. *Journal of Clinical Oncology* 27 (23):3757–3763.

Gorham, Edward, Cedric Garland, Frank Garland, William Grant, Sharif Mohr, Martin Lipkin, Harold Newmark, Edward Giovannucci, Melissa Wei, and Michael Holick. 2005. Vitamin D and prevention of colorectal cancer. *The Journal of Steroid Biochemistry and Molecular Biology* 97 (1–2):179–194.

Gorham, Edward, Cedric Garland, Frank Garland, William Grant, Sharif Mohr, Martin Lipkin, Harold Newmark, Edward Giovannucci, Melissa Wei, and Michael Holick. 2007. Optimal vitamin D status for colorectal cancer prevention: a quantitative meta analysis. *American Journal of Preventive Medicine* 32 (3):210–216.

Grant, William. 2009. How strong is the evidence that solar ultraviolet B and vitamin D reduce the risk of cancer? An examination using Hill's criteria for causality. *Dermato-endocrinology* 1 (1):17–24.

Hanchette, C. L., and G. G. Schwartz. 1992. Geographic patterns of prostate cancer mortality. Evidence for a protective effect of ultraviolet radiation. *Cancer* 70 (12):2861–2869.

Heaney, Robert, and Michael Holick. 2011. Why the IOM recommendations for vitamin D are deficient. *Journal of Bone and Mineral Research* 26 (3):455–457.

Heaney, Robert, K. Michael Davies, Tai Chen, Michael Holick, and M. Janet Barger-Lux. 2003. Human serum 25-hydroxycholecalciferol response to extended oral dosing with cholecalciferol. *The American Journal of Clinical Nutrition* 77 (1):204–210.

Heaney, Robert, Robert Recker, James Grote, Ronald Horst, and Laura A. G. Armas. 2011. Vitamin D(3) is more potent than vitamin D(2) in humans. *The Journal of Clinical Endocrinology and Metabolism* 96 (3):E447–E452.

Heist, Rebecca, Wei Zhou, Zhaoxi Wang, Geoffrey Liu, Donna Neuberg, Li Su, Kofi Asomaning, Bruce Hollis, Thomas Lynch, John Wain, Edward Giovannucci, and David Christiani. 2008. Circulating 25-hydroxyvitamin D, VDR polymorphisms, and survival in advanced non-small-cell lung cancer. *Journal of Clinical Oncology* 26 (34):5596–5602.

Helzlsouer, Kathy. 2010. Overview of the Cohort Consortium Vitamin D Pooling Project of Rarer Cancers. *American Journal of Epidemiology* 172 (1):4–9.

Henry, Helen. 2011. Regulation of vitamin D metabolism. Baillière's best practice and research. *Clinical Endocrinology and Metabolism* 25 (4):531–541.

Hershberger, Pamela, Yu Wei-Dong, Ruth A. Modzelewski, and Robert M. Rueger. 2010. Calcitriol (1,25-dihydroxycholecalciferol) enhances paclitaxel antitumor activity in vitro and in vivo and accelerates paclitaxel-induced apoptosis. *Clinical Cancer Research* 7 (4):1043–1051.

Hershberger, Pamela, Terence McGuire, Wei-Dong Yu, Eleanor Zuhowski, Jan H. M. Schellens, Merrill Egorin, Donald Trump, and Candace Johnson. 2002. Cisplatin potentiates 1,25-dihydroxyvitamin D3-induced apoptosis in association with increased mitogen-activated protein kinase kinase kinase 1 (MEKK-1) expression. *Molecular Cancer Therapeutics* 1 (10):821–829.

Hewison, Martin, Fiona Burke, Katie Evans, David Lammas, David Sansom, Philip Liu, Robert Modlin, John Adams. 2007. Extra-renal 25-hydroxyvitamin D3-1alpha-hydroxylase in human health and disease. *The Journal of Steroid Biochemistry and Molecular Biology* 103 (3–5):316–321.

Holick, Michael. 2008. The vitamin D deficiency pandemic and consequences for nonskeletal health: mechanisms of action. *Molecular Aspects of Medicine* 29 (6):361–368.

Holick, Michael, Rachael Biancuzzo, Tai Chen, Ellen Klein, Azzie Young, Douglass Bibuld, Richard Reitz, Wael Salameh, Allen Ameri, and Andrew Tannenbaum. 2008. Vitamin D2 is as effective as vitamin D3 in maintaining circulating concentrations of 25-hydroxyvitamin D. *The Journal of Clinical Endocrinology and Metabolism* 93 (3):677–681.

Hollick, Michael, Neil Binkley, Heike Bischoff Ferrari, Catherine Gordon, David Hanley, Robert Heaney, M. H. Murad, and Connie Weaver. 2011. Evaluation, treatment, and prevention of vitamin D deficiency: an Endocrine Society clinical practice guideline. *The Journal of Clinical Endocrinology and Metabolism* 96 (7):1911–1930.

Hollis, Bruce. 2009. Nutrition: US recommendations fail to correct vitamin D deficiency. *Nature Reviews. Endocrinology* 5 (10):534–536.

Holt, Sarah, Erika Kwon, Ulrike Peters, Elaine Ostrander, and Janet Stanford. 2009. Vitamin D pathway gene variants and prostate cancer risk. *Cancer Epidemiology, Biomarkers & Prevention* 18 (6):1929–1933.

Holt, Sarah, Erika Kwon, J. Koopmeiners, D. Lin, Z. Feng, Elaine Ostrander, U. Peters, and Janet Stanford. 2010. Vitamin D pathway gene variants and prostate cancer prognosis. *The Prostate* 70:1440–1460.

Jackson, Rebecca, Andrea LaCroix, Margery Gass, Robert Wallace, John Robbins, Cora Lewis, Tamsen Bassford, Shirley A. A. Beresford, Henry Black, Patricia Blanchette, Denise Bonds, Robert Brunner, Robert Brzyski, Bette Caan, Jane Cauley, Rowan Chlebowski, Steven Cummings, Iris Granek, Jennifer Hays, Gerardo Heiss, Susan Hendrix, Barbara Howard, Judith Hsia, F. Allan Hubbell, Karen Johnson, Howard Judd, Jane Kotchen, Lewis Kuller, Robert Langer, Norman Lasser, Marian Limacher, Shari Ludlam, JoAnn Manson, Karen Margolis, Joan McGowan, Judith Ockene, Mary O'Sullivan, Lawrence Phillips, Ross Prentice, Gloria Sarto, Marcia Stefanick, Linda Van Horn, Jean Wactawski-Wende, Evelyn Whitlock, Garnet Anderson, Annlouise Assaf, and David Barad. 2006. Calcium plus vitamin D supplementation and the risk of fractures. *The New England Journal of Medicine* 354 (7):669–683.

Jenab, Mazda, James McKay, Hendrik B. Bueno-de-Mesquita, Franzel J. B. van Duijnhoven, Pietro Ferrari, Nadia Slimani, Eugène H. J. M. Jansen, Tobias Pischon, Sabina Rinaldi, Anne Tjnneland, Anja Olsen, Kim Overvad, Marie-Christine Boutron-Ruault, Francoise Clavel-Chapelon, Pierre Engel, Rudolf Kaaks, Jakob Linseisen, Heiner Boeing, Eva Fisher, Antonia Trichopoulou, Vardis Dilis, Erifili Oustoglou, Franco Berrino, Paolo Vineis, Amalia Mattiello, Giovanna Masala, Rosario Tumino, Alina Vrieling, Carla van Gils, Petra Peeters, Magritt Brustad, Eiliv Lund, Mara-Dolores Chirlaque, Aurelio Barricarte, Laudina Surez, Esther Molina, Miren Dorronsoro, Nria Sala, Gran Hallmans, Richard Palmqvist, Andrew Roddam, Timothy Key, Kay-Tee Khaw, Sheila Bingham, Paolo Boffetta, Philippe Autier, Graham Byrnes, Teresa Norat, and Elio Riboli. 2009. Vitamin D receptor and calcium sensing receptor polymorphisms and the risk of colorectal cancer in European populations. *Cancer Epidemiology, Biomarkers and Prevention* 18 (9):2485–2491.

Jenab, Mazda, H. Bas Bueno-de-Mesquita, Pietro Ferrari, Franzel, J. B. van Duijnhoven, Teresa Norat, Tobias Pischon, Eugène Jansen, Nadia Slimani, Graham Byrnes, Sabina Rinaldi, Anne Tjønneland, Anja Olsen, Kim Overvad, Marie-Christine Boutron-Ruault, Françoise Clavel-Chapelon, Sophie Morois, Kaaks Rudolf, Linseisen Jakob, Boeing Heiner, Manuela M. Bergmann, Antonia Trichopoulou, Gesthimani Misirli, Dimitrios Trichopoulos, Franco Berrino, Paolo Vineis, Salvatore Panico, Domenico Palli, Rosario Tumino, Martine M. Ros, Carla H. van Gils, Petra H. Peeters, Magritt Brustad, Eiliv Lund, María-José Tormo, Eva Ardanaz, Laudina Rodríguez, Maria-José Sánchez, Miren Dorronsoro, Carlos A Gonzalez, Göran Hallmans, Richard Palmqvist, Andrew Roddam, Timothy J. Key, Kay-Tee Khaw, Philippe Autier, Pierre Hainaut, and Ellio Riboli. 2010. Association between pre-diagnostic circulating vitamin D concentration and risk of colorectal cancer in European populations: a nested case-control study. *British Medical Journal* 340. B5500.

Khan, Qamar, Pavan Reddy, Bruce Kimler, Priyanka Sharma, Susan Baxa, Anne O'Dea, Jennifer Klemp, and Carol Fabian. 2010. Effect of vitamin D supplementation on serum 25-hydroxy vitamin D levels, joint pain, and fatigue in women starting adjuvant letrozole treatment for breast cancer. *Breast Cancer Research and Treatment* 119 (1):111–118.

Krishnan, Aruna, and David Feldman. 2011. Mechanisms of the anti-cancer and anti-inflammatory actions of vitamin D. *Annual Review of Pharmacology and Toxicology* 51:311–336.

Krishnan, Aruna, Donald Trump, Candace Johnson, and David Feldman. 2010. The role of vitamin D in cancer prevention and treatment. *Endocrinology and Metabolism Clinics of North America* 39 (2):401–418, table of contents.

Lappe, Joan, Dianne Travers-Gustafson, K. Michael Davies, Robert Recker, and Robert Heaney. 2007. Vitamin D and calcium supplementation reduces cancer risk: results of a randomized trial. *The American Journal of Clinical Nutrition* 85 (6):1586–1591.

Li, Haojie, Meir Stampfer, J. Bruce W. Hollis, Lorelei Mucci, J. Michael Gaziano, David Hunter, Edward Giovannucci, and Jing Ma. 2007. A prospective study of plasma vitamin D metabolites, vitamin D receptor polymorphisms, and prostate cancer. *PLoS Medicine* 4 (3):e103–e103.

Ma, Yanlei, Zhang Peng, Feng Wang, Jianjun Yang, Zhihua Liu, and Huanlong Qin. 2011. Association between vitamin D and risk of colorectal cancer: a systematic review of prospective studies. *Journal of Clinical Oncology* 29 (28):3775–3782.

Ma, Yingyu, Donal Trump, and Candace Johnson. 2010. Vitamin D in combination cancer treatment. *Journal of Cancer* 1:101–107.

McCulough, Marjorie, Robert Bostick, and Tinisha Mayo. 2009. Vitamin D gene pathway polymorphisms and risk of colorectal, breast, and prostate cancer. *Annu Rev Nutr* 29:111–132.

Michael, Yvonne, Evelyn Whitlock, Jennifer Lin, Rongwei Fu, Elizabeth O'Connor, and Rachel Gold. 2010. Primary care-relevant interventions to prevent falling in older adults: a systematic evidence review for the U.S. Preventive Services Task Force. *Annals of Internal Medicine* 153 (12):815–825.

Miller, G. J., G. E. Stapleton, T. E. Hedlund, and K. A. Moffat. 1995. Vitamin D receptor expression, 24-hydroxylase activity, and inhibition of growth by 1alpha,25-dihydroxyvitamin D3 in seven human prostatic carcinoma cell lines. *Clinical Cancer Research* 1 (9):997–1003.

Moffatt, Kirsten A., Widya U. Johannes, and Gary J. Miller. 1999. 1Alpha,25dihydroxyvitamin D3 and platinum drugs act synergistically to inhibit the growth of prostate cancer cell lines. *Clinical Cancer Research* 5 (3):695–703.

Mohr, Sharif, Cedric Garland, Edward Gorham, William Grant, and Frank Garland. 2007. Is ultraviolet B irradiance inversely associated with incidence rates of endometrial cancer: an ecological study of 107 countries. *Preventive Medicine* 45 (5):327–331.

Morris, Michael, Oren Smaletz, David Solit, W. Kevin Kelly, Susan Slovin, Carlos Flombaum, Tracy Curley, Anthony Delacruz, Lawrence Schwartz, Martin Fleisher, Andrew Zhu, Meghan Diani, Mary Fallon, and Howard Scher. 2004. High-dose calcitriol, zoledronate, and dexamethasone for the treatment of progressive prostate carcinoma. *Cancer* 100 (9):1868–1875.

Nagpal, Sunil, Songqing Na, and Radhakrishnan Rathnachalam. 2005. Noncalcemic actions of vitamin D receptor ligands. *Endocrine Reviews* 26 (5):662–687.

Negri, Eva. 2010. Sun exposure, vitamin D, and risk of Hodgkin and non-Hodgkin lymphoma. *Nutrition and Cancer* 62 (7):878–882.

Newton Bishop, Julia, Samantha Beswick, Juliette Randerson Moor, Yu-Mei Chang, Paul Affleck, Faye Elliott, May Chan, Susan Leake, Birute Karpavicius, Sue Haynes, Kairen Kukalizch, Linda Whitaker, Sharon Jackson, Gerry Edwina, Clarissa Nolan, Chandra Bertram, Jerry Marsden, David Elder, Jennifer Barrett, and D. T. Bishop. 2009. Serum 25-hydroxyvitamin D3 levels are associated with breslow thickness at presentation and survival from melanoma. *Journal of Clinical Oncology* 27 (32):5439–5444.

Ng, Kimmie, Jeffrey Meyerhardt, Kana Wu, Diane Feskanich, Bruce Hollis, Edward Giovannucci, and Charles Fuchs. 2008. Circulating 25-hydroxyvitamin d levels and survival in patients with colorectal cancer. *Journal of Clinical Oncology* 26 (18):2984–2991.

Ng, Kimmie, Daniel Sargent, Richard Goldberg, Jeffrey Meyerhardt, Erin Green, Henry Pitot, Bruce Hollis, Michael Pollak, and Charles Fuchs. 2011. Vitamin D status in patients with stage IV colorectal cancer: findings from Intergroup Trial N9741. *Journal of Clinical Oncology* 29 (12):1599–1606.

Pepper, Kara, Suzanne Judd, Mark Nanes, and Vin Tangpricha. 2009. Evaluation of vitamin D repletion regimens to correct vitamin D status in adults. *Endocrine Practice* 15 (2):95–103.

Peppone, Luke J., Aaron S. Rickles, Michelle C. Janelsins, Michael R. Insalaco, and Kristin A. Skinner. 2012. The association between breast cancer prognostic indicators and serum 25-OH vitamin D levels. *Journal of Surgical Oncology* 19 (8):2590–2599.

Pierides, A. M. 1981. Pharmacology and therapeutic use of vitamin D and its analogues. *Drugs* 21 (4):241–256.

Pietras, Sara M., Busayo K. Obayan, Cai H. Mona, and Michael F. Holick. 2009. Vitamin D2 treatment for vitamin D deficiency and insufficiency for up to 6 years. *Arch Intern Med* 169 (19):1806–1808.

Rastelli, Antonella L., Marie E. Taylor, Feng Gao, Reina Armamento-Villareal, Shohreh Jamalabadi-Majidi, Nicola Napoli, and Matthew J. Ellis. 2011. Vitamin D and aromatase inhibitor-induced musculoskeletal symptoms (AIMSS): a phase II, double-blind, placebo-controlled, randomized trial. *Breast Cancer Research and Treatment* 129 (1):107–116.

Rejnmark, Lars, Anna Tietze, Peter Vestergaard, Line Buhl, Melsene Lehbrink, Lene Heickendorff, and Leif Mosekilde. 2009. Reduced prediagnostic 25-hydroxyvitamin D levels in women with breast cancer: a nested case-control study. *Cancer Epidemiology, Biomarkers and Prevention* 18 (10):2655–2660.

Rickels, A., L. Pepperone, A. Houston et al. 2011. Serum 25-hydroxyvitamin D and prognostic tumor characteristics in breast cancer patients. In *American Society of Breast Surgeons 12th Annual Meeting*.

Ross, A. C., JoAnn Manson, Steven Abrams, John Aloia, Patsy Brannon, Steven Clinton, Ramon Durazo-Arvizu, J. C. Gallagher, Richard Gallo, Glenville Jones, Christopher Kovacs, Susan Mayne, Clifford Rosen, and Sue Shapses. 2011. The 2011 report on dietary reference intakes for calcium and vitamin D from the Institute of Medicine: what clinicians need to know. *The Journal of Clinical Endocrinology and Metabolism* 96 (1):53–58.

Saunders, D. E., C. Christensen, N. L. Wappler, Y. L. Cho, W. D. Lawrence, J. M. Malone, V. K. Malviya, and G. Deppe. 1993. Additive inhibition of RL95-2 endometrial carcinoma cell growth by carboplatin and 1,25 dihydroxyvitamin D3. *Gynecologic Oncology* 51 (2):155–159.

Scher, Howard, Jia Xiaoyu, Kim Chi, Ronald de Wit, William Berry, Peter Albers, Brian Henick, David Waterhouse, Dean Ruether, Peterm Rosen, Anthony Meluch, Luke Nordquist, Peter Venner, Axel Heidenreich, Luis Chu, and Glenn Heller. 2011. Randomized, open-label Phase III trial of docetaxel plus high-dose calcitriol versus docetaxel plus prednisone for patients with castration-resistant prostate cancer. *Journal of Clinical Oncology* 29 (16):2191–2198.

Schwartz, Gary, and Carol Hanchette. 2006. UV, latitude, and spatial trends in prostate cancer mortality: all sunlight is not the same (United States). *CCC. Cancer Causes and Control* 17 (8):1091–1101.

Souberbielle, Jean-Claude, Jean-Jacques Body, Joan Lappe, Mario Plebani, Yehuda Shoenfeld, Thomas Wang, Heike Bischoff Ferrari, Etienne Cavalier, Peter Ebeling, Patrice Fardellone, Sara Gandini, Damien Gruson, Alain Gurin, Lene Heickendorff, Bruce Hollis, Sofia Ish Shalom, Guillaume Jean, Philipp von Landenberg, Alvaro Largura, Tomas Olsson, Charles Pierrot Deseilligny, Stefan Pilz, Angela Tincani, Andre Valcour, and Armin Zittermann. 2010. Vitamin D and musculoskeletal health, cardiovascular disease, autoimmunity and cancer: Recommendations for clinical practice. *Autoimmunity Reviews* 9 (11):709–715.

Stalgis Bilinski, Kellie, John Boyages, Elizabeth Salisbury, Colin Dunstan, Stuart Henderson, and Peter Talbot. 2011. Burning daylight: balancing vitamin D requirements with sensible sun exposure. *Medical Journal of Australia* 194 (7):345–348.

Stolzenberg-Solomon, Rachael, Eric Jacobs, Alan Arslan, Dai Qi, Alpa Patel, Kathy Helzlsouer, Stephanie Weinstein, Marjorie McCullough, Mark Purdue, Xiao-Ou Shu, Kirk Snyder, Jarmo Virtamo, Lynn Wilkins, Kai Yu, Anne Zeleniuch-Jacquotte, Wei Zheng, Demetrius Albanes, Qiuyin Cai, Chinonye Harvey, Richard Hayes, Sandra Clipp, Ronald Horst, Lonn Irish, Karen Koenig, Loic Le Marchand, and Laurence Kolonel. 2010. Circulating 25-hydroxyvitamin D and risk of pancreatic cancer: Cohort Consortium Vitamin D Pooling Project of Rarer Cancers. *American Journal of Epidemiology* 172 (1):81–93.

Swami, Srilatha, Aruna Krishnan, Donna Peehl, and David Feldman. 2005. Genistein potentiates the growth inhibitory effects of 1,25-dihydroxyvitamin D3 in DU145 human prostate cancer cells: role of the direct inhibition of CYP24 enzyme activity. *Molecular and Cellular Endocrinology* 241 (1–2):49–61.

Tang, Jean, Teresa Fu, Erin LeBlanc, JoAnn Manson, David Feldman, Eleni Linos, Mara Vitolins, Nathalie Zeitouni, Joseph Larson, Marcia Stefanick. 2011. Calcium plus vitamin D supplementation and the risk of nonmelanoma and melanoma skin cancer: post hoc analyses of the Women's Health Initiative Randomized Controlled Trial. *Journal of Clinical Oncology* 29 (22):3078–3084.

Wactawski-Wende, Jean, Jane Morley Kotchen, Garnet L. Anderson, Annlouise R. Assaf, Robert L. Brunner, Mary Jo O'Sullivan, Karen L. Margolis, Judith K. Ockene, Lawrence Phillips, Linda Pottern, Ross L. Prentice, John Robbins, Thomas E. Rohan, Gloria E. Sarto, Santosh Sharma, Marcia L. Stefanick, Linda Van Horn, Robert B. Wallace, Evelyn Whitlock, Tamsen Bassford, Shirley A. A. Beresford, Henry R. Black, Denise E. Bonds, Robert G. Brzyski, Bette Caan, Rowan T. Chlebowski, Barbara Cochrane, Cedric Garland, Margery Gass, Jennifer Hays, Gerardo Heiss, Susan L. Hendrix, Barbara V. Howard, Judith Hsia, F. Allan Hubbell , Rebecca D. Jackson, Karen C. Johnson, Howard Judd, Charles L. Kooperberg, Lewis H. Kuller, Andrea Z. LaCroix, Dorothy S. Lane, Robert D. Langer, Norman L. Lasser, Cora E. Lewis, Marian C. Limacher, and JoAnn E. Manson. 2006. Calcium plus vitamin D supplementation and the risk of colorectal cancer. *New England Journal of Medicine* 354 (7):684–696.

Wesa, Kathleen, Gria N. Jacobs, Derek Woo, Angel Cronin, Neil H. Segal, Marci I. Coleton, Martin Fleisher, Leonard Saltz, and Barrie Cassileth. 2010. Serum 25-hydroxy vitamin D and survival in colorectal cancer (CRC): a retrospective analysis. In *ASCO* Chicago, Illinois.

Wesa, Kathleen, Simon K. Yeung, Gria N. Jacobs, Marci I. Coleton, and Barrie R. Cassileth. 2011. Serum 25-hydroxy vitamin D testing at Memorial Sloan-Kettering Cancer Center. In *ASCO*. Chicago.

Whiting, Susan, and Mona Calvo. 2010. Correcting poor vitamin D status: do older adults need higher repletion doses of vitamin D3 than younger adults? *Molecular Nutrition & Food Research* 54 (8):1077–1084.

Yao, Song, Lara Sucheston, Amy Millen, Candace Johnson, Donald Trump, Mary Nesline, Warren Davis, Chi-Chen Hong, Susan McCann, Helena Hwang, Swati Kulkarni, Stephen Edge, Tracey O'Connor, and Christine Ambrosone. 2011. Pretreatment serum concentrations of 25-hydroxyvitamin D and breast cancer prognostic characteristics: a case-control and a case-series study. *PLoS ONE* 6 (2):e17251–e17251.

Yin, Lu, Norma Grandi, Elke Raum, Ulrike Haug, Volker Arndt, and Hermann Brenner. 2011. Meta-analysis: circulating vitamin D and ovarian cancer risk. *Gynecologic Oncology* 121 (2):369–375.

Zhou, Wei, Rebecca Heist, Geoffrey Liu, Kofi Asomaning, Donna Neuberg, Bruce Hollis, John Wain, Thomas Lynch, Edward Giovannucci, Li Su, and David Christiani. 2007. Circulating 25-hydroxyvitamin D levels predict survival in early-stage non-small-cell lung cancer patients. *Journal of Clinical Oncology* 25 (5):479–485.

Section V

Omega-3 and Omega-6 Fatty Acids

14 Plant and Marine Sources of Omega-3 Polyunsaturated Fatty Acids, Inflammation, and Cancer Prevention

Julie K. Mason, Ashleigh K. A. Wiggins, and Lilian U. Thompson

CONTENTS

14.1 INTRODUCTION

The most common forms of cancer in the Western world include lung, colorectal, prostate, and breast cancer, and it is well established that modifiable risk factors play a role in the development of these forms of cancer (World Health Organization 2008; World Cancer Research Fund/American Institute for Cancer Research 2007). Interest in the role of diet in the prevention of cancer stems from ecological observations of the increase in cancer incidence and mortality over time within a country, differences of prevalence of subtypes of cancer between countries, and changes in cancer risk with migration. For example, a temporal association is shown between the dramatic rise in colon and breast cancers in Japan with dietary changes toward a most "Westernized" diet (Porter 2008; World Cancer Research Fund/American Institute for Cancer Research 2007). One common feature of cancer, particularly in the most common types in Western countries, is inflammation (Coussens and Werb 2002).

The association between dietary fat intake and cancer risk has been widely debated (Kushi and Giovannucci 2002; Boyd et al. 2003). In recent years, there has been a shift in focus from total fat intake to intake of specific subtypes of fatty acids (FA), in particular, the omega-3 (n-3, ω-3) polyunsaturated FA (PUFA) found in plant and marine sources. This chapter will focus on the role of n-3 PUFA in cancer, with an emphasis on its potential role in influencing the inflammatory process. The properties, common sources, and current intakes in North America of n-3 PUFA will be discussed. Features of the inflammatory process will be outlined, and proposed mechanisms of n-3 PUFA in modulating them will be summarized with support from in vitro, animal, and, when available, human studies. The effect of n-3 PUFA on chemoprevention in observational and randomized controlled trials will be described. Finally, the chapter will conclude with a discussion of the current limitations and gaps that exist in the literature and future directions.

14.2   n-3 PUFA

14.2.1   FA CLASSIFICATION

n-3 PUFA are a class of FA characterized by the presence of multiple double bonds, with the first double bond at the third carbon from the methyl end of the hydrocarbon chain. In contrast, omega-6 (n-6) PUFA have the first double bond at the sixth carbon from the methyl end. The main n-3 PUFA are α-linolenic acid (ALA, 18:3n-3) derived from plants and the long-chain (LC) n-3 PUFA eicosapentaenoic acid (EPA; 20:5n-3) and docosahexaenoic acid (DHA; 22:6n-3) derived from marine sources. Because mammals lack the necessary desaturase enzymes to synthesize ALA and linoleic acid (LA; 18:2n-6), the parent n-3 and n-6 PUFA, these are known as essential FA, and they must be obtained through dietary sources. Both ALA and LA are metabolized to LC-PUFA in a process described in Figure 14.1 and further detailed below. The major metabolites of ALA include EPA and DHA. Arachidonic acid (AA; 20;4n-6) is the major downstream metabolite of LA.

14.2.2   DIETARY SOURCES AND INTAKE

ALA is found primarily in seeds and their oils such as flaxseed (linseed), rapeseed (canola), perilla, chia, soybean, hemp, as well as walnuts. Flaxseed is the richest plant source of ALA, and its oil has up to 57% ALA (Cunnane 2003). EPA and DHA are found in fatty fish such as salmon, herring, and mackerel as well as krill (Siguel 1996). Current intakes of n-3 PUFA in the United States have been estimated using data from the National Health and Nutrition Examination Survey (NHANES), and the 2005–2006 survey showed that US adults are, on average, consuming ~1.5 g/day of ALA and ~135 mg/day of EPA + DHA (United States Department of Agriculture 2010). The Institute of Medicine has set the acceptable macronutrient distribution range (AMDR) for ALA at 0.6% to 1.2% of energy, or 1.3 to 2.7 g/day, on the basis of a 2000 kcal diet. It is further specified that up to 10% of the AMDR for ALA can be consumed as EPA and/or DHA (National Research Council 2005). Evidently, ALA is the predominant n-3 PUFA consumed in the North American diet.

14.2.3   FA METABOLISM

The parent n-3 and n-6 PUFA, ALA and LA, are metabolized to their longer-chain counterparts through an alternating series of elongation (addition of two carbons) via elongase enzymes and desaturation (double-bond insertion) reactions via Δ6 and Δ5 desaturase enzymes (Figure 14.1). There is, therefore, competition between the two classes of FA for the same enzymes. Humans

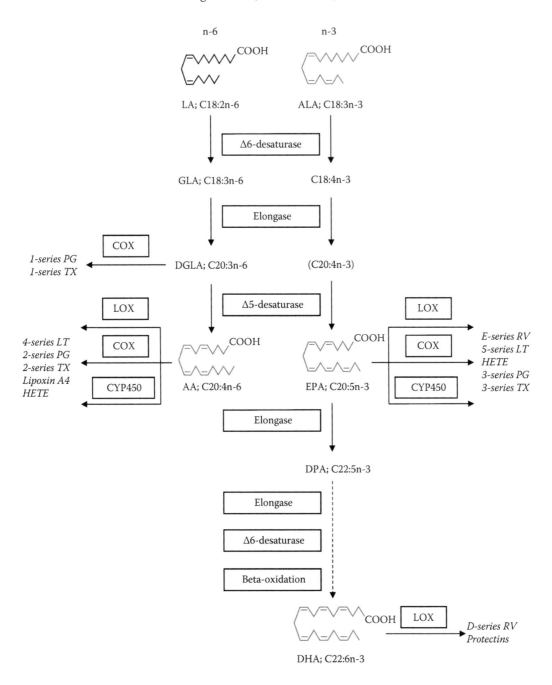

FIGURE 14.1 Metabolism of n-3 and n-6 PUFA and eicosanoid biosynthesis. Metabolic enzymes are in outlined boxes. Enzymes involved in eicosanoid production are in capital letters. Eicosanoids are capitalized and italicized. Dashed lines represent multiple steps. AA, arachidonic acid (18:2n-6); ALA, α-linolenic acid (C18:3n-3); COX, cyclooxygenase; CYP450, cytochrome P450; DGLA, dihomo-γ-linolenic acid (C20:3n-6); DHA, docosahexaaenoic acid (C22:6n-3); DPA, docosapentaaenoic acid (C22:5n-3); EPA, eicosapentaenoic acid (C20:5n-3); GLA, γ-linolenic acid (C18:3n-6); HETE, hydroxyeicosatetraenoic acid; LOX, lipoxygenase; LT, leukotriene; PG, prostaglandin; PUFA, polyunsaturated fatty acid; RV, resolvin; TX, thromboxane.

have functional Δ6 and Δ5 desaturase and elongase enzymes in the liver, gut, and brain and therefore have the ability to convert some ALA to the LC-PUFA. The predominant use of ALA is β-oxidation and carbon recycling to acetate (Miyazaki and Ntambi 2008; Cunnane 2003). Studies conducted in humans have generally shown that even high-dose ALA (up to 40 g/day) increased the plasma levels of EPA but had little effect on DHA (Brenna et al. 2009). The International Society for the Study of Fatty Acids and Lipids (ISSFAL) released a statement in 2009 that concluded that the conversion of ALA to DHA is less than 1% in adults and that the most effective way of increasing the tissue content of a specific n-3 PUFA is through consumption of that specific FA (Brenna et al. 2009).

14.3 INFLAMMATION AND CANCER

Inflammation is a host defense mechanism against an injurious stimulus and the subsequent tissue repair. Acute inflammation is a protective process, whereas chronic inflammation can cause tissue damage. Chronic inflammation develops secondary to persistent infection, repeated episodes of acute inflammation, and the persistence of an injurious agent. At a histopathological level, chronic inflammation is characterized by tissue infiltration with inflammatory cells (e.g., leukocytes, macrophages); tissue destruction; and proliferation of fibroblasts, blood vessels, and fibrosis due to attempts at healing (Kumar et al. 2005). Chronic inflammation is linked to many chronic diseases, including cardiovascular disease, diabetes, and cancer (Coussens and Werb 2002; Kumar et al. Fausto 2005; Roifman et al. 2011; Dandona et al. 2004). The role of inflammation in cancer has been a subject of great interest in recent years.

Inflammation is a multistep process that involves many cells and chemical mediators (Kumar et al. 2005; Clevers 2004). The inflammatory response occurs in vascularized tissues and involves a number of cell types, including mast cells, dendritic cells, fibroblasts, endothelial cells, leukocytes (including lymphocytes, neutrophils, monocytes, eosinophils, and basophils), platelets, and many types of chemical mediators including cytokines, chemokines, and eicosanoids. These cells and mediators work together to coordinate the inflammatory pathway; first, cytokines and chemokines are released at the site of injury or tumor microenvironment; second, inflammatory cells (e.g., mast cells, neutrophils) are activated by chemical mediators, migrate out of the blood vessels into the interstitial fluid, and are attracted to the site of injury; third, inflammatory cells exert their effect to clear up the injurious stimulus. Finally, once the injurious stimulus has been cleared up, inflammatory cells dissipate from the site of injury. Features of this process include (1) hemodynamic alterations to increase blood flow to the site of injury through vasodilation and increased vascular permeability to plasma proteins and leukocytes, (2) activation and transmigration of leukocytes, and (3) activation of the effector inflammatory cells to clear the injurious stimulus.

Anticancer approaches focusing on reducing chronic inflammation target all aspects of the inflammatory process (Demaria et al. 2010). This process is complex, with many interrelated components, and therefore, effects on one part of the process likely have effects on other parts of the inflammatory process. n-3 PUFA are not targeted agents and have pleiotropic effects, which influence multiple portions of the inflammatory pathways. These include hemodynamics; adhesion molecules; production of eicosanoids, chemokines, and cytokines; and the modulation of the immune effector cells (T cells, macrophages). The exact mechanisms of how n-3 PUFA exert these effects are not yet fully understood, but a number of hypothesized avenues will be described below.

14.4 PROPOSED ANTI-INFLAMMATORY AND ANTICANCER MECHANISMS OF n-3 PUFA

Preclinical studies using in vitro and animal models largely support a beneficial effect of n-3 PUFA in chemoprevention. As shown in Figure 14.2, a number of mechanisms have been proposed for

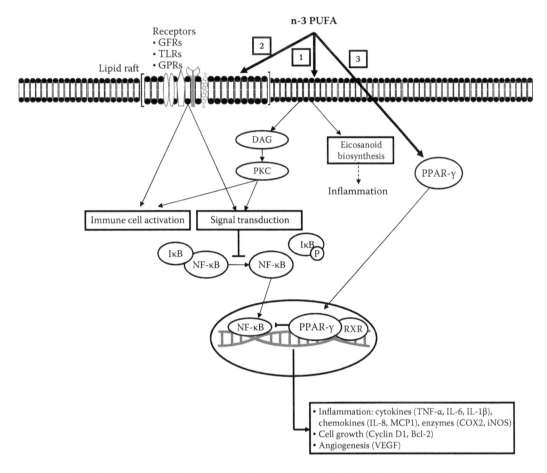

FIGURE 14.2 Proposed anti-inflammatory and anticancer mechanisms of n-3 PUFA. n-3 PUFA exposure results in the following: (1) incorporation into the membrane PL. This alters the synthesis of eicosanoids, resulting in a decrease in n-6 PUFA–derived inflammatory cytokines. The production of the secondary messenger DAG that modulates PKC is also affected. (2) Modulation of lipid raft composition and structure. This modulates expression and downstream signal transduction through GFR, TLR, and GPR and the activation of immune cells. (3) Alteration of transcription factors PPAR-γ and NF-κB. n-3 PUFA act as direct ligands to increase PPAR-γ and RXR expression and heterodimerization, resulting in a decrease in proinflammatory cytokine production, as well as inhibiting NF-κB activity. Inhibition of NF-κB results in a reduction of proinflammatory cytokines, chemokines, enzymes, as well as cell growth and angiogenic factors through (i) n-3 PUFA decreasing the phosphorylation of the inhibitory IκB, preventing the detachment and activation of NF-κB; (ii) n-3 PUFA activating GPR120, which negatively regulates NF-κB; (iii) n-3 PUFA decreasing activity of TLR, leading to a reduction in NF-κB activity; and (iv) n-3 PUFA increasing PPAR-γ activity, which decreases the NF-κB pathway of inflammation and cell growth.

how n-3 PUFA may prevent tumorigenesis and have been the focus of several reviews (Larsson et al. 2004; Sawyer and Field 2010; Calder 2012). This chapter will discuss the most well-studied mechanisms of n-3 effects as they relate to inflammation, including (1) modulation of the cell membrane FA profile, which has effects on (i) eicosanoid biosynthesis, (ii) modulation of cell signaling pathways, and (iii) properties of membrane microdomains, including lipid rafts and caveolae; and (2) regulation of transcription. We acknowledge that a number of other mechanisms exist and refer the readers to the aforementioned review papers.

14.4.1 MODULATION OF THE CELL MEMBRANE

Increased intake of n-3 PUFA results in their incorporation into the cell membrane phospholipids (PL), which has been shown to be associated with a decrease in the membrane n-6 PUFA content (Blonk et al. 1990; Katan et al. 1997; Healy et al. 2000; Dabadie et al. 2006). This alteration in the membrane PL FA profile may affect the inflammatory process through alteration in the substrates available for eicosanoid biosynthesis and cell signaling molecules and through changes in the physical properties of the cell membrane, which may alter the expression of proteins associated with signal transduction.

14.4.1.1 Eicosanoid Biosynthesis

A well-known biological effect of n-3 and n-6 PUFA is the production of hormone-like mediators known as eicosanoids. Eicosanoids are short-lived molecules that are 20 carbons in length and are known to affect many physiological and cellular processes, including inflammation, immune response, platelet aggregation, and cell growth and differentiation. In relation to the inflammatory response, eicosanoids are important regulators of its intensity and duration (Wang and Dubois 2010). PUFA can be enzymatically converted to eicosanoids (Figure 14.1; Voet and Voet 2004). n-3–derived eicosanoids are produced predominantly from EPA, with a small amount coming from DHA, while n-6–derived eicosanoids are generated from AA and from dihomo-γ-linolenic acid (DGLA), an intermediate metabolite in the conversion of LA to AA. The first step in eicosanoid biosynthesis involves the release of the FA from its esterified form in the membrane PL. This is done through the action of phospholipase A2 (PLA_2) and C (PLC). Free EPA, AA, and DGLA are then converted (1) by cyclooxygenases (COX1, the constitutive form, and COX2, the inducible form) to prostaglandins (PG), prostacyclins (PC), and thromboxanes (TX); (2) by lipoxygenases (5-LOX) to leukotrienes (LT), lipoxins, and hydroxy FA; and (3) by cytochrome P450 monooxygenases to hydroxy FA and epoxy FA. Novel anti-inflammatory agents known as resolvins and protectins produced from EPA and DHA in reactions involving COX and LOX enzymes are currently being studied (Serhan et al. 2004). The majority of work done thus far on the effects of protectins and resolvins in mediating inflammation has been in neural tissue; however, these anti-inflammatory mediators may have an important role in cancer.

Eicosanoids derived from n-6 PUFA have different biological effects than those derived from n-3 PUFA. DGLA and AA generate 1- and 2-series PG and TX and 4-series LT, while EPA generates 3-series PG and TX and 5-series LT (Voet and Voet 2004). In general, n-6–derived eicosanoids are proinflammatory while those produced from n-3 PUFA are anti-inflammatory or less potent inflammatory agents (Wang and Dubois 2010; Sawyer and Field 2010; Larsson et al. 2004). One suggested mechanism of the n-3 PUFA anticancer effect is through the suppression of the n-6–derived eicosanoid synthesis. There are multiple ways in which n-3 PUFA can exert this effect. First, the metabolism of n-6 and n-3 PUFA uses the same desaturase and elongase enzymes and therefore occurs in a competitive fashion (de Gomez Dumm and Brenner 1975; Hagve and Christophersen 1984). These enzymes have a higher affinity for n-3 PUFA, and therefore, increased intake of ALA and EPA increases their conversion to DHA and reduces the conversion of LA to AA (Rose and Connolly 1999b; Hagve and Christophersen 1984; Takahashi et al. 1991). This then alters the composition of FA esterified in the PL membrane available for hydrolysis by PLA_2 and PLC, which act indiscriminately (Hagve and Christophersen 1984; Takahashi et al. 1991). Secondly, n-3 PUFA alter the conversion from FA precursors to eicosanoids. n-3 PUFA have been shown to reduce the expression and activity of COX2, thereby reducing the eicosanoid biosynthesis (Hamid et al. 1999; Bhatia et al. 2011). On the other hand, n-6 PUFA have been shown to increase expression of both COX1 and COX2 in rats (Badawi et al. 1998). n-3 and n-6 are both substrates for COX and LOX enzymes; therefore, increased n-3 PUFA reduces the conversion of DGLA and AA to their respective eicosanoids through competitive inhibition (Culp et al. 1979; Marshall and Johnston 1982; Corey et al. 1983). Finally, n-3 PUFA may increase the clearance of eicosanoids. For example, human subjects were fed with a diet rich in n-3 PUFA or a control diet and LTB_4 (AA derived) and LTB_5 (EPA derived), and their metabolites were measured over time. Results showed higher levels of LTB_5 and lower LTB_4 in the n-3 diet as well as constant levels of LTB_4 metabolites over time despite decreasing levels of LTB_4. These results support the role of n-3 PUFA in increasing the synthesis of 5-series and decreasing that of 4-series LT and also accelerating the catabolism of LTB_4. The authors suggest that this catabolism may be due to the induction of peroxisomal enzymes (von Schacky et al. 1993).

Eicosanoids are known to affect the inflammatory process, cell growth, and differentiation and thus have been studied for their role in carcinogenesis. The importance of COX-derived PG and TX in carcinogenesis is supported by evidence showing that COX2, the inducible form of the enzyme, is upregulated in many cancers, including breast, prostate, and colon (Sawyer and Field 2010; Wang and Dubois 2010), yet is undetectable in normal intestine and breast tissue (Rose and Connolly 1999a). Studies support a link between AA-derived PGE_2, LTB_4, TXA_2, and 12-hydroxyeicosatetraenoic acid (12-HETE) and carcinogenesis through effects on cellular proliferation and apoptosis (Larsson et al. 2004; Sawyer and Field 2010). This may occur through the regulation of inflammation through effects on (1) hemodynamics, through effects on vasodilation and angiogenesis (Wang and Dubois 2010; Leahy et al. 2002; Rose et al. 1999); (2) activation and migration of leukocytes through chemoattractant properties and modulation of adhesion molecules (Tull et al. 2009); and (3) activation of the effector inflammatory cells to clear the injurious stimulus (Chapkin et al. 2009).

While many of the studies looking at eicosanoid production have been conducted using EPA and DHA, studies suggest that ALA has potential effects on eicosanoid biosynthesis. Marshall and Johnston (1982) showed that increasing the flaxseed oil content of rat diets reduced n-6 PUFA content of liver and spleen FA, with a reciprocal increase in n-3 PUFA content. They further showed a lower production of PG, including PGE_2, with higher flaxseed oil content of diets (Marshall and Johnston 1982). This effect may be modulated both by the decreased availability of substrate for 2-series PG synthesis and by a reduction in COX2, the enzyme responsible for PG synthesis. In a carcinogen-induced model of colon cancer, a diet rich in canola oil (9% ALA) reduced tumor incidence, multiplicity, and colonic COX2 expression compared to a corn oil diet (1% ALA) (Bhatia et al. 2011). LOX-derived eicosanoid production is also affected by diets rich in ALA. For example, when rats were fed with a diet rich in garden cress seed oil (32% ALA) compared to a sunflower oil (0.5% ALA) control diet, there was a 40% reduction in LTB_4 in peritoneal macrophages (Diwakar et al. 2011). Similarly, an earlier study showed that LTB_4 production was lower and LTB_5 production was higher in stimulated polymorphonuclear leukocytes from rats fed with a diet with ALA-rich perilla seed oil (64% ALA) compared to an LA-rich safflower oil diet (0.05% ALA). Cell membrane PLs also contained higher levels of EPA and DHA (Hashimoto et al. 1988). In contrast, in a rat model of cardiac dysfunction, flaxseed oil–rich diets (0.7%–6.6% energy) had no effect on urinary COX-derived TXB_2, while there were reductions in groups fed with fish oil–rich diets (0.7%–7% energy) (Duda et al. 2009). Although few of these studies look at eicosanoid production in models of cancer, they suggest that dietary sources rich in ALA are capable of modulating cellular levels of EPA and DHA, COX2 expression, and the production of some eicosanoids.

14.4.1.2 Substrate for Formation of Second Messengers

Hydrolysis of membrane PL by PLC produces diacylglycerol (DAG), a lipid mediator that acts as a second messenger in signaling pathways. DAG is linked to carcinogenesis through its activation of some isoforms of PKC. PKC modulates tumorigenesis through activation of the proliferation-inducing mitogen-activated protein kinase (MAPK) pathway and the activation of nuclear transcription factor kappa B (NF-κB), which is associated with the inflammatory response. NF-κB will be discussed in more detail in Section 14.4.2.2. There is a hypothesis that the FA found in the PL that are available for hydrolysis to form DAG alter its actions on PKC (Kishimoto et al. 1980; Miles and Calder 1998; Calder 2012). Interestingly, total DAG production from T cells cultured from the spleens of mice fed with EPA- and DHA-enriched diets was significantly lower compared to those fed with safflower oil- or AA-enriched diets (Jolly et al. 1997). Further studies are required to fully elucidate the effect of n-3 PUFA on DAG-related signaling.

14.4.1.3 Membrane Physical Properties and Signal Transduction

14.4.1.3.1 Properties of Cell Membrane

Alterations in membrane PL FA profile are known to affect properties of the membrane, including fluidity, permeability, compressibility, and microstructure (Calder 2012; Larsson et al. 2004). Due to the multiple double bonds in n-3 PUFA, which cause bends in the hydrocarbon chain, substituting saturated and monounsaturated FA with PUFA will increase steric hindrance within the membrane, causing it to be less tightly packed and thus more fluid. Since ALA, EPA, and DHA have differing degrees of unsaturation, they may have different effects on membrane fluidity, and this has not yet been systematically studied.

The cell membrane is not homogeneous and contains microdomains known as lipid rafts (or membrane rafts) and flask-like invaginations known as caveolae (Staubach and Hanisch 2011). An emerging potential mechanism of n-3 PUFA is through the modulation of the composition of these microdomains. The existence of lipid rafts has been debated; however, improvements in imaging approaches have led to greater confidence that they form a distinct membrane domain. Lipid rafts are characterized by high cholesterol, glycosphingolipid and saturated FA contents, and low membrane fluidity. They act as hubs that colocalize membrane receptors and compartmentalize cellular processes, such as signal transduction. Caveolae are rich in proteins involved in signal transduction as well as the structural protein caveolin-1 (Staubach and Hanisch 2011). Receptors that play important roles in inflammation and carcinogenesis that have been shown to exist in lipid raft and caveolae microdomains include growth factor receptors (Schley et al. 2007), G-protein–coupled receptors (GPR) (Chini and Parenti 2004), and pattern recognition receptors, including toll-like receptors (TLR), which identify inflammatory triggers and initiate the immune response (Chapkin et al. 2009; Fessler and Parks 2011).

There is strong evidence that increased levels of EPA and DHA result in their incorporation into the cell membrane PL and potentially into the lipid rafts. However, a recent review by Calder (2012) states that because of their low affinity for cholesterol, PUFA are not incorporated into the lipid rafts, although they do affect raft formation based on their incorporation into the nonraft membrane. On the other hand, a number of studies have shown EPA and/or DHA incorporation into the lipid rafts of mammary, colon, and lung cancer cells (Schley et al. 2007; Rogers et al. 2010). Nevertheless, exposure of cancer cells to n-3 PUFA has been shown to disrupt lipid rafts by increasing the level of ceramide within the raft due to the hydrolysis of sphingomyelin (Sawyer and Field 2010). This disruption may result in the translocation of receptors from the raft to nonraft domain. Schley et al. (2007) showed that treating breast cancer cells with EPA and DHA resulted in n-3 PUFA enrichment of the lipid raft and a translocation of epidermal growth factor receptor (EGFR) protein from the lipid raft to nonraft domain. With respect to caveolae, Ma et al. (2004) showed that diets rich in n-3 PUFA increased the n-3 content of colonic caveolae and caused displacement of h-ras and endothelial nitric oxide synthase (eNOS) from caveolae. n-3 PUFA have been shown to inhibit specific TLR (Lee et al. 2003) and activate certain GPR (Oh et al. 2010); however, whether this is due to an effect on their localization of TLR and GPR has not yet been established. Little is known on the effect of ALA on the FA composition of lipid rafts or caveolae, and this warrants further study.

The relationship between these membrane changes and the inflammatory pathway are not yet clear. As highlighted above, n-3 PUFA changed the localization of eNOS, which may result in hemodynamic alterations as eNOS is a known vasoregulator associated with increased vascular permeability (Duran et al. 2010). Alterations in lipid rafts may affect signal transduction pathways involved in inflammation. For example, h-ras and EGFR, which were shown to be translocated by n-3 PUFA in studies described above, regulate the MAPK signaling pathway, which has been shown to increase leukocyte recruitment to the site of inflammation (Herlaar and Brown 1999). Alterations in lipid rafts have been shown to affect immune cell activation, which has been the focus of a recent review article (Shaikh et al. 2012). How n-3 PUFA alter the constituent protein and FA of lipid rafts in both cancer cells and immune cells and the consequences of these effects on tumorigenesis require further elucidation.

14.4.2 REGULATION OF TRANSCRIPTION

n-3 PUFA may exert an anti-inflammatory effect through alteration of transcription factors, proteins that control transcription of target genes involved in a variety of cellular processes. To date, n-3 PUFA have been shown to alter a variety of transcription factors, and our review will focus on the anti-inflammatory peroxisome proliferator–activated receptor gamma (PPAR-γ) and proinflammatory nuclear NF-κB. Most research in the area of n-3 PUFA and transcriptional regulation in inflammation and cancer prevention has been conducted on the LC-PUFA EPA and DHA, but many of these effects are likely applicable to ALA and flaxseed oil as well.

14.4.2.1 Peroxisome Proliferator-Activated Receptors

The PPAR are a group of transcription factors that, when activated by ligands, control genes involved in a variety of cellular processes including inflammation, lipid metabolism, and cell differentiation and proliferation (Larsson et al. 2004). There are three isoforms of PPAR: α, β/δ, and γ. Our review will focus on the PPAR-γ isoform, found in a variety of tissues including adipose, heart, skeletal muscle, colon, and intestine (Berger and Moller 2002). PPAR-γ works through heterodimerizing with retinoid x receptors (RXR) and binding to peroxisome proliferator response elements (PPRE) in promoter regions of DNA to increase transcription of specific proteins. Activation of PPAR-γ has been associated with a reduction in proinflammatory cytokines such as tumor necrosis factor α (TNFα), interleukin 6 (IL-6), and IL-1β (Li et al. 2004), but this may be an indirect effect of PPAR-γ decreasing the activity of the inflammatory NF-κB pathway, which upregulates cytokine production (Schmitz and Ecker 2008; Zhao et al. 2005; Su et al. 1999). The NF-κB pathway of inflammation is further discussed below. FA are natural ligands for PPAR, and PUFA ability to bind PPAR-γ may decrease inflammation and lead to a reduction in cancer initiation and progression. Recent studies in both lung (A549) and colon cancer (HT-29) cell lines have shown that EPA, DHA, and AA (25–100 μM) can all suppress cell growth through increasing PPAR-γ activity (Allred et al. 2008; Trombetta et al. 2007). In the colon cancer cell line in particular, the growth reduction from EPA was reversed when a pharmacological PPAR-γ antagonist was supplemented, providing evidence that at least part of the EPA growth-reducing effect is through PPAR-γ upregulation. Similarly, in the THP-1 leukemia cell line, ALA and DHA (0–100 μM) both increased PPAR-γ DNA binding and decreased proinflammatory IL-6, IL-1β, and TNFα expression (Zhao et al. 2005). It is unknown whether these effects are directly from PPAR-γ induction or the result of PPAR-γ inhibiting NF-κB activity as its DNA binding was decreased. The role of n-3 PUFA as PPAR-γ agonists to decrease inflammation is not a clear story, however. One study showed in MCF-7 and MDA-MB-231 breast cancer cell lines that EPA (100 μM), DHA (10 μM), and ALA (10 nM) all decreased PPAR-γ transcriptional activity, while n-6 PUFA γ-linolenic acid (200 μM), AA (250 μM), and LA (250 μM) all increased activity (Thoennes et al. 2000). Similarly in colon (HT-116) and monocytic leukemia (THP-1) cells lines, 100 μM DHA supplementation decreased PPAR-γ transactivation and DNA binding and reduced the production of the PPAR-γ gene product CD26 (Lee et al. 2002). However, in this study, LA was also shown to decrease PPAR-γ expression. These contradictory outcomes regarding n-3 PUFA as PPAR-γ agonists or antagonists may be due in part to variation in doses and cell lines used, and further investigation into the role of n-3 PUFA on PPAR-γ expression and the inflammatory pathway is warranted. Another important aspect of n-3 PUFA control of PPAR-γ is through increased RXR expression. DHA and ALA have been shown to be ligands for RXR (Vanden Heuvel et al. 2006; de Urquiza et al. 2000), which may increase PPAR-γ anticancer effects through increased heterodimerization with RXR. From these studies, ALA as well as the other n-3 PUFA show promise as anti-inflammatory and antineoplastic agents, but more research is necessary to make recommendations.

14.4.2.2 Nuclear Factor-Kappa B

NF-κB is a transcription factor that has been associated with an increase in cancer incidence through regulation of genes involved in the inflammatory response, as well as cell cycle and apoptosis. NF-κB is inactive when attached to the inhibitory IκB protein, but upon IκB phosphorylation by the IκB kinase complex, NF-κB is free to bind regulatory elements on DNA and increase expression of proinflammatory molecules (Kang and Weylandt 2008). Activation of NF-κB has been shown to increase several proinflammatory cytokines (IL-6, IL-1β, TNFα), chemokines (IL-8, MCP-1), as well as COX2 and inducible nitric oxide synthase (iNOS), which produces proinflammatory nitric oxide (NO) (Schmitz and Ecker 2008; Yamada et al. 2012). On top of the inflammatory regulation, NF-κB also plays a role in regulation of cancer-related growth pathways (cellular proliferation, apoptosis, and angiogenesis) through control of molecules such as cyclin D1, bcl-2, and vascular endothelial growth factor (VEGF) (Ghosh and Karin 2002; Karin and Lin 2002; Shibata et al. 2002).

n-3 PUFA have been found to decrease NF-κB activity, and potentially regulate cellular inflammation and cancer development, through (1) decreasing the phosphorylation of NF-κB inhibitor IκB; (2) binding to and increasing activity of GPR120, which negatively regulates NF-κB (Oh et al. 2010); (3) reducing activity of TLR, a receptor that induces inflammation through NF-κB and cytokine regulation (Lee et al. 2003); and (4) indirect NF-κB regulation by PPAR-γ as discussed previously (see Figure 14.2 for a mechanistic overview). In vitro studies of macrophages, leukemia, and breast cancer cells have shown that EPA and DHA decrease NF-κB activity and lower TNFα expression. The reduction in NF-κB activation is likely a result of decreased IκB phosphorylation and NF-κB DNA binding (Schley et al. 2005; Kang and Weylandt 2008; Zhao et al. 2004). One study using an in vitro model of liver inflammation found that peroxidized DHA and EPA reduced NF-κB activation and iNOS and NO expression through alteration of iNOS promoters (transcription effect) and messenger RNA (mRNA) stabilization (posttranscription) (Araki et al. 2011). However, the unoxidized EPA and DHA had no effect. In a similar model using ALA, iNOS mRNA and protein expression was decreased, but there was no effect on NF-κB activation (Yamada et al. 2012). iNOS mRNA stabilization (posttranscription) was decreased, but there was no effect on iNOS promoters as seen with the peroxidized EPA and DHA. These discrepancies are likely a result of the ALA dose being much lower (200 vs. 500 μM) and in an unoxidized form. The fat-1 transgenic mouse is able to convert n-6 to n-3 PUFA at a high efficiency, creating a high n-3 PUFA environment even with a high n-6 diet (Kang and Weylandt 2008). Using this model, it has been shown that a high n-3 PUFA environment decreases inflammation; NF-κB activity; and IL-6, TNFα, and IL-1β expression in a variety of tissues, including the colon (Hudert et al. 2006; Kang and Weylandt 2008).

To investigate the importance of GPR120 in the anti-inflammatory effects of DHA, wild-type and GPR120 knockout mice were treated with a DHA-rich diet; results showed that in the wild-type mice, there was a decrease in inflammation, IL-6, TNFα, MCP-1, IL-1β, and iNOS, but no effect was seen in the GPR120 knockout mice (Oh et al. 2010). This highlights that n-3 PUFA effects on NF-κB activation may be mediated through an increase in GPR120 activity. ALA treatment in a rat model of colitis showed a reduction in colon iNOS, TNFα, NF-κB, and COX2 expression (Hassan et al. 2010). Evidence for n-3 PUFA NF-κB inhibition through TLR was shown in an in vitro study using murine monocytes treated with the TLR4 agonist lipopolysaccharide (Lee et al. 2003). EPA and DHA (0–25 μM) successfully reduced NF-κB and COX2 expression, through inhibition of TLR4. The majority of studies investigating the effects of n-3 PUFA on NF-κB regulation of inflammation have focused on EPA and DHA. In the few ALA- and flaxseed-based studies, however, many similar and beneficial effects on NF-κB have been seen, highlighting the need for further research in this area.

14.4.3 Immunomodulatory Effects

As described above, n-3 PUFA have effects on many compounds known to alter inflammatory response, including a shift from the production of proinflammatory n-6–derived eicosanoids to the less potent n-3-derivatives; altered inflammatory signal transduction pathways through modulation of membrane PL, particularly in lipid raft and caveolae domains; and reduced expression of inflammatory cytokines (TNFα, IL-6, and IL-1β), chemokines (IL-8, MCP-1), and vasoactive factors (iNOS, eNOS). Modulation of these factors may have consequent effects on immune effector cell activation. Cells involved in the mounting of an immune response that have been shown to be affected by n-3 PUFA include T cells (lymphocytes), dendritic cells, macrophages, and neutrophils.

T cells are involved in cell-mediated immunity and are activated by antigen-presenting cells such as dendritic cells. Several studies using rodent models suggest that dietary n-3 PUFA affect the proliferation of CD4 T cells in response to mitogenic and stimulatory agents (Arrington, Chapkin et al. 2001; Arrington, McMurray et al. 2001; Zhang et al. 2005), an effect that appears to be specific to Th1 cells (Zhang et al. 2005). Th1 cells secrete IL-2, and EPA, DHA, and fish oil diets were shown to reduce levels of IL-2 secreted from cultured splenic T- lymphocytes harvested from mice (Arrington, Chapkin et al. 2001; Arrington, McMurray et al. 2001; Jolly et al. 1997). DAG signaling pathways affect T-cell activation. As discussed in Section 14.4.1.2, EPA- and DHA-enriched diets reduced the amount of the second messenger DAG produced from T cells cultured from mouse spleens (Jolly et al. 1997). Alterations in the lipid raft composition in T cells and dendritic cells are also suggested mechanisms of altered activation (Chapkin et al. 2009).

In experimental studies in humans, the story is less clear. For example, in a placebo-controlled, double-blind parallel study, Kew et al. (2003) looked at the effect of five interventions: (1) placebo, (2) 2.5 g ALA/day, (3) 9.5 g ALA/day, (4) 0.77 g EPA+DHA/day, and (5) 1.7 g EPA+DHA/day, given through a combination of fat spreads and pill form for 6 months. None of the treatments showed any effect on the functional activity of lymphocytes, neutrophils, and monocytes (Kew et al. 2003). However, in a cross-sectional study, the same researchers showed that the FA profile of human peripheral blood mononuclear cells (PBMC) extracted from 150 healthy subjects is related to the immune cell functions and that lower n-6:n-3 content is associated with reduced immune cell activation (Kew et al. 2003). No association was reported between dietary intake of classes of FA and immune cell function; however, limitations of the food reporting tool may bias this result. In a small randomized placebo-controlled trial of healthy men, consumption of flaxseed oil (providing 3.5 g/day ALA) or fish oil (providing 0.44, 0.94, or 1.9 g/day EPA+DHA) in pill form did not affect the proliferation of PBMC nor was the production of TNFα, IL-1β, IL-4, or interferon gamma (IFNγ) different between groups (Wallace et al. 2003). IL-6 levels were lower in the medium- and high-dose fish oil groups. As this was a very small study with only eight subjects per group, it may have been underpowered to detect differences. Together, these results suggest that the FA content of immune cells is important in regulating the immune response; however, studies have failed to show an effect of dietary intake of n-3 PUFA on immunoregulation despite their incorporation into the cell PL. Further studies are required to clarify this effect.

14.5   n-3 PUFA AND BREAST AND COLORECTAL CANCER PREVENTION

Preclinical models discussed in Section 14.4 and summarized in reviews (Anderson and Ma 2009; Cockbain et al. 2012) provide evidence that n-3 PUFA may play a role in cancer prevention, and their mechanism of action likely involves a reduction in chronic inflammation. Clinical and epidemiological evidence, however, is conflicting. Focusing on breast and colorectal cancer prevention, human studies of n-3 PUFA and their richest marine and plant sources, fish (EPA and DHA) and flaxseed (ALA), have provided inconsistent results.

14.5.1 Breast Cancer Prevention

To date, several extensive reviews have been conducted on the topic of fish intake and breast cancer risk, and we refer readers to a recent systematic review, which showed that study outcomes varied greatly and failed to establish a consistent relationship (Sala-Vila and Calder 2011). Several clinical studies have also looked specifically at EPA and DHA intake and breast cancer risk and have also provided mixed results. Two studies found that dietary intake and erythrocyte content of EPA and DHA were both associated with a decrease in breast cancer risk and reoccurrence (Kuriki et al. 2007; Patterson et al. 2011), while several have found no association (Witt et al. 2009; Murff et al. 2011).

Although both in vitro and preclinical rodent studies generally have shown that flaxseed and ALA have the ability to decrease breast cancer tumor growth (Bougnoux and Chajes 2003; Saggar et al. 2010a,b; Thompson et al. 1996; Truan et al. 2010; Thompson and Mason 2010; Chen et al. 2011), few clinical studies have investigated them in terms of breast cancer prevention. One clinical trial conducted in postmenopausal newly diagnosed breast cancer patients did find that 25 g/day of flaxseed decreased tumor cell proliferation and increased apoptosis compared to a control diet (Thompson et al. 2005), although this focuses on limiting tumor progression, not prevention. Epidemiological data in the field are also lacking and conflicting. One study concluded that there was an inverse relationship between breast adipose tissue ALA content and breast cancer risk (Klein et al. 2000) but no association with total n-3 PUFA or LC-PUFA content. In agreement with this was a meta-analysis that showed that when separating out the individual n-3 PUFA, ALA was the only one to significantly reduce breast cancer risk (MacLean et al. 2006). Contrary to this, a case-control study in Uruguay found that although total n-3 PUFA intake significantly reduced breast cancer risk, ALA intake caused an increase in risk (De Stefani et al. 1998).

Similar to the clinical evidence for fish, flaxseed, and individual n-3 PUFA, the effects of total n-3 PUFA intake are also conflicting. Three case-control studies showed that dietary n-3 PUFA intake had no significant association with breast cancer risk (Zhang et al. 2011; Chajes et al. 2012; Sulaiman et al. 2011) and are supported by evidence from two prospective cohort studies and a meta-analysis (Witt et al. 2009; Murff et al. 2011; MacLean et al. 2006). Two case-control studies, however, did show a significant decrease in breast cancer risk with increasing PUFA intake and n-3 PUFA erythrocyte content (Kuriki et al. 2007; De Stefani et al. 1998).

14.5.2 Colorectal Cancer Prevention

Similar to breast cancer, several extensive reviews have been conducted on colorectal cancer risk and fish intake, and we refer readers to the review by Sala-Vila and Calder (2011). As seen with breast cancer risk, data on fish consumption and colorectal cancer risk were mixed and failed to provide a clear relationship. One randomized control (West et al. 2010), one cohort (Sasazuki et al. 2011), and several case-control studies (Theodoratou et al. 2007; Kim et al. 2010) have shown an inverse relationship between EPA and DHA consumption and colorectal cancer. Contrary to these promising results, a meta-analysis found no significant association between EPA and DHA and colorectal cancer prevention (MacLean et al. 2006).

Several rodent models of colorectal cancer have provided evidence of a flaxseed and flaxseed oil protective effect and indicate that inflammatory pathways are involved, as there was a reduction in COX1 and COX2 expression (Bommareddy et al. 2006, 2009; Dwivedi et al. 2005; Williams et al. 2007). Despite these findings, there is a lack of clinical studies investigating the relationship between flaxseed and ALA in colorectal cancer prevention. Among the few studies done, one found that there was no significant association between ALA intake and colorectal cancer (Terry et al. 2001), while another study found that ALA intake was associated with a significant increase in colorectal cancer incidence (Theodoratou et al. 2007).

Clinical evidence for a relationship between total n-3 PUFA intake and colorectal cancer incidence is inconsistent. Several case-control studies (Theodoratou et al. 2007; Kim et al. 2010;

Kimura et al. 2007) found a decreased colorectal cancer incidence with increased n-3 PUFA intake; however, meta-analyses failed to support this inverse relationship (MacLean et al. 2006; Geelen et al. 2007).

Although the clinical evidence for the ability of fish, flaxseed, and n-3 PUFA to prevent breast and colorectal cancer is conflicting, further investigation is warranted as preclinical studies have provided promising evidence, and several limitations in the current clinical studies may contribute to the inconsistent results (see Section 14.6). There are currently several ongoing clinical trials that will help to clarify the current disconnect between the fairly consistent preventive effect in in vitro and animal work and the conflicting results seen in human studies. The seAFOod trial is a large multicenter trial in the United Kingdom looking at the effect of fish oil alone and in combination with aspirin for colorectal cancer prevention (trial ISRCTN05926847). Vitamin D and Omega 3 Trial (VITAL) is a large study involving subjects from across the United States investigating the effects of fish oil and vitamin D in cancer prevention (NCT01169259). A smaller trial from Ohio State University will compare dietary fish oil to fish intake and will relate tissue FA levels to the risk of breast cancer (NCT01282580). The effect of flaxseed in the prevention on premenopausal breast cancer is being investigated in a randomized study at the Roswell Park Cancer Institute in Buffalo, New York (NCT00794989). The Center for Botanical Lipids at Wake Forest University is researching the effects of plant-derived n-3 PUFA with a focus on inflammation and cardiovascular disease. Their research will help to determine the effects of ALA on inflammation, which may provide a basis for future work in cancer prevention.

14.6   LIMITATIONS AND FUTURE DIRECTIONS

There are several limitations to the n-3 PUFA cancer prevention clinical studies that are controllable in both in vitro and in vivo work, and these may explain some of the discrepancies between the preclinical and clinical data. Variation in the n-3 PUFA type, source, and amount is likely the largest contributing factor to inconsistencies in the data. Lumping together all n-3 PUFA may nullify potentially significant associations of individual DHA, EPA, and ALA with cancer prevention, as was seen between breast cancer and ALA (MacLean et al. 2006). Furthermore, most studies have focused on EPA and DHA, while flaxseed and ALA are often overlooked even though they have shown significant effects preclinically. The source of n-3 PUFA is also of importance, as fish type (fatty vs. lean) and preparation (raw, dried, fried) and ALA food source (vegetable vs. processed and nuts) have all been shown to modify results (MacLean et al. 2006; Sala-Vila and Calder 2011; Thiebaut et al. 2009). Finally, the actual n-3 PUFA content of marine and plant sources varies greatly, and this is often missed in clinical studies due to a lack of serum and tissue sample FA profiling and lack of specificity in questionnaires.

Distinguishing cancer characteristics has also been limited in clinical trials. In breast cancer, for example, both receptor (estrogen receptor, human epidermal growth factor receptor 2) and menopausal status have been shown to alter n-3 PUFA effects (MacLean et al. 2006). In colorectal cancer, subsite (distal colon, proximal colon, colorectal, rectal) has been shown to modify n-3 PUFA effects (Kim et al. 2010; Sasazuki et al. 2011). It should also be noted that in preclinical models, the focus is often on limiting cancer progression versus prevention, which is the focus of the clinical studies discussed, and this may account for some of the variability. Several other individual characteristics such as genetic predisposition, race, sex, and body mass index (BMI) have also been shown to affect n-3 PUFA breast and colorectal cancer chemoprevention in clinical studies (Signori et al. 2011; Kim et al. 2010; Chajes et al. 2012).

To resolve inconsistencies and establish a more concrete relationship between n-3 PUFA and cancer prevention, future clinical studies should focus attention not only on fish and marine n-3 PUFA but also flaxseed and ALA. As well, steps should be taken to address some of the limitations discussed here such as requiring biological samples to quantify n-3 PUFA content, improving dietary questionnaires to include source and preparation of the foods, evaluating developed tumors for location and molecular receptors, and including detailed personal information such as menopausal status and BMI.

14.7 CONCLUSION

In conclusion, there is a large body of evidence from in vitro and animal models supporting the role of n-3 PUFA in modulating various aspects of the cancer process, including inflammation. The majority of this evidence is for EPA and DHA, and therefore, further studies should aim to clarify the effects of ALA, as it is the most commonly consumed n-3 PUFA in the North American diet. There is inconsistency in the results of observational and experimental studies in humans, which may be due to lumping together of different sources of n-3 PUFA as well as cancer subtypes. Carefully designed clinical trials that take into account these limitations will help to determine the optimum approach to the use of n-3 PUFA for cancer prevention.

REFERENCES

Allred, C. D., D. R. Talbert, R. C. Southard, X. Wang, and M. W. Kilgore. 2008. PPARgamma1 as a molecular target of eicosapentaenoic acid in human colon cancer (HT-29) cells. *J Nutr* 138 (2):250–6.

Anderson, B. M., and D. W. Ma. 2009. Are all n-3 polyunsaturated fatty acids created equal? *Lipids Health Dis* 8:33.

Araki, Y., M. Matsumiya, T. Matsuura et al. 2011. Peroxidation of n-3 polyunsaturated fatty acids inhibits the induction of iNOS gene expression in proinflammatory cytokine-stimulated hepatocytes. *J Nutr Metab* 2011:374542.

Arrington, J. L., R. S. Chapkin, K. C. Switzer, J. S. Morris, and D. N. McMurray. 2001. Dietary n-3 polyunsaturated fatty acids modulate purified murine T-cell subset activation. *Clin Exp Immunol* 125 (3):499–507.

Arrington, J. L., D. N. McMurray, K. C. Switzer, Y. Y. Fan, and R. S. Chapkin. 2001. Docosahexaenoic acid suppresses function of the CD28 costimulatory membrane receptor in primary murine and Jurkat T cells. *J Nutr* 131 (4):1147–53.

Badawi, A. F., A. El-Sohemy, L. L. Stephen, A. K. Ghoshal, and M. C. Archer. 1998. The effect of dietary n-3 and n-6 polyunsaturated fatty acids on the expression of cyclooxygenase 1 and 2 and levels of p21ras in rat mammary glands. *Carcinogenesis* 19 (5):905–10.

Berger, J., and D. E. Moller. 2002. The mechanisms of action of PPARs. *Annu Rev Med* 53:409–35.

Bhatia, E., C. Doddivenaka, X. Zhang et al. 2011. Chemopreventive effects of dietary canola oil on colon cancer development. *Nutr Cancer* 63 (2):242–7.

Blonk, M. C., H. J. Bilo, J. J. Nauta et al. 1990. Dose-response effects of fish-oil supplementation in healthy volunteers. *Am J Clin Nutr* 52 (1):120–7.

Bommareddy, A., B. L. Arasada, D. P. Mathees, and C. Dwivedi. 2006. Chemopreventive effects of dietary flaxseed on colon tumor development. *Nutr Cancer* 54 (2):216–22.

Bommareddy, A., X. Zhang, D. Schrader et al. 2009. Effects of dietary flaxseed on intestinal tumorigenesis in Apc(Min) mouse. *Nutr Cancer* 61 (2):276–83.

Bougnoux, P., and V. Chajes. 2003. Alpha-linolenic acid and cancer. In *Flaxseed in Human Nutrition*, 2nd ed., edited by L. U. Thompson and S. C. Cunnane. Champaign: AOCS Press.

Boyd, N. F., J. Stone, K. N. Vogt et al. 2003. Dietary fat and breast cancer risk revisited: a meta-analysis of the published literature. *Br J Cancer* 89 (9):1672–85.

Brenna, J. T., N. Salem, Jr., A. J. Sinclair, and S. C. Cunnane. 2009. Alpha-linolenic acid supplementation and conversion to n-3 long-chain polyunsaturated fatty acids in humans. *Prostaglandins Leukot Essent Fatty Acids* 80 (2–3):85–91.

Calder, P. C. 2012. Mechanisms of Action of (n-3) Fatty Acids. *J Nutr* 142 (3):592S–9S.

Chajes, V., G. Torres-Mejia, C. Biessy et al. 2012. Omega-3 and omega-6 polyunsaturated fatty acid intakes and the risk of breast cancer in Mexican women: impact of obesity status. *Cancer Epidemiol Biomarkers Prev* 21 (2):319–26.

Chapkin, R. S., W. Kim, J. R. Lupton, and D. N. McMurray. 2009. Dietary docosahexaenoic and eicosapentaenoic acid: emerging mediators of inflammation. *Prostaglandins Leukot Essent Fatty Acids* 81 (2–3):187–91.

Chen, J., J. K. Saggar, P. Corey, and L. U. Thompson. 2011. Flaxseed cotyledon fraction reduces tumour growth and sensitises tamoxifen treatment of human breast cancer xenograft (MCF-7) in athymic mice. *Br J Nutr* 105 (3):339–47.

Chini, B., and M. Parenti. 2004. G-protein coupled receptors in lipid rafts and caveolae: how, when and why do they go there? *J Mol Endocrinol* 32 (2):325–38.

Clevers, H. 2004. At the crossroads of inflammation and cancer. *Cell* 118 (6):671–4.

Cockbain, A. J., G. J. Toogood, and M. A. Hull. 2012. Omega-3 polyunsaturated fatty acids for the treatment and prevention of colorectal cancer. *Gut* 61 (1):135–49.

Corey, E. J., C. Shih, and J. R. Cashman. 1983. Docosahexaenoic acid is a strong inhibitor of prostaglandin but not leukotriene biosynthesis. *Proc Natl Acad Sci U S A* 80 (12):3581–4.

Coussens, L. M., and Z. Werb. 2002. Inflammation and cancer. *Nature* 420 (6917):860–7.

Culp, B. R., B. G. Titus, and W. E. Lands. 1979. Inhibition of prostaglandin biosynthesis by eicosapentaenoic acid. *Prostaglandins Med* 3 (5):269–78.

Cunnane, Stephen C. 2003. Dietary sources and metabolism of α-linolenic acid. In *Flaxseed in Human Nutrition*, 2nd ed., edited by S. C. Cunnane and L. U. Thompson. Champaign: AOCS Press.

Dabadie, H., C. Motta, E. Peuchant, P. LeRuyet, and F. Mendy. 2006. Variations in daily intakes of myristic and alpha-linolenic acids in sn-2 position modify lipid profile and red blood cell membrane fluidity. *Br J Nutr* 96 (2):283–9.

Dandona, P., A. Aljada, and A. Bandyopadhyay. 2004. Inflammation: the link between insulin resistance, obesity and diabetes. *Trends Immunol* 25 (1):4–7.

de Gomez Dumm, I. N., and R. R. Brenner. 1975. Oxidative desaturation of alpha-linoleic, linoleic, and stearic acids by human liver microsomes. *Lipids* 10 (6):315–7.

De Stefani, E., H. Deneo-Pellegrini, M. Mendilaharsu, and A. Ronco. 1998. Essential fatty acids and breast cancer: a case-control study in Uruguay. *Int J Cancer* 76 (4):491–4.

de Urquiza, A. M., S. Liu, M. Sjoberg et al. 2000. Docosahexaenoic acid, a ligand for the retinoid X receptor in mouse brain. *Science* 290 (5499):2140–4.

Demaria, S., E. Pikarsky, M. Karin et al. 2010. Cancer and inflammation: promise for biologic therapy. *J Immunother* 33 (4):335–51.

Diwakar, B. T., B. R. Lokesh, and K. A. Naidu. 2011. Modulatory effect of alpha-linolenic acid-rich garden cress (*Lepidium sativum* L.) seed oil on inflammatory mediators in adult albino rats. *Br J Nutr* 106 (4):530–9.

Duda, M. K., K. M. O'Shea, A. Tintinu et al. 2009. Fish oil, but not flaxseed oil, decreases inflammation and prevents pressure overload-induced cardiac dysfunction. *Cardiovasc Res* 81 (2):319–27.

Duran, W. N., J. W. Breslin, and F. A. Sanchez. 2010. The NO cascade, eNOS location, and microvascular permeability. *Cardiovasc Res* 87 (2):254–61.

Dwivedi, C., K. Natarajan, and D. P. Matthees. 2005. Chemopreventive effects of dietary flaxseed oil on colon tumor development. *Nutr Cancer* 51 (1):52–8.

Fessler, M. B., and J. S. Parks. 2011. Intracellular lipid flux and membrane microdomains as organizing principles in inflammatory cell signaling. *J Immunol* 187 (4):1529–35.

Geelen, A., J. M. Schouten, C. Kamphuis et al. 2007. Fish consumption, n-3 fatty acids, and colorectal cancer: a meta-analysis of prospective cohort studies. *Am J Epidemiol* 166 (10):1116–25.

Ghosh, S., and M. Karin. 2002. Missing pieces in the NF-kappaB puzzle. *Cell* 109 Suppl:S81–96.

Hagve, T. A., and B. O. Christophersen. 1984. Effect of dietary fats on arachidonic acid and eicosapentaenoic acid biosynthesis and conversion to C22 fatty acids in isolated rat liver cells. *Biochim Biophys Acta* 796 (2):205–17.

Hamid, R., J. Singh, B. S. Reddy, and L. A. Cohen. 1999. Inhibition by dietary menhaden oil of cyclooxygenase-1 and -2 in N-nitrosomethylurea-induced rat mammary tumors. *Int J Oncol* 14 (3):523–8.

Hashimoto, A., M. Katagiri, S. Torii et al. 1988. Effect of the dietary alpha-linolenate/linoleate balance on leukotriene production and histamine release in rats. *Prostaglandins* 36 (1):3–16.

Hassan, A., A. Ibrahim, K. Mbodji et al. 2010. An alpha-linolenic acid-rich formula reduces oxidative stress and inflammation by regulating NF-kappaB in rats with TNBS-induced colitis. *J Nutr* 140 (10):1714–21.

Healy, D. A., F. A. Wallace, E. A. Miles, P. C. Calder, and P. Newsholm. 2000. Effect of low-to-moderate amounts of dietary fish oil on neutrophil lipid composition and function. *Lipids* 35 (7):763–8.

Herlaar, E., and Z. Brown. 1999. p38 MAPK signalling cascades in inflammatory disease. *Mol Med Today* 5 (10):439–47.

Hudert, C. A., K. H. Weylandt, Y. Lu et al. 2006. Transgenic mice rich in endogenous omega-3 fatty acids are protected from colitis. *Proc Natl Acad Sci U S A* 103 (30):11276–81.

Jolly, C. A., Y. H. Jiang, R. S. Chapkin, and D. N. McMurray. 1997. Dietary (n-3) polyunsaturated fatty acids suppress murine lymphoproliferation, interleukin-2 secretion, and the formation of diacylglycerol and ceramide. *J Nutr* 127 (1):37–43.

Kang, J. X., and K. H. Weylandt. 2008. Modulation of inflammatory cytokines by omega-3 fatty acids. In *Lipids in Health and Disease*, edited by P. W. X. Quinn. New York: Springer.

Karin, M., and A. Lin. 2002. NF-kappaB at the crossroads of life and death. *Nat Immunol* 3 (3):221–7.

Katan, M. B., J. P. Deslypere, A. P. van Birgelen, M. Penders, and M. Zegwaard. 1997. Kinetics of the incorporation of dietary fatty acids into serum cholesteryl esters, erythrocyte membranes, and adipose tissue: an 18-month controlled study. *J Lipid Res* 38 (10):2012–22.

Kew, S., T. Banerjee, A. M. Minihane et al. 2003. Lack of effect of foods enriched with plant- or marine-derived n-3 fatty acids on human immune function. *Am J Clin Nutr* 77 (5):1287–95.

Kim, S., D. P. Sandler, J. Galanko, C. Martin, and R. S. Sandler. 2010. Intake of polyunsaturated fatty acids and distal large bowel cancer risk in whites and African Americans. *Am J Epidemiol* 171 (9):969–79.

Kimura, Y., S. Kono, K. Toyomura et al. 2007. Meat, fish and fat intake in relation to subsite-specific risk of colorectal cancer: The Fukuoka Colorectal Cancer Study. *Cancer Sci* 98 (4):590–7.

Kishimoto, A., Y. Takai, T. Mori, U. Kikkawa, and Y. Nishizuka. 1980. Activation of calcium and phospholipid-dependent protein kinase by diacylglycerol, its possible relation to phosphatidylinositol turnover. *J Biol Chem* 255 (6):2273–6.

Klein, V., V. Chajes, E. Germain et al. 2000. Low alpha-linolenic acid content of adipose breast tissue is associated with an increased risk of breast cancer. *Eur J Cancer* 36 (3):335–40.

Kumar, V., A. K. Abbas, and N. Fausto. 2005. Acute and chronic inflammation. In *Robbins and Cotran Pathologic Basis of Disease*, edited by V. Kumar, A. K. Abbas, N. Fausto, S. L. Robbins and R. S. Cotran. Philadelphia: Elsevier Saunders.

Kuriki, K., K. Hirose, K. Wakai et al. 2007. Breast cancer risk and erythrocyte compositions of n-3 highly unsaturated fatty acids in Japanese. *Int J Cancer* 121 (2):377–85.

Kushi, L., and E. Giovannucci. 2002. Dietary fat and cancer. *Am J Med* 113 Suppl 9B:63S–70S.

Larsson, S. C., M. Kumlin, M. Ingelman-Sundberg, and A. Wolk. 2004. Dietary long-chain n-3 fatty acids for the prevention of cancer: a review of potential mechanisms. *Am J Clin Nutr* 79 (6):935–45.

Leahy, K. M., R. L. Ornberg, Y. Wang et al. 2002. Cyclooxygenase-2 inhibition by celecoxib reduces proliferation and induces apoptosis in angiogenic endothelial cells in vivo. *Cancer Res* 62 (3):625–31.

Lee, J. Y., and D. H. Hwang. 2002. Docosahexaenoic acid suppresses the activity of peroxisome proliferator-activated receptors in a colon tumor cell line. *Biochem Biophys Res Commun* 298 (5):667–74.

Lee, J. Y., A. Plakidas, W. H. Lee et al. 2003. Differential modulation of Toll-like receptors by fatty acids: preferential inhibition by n-3 polyunsaturated fatty acids. *J Lipid Res* 44 (3):479–86.

Li, A. C., C. J. Binder, A. Gutierrez et al. 2004. Differential inhibition of macrophage foam-cell formation and atherosclerosis in mice by PPARalpha, beta/delta, and gamma. *J Clin Invest* 114 (11):1564–76.

Ma, D. W., J. Seo, L. A. Davidson et al. 2004. n-3 PUFA alter caveolae lipid composition and resident protein localization in mouse colon. *FASEB J* 18 (9):1040–2.

MacLean, C. H., S. J. Newberry, W. A. Mojica et al. 2006. Effects of omega-3 fatty acids on cancer risk: a systematic review. *JAMA* 295 (4):403–15.

Marshall, L. A., and P. V. Johnston. 1982. Modulation of tissue prostaglandin synthesizing capacity by increased ratios of dietary alpha-linolenic acid to linoleic acid. *Lipids* 17 (12):905–13.

Miles, E. A., and P. C. Calder. 1998. Modulation of immune function by dietary fatty acids. *Proc Nutr Soc* 57 (2):277–92.

Miyazaki, M., and J. M. Ntambi. 2008. Fatty acid desaturation and chain elongation in mammals. In *Biochemistry of Lipids, Lipoproteins and Membranes*, 5th ed., edited by D. E. Vance and J. E. Vance. San Diego: Elsevier.

Murff, H. J., X. O. Shu, H. Li et al. 2011. Dietary polyunsaturated fatty acids and breast cancer risk in Chinese women: a prospective cohort study. *Int J Cancer* 128 (6):1434–41.

National Research Council. 2005. *Dietary Reference Intakes for Energy, Carbohydrate, Fiber, Fat, Fatty Acids, Cholesterol, Protein, and Amino Acids (Macronutrients)*. Washington, DC: The National Academies Press.

Oh, D. Y., S. Talukdar, E. J. Bae et al. 2010. GPR120 is an omega-3 fatty acid receptor mediating potent anti-inflammatory and insulin-sensitizing effects. *Cell* 142 (5):687–98.

Patterson, R. E., S. W. Flatt, V. A. Newman et al. 2011. Marine fatty acid intake is associated with breast cancer prognosis. *J Nutr* 141 (2):201–6.

Porter, P. 2008. "Westernizing" women's risks? Breast cancer in lower-income countries. *N Engl J Med* 358 (3):213–6.

Rogers, K. R., K. D. Kikawa, M. Mouradian et al. 2010. Docosahexaenoic acid alters epidermal growth factor receptor-related signaling by disrupting its lipid raft association. *Carcinogenesis* 31 (9):1523–30.

Roifman, I., P. L. Beck, T. J. Anderson, M. J. Eisenberg, and J. Genest. 2011. Chronic inflammatory diseases and cardiovascular risk: a systematic review. *Can J Cardiol* 27 (2):174–82.

Rose, D. P., and J. M. Connolly. 1999a. Antiangiogenicity of docosahexaenoic acid and its role in the suppression of breast cancer cell growth in nude mice. *Int J Oncol* 15 (5):1011–5.

Rose, D. P., and J. M. Connolly. 1999b. Omega-3 fatty acids as cancer chemopreventive agents. *Pharmacol Ther* 83 (3):217–44.

Saggar, J. K., J. Chen, P. Corey, and L. U. Thompson. 2010a. Dietary flaxseed lignan or oil combined with tamoxifen treatment affects MCF-7 tumor growth through estrogen receptor- and growth factor-signaling pathways. *Mol Nutr Food Res* 54 (3):415–425.

Saggar, J. K., J. Chen, P. Corey, and L. U. Thompson. 2010b. The effect of secoisolariciresinol diglucoside and flaxseed oil, alone and in combination, on MCF-7 tumor growth and signaling pathways. *Nutr Cancer* 62 (4):533–542.

Sala-Vila, A., and P. C. Calder. 2011. Update on the relationship of fish intake with prostate, breast, and colorectal cancers. *Crit Rev Food Sci Nutr* 51 (9):855–71.

Sasazuki, S., M. Inoue, M. Iwasaki et al. 2011. Intake of n-3 and n-6 polyunsaturated fatty acids and development of colorectal cancer by subsite: Japan Public Health Center-based prospective study. *Int J Cancer* 129 (7):1718–29.

Sawyer, M. B., and C. J. Field. 2010. Possible mechanisms of n-3 PUFA anti-tumor action. In *Dietary n-3 Polyunsaturated Fatty Acids and Cancer*, edited by G. Calviello and S. Serini. New York: Springer Science.

Schley, P. D., D. N. Brindley, and C. J. Field. 2007. (n-3) PUFA alter raft lipid composition and decrease epidermal growth factor receptor levels in lipid rafts of human breast cancer cells. *J Nutr* 137 (3):548–53.

Schley, P. D., H. B. Jijon, L. E. Robinson, and C. J. Field. 2005. Mechanisms of omega-3 fatty acid-induced growth inhibition in MDA-MB-231 human breast cancer cells. *Breast Cancer Res Treat* 92 (2):187–95.

Schmitz, G., and J. Ecker. 2008. The opposing effects of n-3 and n-6 fatty acids. *Prog Lipid Res* 47 (2):147–55.

Serhan, C. N., M. Arita, S. Hong, and K. Gotlinger. 2004. Resolvins, docosatrienes, and neuroprotectins, novel omega-3-derived mediators, and their endogenous aspirin-triggered epimers. *Lipids* 39 (11):1125–32.

Shaikh, S. R., C. A. Jolly, and R. S. Chapkin. 2012. n-3 Polyunsaturated fatty acids exert immunomodulatory effects on lymphocytes by targeting plasma membrane molecular organization. *Mol Aspects Med* 33 (1):46–54.

Shibata, A., T. Nagaya, T. Imai et al. 2002. Inhibition of NF-kappaB activity decreases the VEGF mRNA expression in MDA-MB-231 breast cancer cells. *Breast Cancer Res Treat* 73 (3):237–43.

Signori, C., K. El-Bayoumy, J. Russo et al. 2011. Chemoprevention of breast cancer by fish oil in preclinical models: trials and tribulations. *Cancer Res* 71 (19):6091–6.

Siguel, E. N. 1996. Dietary sources of long-chain n-3 polyunsaturated fatty acids. *JAMA* 275 (11):836–7.

Staubach, S., and F. G. Hanisch. 2011. Lipid rafts: signaling and sorting platforms of cells and their roles in cancer. *Expert Rev Proteomics* 8 (2):263–77.

Su, C. G., X. Wen, S. T. Bailey et al. 1999. A novel therapy for colitis utilizing PPAR-gamma ligands to inhibit the epithelial inflammatory response. *J Clin Invest* 104 (4):383–9.

Sulaiman, S., M. R. Shahril, S. H. Shaharudin et al. 2011. Fat intake and its relationship with pre- and postmenopausal breast cancer risk: a case-control study in Malaysia. *Asian Pac J Cancer Prev* 12 (9):2167–78.

Takahashi, R., M. E. Begin, G. Ells, and D. F. Horrobin. 1991. Effects of eicosapentaenoic acid and arachidonic acid on incorporation and metabolism of radioactive linoleic acid in cultured human fibroblasts. *Prostaglandins Leukot Essent Fatty Acids* 42 (2):113–7.

Terry, P., L. Bergkvist, L. Holmberg, and A. Wolk. 2001. No association between fat and fatty acids intake and risk of colorectal cancer. *Cancer Epidemiol Biomarkers Prev* 10 (8):913–4.

Theodoratou, E., G. McNeill, R. Cetnarskyj et al. 2007. Dietary fatty acids and colorectal cancer: a case-control study. *Am J Epidemiol* 166 (2):181–95.

Thiebaut, A. C., V. Chajes, M. Gerber et al. 2009. Dietary intakes of omega-6 and omega-3 polyunsaturated fatty acids and the risk of breast cancer. *Int J Cancer* 124 (4):924–31.

Thoennes, S. R., P. L. Tate, T. M. Price, and M. W. Kilgore. 2000. Differential transcriptional activation of peroxisome proliferator-activated receptor gamma by omega-3 and omega-6 fatty acids in MCF-7 cells. *Mol Cell Endocrinol* 160 (1–2):67–73.

Thompson, L. U., and J. K. Mason. 2010. Flaxseed. In *Encyclopedia of Dietary Supplements*, edited by P. M. Coates. London: Informa Healthcare.

Thompson, L. U., J. M. Chen, T. Li, K. Strasser-Weippl, and P. E. Goss. 2005. Dietary flaxseed alters tumor biological markers in postmenopausal breast cancer. *Clin Cancer Res* 11 (10):3828–35.

Thompson, L. U., S. E. Rickard, L. J. Orcheson, and M. M. Seidl. 1996. Flaxseed and its lignan and oil components reduce mammary tumor growth at a late stage of carcinogenesis. *Carcinogenesis* 17 (6):1373–6.

Trombetta, A., M. Maggiora, G. Martinasso et al. 2007. Arachidonic and docosahexaenoic acids reduce the growth of A549 human lung-tumor cells increasing lipid peroxidation and PPARs. *Chem Biol Interact* 165 (3):239–50.

Truan, J. S., J. M. Chen, and L. U. Thompson. 2010. Flaxseed oil reduces the growth of human breast tumors (MCF-7) at high levels of circulating estrogen. *Mol Nutr Food Res* 54 (10):1414–21.

Tull, S. P., C. M. Yates, B. H. Maskrey et al. 2009. Omega-3 fatty acids and inflammation: novel interactions reveal a new step in neutrophil recruitment. *PLoS Biol* 7 (8):e1000177.

United States Department of Agriculture. 2010. *Nutrient Intakes from Food: Mean Amounts Consumed per Individual by Gender and Age, What We Eat in America, NHANES 2007–2008*, August 2010 [cited February 22, 2012]. Available from www.ars.usda.gov/ba/bhnrc/fsrg.

Vanden Heuvel, J. P., J. T. Thompson, S. R. Frame, and P. J. Gillies. 2006. Differential activation of nuclear receptors by perfluorinated fatty acid analogs and natural fatty acids: a comparison of human, mouse, and rat peroxisome proliferator-activated receptor-alpha, -beta, and -gamma, liver X receptor-beta, and retinoid X receptor-alpha. *Toxicol Sci* 92 (2):476–89.

Voet, D., and J. G. Voet. 2004. Lipid Metabolism. In *Biochemistry*. Hoboken, NJ: John Wiley & Sons, Inc.

von Schacky, C., R. Kiefl, A. J. Marcus, M. J. Broekman, and W. E. Kaminski. 1993. Dietary n-3 fatty acids accelerate catabolism of leukotriene B4 in human granulocytes. *Biochim Biophys Acta* 1166 (1):20–4.

Wallace, F. A., E. A. Miles, and P. C. Calder. 2003. Comparison of the effects of linseed oil and different doses of fish oil on mononuclear cell function in healthy human subjects. *Br J Nutr* 89 (5):679–89.

Wang, D., and R. N. Dubois. 2010. Eicosanoids and cancer. *Nat Rev Cancer* 10 (3):181–93.

West, N. J., S. K. Clark, R. K. Phillips et al. 2010. Eicosapentaenoic acid reduces rectal polyp number and size in familial adenomatous polyposis. *Gut* 59 (7):918–25.

Williams, D., M. Verghese, L. T. Walker et al. 2007. Flax seed oil and flax seed meal reduce the formation of aberrant crypt foci (ACF) in azoxymethane-induced colon cancer in Fisher 344 male rats. *Food Chem Toxicol* 45 (1):153–9.

Witt, P. M., J. H. Christensen, E. B. Schmidt et al. 2009. Marine n-3 polyunsaturated fatty acids in adipose tissue and breast cancer risk: a case-cohort study from Denmark. *Cancer Causes Control* 20 (9):1715–21.

World Cancer Research Fund/American Institute for Cancer Research. 2007. *Food, Nutrition, Physical Activity, and the Prevention of Cancer: a Global Perspective.*. Washington, DC: AICR.

World Health Organization. 2008. *World Cancer Report 2008*. Lyon: World Health Organization.

Yamada, M., M. Kaibori, H. Tanaka et al. 2012. Alpha-lipoic acid prevents the induction of inos gene expression through destabilization of its mRNA in proinflammatory cytokine-stimulated hepatocytes. *Dig Dis Sci* 57 (4):943–51.

Zhang, C. X., S. C. Ho, F. Y. Lin et al. 2011. Dietary fat intake and risk of breast cancer: a case-control study in China. *Eur J Cancer Prev* 20 (3):199–206.

Zhang, P., R. Smith, R. S. Chapkin, and D. N. McMurray. 2005. Dietary (n-3) polyunsaturated fatty acids modulate murine Th1/Th2 balance toward the Th2 pole by suppression of Th1 development. *J Nutr* 135 (7):1745–51.

Zhao, G., T. D. Etherton, K. R. Martin et al. 2005. Anti-inflammatory effects of polyunsaturated fatty acids in THP-1 cells. *Biochem Biophys Res Commun* 336 (3):909–17.

Zhao, Y., S. Joshi-Barve, S. Barve, and L. H. Chen. 2004. Eicosapentaenoic acid prevents LPS-induced TNF-alpha expression by preventing NF-kappaB activation. *J Am Coll Nutr* 23 (1):71–8.

15 Polyunsaturated Fatty Acids and Cancer Prevention

Janel Suburu and Yong Q. Chen

CONTENTS

15.1 INTRODUCTION

Investigations of dietary fat consumption and cancer risk and progression point to a critical role for both the quantity and the quality of dietary fat in modulating cancer. In particular, omega-6 (ω-6) polyunsaturated fatty acids (PUFAs) are highly suspect to be the underlying culprits for dietary promotion of cancer. Conversely, evidence suggests that omega-3 (ω-3) PUFAs oppose the effects of ω-6 PUFAs. Clinical studies, although with some mixed results, have largely supported these claims. Animal studies investigating the effects of dietary PUFAs have consistently demonstrated the cancer-promoting and -protective effects of ω-6 and ω-3 PUFA, respectively, in a variety of cancer types. Although the mechanisms underlying these apparent cancer-modulating phenotypes by PUFAs remain to be further clarified, several hypotheses have been postulated, including regulation of membrane signaling, oxidative stress, production of proinflammatory and anti-inflammatory signaling molecules, and immune regulation. In this chapter, we will review PUFA metabolism to various downstream metabolites and their potential roles in modulating cancer risk and progression.

15.2 TYPES AND SOURCES OF PUFAs

Fatty acids are lipid molecules typically consisting of a single carbon chain with a carboxylic acid functional group at the alpha carbon. Saturated fatty acids (SAFAs) contain completely hydrogenated carbons with no double bonds, whereas monounsaturated fatty acids (MUFAs) and PUFAs contain one or more than one double bond, respectively. There are two main types of PUFAs: ω-3 and ω-6. Each group is characterized by the placement of the first double bond in the carbon chain counting from the omega carbon; for example, the first double bond in an ω-3 PUFA is positioned between the third and fourth carbons, whereas an ω-6 PUFA contains its first double bond between the sixth and seventh carbons. Unlike SAFAs and MUFAs, ω-3 or ω-6 PUFAs cannot be synthesized in humans and are therefore considered essential fatty acids that must be acquired through the diet. ω-3 and ω-6 PUFAs are essential for a number of biological processes, including brain development, parturition, vision, prevention of water loss by the skin's lipid barrier, and maintenance of cellular lipid membrane fluidity (Lauritzen et al. 2001). PUFAs are the precursors of eicosanoids: prostaglandins, leukotrienes, thromboxanes, and hydroxyeicosatetraenoic or hydroxyeicosapentaenoic acids. In contrast to a hormone, which is usually produced in a specialized tissue and acts systemically, eicosanoids are produced throughout the body and act locally in a paracrine or autocrine manner. Eicosanoids are known to modulate hemostasis, smooth muscle contraction and relaxation, and most notably, immune responses (Lauritzen et al. 2001; Wymann and Schneiter 2008). The source of fatty acids has been the topic of several reviews (Suburu and Chen 2012; Berquin et al. 2011; Berquin, Edwards, and Chen 2008; Chen et al. 2007).

15.3 PUFAs IN CANCER RISK AND PROGRESSION

A large body of evidence suggests that dietary PUFAs significantly affect cancer risk and progression. Implications of PUFA effects on cancer were originally revealed by epidemiological studies depicting a negative correlation between cancer risk and fish consumption, an ω-3–enriched food. Indeed, studies have identified opposing roles for ω-3 and ω-6 PUFAs in cancer. While ω-6 PUFAs increase cancer risk and promote its progression, ω-3 PUFAs show a protective effect. Although the topic is still controversial, investigations continue to highlight PUFA modulation of cancer (Chen et al. 2007; Berquin, Edwards, and Chen 2008; Berquin et al. 2011).

Nonsteroidal anti-inflammatory drugs (NSAIDs) are inhibitors of the proinflammatory cyclooxygenase enzymes (COX), which regulate the conversion of PUFAs to eicosanoids. NSAIDs can be selective for COX2 or nonselective, thereby inhibiting both COX1 and COX2. Clinical and preclinical data clearly demonstrate a potential use for NSAIDs in cancer prevention. Although the potential for NSAIDs use may lie in numerous cancer types including breast, lung, prostate, and ovarian, evidence is particularly overwhelming for colorectal cancer prevention. Unfortunately, their adverse side effects, such as intestinal bleeding and adverse cardiac events, observed following their prolonged use, pose a threat to the risk–benefit analysis of using NSAIDs as anticancer agents (Harris et al. 2005; Ulrich, Bigler, and Potter 2006; Pereg and Lishner 2005; Cuzick et al. 2009; Gupta and Dubois 2001).

Renewed interest in NSAID-mediated cancer prevention has emerged with a very recent double-blind clinical trial study where over 800 participants carrying Lynch syndrome, a form of hereditary colorectal cancer, were followed over a course of approximately 4 years. Patients randomized to a group taking a daily low dose of aspirin showed significantly reduced incidence of colorectal cancer compared to placebo (Burn et al. 2011). This is the first study to monitor aspirin use with cancer incidence as the primary end point. Among NSAIDs, aspirin is unique in that it is the only irreversible inhibitor, suggesting that its mechanisms of cancer prevention may vary from other NSAIDs.

15.3.1 CLINICAL STUDIES OF PUFAs AND CANCER

A number of clinical studies demonstrate a significant role for dietary PUFAs in cancer risk or progression. Consumption of ω-3 PUFAs from fish or fish oil has shown negative correlations with the risk of developing many cancers, including prostate, breast, colorectal, bladder, esophageal, lung, and pancreatic cancers, with particular emphasis on metastatic or advanced disease (reviewed in Chen et al. 2007; Murphy, Mourtzakis, and Mazurak 2012). Unfortunately, human studies of PUFAs in cancer show considerable variance, resulting in controversy over the association between the two (Szymanski, Wheeler, and Mucci 2010; Wu et al. 2011). Thus, more stringent control will be required in the design of future studies.

15.3.2 Preclinical Studies of PUFAs and Cancer

Research on dietary interventions in murine cancer models has greatly increased our knowledge on PUFA modulation of cancer. Animal studies in various prostate, breast, and colorectal cancer models have clearly demonstrated protective effects from an ω-3–enriched diet and cancer-promoting effects from an ω-6–enriched diet (reviewed in Chen et al. 2007; Berquin, Edwards, and Chen 2008). Additional studies comparing a high-fat to a low-fat diet in murine cancer models suggest that low-fat diet consumption delays tumor progression (Kobayashi et al. 2008; Kim et al. 2011). Although a low-fat diet may in fact prevent cancer progression, such studies have often used corn oil or lard as a dietary fat source. Therefore, these studies may provide further evidence for a cancer-promoting effect of ω-6 PUFAs due to the enrichment of ω-6 PUFAs in these dietary fat sources, which is likely exacerbating the effects of a high-fat diet by skewing the ratio of ω-6 to ω-3 PUFA toward ω-6 PUFA. Indeed, we and others have shown that the quality, rather than simply the quantity, of dietary fat significantly affects cancer growth and progression (Escobar, Gomes-Marcondes, and Carvalho 2009; Berquin et al. 2007). Additionally, our data suggest that a diet with a disproportionately high (greater than 20:1) ratio of ω-6 to ω-3 PUFAs, similar to a modern Western diet, may have cancer-promoting effects compared to a diet with a more balanced ratio of ω-6 to ω-3 PUFAs (Berquin et al. 2007; Wang et al. 2012). In line with these observations, arachidonic acid (AA, 20:4n-6) metabolism in cancer cells in vitro increases growth, proliferation, and resistance to apoptosis (Tang, Chen, and Honn 1996; Wang and Dubois 2010), while treatment of cancer cells with ω-3 PUFAs sensitizes cells to growth inhibition (Cavazos et al. 2011; Friedrichs et al. 2011).

Due to the diet complexity, the development of transgenic mice bearing the *fat-1* transgene, a *Caenorhabditis elegans* gene encoding a desaturase enzyme that converts ω-6 PUFAs to ω-3 PUFAs, paved the way for genetically modeling the role of ω-3 PUFAs in cancer suppression (Kang et al. 2004). This transgenic mouse model has been successfully used with prostate, liver, colorectal, melanoma, and pancreatic cancer models to illustrate the positive effects of ω-3 PUFAs in modulating cancer (Jia et al. 2008; Berquin et al. 2007; Xia et al. 2006; Griffitts et al. 2010; Song et al. 2011). With promising outcomes highlighting the effects of ω-3 PUFAs on cancer mouse models, a number of clinical trials have initiated the investigation of ω-3 PUFAs as a potential adjuvant therapy in cancer patients (reviewed in Berquin, Edwards, and Chen 2008; Murphy, Mourtzakis, and Mazurak 2012).

15.4 MECHANISMS OF PUFA-MEDIATED CANCER MODULATION

The consensus is fairly clear from animal studies that PUFAs modulate cancer progression, with ω-6 PUFAs demonstrating cancer-promoting effects, while ω-3 PUFAs show a protective effect. Several hypotheses have been advanced to explain the mechanisms by which PUFAs exert their cancer regulation, including regulation of oxidative stress, intracellular signaling, and inflammation (Chen et al. 2007; Berquin, Edwards, and Chen 2008; Berquin et al. 2011). Fatty acids are critical components of membrane, and the presence of PUFA in membrane phospholipids may have numerous cellular effects. The multiple double bonds in PUFA are particularly susceptible to peroxidation by free radicals. Lipid peroxidation by reactive oxygen species (ROS) can initiate a cascade of membrane damage, culminating in cell death if the cell does not produce enough reducing power to stop the process. Cellular signaling molecules localize at special microdomains of the membrane known as lipid rafts, which are enriched with cholesterol and sphingolipids. Here, signaling proteins and scaffolds combine to form complex structures to mediate intercellular signaling. The highly polyunsaturated structure of docosahexaenoic acid (DHA) prevents its association with the tightly packed and ordered SAFAs, sphingolipids, and cholesterol found in lipid rafts (Wassall and Stillwell 2008). Thus, incorporation of ω-3 PUFAs, in lieu of ω-6 PUFA, into phospholipids may hinder raft formation and alter signaling patterns (Chapkin et al. 2008, 2009). Finally, membrane phospholipids are the source of PUFAs for eicosanoid production and related lipid signaling molecules, which are critical inflammatory mediators

(Bozza et al. 2011). Recent evidence suggests that eicosanoids can be produced from the membrane of unique intracellular lipid body compartments, formerly described as lipid droplets, and formation of lipid bodies is associated with cancer progression (Bozza and Viola 2010; Bozza et al. 2011).

15.4.1 ROLE OF PUFAs IN OXIDATIVE STRESS

One mechanism by which PUFAs may exert their antineoplastic effects is through increased oxidative stress, which is often followed by apoptosis, a process of programmed cell death. Oxidative stress is common in cancer cells, which often respond with increased production of reducing agents, such as nicotinamide adenine dinucleotide phosphate (NADPH), to maintain redox homeostasis. Exceeding the threshold of oxidative stress in a cancer cell can push the cell toward apoptosis (Halliwell 2007). Due to their chemical structure containing a high number of double bonds, ω-3 PUFAs are particularly sensitive to lipid peroxidation by ROS, leading to significant damage of the cellular membrane. Increased *de novo* fatty acid synthesis, a very common event in cancer cells (Swinnen et al. 2002), dilutes PUFA-containing phospholipids and provides protection from oxidative stress (Rysman et al. 2011). A recent study showed that inhibition of *de novo* SAFA synthesis increased the concentration of PUFA-containing phospholipids; this was accompanied by increased lipid peroxidation and cell death in the cancer cells. Incubation with H_2O_2 exacerbated the effects of inhibiting fatty acid synthesis, an effect that was rescued by exogenous SAFAs (Rysman et al. 2011). Several other studies have described similar effects of increased lipid peroxidation upon ω-3 PUFA treatment, followed by enhanced cell death that was rescued by antioxidants (Chen et al. 2007). Interestingly, treatment of colon cancer cells with DHA increased lipid peroxidation and decreased expression of sterol response element binding protein-1 (SREBP-1), a positive transcriptional regulator of SAFA production. Moreover, DHA-mediated lipid peroxidation was rescued by the antioxidant vitamin E (Schonberg et al. 2006).

15.4.2 ROLE OF PUFAs IN PHOSPHOLIPIDS

Increased endogenous SAFA production in cancer cells also supplies SAFAs for phospholipid production and facilitates membrane raft formation (Swinnen et al. 2003), as PUFAs do not colocalize with the tightly ordered lipid rafts (Wassall and Stillwell 2008). Indeed, depletion of *de novo* synthesized SAFAs changed the dynamic properties of the plasma membrane in cancer cells, including increased flip-flop and uptake of chemotherapeutic drug (Rysman et al. 2011). A diet enriched with PUFAs, particularly the highly unsaturated DHA, may facilitate PUFA incorporation into phospholipids, thereby decreasing lipid raft formation and oncogenic signaling. Cellular phospholipids typically contain a SAFA or MUFA in the *sn*-1 position and a MUFA or PUFA in the *sn*-2 position. Preliminary data from our lab suggest that DHA treatment significantly alters the phospholipid profile of prostate cancer cells. We observed an increase in DHA-containing phospholipids in all four phospholipid classes: phosphatidylcholine, phosphatidylserine, phosphatidylinositol, and phosphatidylethanolamine. AKT, a well-known regulator of cancer proliferation and survival, is activated by phosphatidylinositol-3,4,5-triphosphate (PIP_3). This shift in lipid profile changes the localization and activation of AKT, suggesting that the lipid modification of PIP_3 or lipid rafts may directly affect AKT activation and cancer cell survival (Chen, unpublished data).

15.4.3 PUFA METABOLITES AND CANCER

PUFAs are essential for the synthesis of a wide variety of lipid signaling mediators, including prostaglandins, leukotrienes, lipoxins, resolvins, protectins, and most recently identified, maresins. These lipid signals are responsible for regulating the initiation, propagation, and resolution of an inflammatory response. Inflammation is a well-characterized attribute of the tumor microenvironment and considered an enabling feature in cancer development (Hanahan and Weinberg 2011).

Therefore, the synthesis and downstream effects of these PUFA-derived inflammatory modulators are critical components of cancer biology. The production of the various eicosanoids is dependent upon the PUFA precursor, which is subject to the fatty acids available in the membrane. Among these classes of lipids are both proinflammatory and anti-inflammatory mediators that regulate the activity of tumor cells, stromal cells, and infiltrating leukocytes (Wang and Dubois 2010; Panigrahy et al. 2010; Serhan and Petasis 2011; Berquin et al. 2011).

15.4.4 Proinflammatory PUFA Metabolites

AA is the primary precursor for the synthesis of proinflammatory eicosanoids. AA metabolism produces the 2-series prostaglandins, 4-series leukotrienes, and epoxyeicosatrienoic/hydroxyeicosatetraenoic acids (EET/HETEs) through COX, lipoxygenase (LOX), and cytochrome P450 (CYP) enzymes, respectively. Literature strongly supports the notion that increased production of proinflammatory AA metabolites, such as prostaglandin E2 (PGE_2), $PGF_{2\alpha}$, leukotriene B4 (LTB_4), LTD_4, and 20-HETE, and increased expression of their corresponding receptors, promotes cancer progression by activating tumor survival, proliferation, migration, invasion, angiogenesis, and inflammation. These functions have been extensively reviewed (Wang and Dubois 2010; Panigrahy et al. 2010; Berquin et al. 2011).

15.4.5 Anti-Inflammatory PUFA Metabolites

Although our understanding of PUFA metabolism continues to evolve, significant headway has been made in revealing their role as precursors to anti-inflammatory mediators, particularly those active during the resolution phase of inflammation. Much of our current understanding of the anti-inflammatory eicosanoids and docosanoids and the active process of inflammatory resolution was pioneered by the work of Serhan, Chiang, and Van Dyke (2008). The anti-inflammatory PUFA metabolites include the AA-derived lipoxins; eicosapentaenoic acid (EPA)–derived 3-series prostaglandins, 5-series leukotrienes, and E-resolvins; and the DHA-derived D-resolvins, protectins, and maresins. Each of these metabolites has been fairly well characterized in the context of acute inflammation, and we direct the reader to other reviews (Serhan, Chiang, and Van Dyke 2008; Zhang and Spite 2012; Serhan and Petasis 2011; Serhan 2007); however, their role in cancer suppression is less clear.

Despite their propensity for proinflammatory metabolism, AA can also be metabolized into an anti-inflammatory signal, in the form of lipoxins. Unlike other AA-derived eicosanoids, lipoxins are produced at the resolution of inflammation (Serhan, Hamberg, and Samuelsson 1984). Lipoxins are produced by leukocytes through the LOX enzymes. Alternatively, lipoxins can be created by aspirin-modified COX2, often referred to as aspirin-triggered lipoxin, demonstrating an anticancer property of aspirin (Chiang, Arita, and Serhan 2005). Indeed, lipoxin A4 was shown to block cancer cell proliferation, migration, and angiogenesis induced by activated macrophages (Hao et al. 2011; Greene et al. 2011).

Evidence suggests competition between ω-3 and ω-6 PUFAs for substrate binding to enzymes (Larsson et al. 2004). Metabolism of EPA by COX1 and COX2 produces the 3-series of prostaglandins, and metabolism by 5-LOX creates the 5-series of leukotrienes (Terano et al. 1986). Although the 3- and 5-series eicosanoids may act on the same receptors as their proinflammatory counterparts, their competitive inhibition against the 2- and 4-series supports their anti-inflammatory role. Indeed, PGE_3 has a lower affinity for the prostaglandin E receptor 4 (EP4) receptor but acts as a competitive antagonist to PGE_2 to decrease EP4-mediated signaling (Hawcroft et al. 2010). Despite lower affinity, decreased potency of these ω-3 PUFA metabolites may be another explanation for their antitumorigenic properties. Both PGE_3 and LTB_5 have demonstrated antiangiogenic and tumor suppressing properties (Bachi et al. 2009; Yang et al. 2004; Vanamala et al. 2008; Szymczak, Murray, and Petrovic 2008).

Emerging evidence suggests that PUFAs strongly influence the resolution phase of the inflammatory process. Upon an acute inflammatory response, propagation of the signaling cascade subsides only through a reciprocal response between activated fibroblasts, epithelial cells, and immune cells. In the absence of the resolution phase, a state of chronic inflammation ensues (Serhan 2007). Ω-3 PUFA–derived lipid mediators of the resolution process were first identified through examination of exudates collected during acute inflammation resolution from mice treated with aspirin and ω-3 PUFAs. These studies identified the conversion of EPA to E-resolvins and DHA to D-resolvins, protectins, and maresins (Serhan et al. 2000, 2002, 2009).

Resolvins and protectins act in concert to regulate inflammatory resolution by promoting wound healing and tissue preservation. Resolvins are known to reduce leukocyte infiltration and clear the site of inflammation by increasing phagocytosis of apoptotic cells (Zhang and Spite 2012; Janakiram, Mohammed, and Rao 2011; Serhan 2007). Protectins, originally identified as neuroprotectins due to their role in preventing neuronal damage (Marcheselli et al. 2003), have been shown to protect against tissue injury in other disease models as well, including asthma, atherosclerosis, and renal injury (Weylandt et al. 2012; Serhan 2007). While the role of resolvins and protectins has been described in acute inflammation, very little research has investigated their role, or absence in cancer. One study showed that normal neurons actively metabolize DHA into resolvins and protectins, while neuroblastoma cells displayed no production of either (Gleissman et al. 2010). Whether this was a result of genetic or epigenetic changes in the cancer cells, or an issue of undetectable levels, is unknown.

Maresins are the most recently identified proresolving molecules. They were identified from DHA-derived proresolving metabolites in macrophages. Hence, the name was coined as maresin (macrophage mediator in resolving inflammation) (Serhan et al. 2009). Very little is known about maresins, although a very recent study showed that maresin 1 (MaR1) decreased neutrophil infiltration and enhanced apoptotic cell phagocytosis similar to resolvin D1, induced tissue regeneration in *Planaria*, and reduced inflammatory pain in mice (Serhan et al. 2012). Resolvins and protectins have also shown efficacy in reducing inflammatory pain (Xu et al. 2010), highlighting the redundancy of these anti-inflammatory mediators.

Because resolvins, protectins, and maresins are derived from ω-3 PUFAs and play a critical role in inflammatory resolution, a diet lacking sufficient ω-3 PUFAs may thwart the natural process of inflammatory resolution, leading to a state of chronic inflammation. This, in conjunction with other known oncogenic events, may be sufficient for tumorigenesis. Furthermore, the lack of inflammatory resolving power in the cancer microenvironment may promote progression to advanced disease. Therefore, reintroduction of these eicosanoids by synthetic analogs or dietary ω-3 PUFAs may be a therapeutic approach to prevent cancer initiation and/or progression. Overall, observations of ω-3 PUFA–mediated cancer suppression may be due, in part, to their production of proresolving inflammatory mediators and prevention of chronic inflammation.

15.4.6 IMMUNOREGULATION BY PUFAS

Our current understanding of PUFA metabolism clearly highlights their immunoregulatory role, with ω-6 PUFAs being predominantly proinflammatory and ω-3 PUFAs anti-inflammatory. Because we know inflammation and evasion from the immune system is an integral component of cancer biology (Hanahan and Weinberg 2011), research to identify the mechanisms of PUFA's effects in cancer has turned to investigate their ability to regulate the tumor immune response.

Toll-like receptors (TLRs) located on the plasma membrane of innate immune cells regulate the production of proinflammatory cytokines and chemokines. Activation of TLRs by pathogen-derived ligands initiates this immune response. Interestingly, in the absence of pathogenic antigens, SAFAs can activate certain TLRs in macrophages to induce COX2 and nuclear factor kappaB (NF-κB) expression, and ω-3 PUFAs can inhibit SAFA-induced TLR activation, suggesting one mechanism by which ω-3 PUFAs exert their anti-inflammatory effects (Lee et al. 2001, 2004). Evidence suggests that cancer cells also express TLRs and that their activation by endogenous ligands promotes cancer growth and progression; this topic has been extensively reviewed (Rakoff-Nahoum and Medzhitov 2009). In short, a diet enriched with ω-3 PUFAs may be beneficial by inhibiting endogenous activation of TLR-mediated inflammation.

Regulation of innate immune cells, including natural killer (NK) cells and, particularly, the professional antigen-presenting dendritic cells (DCs) and macrophages by tumor-derived signaling molecules influences the adaptive immune response to the tumor. Literature suggests that tumor cells manipulate the innate immune system in order to suppress type-1 immunity and promote Th2/Th17 polarization. This encourages an immune-tolerant rather than cytotoxic response (Wang and Dubois 2010).

The most widely studied PUFA metabolite known to mediate these effects is PGE_2. PGE_2 is a stimulant commonly used during DC priming for vaccines due to its enhancement of C-C chemokine receptor type 7 (CCR7) expression, a critical regulator of T-cell recruitment. However, PGE_2-primed DCs show depressed expression of Th1-polarizing cytokines—C-C chemokine ligand 5 (CCL5), C-X-C motif chemokine ligand 9 (CXCL9), CXCL10, CXCL11, and CCL19—resulting in decreased recruitment and activation of NK cells (Van Elssen et al. 2011) and naive and memory T cells (Muthuswamy et al. 2010), whereas increased CCL22 secretion stimulated by PGE_2 leads to recruitment of regulatory T cells (Muthuswamy et al. 2008).

The effect of PGE_2 on DC in the tumor microenvironment appears to support cancer growth and progression and is a critical regulator of the DC and macrophage phenotypes. Tumor-derived PGE_2 promotes monocyte differentiation into the tumor-promoting M2 macrophage and orchestrates a phenotypic switch in immunocompetent DC to bear an immunosuppressive role, including a markedly impaired ability for these immune cells to induce a tumor-reactive T-cell response (Scarlett et al. 2012; Heusinkveld et al. 2011). Interestingly, inhibition of COX2 by a selective or nonselective COX inhibitor helps restore normal monocyte differentiation to the antitumor M1 macrophage (Heusinkveld et al. 2011). Indeed, the consensus of literature suggests that PGE_2 is a major contributor to Th1 suppression and Th2 polarization. This PGE_2-regulated immune response has recently been reviewed (Kalinski 2012). In short, PGE_2 promotes the recruitment of macrophages, mast cells, and neutrophils but impairs their ability to elicit a cytotoxic response. These PGE_2-primed cells represent a myeloid-derived suppressor cell (MDSC) population that promotes tissue preservation. Moreover, tumor-derived PGE_2 induces expression of COX2 and secretion of PGE_2 in MDSCs, providing a feed-forward loop that exacerbates the Th2 immune response (Kalinski 2012).

Supporting the anti-inflammatory properties of ω-3 PUFA, a number of studies have identified immunosuppressive phenotypes in *fat-1* transgenic models. Splenocytes from *fat-1* mice on a calorie-restricted diet displayed a decreased ratio of ω-6 to ω-3 and an impaired capacity to mediate an inflammatory response to exogenous stimuli (Bhattacharya et al. 2006). A study from Chapkins' group showed that *fat-1* mice were less sensitive to azomethane-induced colon carcinogenesis and had significantly decreased immune infiltration, suggesting that ω-3 PUFA decreases progression to cancer by suppressing inflammation (Jia et al. 2008). This was followed by a very recent study from the same group showing that *fat-1* mice had decreased levels of Th17 chemokine receptors on colonocytes and decreased infiltration of Th17 T cells in the colon and spleen following either acute or chronic inflammation (Monk et al. 2012). In prostate cancer, evidence indicates that tumors foster a proinflammatory environment, for example, upregulation of COX2 protein, and tumors have significantly higher numbers of infiltrating T and B lymphocytes than normal prostate. Knockout of *Rag1*, which disables the formation of mature B and T lymphocytes, in prostate-specific *Pten*-null mice significantly reduces tumor growth, and adoptive transfer of *Rag1*$^{+/+}$, but not *Rag1*$^{-/-}$, bone marrow into the *Rag1* knockout mice reverses the phenotype. Additionally, the number of tumor-infiltrating lymphocytes is modulated by dietary PUFA; that is, prostate tumors have higher numbers of infiltrating lymphocytes from mice on ω-6 PUFAs than in mice on a ω-3 PUFA diet (Chen et al., unpublished). This suggests that the modification of immune and epithelial cells by PUFA may regulate the progression from chronic inflammation to cancer. A diet with excessive ω-6 PUFA intake and insufficient ω-3 PUFAs may impair the switch to turn off inflammation, thereby facilitating progression to cancer. Conversely, a diet with excessive consumption of ω-3 PUFAs may render the consumer susceptible to infection due to a reduced immune response.

15.5 CONCLUSIONS AND PERSPECTIVES

Evidence clearly demonstrates an active contribution of ω-6 and ω-3 PUFA in modulating cancer. A diet enriched with ω-6 PUFA increases cancer risk by altering the cellular lipid profile to a cancer-promoting environment. These changes may include increased oncogenic signaling at the plasma membrane, increased production of proinflammatory signals leading to a microenvironment conducive to tumor growth and survival, and promotion of tumor cell immunotolerance. Conversely, these ω-6 PUFA effects may be ameliorated by ω-3 PUFA. Hence, a diet rich in ω-3 PUFA protects against chronic inflammation and promotion of tumor cell survival. ω-6 and ω-3 PUFA are nonetheless both essential fatty acids required for normal cell biology; therefore, one cannot simply remove them from the diet. However, a diet balanced in ω-6 and ω-3 PUFA may be beneficial in reducing cancer risk and progression, compared to a heavily weighted ω-6 PUFA diet.

ACKNOWLEDGMENT

The authors' work cited in this review article was funded by grants from the National Institutes of Health (R01CA107668, P01CA106742, and R01CA163273).

REFERENCES

Bachi, A. L., F. J. Kim, S. Nonogaki et al. 2009. Leukotriene B4 creates a favorable microenvironment for murine melanoma growth. *Mol Cancer Res* 7 (9):1417–24.

Berquin, I. M., I. J. Edwards, and Y. Q. Chen. 2008. Multi-targeted therapy of cancer by omega-3 fatty acids. *Cancer Lett* 269 (2):363–77.

Berquin, I. M., I. J. Edwards, S. J. Kridel, and Y. Q. Chen. 2011. Polyunsaturated fatty acid metabolism in prostate cancer. *Cancer Metastasis Rev* 30 (3–4):295–309.

Berquin, I. M., Y. Min, R. Wu et al. 2007. Modulation of prostate cancer genetic risk by omega-3 and omega-6 fatty acids. *J Clin Invest* 117 (7):1866–75.

Bhattacharya, A., B. Chandrasekar, M. M. Rahman, J. Banu, J. X. Kang, and G. Fernandes. 2006. Inhibition of inflammatory response in transgenic fat-1 mice on a calorie-restricted diet. *Biochem Biophys Res Commun* 349 (3):925–30.

Bozza, P. T., I. Bakker-Abreu, R. A. Navarro-Xavier, and C. Bandeira-Melo. 2011. Lipid body function in eicosanoid synthesis: an update. *Prostaglandins Leukot Essent Fatty Acids* 85 (5):205–13.

Bozza, P. T., and J. P. Viola. 2010. Lipid droplets in inflammation and cancer. *Prostaglandins Leukot Essent Fatty Acids* 82 (4–6):243–50.

Burn, J., A. M. Gerdes, F. Macrae et al. 2011. Long-term effect of aspirin on cancer risk in carriers of hereditary colorectal cancer: an analysis from the CAPP2 randomised controlled trial. *Lancet* 378 (9809):2081–7.

Cavazos, D. A., R. S. Price, S. S. Apte, and L. A. deGraffenried. 2011. Docosahexaenoic acid selectively induces human prostate cancer cell sensitivity to oxidative stress through modulation of NF-kappaB. *Prostate* 71 (13):1420–8.

Chapkin, R. S., W. Kim, J. R. Lupton, and D. N. McMurray. 2009. Dietary docosahexaenoic and eicosapentaenoic acid: emerging mediators of inflammation. *Prostaglandins Leukot Essent Fatty Acids* 81 (2–3):187–91.

Chapkin, R. S., N. Wang, Y. Y. Fan, J. R. Lupton, and I. A. Prior. 2008. Docosahexaenoic acid alters the size and distribution of cell surface microdomains. *Biochim Biophys Acta* 1778 (2):466–71.

Chen, Y. Q., I. J. Edwards, S. J. Kridel, T. Thornburg, and I. M. Berquin. 2007. Dietary fat-gene interactions in cancer. *Cancer Metastasis Rev* 26 (3–4):535–51.

Chiang, N., M. Arita, and C. N. Serhan. 2005. Anti-inflammatory circuitry: lipoxin, aspirin-triggered lipoxins and their receptor ALX. *Prostaglandins Leukot Essent Fatty Acids* 73 (3–4):163–77.

Cuzick, J., F. Otto, J. A. Baron et al. 2009. Aspirin and non-steroidal anti-inflammatory drugs for cancer prevention: an international consensus statement. *Lancet Oncol* 10 (5):501–7.

Escobar, E. L., M. C. Gomes-Marcondes, and H. F. Carvalho. 2009. Dietary fatty acid quality affects AR and PPARgamma levels and prostate growth. *Prostate* 69 (5):548–58.

Friedrichs, W., S. B. Ruparel, R. A. Marciniak, and L. deGraffenried. 2011. Omega-3 fatty acid inhibition of prostate cancer progression to hormone independence is associated with suppression of mTOR signaling and androgen receptor expression. *Nutr Cancer* 63 (5):771–7.

Gleissman, H., R. Yang, K. Martinod et al. 2010. Docosahexaenoic acid metabolome in neural tumors: identification of cytotoxic intermediates. *FASEB J* 24 (3):906–15.

Greene, E. R., S. Huang, C. N. Serhan, and D. Panigrahy. 2011. Regulation of inflammation in cancer by eicosanoids. *Prostaglandins Other Lipid Mediat* 96 (1–4):27–36.

Griffitts, J., D. Saunders, Y. A. Tesiram et al. 2010. Non-mammalian fat-1 gene prevents neoplasia when introduced to a mouse hepatocarcinogenesis model: Omega-3 fatty acids prevent liver neoplasia. *Biochim Biophys Acta* 1801 (10):1133–44.

Gupta, R. A., and R. N. Dubois. 2001. Colorectal cancer prevention and treatment by inhibition of cyclooxygenase-2. *Nat Rev Cancer* 1 (1):11–21.

Halliwell, B. 2007. Oxidative stress and cancer: have we moved forward? *Biochem J* 401 (1):1–11.

Hanahan, D., and R. A. Weinberg. 2011. Hallmarks of cancer: the next generation. *Cell* 144 (5):646–74.

Hao, H., M. Liu, P. Wu et al. 2011. Lipoxin A4 and its analog suppress hepatocellular carcinoma via remodeling tumor microenvironment. *Cancer Lett* 309 (1):85–94.

Harris, R. E., J. Beebe-Donk, H. Doss, and D. Burr Doss. 2005. Aspirin, ibuprofen, and other non-steroidal anti-inflammatory drugs in cancer prevention: a critical review of non-selective COX-2 blockade (review). *Oncol Rep* 13 (4):559–83.

Hawcroft, G., P. M. Loadman, A. Belluzzi, and M. A. Hull. 2010. Effect of eicosapentaenoic acid on E-type prostaglandin synthesis and EP4 receptor signaling in human colorectal cancer cells. *Neoplasia* 12 (8):618–27.

Heusinkveld, M., P. J. de Vos van Steenwijk, R. Goedemans et al. 2011. M2 macrophages induced by prostaglandin E2 and IL-6 from cervical carcinoma are switched to activated M1 macrophages by CD4+ Th1 cells. *J Immunol* 187 (3):1157–65.

Janakiram, N. B., A. Mohammed, and C. V. Rao. 2011. Role of lipoxins, resolvins, and other bioactive lipids in colon and pancreatic cancer. *Cancer Metastasis Rev* 30 (3–4):507–23.

Jia, Q., J. R. Lupton, R. Smith et al. 2008. Reduced colitis-associated colon cancer in Fat-1 (n-3 fatty acid desaturase) transgenic mice. *Cancer Res* 68 (10):3985–91.

Kalinski, P. 2012. Regulation of immune responses by prostaglandin E2. *J Immunol* 188 (1):21–8.

Kang, J. X., J. Wang, L. Wu, and Z. B. Kang. 2004. Transgenic mice: fat-1 mice convert n-6 to n-3 fatty acids. *Nature* 427 (6974):504.

Kim, E. J., M. R. Choi, H. Park et al. 2011. Dietary fat increases solid tumor growth and metastasis of 4T1 murine mammary carcinoma cells and mortality in obesity-resistant BALB/c mice. *Breast Cancer Res* 13 (4):R78.

Kobayashi, N., R. J. Barnard, J. Said et al. 2008. Effect of low-fat diet on development of prostate cancer and Akt phosphorylation in the Hi-Myc transgenic mouse model. *Cancer Res* 68 (8):3066–73.

Larsson, S. C., M. Kumlin, M. Ingelman-Sundberg, and A. Wolk. 2004. Dietary long-chain n-3 fatty acids for the prevention of cancer: a review of potential mechanisms. *Am J Clin Nutr* 79 (6):935–45.

Lauritzen, L., H. S. Hansen, M. H. Jorgensen, and K. F. Michaelsen. 2001. The essentiality of long chain n-3 fatty acids in relation to development and function of the brain and retina. *Prog Lipid Res* 40 (1–2):1–94.

Lee, J. Y., K. H. Sohn, S. H. Rhee, and D. Hwang. 2001. Saturated fatty acids, but not unsaturated fatty acids, induce the expression of cyclooxygenase-2 mediated through Toll-like receptor 4. *J Biol Chem* 276 (20):16683–9.

Lee, J. Y., L. Zhao, H. S. Youn et al. 2004. Saturated fatty acid activates but polyunsaturated fatty acid inhibits Toll-like receptor 2 dimerized with Toll-like receptor 6 or 1. *J Biol Chem* 279 (17):16971–9.

Marcheselli, V. L., S. Hong, W. J. Lukiw et al. 2003. Novel docosanoids inhibit brain ischemia-reperfusion-mediated leukocyte infiltration and pro-inflammatory gene expression. *J Biol Chem* 278 (44):43807–17.

Monk, J. M., Q. Jia, E. Callaway et al. 2012. Th17 cell accumulation is decreased during chronic experimental colitis by (n-3) PUFA in Fat-1 mice. *J Nutr* 142 (1):117–24.

Murphy, R. A., M. Mourtzakis, and V. C. Mazurak. 2012. n-3 polyunsaturated fatty acids: the potential role for supplementation in cancer. *Curr Opin Clin Nutr Metab Care* 15 (3):246–51.

Muthuswamy, R., J. Mueller-Berghaus, U. Haberkorn, T. A. Reinhart, D. Schadendorf, and P. Kalinski. 2010. PGE(2) transiently enhances DC expression of CCR7 but inhibits the ability of DCs to produce CCL19 and attract naive T cells. *Blood* 116 (9):1454–9.

Muthuswamy, R., J. Urban, J. J. Lee, T. A. Reinhart, D. Bartlett, and P. Kalinski. 2008. Ability of mature dendritic cells to interact with regulatory T cells is imprinted during maturation. *Cancer Res* 68 (14):5972–8.

Panigrahy, D., A. Kaipainen, E. R. Greene, and S. Huang. 2010. Cytochrome P450-derived eicosanoids: the neglected pathway in cancer. *Cancer Metastasis Rev* 29 (4):723–35.

Pereg, D., and M. Lishner. 2005. Non-steroidal anti-inflammatory drugs for the prevention and treatment of cancer. *J Intern Med* 258 (2):115–23.

Rakoff-Nahoum, S., and R. Medzhitov. 2009. Toll-like receptors and cancer. *Nat Rev Cancer* 9 (1):57–63.

Rysman, E., K. Brusselmans, K. Scheys et al. 2011. De novo lipogenesis protects cancer cells from free radicals and chemotherapeutics by promoting membrane lipid saturation. *Cancer Res* 70 (20):8117–26.

Scarlett, U. K., M. R. Rutkowski, A. M. Rauwerdink et al. 2012. Ovarian cancer progression is controlled by phenotypic changes in dendritic cells. *J Exp Med* 209 (3):495–506.

Schonberg, S. A., A. G. Lundemo, T. Fladvad et al. 2006. Closely related colon cancer cell lines display different sensitivity to polyunsaturated fatty acids, accumulate different lipid classes and downregulate sterol regulatory element-binding protein 1. *FEBS J* 273 (12):2749–65.

Serhan, C. N. 2007. Resolution phase of inflammation: novel endogenous anti-inflammatory and proresolving lipid mediators and pathways. *Annu Rev Immunol* 25:101–37.

Serhan, C. N., N. Chiang, and T. E. Van Dyke. 2008. Resolving inflammation: dual anti-inflammatory and pro-resolution lipid mediators. *Nat Rev Immunol* 8 (5):349–61.

Serhan, C. N., C. B. Clish, J. Brannon, S. P. Colgan, N. Chiang, and K. Gronert. 2000. Novel functional sets of lipid-derived mediators with antiinflammatory actions generated from omega-3 fatty acids via cyclooxygenase 2-nonsteroidal antiinflammatory drugs and transcellular processing. *J Exp Med* 192 (8):1197–204.

Serhan, C. N., J. Dalli, S. Karamnov et al. 2012. Macrophage proresolving mediator maresin 1 stimulates tissue regeneration and controls pain. *FASEB J* 26 (4):1755–1765.

Serhan, C. N., M. Hamberg, and B. Samuelsson. 1984. Lipoxins: novel series of biologically active compounds formed from arachidonic acid in human leukocytes. *Proc Natl Acad Sci U S A* 81 (17):5335–9.

Serhan, C. N., S. Hong, K. Gronert et al. 2002. Resolvins: a family of bioactive products of omega-3 fatty acid transformation circuits initiated by aspirin treatment that counter proinflammation signals. *J Exp Med* 196 (8):1025–37.

Serhan, C. N., and N. A. Petasis. 2011. Resolvins and protectins in inflammation resolution. *Chem Rev* 111 (10):5922–43.

Serhan, C. N., R. Yang, K. Martinod et al. 2009. Maresins: novel macrophage mediators with potent antiinflammatory and proresolving actions. *J Exp Med* 206 (1):15–23.

Song, K. S., K. Jing, J. S. Kim et al. 2011. Omega-3-polyunsaturated fatty acids suppress pancreatic cancer cell growth in vitro and in vivo via downregulation of Wnt/Beta-catenin signaling. *Pancreatology* 11 (6):574–84.

Suburu, J., and Y. Q. Chen. 2012. Lipids and prostate cancer. *Prostaglandins Other Lipid Mediat* 98 (1–2):1–10.

Swinnen, J. V., T. Roskams, S. Joniau et al. 2002. Overexpression of fatty acid synthase is an early and common event in the development of prostate cancer. *Int J Cancer* 98 (1):19–22.

Swinnen, J. V., P. P. Van Veldhoven, L. Timmermans et al. 2003. Fatty acid synthase drives the synthesis of phospholipids partitioning into detergent-resistant membrane microdomains. *Biochem Biophys Res Commun* 302 (4):898–903.

Szymanski, K. M., D. C. Wheeler, and L. A. Mucci. 2010. Fish consumption and prostate cancer risk: a review and meta-analysis. *Am J Clin Nutr* 92 (5):1223–33.

Szymczak, M., M. Murray, and N. Petrovic. 2008. Modulation of angiogenesis by omega-3 polyunsaturated fatty acids is mediated by cyclooxygenases. *Blood* 111 (7):3514–21.

Tang, D. G., Y. Q. Chen, and K. V. Honn. 1996. Arachidonate lipoxygenases as essential regulators of cell survival and apoptosis. *Proc Natl Acad Sci U S A* 93 (11):5241–6.

Terano, T., J. A. Salmon, G. A. Higgs, and S. Moncada. 1986. Eicosapentaenoic acid as a modulator of inflammation. Effect on prostaglandin and leukotriene synthesis. *Biochem Pharmacol* 35 (5):779–85.

Ulrich, C. M., J. Bigler, and J. D. Potter. 2006. Non-steroidal anti-inflammatory drugs for cancer prevention: promise, perils and pharmacogenetics. *Nat Rev Cancer* 6 (2):130–40.

Van Elssen, C. H., J. Vanderlocht, T. Oth, B. L. Senden-Gijsbers, W. T. Germeraad, and G. M. Bos. 2011. Inflammation-restraining effects of prostaglandin E2 on natural killer-dendritic cell (NK-DC) interaction are imprinted during DC maturation. *Blood* 118 (9):2473–82.

Vanamala, J., A. Glagolenko, P. Yang et al. 2008. Dietary fish oil and pectin enhance colonocyte apoptosis in part through suppression of PPARdelta/PGE2 and elevation of PGE3. *Carcinogenesis* 29 (4):790–6.

Wang, D., and R. N. Dubois. 2010. Eicosanoids and cancer. *Nat Rev Cancer* 10 (3):181–93.

Wang, S., J. Wu, J. Suburu et al. 2012. Effect of dietary polyunsaturated fatty acids on castration-resistant Pten-null prostate cancer. *Carcinogenesis* 33 (2):404–12.

Wassall, S. R., and W. Stillwell. 2008. Docosahexaenoic acid domains: the ultimate non-raft membrane domain. *Chem Phys Lipids* 153 (1):57–63.

Weylandt, K. H., C. Y. Chiu, B. Gomolka, S. F. Waechter, and B. Wiedenmann. 2012. Omega-3 fatty acids and their lipid mediators: Towards an understanding of resolvin and protectin formation. *Prostaglandins Other Lipid Mediat* 97 (3–4):73–82.

Wu, S., J. Liang, L. Zhang, X. Zhu, X. Liu, and D. Miao. 2011. Fish consumption and the risk of gastric cancer: systematic review and meta-analysis. *BMC Cancer* 11:26.

Wymann, M. P., and R. Schneiter. 2008. Lipid signalling in disease. *Nat Rev Mol Cell Biol* 9 (2):162–76.

Xia, S., Y. Lu, J. Wang et al. 2006. Melanoma growth is reduced in fat-1 transgenic mice: impact of omega-6/omega-3 essential fatty acids. *Proc Natl Acad Sci U S A* 103 (33):12499–504.

Xu, Z. Z., L. Zhang, T. Liu et al. 2010. Resolvins RvE1 and RvD1 attenuate inflammatory pain via central and peripheral actions. *Nat Med* 16 (5):592–7, 1 p. following 597.

Yang, P., D. Chan, E. Felix et al. 2004. Formation and antiproliferative effect of prostaglandin E(3) from eicosapentaenoic acid in human lung cancer cells. *J Lipid Res* 45 (6):1030–9.

Zhang, Michael J., and Matthew Spite. 2012. Resolvins: Anti-inflammatory and proresolving mediators derived from omega-3 polyunsaturated fatty acids. *Annual Review of Nutrition* 32:7.1–7.25.

16 Anti-Inflammatory and Proresolving Effects of Docosahexaenoic Acid
Implications for Its Chemopreventive Potential

Young-Joon Surh, Na-Young Song,
Ha-Na Lee, and Hye-Kyung Na

CONTENTS

16.1 INTRODUCTION

Inflammation underlies many common physiologic and pathogenic conditions. While acute inflammation is protective against infection and injury, the failure to resolve the inflammation at an early stage can cause pathologic conditions, such as rheumatoid arthritis, Crohn's disease, diabetes, obesity, asthma, cardiovascular diseases, and neurodegenerative disorders (Chapkin et al. 2009). Chronic inflammation is also closely linked to some types of human cancer. The emerging role of inflammation in multistage carcinogenesis has been extensively investigated in recent years at the cellular and molecular levels (Kundu and Surh 2012). It is becoming more evident that the classical mediators of inflammation, such as eicosanoids and cytokines, contribute to carcinogenesis, especially in the promotion stage.

16.2 ROLE OF POLYUNSATURATED FATTY ACIDS IN INFLAMMATION

Polyunsaturated fatty acids (PUFAs) are precursors of potent lipid mediators, termed eicosanoids, which play an important role in modulating overall inflammatory events. Inflammation is mediated by a distinct set of proinflammatory lipid mediators derived from arachidonic acid (AA; 20:4n-6), a key member of the omega-6 (n-6) PUFA. These include prostaglandins (PGs, e.g., PGD_2 and PGE_2), leukotrienes (LTs, e.g., LTB_4 and LTC_4), and thromboxanes (TXs, e.g., TXB_2) (Calder 2006). However, eicosanoids produced from n-3 PUFAs have opposing effects. Major dietary sources of anti-inflammatory n-3 PUFAs are fish oils containing eicosapentaenoic acid (EPA, 20:5n-3) and docosahexaenoic acid (DHA, 22:6n-3) as well as nuts, seeds, and vegetable oils containing their precursor form α-linolenic acid (ALA). Figure 16.1 illustrates the differential effects of n-6 and n-3 PUFAs on inflammation.

Long-chain PUFAs modulate inflammatory processes through multiple mechanisms, some of which are mediated by changing the fatty acid composition of cell membranes (Calder 2010). Cells involved in the inflammatory response are typically rich in the n-6 fatty acid AA, but the contents of AA can be altered through oral administration of n-3 PUFAs. DHA and EPA, when consumed as part of the human diet, are incorporated into membrane phospholipids of inflammatory cells at the expense of AA. As a result, there is less AA available as a substrate for the synthesis of proinflammatory eicosanoids. Thus, dietary supplementation with n-3 PUFAs, such as EPA and DHA, can modify the lipid mediator profile, resulting in reduced production of TXB_2, LTB_4, and so forth by inflammatory cells (Calder 2008, 2009). Changing the fatty acid composition of cells involved in the inflammatory response also affects production of peptide mediators of inflammation (e.g., adhesion molecules, cytokines, etc.). Besides exerting anti-inflammatory actions by inhibiting AA metabolism to proinflammatory eicosanoids (Wall et al. 2010), fish oil supplementation enriched with EPA and DHA remarkably reduces the expression of inflammatory markers and concomitantly induces anti-inflammatory gene expression (Bouwens et al. 2009; Deike et al. 2012). Thus, the fatty acid composition of human inflammatory cells influences their function.

Of the two major n-3 fatty acids present in fish oil, DHA is generally known to be more effective than EPA in terms of the health beneficial effects (Serini et al. 2011), as evidenced by better capability of decreasing blood pressure, heart rate, and platelet aggregation (Cottin, Sanders, and Hall 2011; Ibrahim et al. 2011). This chapter focuses mainly on the anti-inflammatory and inflammation-resolving activity of DHA in the context of its chemopreventive potential.

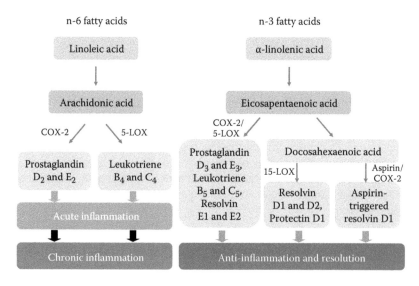

FIGURE 16.1 General overview of the synthesis of DHA and its metabolites. ALA, the precursor form of the n-3 PUFAs, undergoes metabolism to produce EPA and, subsequently, DHA. DHA can be further metabolized by COX and LOX to form D-series resolvins and protectin D1.

16.3 ANTI-INFLAMMATORY EFFECTS OF DHA

The health beneficial effects associated with fish oil consumption have been ascribed to the long-chain PUFAs, predominantly DHA (Figure 16.2).

16.3.1 CLINICAL DATA

Numerous studies have demonstrated the benefits of dietary supplementation with fish oils and its constituents, n-3 PUFAs, in several inflammatory and autoimmune diseases in humans, including rheumatoid arthritis, Crohn's disease, ulcerative colitis, psoriasis, lupus erythematosus, multiple sclerosis, and migraine headaches. Many placebo-controlled trials with fish oil in chronic inflammatory diseases reveal significant benefits, including decreased disease activity and a lowered use of anti-inflammatory drugs (Simopoulos 2002). There are a number of randomized, placebo-controlled, double-blind intervention trials evaluating the effects of n-3 PUFAs as well as fish oil on inflammatory bowel disease (IBD) (reviewed in Calder 2008). Long-chain n-3 PUFAs consumed as a supplement by patients with IBD are incorporated into gut mucosal tissue. This results in anti-inflammatory effects as evidenced by reduced LTB_4 production by neutrophils and colonic mucosa, decreased production of PGE_2 and TXB_2 by colonic mucosa, and decreased production of PGE_2 and interferon gamma (IFNγ) by blood mononuclear cells (Calder 2008 and references therein).

PUFAs from fish oil appear to have anti-inflammatory and antioxidative effects and may hence improve nutritional status in cancer patients. In a multicenter, randomized, double-blind trial, there was a progressive decrease in the levels of two inflammatory markers, C-reactive protein (CRP) and interleukin 6 (IL-6), during chemotherapy in patients with advanced non–small cell lung cancer who received four capsules per day containing 340 mg of DHA and 510 mg of EPA for 66 days. In addition, plasma reactive oxygen species (ROS) levels increased in the placebo group as compared to the n-3 PUFA group at the later treatment times. The levels of hydroxynonenal, a hallmark of oxidative stress, increased in the placebo group during the study, while they stabilized in the n-3 PUFA treatment group. The consumption of n-3 PUFAs is hence likely to potentiate the body's anti-inflammatory and antioxidative defense, which could be considered as an alternative choice for anticachectic therapy (Finocchiaro et al. 2011). Likewise, patients supplemented with fish oil containing 600 mg of

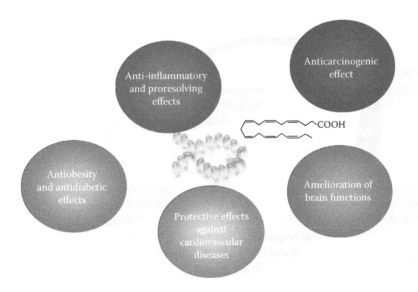

FIGURE 16.2 Health beneficial effects of DHA.

DHA and EPA for 9 weeks showed a clinically relevant decrease in the plasma CRP/albumin ratio, which reflects nutritional and inflammatory status (Silva Jde et al. 2012).

Dietary supplementation with DHA and EPA significantly increased their levels in red blood cells (RBCs) in patients with chronic renal failure on maintenance hemodialysis. There was a marked decrease in the levels of inflammatory markers, such as tumor necrosis factor α (TNFα), IL-6, and high-sensitivity CRP (Rasic-Milutinovic et al. 2007). In another study, DHA supplementation reduced circulating concentrations of CRP, IL-6, and granulocyte monocyte colony-stimulating factor (Kelley et al. 2009).

Chronic wounds often result from prolonged inflammation involving excessive polymorphonuclear (PMN) leukocyte activity. DHA plus EPA supplementation significantly elevated the plasma levels of each n-3 PUFA compared with those in the placebo control group and lowered wound fluid levels of two 15-lipoxygenase (15-LOX) products of n-6 PUFAs, 9-hydroxyoctadecadienoic acid and 15-hydroxyeicosatrienoic acid, at 24 h postwounding. The individuals supplemented with DHA and EPA also had lower mean levels of myeloperoxidase (MPO), a leukocyte marker, at 12 h and significantly more reepithelialization on day 5 postwounding. These findings suggest that lipid mediator profiles can be manipulated by altering PUFA intake to create a wound microenvironment more conducive to healing (McDaniel, Massey, and Nicolaou 2011).

16.3.2 ANIMAL DATA

DHA as well as EPA found in fish oils generate bioactive lipid mediators that reduce inflammation and PMN leukocyte recruitment in several inflammatory disease models, including one that mimics human IBD. IBD increases the risk of developing colorectal cancer. Dietary supplementation with n-3 PUFAs containing DHA was effective in alleviating colitis in Balb/c mice induced by 5% dextran sulfate sodium (DSS) in drinking water for 7 days. Oral administration of DHA (30 mg/kg per day) attenuated DSS-induced colitis as assessed by the use of symptomatic markers (colon length, stool consistency, and diarrhea); histopathological scores (inflammation score, crypt destruction, and infiltration of neutrophils); and MPO activity (Cho, Chi, and Chun 2011). Furthermore, the microarray analysis showed downregulation of DSS-responsive genes encoding inflammatory cytokines (e.g., IL-1β, cluster of differentiation 14 [CD14] antigen, and TNF receptor superfamily member 1β) (Cho, Chi, and Chun 2011).

The role of endothelial cells in IBD has been recently emphasized. Migration of leucocytes is a key process in inflammation that involves adhesion molecules, such as intercellular adhesion molecule 1 (ICAM-1) and vascular adhesion molecule 1 (VCAM-1). Dietary intervention with fish oil rich in EPA and DHA significantly decreased colon production of PGE_2 and LTB_4 and endothelial expression of VCAM-1 and vascular endothelial growth factor receptor 2 (VEGFR2) in rats with colitis induced by intrarectal injection of 2-4-6-trinitrobenzen sulfonic acid (Ibrahim et al. 2011).

Balb/c mice fed with diets enriched with DHA for 3 weeks were subjected to a contact dermatitis induced in the ears. DHA attenuated ear inflammation, as demonstrated by reduced neutrophil infiltration. There was also attenuation of the systemic macrophage inflammatory response and T-helper type 2 response with increased production of IL-10 (Sierra et al. 2008). A DHA-enriched diet also attenuated inflammatory edema in 2,4-dinitro-1-fluorobenzene–induced contact hypersensitivity in mice and carrageenan-induced rat paw edema (Tomobe et al. 2000; Nakamura et al. 1994). These findings suggest the immunosuppressive and anti-inflammatory effects of DHA. Topical application of DHA attenuated cyclooxygenase 2 (COX2) expression in hairless mouse skin irradiated with ultraviolet B (UVB) (Rahman et al. 2011). NADP(H) oxidases (NOXs) play a major role in cellular generation of ROS. While ROS act as a second messenger in the cellular signal transduction, the excess amounts can cause inflammation as well as oxidative stress. DHA downregulates overexpression of NOX4 in various types of cells, which may account for its anti-inflammatory effect (Massaro et al. 2006; Richard et al. 2009; Rahman et al. 2011).

The effects of n-3 PUFAs on sudden cardiac death and vascular inflammation were examined by utilizing a rat coronary ligation model and a mouse femoral artery ligation model, respectively. n-3 PUFAs improved animal survival after myocardial infarction, prevented development of atherosclerotic lesions, and stimulated compensatory vascular remodeling (Siddiqui et al. 2009).

Fish oil enriched with DHA dramatically extended the life span of mice and lowered lipopolysaccharide (LPS)-mediated increases in serum IL-18 levels and activation of nuclear factor kappaB (NF-κB) as well as cleavage of pro–IL-18 to mature IL-18 in the kidney. Based on these findings, it was suggested that DHA suppresses glomerulonephritis and extends the life span of systemic lupus erythematosus–prone short-lived F1 hybrid of New Zealand Black × New Zealand White (NZB × NZW) F1 mice, and that these effects are likely to be mediated via inhibition of IL-18 production and IL-18–dependent inflammatory signaling (Halade et al. 2010).

Rats fed choline-deficient high-fat diets developed severe steatohepatitis and liver fibrosis. Treatment with DHA significantly decreased the n-6/n-3 ratio in the liver and increased plasma superoxide dismutase–like activity compared with rats developing nonalcoholic steatohepatitis. In addition, DHA attenuated liver fibrosis during the development of nonalcoholic steatohepatitis. Therefore, a higher DHA ratio in the liver of nonalcoholic steatohepatitis rats might regulate the inflammatory response through a low n-6 ratio and diminished oxidative stress, effectively inhibiting liver fibrosis during steatohepatitis progression (Takayama et al. 2010).

Pregnant C3H/HeN dams were fed purified control or DHA-supplemented diets (~0.25% of total fat) at embryonic day 16, and they consumed these diets throughout the study. There were fewer neutrophils and macrophages in pulmonary tissues from pups nursed by DHA-supplemented dams than in those nursed by dams fed the control diet at day 7 of hyperoxia exposure. In mice, maternal DHA supplementation decreased leukocyte infiltration in the offspring exposed to hyperoxia, suggesting a potential role for DHA supplementation as a therapy to reduce inflammation in preterm infants (Rogers et al. 2011).

Necrotizing enterocolitis (NEC) is a devastating gastrointestinal disease of premature infants. Mother Sprague-Dawley rats were fed a DHA-enriched diet from 7 to 20 days of gestation. In a neonatal Sprague-Dawley rat model of NEC, the incidence of NEC-like colitis was markedly reduced in the pups of the DHA-enriched diet group. The expression of peroxisome proliferator–activated receptor-gamma (PPAR-γ) was significantly increased, whereas the inhibitor of NF-κB (IκB) α/β decreased in the intestines of DHA-treated animals (Ohtsuka et al. 2011). In another study, DHA given to neonatal rats also exerted a protective effect on experimentally induced NEC in rats and inhibited intestinal expression of toll-like receptor 4 (TLR4) and platelet-activating factor receptor, molecules that are important in the pathogenesis of NEC in epithelial cells (Lu et al. 2007).

Bile duct obstruction and subsequent cholestasis are associated with hepatocellular injury, cholangiocyte proliferation, stellate cell activation, Kupffer cell activation, oxidative stress, and fibrosis as well as inflammation. Cholestasis was produced by bile duct ligation (BDL) in male Sprague-Dawley rats for 3 weeks. The BDL group showed elevated ductular reaction, fibrosis, inflammation, and oxidative stress. These pathophysiological changes were attenuated by DHA supplementation, which started 2 weeks before injury and lasted for 5 weeks. DHA also alleviated BDL-induced expression of transforming growth factor β1, IL-1β, connective tissue growth factor, and collagen. DHA also attenuated BDL-induced leukocyte accumulation and NF-κB activation (Chen et al. 2012).

Plasma concentrations of IL-6, TNFα, and CRP were significantly greater in n-3-PUFA–deficient rats relative to controls. Changes in the membrane n-3 and n-6 PUFA composition and elevations in plasma IL-6 and TNFα were all prevented by normalization of n-3 fatty acid status. Erythrocyte DHA was inversely correlated, and the AA/DHA ratio was positively correlated with plasma levels of IL-6, TNFα, and CRP. These preclinical data provide evidence for a functional link between n-3 fatty acid deficiency and elevated peripheral inflammatory signaling (McNamara et al. 2010).

Acute and chronic inflammation plays essential roles in inflammatory/autoimmune conditions. Dendritic cells (DCs) represent the essential cellular link between innate and adaptive immunity and have a prominent role in tolerance to self-antigens. Dietary DHA exerted an inhibitory effect on expression of proinflammatory IL-12–family cytokines in splenic DCs from LPS-inoculated mice (Kong et al. 2010).

Chronic macrophage-mediated tissue inflammation is a key mechanism for insulin resistance in obesity. n-3 PUFAs ameliorate obesity-induced adipose tissue inflammation and insulin resistance. G-protein–coupled receptor 120 (GPCR120), as a putative functional n-3 PUFA receptor/sensor, may mediate insulin-sensitizing and antidiabetic effects by repressing macrophage-induced tissue inflammation. The n-3 PUFA supplementation inhibited inflammation and enhanced systemic insulin sensitivity in obese wild-type mice but not in GPCR120 knockout animals (Oh et al. 2010).

In another study, inflamed adipose tissue from high fat-diet–induced obese mice showed increased F4/80 and CD11b double-positive macrophage staining and elevated IL-6 and monocyte chemotactic protein-1 (MCP-1) levels. DHA (4 µg/g) did not change the total number of macrophages but significantly reduced the proportion of high-CD11b/F4/80-expressing cells in parallel with the emergence of low-expressing CD11b/F4/80 macrophages in the adipose tissue. This effect was associated with downregulation of proinflammatory adipokines in parallel with increased expression of IL-10, CD206, arginase 1, resistin-like molecule α, and chitinase-3–like protein, indicative of a phenotypic switch in macrophage polarization toward an M2-like phenotype. This shift was confined to the stromal vascular cell fraction, in which secretion of Th1 cytokines (IL-6, MCP-1, and TNFα) was blocked by DHA (Titos et al. 2011).

A *fat-1* transgenic mouse rich in endogenous n-3 fatty acids was generated by knocking-in of the *Caenorhabditis elegans fat-1* gene that encodes the n-3 fatty acid desaturase able to convert the n-6 into the n-3 PUFAs (Kang et al. 2004). Consequently, *fat-1* mice exhibit relatively low expression levels of those proinflammatory genes that encode COX2, PGE$_2$, and ILs (Gravaghi et al. 2011). The *fat-1* mice are less susceptible to inflammation-associated abnormalities, such as DSS-induced colitis (Hudert et al. 2006), cerulein-induced pancreatitis (Weylandt et al. 2008), and experimentally induced acute lung injury (Mayer et al. 2009).

16.3.3 In Vitro Data

n-3 and n-6 PUFAs have opposing effects on inflammation. LPS-induced cytokine release by human alveolar cells was affected by changes in the n-3/n-6 ratio of cell membranes induced by different supplies of PUFAs. Thus, the supply of 1:1 and 1:2 DHA/AA ratios reversed the baseline predominance of n-6 over n-3 in cell membranes. The release of proinflammatory cytokines (TNFα, IL-6, and IL-8) was also reduced by 1:1 and 1:2 DHA/AA ratios but increased by 1:4 and 1:7 DHA/AA ratios versus control. The 1:1 and 1:2 ratios increased the release of anti-inflammatory IL-10. This study showed that proinflammatory cytokine release was dependent on the proportion of n-3 in the n-3/n-6 ratio of alveolar cell membranes, being reduced with the supply of a high proportion of DHA and increased with a high proportion of AA. These results support the biochemical basis for current recommendations to shift the PUFA supply from n-6 to n-3 PUFAs in nutrition support of patients with acute lung injury (Cotogni et al. 2011).

Activated immune cells produce various proinflammatory cytokines that circulate in the bloodstream and provoke inflammatory responses in the peripheries. There is accumulating evidence that n-3 PUFAs reduce proinflammatory responses, in part, by modulating immune responses. These include abrogation of T-cell proliferative capacity in response to mitogenic stimuli and antigenic stimulation. Similar suppressive effects were observed with respect to the DC, endothelial cell, macrophage, and neutrophil components of the inflammatory response (Chapkin et al. 2009). Likewise, the anti-inflammatory effects of DHA might be attributed to its direct influence on immune cells. DHA prevents adhesion of neutrophils to endothelial cells, the initial phase of inflammation, via downregulation of adhesion molecules, such as VCAM-1 and P-selectin (Wang et al. 2011; Wang, Liu, and Thorlacius 2003; Yates et al. 2011).

DHA attenuates maturation and cytokine secretion of DCs, the antigen-presenting cells that link between innate and adaptive immunity (Kong, Yen, and Ganea 2011; Kong et al. 2010). DHA maintained the immature phenotype in murine bone marrow–derived DCs by preventing the upregulation of major histocompatibilty complex II (MHCII) and costimulatory molecules (CD40, CD80, and CD86). DHA inhibited the production of proinflammatory cytokines, including the IL-12 cytokine–family proteins, by DCs stimulated with various TLR ligands. DHA inhibition of IL-12–family cytokine expression was mediated through activation of PPAR-γ and inhibition of NF-κB/p65 nuclear translocation (Kong et al. 2010). Mature DCs treated with DHA showed inhibition of IL-6 expression and IL-12 secretion, and their lymphoproliferative stimulation capacity was impaired. Moreover, DHA induced the expression of PPAR-γ target genes pyruvate dehydrogenase kinase-4 and adipocyte protein-2 in immature DCs (Zapata-Gonzalez et al. 2008). Likewise, DHA attenuates production of IL-12, a proinflammatory cytokine, in murine DCs, while secretion of the anti-inflammatory cytokine IL-10 is enhanced (Draper et al. 2011). Treatment of human DCs with DHA downregulated the LPS-induced production of TNFα (Marion-Letellier et al. 2008).

A number of studies have investigated the effects of fish oil on the production of proinflammatory cytokines using peripheral blood mononuclear cell (PBMC) models. The majority of these studies have employed heterogeneous blends of long-chain n-3 PUFAs, EPA and DHA, which preclude examination of the individual effects of n-3 PUFAs. LPS-stimulated secretion of IL-1β and TNFα in PBMCs was inhibited, with apparent relative potencies of DHA > EPA (Nauroth et al. 2010).

Inflammation elicited by macrophages is increasingly recognized in the etiology of metabolic syndrome. GPCR120 functions as an n-3 PUFA receptor/sensor. Stimulation of GPCR120 with n-3 PUFAs or a chemical agonist causes broad anti-inflammatory effects in monocytic RAW 264.7 cells and in primary intraperitoneal macrophages. All of these effects are abrogated by GPCR120 knockdown (Oh et al. 2010). EPA and DHA downregulated the production of proinflammatory cytokines (e.g., IL-1β, IL-6, and TNFα), NF-κB transcriptional activity, and upstream cytoplasmic signaling events (Mullen, Loscher, and Roche 2010). The differential effects of pure EPA and DHA on cytokine expression and NF-κB activation in human THP-1 monocyte-derived macrophages were investigated. Pretreatment of human THP-1 monocyte-derived macrophages with the same concentration (i.e., 100 μM) each of EPA and DHA significantly decreased LPS-induced production as well as messenger RNA (mRNA) expression of TNFα, IL-1β, and IL-6, compared to control cells. In all cases, the effect of DHA was significantly more potent than that of EPA. DHA markedly reduced LPS-induced nuclear localization and DNA binding of NF-κB in THP-1 macrophages, which was mediated by blocking the degradation of cytoplasmic IκBα (Weldon et al. 2007). The inhibitory effect of DHA on expression of TLR4 and COX2 as well as NF-κB activation was also more pronounced than that of EPA in macrophages (Lee et al. 2003).

Obesity leads to several chronic morbidities, including type 2 diabetes, dyslipidemia, atherosclerosis, and hypertension, which are major components of the metabolic syndrome. Adipocyte-derived adipokines including leptin and visfatin play a key role in the development of obesity-associated metabolic disturbances by causing systemic low-grade inflammation. The n-3 PUFAs, including DHA, have been shown to ameliorate low-grade inflammation in adipose tissue associated with obesity by regulating adipokine gene expression and secretion (Moreno-Aliaga, Lorente-Cebrian, and Martinez 2010).

Adipose tissue inflammation with immune cell recruitment plays a key role in obesity-induced IR. EPA and DHA have anti-inflammatory potential, but their individual effects on adipose IR remain poorly defined. It has been speculated that EPA and DHA may differentially affect macrophage-induced IR in adipocytes. J774.2 macrophages pretreated with EPA or DHA (50 μM for 5 days) were stimulated with LPS. As observed in other studies, DHA had more potent anti-inflammatory effects than EPA, with marked attenuation of LPS-induced NF-κB activation and TNFα secretion in macrophages. DHA specifically enhanced anti-inflammatory IL-10 secretion and reduced the expression of proinflammatory M1 [F4/80(+)/CD11(+)] macrophages. Coculture of DHA-enriched macrophages with adipocytes attenuated IL-6 and TNFα secretion while it enhanced IL-10 secretion. Conditioned media (CM) from DHA-enriched macrophages attenuated adipocyte NF-κB activation. Adipocytes cocultured with DHA-enriched macrophages maintained insulin sensitivity with enhanced insulin-stimulated ^{3}H-glucose transport, glucose transporter 4 (GLUT4) translocation, and preservation of insulin receptor substrate-1 expression compared to coculture with untreated macrophages. Thus, IL-10 expressed by DHA-enriched macrophages attenuates manifestation of the CM-induced proinflammatory IR phenotype in adipocytes (Oliver et al. 2011).

PPAR-γ regulates the expression of numerous genes. In addition to their antidiabetic activity, PPAR-γ agonists have been reported to have beneficial effects for IBD, atherosclerosis, brain inflammation, bone turnover as well as cancer (Itoh and Yamamoto 2008). The role of PPAR-γ in the regulation of intestinal inflammation was investigated in the human enterocyte-like cell line Caco-2 and human DCs stimulated by IL-1β and LPS, respectively. In Caco-2 cells, production of IL-6 and IL-8 as well as PPAR-γ expression was significantly decreased by DHA, EPA, and the synthetic PPAR-γ agonist troglitazone. Inducible nitric oxide synthase (iNOS) expression was similarly inhibited by these compounds. EPA and DHA also modulated the DC response to LPS (Marion-Letellier et al. 2008).

Fish oil rich in n-3 PUFAs, especially EPA and DHA, protects against bone loss in chronic inflammatory diseases like rheumatoid arthritis, periodontitis, and osteoporosis. One of the risk factors for bone loss implicated in inflammatory bone disorders is the elevation of bone-resorbing osteoclasts, and the protective effects of n-3 PUFAs against bone loss may be attributed to their attenuation of osteoclastogenesis. Receptor activator of NF-κB ligand (RANKL) is known to be the most critical mediator of osteoclastogenesis. The differential effects of EPA and DHA on RANKL-stimulated osteoclastogenesis and RANKL signaling were examined using a murine monocytic cell line, RAW 264.7. DHA was found to be more effective than EPA in alleviating RANKL-induced proinflammatory cytokine production. DHA blocked NF-κB–mediated intracellular signaling activation, thereby decreasing osteoclast activation/differentiation and bone resorption (Rahman, Bhattacharya, and Fernandes 2008). Likewise, DHA inhibited cytokine production to a greater extent than did EPA in human intestinal epithelial cells stimulated with IL-1β (Marion-Letellier et al. 2008).

Although supplementation of preterm formula with PUFAs has been shown to reduce the incidence of NEC in animal models and clinical trials, the mechanisms remain elusive. To validate the in vivo observations, IEC-6 cells were exposed to platelet-activating factor (PAF) after pretreatment with DHA. DHA pretreatment blocked PAF-induced TLR4 and PAF receptor (PAFR) mRNA expression in these enterocytes. These effects might, in part, account for the protective effect of DHA and other PUFAs on neonatal NEC (Lu et al. 2007; Ohtsuka et al. 2011). The cytosolic phospholipase A$_2$ (cPLA$_2$)–dependent release of AA from the intraepithelial lymphocytes plays a pivotal role in arming lymphocytes to cytolysis in the immune response of celiac disease. A human intestinal epithelial cell line (Caco-2) was exposed to gliadin peptides (PT-gl) (500 μg/mL) and DHA (2 μg/mL), both alone and simultaneously for up to 24 h. The exposure of those cells to PT-gl alone resulted in increased AA release, COX2 expression, cPLA$_2$ activity, and release of PGE$_2$ and IL-8 in the culture medium, whereas the simultaneous exposure of the cells to DHA and PT-gl prevented the above-mentioned increases (Vincentini et al. 2011).

Oxidative stress is causally associated with inflammation. DHA suppressed the generation of ROS from AA via the COX2 and xanthine oxidase pathways in rat renal epithelial cells and murine macrophages, while it enhanced the levels of reduced glutathione (GSH) and antioxidative enzyme activities. Furthermore, production of inflammatory mediators (TXB$_2$, PGE$_2$, and 6-keto-PGF$_{1\alpha}$) and nitrite in LPS-stimulated murine macrophages (RAW 264.7) was effectively inhibited by DHA. These results strongly indicate that DHA exerts antioxidative and anti-inflammatory actions by reducing the intracellular production/accumulation of ROS, proinflammatory mediators, and nitrite and by maintaining levels of GSH and antioxidative enzymes (Kim and Chung 2007). DHA has been reported to block production of nitric oxide (NO) as well as ROS in murine macrophages (Ambrozova, Pekarova, and Lojek 2010; Komatsu et al. 2003). DHA significantly suppressed

TNFα and IL-1β mRNA expression and the production of LTB_4, PGD_2, TNFα, and IL-1β in LPS-stimulated primary human asthmatic alveolar macrophages (Mickleborough et al. 2009).

Oxidative stress is regarded as a major pathogenic factor in acute pancreatitis. Inflammation and apoptosis linked to oxidative stress have been implicated in cerulein-induced pancreatitis. ROS have been found to mediate inflammatory cytokine expression and apoptosis in pancreatic acinar cells stimulated with cerulein. DHA and its precursor ALA suppressed the expression of inflammatory cytokines (IL-1β and IL-6) and inhibited the activation of transcription factor activator protein 1 (AP-1) in cerulein-stimulated pancreatic acinar cells. Both DHA and ALA inhibited induced DNA fragmentation and inhibited the expression of proapoptotic genes (p53, Bax, and apoptosis-inducing factor) in pancreatic acinar cells exposed to hydrogen peroxide (Park, Lim, and Kim 2009).

The anti-inflammatory and antioxidant activities of DHA were evaluated in terms of its modulation of endothelial secreted phospholipase A_2 ($sPLA_2$) and NOX4, the two key enzymes involved in vascular inflammation. Exposure of human aortic endothelial cells to DHA led to its preferential incorporation into outer leaflet phospholipids and abolished stimulation of these cells induced by A23187 and angiotensin. In addition, DHA decreased NOX4 expression and activity; this effect was associated with reduced production of ROS. Further, the use of specific inhibitors has revealed that group V $sPLA_2$ is involved in the downregulation of NOX4 expression and activity by DHA (Richard et al. 2009).

Vascular inflammation is implicated in pathogenesis of diabetic retinopathy. DHA, the principal n-3 PUFA in the retina, markedly inhibited cytokine-induced adhesion molecule (CAM) expression in primary human retinal vascular endothelial (hRVE) cells, the target tissue affected by diabetic retinopathy, most likely through suppression of phosphorylation and degradation of IκBα and subsequent NF-κB nuclear translocation (Chen et al. 2005). DHA also inhibited expression of adhesion molecules in retinal endothelial cells (Chen et al. 2005) and human umbilical vein endothelial cells (HUVECs) (Collie-Duguid and Wahle 1996). In another study, DHA inhibited VCAM-1 expression induced by IL-1, IL-4, TNF, or LPS in human saphenous vein endothelial cells, but EPA failed to. DHA also limited cytokine-stimulated endothelial cell expression of E-selectin and ICAM-1 and the secretion of IL-6 and IL-8 into the medium but not the surface expression of constitutive surface molecules. In parallel with reduced surface VCAM-1 protein expression, DHA reduced VCAM-1 mRNA induction by IL-1 or TNF. DHA treatment also reduced the adhesion of human monocytes and of monocytic U937 cells to cytokine-stimulated endothelial cells. These properties of DHA may contribute to its antiatherogenic and anti-inflammatory effects (De Caterina et al. 1994).

DHA is thought to modulate the vascular inflammatory response. However, there are limited data on the interactions of DHA with the vascular endothelium, the cells that regulate the trafficking of leukocytes from the blood into inflamed tissue. DHA inhibited recruitment of neutrophils to the endothelial cell surface, although cells that became adherent were activated and could migrate across the HUVEC monolayer normally. In contrast, EPA had no effect on the levels of neutrophil adhesion in this assay. Analysis of adhesion receptor expression by quantitative polymerase chain reaction demonstrated that DHA did not alter the transcriptional activity of HUVEC. However, DHA did significantly reduce E-selectin expression at the HUVEC surface without altering the total cellular pool of this adhesion receptor. These results provide a novel mechanism by which DHA alters the trafficking of leukocytes during inflammation through disruption of intracellular transport machinery used to present adhesion molecules on the surface of cytokine-stimulated endothelial cells (Yates et al. 2011). In another study, DHA reduced rolling, adhesion, and transmigration of monocytes through inflammatory-activated HUVEC which was in part phosphatidylinositol-3-kinase (PI3-K) dependent. PI3-K–driven phosphorylation of Akt and apoptosis of HUVEC was modulated by DHA (Schaefer et al. 2008).

Microvascular endothelial cells regulate the migration of leukocytes from the intravascular compartment into the inflammatory tissue. Endothelial activation and expression of adhesion molecules are critical for leukocyte recruitment into the inflammatory wall. DHA pretreatment attenuated expression of VCAM-1, TLR4, COX2, and VEGFR2 and production of IL-6 and IL-8 as well as granulocyte-macrophage colony-stimulating factor, PGE$_2$, and LTB$_4$ in primary cultures of human intestinal microvascular endothelial cells stimulated with IL-1β (Ibrahim et al. 2011). Human aortic endothelial cells treated with DHA showed significantly reduced expression of ICAM-1 and nitrosylation of cellular proteins (Siddiqui et al. 2009). COX2 is one of the most well-known proteins induced in the inflammatory reactions (Morteau 2000). It has been reported that DHA inhibits IL-1α–induced expression as well as activity of COX2 in human saphenous vein endothelial cells (Massaro et al. 2006).

Sphingolipids represent a major component of membrane microdomains, and ceramide-enriched microdomains appear to be a prerequisite for inflammatory cytokine signaling. Acid sphingomyelinase (ASMase) and neutral sphingomyelinase (NSMase) are key regulatory enzymes of sphingolipid metabolism, promoting sphingomyelin hydrolysis to proinflammatory ceramide. DHA downregulated the basal and cytokine-induced expression of ASMase and NSMase and their activity in human retinal endothelial cells, thereby inhibiting cytokine-induced inflammatory signaling (Opreanu et al. 2010).

n-3 PUFAs have been shown to inhibit UVB-induced inflammation and other inflammatory states in vivo. Pretreatment of keratinocytes (HaCaT) and fibroblasts with DHA reduced both basal and UVB-induced secretion of IL-8, a chemokine pivotal to skin inflammation. In addition, TNFα-induced IL-8 secretion by keratinocytes was reduced by DHA (Storey et al. 2005).

PUFAs are highly abundant in brain tissue, and DHA might protect cells from oxidative stress during inflammation and demyelinating disorders. The effects of PUFA supplements on heat shock protein induction, cell survival, and stress responses to hydrogen peroxide–induced oxidative stress were investigated in oligodendroglial OLN-93 cells. Depending on the degree of desaturation, PUFA supplements caused the upregulation of heme oxygenase 1 (HO-1; HSP32), a stress responsive protein, and an increase in sensitivity to hydrogen peroxide treatment. DHA, with the highest number of double bonds, was most effective among the PUFAs tested (Brand et al. 2010).

Accumulating evidence suggests that the pathophysiology of depression might be associated with neuroinflammation. n-3 PUFAs are anti-inflammatory and exert antidepressant effects. When treated to BV-2 microglia, DHA reduced expression of TNFα, IL-6, NOS, and COX2 induced by IFNγ, and induced upregulation of HO-1 expression. The inhibitory effect of DHA on NO production was abolished by the HO-1 inhibitor zinc protoporphyrin IX. In addition, DHA caused Akt and extracellular signal–regulated kinase (ERK) activation in a time-dependent manner, and the DHA-induced HO-1 upregulation could be attenuated by PI3-K/AKT and mitogen-activated protein kinase kinase (MEK)/ERK inhibitors. DHA also increased IκB kinase α/β (IKKα/β) phosphorylation, IκBα phosphorylation, and IκBα degradation, whereas both NF-κB and IκB protease inhibitors could suppress DHA-induced HO-1 expression (Lu et al. 2010).

16.4 MOLECULAR MECHANISMS OF DHA-INDUCED ANTI-INFLAMMATORY EFFECTS

DHA possesses potent anti-inflammatory properties and has shown therapeutic benefit in numerous inflammatory diseases. However, the molecular mechanisms of these anti-inflammatory properties are poorly understood. Some of the effects of n-3 PUFAs are brought about by modulation of the amount and types of eicosanoids made, while other effects are elicited by eicosanoid-independent mechanisms, including actions upon intracellular signaling pathways, transcription factor activity, and gene expression (Chapkin et al. 2009).

The primary molecular target for the anti-inflammatory effects of DHA is NF-κB, a key transcription factor responsible for expression of proteins mediating inflammation and immune responses. NF-κB normally exists as a dimer, is mainly composed of p50 and p65, and is sequestered in the cytoplasm as an inactive complex with its negative regulator, IκBα (Surh 2003). When the IκB is phosphorylated by IKK, the IκB undergoes proteasome-mediated degradation, liberating NF-κB for translocation into the nucleus, where it transactivates target genes (Surh 2003). DHA attenuates TNFα-induced degradation of IκBα and nuclear accumulation of the p50 and p65 subunits in human aortic endothelial cells (Wang et al. 2011). DHA shows the consistent effects on IκBα, p50, and p65 in LPS-treated THP-1 macrophages (Mullen, Loscher, and Roche 2010). Furthermore, DHA inhibits NF-κB p65 DNA-binding activity provoked by LPS in THP-1 macrophages and human kidney cells (Li et al. 2005; Martinez-Micaelo et al. 2012).

Transcription factors other than NF-κB have been proposed as alternative molecular targets of DHA in exerting its anti-inflammatory effects. PPARs are transcription factors that regulate transcription of genes involved in metabolism and immunomodulation. It has been reported that DHA-induced PPAR-γ activation leads to inhibition of NF-κB as well as cytokine secretion (Li et al. 2005; Zapata-Gonzalez et al. 2008). Moreover, the n-3 fatty acid–enriched supplementation activates PPAR-α that subsequently interacts with the p65 subunit of NF-κB, hampering NF-κB–dependent transcription of the proinflammatory mediators (Zuniga et al. 2011). Suppression of AP-1 and cyclic adenosine monophosphate (cAMP) response element–binding protein is also responsible for the anti-inflammatory effect of DHA (Shi and Pestka 2009; Wang et al. 2011).

Nuclear factor erythroid 2 p45 (NF-E2)–related factor 2 (Nrf2), a redox-sensitive transcription factor, mediates DHA suppression of COX2, IL-1β, IL-6, and TNFα, possibly by reducing the levels of ROS and NO (Wang et al. 2010). The role of Nrf2 in suppressing LPS-mediated inflammation by DHA and EPA was investigated ex vivo with primary peritoneal macrophages from Nrf2 wild-type and knockout mice. Quantitative real-time PCR analyses showed that LPS potently induced expression of COX2, iNOS, IL-1β, IL-6, and TNFα in the macrophages collected from Nrf2 wild-type mice. DHA and EPA inhibited LPS-induced expression of COX2, iNOS, IL-1β, IL-6, and TNFα but increased HO-1 expression. DHA was found to be more potent than EPA in inhibiting COX2, iNOS, IL-1β, IL-6, and TNFα mRNA expression. DHA and EPA were also found to induce HO-1 and Nrf2 mRNA with a different dose response. However, in the macrophages collected from Nrf2 knockout mice, DHA and EPA suppression of LPS-induced expression of COX2, iNOS, IL-1β, IL-6, and TNFα was attenuated as compared to that in Nrf2 wild-type macrophages. These results suggest that Nrf2 plays a role in DHA/EPA suppression of LPS-induced inflammation (Wang et al. 2010).

16.5 PRORESOLVING METABOLITES OF DHA

Inflammation is the main defense mechanism against infection and various deleterious insults. Once the acute inflammation is initiated, the proinflammatory cytokines are released to recruit neutrophils to the inflammatory site. Subsequently, monocytes and macrophages are further engaged for effective phagocytosis (Serhan and Petasis 2011). During this process, a lipid mediator class switching occurs, from the initial proinflammatory mediators to the proresolving mediators, in order to promote the resolution phase that returns the body to homeostasis (Serhan 2007). If the acute inflammation is not completely resolved, the inflammatory responses might be prolonged and aggravated, leading to chronic inflammation (Serhan, Chiang, and Van Dyke 2008).

In recent years, a series of novel lipid metabolites derived from EPA and DHA were found to play an active role in stimulating the resolution of self-limited acute inflammation. Members of each limit neutrophilic infiltration, suppress release of local mediators (chemokines, cytokines) in inflamed sites, and/or stimulate monocyte/macrophage-enhanced clearance of apoptotic PMN, cellular debris, and microbes (Oh, Vickery, and Serhan 2011). Among the proresolving molecules, resolvins, including those of the D and E series, are endogenous lipid mediators generated from DHA and EPA, respectively, during the resolution phase of acute inflammation. Resolvins have been shown to possess both anti-inflammatory and proresolving actions in several animal models of inflammation. Resolvins act on their receptors in immune cells and neurons to normalize exaggerated pain via regulation of inflammatory mediators, transient receptor potential ion channels, and spinal cord synaptic transmission (Ji et al. 2011).

Notably, resolvin D1, an anti-inflammatory and proresolving mediator biosynthesized from DHA, markedly attenuated IFNγ/LPS-induced Th1 cytokines while upregulating arginase 1 expression in a concentration-dependent manner. Resolvin D1 also stimulated nonphlogistic phagocytosis in adipose stromal vascular cell macrophages by increasing both the number of macrophages containing ingested particles and the number of phagocytosed particles and by reducing macrophage ROS production. No changes in the adipocyte area and the phosphorylation of hormone-sensitive lipase, a rate-limiting enzyme regulating adipocyte lipolysis, were observed. These findings illustrate novel mechanisms by which resolvin D1 and its precursor DHA confer anti-inflammatory and proresolving actions in inflamed adipose tissue (Titos et al. 2011).

DHA is also a substrate for other anti-inflammatory mediators, such as neuroprotectin and maresin. They are formed in cooperating cells present in the region of inflammation in a process called transcellular biosynthesis, with the aid of specific LOX and COX. Proresolving anti-inflammatory mediators exert their biological activities in a receptor-dependent manner in the resolution phase of inflammation (Nowak 2010). Figure 16.3 depicts the chemical structures of some representative DHA-derived bioactive lipid mediators with potent proresolving/anti-inflammatory activity.

16.6 CHEMOPREVENTIVE POTENTIAL

A combination of curcumin, an anti-inflammatory phytochemical, and DHA had synergistic effects on endogenous or LPS-stimulated production of NO in RAW 264.7 cells. Curcumin and DHA also synergistically suppressed the LPS-induced PGE_2 production. The combinations were also found to suppress the expression of iNOS, COX2, 5-LOX, and $cPLA_2$ while inducing the anti-inflammatory enzyme HO-1 (Saw, Huang, and Kong 2010).

Epidemiological studies suggest that high fish intake is associated with a reduced risk of colorectal cancer, which has been linked to the high content of the n-3 PUFAs, including DHA. Gene expression profiles in preneoplastic LT97 colon adenoma cells were analyzed in response to DHA as well as EPA treatment by utilizing custom-designed cDNA arrays. DHA and EPA generally modulated different sets of genes, although a few common effects were noted (Habermann et al. 2009).

Infection with *Helicobacter pylori* is linked to inflammation and is the main cause of peptic ulcer, gastritis, and gastric malignancies. To examine associations between the gastric cancer risk and the erythrocyte composition of DHA, a case-control study of 179 incident gastric cancer cases and 357 noncancer controls (matched by age, sex, and season of sample collection) was conducted. The gastric cancer risk did not seem to be directly associated with dietary intake of fish oil and n-3 PUFA. However, the erythrocyte composition of DHA was found to be negatively linked to the risk of gastric cancer, especially of well-differentiated adenocarcinoma (Kuriki et al. 2007).

The antitumor effects of DHA, alone or in combination with cisplatin (CP), were evaluated in the Ehrlich ascites carcinoma solid tumor mouse model, with concomitant monitoring of changes in serum levels of CRP; lipid peroxidation (measured as malondialdehyde [MDA]); and leukocytic count (LC). DHA (125 or 250 mg/kg) elicited significant, dose-dependent reductions in the tumor size as well as in LC, CRP, and MDA levels. Interestingly, DHA (125 mg/kg) markedly enhanced the chemopreventive effects of CP and boosted its ability to reduce serum CRP and MDA levels. Rats treated with DHA (250 mg/kg, but not 125 mg/kg) survived the lethal effects of CP and showed a significant recovery of glomerular filtration rate, while their homogenates had markedly reduced MDA and TNFα but increased GSH levels. This study reveals that DHA can obliterate the lethal CP-induced renal tissue injury (El-Mesery et al. 2009).

Recently, resolvins have become the topic of intense interest because of expanding views on their action, particularly in chronic disorders where unresolved inflammation is a key pathogenic factor. Resolvins are biosynthesized from DHA via COX2/LOX pathways. They are shown to dramatically reduce dermal inflammation, peritonitis, DC migration, and IL production. Resolvins are endogenously generated during the spontaneous resolution phase. The role of proresolving mediators

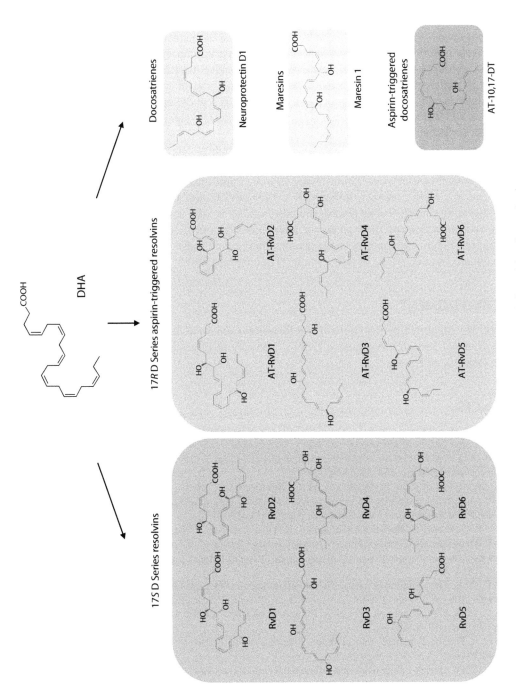

FIGURE 16.3 Major bioactive products derived from DHA: resolvins, docosatrienes, and their aspirin-triggered epimers.

in preventing chronic inflammation, which leads to carcinogenesis, need further investigation (Janakiram and Rao 2009).

16.7 CONCLUDING REMARKS

Low-grade systemic inflammation is a common denominator of the metabolic syndrome and implicated in diverse pathological conditions such as obesity, hypertension, type 2 diabetes mellitus, atherosclerosis, coronary artery disease, lupus, neurodegenerative disorders, nonalcoholic fatty liver disease, and some types of cancer. There has been a growing body of epidemiological, clinical, and experimental evidence underscoring protective effects of DHA or dietary fish oil enriched with this long-chain n-3 PUFA against pathogenesis of some cancers. The pleiotropic effects of DHA have largely been attributed to its anti-inflammatory property.

Recent studies on the formation of a distinct set of metabolites derived from DHA have revealed the endogenous formation of several novel lipid mediators called resolvins, especially those of the D series, and protectins, which have proresolving as well as anti-inflammatory effects. If not resolved properly and in a timely manner, inflammation becomes chronic and can cause various human diseases including cancer. In this regard, the proresolving as well as anti-inflammatory effects of resolvins and protectins and their precursor DHA merit therapeutic applications in the management of cancer. Future development of therapeutically relevant, stable analogs capable of activating inflammation resolution will be of prime interest (Bannenberg 2009).

ACKNOWLEDGMENT

This work was supported by the Global Core Research Center (GCRC) grant (no. 2012-0001184) from the National Research Foundation (NRF), Ministry of Education, Science and Technology (MEST), Republic of Korea.

REFERENCES

Ambrozova, G., M. Pekarova, and A. Lojek. 2010. Effect of polyunsaturated fatty acids on the reactive oxygen and nitrogen species production by raw 264.7 macrophages. *Eur J Nutr* 49 (3):133–9.

Bannenberg, G. L. 2009. Resolvins: Current understanding and future potential in the control of inflammation. *Curr Opin Drug Discov Dev* 12 (5):644–58.

Bouwens, M., O. van de Rest, N. Dellschaft, M. G. Bromhaar, L. C. de Groot, J. M. Geleijnse, M. Muller, and L. A. Afman. 2009. Fish-oil supplementation induces antiinflammatory gene expression profiles in human blood mononuclear cells. *Am J Clin Nutr* 90 (2):415–24.

Brand, A., N. G. Bauer, A. Hallott, O. Goldbaum, K. Ghebremeskel, R. Reifen, and C. Richter-Landsberg. 2010. Membrane lipid modification by polyunsaturated fatty acids sensitizes oligodendroglial OLN-93 cells against oxidative stress and promotes up-regulation of heme oxygenase-1 (HSP32). *J Neurochem* 113 (2):465–76.

Calder, P. C. 2006. Polyunsaturated fatty acids and inflammation. *Prostaglandins Leukot Essent Fatty Acids* 75 (3):197–202.

Calder, P. C. 2008. Polyunsaturated fatty acids, inflammatory processes and inflammatory bowel diseases. *Mol Nutr Food Res* 52 (8):885–97.

Calder, P. C. 2009. Polyunsaturated fatty acids and inflammatory processes: New twists in an old tale. *Biochimie* 91 (6):791–5.

Calder, P. C. 2010. Omega-3 fatty acids and inflammatory processes. *Nutrients* 2 (3):355–74.

Chapkin, R. S., W. Kim, J. R. Lupton, and D. N. McMurray. 2009. Dietary docosahexaenoic and eicosapentaenoic acid: emerging mediators of inflammation. *Prostaglandins Leukot Essent Fatty Acids* 81 (2–3):187–91.

Chen, W., W. J. Esselman, D. B. Jump, and J. V. Busik. 2005. Anti-inflammatory effect of docosahexaenoic acid on cytokine-induced adhesion molecule expression in human retinal vascular endothelial cells. *Invest Ophthalmol Vis Sci* 46 (11):4342–7.

Chen, W. Y., S. Y. Lin, H. C. Pan, S. L. Liao, Y. H. Chuang, Y. J. Yen, and C. J. Chen. 2012. Beneficial effect of docosahexaenoic acid on cholestatic liver injury in rats. *J Nutr Biochem* 23 (3):252–64.

Cho, J. Y., S. G. Chi, and H. S. Chun. 2011. Oral administration of docosahexaenoic acid attenuates colitis induced by dextran sulfate sodium in mice. *Mol Nutr Food Res* 55 (2):239–46.

Collie-Duguid, E. S., and K. W. Wahle. 1996. Inhibitory effect of fish oil N-3 polyunsaturated fatty acids on the expression of endothelial cell adhesion molecules. *Biochem Biophys Res Commun* 220 (3):969–74.

Cotogni, P., G. Muzio, A. Trombetta, V. M. Ranieri, and R. A. Canuto. 2011. Impact of the omega-3 to omega-6 polyunsaturated fatty acid ratio on cytokine release in human alveolar cells. *JPEN J Parenter Enteral Nutr* 35 (1):114–21.

Cottin, S. C., T. A. Sanders, and W. L. Hall. 2011. The differential effects of EPA and DHA on cardiovascular risk factors. *Proc Nutr Soc* 70 (2):215–31.

De Caterina, R., M. I. Cybulsky, S. K. Clinton, M. A. Gimbrone, Jr., and P. Libby. 1994. The omega-3 fatty acid docosahexaenoate reduces cytokine-induced expression of proatherogenic and proinflammatory proteins in human endothelial cells. *Arterioscler Thromb* 14 (11):1829–36.

Deike, E., R. G. Bowden, J. J. Moreillon, J. O. Griggs, R. L. Wilson, M. Cooke, B. D. Shelmadine, and A. A. Beaujean. 2012. The effects of fish oil supplementation on markers of inflammation in chronic kidney disease patients. *J Ren Nutr* 22 (6):572–7.

Draper, E., C. M. Reynolds, M. Canavan, K. H. Mills, C. E. Loscher, and H. M. Roche. 2011. Omega-3 fatty acids attenuate dendritic cell function via NF-kappaB independent of PPARgamma. *J Nutr Biochem* 22 (8):784–90.

El-Mesery, M., M. Al-Gayyar, H. Salem, M. Darweish, and A. El-Mowafy. 2009. Chemopreventive and renal protective effects for docosahexaenoic acid (DHA): implications of CRP and lipid peroxides. *Cell Div* 4:6.

Finocchiaro, C., O. Segre, M. Fadda, T. Monge, M. Scigliano, M. Schena, M. Tinivella, E. Tiozzo, M. G. Catalano, M. Pugliese, N. Fortunati, M. Aragno, G. Muzio, M. Maggiora, M. Oraldi, and R. A. Canuto. 2011. Effect of n-3 fatty acids on patients with advanced lung cancer: A double-blind, placebo-controlled study. *Br J Nutr* 1–7.

Gravaghi, C., K. M. La Perle, P. Ogrodwski, J. X. Kang, F. Quimby, M. Lipkin, and S. A. Lamprecht. 2011. Cox-2 expression, PGE(2) and cytokines production are inhibited by endogenously synthesized n-3 PUFAs in inflamed colon of fat-1 mice. *J Nutr Biochem* 22 (4):360–5.

Habermann, N., E. K. Lund, B. L. Pool-Zobel, and M. Glei. 2009. Modulation of gene expression in eicosapentaenoic acid and docosahexaenoic acid treated human colon adenoma cells. *Genes Nutr* 4 (1):73–6.

Halade, G. V., M. M. Rahman, A. Bhattacharya, J. L. Barnes, B. Chandrasekar, and G. Fernandes. 2010. Docosahexaenoic acid-enriched fish oil attenuates kidney disease and prolongs median and maximal life span of autoimmune lupus-prone mice. *J Immunol* 184 (9):5280–6.

Hudert, C. A., K. H. Weylandt, Y. Lu, J. Wang, S. Hong, A. Dignass, C. N. Serhan, and J. X. Kang. 2006. Transgenic mice rich in endogenous omega-3 fatty acids are protected from colitis. *Proc Natl Acad Sci U S A* 103 (30):11276–81.

Ibrahim, A., K. Mbodji, A. Hassan, M. Aziz, N. Boukhettala, M. Coeffier, G. Savoye, P. Dechelotte, and R. Marion-Letellier. 2011. Anti-inflammatory and anti-angiogenic effect of long chain n-3 polyunsaturated fatty acids in intestinal microvascular endothelium. *Clin Nutr* 30 (5):678–87.

Itoh, T., and K. Yamamoto. 2008. Peroxisome proliferator activated receptor gamma and oxidized docosahexaenoic acids as new class of ligand. *Naunyn Schmiedebergs Arch Pharmacol* 377 (4–6):541–7.

Janakiram, N. B., and C. V. Rao. 2009. Role of lipoxins and resolvins as anti-inflammatory and proresolving mediators in colon cancer. *Curr Mol Med* 9 (5):565–79.

Ji, R. R., Z. Z. Xu, G. Strichartz, and C. N. Serhan. 2011. Emerging roles of resolvins in the resolution of inflammation and pain. *Trends Neurosci* 34 (11):599–609.

Kang, J. X., J. Wang, L. Wu, and Z. B. Kang. 2004. Transgenic mice: fat-1 mice convert n-6 to n-3 fatty acids. *Nature* 427 (6974):504.

Kelley, D. S., D. Siegel, D. M. Fedor, Y. Adkins, and B. E. Mackey. 2009. DHA supplementation decreases serum C-reactive protein and other markers of inflammation in hypertriglyceridemic men. *J Nutr* 139 (3):495–501.

Kim, Y. J., and H. Y. Chung. 2007. Antioxidative and anti-inflammatory actions of docosahexaenoic acid and eicosapentaenoic acid in renal epithelial cells and macrophages. *J Med Food* 10 (2):225–31.

Komatsu, W., K. Ishihara, M. Murata, H. Saito, and K. Shinohara. 2003. Docosahexaenoic acid suppresses nitric oxide production and inducible nitric oxide synthase expression in interferon-gamma plus lipopolysaccharide-stimulated murine macrophages by inhibiting the oxidative stress. *Free Radic Biol Med* 34 (8):1006–16.

Kong, W., J. H. Yen, E. Vassiliou, S. Adhikary, M. G. Toscano, and D. Ganea. 2010. Docosahexaenoic acid prevents dendritic cell maturation and in vitro and in vivo expression of the IL-12 cytokine family. *Lipids Health Dis* 9:12.

Kong, W., J. H. Yen, and D. Ganea. 2011. Docosahexaenoic acid prevents dendritic cell maturation, inhibits antigen-specific Th1/Th17 differentiation and suppresses experimental autoimmune encephalomyelitis. *Brain Behav Immun* 25 (5):872–82.

Kundu, J. K., and Y. J. Surh. 2012. Emerging avenues linking inflammation and cancer. *Free Radic Biol Med* 52 (9):2013–37.

Kuriki, K., K. Wakai, K. Matsuo, A. Hiraki, T. Suzuki, Y. Yamamura, K. Yamao, T. Nakamura, M. Tatematsu, and K. Tajima. 2007. Gastric cancer risk and erythrocyte composition of docosahexaenoic acid with anti-inflammatory effects. *Cancer Epidemiol Biomarkers Prev* 16 (11):2406–15.

Lee, J. Y., A. Plakidas, W. H. Lee, A. Heikkinen, P. Chanmugam, G. Bray, and D. H. Hwang. 2003. Differential modulation of Toll-like receptors by fatty acids: Preferential inhibition by n-3 polyunsaturated fatty acids. *J Lipid Res* 44 (3):479–86.

Li, H., X. Z. Ruan, S. H. Powis, R. Fernando, W. Y. Mon, D. C. Wheeler, J. F. Moorhead, and Z. Varghese. 2005. EPA and DHA reduce LPS-induced inflammation responses in HK-2 cells: Evidence for a PPAR-gamma-dependent mechanism. *Kidney Int* 67 (3):867–74.

Lu, D. Y., Y. Y. Tsao, Y. M. Leung, and K. P. Su. 2010. Docosahexaenoic acid suppresses neuroinflammatory responses and induces heme oxygenase-1 expression in BV-2 microglia: Implications of antidepressant effects for omega-3 fatty acids. *Neuropsychopharmacology* 35 (11):2238–48.

Lu, J., T. Jilling, D. Li, and M. S. Caplan. 2007. Polyunsaturated fatty acid supplementation alters proinflammatory gene expression and reduces the incidence of necrotizing enterocolitis in a neonatal rat model. *Pediatr Res* 61 (4):427–32.

Marion-Letellier, R., M. Butler, P. Dechelotte, R. J. Playford, and S. Ghosh. 2008. Comparison of cytokine modulation by natural peroxisome proliferator-activated receptor gamma ligands with synthetic ligands in intestinal-like Caco-2 cells and human dendritic cells—potential for dietary modulation of peroxisome proliferator-activated receptor gamma in intestinal inflammation. *Am J Clin Nutr* 87 (4):939–48.

Martinez-Micaelo, N., N. Gonzalez-Abuin, X. Terra, C. Richart, A. Ardevol, M. Pinent, and M. Blay. 2012. Omega-3 docosahexaenoic acid and procyanidins inhibit cyclo-oxygenase activity and attenuate NF-kappaB activation through a p105/p50 regulatory mechanism in macrophage inflammation. *Biochem J* 441 (2):653–63.

Massaro, M., A. Habib, L. Lubrano, S. Del Turco, G. Lazzerini, T. Bourcier, B. B. Weksler, and R. De Caterina. 2006. The omega-3 fatty acid docosahexaenoate attenuates endothelial cyclooxygenase-2 induction through both NADP(H) oxidase and PKC epsilon inhibition. *Proc Natl Acad Sci U S A* 103 (41):15184–9.

Mayer, K., A. Kiessling, J. Ott, M. B. Schaefer, M. Hecker, I. Henneke, R. Schulz, A. Gunther, J. Wang, L. Wu, J. Roth, W. Seeger, and J. X. Kang. 2009. Acute lung injury is reduced in fat-1 mice endogenously synthesizing n-3 fatty acids. *Am J Respir Crit Care Med* 179 (6):474–83.

McDaniel, J. C., K. Massey, and A. Nicolaou. 2011. Fish oil supplementation alters levels of lipid mediators of inflammation in microenvironment of acute human wounds. *Wound Repair Regen* 19 (2):189–200.

McNamara, R. K., R. Jandacek, T. Rider, P. Tso, A. Cole-Strauss, and J. W. Lipton. 2010. Omega-3 fatty acid deficiency increases constitutive pro-inflammatory cytokine production in rats: Relationship with central serotonin turnover. *Prostaglandins Leukot Essent Fatty Acids* 83 (4-6):185–91.

Mickleborough, T. D., S. L. Tecklenburg, G. S. Montgomery, and M. R. Lindley. 2009. Eicosapentaenoic acid is more effective than docosahexaenoic acid in inhibiting proinflammatory mediator production and transcription from LPS-induced human asthmatic alveolar macrophage cells. *Clin Nutr* 28 (1):71–7.

Moreno-Aliaga, M. J., S. Lorente-Cebrian, and J. A. Martinez. 2010. Regulation of adipokine secretion by n-3 fatty acids. *Proc Nutr Soc* 69 (3):324–32.

Morteau, O. 2000. Prostaglandins and inflammation: The cyclooxygenase controversy. *Arch Immunol Ther Exp (Warsz)* 48 (6):473–80.

Mullen, A., C. E. Loscher, and H. M. Roche. 2010. Anti-inflammatory effects of EPA and DHA are dependent upon time and dose-response elements associated with LPS stimulation in THP-1-derived macrophages. *J Nutr Biochem* 21 (5):444–50.

Nakamura, N., T. Hamazaki, M. Kobayashi, and K. Yazawa. 1994. The effect of oral administration of eicosapentaenoic and docosahexaenoic acids on acute inflammation and fatty acid composition in rats. *J Nutr Sci Vitaminol (Tokyo)* 40 (2):161–70.

Nauroth, J. M., Y. C. Liu, M. Van Elswyk, R. Bell, E. B. Hall, G. Chung, and L. M. Arterburn. 2010. Docosahexaenoic acid (DHA) and docosapentaenoic acid (DPAn-6) algal oils reduce inflammatory mediators in human peripheral mononuclear cells in vitro and paw edema in vivo. *Lipids* 45 (5):375–84.

Nowak, J. Z. 2010. [Anti-inflammatory pro-resolving derivatives of omega-3 and omega-6 polyunsaturated fatty acids]. *Postepy Hig Med Dosw (Online)* 64:115–32.

Oh, D. Y., S. Talukdar, E. J. Bae, T. Imamura, H. Morinaga, W. Fan, P. Li, W. J. Lu, S. M. Watkins, and J. M. Olefsky. 2010. GPR120 is an omega-3 fatty acid receptor mediating potent anti-inflammatory and insulin-sensitizing effects. *Cell* 142 (5):687–98.

Oh, S. F., T. W. Vickery, and C. N. Serhan. 2011. Chiral lipidomics of E-series resolvins: Aspirin and the biosynthesis of novel mediators. *Biochim Biophys Acta* 1811 (11):737–47.

Ohtsuka, Y., K. Okada, Y. Yamakawa, T. Ikuse, Y. Baba, E. Inage, T. Fujii, H. Izumi, K. Oshida, S. Nagata, Y. Yamashiro, and T. Shimizu. 2011. omega-3 fatty acids attenuate mucosal inflammation in premature rat pups. *J Pediatr Surg* 46 (3):489–95.

Oliver, E., F. C. McGillicuddy, K. A. Harford, C. M. Reynolds, C. M. Phillips, J. F. Ferguson, and H. M. Roche. 2011. Docosahexaenoic acid attenuates macrophage-induced inflammation and improves insulin sensitivity in adipocytes-specific differential effects between LC n-3 PUFA. *J Nutr Biochem* 23 (9):1192–200.

Opreanu, M., T. A. Lydic, G. E. Reid, K. M. McSorley, W. J. Esselman, and J. V. Busik. 2010. Inhibition of cytokine signaling in human retinal endothelial cells through downregulation of sphingomyelinases by docosahexaenoic acid. *Invest Ophthalmol Vis Sci* 51 (6):3253–63.

Park, K. S., J. W. Lim, and H. Kim. 2009. Inhibitory mechanism of omega-3 fatty acids in pancreatic inflammation and apoptosis. *Ann N Y Acad Sci* 1171:421–7.

Rahman, M. M., A. Bhattacharya, and G. Fernandes. 2008. Docosahexaenoic acid is more potent inhibitor of osteoclast differentiation in RAW 264.7 cells than eicosapentaenoic acid. *J Cell Physiol* 214 (1):201–9.

Rahman, M., J. K. Kundu, J. W. Shin, H. K. Na, and Y. J. Surh. 2011. Docosahexaenoic acid inhibits UVB-induced activation of NF-kappaB and expression of COX-2 and NOX-4 in HR-1 hairless mouse skin by blocking MSK1 signaling. *PLoS One* 6 (11):e28065.

Rasic-Milutinovic, Z., G. Perunicic, S. Pljesa, Z. Gluvic, S. Sobajic, I. Djuric, and D. Ristic. 2007. Effects of N-3 PUFAs supplementation on insulin resistance and inflammatory biomarkers in hemodialysis patients. *Ren Fail* 29 (3):321–9.

Richard, D., C. Wolf, U. Barbe, K. Kefi, P. Bausero, and F. Visioli. 2009. Docosahexaenoic acid down-regulates endothelial Nox 4 through a sPLA2 signalling pathway. *Biochem Biophys Res Commun* 389 (3):516–22.

Rogers, L. K., C. J. Valentine, M. Pennell, M. Velten, R. D. Britt, K. Dingess, X. Zhao, S. E. Welty, and T. E. Tipple. 2011. Maternal docosahexaenoic acid supplementation decreases lung inflammation in hyperoxia-exposed newborn mice. *J Nutr* 141 (2):214–22.

Saw, C. L., Y. Huang, and A. N. Kong. 2010. Synergistic anti-inflammatory effects of low doses of curcumin in combination with polyunsaturated fatty acids: docosahexaenoic acid or eicosapentaenoic acid. *Biochem Pharmacol* 79 (3):421–30.

Schaefer, M. B., A. Wenzel, T. Fischer, R. C. Braun-Dullaeus, F. Renner, H. Dietrich, C. A. Schaefer, W. Seeger, and K. Mayer. 2008. Fatty acids differentially influence phosphatidylinositol 3-kinase signal transduction in endothelial cells: Impact on adhesion and apoptosis. *Atherosclerosis* 197 (2):630–7.

Serhan, C. N. 2007. Resolution phase of inflammation: Novel endogenous anti-inflammatory and proresolving lipid mediators and pathways. *Annu Rev Immunol* 25:101–37.

Serhan, C. N., and N. A. Petasis. 2011. Resolvins and protectins in inflammation resolution. *Chem Rev* 111 (10):5922–43.

Serhan, C. N., N. Chiang, and T. E. Van Dyke. 2008. Resolving inflammation: Dual anti-inflammatory and pro-resolution lipid mediators. *Nat Rev Immunol* 8 (5):349–61.

Serini, S., E. Fasano, E. Piccioni, A. R. Cittadini, and G. Calviello. 2011. Differential anti-cancer effects of purified EPA and DHA and possible mechanisms involved. *Curr Med Chem* 18 (26):4065–75.

Shi, Y., and J. J. Pestka. 2009. Mechanisms for suppression of interleukin-6 expression in peritoneal macrophages from docosahexaenoic acid-fed mice. *J Nutr Biochem* 20 (5):358–68.

Siddiqui, R. A., K. A. Harvey, N. Ruzmetov, S. J. Miller, and G. P. Zaloga. 2009. n-3 fatty acids prevent whereas trans-fatty acids induce vascular inflammation and sudden cardiac death. *Br J Nutr* 102 (12):1811–9.

Sierra, S., F. Lara-Villoslada, M. Comalada, M. Olivares, and J. Xaus. 2008. Dietary eicosapentaenoic acid and docosahexaenoic acid equally incorporate as decosahexaenoic acid but differ in inflammatory effects. *Nutrition* 24 (3):245–54.

Silva Jde, A., E. B. Trindade, M. E. Fabre, V. M. Menegotto, S. Gevaerd, S. Buss Zda, and T. S. Frode. 2012. Fish oil supplement alters markers of inflammatory and nutritional status in colorectal cancer patients. *Nutr Cancer* 64 (2):267–73.

Simopoulos, A. P. 2002. The importance of the ratio of omega-6/omega-3 essential fatty acids. *Biomed Pharmacother* 56 (8):365–79.

Storey, A., F. McArdle, P. S. Friedmann, M. J. Jackson, and L. E. Rhodes. 2005. Eicosapentaenoic acid and docosahexaenoic acid reduce UVB- and TNF-alpha-induced IL-8 secretion in keratinocytes and UVB-induced IL-8 in fibroblasts. *J Invest Dermatol* 124 (1):248–55.

Surh, Y. J. 2003. Cancer chemoprevention with dietary phytochemicals. *Nat Rev Cancer* 3 (10):768–80.

Takayama, F., K. Nakamoto, N. Totani, T. Yamanushi, H. Kabuto, T. Kaneyuki, and M. Mankura. 2010. Effects of docosahexaenoic acid in an experimental rat model of nonalcoholic steatohepatitis. *J Oleo Sci* 59 (8):407–14.

Titos, E., B. Rius, A. Gonzalez-Periz, C. Lopez-Vicario, E. Moran-Salvador, M. Martinez-Clemente, V. Arroyo, and J. Claria. 2011. Resolvin D1 and its precursor docosahexaenoic acid promote resolution of adipose tissue inflammation by eliciting macrophage polarization toward an M2-like phenotype. *J Immunol* 187 (10):5408–18.

Tomobe, Y. I., K. Morizawa, M. Tsuchida, H. Hibino, Y. Nakano, and Y. Tanaka. 2000. Dietary docosahexaenoic acid suppresses inflammation and immunoresponses in contact hypersensitivity reaction in mice. *Lipids* 35 (1):61–9.

Vincentini, O., M. G. Quaranta, M. Viora, C. Agostoni, and M. Silano. 2011. Docosahexaenoic acid modulates in vitro the inflammation of celiac disease in intestinal epithelial cells via the inhibition of cPLA2. *Clin Nutr* 30 (4):541–6.

Wall, R., R. P. Ross, G. F. Fitzgerald, and C. Stanton. 2010. Fatty acids from fish: The anti-inflammatory potential of long-chain omega-3 fatty acids. *Nutr Rev* 68 (5):280–9.

Wang, H., T. O. Khor, C. L. Saw, W. Lin, T. Wu, Y. Huang, and A. N. Kong. 2010. Role of Nrf2 in suppressing LPS-induced inflammation in mouse peritoneal macrophages by polyunsaturated fatty acids docosahexaenoic acid and eicosapentaenoic acid. *Mol Pharm* 7 (6):2185–93.

Wang, T. M., C. J. Chen, T. S. Lee, H. Y. Chao, W. H. Wu, S. C. Hsieh, H. H. Sheu, and A. N. Chiang. 2011. Docosahexaenoic acid attenuates VCAM-1 expression and NF-kappaB activation in TNF-alpha-treated human aortic endothelial cells. *J Nutr Biochem* 22 (2):187–94.

Wang, Y., Q. Liu, and H. Thorlacius. 2003. Docosahexaenoic acid inhibits cytokine-induced expression of P-selectin and neutrophil adhesion to endothelial cells. *Eur J Pharmacol* 459 (2–3):269–73.

Weldon, S. M., A. C. Mullen, C. E. Loscher, L. A. Hurley, and H. M. Roche. 2007. Docosahexaenoic acid induces an anti-inflammatory profile in lipopolysaccharide-stimulated human THP-1 macrophages more effectively than eicosapentaenoic acid. *J Nutr Biochem* 18 (4):250–8.

Weylandt, K. H., A. Nadolny, L. Kahlke, T. Kohnke, C. Schmocker, J. Wang, G. Y. Lauwers, J. N. Glickman, and J. X. Kang. 2008. Reduction of inflammation and chronic tissue damage by omega-3 fatty acids in fat-1 transgenic mice with pancreatitis. *Biochim Biophys Acta* 1782 (11):634–41.

Yates, C. M., S. P. Tull, J. Madden, P. C. Calder, R. F. Grimble, G. B. Nash, and G. E. Rainger. 2011. Docosahexaenoic acid inhibits the adhesion of flowing neutrophils to cytokine stimulated human umbilical vein endothelial cells. *J Nutr* 141 (7):1331–4.

Zapata-Gonzalez, F., F. Rueda, J. Petriz, P. Domingo, F. Villarroya, J. Diaz-Delfin, M. A. de Madariaga, and J. C. Domingo. 2008. Human dendritic cell activities are modulated by the omega-3 fatty acid, docosahexaenoic acid, mainly through PPAR(gamma):RXR heterodimers: Comparison with other polyunsaturated fatty acids. *J Leukoc Biol* 84 (4):1172–82.

Zuniga, J., M. Cancino, F. Medina, P. Varela, R. Vargas, G. Tapia, L. A. Videla, and V. Fernandez. 2011. N-3 PUFA supplementation triggers PPAR-alpha activation and PPAR-alpha/NF-kappaB interaction: Anti-inflammatory implications in liver ischemia-reperfusion injury. *PLoS One* 6 (12):e28502.

Section VI

Flavonoids and Polyphenols

17 Green Tea and Cancer Prevention

Naghma Khan and Hasan Mukhtar

CONTENTS

17.1 INTRODUCTION

Tea is the most consumed beverage in the world, next to water. Of the total amount of tea undergoing different manufacturing processes produced and consumed globally, 78% is black tea, 20% is green tea, and <2% is oolong tea (Ju et al. 2007). Black tea is fully fermented, oolong tea is partially fermented, and green tea is not at all fermented but only steamed. Green tea is consumed mostly in China, Japan, India, and a few countries in North Africa and the Middle East, black tea is consumed primarily in Western countries and in some Asian countries, while oolong tea consumption is limited to southeastern China and Taiwan (Khan et al. 2008). Green tea was always considered as a healthy beverage in ancient Chinese medicine. In the past few years, the chemical constituents of green tea received great scientific attention for their beneficial health effects and lack of toxicity. The intake of green tea has been shown to lower blood pressure and the risk of cardiovascular diseases, prevent the development of atherosclerosis, improve lipid profile, and have antithrombotic and anti-inflammatory properties. Green tea contains characteristic polyphenolic compounds, (–)-epigallocatechin-3-gallate (EGCG), (–)-epigallocatechin (EGC), (–)-epicatechin-3-gallate (ECG), and (–)-epicatechin (EC). These compounds are commonly known as catechins. Most of the studies carried out with green tea are with green tea polyphenols (GTPs) or individual catechins, especially EGCG. Green tea has received considerable attention due to its plentiful, scientifically proven, favorable effects on the health of humans. One cup of green tea contains 200 mg of EGCG, which has been reported to have chemopreventive effects against numerous cancers (Yang et al. 2002, 2009). Appropriate drinking of green tea is 3 to 5 cups per day, which provides a minimum of 250 mg per day of catechins (Boehm et al. 2009). The effects of green tea on the activities of various receptor tyrosine kinases and pathways of signal transduction have also been reported (Khan and Mukhtar 2008). EGCG has also been shown to inhibit tumor invasion and angiogenesis, critical for tumor growth and metastasis (Khan and Mukhtar 2010). In this chapter, we will discuss the effects of green tea and its polyphenols against cancers of the prostate, skin, lung, liver, breast, and gastrointestinal tract.

17.2 GREEN TEA AND PREVENTION OF CANCER

17.2.1 EFFECT OF GREEN TEA ON PROSTATE CANCER

It has been recently reported that GTP treatment of human prostate cancer (PCa) LNCaP cells (harboring wild-type p53) and PC-3 cells (lacking p53) caused inhibition of class I histone deacetylase (HDAC) enzyme activity and its protein expression with accumulation of acetylated histone H3 in total cellular chromatin, resulting in increased accessibility to bind with the promoter sequences of WAF1/p21 and Bax, similar to the effects elicited by an HDAC inhibitor, trichostatin A. GTP and proteasome inhibitor MG132 treatment of cells prevented degradation of class I HDACs, demonstrating increased proteasomal degradation of class I HDACs by GTP. There was also G(0)–G(1)–phase cell-cycle arrest and induction of apoptosis in both LNCaP and PC-3 cell lines (Thakur et al. 2011). A study from our lab has recently shown that EGCG is a direct antagonist of androgen action. EGCG was found to physically interact with the ligand-binding domain of the androgen receptor (AR) by replacing a high-affinity labeled ligand by in silico modeling and fluorescence resonance energy transfer (FRET)-based competition assay. EGCG was also found to inhibit AR nuclear translocation and protein expression in a xenograft model with downregulation of androgen-regulated microRNA 21 (miRNA-21) and upregulation of a tumor suppressor, miRNA-330, in tumors of mice treated with EGCG (Siddiqui et al. 2011). Patients with positive prostate biopsies and scheduled for radical prostatectomy were given daily doses of polyphenon E (PPE), containing 800 mg of EGCG and lesser amounts of EC, EGC, and ECG until the time of radical prostatectomy. There was a significant reduction in serum levels of prostate-specific antigen (PSA), hepatocyte growth factor (HGF), and vascular endothelial growth factor (VEGF) without the elevation of liver enzymes (McLarty et al. 2009). The consumption of GTP was found to significantly inhibit PCa development and metastasis in a transgenic adenocarcinoma of the mouse prostate (TRAMP) model. This was achieved by an oral infusion of GTP equivalent to six cups of green tea a day, that is, at an achievable dose in humans (Gupta et al. 2001). A study from our lab has identified the stage of PCa that is most vulnerable to chemopreventive intervention by GTP in TRAMP mice. The animals were selected at different ages representing different stages of the disease and initiated with oral feeding of GTP (0.1% in drinking water ad libitum) as follows: (1) 6 weeks, mice with normal prostate pathology; (2) 12 weeks, when mice histologically display hyperplasia; (3) 18 weeks, when well-differentiated adenocarcinoma was observed and; (4) 28 weeks, when mice display moderately differentiated adenocarcinoma. It was found that chemopreventive potential of GTP decreases with advancing age (Adhami et al. 2009). It has been shown that EGCG induced apoptosis in human PCa cells via stabilization of p53 by phosphorylation on critical serine residues and p14alternate reading frame (p14ARF)-mediated downregulation of murine double minute 2 (MDM2) protein, negative regulation of nuclear factor kappaB (NF-κB) activity, and activation of caspases, causing a change in the ratio of Bax/Bcl-2, favoring apoptosis (Hastak et al. 2003). Treatment with GTP was found to reduce the levels of insulin-like growth factor-I (IGF-I) and concomitantly increase insulin-like growth factor binding protein-3 (IGFBP-3), with inhibition of markers of angiogenesis and metastasis causing reduction in the downstream signaling and inhibition of PCa development and progression (Adhami et al. 2004). EGCG was found to inhibit early-stage but not late-stage PCa in TRAMP mice. In the ventrolateral prostate, EGCG significantly reduced cell proliferation, induced apoptosis, and decreased AR, IGF-I, IGF-I receptor (IGF-IR), phosphoextracellular signal–regulated kinases 1 and 2 (ERK1/2), cyclooxygenase 2 (COX2), and inducible nitric oxide synthase (iNOS) (Harper et al. 2007). The treatment of human PCa cells with a combination of EGCG and COX2 inhibitor resulted in enhanced cell growth inhibition, apoptosis induction, and inhibition of NF-κB. In athymic nude mice implanted with CWR22Rν1 cells, combination treatment with GTP and celecoxib resulted in enhanced tumor growth inhibition, lowering of PSA and IGF-I levels, and an increase in IGFBP-3 levels (Adhami et al. 2007).

17.2.2 Effect of Green Tea on Skin Cancer

Ellis et al. (2011) have recently reported that EGCG inhibits melanoma cell growth at physiological doses and inhibits NF-κB, which was associated with decreased interleukin 1β (IL-1β) secretion from melanoma cells. Treatment with EGCG also led to downregulation of the inflammasome component, nucleotide-binding oligomerization domain-like receptors P1 (NLRP1), and reduced caspase-1 activation. When the expression of NLRP1 was silenced, it abolished EGCG-induced inhibition of tumor cell proliferation (Ellis et al. 2011). Treatment with EGCG decreased global DNA methylation levels in A431 cells and decreased HDAC activity; the levels of 5-methylcytosine, DNA methyltransferase (DNMT) activity, and messenger RNA (mRNA); and protein levels of DNMT1, DNMT3a, and DNMT3b. It also increased levels of acetylated lysine 9 and 14 on histone H3 (H3-Lys 9 and 14) and acetylated lysine 5, 12, and 16 on histone H4 but decreased levels of methylated H3-Lys 9 and caused reexpression of the mRNA and proteins of silenced tumor suppressor genes, p16INK4a and Cip1/p21 (Nandakumar et al. 2011).

GTP in drinking water reduced UV-induced suppression of contact hypersensitivity (CHS) in response to a contact sensitizer in local CHS and models of CHS. GTP-treated mice had a reduced number of cyclobutane pyrimidine dimer–positive [CPD(+)] cells in the skin, showing faster repair of ultraviolet (UV)-induced DNA damage, and had a twofold reduced migration of CPD(+) cells from the skin to draining lymph nodes, which was associated with elevated levels of nucleotide excision repair (NER) genes as compared with untreated mice. Treatment with GTP did not prevent UV-induced immunosuppression in NER-deficient mice but prevented it in NER-proficient mice. GTP supplementation also repaired UV-induced CPDs in xeroderma pigmentosum complementation group A (XPA)–proficient cells of a healthy person but did not in XPA-deficient cells obtained from XPA patients, indicating that an NER mechanism is involved in DNA repair (Katiyar et al. 2010). We have reported that topical application of GTP resulted in a decrease in UVB-induced bifold skin thickness, skin edema, infiltration of leukocytes, and inhibition of mitogen-activated protein kinases (MAPKs) and NF-κB pathways in SKH-1 hairless mice (Afaq et al. 2003). We have earlier shown that GTP acts as anti-initiating agent against the skin tumorigenicity induced by polycyclic aromatic hydrocarbons in mice. Topical application of GTP to female BALB/c mice resulted in substantial protection against the onset and subsequent development of tumors. Topical application of GTP to female sensitivity to carcinogenesis (SENCAR) mice afforded significant protection against skin tumorigenicity in the two-stage 7,12-dimethylbenz(a)anthracene (DMBA)–2-O-tetradecanoylphorbol-13-acetate (TPA) skin tumorigenesis protocol. Oral feeding of GTP in drinking water to female SENCAR mice also protected against skin tumorigenesis (Wang et al. 1989). Topical application of a GTP fraction to the skin of DMBA-initiated mice, prior to that of TPA or mezerein, resulted in protection against skin tumor promotion and a decrease in tumor incidence, tumor multiplicity, and tumor volume. GTP treatment also protected against the malignant conversion of papillomas to squamous cell carcinomas (Katiyar et al. 1997). There was enhancement in the rate and extent of disappearance of the mutant p53-positive patches by the oral administration of green tea as the sole source of drinking fluid starting immediately after discontinuation of UVB treatment in SKH-1 mice (Lu et al. 2005). Using IL-12p40 knockout (KO) mice and their wild-type counterparts, it has been reported that although administration of GTP (0.2%, w/v) in drinking water significantly reduced UVB-induced tumor development in wild-type mice, this treatment had a nonsignificant effect in IL-12–KO mice. Treatment with GTP resulted in reduction in the levels of markers of inflammation and proinflammatory cytokines in chronically UVB-exposed skin and skin tumors of wild-type mice but was less effective in IL-12p40–KO mice. The DNA damage induced by UVB was resolved more rapidly in wild-type mice treated with GTP than in untreated wild-type mice, and this resolution followed the same time course as the GTP-induced reduction in the levels of inflammatory responses, with the effect of GTP less pronounced in IL-12–KO mice (Meeran et al. 2009). Hsu et al. (2007) recently determined whether MAPK pathways are required for GTP-induced caspase-14 expression in normal human epidermal keratinocytes (NHEKs) and whether GTP can modulate the expression of pathological markers in the psoriasiform lesions that develop in the flaky skin mouse. It was shown that p38 and c-Jun NH_2-terminal kinase (JNK) MAPK pathways are required for EGCG-induced expression of caspase-14 in NHEKs. The topical application of GTP significantly reduced the symptoms of epidermal pathology in the flaky skin mice, associated with efficient caspase-14 processing and reduction in proliferating cell nuclear antigen (PCNA) levels, suggesting that GTP-activated pathways may be potential targets for novel therapeutic approaches to the treatment of some psoriasiform skin disorders (Hsu et al. 2007). Oral administration of GTP reduced UVB-induced skin tumor incidence, tumor multiplicity, and tumor growth in SKH-1 mice. On treatment with GTP, there was a decrease in the expression of matrix metalloproteinase 2 (MMP-2), MMP-9, cluster of differentiation 31 (CD31), VEGF, and PCNA. In the tumors of the group that orally administered GTP, there was an increase in cytotoxic CD8(+) T cells and in the activation of caspase-3 (Mantena et al. 2005).

17.2.3 EFFECT OF GREEN TEA ON LIVER CANCER

Recently, it has been shown that in C57BL/KsJ-db/db (db/db) obese mice, drinking water with EGCG significantly inhibited the development of liver cell adenomas in comparison with the control EGCG-untreated group. Consumption of EGCG inhibited the phosphorylation of the IGF-IR, ERK, Akt, glycogen synthase kinase-3β (GSK-3β), signal transduction and activators of transcription (STAT)3, and JNK proteins in the livers of experimental mice. There was also a decrease in the serum levels of insulin, IGF-I, IGF-II, free fatty acid, and tumor necrosis factor α (TNFα). There was improvement in the liver steatosis and adenosine monophosphate (AMP)-activated kinase protein in the liver, suggesting that EGCG prevents obesity-related liver tumorigenesis by inhibiting the IGF/IGF-IR axis, improving hyperinsulinemia, and attenuating chronic inflammation (Shimizu et al. 2011). ECG and EGCG are the most abundant polyphenolic compounds in green tea. Liang et al. (2010) have reported that ECG or EGCG at higher doses had a slight inhibitory effect on cell proliferation in the resistant human hepatocellular carcinoma (HCC) cell line BEL-7404/doxorubicin (DOX) in vitro and in vivo. In a xenograft mouse model, the administration of DOX with these compounds at lower doses significantly inhibited HCC cell proliferation in vitro and hepatoma growth as compared with treatment with either ECG or EGCG at the same dose (Liang et al. 2010). The effects of EGCG on the activity of the VEGF–Vascular endothelial growth factor (VEGFR) axis in human HCC cells were examined. It was noted that the levels of total and phosphorylated forms of VEGFR-2 protein were increased in a series of human HCC cell lines in comparison to the normal Hc human hepatocytes. Treatment with EGCG inhibited the growth of HuH7 HCC cells, which express constitutive activation of the VEGF–VEGFR axis, in comparison to Hc cells, with a time- and dose-dependent decrease in the expression of VEGFR-2 and phospho-vascular endothelial growth factor 2 (p-VEGFR-2) proteins. In athymic nude mice, treatment with EGCG in drinking water inhibited the growth of HuH7 xenografts and was associated with inhibition of the activation of VEGFR-2, ERK, Akt, Bcl-xL, and VEGF mRNA in the xenografts (Shirakami et al. 2009). EGCG inhibited the growth of hepatocellular carcinoma cell lines, induced apoptosis, and downregulated Bcl-2 and Bcl-xL by inactivation of NF-κB. In xenograft tumors, oral treatment with EGCG showed similar effects. Cotreatment with EGCG and TNF-related apoptosis-inducing ligand (TRAIL) synergistically induced apoptosis in HLE cells (Nishikawa et al. 2006). Treatment with green tea prevented the increase in incidences and multiplicities of diethylnitrosamine (DEN)-induced hepatocellular tumors and also arrested the progression of cholangiocellular tumors in mice (Umemura et al. 2003). Administration of green tea inhibited the number of glutathione S-transferase placental form- and gamma-glutamyl transpeptidase–positive hepatic foci in male Fischer rats treated with aflatoxin B1 (AFB1) and carbon tetrachloride (CCl4). There was also inhibition of cell proliferation, suggesting that green tea inhibited initiation and promotion steps of AFB1 hepatocarcinogenesis and that the inhibition of cell proliferation is responsible for the inhibition of promotion (Qin et al. 2000).

17.2.4 Effect of Green Tea on Lung Cancer

EGCG has been shown to suppress the invasion and migration of highly invasive CL1-5 lung cancer cells. On treatment with EGCG, there was decrease in MMP-2 expression at the transcriptional level in CL1-5 cells with downregulation of JNK, resulting in repression of the translocation of transcriptional factors, Sp1, and NF-κB, from the cytosol into the nucleus. EGCG also enhanced the antitumor effects of docetaxel in CL1-5 cells, signifying that a combination of EGCG and docetaxel may increase the efficacy of docetaxel in suppressing metastasis in lung cancer cells (Deng and Lin 2011). EGCG upregulated the expression of microRNA-210 (miR-210), a major miRNA regulated by hypoxia inducible factor-1α (HIF-1α) in both human and mouse lung cancer cells, and overexpression of miR-210 led to reduced cell proliferation rate and anchorage-independent growth as well as reduced sensitivity to EGCG. The regulation was mediated through the hypoxia response element in miR-210 promoter, and the upregulation of miR-210 was found to be correlated with the stabilized HIF-1α in lung cancer cell lines after EGCG treatment. This EGCG-induced stabilization of HIF-1α was further shown by the stabilization of human influenza hemagglutinin (HA)-tagged HIF-1α but not the P402A/P564A-mutated HIF-1α by EGCG, suggesting that EGCG targets the oxygen-dependent degradation domain (Wang et al. 2011). Treatment with a standardized GTP preparation, PPE, significantly reduced the 4-(methylnitrosamino)-1-(3-pyridyl)-1-butanone (NNK)-induced lung tumor incidence and multiplicity in female A/J mice. PPE treatment inhibited cell proliferation and enhanced apoptosis in adenocarcinomas and adenomas and lowered levels of c-Jun and ERK1/2 phosphorylation (Lu et al. 2006). EGCG interacted with the Ras-GTPase–activating protein SH3 domain-binding protein 1 (G3BP1), with high binding affinity and suppressed anchorage-independent growth of H1299 and CL13 lung cancer cells containing an abundance of the G3BP1 protein. Knockdown shG3BP1-transfected H1299 cells had decreased proliferation and anchorage-independent growth, and shG3BP1 H1299 cells were resistant to the inhibitory effects of EGCG on growth and colony formation compared with shMock-transfected H1299 cells. Treatment with EGCG affected the interaction of shG3BP1 with the Ras-GTPase–activating protein and suppressed the activation of Ras (Shim et al. 2010). We reported that treatment with EGCG caused inhibition of NF-κB/phosphatidylinositol 3-kinase (PI3-K)/AKT/mammalian target of rapamycin (mTOR) and MAPKs in normal human bronchial epithelial (NHBE) cells, contributing to its capacity to suppress inflammation, proliferation, and angiogenesis induced by cigarette smoke (Syed et al. 2007). Green tea significantly reduced tumor incidence and multiplicity in N-methyl-N9-nitro-N-nitrosoguanidine (MNNG)-induced lung cancers and precancerous lesions in laboratory animal center A-strain mice (LACA) mice (Luo and Li 1992). The effect of EGCG on the inhibition of cell proliferation, c-Met receptor, and epidermal growth factor (EGF) receptor (EGFR) kinase activation in several non-small-cell lung cancer (NSCLC) cell lines was investigated by Milligan et al. (2009). It was reported that EGCG inhibited cell proliferation in erlotinib-sensitive and -resistant cell lines, including those with c-Met overexpression, and acquired resistance to erlotinib. There was greater inhibition of cell proliferation and colony formation by the combination of erlotinib and EGCG than either agent alone, and EGCG completely inhibited ligand-induced c-Met phosphorylation and partially inhibited EGFR phosphorylation. There was greater inhibition of proliferation by the triple combination of EGCG/erlotinib/SU11274 than EGCG with erlotinib, and the combination of EGCG and erlotinib considerably slowed the growth rate of H460 xenografts (Milligan et al. 2009). ECG, EGC, and a catechin mixture, in addition to EGCG, decreased cell viability in A549 human lung carcinoma cells. EGCG treatment specifically induced the activities of caspases-3 and -7. Catechin mixture only upregulated the p53 reporter, as shown by luciferase-based reporter assays. EGCG was found to be a more potent inducer of p53-dependent transcription, as demonstrated by the induced level of p53 protein. EGCG-induced apoptosis was completely eliminated by RNA interference–mediated p53 knockdown, suggesting that EGCG, among several GTPs, is a potent inducer of apoptosis that functions exclusively through a p53-dependent pathway in A549 cells (Yamauchi et al. 2009). Lu et al. (2008) investigated the possible synergistic inhibitory effect of a novel combination of PPE, a standardized

GTP preparation, and atorvastatin in a mouse tumorigenesis model and in human lung cancer H1299 and H460 cell lines. Lung tumorigenesis induced by NNK was not inhibited by PPE or atorvastatin, when given alone. However, tumor multiplicity and tumor burden were significantly reduced by a low-dose combination of PPE and atorvastatin, which was associated with enhanced apoptosis and suppressed myeloid cell leukemia 1 (Mcl-1) level in lung adenomas. There was a decrease in the number of viable H1299 and H460 cells, induction of apoptosis as determined by the terminal deoxyribonucleotide transferase-mediated nick-end labeling assay, reduction in the antiapoptotic protein Mcl-1 level, and an increase in the cleaved caspase-3 and cleaved polyadenosine diphosphate (ADP)-ribose polymerase (PARP) levels on treatment with combination of PPE and atorvastatin compared with the single-agent treatment (Lu et al. 2008). In drug-sensitive (H69) and drug-resistant (H69VP) small-cell lung carcinoma cells, treatment with EGCG caused reduced telomerase activity as measured by a polymerase chain reaction (PCR)-based assay for telomeric repeats and a decrease in the activities of caspases-3 and -9 but not caspase-8, indicating induction of apoptosis. EGCG also caused DNA fragmentation and S-phase arrest of the cell cycle in these cells (Sadava et al. 2007). It has been shown that cotreatment with EGCG plus celecoxib strongly induced the expression of both DNA damage-inducible 153 (GADD153) mRNA and protein and caused induction of apoptosis in human lung cancer PC-9 cells, whereas EGCG or celecoxib given alone had no effect. However, cotreatment with EGCG plus celecoxib did not induce expression of other apoptosis-related genes such as WAF1/p21 and GADD45. Synergistic effects with this combination were also observed in A549 and ChaGo K-1 lung cancer cell lines. EGCG treatment did not enhance GADD153 gene expression or induction of apoptosis in PC-9 cells in combination with N-(4-hydroxyphenyl) retinamide or with aspirin, indicating that upregulation of GADD153 is closely correlated with synergistic enhancement of apoptosis with EGCG. Cotreatment with EGCG plus celecoxib also activated ERK1/2 and p38. Pretreatment with PD98059 (ERK1/2 inhibitor) and UO126 (selective MEK inhibitor) abrogated both upregulation of GADD153 and synergistic induction of apoptosis of PC-9 cells, but pretreatment with SB203580 (p38 MAPK inhibitor) did not, indicating that GADD153 expression was mediated through the ERK signaling pathway (Suganuma et al. 2006).

17.2.5 Effect of Green Tea on Gastrointestinal Tract Cancer

EGCG treatment of gastric cancer cell line NUGC-3 cells induced apoptosis, decreased the expression of survivin, and increased Bax and TRAIL expression with induction of p73 activation. Small interfering RNA against p73 diminished EGCG effects on survivin expression and cell viability, suggesting that EGCG induced cell death in gastric cancer cells by apoptosis via inhibition of survivin expression downstream of p73 (Onoda et al. 2011). Extended exposure to EGCG caused EGFR degradation in SW480 colon cancer cells, but EGCG required neither a ubiquitin ligase binding to EGFR nor a phosphorylation of EGFR at tyrosine residues, both of which are reportedly necessary for EGFR degradation induced by EGF. EGCG also caused induction of the phosphorylation of p38 MAPK, and gene silencing using p38 MAPK small interfering RNA (siRNA) suppressed the internalization and subsequent degradation of EGFR induced by EGCG. Treatment with EGCG also caused phosphorylation of EGFR at Ser[1046/1047], sites critical for its downregulation, and this was also suppressed by p38 MAPK siRNA (Adachi et al. 2009). The mechanisms of inhibition of colorectal carcinogenesis by green tea in azoxymethane (AOM)-treated Apc(Min/+) mice were investigated. Treatment with green tea to AOM-treated Apc(Min/+) mice caused a statistically significant reduction in the number of newly formed tumors and decreased the levels of β-catenin, cyclin D1, and retinoid X receptor alpha (RXRα), with an increase in the levels of RXRα mRNA. Green tea treatment also caused a significant decrease in CpG methylation as shown by genomic bisulfite treatment of colonic DNA followed by pyrosequencing of 24 CpG sites in the promoter region of the RXRα gene (Volate et al. 2009). EGCG given in drinking fluid inhibited small intestinal tumorigenesis in ApcMin/+ mice and resulted in increased levels of E-cadherin as well as decreased levels of β-catechin in the nucleus and c-Myc, phospho-Akt, and phospho-Erk in the tumors (Ju et al. 2005). In an AOM-induced rat colon cancer model using aberrant crypt foci (ACF) as an end point, dietary PPE administration was found to dose-dependently decrease the total number of ACF per rat and the total number of aberrant crypts per rat. Treatment with PPE also significantly decreased the percentage of large ACF and the percentage of ACF with high-grade dysplasia in total ACF, with an increase in apoptosis and decrease in nuclear expression levels of β-catenin and cyclin D1. There was a decrease in the expression of RXRα in high-grade dysplastic ACF, adenoma, and adenocarcinoma during AOM-induced colon carcinogenesis, and the PPE treatment partially prevented the loss of RXRα expression in high-grade dysplastic ACF (Xiao et al. 2008). The cancer-preventive activities of PPE given in the diet versus drinking fluid as well as the activities of PPE versus individual catechins were compared. There was a decrease in tumor multiplicity with the supplementation of dietary PPE and EGCG in drinking fluid in Apc(Min/+) mice. Dietary PPE delivered twice more EGCG to the small intestine as compared to PPE in drinking fluid. There was decreased cell proliferation, β-catenin nuclear expression, and phospho-Akt levels and higher cleaved caspase-3 and retinoic acid receptor α (RARα) expression in adenomas of groups treated with PPE and EGCG (Hao et al. 2007). Treatment of SW837 human colon cancer cells with EGCG resulted in a decrease in the phosphorylated forms of EGFR, human epidermal growth factor receptor 2 (HER2), and HER3; inhibition of the transcriptional activities of COX2, activator protein 1 (AP-1), and NF-κB promoters; and a decrease in the production of prostaglandin E2 (PGE$_2$), a major product of COX2. There was also inhibition of cell growth; inhibition of the activation of EGFR, HER2, and HER3; a decrease in the levels of COX2 and Bcl-xL proteins; and apoptosis (Shimizu et al. 2005). In HT-29 human colorectal cancer cells, treatment with EGCG increased both intracellular and extracellular pro–MMP-7 protein levels and upregulation of its mRNA expression. EGCG also caused increased expression of ERK1/2, JNK1/2, and p38; phosphorylation of c-Jun; induction of c-Jun/c-Fos; and increase in the DNA binding activity of AP-1. EGCG-induced pro–MMP-7 production was diminished by N-acetyl-L-cysteine, superoxide (O^{2-}) dismutase, and catalase. There was also spontaneous generation of O^{2-} in a cell-free system that utilized a cytochrome c reduction method. Pro–MMP-7 expression was induced by ECG and GTP but not by EC and EGC (Kim et al. 2005). Ohishi et al. (2002) investigated the effects of the combination of EGCG and sulindac against rat colon carcinogenesis induced by AOM. There was significant reduction in the number of ACFs representing preneoplastic lesions and a decrease in cell proliferation and enhancement of apoptosis in groups treated with EGCG and sulindac as compared with the AOM-treated group (Ohishi et al. 2002).

17.2.6 EFFECT OF GREEN TEA ON BREAST CANCER

Luo et al. (2010) reported that EGCG synergistically sensitized breast cancer cells to paclitaxel in vitro and in vivo. Treatment with EGCG in combination with paclitaxel significantly induced 4T1 breast cancer cell apoptosis compared with each single treatment. In BALB/c mice treated with paclitaxel and EGCG, there was significant inhibition of tumor growth, whereas the single-agent activity for paclitaxel or EGCG was poor. EGCG also overcame paclitaxel-induced GRP78 expression and potentiated paclitaxel-induced JNK phosphorylation in 4T1 cells both in vitro and in vivo. It was concluded that EGCG may be used as a sensitizer to enhance the cytotoxicity of paclitaxel (Luo et al. 2010). It has been shown that EGCG decreased the migratory and invasive potential of MCF-7 cells with a concomitant downregulation of vasodilator-stimulated phosphoprotein (VASP) expression and Rac1 activity in a dose-dependent manner. The regulation of cell migration and invasion was associated with Rac1 activity and VASP expression when specific siRNAs were used to block the expression of VASP and Rac1 in MCF-7 cells treated with EGF. In MCF-7 cells, siRNA-mediated knockdown of Rac1 decreased the amount of VASP expression at the mRNA level, while VASP-specific siRNA had no effect on the expression of Rac1, suggesting that the downregulation of VASP expression via the Rac1 pathway is responsible for the inhibitory effect of EGCG on MCF-7 cell migration and invasion (Zhang et al. 2009). Treatment with EGCG caused a decrease in the activity, protein expression, and mRNA expression level of MMP-2, focal adhesion kinase (FAK), membrane type-1–MMP (MT1-MMP), NF-κB, and VEGF and reduced the adhesion of MCF-7 cells to ECM, fibronectin, and vitronectin, with reduction in the expression of integrin receptors α5, β1, αv, and β3 (Sen et al. 2009). It has been shown that treatment of HER2/neu-driven mammary tumor cells with EGCG altered the expression of key regulators in the epithelial-to-mesenchymal transition (EMT) pathway, reducing invasive phenotype. Treatment with EGCG upregulated E-cadherin, γ-catenin, metastasis-associated protein (MTA3), and estrogen receptor α (ERα), downregulated the proinvasive snail gene, and inhibited colony growth and invasion in Matrigel. There was also inhibition of the invasive phenotype of mouse mammary tumor cells driven by NF-κB, c-Rel, and protein kinase CK2 on EGCG treatment. It was also found that forkhead box O3 α (FOXO3α) was also activated by EGCG and that ectopic expression of a constitutively active FOXO3α overrode transforming growth factor beta 1 (TGF-β1)–mediated invasive phenotype and induced a more epithelial phenotype, which was dependent on ERα expression and signaling, while there was a reduced epithelial phenotype of ERα-low breast cancer cells by a dominant negative FOXO3α (Belguise et al. 2007). Pan et al. (2007) have demonstrated that EGCG treatment of MCF-7 cells caused inhibition of heregulin-β1 (HRG-β1) dependent induction of mRNA and protein expression of FAS and also decreased the phosphorylation of Akt and ERK1/2. It was found that growth inhibition of HRG-β1-treated cells was parallel to suppression of FAS by EGCG. It was concluded in this study that EGCG may be useful in the chemoprevention of breast carcinoma in which FAS overexpression results from HER2 or/and HER3 signaling (Pan et al. 2007). Treatment with green tea improved the inhibitory effect of tamoxifen on the proliferation of ER-positive MCF-7, ZR75, and T47D human breast cancer cells in vitro. The combination of green tea and tamoxifen was also more potent than either agent alone in inducing apoptosis in these cells. Treatment of mice with both green tea and tamoxifen was associated with the smallest MCF-7 xenograft tumor size and the highest levels of apoptosis in tumor tissues as compared with either agent administered alone. In treated xenograft tissues, the suppression of angiogenesis correlated with larger areas of necrosis and lower tumor blood vessel density. Green tea decreased levels of ER-α in tumors. Treatment with green tea blocked ER-dependent transcription, estradiol-induced phosphorylation, and nuclear localization of MAPK (Sartippour et al. 2006). It has been reported that GTP and EGCG treatment inhibited proliferation and induced apoptosis of MDA-MB-231 cells in vitro and in vivo. Treatment with both GTP and EGCG caused G1-phase cell-cycle arrest and downregulated the expression of cyclin D, cyclin E, cyclin-dependent kinase (cdk)4, cdk1, and PCNA. In athymic nude mice implanted with human breast cancer MDA-MB-231 cells, there was a delay in tumor incidence and decrease in tumor burden in GTP- and EGCG-treated mice as compared to the water-fed control group. In tumor tissues of mice treated with GTP and EGCG, there was induction of apoptosis and inhibition of proliferation as compared to tissues from control-group mice (Thangapazham et al. 2007). There was dose-dependent inhibition of colony formation and a decrease in cell viability on treatment with EGCG in human breast carcinoma MCF-7 cells, but treatment had no adverse effect on the growth of normal mammary cells. Treatment with EGCG also increased the percentage of apoptotic cells in MCF-7 cells compared to that of non-EGCG-treated cells and inhibited telomerase activity and protein and mRNA expression of human telomerase reverse transcriptase (hTERT), a catalytic subunit of telomerase, suggesting that inhibition of telomerase was associated with downregulation of hTERT (Mittal et al. 2004).

Treatment with green tea extract (GTE) or EGCG significantly decreased the levels of the VEGF peptide secreted into conditioned media in both human umbilical vein endothelial cells (HUVECs) and human breast cancer cells. GTE and EGCG also caused a decrease in the RNA levels and promoter activity of VEGF in human breast cancer cells. There was also decreased c-fos and c-jun RNA transcripts, suggesting that AP-1-responsive regions present in the human VEGF promoter may be involved in the inhibitory effect of GTE and suppression of the expression of protein kinase C in breast cancer cells (Sartippour et al. 2002).

17.3 CONCLUSIONS AND PERSPECTIVES

Remarkable cancer chemopreventive as well as some anticancer effects of green tea and its constituents have been reported in several laboratory and animal model systems. In some clinical trials, these effects have been verified in human patients with disease or in geographical and/or epidemiological observations. Due to the strong evidence for the cancer-preventive and therapeutic effects of green tea emerging from laboratory and animal studies, more carefully planned epidemiological studies and clinical trials are required to further establish the role of green tea in the prevention of cancer in human subjects. Identification of new molecular targets for green tea is essential for improving the design of trials and leading to further elucidation of the mechanisms responsible for the anticancer effects. Multiple mechanisms for the cancer-preventive effects of green tea are likely to be involved, depending on the organ site involved.

REFERENCES

Adachi, S., M. Shimizu, Y. Shirakami et al. 2009. (−)-Epigallocatechin gallate downregulates EGF receptor via phosphorylation at Ser1046/1047 by p38 MAPK in colon cancer cells. *Carcinogenesis* 30: 1544–52.

Adhami, V. M., A. Malik, N. Zaman et al. 2007. Combined inhibitory effects of green tea polyphenols and selective cyclooxygenase-2 inhibitors on the growth of human prostate cancer cells both in vitro and in vivo. *Clin Cancer Res* 13: 1611–9.

Adhami, V. M., I. A. Siddiqui, N. Ahmad, S. Gupta, and H. Mukhtar. 2004. Oral consumption of green tea polyphenols inhibits insulin-like growth factor-I-induced signaling in an autochthonous mouse model of prostate cancer. *Cancer Res* 64: 8715–22.

Adhami, V. M., I. A. Siddiqui, S. Sarfaraz et al. 2009. Effective prostate cancer chemopreventive intervention with green tea polyphenols in the TRAMP model depends on the stage of the disease. *Clin Cancer Res* 15: 1947–53.

Afaq, F., N. Ahmad, and H. Mukhtar. 2003. Suppression of UVB-induced phosphorylation of mitogen-activated protein kinases and nuclear factor kappa B by green tea polyphenol in SKH-1 hairless mice. *Oncogene* 22: 9254–64.

Belguise, K., S. Guo, and G. E. Sonenshein. 2007. Activation of FOXO3a by the green tea polyphenol epigallocatechin-3-gallate induces estrogen receptor alpha expression reversing invasive phenotype of breast cancer cells. *Cancer Res* 67: 5763–70.

Boehm, K., F. Borrelli, E. Ernst et al. 2009. Green tea (Camellia sinensis) for the prevention of cancer. *Cochrane Database Syst Rev* CD005004.

Deng, Y. T. and J. K. Lin. 2011. EGCG inhibits the invasion of highly invasive CL1-5 lung cancer cells through suppressing MMP-2 expression via JNK signaling and induces G2/M arrest. *J Agric Food Chem* 59: 13318–27.

Ellis, L. Z., W. Liu, Y. Luo et al. 2011. Green tea polyphenol epigallocatechin-3-gallate suppresses melanoma growth by inhibiting inflammasome and IL-1beta secretion. *Biochem Biophys Res Commun* 414: 551–6.

Gupta, S., K. Hastak, N. Ahmad, J. S. Lewin, and H. Mukhtar. 2001. Inhibition of prostate carcinogenesis in TRAMP mice by oral infusion of green tea polyphenols. *Proc Natl Acad Sci U S A* 98: 10350–5.

Hao, X., Y. Sun, C. S. Yang et al. 2007. Inhibition of intestinal tumorigenesis in Apc(min/+) mice by green tea polyphenols (polyphenon E) and individual catechins. *Nutr Cancer* 59: 62–9.

Harper, C. E., B. B. Patel, J. Wang, I. A. Eltoum, and C. A. Lamartiniere. 2007. Epigallocatechin-3-gallate suppresses early stage, but not late stage prostate cancer in TRAMP mice: mechanisms of action. *Prostate* 67: 1576–89.

Hastak, K., S. Gupta, N. Ahmad, M. K. Agarwal, M. L. Agarwal, and H. Mukhtar. 2003. Role of p53 and NF-kappaB in epigallocatechin-3-gallate-induced apoptosis of LNCaP cells. *Oncogene* 22: 4851–9.

Hsu, S., D. Dickinson, J. Borke et al. 2007. Green tea polyphenol induces caspase 14 in epidermal keratinocytes via MAPK pathways and reduces psoriasiform lesions in the flaky skin mouse model. *Exp Dermatol* 16: 678–84.

Ju, J., J. Hong, J. N. Zhou et al. 2005. Inhibition of intestinal tumorigenesis in Apcmin/+ mice by (−)-epigallocatechin-3-gallate, the major catechin in green tea. *Cancer Res* 65: 10623–31.

Ju, J., G. Lu, J. D. Lambert, and C. S. Yang. 2007. Inhibition of carcinogenesis by tea constituents. *Sem Cancer Biol* 17: 395–402.

Katiyar, S. K., R. R. Mohan, R. Agarwal, and H. Mukhtar. 1997. Protection against induction of mouse skin papillomas with low and high risk of conversion to malignancy by green tea polyphenols. *Carcinogenesis* 18: 497–502.

Katiyar, S. K., M. Vaid, H. van Steeg, and S. M. Meeran. 2010. Green tea polyphenols prevent UV-induced immunosuppression by rapid repair of DNA damage and enhancement of nucleotide excision repair genes. *Cancer Prev Res (Phila)* 3: 179–89.

Khan, N., F. Afaq and H. Mukhtar. 2008. Cancer chemoprevention through dietary antioxidants: progress and promise. *Antioxid Redox Signal* 10: 475–510.

Khan, N. and H. Mukhtar. 2010. Cancer and metastasis: prevention and treatment by green tea. *Cancer Metastasis Rev* 29: 435–45.

Khan, N. and H. Mukhtar. 2008. Multitargeted therapy of cancer by green tea polyphenols. *Cancer Lett* 269: 269–80.

Kim, M., A. Murakami, K. Kawabata, and H. Ohigashi. 2005. (–)-Epigallocatechin-3-gallate promotes pro-matrix metalloproteinase-7 production via activation of the JNK1/2 pathway in HT-29 human colorectal cancer cells. *Carcinogenesis* 26: 1553–62.

Liang, G., A. Tang, X. Lin et al. 2010. Green tea catechins augment the antitumor activity of doxorubicin in an in vivo mouse model for chemoresistant liver cancer. *Int J Oncol* 37: 111–23.

Lu, G., J. Liao, G. Yang, K. R. Reuhl, X. Hao, and C. S. Yang. 2006. Inhibition of adenoma progression to ade-nocarcinoma in a 4-(methylnitrosamino)-1-(3-pyridyl)-1-butanone-induced lung tumorigenesis model in A/J mice by tea polyphenols and caffeine. *Cancer Res* 66: 11494–501.

Lu, G., H. Xiao, H. You et al. 2008. Synergistic inhibition of lung tumorigenesis by a combination of green tea polyphenols and atorvastatin. *Clin Cancer Res* 14: 4981–8.

Lu, Y. P., Y. R. Lou, J. Liao et al. 2005. Administration of green tea or caffeine enhances the disappearance of UVB-induced patches of mutant p53 positive epidermal cells in SKH-1 mice. *Carcinogenesis* 26: 1465–72.

Luo, D. and Y. Li. 1992. [Preventive effect of green tea on MNNG-induced lung cancers and precancerous lesions in LACA mice]. *Hua Xi Yi Ke Da Xue Xue Bao* 23: 433–7.

Luo, T., J. Wang, Y. Yin et al. 2010. (–)-Epigallocatechin gallate sensitizes breast cancer cells to paclitaxel in a murine model of breast carcinoma. *Breast Cancer Res* 12: R8.

Mantena, S. K., S. M. Meeran, C. A. Elmets, and S. K. Katiyar. 2005. Orally administered green tea polyphe-nols prevent ultraviolet radiation-induced skin cancer in mice through activation of cytotoxic T cells and inhibition of angiogenesis in tumors. *J Nutr* 135: 2871–7.

McLarty, J., R. L. Bigelow, M. Smith, D. Elmajian, M. Ankem, and J. A. Cardelli. 2009. Tea polyphenols decrease serum levels of prostate-specific antigen, hepatocyte growth factor, and vascular endothelial growth factor in prostate cancer patients and inhibit production of hepatocyte growth factor and vascular endothelial growth factor in vitro. *Cancer Prev Res (Phila Pa)* 2: 673–82.

Meeran, S. M., S. Akhtar, and S. K. Katiyar. 2009. Inhibition of UVB-induced skin tumor development by drinking green tea polyphenols is mediated through DNA repair and subsequent inhibition of inflamma-tion. *J Invest Dermatol* 129: 1258–70.

Milligan, S. A., P. Burke, D. T. Coleman et al. 2009. The green tea polyphenol EGCG potentiates the antipro-liferative activity of c-Met and epidermal growth factor receptor inhibitors in non-small cell lung cancer cells. *Clin Cancer Res* 15: 4885–94.

Mittal, A., M. S. Pate, R. C. Wylie, T. O. Tollefsbol, and S. K. Katiyar. 2004. EGCG down-regulates telomerase in human breast carcinoma MCF-7 cells, leading to suppression of cell viability and induction of apop-tosis. *Int J Oncol* 24: 703–10.

Nandakumar, V., M. Vaid, and S. K. Katiyar. 2011. (–)-Epigallocatechin-3-gallate reactivates silenced tumor suppressor genes, Cip1/p21 and p16INK4a, by reducing DNA methylation and increasing histones acety-lation in human skin cancer cells. *Carcinogenesis* 32: 537–44.

Nishikawa, T., T. Nakajima, M. Moriguchi et al. 2006. A green tea polyphenol, epigalocatechin-3-gallate, induces apoptosis of human hepatocellular carcinoma, possibly through inhibition of Bcl-2 family pro-teins. *J Hepatol* 44: 1074–82.

Ohishi, T., Y. Kishimoto, N. Miura et al. 2002. Synergistic effects of (–)-epigallocatechin gallate with sulindac against colon carcinogenesis of rats treated with azoxymethane. *Cancer Lett* 177: 49–56.

Onoda, C., K. Kuribayashi, S. Nirasawa et al. 2011. (–)-Epigallocatechin-3-gallate induces apoptosis in gastric cancer cell lines by down-regulating survivin expression. *Int J Oncol* 38: 1403–8.

Pan, M. H., C. C. Lin, J. K. Lin, and W. J. Chen. 2007. Tea polyphenol (–)-epigallocatechin 3-gallate sup-presses heregulin-beta1-induced fatty acid synthase expression in human breast cancer cells by inhibiting phosphatidylinositol 3-kinase/Akt and mitogen-activated protein kinase cascade signaling. *J Agric Food Chem* 55: 5030–7.

Qin, G., Y. Ning, and P. D. Lotlikar. 2000. Chemoprevention of aflatoxin B1-initiated and carbon tetrachloride-promoted hepatocarcinogenesis in the rat by green tea. *Nutr Cancer* 38: 215–22.

Sadava, D., E. Whitlock and S. E. Kane. 2007. The green tea polyphenol, epigallocatechin-3-gallate inhibits telomerase and induces apoptosis in drug-resistant lung cancer cells. *Biochem Biophys Res Commun* 360: 233–7.

Sartippour, M. R., R. Pietras, D. C. Marquez-Garban et al. 2006. The combination of green tea and tamoxifen is effective against breast cancer. *Carcinogenesis* 27: 2424–33.

Sartippour, M. R., Z. M. Shao, D. Heber et al. 2002. Green tea inhibits vascular endothelial growth factor (VEGF) induction in human breast cancer cells. *J Nutr* 132: 2307–11.

Sen, T., S. Moulik, A. Dutta et al. 2009. Multifunctional effect of epigallocatechin-3-gallate (EGCG) in down-regulation of gelatinase-A (MMP-2) in human breast cancer cell line MCF-7. *Life Sci* 84: 194–204.

Shim, J. H., Z. Y. Su, J. I. Chae et al. 2010. Epigallocatechin gallate suppresses lung cancer cell growth through Ras-GTPase-activating protein SH3 domain-binding protein 1. *Cancer Prev Res (Phila)* 3: 670–9.

Shimizu, M., A. Deguchi, A. K. Joe, J. F. McKoy, H. Moriwaki, and I. B. Weinstein. 2005. EGCG inhibits activation of HER3 and expression of cyclooxygenase-2 in human colon cancer cells. *J Exp Ther Oncol* 5: 69–78.

Shimizu, M., H. Sakai, Y. Shirakami et al. 2011. Preventive effects of (–)-epigallocatechin gallate on diethylnitrosamine-induced liver tumorigenesis in obese and diabetic C57BL/KsJ-db/db Mice. *Cancer Prev Res (Phila)* 4: 396–403.

Shirakami, Y., M. Shimizu, S. Adachi et al. 2009. (–)-Epigallocatechin gallate suppresses the growth of human hepatocellular carcinoma cells by inhibiting activation of the vascular endothelial growth factor-vascular endothelial growth factor receptor axis. *Cancer Sci* 100: 1957–62.

Siddiqui, I. A., M. Asim, B. B. Hafeez, V. M. Adhami, R. S. Tarapore, and H. Mukhtar. 2011. Green tea polyphenol EGCG blunts androgen receptor function in prostate cancer. *FASEB J* 25: 1198–207.

Suganuma, M., M. Kurusu, K. Suzuki, E. Tasaki, and H. Fujiki. 2006. Green tea polyphenol stimulates cancer preventive effects of celecoxib in human lung cancer cells by upregulation of GADD153 gene. *Int J Cancer* 119: 33–40.

Syed, D. N., F. Afaq, M. H. Kweon et al. 2007. Green tea polyphenol EGCG suppresses cigarette smoke condensate-induced NF-kappaB activation in normal human bronchial epithelial cells. *Oncogene* 26: 673–82.

Thakur, V. S., K. Gupta, and S. Gupta. 2012. Green tea polyphenols causes cell cycle arrest and apoptosis in prostate cancer cells by suppressing class I histone deacetylases. *Carcinogenesis* 33: 377–84.

Thangapazham, R. L., N. Passi, and R. K. Maheshwari. 2007. Green tea polyphenol and epigallocatechin gallate induce apoptosis and inhibit invasion in human breast cancer cells. *Cancer Biol Ther* 6: 1938–43.

Umemura, T., S. Kai, R. Hasegawa et al. 2003. Prevention of dual promoting effects of pentachlorophenol, an environmental pollutant, on diethylnitrosamine-induced hepato- and cholangiocarcinogenesis in mice by green tea infusion. *Carcinogenesis* 24: 1105–9.

Volate, S. R., S. J. Muga, A. Y. Issa, D. Nitcheva, T. Smith, and M. J. Wargovich. 2009. Epigenetic modulation of the retinoid X receptor alpha by green tea in the azoxymethane-Apc Min/+ mouse model of intestinal cancer. *Mol Carcinog* 48: 920–33.

Wang, H., S. Bian, and C. S. Yang. 2011. Green tea polyphenol EGCG suppresses lung cancer cell growth through upregulating miR-210 expression caused by stabilizing HIF-1alpha. *Carcinogenesis* 32: 1881–9.

Wang, Z. Y., W. A. Khan, D. R. Bickers, and H. Mukhtar. 1989. Protection against polycyclic aromatic hydrocarbon-induced skin tumor initiation in mice by green tea polyphenols. *Carcinogenesis* 10: 411–5.

Xiao, H., X. Hao, B. Simi et al. 2008. Green tea polyphenols inhibit colorectal aberrant crypt foci (ACF) formation and prevent oncogenic changes in dysplastic ACF in azoxymethane-treated F344 rats. *Carcinogenesis* 29: 113–9.

Yamauchi, R., K. Sasaki, and K. Yoshida. 2009. Identification of epigallocatechin-3-gallate in green tea polyphenols as a potent inducer of p53-dependent apoptosis in the human lung cancer cell line A549. *Toxicol In Vitro* 23: 834–9.

Yang, C. S., P. Maliakal, and X. Meng. 2002. Inhibition of carcinogenesis by tea. *Annu Rev Pharmacol Toxicol* 42: 25–54.

Yang, C. S., X. Wang, G. Lu, and S. C. Picinich. 2009. Cancer prevention by tea: animal studies, molecular mechanisms and human relevance. *Nat Rev Cancer* 9: 429–39.

Zhang, Y., G. Han, B. Fan et al. 2009. Green tea (–)-epigallocatechin-3-gallate down-regulates VASP expression and inhibits breast cancer cell migration and invasion by attenuating Rac1 activity. *Eur J Pharmacol* 606: 172–9.

18 Curcumin from Turmeric Spice, Anti-Inflammatory and Antioxidant Phytochemical, and Cancer Prevention

Tin Oo Khor and Ah-Ng Tony Kong

CONTENTS

18.1 INTRODUCTION

Turmeric from the rhizome of plant *Curcuma longa* has been widely used as a spice for centuries in India and many other parts of Asia. In addition to its utilization as food flavoring and coloring, turmeric has also been used as an herbal remedy to treat many different types of diseases, possibly due to its effectiveness and low toxicity (Aggarwal et al. 2007). Curcuminoids have been identified as the major active components from turmeric that contribute to its therapeutic properties. Curcumin (curcumin I), demethoxycurcumin (curcumin II), and bisdemethoxycurcumin (curcumin III) are three major curcuminoids found in turmeric (Figure 18.1). Among them, curcumin is considered as one of the most extensively studied dietary compounds for its anticancer, anti-inflammatory, and antioxidant activities (Aggarwal et al. 2007). Curcumin is a multitargeting compound that modulates a wide variety of signaling pathways either through direct or indirect interaction with different molecules. The cancer chemopreventive or therapeutic effect of curcumin has been demonstrated in almost all kinds of cancers using in vitro or in vivo assays. There are 67 ongoing clinical trials being conducted on curcumin for various diseases, including cancers, asthma, dermatitis, irritable bowel syndrome, mild cognitive impairment, diabetes, chronic obstructive pulmonary disease, rheumatoid arthritis, depressive disorder, ulcerative colitis, and neurodegenerative Alzheimer's disease (listed in http://clinicaltrials.gov, last accessed in February 2012). In this chapter, we will discuss the underlying mechanisms, the potential, and the challenges of developing curcumin as a cancer chemopreventive or therapeutic agent.

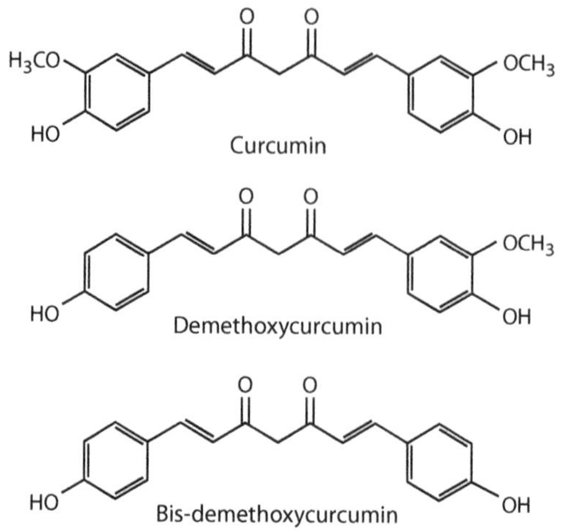

FIGURE 18.1   Chemical structure of the curcuminoids.

18.2   ANTI-INFLAMMATORY EFFECT OF CURCUMIN

The withdrawal of rofecoxib (Vioxx) from the market due to cardiac toxicity and the adverse side effects associated with nonsteroidal anti-inflammatory drugs (NSAIDs) has alerted scientists to the need to search for an anti-inflammatory agent that is safer than the conventional drugs. Hailed as one of the "natural-occurring COX2 inhibitors," curcumin has been used as an anti-inflammatory agent for centuries. Inflammation has been identified as the seventh feature of cancer recently (Mantovani 2009). In fact, chronic inflammation has been linked to increased risk of the development of many diseases, including cancers (Mantovani 2009; Coussens and Werb 2002). Therefore, suppression of chronic inflammation is an important strategy for the prevention as well as treatment of proin-flammatory diseases including cancer. The anti-inflammatory property of curcumin has been exten-sively investigated in preclinical and clinical studies (Jurenka 2009; Basnet and Skalko-Basnet 2011; Aggarwal and Sung 2009). Previous studies have shown that curcumin mediates its anti-inflammatory effects through the suppression of inflammatory transcription factors (nuclear factor kappaB [NF-κB], enzymes like cyclooxygenase 2 [COX2], and 5-lipoxygenase [5-Lox]); proinflammatory cytokines (tumor necrosis factor α [TNFα], interleukin 1 [IL-1], IL-2, IL-6, IL-8, and IL-12); migration inhibi-tory protein; and mitogen-activated kinases (MAPKs) (Goel et al. 2008; Abe et al. 1999). NF-κB is a transcription factor that plays an essential role in response to various inflammatory signaling. Previous studies showed that curcumin is a potent inhibitor of NF-κB activation through the inhibition of IκB kinase (IKK) (Singh and Aggarwal 1995; Bharti et al. 2003). The anti-NF-κB and antiproliferative activity of curcumin have been reported in breast cancer, ovarian cancer, pancreatic cancer, leukemia and multiple myeloma, oral cancer, bladder cancer, and prostate cancer (Bachmeier et al. 2007; Lin et al. 2007; Kunnumakkara et al. 2007; Alaikov et al. 2007; Sharma et al. 2006; Kamat et al. 2007; Deeb et al. 2004). Treatment of human myeloid ML-1a cells with curcumin attenuates TNF-, phorbol ester–, and hydrogen peroxide–mediated activation of NF-κB (Singh and Aggarwal 1995). Curcumin also suppresses activator protein 1 (AP-1) and NF-κB activation by IL-1α or TNFα in bone marrow stromal cells (Xu et al. 1997). Similarly, Kumar et al. (1998) reported that curcumin inhibited the adhesion of monocytes to human umbilical vein endothelial cells (HUVECs) through suppression of NF-κB. In our laboratory, we have previously shown that curcumin inhibits lipopolysaccharide (LPS)-induced NF-κB activation through suppression of IkB phosphorylation in HT29 cells (Jeong et al. 2004). In addition to the direct inhibition of NF-κB, curcumin could also modulate inflammation through targeting the upstream Akt/MAPK pathway or downstream COX2/arachidonic acid metabo-lism pathway. Curcumin was previously reported to be able, either directly or indirectly, to modulate one of three independent inflammation-induced MAPK pathways (Goel et al. 2008). Cho et al. (2005)

demonstrated that curcumin inhibits COX2 expression by suppressing p38 MAPK and c-Jun NH_2-terminal kinase (JNK) activities in ultraviolet B (UVB)–irradiated HaCaT cells. Additionally, inhibition of p38 MAPK signaling by curcumin could lead to suppression of COX2 and inducible nitric oxide synthase (iNOS) expression as well as the nitrite production in colonic mucosa during the development of chronic experimental colitis (Camacho-Barquero et al. 2007). Kim et al. (2007) found that treatment of HUVECs with curcumin could inhibit the adverse vascular effect of the proinflammatory response through modulation of p38 and signal transducer and activator of transcription 3 (STAT3) in addition to NF-κB and JNK. Interestingly, curcumin has been reported to inhibit cyclooxygenase and lipoxygenase activities in a variety of different cell lines and tissues. Huang et al. (1991) reported that curcumin inhibited 12-O-tetradecanoylphorbol-13-acetate (TPA)–induced tumor promotion in mouse epidermis through inhibition of TPA-induced epidermal inflammation and epidermal lipoxygenase and cyclooxygenase activities. In addition, Zhang et al. (1999) found that curcumin could suppress chenodeoxycholate (CD)- or phorbol ester (phorbol myristate acetate [PMA])–mediated induction of COX2 protein and synthesis of prostaglandin E2 (PGE_2) in several gastrointestinal cell lines. They found that curcumin inhibited the binding of AP-1 to DNA as well as directly inhibited the activity of COX2. Likewise, curcumin was found to inhibit COX2 induction by the TNFα or fecapentaene-12 in human colon epithelial cells via inhibition of IKK activity (Plummer et al. 1999). Moriyuki et al. (2010) reported that curcumin inhibits the protease activated receptor 2 (PAR2)-triggered PGE_2 production by suppressing COX2 upregulation and Akt/NF-κB signals in A549 cells. In our laboratory, we have reported that low doses of curcumin in combination with polyunsaturated fatty acids (docosahexaenoic acid [DHA] or eicosapentaenoic acid [EPA]) as well as isothiocynates (sulforaphane and phenethyl isothiocyanate [PEITC]) synergistically suppressed LPS-induced inflammatory markers in RAW 264.7 cells (Saw et al. 2010; Cheung et al. 2009).

As a strong anti-inflammatory agent with relatively low toxicity, the chemopreventive and therapeutic effect of curcumin against proinflammatory diseases has been investigated in many preclinical studies (reviewed in Jurenka 2009; Goel et al. 2008). The efficacy of curcumin for the prevention of inflammatory bowel disease (IBD) has been previously tested using an experimental colitis model in mice (Ukil et al. 2003). Pretreatment of mice with curcumin (50, 100, 300 mg/kg daily i.g. for 10 days) significantly inhibited trinitrobenzene sulfonic acid–induced colitis as evidenced by amelioration of the appearance of diarrhea and the disruption of colonic architecture. More importantly, curcumin treatment also suppresses neutrophil infiltration, lipid peroxidation, levels of nitric oxide production, as well NF-κB activation in colonic mucosa. The protective effect of curcumin against experimentally induced colitis was also reported by other groups (Sugimoto et al. 2002; Salh et al. 2003; Venkataranganna et al. 2007).

In addition to in vitro cell culture assays and preclinical animal models, the anti-inflammatory effects of curcumin were also tested in various clinical trials to treat proinflammatory diseases (reviewed in Goel et al. 2008). The efficacy of curcumin as an antirheumatic agent was tested in short-term, double-blind, crossover study involving 18 subjects (Deodhar et al. 1980). The results showed that curcumin (1200 mg/day) is well tolerated by patients without any significant side effect. Interestingly, antirheumatic activity of curcumin was comparable to that of phenylbutazone. In another crossover randomized controlled trial, the effect of turmeric extract (50 mg/capsule) in combination with zinc complex (50 mg/capsule) and other *Withania somnifera* (450 mg/capsule) and *Boswellia serrata* (100 mg/capsule) on osteoarthritis was tested in 42 patients (Kulkarni et al. 1991). Although treatment with the herbomineral formulation produced a significant drop in severity of pain and disability score, no significant changes were observed in radiological assessment. Likewise, curcumin was also found to be effective in treating chronic anterior uveitis (CAU), idiopathic inflammatory orbital pseudotumors (IIOTs), psoriasis, pancreatitis, and IBDs (Lal et al. 1999, 2000; Heng et al. 2000; Durgaprasad et al. 2005; Holt et al. 2005).

18.3 THE CANCER CHEMOPREVENTIVE EFFECT OF CURCUMIN

The cancer chemopreventive and therapeutic effect of curcumin has been demonstrated in various in vitro and in vivo studies. As a highly pleiotropic molecule, curcumin interacts physically with a variety of different targets such as transcriptional factors; growth factors and their receptors; cytokines; enzymes; adhesion proteins; and genes regulating cell proliferation, cell cycle, and apoptosis (reviewed in Goel et al. 2008; Surh and Chun 2007; Khor et al. 2008; Aggarwal 2008). As shown in Table 18.1, curcumin has been used for treatment and chemoprevention of a variety of different malignancies and is currently in different phases of clinical trials.

TABLE 18.1
Clinical Trials of Curcumin on Various Human Malignancies

Study That Involves Curcumin	Status	Phase
Colorectal Cancer		
Curcumin in Preventing Colon Cancer in Smokers with Aberrant Crypt Foci	Active, not recruiting	II
Curcumin in Preventing Colorectal Cancer in Patients Undergoing Colorectal Endoscopy or Colorectal Surgery	Unknown	I
Study Investigating the Ability of Plant Exosomes to Deliver Curcumin to Normal and Colon Cancer Tissue	Recruiting	I
Curcumin with Preoperative Capecitabine and Radiation Therapy Followed by Surgery for Rectal Cancer	Active, not recruiting	II
Combining Curcumin with FOLFOX Chemotherapy in Patients with Inoperable Colorectal Cancer (CUFOX)	Not yet recruiting	I and II
Curcumin Biomarkers	Active, not recruiting	I
Phase III Trial of Gemcitabine, Curcumin, and Celebrex in Patients with Metastatic Colon Cancer	Unknown	III
Curcumin for the Prevention of Colon Cancer	Completed	I
Sulindac and Plant Compounds in Preventing Colon Cancer	Terminated	
Curcumin for the Chemoprevention of Colorectal Cancer	Active, not recruiting	II
Pancreatic Cancer		
Trial of Curcumin in Advanced Pancreatic Cancer	Active, not recruiting	II
Gemcitabine with Curcumin for Pancreatic Cancer	Completed	II
Phase III Trial of Gemcitabine, Curcumin, and Celebrex in Patients with Advanced or noperable Pancreatic Cancer	Unknown	III
Breast Cancer		
Curcumin in Treating Dermatitis Caused by Radiation Therapy in Patients with Breast Cancer	Not yet recruiting	II and III
Curcumin for the Prevention of Radiation-Induced Dermatitis in Breast Cancer Patients	Completed	II
Other Malignancies		
Curcumin Biomarker Trial in Head and Neck Cancer	Recruiting	0
Reducing Symptom Burden—Non-small Cell Lung Cancer (NSCLC)	Not yet recruiting	I and II
Symptom Burden in Head and Neck Cancer	Not yet recruiting	I and II
Oral Curcumin for Radiation Dermatitis	Recruiting	II and III
Efficacy of NF-κB Inhibition for Reducing Symptoms during Maintenance Therapy in Multiple Myeloma Patients	Not yet recruiting	II
Curcumin (Diferuloylmethane Derivative) with or without Bioperine in Patients with Multiple Myeloma	Completed	–
Trial of Curcumin in Cutaneous T-cell Lymphoma Patients	Not yet recruiting	II
Pilot Study of Curcumin Formulation and Ashwagandha Extract in Advanced Osteosarcoma (OSCAT)	Recruiting	I and II
Turmeric Effect on Reduction of Serum Prolactin and Related Hormonal Change and Adenoma Size in Prolactinoma Patients	Recruiting	I

18.3.1 Colorectal Cancer

Curcumin has been reported to be able to prevent colon carcinogenesis at the initiation, promotion, and progression stages in rodent models. A dietary supplement of curcumin inhibited the azoxymethane-induced aberrant crypt foci and adenocarcinoma in the rat colon (Rao et al. 1993, 1995; Pereira et al. 1996). In addition to carcinogen-induced colorectal cancer models, curcumin was also reported to prevent adenoma development in the intestinal tract of adenomatous polypopsis coli (APC)Min/+ mice (Perkins et al. 2002). Much of the cancer chemopreventive effect of curcumin has been linked with its inhibitory effect on prostaglandin synthesis (Reddy et al. 2006; Goel et al. 2001). Curcumin was also found to be able to inhibit cell proliferation and induce cell-cycle changes in colon adenocarcinoma cell lines by a prostaglandin-independent pathway (Hanif et al. 1997). Jaiswal et al. (2002) found that curcumin can exert its chemopreventive effect against colorectal cancer through suppression of transcriptional activity of β-catenin. We have previously shown that AP-1 could be a target of curcumin in exerting its cancer chemoprevention effect (Jeong et al. 2004). Additionally, epidermal growth factor receptor (EGFR) has also been reported to be a target of curcumin in colon cancer cells (Chen et al. 2006; Reddy et al. 2006). Furthermore, curcumin has also been reported to induce apoptosis and suppress colon cancer cell proliferation through interaction with p53, p21, cyclins, and MAPKs (reviewed in Ravindran et al. 2009).

Curcumin is also used as a chemosensitizer and radiosensitizer in adjuvant therapies to treat or prevent colorectal cancer (reviewed in Goel and Aggarwal 2010). The combination of curcumin with some of the conventional chemotherapy drugs such as 5-fluorouracil (5-FU) and oxaliplatin has generated some exciting results and will be tested in a clinical trial on patients with inoperable colorectal cancer, a study that will be conducted in the United Kingdom by the University of Leicester (http://clinicaltrials.gov). In addition to the above-mentioned clinical trial, there are at least 14 ongoing clinical trials that use curcumin alone or in combination with other drugs to treat or prevent colorectal cancer (Table 18.1).

18.3.2 Pancreatic Cancer

Pancreatic cancer is one of the most deadly cancers across the world due to its highly invasive tumor phenotype and relatively fewer available treatment options. The efficacy of curcumin to treat and prevent pancreatic cancers has been tested in in vitro; in vivo; and phase I, II, and III clinical trials. In vitro studies using pancreatic cancer cell lines demonstrated that NF-κB, COX2, EGFR, Notch1, STAT3, and more recently, microRNA (miRNA), and phosphatase and tensin homolog (PTEN) are the possible targets of curcumin in exerting its anticancer effects (Li et al. 2004; Lev-Ari et al. 2006; Wang et al. 2006; Bao et al. 2011; Glienke et al. 2010).

A phase I/II study of gemcitabine-based chemotherapy plus curcumin for patients with gemcitabine-resistant pancreatic cancer has been previously carried out in Japan involving 21 patients (Kanai et al. 2011). They found that the combination therapy using 8 g oral curcumin daily with gemcitabine-based chemotherapy is safe and feasible in patients with pancreatic cancer. Another study conducted by Epelbaum et al. (2010), involving 17 patients treated with a combination of curcumin and gemcitabine, demonstrated that although the combined treatment option is tolerable, a reduction in the oral dose of 8 g/day of curcumin was recommended. A phase II study was also conducted by Dhillon et al. (2008) that involved 25 patients. Despite its poor oral availability, curcumin was found to be well tolerated and showed biological activity in some patients with pancreatic cancer. A phase III clinical trial of curcumin is being conducted at the Tev-Aviv Sourasky Medical Center in Israel on patients with advanced or inoperable pancreatic cancer (Table 18.1).

18.3.3 Prostate Cancer

In our laboratory, we have previously shown that curcumin inhibited the phosphorylation of Akt, mammalian target of rapamycin (mTOR), and their downstream substrates in human prostate cancer

PC-3 cells in a concentration- and time-dependent manner (Li et al. 2008). We have also reported curcumin and PEITC simultaneously targeting EGFR, Akt, and NF-κB signaling pathways in exerting their additive inhibitory effects on cell proliferation and apoptosis of PC-3 cells (Khor et al. 2006). Deeb et al. (2007) reported that curcumin sensitizes prostate cancer cells to TNF-related apoptosis-inducing ligand (TRAIL)–induced apoptosis by inhibiting Akt-regulated NF-κB and its downstream antiapoptotic genes such as Bcl-2, Bcl-xL, and x-linked inhibitor of apoptosis (XIAP). A similar effect was also reported by Shankar et al. (2007). Additionally, curcumin was found to inhibit methyltrienolone- and IL-6–mediated PSA gene expression in LNCaP cells through down-regulation of the expression and activity of androgen receptors (ARs) (Tsui et al. 2008). Curcumin was also reported to modulate the proliferation of androgen-dependent prostate cancer cells by targeting the Wnt signaling pathway. Curcumin decreases the level of transcription factor-4 (Tcf-4), CBP, and p300 proteins, leading to the suppression of β-catenin/Tcf-4 transcriptional activity and of the expression of β-catenin target genes and, ultimately, autophagy of the cells (Teiten et al. 2011). Choi et al. (2010) demonstrated that the suppression of the Wnt signaling pathway in LNCaP cells was through inhibition of akt and glycogen synthase kinase-3 beta (GSK-3β) phosphorylation and increased β-catenin phosphorylation by curcumin. Hilchie et al. (2010) suggested that cur-cumin-induced apoptosis in PC-3 cells was due to cellular ceramide accumulation and damage to mitochondria in a caspase-independent pathway. Curcumin was also found to suppress the transac-tivation and expression of AR and AR-related cofactors (AP-1, NF-κB, CBP) in prostate cancer cell lines (Nakamura et al. 2002). Downregulation of AR by curcumin was also reported to suppress NKX3.1 expression in LNCaP cells (Zhang et al. 2007).

In addition to the in vitro findings, the prostate cancer chemopreventive and therapeutic effects of curcumin have been investigated in many preclinical models for human prostate cancer. We have previ-ously demonstrated that PEITC and curcumin alone or in combination possess strong cancer-preventive activities in the PC-3 prostate tumor xenografts (Khor et al. 2006). Curcumin was also found to inhibit the growth of LNCaP and DU145 xenografts in nude mice and severe combined immunodeficiency (SCID) mice, respectively (Dorai et al. 2001; Hong et al. 2006). Besides cancer cell xenograft models, we also reported the efficacy of curcumin in suppressing the development and progression of prostate tumors in a transgenic adenocarcinoma of the mouse prostate (TRAMP) model (Barve et al. 2008).

18.4 CURCUMIN AS EPIGENETIC MODIFIER FOR CANCER CHEMOPREVENTION AND THERAPY

Experimental evidence indicates that curcumin may exert its chemopreventive/therapeutic effect through epigenetic modifications (Aggarwal and Sung 2009). Curcumin has been shown to pos-sess inhibitory effects on histone deacetylase (HDACs), histone acetyltransferase (HATs), and more recently, DNA methyltransferase (DNMT) activity (Bora-Tatar et al. 2009; Chen et al. 2007; Liu et al. 2005; Meja et al. 2008; Balasubramanyam et al. 2004; Medina-Franco et al. 2011). We have shown that curcumin can reverse the nuclear factor erythroid 2 p45–related factor 2 (Nrf2) promoter hypermeth-ylation in TRAMP C1 cells (Khor et al. 2011). Demethylation of Nrf2 was found to be associated with the reexpression of Nrf2 and one of its downstream target genes, NAD(P)H dehydrogenace quinone 1 (NQO1). We also found that treatment of LNCaP cells with curcumin reverses DNA methylation of the Neurog1 gene (Shu et al. 2011). Although curcumin has no effect on the expression of DNMTs, curcumin significantly inhibited the enzymatic activity of CpG methylase M.SssI in a dose-dependent manner (Khor et al. 2011). Similarly, a recent report from Jha et al. (2010) showed that treatment of cervical cancer cell lines with curcumin can reverse the hypermethylation of the RARβ2 gene leading to its activation. Although the exact mechanisms by which curcumin exerts its DNA demethylation effect remain elusive, a recent report by Liu et al. (2009) indicated that curcumin may covalently block the catalytic thiolate of C1226 of DNMT1. They also found that curcumin but not hexahydrocurcumin can inhibit the activity of M.SssI with an inhibition concentration 50 (IC50) of 30 nM. Curcumin can also induce global DNA hypomethylation in a leukemia cell line. These findings indicate that curcumin can be used as a DNA hypomethylation agent for cancer chemoprevention or therapy.

In vitro studies indicate that curcumin is also a strong HDAC and HAT inhibitor. Curcumin was found to inhibit the expression of HDAC1, HDAC3, and HDAC8 but increase the expression of Ac-histone H4 in Raji cells (Liu et al. 2005). Meja et al. (2008) reported that curcumin maintains both HDAC2 activity and expression at a posttranslational level, leading to the restoration of corticosteroid function in monocytes exposed to oxidants.

In addition to DNA demethylation and histone modification effects, curcumin was found to be able to modulate miRNAs. miRNA 22 and miRNA 199a* were previously identified as targets for curcumin in human pancreatic cell lines (Sun et al. 2008). Curcumin upregulated the expression of miRNA 22 in the PxBC-3 pancreatic cancer cell line, leading to the suppression of the expression of its target genes, specificity protein 1 (SP1) transcription factor (SP1) and estrogen receptor 1 (ESR1). Similarly, Yang et al. (2010) reported that curcumin reduced the expression of Bcl-2 by upregulating the expression of microRNA (miR)-15a and miR-16 in MCF-7 cells. Additionally, curcumin was also found to sensitize gemcitabine-resistant pancreatic cancer cells via modulation of miR-200 and miR-21 expression (Ali et al. 2010). A recent report from Mudduluru et al. (2011) found that curcumin can reduce miR-21 promoter activity and expression by inhibiting AP-1 binding to the promoter in colorectal cancer.

18.5 CHALLENGES AND FUTURE DIRECTION

One of the major obstacles of developing curcumin as a therapeutic or chemopreventive agent for various diseases is its low bioavailability. Its poor absorption and rapid metabolism resulted in low serum concentration and ultimately poor target tissue distribution. It is estimated that approximately 60% to 70% of an oral dose of curcumin will be eliminated from the body (Pan et al. 1999). The liver and intestine are two major organs responsible for the metabolism of curcumin (Anand et al. 2007). Curcumin glucuronides and curcumin sulfates are two major metabolites formed in the intestine and liver. Numerous approaches have been implemented in order to improve the bioavailability of curcumin. Shoba et al. (1998) demonstrated that combined administration of piperine, a known inhibitor of hepatic and intestinal glucuronidation, enhances the serum concentration, extent of absorption, and bioavailability of curcumin in both rats and humans. They found that concomitant administration of piperine increased the bioavailability of curcumin by 154% and 2000% in rats and humans, respectively. Novel drug delivery systems have also been developed to overcome the bioavailability problem of curcumin (Bansal et al. 2011). Encapsulation of curcumin in liposomes using dimyristoyl-sn-glycero-3-phosphocholine was found to be able to inhibit the growth of pancreatic carcinoma cells and pancreatic tumor xenograft (Li et al. 2005). Thangapazham et al. (2008) reported that treatment of prostate cancer cells with liposomal curcumin (5–10 µM) resulted in at least 70% to 80% inhibition of cellular proliferation without affecting their viability. In contrast, to achieve similar inhibitory effect, a 10-fold higher dose of free curcumin is needed (Thangapazham et al. 2008). In addition to liposome encapsulation, a nanoparticle-based curcumin delivery system has also been tested. Anand et al. (2010) demonstrate that curcumin-loaded poly(lactic-co-glycolic acid) (PLGA) nanoparticle formulation has enhanced cellular uptake, increased bioactivity in vitro, and improved bioavailability in vivo as compared to free curcumin. These promising results from in vitro and preclinical in vivo studies utilizing advanced delivery systems will serve as a platform for the future clinical development of curcumin as a cancer chemopreventive and therapeutic drug.

REFERENCES

Abe, Y., S. Hashimoto, and T. Horie. 1999. Curcumin inhibition of inflammatory cytokine production by human peripheral blood monocytes and alveolar macrophages. *Pharmacol Res* 39 (1):41–7.

Aggarwal, B. B. 2008. Prostate cancer and curcumin: add spice to your life. *Cancer Biol Ther* 7 (9):1436–40.

Aggarwal, B. B., C. Sundaram, N. Malani, and H. Ichikawa. 2007. Curcumin: the Indian solid gold. *Adv Exp Med Biol* 595:1–75.

Aggarwal, B. B., and B. Sung. 2009. Pharmacological basis for the role of curcumin in chronic diseases: an age-old spice with modern targets. *Trends Pharmacol Sci* 30 (2):85–94.

Alaikov, T., S. M. Konstantinov, T. Tzanova, K. Dinev, M. Topashka-Ancheva, and M. R. Berger. 2007. Antineoplastic and anticlastogenic properties of curcumin. *Ann N Y Acad Sci* 1095:355–70.

Ali, S., A. Ahmad, S. Banerjee, S. Padhye, K. Dominiak, J. M. Schaffert, Z. Wang, P. A. Philip, and F. H. Sarkar. 2010. Gemcitabine sensitivity can be induced in pancreatic cancer cells through modulation of miR-200 and miR-21 expression by curcumin or its analogue CDF. *Cancer Res* 70 (9):3606–17.

Anand, P., A. B. Kunnumakkara, R. A. Newman, and B. B. Aggarwal. 2007. Bioavailability of curcumin: problems and promises. *Mol Pharm* 4 (6):807–18.

Anand, P., H. B. Nair, B. Sung, A. B. Kunnumakkara, V. R. Yadav, R. R. Tekmal, and B. B. Aggarwal. 2010. Design of curcumin-loaded PLGA nanoparticles formulation with enhanced cellular uptake, and increased bioactivity in vitro and superior bioavailability in vivo. *Biochem Pharmacol* 79 (3):330–8.

Bachmeier, B., A. G. Nerlich, C. M. Iancu, M. Cilli, E. Schleicher, R. Vene, R. Dell'Eva, M. Jochum, A. Albini, and U. Pfeffer. 2007. The chemopreventive polyphenol Curcumin prevents hematogenous breast cancer metastases in immunodeficient mice. *Cell Physiol Biochem* 19 (1–4):137–52.

Balasubramanyam, K., R. A. Varier, M. Altaf, V. Swaminathan, N. B. Siddappa, U. Ranga, and T. K. Kundu. 2004. Curcumin, a novel p300/CREB-binding protein-specific inhibitor of acetyltransferase, represses the acetylation of histone/nonhistone proteins and histone acetyltransferase-dependent chromatin transcription. *J Biol Chem* 279 (49):51163–71.

Bansal, S. S., M. Goel, F. Aqil, M. V. Vadhanam, and R. C. Gupta. 2011. Advanced drug delivery systems of curcumin for cancer chemoprevention. *Cancer Prev Res (Phila)* 4 (8):1158–71.

Bao, B., S. Ali, D. Kong, S. H. Sarkar, Z. Wang, S. Banerjee, A. Aboukameel, S. Padhye, P. A. Philip, and F. H. Sarkar. 2011. Anti-tumor activity of a novel compound-CDF is mediated by regulating miR-21, miR-200, and PTEN in pancreatic cancer. *PLoS One* 6 (3):e17850.

Barve, A., T. O. Khor, X. Hao, Y. S. Keum, C. S. Yang, B. Reddy, and A. N. Kong. 2008. Murine prostate cancer inhibition by dietary phytochemicals—curcumin and phenyethylisothiocyanate. *Pharm Res* 25 (9):2181–9.

Basnet, P., and N. Skalko-Basnet. 2011. Curcumin: an anti-inflammatory molecule from a curry spice on the path to cancer treatment. *Molecules* 16 (6):4567–98.

Bharti, A. C., N. Donato, S. Singh, and B. B. Aggarwal. 2003. Curcumin (diferuloylmethane) down-regulates the constitutive activation of nuclear factor-kappa B and IkappaBalpha kinase in human multiple myeloma cells, leading to suppression of proliferation and induction of apoptosis. *Blood* 101 (3):1053–62.

Bora-Tatar, G., D. Dayangac-Erden, A. S. Demir, S. Dalkara, K. Yelekci, and H. Erdem-Yurter. 2009. Molecular modifications on carboxylic acid derivatives as potent histone deacetylase inhibitors: Activity and docking studies. *Bioorg Med Chem* 17 (14):5219–28.

Camacho-Barquero, L., I. Villegas, J. M. Sanchez-Calvo, E. Talero, S. Sanchez-Fidalgo, V. Motilva, and C. Alarcon de la Lastra. 2007. Curcumin, a Curcuma longa constituent, acts on MAPK p38 pathway modulating COX-2 and iNOS expression in chronic experimental colitis. *Int Immunopharmacol* 7 (3):333–42.

Chen, A., J. Xu, and A. C. Johnson. 2006. Curcumin inhibits human colon cancer cell growth by suppressing gene expression of epidermal growth factor receptor through reducing the activity of the transcription factor Egr-1. *Oncogene* 25 (2):278–87.

Chen, Y., W. Shu, W. Chen, Q. Wu, H. Liu, and G. Cui. 2007. Curcumin, both histone deacetylase and p300/CBP-specific inhibitor, represses the activity of nuclear factor kappa B and Notch 1 in Raji cells. *Basic Clin Pharmacol Toxicol* 101 (6):427–33.

Cheung, K. L., T. O. Khor, and A. N. Kong. 2009. Synergistic effect of combination of phenethyl isothiocyanate and sulforaphane or curcumin and sulforaphane in the inhibition of inflammation. *Pharm Res* 26 (1):224–31.

Cho, J. W., K. Park, G. R. Kweon, B. C. Jang, W. K. Baek, M. H. Suh, C. W. Kim, K. S. Lee, and S. I. Suh. 2005. Curcumin inhibits the expression of COX-2 in UVB-irradiated human keratinocytes (HaCaT) by inhibiting activation of AP-1: p38 MAP kinase and JNK as potential upstream targets. *Exp Mol Med* 37 (3):186–92.

Choi, H. Y., J. E. Lim, and J. H. Hong. 2010. Curcumin interrupts the interaction between the androgen receptor and Wnt/beta-catenin signaling pathway in LNCaP prostate cancer cells. *Prostate Cancer Prostatic Dis* 13 (4):343–9.

Coussens, L. M., and Z. Werb. 2002. Inflammation and cancer. *Nature* 420 (6917):860–7.

Deeb, D., H. Jiang, X. Gao, S. Al-Holou, A. L. Danyluk, S. A. Dulchavsky, and S. C. Gautam. 2007. Curcumin [1,7-bis(4-hydroxy-3-methoxyphenyl)-1-6-heptadine-3,5-dione; C21H20O6] sensitizes human prostate cancer cells to tumor necrosis factor-related apoptosis-inducing ligand/Apo2L-induced apoptosis by suppressing nuclear factor-kappaB via inhibition of the prosurvival Akt signaling pathway. *J Pharmacol Exp Ther* 321 (2):616–25.

Deeb, D., H. Jiang, X. Gao, M. S. Hafner, H. Wong, G. Divine, R. A. Chapman, S. A. Dulchavsky, and S. C. Gautam. 2004. Curcumin sensitizes prostate cancer cells to tumor necrosis factor-related apoptosis-inducing ligand/Apo2L by inhibiting nuclear factor-kappaB through suppression of IkappaBalpha phosphorylation. *Mol Cancer Ther* 3 (7):803–12.

Deodhar, S. D., R. Sethi, and R. C. Srimal. 1980. Preliminary study on antirheumatic activity of curcumin (diferuloyl methane). *Indian J Med Res* 71:632–4.

Dhillon, N., B. B. Aggarwal, R. A. Newman, R. A. Wolff, A. B. Kunnumakkara, J. L. Abbruzzese, C. S. Ng, V. Badmaev, and R. Kurzrock. 2008. Phase II trial of curcumin in patients with advanced pancreatic cancer. *Clin Cancer Res* 14 (14):4491–9.

Dorai, T., Y. C. Cao, B. Dorai, R. Buttyan, and A. E. Katz. 2001. Therapeutic potential of curcumin in human prostate cancer. III. Curcumin inhibits proliferation, induces apoptosis, and inhibits angiogenesis of LNCaP prostate cancer cells in vivo. *Prostate* 47 (4):293–303.

Durgaprasad, S., C. G. Pai, Vasanthkumar, J. F. Alvres, and S. Namitha. 2005. A pilot study of the antioxidant effect of curcumin in tropical pancreatitis. *Indian J Med Res* 122 (4):315–8.

Epelbaum, R., M. Schaffer, B. Vizel, V. Badmaev, and G. Bar-Sela. 2010. Curcumin and gemcitabine in patients with advanced pancreatic cancer. *Nutr Cancer* 62 (8):1137–41.

Glienke, W., L. Maute, J. Wicht, and L. Bergmann. 2010. Curcumin inhibits constitutive STAT3 phosphorylation in human pancreatic cancer cell lines and downregulation of survivin/BIRC5 gene expression. *Cancer Invest* 28 (2):166–71.

Goel, A., and B. B. Aggarwal. 2010. Curcumin, the golden spice from Indian saffron, is a chemosensitizer and radiosensitizer for tumors and chemoprotector and radioprotector for normal organs. *Nutr Cancer* 62 (7):919–30.

Goel, A., C. R. Boland, and D. P. Chauhan. 2001. Specific inhibition of cyclooxygenase-2 (COX-2) expression by dietary curcumin in HT-29 human colon cancer cells. *Cancer Lett* 172 (2):111–8.

Goel, A., A. B. Kunnumakkara, and B. B. Aggarwal. 2008. Curcumin as "Curecumin": from kitchen to clinic. *Biochem Pharmacol* 75 (4):787–809.

Hanif, R., L. Qiao, S. J. Shiff, and B. Rigas. 1997. Curcumin, a natural plant phenolic food additive, inhibits cell proliferation and induces cell cycle changes in colon adenocarcinoma cell lines by a prostaglandin-independent pathway. *J Lab Clin Med* 130 (6):576–84.

Heng, M. C., M. K. Song, J. Harker, and M. K. Heng. 2000. Drug-induced suppression of phosphorylase kinase activity correlates with resolution of psoriasis as assessed by clinical, histological and immunohistochemical parameters. *Br J Dermatol* 143 (5):937–49.

Hilchie, A. L., S. J. Furlong, K. Sutton, A. Richardson, M. R. Robichaud, C. A. Giacomantonio, N. D. Ridgway, and D. W. Hoskin. 2010. Curcumin-induced apoptosis in PC3 prostate carcinoma cells is caspase-independent and involves cellular ceramide accumulation and damage to mitochondria. *Nutr Cancer* 62 (3):379–89.

Holt, P. R., S. Katz, and R. Kirshoff. 2005. Curcumin therapy in inflammatory bowel disease: a pilot study. *Dig Dis Sci* 50 (11):2191–3.

Hong, J. H., K. S. Ahn, E. Bae, S. S. Jeon, and H. Y. Choi. 2006. The effects of curcumin on the invasiveness of prostate cancer in vitro and in vivo. *Prostate Cancer Prostatic Dis* 9 (2):147–52.

Huang, M. T., T. Lysz, T. Ferraro, T. F. Abidi, J. D. Laskin, and A. H. Conney. 1991. Inhibitory effects of curcumin on in vitro lipoxygenase and cyclooxygenase activities in mouse epidermis. *Cancer Res* 51 (3):813–9.

Jaiswal, A. S., B. P. Marlow, N. Gupta, and S. Narayan. 2002. Beta-catenin-mediated transactivation and cell-cell adhesion pathways are important in curcumin (diferuylmethane)-induced growth arrest and apoptosis in colon cancer cells. *Oncogene* 21 (55):8414–27.

Jeong, W. S., I. W. Kim, R. Hu, and A. N. Kong. 2004. Modulation of AP-1 by natural chemopreventive compounds in human colon HT-29 cancer cell line. *Pharm Res* 21 (4):649–60.

Jeong, W. S., I. W. Kim, R. Hu, and A. N. Kong. 2004. Modulatory properties of various natural chemopreventive agents on the activation of NF-kappaB signaling pathway. *Pharm Res* 21 (4):661–70.

Jha, A. K., M. Nikbakht, G. Parashar, A. Shrivastava, N. Capalash, and J. Kaur. 2010. Reversal of hypermethylation and reactivation of the RARbeta2 gene by natural compounds in cervical cancer cell lines. *Folia Biol (Praha)* 56 (5):195–200.

Jurenka, J. S. 2009. Anti-inflammatory properties of curcumin, a major constituent of Curcuma longa: a review of preclinical and clinical research. *Altern Med Rev* 14 (2):141–53.

Kamat, A. M., G. Sethi, and B. B. Aggarwal. 2007. Curcumin potentiates the apoptotic effects of chemotherapeutic agents and cytokines through down-regulation of nuclear factor-kappaB and nuclear factor-kappaB-regulated gene products in IFN-alpha-sensitive and IFN-alpha-resistant human bladder cancer cells. *Mol Cancer Ther* 6 (3):1022–30.

Kanai, M., K. Yoshimura, M. Asada, A. Imaizumi, C. Suzuki, S. Matsumoto, T. Nishimura, Y. Mori, T. Masui, Y. Kawaguchi, K. Yanagihara, S. Yazumi, T. Chiba, S. Guha, and B. B. Aggarwal. 2011. A phase I/II study of gemcitabine-based chemotherapy plus curcumin for patients with gemcitabine-resistant pancreatic cancer. *Cancer Chemother Pharmacol* 68 (1):157–64.

Khor, T. O., Y. Huang, T. Y. Wu, L. Shu, J. Lee, and A. N. Kong. 2011. Pharmacodynamics of curcumin as DNA hypomethylation agent in restoring the expression of Nrf2 via promoter CpGs demethylation. *Biochem Pharmacol* 82 (9):1073–8.

Khor, T. O., Y. S. Keum, W. Lin, J. H. Kim, R. Hu, G. Shen, C. Xu, A. Gopalakrishnan, B. Reddy, X. Zheng, A. H. Conney, and A. N. Kong. 2006. Combined inhibitory effects of curcumin and phenethyl isothiocyanate on the growth of human PC-3 prostate xenografts in immunodeficient mice. *Cancer Res* 66 (2):613–21.

Khor, T. O., S. Yu, and A. N. Kong. 2008. Dietary cancer chemopreventive agents—targeting inflammation and Nrf2 signaling pathway. *Planta Med* 74 (13):1540–7.

Kim, Y. S., Y. Ahn, M. H. Hong, S. Y. Joo, K. H. Kim, I. S. Sohn, H. W. Park, Y. J. Hong, J. H. Kim, W. Kim, M. H. Jeong, J. G. Cho, J. C. Park, and J. C. Kang. 2007. Curcumin attenuates inflammatory responses of TNF-alpha-stimulated human endothelial cells. *J Cardiovasc Pharmacol* 50 (1):41–9.

Kulkarni, R. R., P. S. Patki, V. P. Jog, S. G. Gandage, and B. Patwardhan. 1991. Treatment of osteoarthritis with a herbomineral formulation: a double-blind, placebo-controlled, cross-over study. *J Ethnopharmacol* 33 (1–2):91–5.

Kumar, A., S. Dhawan, N. J. Hardegen, and B. B. Aggarwal. 1998. Curcumin (Diferuloylmethane) inhibition of tumor necrosis factor (TNF)-mediated adhesion of monocytes to endothelial cells by suppression of cell surface expression of adhesion molecules and of nuclear factor-kappaB activation. *Biochem Pharmacol* 55 (6):775–83.

Kunnumakkara, A. B., S. Guha, S. Krishnan, P. Diagaradjane, J. Gelovani, and B. B. Aggarwal. 2007. Curcumin potentiates antitumor activity of gemcitabine in an orthotopic model of pancreatic cancer through suppression of proliferation, angiogenesis, and inhibition of nuclear factor-kappaB-regulated gene products. *Cancer Res* 67 (8):3853–61.

Lal, B., A. K. Kapoor, P. K. Agrawal, O. P. Asthana, and R. C. Srimal. 2000. Role of curcumin in idiopathic inflammatory orbital pseudotumours. *Phytother Res* 14 (6):443–7.

Lal, B., A. K. Kapoor, O. P. Asthana, P. K. Agrawal, R. Prasad, P. Kumar, and R. C. Srimal. 1999. Efficacy of curcumin in the management of chronic anterior uveitis. *Phytother Res* 13 (4):318–22.

Lev-Ari, S., A. Starr, A. Vexler, V. Karaush, V. Loew, J. Greif, E. Fenig, D. Aderka, and R. Ben-Yosef. 2006. Inhibition of pancreatic and lung adenocarcinoma cell survival by curcumin is associated with increased apoptosis, down-regulation of COX-2 and EGFR and inhibition of Erk1/2 activity. *Anticancer Res* 26 (6B):4423–30.

Li, L., B. B. Aggarwal, S. Shishodia, J. Abbruzzese, and R. Kurzrock. 2004. Nuclear factor-kappaB and IkappaB kinase are constitutively active in human pancreatic cells, and their down-regulation by curcumin (diferuloylmethane) is associated with the suppression of proliferation and the induction of apoptosis. *Cancer* 101 (10):2351–62.

Li, L., F. S. Braiteh, and R. Kurzrock. 2005. Liposome-encapsulated curcumin: in vitro and in vivo effects on proliferation, apoptosis, signaling, and angiogenesis. *Cancer* 104 (6):1322–31.

Li, W., T. O. Khor, C. Xu, G. Shen, W. S. Jeong, S. Yu, and A. N. Kong. 2008. Activation of Nrf2-antioxidant signaling attenuates NFkappaB-inflammatory response and elicits apoptosis. *Biochem Pharmacol* 76 (11):1485–9.

Lin, Y. G., A. B. Kunnumakkara, A. Nair, W. M. Merritt, L. Y. Han, G. N. Armaiz-Pena, A. A. Kamat, W. A. Spannuth, D. M. Gershenson, S. K. Lutgendorf, B. B. Aggarwal, and A. K. Sood. 2007. Curcumin inhibits tumor growth and angiogenesis in ovarian carcinoma by targeting the nuclear factor-kappaB pathway. *Clin Cancer Res* 13 (11):3423–30.

Liu, H. L., Y. Chen, G. H. Cui, and J. F. Zhou. 2005. Curcumin, a potent anti-tumor reagent, is a novel histone deacetylase inhibitor regulating B-NHL cell line Raji proliferation. *Acta Pharmacol Sin* 26 (5):603–9.

Liu, Z., Z. Xie, W. Jones, R. E. Pavlovicz, S. Liu, J. Yu, P. K. Li, J. Lin, J. R. Fuchs, G. Marcucci, C. Li, and K. K. Chan. 2009. Curcumin is a potent DNA hypomethylation agent. *Bioorg Med Chem Lett* 19 (3):706–9.

Mantovani, A. 2009. Cancer: inflaming metastasis. *Nature* 457 (7225):36–7.

Medina-Franco, J. L., F. Lopez-Vallejo, D. Kuck, and F. Lyko. 2011. Natural products as DNA methyltransferase inhibitors: a computer-aided discovery approach. *Mol Divers* 15 (2):293–304.

Meja, K. K., S. Rajendrasozhan, D. Adenuga, S. K. Biswas, I. K. Sundar, G. Spooner, J. A. Marwick, P. Chakravarty, D. Fletcher, P. Whittaker, I. L. Megson, P. A. Kirkham, and I. Rahman. 2008. Curcumin restores corticosteroid function in monocytes exposed to oxidants by maintaining HDAC2. *Am J Respir Cell Mol Biol* 39 (3):312–23.

Moriyuki, K., F. Sekiguchi, K. Matsubara, H. Nishikawa, and A. Kawabata. 2010. Curcumin Inhibits the proteinase-activated receptor-2-triggered prostaglandin E2 production by suppressing cyclooxygenase-2 upregulation and Akt-dependent activation of nuclear factor-kappaB in human lung epithelial cells. *J Pharmacol Sci* 114 (2):225–9.

Mudduluru, G., J. N. George-William, S. Muppala, I. A. Asangani, R. Kumarswamy, L. D. Nelson, and H. Allgayer. 2011. Curcumin regulates miR-21 expression and inhibits invasion and metastasis in colorectal cancer. *Biosci Rep* 31 (3):185–97.

Nakamura, K., Y. Yasunaga, T. Segawa, D. Ko, J. W. Moul, S. Srivastava, and J. S. Rhim. 2002. Curcumin downregulates AR gene expression and activation in prostate cancer cell lines. *Int J Oncol* 21 (4):825–30.

Pan, M. H., T. M. Huang, and J. K. Lin. 1999. Biotransformation of curcumin through reduction and glucuronidation in mice. *Drug Metab Dispos* 27 (4):486–94.

Pereira, M. A., C. J. Grubbs, L. H. Barnes, H. Li, G. R. Olson, I. Eto, M. Juliana, L. M. Whitaker, G. J. Kelloff, V. E. Steele, and R. A. Lubet. 1996. Effects of the phytochemicals, curcumin and quercetin, upon azoxymethane-induced colon cancer and 7,12-dimethylbenz[a]anthracene-induced mammary cancer in rats. *Carcinogenesis* 17 (6):1305–11.

Perkins, S., R. D. Verschoyle, K. Hill, I. Parveen, M. D. Threadgill, R. A. Sharma, M. L. Williams, W. P. Steward, and A. J. Gescher. 2002. Chemopreventive efficacy and pharmacokinetics of curcumin in the min/+ mouse, a model of familial adenomatous polyposis. *Cancer Epidemiol Biomarkers Prev* 11 (6): 535–40.

Plummer, S. M., K. A. Holloway, M. M. Manson, R. J. Munks, A. Kaptein, S. Farrow, and L. Howells. 1999. Inhibition of cyclo-oxygenase 2 expression in colon cells by the chemopreventive agent curcumin involves inhibition of NF-kappaB activation via the NIK/IKK signalling complex. *Oncogene* 18 (44):6013–20.

Rao, C. V., A. Rivenson, B. Simi, and B. S. Reddy. 1995. Chemoprevention of colon carcinogenesis by dietary curcumin, a naturally occurring plant phenolic compound. *Cancer Res* 55 (2):259–66.

Rao, C. V., B. Simi, and B. S. Reddy. 1993. Inhibition by dietary curcumin of azoxymethane-induced ornithine decarboxylase, tyrosine protein kinase, arachidonic acid metabolism and aberrant crypt foci formation in the rat colon. *Carcinogenesis* 14 (11):2219–25.

Ravindran, J., S. Prasad, and B. B. Aggarwal. 2009. Curcumin and cancer cells: how many ways can curry kill tumor cells selectively? *AAPS J* 11 (3):495–510.

Reddy, S., A. K. Rishi, H. Xu, E. Levi, F. H. Sarkar, and A. P. Majumdar. 2006. Mechanisms of curcumin- and EGF-receptor related protein (ERRP)-dependent growth inhibition of colon cancer cells. *Nutr Cancer* 55 (2):185–94.

Salh, B., K. Assi, V. Templeman, K. Parhar, D. Owen, A. Gomez-Munoz, and K. Jacobson. 2003. Curcumin attenuates DNB-induced murine colitis. *Am J Physiol Gastrointest Liver Physiol* 285 (1):G235–43.

Saw, C. L., Y. Huang, and A. N. Kong. 2010. Synergistic anti-inflammatory effects of low doses of curcumin in combination with polyunsaturated fatty acids: docosahexaenoic acid or eicosapentaenoic acid. *Biochem Pharmacol* 79 (3):421–30.

Shankar, S., Q. Chen, K. Sarva, I. Siddiqui, and R. K. Srivastava. 2007. Curcumin enhances the apoptosis-inducing potential of TRAIL in prostate cancer cells: molecular mechanisms of apoptosis, migration and angiogenesis. *J Mol Signal* 2:10.

Sharma, C., J. Kaur, S. Shishodia, B. B. Aggarwal, and R. Ralhan. 2006. Curcumin down regulates smokeless tobacco-induced NF-kappaB activation and COX-2 expression in human oral premalignant and cancer cells. *Toxicology* 228 (1):1–15.

Shoba, G., D. Joy, T. Joseph, M. Majeed, R. Rajendran, and P. S. Srinivas. 1998. Influence of piperine on the pharmacokinetics of curcumin in animals and human volunteers. *Planta Med* 64 (4):353–6.

Shu, L., T. O. Khor, J. H. Lee, S. S. Boyanapalli, Y. Huang, T. Y. Wu, C. L. Saw, K. L. Cheung, and A. N. Kong. 2011. Epigenetic CpG demethylation of the promoter and reactivation of the expression of Neurog1 by curcumin in prostate LNCaP cells. *AAPS J* 13 (4):606–14.

Singh, S., and B. B. Aggarwal. 1995. Activation of transcription factor NF-kappa B is suppressed by curcumin (diferuloylmethane) [corrected]. *J Biol Chem* 270 (42):24995–5000.

Sugimoto, K., H. Hanai, K. Tozawa, T. Aoshi, M. Uchijima, T. Nagata, and Y. Koide. 2002. Curcumin prevents and ameliorates trinitrobenzene sulfonic acid-induced colitis in mice. *Gastroenterology* 123 (6):1912–22.

Sun, M., Z. Estrov, Y. Ji, K. R. Coombes, D. H. Harris, and R. Kurzrock. 2008. Curcumin (diferuloylmeth-ane) alters the expression profiles of microRNAs in human pancreatic cancer cells. *Mol Cancer Ther* 7 (3):464–73.

Surh, Y. J., and K. S. Chun. 2007. Cancer chemopreventive effects of curcumin. *Adv Exp Med Biol* 595:149–72.

Teiten, M. H., F. Gaascht, M. Cronauer, E. Henry, M. Dicato, and M. Diederich. 2011. Anti-proliferative poten-tial of curcumin in androgen-dependent prostate cancer cells occurs through modulation of the Wingless signaling pathway. *Int J Oncol* 38 (3):603–11.

Thangapazham, R. L., A. Puri, S. Tele, R. Blumenthal, and R. K. Maheshwari. 2008. Evaluation of a nano-technology-based carrier for delivery of curcumin in prostate cancer cells. *Int J Oncol* 32 (5):1119–23.

Tsui, K. H., T. H. Feng, C. M. Lin, P. L. Chang, and H. H. Juang. 2008. Curcumin blocks the activation of androgen and interleukin-6 on prostate-specific antigen expression in human prostatic carcinoma cells. *J Androl* 29 (6):661–8.

Ukil, A., S. Maity, S. Karmakar, N. Datta, J. R. Vedasiromoni, and P. K. Das. 2003. Curcumin, the major component of food flavour turmeric, reduces mucosal injury in trinitrobenzene sulphonic acid-induced colitis. *Br J Pharmacol* 139 (2):209–18.

Venkataranganna, M. V., M. Rafiq, S. Gopumadhavan, G. Peer, U. V. Babu, and S. K. Mitra. 2007. NCB-02 (standardized Curcumin preparation) protects dinitrochlorobenzene-induced colitis through down-regulation of NFkappa-B and iNOS. *World J Gastroenterol* 13 (7):1103–7.

Wang, Z., Y. Zhang, S. Banerjee, Y. Li, and F. H. Sarkar. 2006. Notch-1 down-regulation by curcumin is associ-ated with the inhibition of cell growth and the induction of apoptosis in pancreatic cancer cells. *Cancer* 106 (11):2503–13.

Xu, Y. X., K. R. Pindolia, N. Janakiraman, R. A. Chapman, and S. C. Gautam. 1997. Curcumin inhibits IL1 alpha and TNF-alpha induction of AP-1 and NF-kB DNA-binding activity in bone marrow stromal cells. *Hematopathol Mol Hematol* 11 (1):49–62.

Yang, J., Y. Cao, J. Sun, and Y. Zhang. 2010. Curcumin reduces the expression of Bcl-2 by upregulating miR-15a and miR-16 in MCF-7 cells. *Med Oncol* 27 (4):1114–8.

Zhang, F., N. K. Altorki, J. R. Mestre, K. Subbaramaiah, and A. J. Dannenberg. 1999. Curcumin inhibits cyclo-oxygenase-2 transcription in bile acid- and phorbol ester-treated human gastrointestinal epithelial cells. *Carcinogenesis* 20 (3):445–51.

Zhang, H. N., C. X. Yu, P. J. Zhang, W. W. Chen, A. L. Jiang, F. Kong, J. T. Deng, J. Y. Zhang, and C. Y. Young. 2007. Curcumin downregulates homeobox gene NKX3.1 in prostate cancer cell LNCaP. *Acta Pharmacol Sin* 28 (3):423–30.

19 Flavonoids
Impact on Prostate Cancer and Breast Cancer

James Cardelli, David Coleman, and Katherine D. Crew

CONTENTS

19.1 INTRODUCTION

Plant-derived compounds (phytochemicals) are being studied as chemopreventive and anticancer agents (Surh 2003). This trend is driven by the huge cost to develop anticancer drugs and the low probability that drugs are either approved or remain on the market because of a lack of efficacy or unexpected toxicity. Population studies support the idea that a diet rich in phytochemicals can have a dramatic effect on health and carcinogenesis (Scalbert et al. 2005). Preclinical studies have demonstrated that natural products can inhibit all stages of cancer progression (Gupta et al. 2010).

Unfortunately, natural products are not routinely used as chemopreventive or anticancer agents for a variety of reasons. This is due in large part to the inability to commercialize these agents. Barriers to clinical use of phytochemicals include the following: (1) research that involves in vitro approaches using cultured cell lines and concentrations of agents that are not achievable in vivo; (2) many of the better-studied components appear to impact multiple cellular processes and proteins, compounding the attempts at defining molecular mechanisms and thereby limiting clinical predictability; (3) there is a lack of human clinical trials using phytochemicals demonstrating that these agents work to slow or stop the progression of cancer in patients; and (4) there is a lack of patent space for most phytochemicals, so drug company-sponsored research, development, and marketing are wanting.

The main goal of this chapter will be to review the preclinical and clinical evidence that polyphenols, in the flavonoid class, act as anticancer agents. We will also discuss the idea that these agents might share common mechanisms of action, although their molecular targets may vary. Polyphenols are defined as substances found in plants that are characterized by the presence of at least one hydroxylated phenol group, and they are classified as belonging to the flavonoid, chalcone, stilbene, or phenolic acid/alcohol subclasses (Kang et al. 2011). The flavonoid class of polyphenols can be divided into the anthocyanins (e.g., malvidin and cyanidin), flavan-3-ols (e.g., catechins epigallocatechin-3-gallate [EGCG] and theaflavin), flavanones (e.g., taxifolin and hesperetin), flavones (e.g., luteolin and apigenin), isoflavones (e.g., genistein), and flavonols (e.g., quercetin and myricetin). These substances are found in a rich array of fruits and vegetables.

Flavonoids target many downstream signaling components including, but not limited to, receptor tyrosine kinases (RTKs), cell-cycle modulators, and apoptosis regulators in a variety of human cancers (Kang et al. 2011). Current research focuses on defining which of the many targets affected by flavonoids are critical in cancer progression. We will limit our discussion to preclinical and clinical studies of the targets and mechanisms of action of flavonoids in breast and prostate cancer.

19.2 FLAVONOID FAMILY OF POLYPHENOLS: PRECLINICAL STUDIES

Flavonoids are one of the largest groups of antioxidants and are responsible for the vibrant colors found in petals of flowers and fruits. Their distribution is widespread and includes apples, grapes, walnuts, onions, blueberries, soybeans, citrus fruits, and many vegetables. Flavonoids are polyphenol compounds characterized by two or more aromatic rings with at least one hydroxyl group. Within this subclass, individual flavonoids are distinguished by the extent of hydroxylation and saturation (Figure 19.1). Members in each of the subclasses described below have been demonstrated as potent inhibitors against a wide range of molecular targets (Kang et al. 2011). In this section, we will review the best-studied flavonoids and summarize preclinical research that demonstrates their anticancer properties.

19.2.1 PROSTATE CANCER AND ISOFLAVONES

Genistein, a compound highly enriched in soy products, is the most prevalently studied of the isoflavone class of flavonoids. This particular isoflavone is commonly referred to as a general RTK inhibitor, although caution should be taken with this consideration (Akiyama et al. 1987). Genistein, like the other flavonoids discussed in this review, is a highly reactive compound affecting numerous proteins and pathways as well as the oxidation status of cells (Williams et al. 2004). This isoflavone has been shown to induce cell cycle arrest and apoptosis in a panel of prostate cancer cells by the upregulation of p21 and subsequent downregulation of polo-like kinase 1 (PLK-1) (Seo et al. 2011). The antioxidant effects of genistein lead to activation of activated protein kinase (AMPK), subsequent upregulation of phosphatase and tensin homolog (PTEN) expression, and ultimately, reversal of the phosphoinositide 3-kinase (PI3-K) pathway (Park et al. 2010). Genistein has been demonstrated to prevent angiogenesis through downregulation of vascular endothelial growth factor (VEGF) as well as inhibition of hypoxia-inducible factor-1 alpha (HIF-1α) in prostate cancer cell lines (Cao et al. 2006; Guo et al. 2007; Singh-Gupta et al. 2009). Prostate cancer is an androgen-sensitive disease that can often be kept in control by androgen antagonists during the early stages. The androgen receptor (AR) is reported to be transcriptionally downregulated in prostate cancer

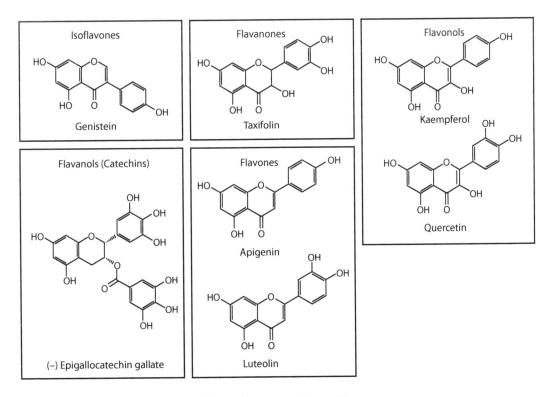

FIGURE 19.1 Chemical structures of the main groups of flavonoids.

cell lines following genistein treatment, suggesting a possible role for genistein at slowing tumor progression at early stages (Davis et al. 2000).

Despite these findings, caution is warranted with the use of genistein as a therapeutic treatment. A report by Wang et al. (2010) reveals that 80–400 mg/kg/day genistein treatment of immunologically deficient mice with prostate xenografts actually increased the frequency of lymph node and distant tissue metastasis (Nakamura et al. 2011). An important point with regard to the physiological relevance of many of these experiments is that oral consumption of genistein leads to the vast majority being conjugated to sulfate or glucuronide moieties in the liver and intestine (Setchell et al. 2001). These conjugated metabolites are orders of magnitude less potent as determined by in vitro experiments (Schwartz et al. 1998).

19.2.2 Breast Cancer and Isoflavones

A number of studies have shown that genistein can induce apoptosis in breast cancer cell lines and can act synergistically with traditional chemotherapeutic agents such as adriamycin and docetaxel, albeit at relatively high concentrations (10–100 μM) (Satoh et al. 2003; Li et al. 2005). This isoflavone was determined to act synergistically with tamoxifen to induce apoptosis in the human epidermal growth factor receptor 2 (HER2)–overexpressing and tamoxifen-resistant cell line BT-474 (Mai et al. 2007). Additionally, genistein was shown to increase the expression of the tumor suppressor proteins BRCA1 and BRCA2 in breast cancer cells (Fan et al. 2006).

The estrogen receptors (ERs) are members of a family of intracellular receptors that are important in the progression of breast cancer. These receptors are activated by the hormone 17β-estradiol and function as transcription factors. ERα and ERβ have pleiotropic effects depending on the ligand and tissue context. ERα and ERβ are expressed in different tissues throughout the body and have unique affinities for different ligands (Weatherman et al. 1999; Rich et al. 2002). Genistein has been shown to have a much greater affinity for ERβ and, through this antagonistic interaction, restrict the expression of estrogen-responsive genes that regulate breast cancer cell proliferation (Kuiper et al. 1998; Kinjo et al. 2004). Conversely, there is some evidence that genistein can actually be mitogenic in ER-positive MCF-7 breast cells through its limited affinity toward ERα (Hsieh et al. 1998; Du et al. 2012). However, growth of tamoxifen-insensitive ER-negative breast cancer cells was either stunted or unaffected with genistein treatment (Seo et al. 2006).

In vivo, genistein was shown to reduce the carcinogenic effects of 7,12-dimethylbenz(a)anthracene (DMBA) on mammary tumor formation when given to early neonatal rats, suggesting that early exposure to genistein could be protective against breast cancer (Constantinou et al. 2001). In a very interesting study performed by the Simmen laboratory, sera collected from mice consuming genistein in the diet at 250 mg/kg food was used to treat MCF-7 and MBA-MB-231 breast cells growing as mammospheres. The sera from genistein-treated mice was able to limit mammosphere formation from both cell types, indicating that this isoflavone, at concentrations obtainable in sera, can target the tumor stem/initiating cells of this population (Montales et al. 2012).

19.2.3 PROSTATE CANCER AND TEA CATECHINS

Studies of tea catechins and prostate cancer have been fairly extensive over the years and yielded a wealth of information. Hassan Mukhtar has been one of the leaders in this area and has published a number of recent reviews that summarize studies over the last two decades (Khan et al. 2009; Johnson et al. 2010). This section will summarize some of the recent studies done with tea catechins, primarily EGCG, with an emphasis on new molecular mechanisms of action and delivery approaches (Table 19.1).

A recent study demonstrated that human prostate cancer cells contain a limited number of cancer stem cells and that EGCG inhibited the self-renewal capacity of these cells (Tang et al. 2010). EGCG also induced apoptosis and inhibited an epithelial-to-mesenchymal transition (EMT) by blocking expression of Slug and Snail, thereby blocking invasion and migration. Interestingly, hepatocyte growth factor (HGF) stimulates the appearance of cancer stem cells (Van Leenders et al. 2011), and we have published that EGCG is a potent inhibitor of c-Met activation in prostate cancer cells, primarily by disrupting lipid rafts (Duhon et al. 2010). Furthermore, EGCG reduces expression of HGF from cancer-associated fibroblasts both in prostate cancer patients and in cell culture (Mclarty et al. 2009).

Additional recent studies suggest that EGCG could act to slow the appearance of castrate-resistant prostate cancer (CRPC) to slow metastatic disease. The AR mediates the biological activities of androgens in normal and cancerous prostate tissue. This transcription factor is a major target in slowing progression of prostate cancer. For instance, it has been published by the Mukhtar group that EGCG interacts with the AR to blunt its activity (Siddiqui et al. 2011). The AR is still expressed in CRPC cells, and inhibitors of this transcription factor have been proposed to still block progression of CRPC. EGCG binds to the ligand-binding domain of AR, thus decreasing transcriptional activity. Recent studies have demonstrated that EGCG synergistically acts with taxanes in vitro and in vivo to stimulate apoptosis and slow tumor cell proliferation (Stearns et al. 2010; Stearns and Wang 2011). This is important since taxanes are used in the clinic to slow progression of CRPC; however, effects are often short acting, and resistance rapidly develops.

A number of studies have recently appeared describing the use of nanoparticles (NPs) loaded with EGCG to treat prostate tumor cells (Shutava et al. 2009; Rocha et al. 2010; Sanna et al. 2011). The Cardelli laboratory has published that EGCG could be loaded into NPs built using a layer-by-layer approach, and these particles were active in vitro to block c-Met activation in prostate tumor cells (Shutava et al. 2009). Rocha et al. (2010) demonstrated that EGCG could be incorporated into a carbohydrate matrix of gum arabic and maltodextrin while retaining its biological activity. This activity included inducing apoptosis and inhibiting cell proliferation at concentrations even lower than free EGCG. Sanna et al. (2011) published an interesting paper demonstrating targeted delivery of EGCG

TABLE 19.1

Ongoing Trials of Isoflavones or Tea Catechins for Prostate or Breast Cancer Prevention

Study Design (ClinicalTrials.gov number)	Study Population (N)	Study Intervention	Study End points
	Prostate: Isoflavone		
Presurgical (NCT00345813): randomized double-blind placebo-controlled	Men with localized prostate cancer scheduled for radical prostatectomy (N = 80)	Oral soy supplementation daily for 4 weeks versus placebo	Expression of proliferation markers (Ki-67), biomarkers of cell cycle regulation, differentiation, apoptosis, and signaling pathways in normal and prostate tumor tissue
Presurgical (NCT00255125): randomized double-blind placebo-controlled	Men with localized prostate cancer and candidate for radical prostatectomy (N = 87)	Soy supplement, four capsules twice daily for 2–4 weeks, versus placebo	Serum PSA, hormonal levels; tissue levels of ER, biomarkers of cell cycle regulation
Presurgical (NCT01036321): randomized double-blind placebo-controlled	Men with localized prostate cancer scheduled for prostatectomy (N = 260)	Purified isoflavones, two capsules (40 mg) daily for 4–6 weeks, versus placebo	Ki-67 in prostate tumor tissue; biomarkers of disease progression (serum steroid hormones, PSA, apoptotic index, tumor volume, Gleason score, urinary symptoms); toxicity
Presurgical (NCT01325311): randomized double-blind placebo-controlled	Men with localized prostate cancer who are candidates for prostatectomy (N = 50)	Genistein 600 mg (G-2535) daily for 3–4 weeks + vitamin D_3 200,000 IU on day 1 versus placebo	Plasma/tissue levels of vitamin D/metabolites and genistein, various tissue biomarkers
Presurgical (NCT01009736): single-arm open-label	Men with biopsy-proven prostate carcinoma who have chosen to undergo radical prostatectomy (N = 80)	Tomato–soy juice daily for 4 weeks	Toxicity, tissue/blood/urine levels of soy isoflavones and tomato phytochemicals, oxidative stress biomarkers, systemic hormones, tumor proliferation index, apoptosis, and angiogenesis/vascularity
Presurgical (NCT00042731): randomized double-blind dose-finding	Men with stage I–II prostate cancer scheduled for prostatectomy (N = 87)	*Arm I–III:* 3 doses of oral isoflavones twice daily + multivitamin (MVI) *Arm IV–VI:* 3 doses of oral lycopene twice + MVI *Arm VII:* MVI alone for 4–6 weeks	Tissue biomarkers of proliferation, apoptosis; serum PSA, sex steroid hormones
Presurgical/secondary prevention (NCT01126879): randomized double-blind placebo-controlled	Men with stage I–III prostate cancer undergoing radical prostatectomy with detectable circulating prostate cancer cells (CPCs) (N = 36)	Oral genistein once daily for 3 months starting 1 month prior to radical prostatectomy versus placebo	CPCs in blood, serum PSA, prostate tissue biomarkers (HSP27, MMP-2, ALK-2, BASP1, HCF2)

(continued)

TABLE 19.1 (Continued)
Ongoing Trials of Isoflavones or Tea Catechins for Prostate or Breast Cancer Prevention

Study Design (ClinicalTrials.gov number)	Study Population (N)	Study Intervention	Study End points
Secondary prevention/active surveillance (NCT00027950): randomized double-blind placebo-controlled	Men with stage I–II prostate cancer, Gleason score 2–6 (N = 148)	Oral isoflavones twice daily for 12 weeks versus placebo	Serum PSA, steroid hormones, anthropometric measures, nutritional intake
Secondary prevention/PSA relapse (NCT00499408): single-arm open-label	Men with localized prostate cancer following definitive therapy with PSA relapse (N = 36)	Soy supplement (bar or shake) once daily + vitamin D₃ twice daily for 3–12 months until disease progression	Serum PSA/slope/doubling time, time to progression, vitamin D receptor signaling, p21 and p27 expression in peripheral blood lymphocytes, toxicity
Secondary prevention (NCT00765479): Randomized double-blind placebo-controlled	Men with stage II prostate cancer who have undergone radical prostatectomy within 4 months (N = 284)	Soy protein isolate beverage once daily versus placebo	PSA relapse, serum cholesterol, steroid hormones, apoptotic activity, angiogenesis, oxidative stress, IGF axis
Primary prevention (NCT01174953): single-arm open-label	Men at high risk for prostate cancer (>25% risk) (N = 40)	Isoflavones, four capsules twice daily (240 mg) + finasteride 5 mg daily	Serum and tissue biomarkers of prostate cancer risk, safety
Primary prevention (NCT01538316): randomized double-blind placebo-controlled crossover	Healthy men, age 18–65 years (N = 60)	Genistein 100 mg daily versus quercetin 500 mg daily versus placebo for 6 months	Serum PSA, prostate cancer incidence, International Prostate Symptom Score (IPSS), quality of life
Prostate: Tea Catechins			
Presurgical (NCT00685516): randomized controlled open-label	Men with prostate adenocarcinoma scheduled for radical prostatectomy (N = 160)	Green tea 6 cups daily versus water for 2–8 weeks	Prostate tumor grade, stage, serum PSA, proliferation, apoptosis, inflammation, oxidative stress, IGF axis, sex steroids, *COMT/UGT1A1/SULT1A1* genotype, serum/urine/prostate tissue total, free tea polyphenols
Presurgical (NCT00844792): randomized double-blind placebo-controlled	Men with localized prostate cancer with planned radical prostatectomy (N = 48)	Dietary supplement (with green tea extract 75 mg, lycopene 20 mg, vitamin D₃ 200 IU, selenium 100 μg, vitamin E 50 IU) twice daily versus placebo for 6–8 weeks	Tumor size, blood and prostate tissue biomarkers

Secondary prevention/active surveillance (NCT00744549): randomized double-blind placebo-controlled, crossover	Men with magnetic resonance imaging (MRI)–detectable localized prostate cancer ($N = 40$)	Dietary supplement (with green tea extract 75 mg, lycopene 20 mg, vitamin D_3 200 IU, selenium 100 µg, vitamin E 50 IU) twice daily versus placebo for 1 year	Tumor size, tumor blood flow
Secondary prevention/PSA relapse (NCT00669656): single-arm open-label	Men with prostate cancer treated with local therapy, evidence of PSA recurrence ($N = 45$)	Prostate Health Cocktail (green tea extract, vitamin D_3, vitamin E, selenium, saw palmetto, lycopene, soy derivatives), three capsules daily for 1 year	PSA response/doubling time, tissue GFP78, serum neuroendocrine markers, circulating tumor cells, toxicity
Primary prevention (NCT00596011): randomized double-blind placebo-controlled	Men with HGPIN or ASAP on prostate biopsy within the past 6 months ($N = 272$)	Poly E 200 mg bid versus placebo for 12 months	Rate of progression to prostate cancer at 1 year, serum prostate cancer-associated diagnostic marker-1 (PCADM-1), urine ABCA5, quality of life, safety
Primary prevention (NCT01105338): randomized double-blind placebo-controlled	Men with abnormal PSA and negative prostate biopsy, age 50–69 years ($N = 126$)	Oral green tea capsules once daily versus lycopene supplement once daily for 6 months	Serum PSA, lycopene and EGCG levels, blood pressure, anthropometric measures, urinary symptoms, tolerability
Primary prevention (NCT00253643): randomized double-blind placebo-controlled	Men without prostate cancer requiring repeat prostate biopsy ($N = 144$)	Oral green tea extract daily versus omega-3 fatty acid three times daily, either alone or in combination, versus placebo for up to 20 weeks	Tissue expression of fatty acid synthase, Ki-67, apoptosis index, phospholipid membrane composition, sterol regulatory element binding protein, bone formation/loss
Breast: Isoflavones			
Presurgical (NCT00036686): randomized double-blind placebo-controlled	Women with early-stage breast cancer scheduled for definitive breast surgery ($N = 106$)	Oral soy protein isolate twice daily versus placebo for 2–4 weeks	Tissue markers of cell proliferation and apoptosis, serum steroid hormones, isoflavone levels
Primary and secondary prevention (NCT01219075): randomized double-blind placebo-controlled	High-risk women (5-year Gail risk >1.7%, Lobular carcinoma in situ (LCIS), BRCA mutation carrier) or breast cancer survivors ($N = 100$)	Oral soy isoflavone supplement once daily versus placebo for 12 months	Breast MRI volume, breast tissue markers of cell proliferation, apoptosis, ER-α and ER-β
Primary prevention (NCT00099008): randomized double-blind placebo-controlled	Healthy postmenopausal women ($N = 30$)	Oral genistein twice daily versus placebo for 84 days	DNA damage and apoptosis, serum steroid hormones, side effects
Primary prevention (NCT00555386): randomized double-blind placebo-controlled	Moderate- to high-risk premenopausal women ($N = 30$)	Soy protein isolate 50 mg + selenium 200 µg daily versus placebo for one menstrual cycle (25–35 days)	Metabolomics analysis

(continued)

TABLE 19.1 (Continued)
Ongoing Trials of Isoflavones or Tea Catechins for Prostate or Breast Cancer Prevention

Study Design (ClinicalTrials.gov number)	Study Population (N)	Study Intervention	Study End points
Primary prevention (NCT00204490): randomized double-blind placebo-controlled	Healthy premenopausal women (N = 200)	Soy isoflavones (containing 246 mg Novasoy), two tablets daily, versus placebo for 2 years	MD, bone density, blood/urine/breast fluid biomarkers
Metastatic setting (NCT00244933): single-arm open-label	Women with metastatic breast cancer (N = 19)	Gemcitabine chemotherapy + genistein	Objective response rate, time to progression, overall survival, toxicities, breast tumor tissue biomarkers, toxicities
Supportive care (NCT00262184): randomized double-blind placebo-controlled	Postmenopausal women with osteopenia (N = 420)	Isoflavone aglycone 300 mg daily versus placebo for 2 years	Bone mineral density, metabolic indicators of osteoporosis, blood pressure, blood sugar, insulin, insulin resistance (HOMA-IR), lipid profile, adiponectin, high sensitivity C-reactive protein (hsCRP)
Breast: Tea Catechins			
Presurgical (NCT01060345): single-arm open-label	Women with DCIS prior to surgical resection (N = 50)	Poly E 600 mg daily for 4-6 weeks	Ki-67, breast MRI tumor volume and signal enhancement ratio (SER), tissue expression of cluster determinant 68 (CD68), CD31, VEGF, serum IGF-I, safety
Primary prevention (NCT00917735): randomized double-blind placebo-controlled	Postmenopausal women with dense breasts on mammography (N = 800)	Green tea extract, two capsules (CORBAN GTB-3D) twice daily, versus placebo for 1 year	MD, serum IGF-I, IGFBP-3, steroid hormones, urine estrogen metabolites, F2 isoprostanes, COMT genotype

to prostate cancer cells. The prostate-specific membrane antigen (PSMA) is overexpressed in prostate tumor cells and represents a useful target. The authors incorporated EGCG into NPs functionalized with small molecules that allowed for targeting of the NPs to PSMA-expressing cells. We have proposed that c-Met could be a useful target for directed NPs, since it is often overexpressed in prostate cancer cells and plays an important role in the progression of CRPC (Varkaris et al. 2011).

As promising as natural products appear to be as anticancer and chemopreventive agents, a recent paper was published suggesting that EGCG actually reduced the effectiveness of radiotherapy to kill prostate tumor cells (Thomas et al. 2011). Others have shown that EGCG blunted the effectiveness of bortezomib, a proteasomal inhibitor used to treat multiple myeloma (Golden et al. 2009). Therefore, future studies will have to be done to test the effectiveness of EGCG and other flavonoids in combinations with more traditional anticancer therapies.

19.2.4 BREAST CANCER AND TEA CATECHINS

The incidence of breast cancer is lower in Asian women as compared to women living in Western countries, and this protective effect is attributed to the Asian diet, rich in soy-based products and green tea. Studies examining the correlation between tea consumption and breast cancer incidence are unfortunately inconclusive. A meta-analysis of eight epidemiological studies suggested that consumption of tea provided a marginal trend toward prevention of breast cancer incidence and recurrence in early stages (Seely et al. 2005). A second study determined that consumption of high levels of tea significantly reduced the risk of breast cancer (Sun et al. 2006). Finally, a recent study done in Japan found no significant association between plasma levels of catechins and breast cancer occurrence (Iwasaki et al. 2010).

A possible explanation for these conflicting results may be that certain women who possess low levels of the catechol-O-methyltransferase (COMT) allele may demonstrate higher serum levels of catechins (Wu et al. 2003). COMT may inactivate the biological functions of tea catechins such as EGCG.

The epidermal growth factor (EGF) receptor (EGFR)/Her (EGFR, Her2, Her3, and Her4) family of growth factor receptors mediate various aspects of breast cancer development, growth, survival, invasion, and metastasis. The receptors mediate their effects via homodimerization and heterodimerization, transphosphorylation, and subsequent activation of downstream signaling pathways, including the PI3-K/AKT, p38/mitogen-activated protein kinase (MAPK), and extracellular signal-regulated kinases 1 and 2 (ERK1/2) pathways. Her2 plays a prominent role in breast cancer development, being overexpressed or mutated in approximately 25% of all breast cancer patients, leading to a more aggressive phenotype and conveying resistance to common chemotherapeutic regimens. Her2 does not have a natural ligand; therefore, signaling via Her2 is dependent on dimerization with other EGFR family members including EGFR and Her3, which are also overexpressed in a high proportion of breast cancer patients (Sebastian et al. 2006). EGCG inhibited the growth of Her2-overexpressing breast cancer cells, and this may be due to a decrease in PI-3K and nuclear factor kappaB (NF-κB) activity via inhibition of Her2 phosphorylation (Pianetti et al. 2002; Masuda et al. 2003). Herceptin is a humanized monoclonal antibody that targets Her2 as many patients demonstrate stabilization and regression of disease. Unfortunately, many patients become resistant to therapy, and metastatic disease is often the outcome. Interestingly, EGCG also inhibits the growth and survival of Herceptin-resistant breast cancer cells (Eddy et al. 2007).

The c-Met receptor is often overexpressed in breast cancer patients, and this is associated with poor prognosis and low survival, especially in women with triple-negative breast cancer. Overexpression of c-Met or its only known ligand, HGF, leads to the activation of a number of downstream signaling pathways, leading to tumor cell survival, growth, invasion, and metastasis (Gastaldi et al. 2010). EGCG at physiologically relevant concentrations inhibited HGF-induced activation of the c-Met receptor in the invasive breast cancer cell line MDA-MB-231, leading to a reduction in activation of the PI-3K and MAPK pathways (Bigelow and Cardelli 2006). Green tea is also composed of the additional catechins, (–)-epicatechin (EC), (–)-epigallocatechin (EGC), and

(–)-epicatechin-3-gallate (ECG). Only EGCG and ECG were active, suggesting that the R1 galloyl and R2 hydroxyl groups play an important role in mediating the effects of tea catechins on c-Met signaling (Bigelow and Cardelli 2006).

The VEGF signaling pathway includes two transmembrane receptors, VEGFR1 and VEGFR2, and a soluble form of VEGFR1, sVEGFR. The ligand, VEGF, is capable of binding both transmembrane receptors, as well as the soluble receptor. The receptors are primarily expressed on endothelium, and activation of the pathway leads to endothelial growth and subsequent increased tumoral microvessel density, invasion, and metastasis. Numerous studies have demonstrated that high serum and intratumoral levels of VEGF are associated with poor prognosis, high recurrence, and increased risk of metastatic disease (Fox et al. 2007). Several studies have shown that EGCG inhibited growth and survival of endothelial cells through inhibition of VEGF signaling. This appears to occur at multiple levels since EGCG blocks VEGF secretion (Sartippour et al. 2002) by blocking transcription.

Insulin-like growth factor-I receptor (IGF-IR) is a heterotetrameric glycoprotein that, upon binding by its ligands, insulin-like growth factor I (IGF-I) or II (IGF-II), becomes autophosphorylated, stimulating downstream proteins including PI-3K/AKT, Ras/Raf, and MAPK/ERK. Activation of this pathway leads to increased proliferation, transformation, and survival and is associated with breast cancer development and poor prognosis. EGCG was shown to lower IGF-IR kinase activity, perhaps by direct association (Li et al. 2007).

As is true for most flavonoids, EGCG is a potent cytotoxic agent, particularly at high concentrations in vitro, and has well-documented activity as an apoptosis-inducing agent. It has been known for over 15 years that tea catechins inhibit cell growth and induce cell death in tumor but not normal cells (Chen et al. 1998). This has been well studied in both ER-positive and ER-negative breast tumor cells (Mittal et al. 2004). It has been published that treatment of the ER-negative cell line MDA-MB-468 with EGCG inhibited cell proliferation and stimulated apoptosis (Roy et al. 2005). EGCG increased the expression of the tumor suppressor protein p53 and the proapoptotic protein Bax while reducing the levels of the antiapoptotic protein Bcl-2 (Roy et al. 2005).

MDA-MB-231 cells treated with EGCG were arrested at stage G1 in the cell cycle (Thangapazham et al. 2007). This was accompanied by a decrease in the expression of the cell cycle regulatory proteins cyclin D, cyclin E, cyclin-dependent kinase 4 (CDK4), CDK1, and proliferating cell nuclear antigen (PCNA). MDA-MB-231 xenograph experiments also demonstrated that EGCG acted as a growth inhibitory/apoptotic agent in vivo. Nude mice treated with green tea polyphenols or EGCG alone had a significantly reduced tumor incidence and burden compared to control mice (Thangapazham et al. 2007).

Reduced levels of p27 and p21 correlate with poor prognosis in breast cancer patients. Interestingly, EGCG increased expression of these proteins in MCF-7 cells (Liang et al. 1999). Others have demonstrated that EGCG treatment of MCF-7 cells resulted in decreased Skp2 levels, potentially through posttranslational degradation (Huang et al. 2008). Lower levels of Skp2 lead to a loss of the negative regulatory degradative pathway and a subsequent increase in p27 levels.

Cancer cell invasion leading to metastasis is the main cause of death of cancer patients. Invasion requires a plethora of signaling pathways, including changes in integrins, downregulation of cadherins, and upregulation of proteins, including Rho GTPases, focal adhesion kinase (FAK), and Erk. Recent studies have demonstrated that tea flavonoids block many of these events to lower tumor invasion. EMT leads to increases in cell invasion and motility. This is preceded by reductions in E-cadherin and increases in mesenchymal protein such as Snail, N-cadherin, vimentin, and fibronectin (Micalizzi et al. 2010). Blocking EMT could reduce invasion and metastasis. The Sonenshein laboratory demonstrated that EGCG reversed the EMT phenotype in the mouse mammary tumor Her2-overexpressing cell line, NF639 (Belguise et al. 2007), although relatively high concentrations of EGCG were used. Notably, E-cadherin expression increased, while Snail levels dropped. This was accompanied by an increase in the epithelial phenotype and a reduction in invasion. The authors suggest that EGCG works by inducing FOXO3A activity, leading to changes in a transcriptional profile, reversing the EMT phenotype.

Others have reported that EGCG decreased levels of matrix metallopeptidase 9 (MMP-9), a protease associated with poor prognosis in breast cancer (Sen et al. 2010). The authors speculate that the lower levels of MMP-9 RNA were due to decreased NF-κB and activator protein 1 (AP-1) transcription factor binding to the MMP-9 promoter. Expression of integrins that facilitate adhesion and motility through binding of fibronection and vitronectin was also decreased by EGCG treatment of MDA-MB-231 cells (Sen et al. 2010). The Orlandi laboratory reported similar results in an MCF-7 breast carcinoma cell line resistant to tamoxifen. EGCG treatment significantly reduced levels of the gelatinases, MMP-2 and MMP-9, and also increased levels of their natural inhibitors, tissue inhibitor of metalloprotease (TIMP-1) and TIMP-2 (Farabegoli et al. 2011).

Rho GTPase members regulate changes in the actin cytoskeleton and play key roles in tumor cell motility and invasion. Rac GTPases (a subgroup) are activated by growth factors and cell attachments via integrins. This leads to the formation of lamellipodia and membrane ruffles, which help to propel cells forward. For instance, EGF activates Rac1 in breast cancer cells, resulting in increased motility and invasion (Zhang et al. 2009). EGCG dose-dependently inhibited basal and EGF-stimulated migration and invasion of MCF-7 cells, potentially through its ability to inhibit Rac1 activity under these conditions (Zhang et al. 2009).

Given the multitude of EGCG effects, it remains to be explored if EGCG acts through one or more mechanisms. These mechanisms include (1) inhibition of or even promotion of reactive oxygen species (ROS) formation, (2) direct binding and inhibition of enzyme or receptor activity, and (3) binding to cell surface domains or proteins, including lipid rafts, laminin, and so forth. All of these mechanisms are discussed in a recent review (Bigelow and Cardelli, in press).

19.2.5 Prostate Cancer and Flavonols

Research involving quercetin and related flavonoids belonging to the flavonol class has been less extensive than studies involving tea catechin. Interestingly, most of the studies have focused on quercetin and the impact it has on hormone-resistant prostate cancer cells (HRPCs).

A number of studies have been published that test quercetin as an anticancer agent using PC3 prostate tumor cells that are no longer responsive to androgens. The Arunakaran laboratory published a study demonstrating that quercetin inhibited cell invasion, migration, and signaling pathways involved in cell survival and proliferation (Senthilkumar et al. 2011). The authors demonstrate that quercetin lowers urokinase and urokinase receptor messenger RNA (mRNA) levels, which might partially explain the decrease in tumor cell invasion. In addition to inhibiting EGFR activation, quercetin lowered EGF and EGFR mRNA levels. Finally, this group demonstrated the quercetin-reduced signaling through NF-κB. The Arunakaran laboratory also published findings demonstrating that quercetin interferes with IGF signaling pathways, leading to an increase in apoptosis and signaling molecules regulating this process (Senthilkumar et al. 2010). Unfortunately, these experiments were performed at fairly high concentrations of quercetin exceeding 50 μM, which calls into question the physiological relevance.

In a related study, the Hashemi group analyzed the effects of quercetin on cell cytotoxicity, proliferation, and gene expression. This flavonoid modulated the expression of genes regulating DNA repair, invasion, angiogenesis, apoptosis, and cell cycle. Again unrealistically high concentrations exceeding 100 μM were used (Noori-Daloii et al. 2011).

Hsieh and Wu (2009) demonstrated that quercetin inhibited proliferation of the androgen-independent prostate cancer cell line CWR22Rv1 and that it acted synergistically with EGCG and genistein. This paper supports the idea that combinations of flavonoids may be more effective as anticancer agents than single compounds (Hsieh and Wu 2009).

The Chung group also used PC3 tumor cells to explore the role of ER stress in regulating quercetin-induced apoptosis. They concluded that quercetin may induce apoptosis via mitochondrial and ER stress–mediated activation of the caspase cascade (Liu et al. 2012).

Slusarz et al. (2010) presented findings suggesting that quercetin may inhibit the hedgehog signaling pathway. GLI-1 is one of three transcription factors activated by hedgehog signaling, and quercetin reduced levels of mRNA encoding this factor. Quercetin, especially in combination with other botanicals, slowed progression of tumors in the transgenic adenocarcinoma of the mouse prostate (TRAMP) model of prostate cancer development (Slusarz et al. 2010).

An interesting study has recently been published showing that quercetin enhanced the action of EGCG in inhibiting multiple signaling pathways in prostate cancer stem cells. These pathways included cell viability, migration, colony formation, invasion, and apoptosis (Tang et al. 2010). Given the apparent importance of cancer stem cells in tumor progression, these studies support an increased effort in determining if flavonoids impact stem cells and through what mechanism.

The Lou laboratory demonstrated that c-Jun expression is induced by quercetin, and this inhibited AR transactivation (Xing et al. 2001; Yuan et al. 2004, 2005). They also showed that the transcription factor Sp-1 was involved in AR activation. In a subsequent paper, they demonstrated that quercetin induced a physical association between c-Jun, Sp-1, and AR via c-Jun NH_2-terminal kinases (JNK) activation, which led to suppression of AR activity (Yuan et al. 2010).

19.2.6 Breast Cancer and Flavonols

Recent reports suggest that quercetin and related flavonoids can act as anti-breast cancer agents, and as observed for prostate cancer, there appear to be a number of different targets. A recent report demonstrated that quercetin inhibits breast cancer cell proliferation and induces apoptosis via Bcl-2 and Bax regulation in MCF-7 cells (Duo et al. 2012). It was also demonstrated that quercetin inhibited tumor invasion by suppressing MMP-9 activation. Biochemical studies indicated that the protein kinase C (PKC) and AP-1 signaling cascade was required for MMP-9 activation and was the target of this flavonoid (Lin et al. 2008).

Recent studies have reported that aromatase, a key enzyme in estrogen biosynthesis, is overexpressed locally in many breast cancers and is considered a potential target for endocrine treatment. Some evidence has been presented that quercetin and other related flavonoids can inhibit aromatase activity (Khan et al. 2011).

A cautionary note was recently published suggesting that quercetin can actually increase the development of estrogen-induced breast tumors in a rat model (Singh et al. 2010). The authors revealed that latency for tumor formation was actually shortened by quercetin. The results are worthy of consideration since many in the phytochemical field often assume that if a small amount of phytochemicals is good, a lot is even better.

An evolving approach is to combine natural products with targeted agents or chemotherapeutic agents, with the end result being an additive or synergistic reduction in tumor size and/or incidence. For instance, it has been reported that quercetin consumed in a diet combined with doxorubicin synergistically reduces breast cancer in mice (Du et al. 2012). Quercetin treatment was reported to stimulate lymphocyte proliferation and induced a tumor-specific T-cell response. This is an area of phytochemical research that remains underexplored, namely, the effect of phytochemicals on the immune system and anticancer responses. Another laboratory reported in vitro results that demonstrated that quercetin with doxorubicin potentiated antitumor effects (Staedler et al. 2011). Quercetin specifically interfered with invasive properties of tumor cells as compared to changes observed with the actin cytoskeleton of nontumor breast cells. Doxorubicin increased DNA damage in tumor and normal cells, but the addition of quercetin prevented damage to nontumor cells, suggesting a potential role as adjuvant therapy to limit off-target toxicity.

Options for treatment of hormone- and trastuzumab-insensitive breast cancers are limited. The Chiu laboratory developed a liposome formulation that contains quercetin and vincristine to prolong circulation times and coordinate drug release. They reported that liposome encapsulation was effective at reducing tumor growth compared to single agents. Importantly, reduced levels of vincristine were required for this effect in animal models, thereby reducing the typical toxic side effects caused by this chemotherapeutic agent (Wong et al. 2011).

19.2.7 PROSTATE CANCER AND FLAVONES

The efficacy of apigenin and luteolin toward many known prostate cancer targets has been tested thoroughly in vitro as well as in several in vivo models. As mentioned, prostate cancer is driven, especially at early stages, by the signaling of androgens regulated by both androgen synthesis as well as AR expression. The Lin laboratory has published that luteolin can downregulate AR expression in the androgen-sensitive prostate cancer cell line LNCaP. This effect contributes to repression of cell proliferation and tumor growth in a xenograft model (Chiu and Lin 2008).

Flavones, particularly luteolin, are potent inhibitors of PI3-K activity, thereby shutting down a pathway commonly hyperactive in prostate cancer due to loss of PTEN. Inhibition of Akt phosphorylation downstream of PI3-K can lead to cell cycle arrest and apoptosis (Kaur et al. 2008). The Rodriguez laboratory has published work showing that an array of cell cycle genes, including CCNA2, CCNE2, CDC25A, CDKN1B, and PLK-1, are affected by luteolin treatment in PC3 prostate cancer cells, which their follow-up work attributes to blocks along the EGFR signaling pathway (Markaverich et al. 2010). Shukla and Gupta (2004) have shown that apigenin treatment results in downregulation of cyclins D1, D2, and E and CDK2, CDK4, and CDK6 and upregulation of WAF1/p21, resulting in growth inhibition of DU145 prostate cancer cells. Moreover, a multitude of reports have shown the ability of flavones to induce apoptosis in prostate cancer cell lines by influencing the balance of proapoptotic and antiapoptotic proteins, including Bax and Bcl-2 (Gupta et al. 2002; Pandey et al. 2011).

Flavones, especially luteolin, have been shown to have exceptional inhibitory activity toward fatty acid synthase (FASN), which supports cancer growth by providing fatty acids to maintain cell membrane growth and integrity, to stabilize and regulate trafficking of proteins, and as an alternate energy source (Brusselmans et al. 2005; Menendez and Lupu 2007). Inhibition of FASN is selectively cytotoxic to cancer cells and restricts the growth of prostate cancer xenografts (Brusselmans et al. 2003; Zhou et al. 2003; Kridel et al. 2004; Menendez et al. 2005). Luteolin has been shown to posttranslationally downregulate the expression of the c-Met receptor, which seems to play a major role in prostate cancer bone metastases, as evidenced by the efficacy of the targeted therapy cabozantinib (Coleman et al. 2009; Dayyani et al. 2011). Furthermore, in vitro, apigenin can inhibit IGF-IR autophosphorylation and its downstream signaling, including PI3-K and glycogen synthase kinase-3 (Fang et al. 2006; Shukla and Gupta 2009). In addition to receptor signaling, more downstream targets can also be modulated by the flavones. Proteins such as FAK and Src, involved in cell motility and invasion, were inhibited by micromolar concentrations of apigenin in PC3-M metastatic prostate cancer cells (Franzen et al. 2009). In addition, luteolin upregulates the expression of E-cadherin through the Akt/mdm2 pathway, thereby preventing prostate cancer cell motility and invasion (Zhou et al. 2009). Inhibition of angiogenesis by apigenin has been demonstrated through the downregulation of HIF-1α as well as VEGF in PC3-M cells under both normoxic and hypoxic conditions (Mirzoeva et al. 2008).

In the TRAMP model of prostate cancer progression, apigenin was shown to reduce the serum levels of IGF-I, VEGF, and urokinase (uPA), as well as tumor phosphorylated Akt and ERK1/2 levels, when delivered orally at 20–50 µg/day for 20 weeks (Shukla et al. 2012). In another TRAMP model study, it was shown that 20 weeks of oral apigenin intake of 20–50 µg/day resulted in increased E-cadherin levels, reduced nuclear β-catenin and c-Myc, and reduced cytoplasmic cyclin D1 in the dorsolateral prostates (Shukla et al. 2007).

19.2.8 BREAST CANCER AND FLAVONES

Numerous established targets of the flavones apigenin and luteolin are important in breast cancer as well. In vitro studies provide strong rationale for testing this class of flavonoids in a chemopreventive and clinical therapy setting. Like prostate cancer, androgen synthesis and signaling is of great importance in the progression of breast cancer. A major dilemma with breast cancer therapy is developed resistance to antiestrogen therapy such as tamoxifen and fulvestrant (Musgrove and Sutherland 2009). A report by Long et al. (2008) suggests that apigenin, at concentrations greater than 10 μM, can resensitize antiestrogen-resistant cell lines to these therapies through inhibition of ERα activity. Of note, in this study, low concentrations of apigenin (1 μM) actually mimicked estrogen in inducing growth of the antiestrogen-sensitive cell line MCF-7 (Long et al. 2008).

RTK-activating mutations or amplification commonly drives breast cancer progression, and targeted therapy has shown substantial efficacy in the clinic. Flavones can restrict RTK stability and/or activity in a number of ways, many of which were mentioned above. Apigenin has been shown to have potent inhibitory effects on the growth of breast cancer cells with amplified expression of Her2/neu (Way et al. 2004). Similar to other flavonoids, apigenin could be affecting Her2/neu and other RTKs, including c-Met, IGFR, and EGFR, through a number of proposed mechanisms, including inhibition of fatty acid synthase, downregulation of heat shock protein expression and stability, lowering receptor expression by blocking PI3-K activity, or disruption of membrane microdomain integrity required for efficient activation (Tarahovsky et al. 2008; Teillet et al. 2008). The PI3-K pathway, which plays a role in cell survival, proliferation, and motility, is commonly hyperactive either through RTK signaling or PTEN loss in breast cancer (Gonzalez-Angulo et al. 2011). As discussed with prostate cancer, flavones are potent PI3-K inhibitors in vitro.

Phenotypes associated with later stages of breast cancer, including invasion, motility, and metastasis, have also been shown to be inhibited by flavones. Apigenin and luteolin both inhibit breast cancer cell motility and invasion through proposed mechanisms, including inhibition of the PI3-K and MAPK pathways as well as inhibition of small GTPases like RhoA and the tyrosine kinase FAK involved in essential steps of cell motility and adhesion (Lee et al. 2004; Huang et al. 2005). A report by Lee et al. (2008) determined that apigenin can prevent HGF-induced in vitro and in vivo invasion and metastasis, at least partly, through prevention of integrin β4 clustering at adhesion sites. Apigenin and luteolin can prevent vessel formation by endothelial cells representative of angiogenesis through downregulation of VEGF, inhibition of platelet-derived growth factor receptor-β (PDGFR-β) activity, and impairment of smooth muscle cell migration (Lamy et al. 2008; Mafuvadze et al. 2010).

19.3 FLAVONOID FAMILY OF POLYPHENOLS: CLINICAL TRIALS

A major challenge is translating these preclinical findings into human intervention trials. Geographic variation in the incidence of prostate and breast cancer between high-risk regions (e.g., North America and Europe) and low-risk regions (e.g., Asia) is often attributed to the Asian diet, which is rich in soy-based products and antioxidant-containing foods and beverages, such as green tea. A growing body of epidemiologic data supports an inverse association of soy and green tea intake with prostate and breast cancer risk. However, observational findings have not always translated into positive results in randomized controlled trials for cancer chemoprevention (Group 1994; Omenn et al. 1994; Albanes et al. 1996; Cole et al. 2007; Klein et al. 2011). Therefore, these agents need to be rigorously tested in clinical trials before widespread adoption in the prevention setting.

The high costs of large-scale chemoprevention studies have prompted the search for intermediate markers of cancer development. An emphasis has been placed on developing novel clinical trial designs, which use surrogate end point biomarkers in lieu of cancer occurrence in order to improve the efficiency and reduce the cost of chemoprevention trials. This section will review the data on isoflavones and tea catechins in early-phase chemoprevention trials for prostate and breast cancer.

19.3.1 PROSTATE CANCER: ISOFLAVONES

For prostate cancer, a number of study designs have been adopted to test novel chemopreventive agents in the clinical setting. Presurgical or "window-of-opportunity" trials involve short-term drug interventions in patients with localized prostate cancer who are scheduled for prostatectomy. Prostate tissue from the diagnostic core biopsy and surgical excision may be used to assess tissue-based biomarkers of response. Secondary prevention trials have used study populations of prostate cancer patients opting for active surveillance or "watchful waiting" or those with serum prostate-specific antigen (PSA) relapse following definitive treatment. The main end point in these trials is change in serum PSA. Finally, primary prevention trials in high-risk populations such as men with high-grade prostatic intraepithelial neoplasia (HGPIN), atypical small acinar proliferation (ASAP), or an elevated PSA without evidence of prostate cancer are also being utilized.

Three presurgical trials of oral soy supplements given for up to 2 weeks in men with early-stage prostate cancer prior to prostatectomy found high concentrations of isoflavones and their metabolites in prostate tissue and plasma (Rannikko et al. 2006; Guy et al. 2008; Gardner et al. 2009). Other clinical trials in the presurgical setting have noted other biological effects of soy, including reduced serum PSA and total cholesterol (Lazarevic et al. 2011), increased apoptosis (Jarred et al. 2002), decreased cyclooxygenase 2 (COX2) and increased p21 mRNA expression in prostate tissue (Swami et al. 2009), and a nonsignificant reduction in androgen and cell cycle-related biomarkers (Lazarevic et al. 2012). These short-term intervention trials serve as proof-of-principle studies to document a biological effect of the chemopreventive agent prior to embarking on clinical trials with longer interventions.

Secondary prevention trials of various formulations of soy isoflavones given for 3–12 months in prostate cancer patients with a PSA relapse or undergoing active surveillance have yielded inconsistent results. Four trials showed no significant effect of soy supplementation on serum PSA (deVere White et al. 2004, 2010; Fischer et al. 2004; Kwan et al. 2010), whereas two trials reported a decline in serum PSA (Kumar et al. 2004; Pendleton et al. 2008). Two trials demonstrated a significant decrease in serum testosterone and dehydroepiandrosterone (DHEA) with 3 months of soy isoflavones (Fischer et al. 2004; Kumar et al. 2004); however, another trial found no difference in serum steroid hormone levels compared to placebo (Kumar et al. 2007). Clinical trials in the primary prevention setting among men at high risk for prostate cancer observed no difference in serum PSA among soy-treated groups (Urban et al. 2001; Hamilton-Reeves et al. 2007a; Miyanaga et al. 2012). However, two trials reported a lower rate of prostate cancer development in the isoflavone group compared to placebo, particularly among older men (Urban et al. 2001; Hamilton-Reeves et al. 2007b). One study demonstrated suppressed AR expression in the prostate (Hamilton-Reeves et al. 2007b), and another reported decreases in dihydrotestosterone (DHT) and DHT/testosterone levels among healthy young men with soy protein consumption (Dillingham et al. 2005).

Differences in the isoflavone formulations and dosing used in these clinical trials have made it difficult to compare results across studies. Given that individual dietary components have not been successful in preventing cancer (Group 1994; Omenn et al. 1994; Albanes 1996; Cole et al. 2007; Klein et al. 2011), dietary interventions enriched for soy have also been tested in prostate cancer patients and demonstrated favorable effects on serum PSA levels (Dalais et al. 2004; Maskarinec et al. 2006; Grainger et al. 2008). Soy isoflavones have also been evaluated in combination with lycopene (Vaishampayan et al. 2007), selenium and vitamin E (Joniau et al. 2007), and curcumin (Ide et al. 2010), with evidence of a decrease or stabilization in serum PSA.

For supportive care, soy isoflavones have been shown to reduce urinary symptoms in randomized placebo-controlled trials among men with benign prostatic hyperplasia (BPH) (Wong et al. 2012) and prostate cancer patients undergoing external beam radiation therapy (Ahmad et al. 2010). However, high-dose isoflavones did not improve vasomotor symptoms, cognition, or quality of life among men undergoing androgen deprivation therapy for prostate cancer (Sharma et al. 2009).

In summary, soy isoflavones have shown some promising biological activity in early-phase prostate cancer prevention trials. However, the optimal formulation, dose, and duration of soy supplementation for chemoprevention have yet to be determined.

19.3.2   Prostate Cancer: Tea Catechins

The most abundant and possibly most potent polyphenol in green tea is EGCG (Yang et al. 1993; Yang 1997). A well-defined oral green tea extract has been studied in several clinical trials for cancer prevention. Polyphenon E (Poly E) is a pharmaceutical-grade decaffeinated green tea catechin (GTC) mixture, including epicatechin (EC), epigallocatechin (EGC), epicatechin gallate (ECG), and most abundantly, ~65% EGCG (Chang et al. 2003). Each capsule contains 200 mg of EGCG, which is equivalent to about 2–3 cups of brewed green tea. In phase I pharmacokinetic trials of Poly E 200–800 mg daily given as a single dose or 4-week administration in healthy individuals, high plasma EGCG levels were achieved (Chow et al. 2001, 2003). All adverse events were rated as mild and mainly gastrointestinal (GI) in nature (Chow et al. 2003).

Two clinical trials of Poly E 800 mg daily for 3–6 weeks in men with prostate cancer scheduled to undergo radical prostatectomy were completed. The first was a single-arm open-label trial conducted by our group at Louisiana State University, which demonstrated a significant reduction in serum PSA HGF, and VEGF levels (Mclarty et al. 2009). The second was a randomized, double-blind, placebo-controlled trial, in which the Poly E intervention led to favorable but nonsignificant changes in serum PSA, Gleason score, IGF axis, and oxidative damage biomarkers (Nguyen et al. 2012). Notably, green tea polyphenol levels in prostate tissue were low to undetectable following the intervention. However, two prostate cancer trials involving consumption of up to 6 cups of green tea daily in the presurgical setting demonstrated bioavailable levels of EGCG and other tea polyphenols in prostate tissue (Henning et al. 2006; Wang et al. 2010).

The most compelling evidence of green tea for prostate cancer prevention came from a randomized, double-blind, placebo-controlled trial of GTCs 600 mg daily in 60 men with HGPIN (Bettuzzi et al. 2006). Men with these high-risk lesions have up to a 30% risk of developing prostate cancer within a year. After 2 years of follow-up, only 2 prostate cancers were detected in the GTC-treated arm compared to 11 with placebo (Brausi et al. 2008). Although PSA did not change significantly, International Prostate Symptom Scores and quality of life improved in GTC-treated men with BPH (Bettuzzi et al. 2006). A larger confirmatory trial is currently underway, which will randomize 272 men with HGPIN or ASAP to Poly E 200 mg bid versus placebo for 12 months (NCT00596011).

In phase II trials of men with castration-resistant metastatic prostate cancer, green tea extract had limited clinical activity, as assessed by serum PSA and measurable disease progression (Jatoi et al. 2003; Choan et al. 2005). Therefore, tea catechins may be most useful in the prevention setting or in combination with other antineoplastic agents for prostate cancer treatment.

19.3.3   Breast Cancer: Isoflavones

The short-term presurgical study design is also commonly used for the early assessment of drugs for breast cancer treatment and prevention, particularly hormonal interventions (Dowsett et al. 2000, 2001; Bundred et al. 2002). Early changes in tumor expression of the Ki-67 proliferation index within 2 weeks of treatment serve as a pharmacodynamic marker that is associated with long-term clinical outcomes in breast cancer patients (Dowsett et al. 2007). Therefore, Ki-67 expression in tumor tissue may serve as a useful surrogate end point for clinical efficacy in these presurgical trials. In two clinical trials of women with benign or malignant breast disease given 14 days of soy supplementation prior to breast surgery (Hargreaves et al. 1999), dietary soy demonstrated weak estrogenic effects with increased progesterone receptor expression and proliferation of breast lobular epithelium. There are conflicting reports about whether bioavailable levels of isoflavones are achieved in breast tissue following short-term presurgical administration of soy-based food supplements (Maubach et al. 2004; Bolca et al. 2010).

In addition to Ki-67, another potential modifiable biomarker of breast cancer risk is mammographic density (MD), which refers to the relative proportions of radiolucent fat and radiodense connective tissue and glandular epithelium within the breast seen on mammogram (Wolfe 1976).

In observational studies, women in the highest quartile of MD demonstrated a 4- to 6-fold increase in breast cancer incidence compared to women in the lowest quartile (Boyd et al. 1995, 1998, 2007; Mccormack and dos Santos Silva 2006). Recent data from the International Breast Cancer Intervention Study (IBIS-I) demonstrated that only women who had at least a 10% decrease in MD within a year of starting tamoxifen derived benefits in terms of lowering breast cancer incidence (Cuzick et al. 2011). Since tamoxifen decreases breast cancer risk as well as breast density (Brisson et al. 2000; Chow et al. 2000; Cuzick et al. 2004), change in MD may be a useful surrogate end point biomarker for breast cancer chemoprevention. A recent meta-analysis of eight randomized controlled trials found that isoflavone intake did not alter MD in postmenopausal women but was associated with a small increase in premenopausal women (Hooper et al. 2010).

Various early-phase chemoprevention trials have also incorporated breast tissue sampling with random periareolar fine needle aspiration (RPFNA) or nipple aspirate fluid (NAF) to assess tissue-based risk biomarkers. Among healthy premenopausal women, 1 month of isoflavones induced dose-specific changes in retinoic acid receptor-beta 2 (*RARβ2*) and *CCND2* gene methylation (Qin et al. 2009). Another trial found a trend toward lower estrogen levels in NAF after a high-soy diet ($P = .07$) (Maskarinec et al. 2011). However, a randomized placebo-controlled trial of a 6-month intervention of mixed soy isoflavones (PTIG-2535) among 126 healthy high-risk women found no significant change in breast epithelial proliferation, apoptosis, or estrogenic effects (Khan et al. 2012).

The hormonal effects of soy and isoflavones have been investigated in numerous trials with equivocal findings. A recent meta-analysis of 47 trials of soy isoflavones given for 4 or more weeks found that isoflavone-rich soy products decreased serum follicle-stimulating hormone (FSH) and luteinizing hormone (LH) by 20% in premenopausal women, and there was a trend toward an increase in serum estradiol levels by 14% ($P = .07$) among postmenopausal women (Hooper et al. 2009). However, two other soy intervention trials reported significant improvements in the ratio of urinary 2-hydroxyestrone to 16α-hydroxyestrone [2:16α-OH E(1)], a proposed biomarker of breast cancer risk (Lukaczer et al. 2005; Morimoto et al. 2012).

Other biomarkers that have been correlated with breast cancer risk and incorporated into clinical trials include serum-based markers of the IGF axis, inflammation, and oxidative stress. In randomized controlled trials, soy consumption led to an increase in IGF-I, decrease in IGF binding protein-3 (IGFBP-3), and increase in IGF-I:IGFBP-3 ratio, which have been hypothesized to promote rather than prevent cancer growth (Gann et al. 2005; Maskarinec et al. 2005; Mclaughlin et al. 2011; Teas et al. 2011). Dietary soy did not modify inflammatory serum markers, such as C-reactive protein (CRP), interleukin 6 (IL-6), leptin, and adiponectin (Maskarinec et al. 2009), and had no effects on lipids, lipoproteins, or insulin sensitivity (Nikander et al. 2004b). Results on the effects of soy on oxidative stress, as measured by urinary isoprostane levels, are mixed (Nhan et al. 2005; Sen et al. 2012).

Isoflavones have also been evaluated for the management of hot flashes and prevention of bone loss, chronic conditions that are relevant to breast cancer survivors. Two trials of soy isoflavone in postmenopausal women with frequent hot flashes reported improvement in vasomotor and other menopausal symptoms (Faure et al. 2002; Basaria et al. 2009). However, four randomized controlled trials of soy products in breast cancer survivors with substantial hot flashes yielded negative results (Quella et al. 2000; Van Patten et al. 2002; Nikander et al. 2003; Macgregor et al. 2005). Randomized studies have demonstrated inconsistent results on the effects of isoflavones on bone turnover and the prevention of bone loss (Nikander et al. 2004a; Brink et al. 2008; Marini et al. 2008).

In conclusion, the weak estrogenic effects of soy isoflavones have raised some concerns that this naturally occurring phytochemical may increase breast cancer risk. These breast cancer trials suffer from the same limitations of the soy intervention trials in prostate cancer, in terms of small sample sizes and the lack of consistency in isoflavone formulations. Therefore, the clinical efficacy of soy isoflavones for breast cancer chemoprevention remains uncertain.

19.3.4 Breast Cancer: Tea Catechins

There are currently limited data on the effects of tea catechins for breast cancer prevention from human intervention trials. In the presurgical setting, we conducted a phase II single-arm trial of the oral green tea extract, Poly E, 800 mg daily, for 2–4 weeks in 27 women with newly diagnosed breast cancer prior to surgical resection. Similar to the prostate cancer trials of Poly E (Mclarty et al. 2009; Nguyen et al. 2012), we found a trend toward a decrease in serum HGF levels but no change in Ki-67 tumor expression compared to historical controls (Campbell et al. 2010). A trial of Poly E 600 mg daily for 4–6 weeks in 50 women with ductal carcinoma in situ (DCIS) prior to breast surgery is currently ongoing (NCT01060345).

For secondary prevention, we conducted a phase I dose escalation trial of Poly E 400–800 mg twice daily for 6 months in 40 women with a history of ER-negative breast cancer (Crew et al. 2011). The primary objective of this study was to assess long-term toxicity and determine the optimal dose of a potential chemopreventive agent being developed for chronic use in healthy individuals. Dose-limiting toxicities included an episode of rectal bleeding and transient elevation in liver function tests. Although the pervading public perception is that dietary supplements are generally safe, these toxicities need to be taken into account when weighing the risks and benefits of any chemopreventive agent.

In a randomized controlled trial of Poly E 400 mg or 800 mg daily (equivalent to 5–10 cups of green tea) for 2 months in 103 healthy postmenopausal women, LDL cholesterol, glucose, and insulin decreased significantly with Poly E compared to placebo (Wu et al. 2012). To determine the effects of green tea on metabolic parameters, weight, and body composition, 54 overweight breast cancer survivors were randomized to 6 months of daily decaffeinated green tea versus placebo tea (Stendell-Hollis et al. 2010). Green tea intake was associated with a decrease in body weight, improved HDL cholesterol, and glucose homeostasis. Therefore, a potential mechanism of tea catechins for breast cancer prevention may be through targeting insulin resistance and the metabolic syndrome.

An ongoing randomized double-blind placebo-controlled trial is examining the effects of a 1-year intervention of an oral green tea extract in 800 postmenopausal women on MD and other circulating biomarkers of breast cancer risk (NCT00917735). These trials highlight the importance of understanding the biology of potential chemopreventive agents prior to embarking in large-scale clinical trials. Drug development for cancer prevention has been hampered by the need for expensive, long-term clinical trials with cancer incidence as the main outcome. If modifiable biomarkers of cancer risk can be validated and shown to reliably predict response in early-phase chemoprevention trials, this will dramatically reduce the time and expense associated with the development of new prevention drugs and may elucidate novel mechanisms of action for cancer prevention.

19.4 FUTURE DIRECTIONS

19.4.1 Enhancing Bioavailability

The major issue limiting progress into the development of flavonoids as true anticancer agents is not only predictability, due to the multitude of targets, but also how well in vitro findings can be translated into in vivo efficacy. The majority of published in vitro reports demonstrate effects using concentrations orders of magnitudes greater than that currently achievable in vivo. Translating the overwhelming number of molecular findings into true clinical reward has been hampered by this disconnect. Commonly, the polyphenol curcumin is used at micromolar concentrations for in vitro studies despite recent human studies reporting that only submicromolar levels are achieved in serum following very large doses (Goel et al. 2008; Shehzad et al. 2010). This disconnect emphasizes that in vivo targets may not be predictable based on in vitro studies; however, it does not rule out cancer-targeting effects. Here we discuss proposed means of increasing flavonoid bioavailability that is characterized by poor adsorption and rapid metabolism.

19.4.2 USING POLYPHENOLS MORE EFFECTIVELY

It was concluded in a recent publication analyzing nearly 100 studies covering 18 common polyphenols that most only reached submicromolar concentrations in serum (Manach et al. 2005). Unfortunately, these polyphenols typically have little to no activity at submicromolar concentrations as shown with in vitro experiments. This major issue impedes progress in the field yet continues to be avoided or ignored; however, we believe it should be an absolute priority of future work. In the following sections, we will discuss possible means of addressing the bioavailability problems that have kept the immense amount of in vitro work from being translated into prevalent clinical use.

19.4.3 NPS TO DELIVER POLYPHENOLS

One area of research aimed at increasing bioavailability that is applicable to polyphenol delivery is NP technology. NPs have the potential to increase solubility, slow the rate of metabolic breakdown, and even directly deliver chemicals to specific target sites. A recent review summarizes the use of nanotechnology to more effectively deliver polyphenols and other nutraceuticals that have poor solubility and low bioavailability (Nair et al. 2010). Reports have already demonstrated the use of nanotechnology with nutraceuticals including resveratrol, genistein, ellagic acid, eugenol, curcumin, and EGCG, among others. A 9-fold improvement in oral bioavailability was observed in one study of NPs containing curcumin, and other studies have shown that this modification can increase its anticancer activity (Bansal et al. 2011). Studies have experimented with EGCG encapsulated in a few different formats, including a layer-by-layer engineered particle that increased efficacy in vitro and another using poly(lactic acid)-poly(ethylene glycol) (PLA-PEG) NPs to enhance chemoprevention in animal models (Shutava et al. 2009; Siddiqui et al. 2009; Siddiqui and Mukhtar 2010). NPs that can be targeted to cell surface proteins overexpressed on cancer cells have also been reported as a means of concentrating the compounds at the intended site of action (Sanna et al. 2011).

Many of these in vivo studies administered the polyphenol NP by i.v. injection. Maintaining high serum levels of the active polyphenol with oral administration will be an important goal for future work.

19.4.4 COMBINATION THERAPY

Another strategy for increasing the overall in vivo efficacy of flavonoids is to combine them into formulations or as adjuvants with other targeted therapies. Milligan et al. (2009) recently published data showing that EGCG could increase the effect of erlotinib on lung cancer cells in vitro and in vivo. More specifically, EGCG seemed to resensitize cell lines that were completely resistant to these targeted therapies. Other studies have demonstrated that flavonoids can enhance the cancer-killing effect of traditional chemotherapies and radiotherapies through several proposed mechanisms (Suganuma et al. 2011; Yunos et al. 2011).

It is conceivable that combinations of flavonoids could have synergistic activity and thereby be effective at much lower concentrations, those achievable in vivo, when compared to individual compounds alone. Considering that bioavailability is such an obstructing issue, low serum/tissue levels of these compounds might not be limiting if multiple flavonoids were present and combinations were more effective than single agents. The authors predict that studies addressing possible additivity and/or synergy of flavonoid combinations will become more common in the near future.

19.4.5 The Long Road to Clinical Use

The use of flavonoids in a true clinical setting is a commendable goal, yet despite abounding laboratory data demonstrating anticancer activity, as well as other health benefits, this goal lies stagnant and unreached. We propose the emphasis of flavonoid research be redirected from the identification of molecular targets in cell culture to addressing bioavailability, formulation development, clinical trial evaluation, and eventual commercialization. There are multiple reasons for the slow progression along this line of research, including the difficulty in gaining approval for use of flavonoids in a clinical setting given the high cost, time and effort, lack of access to drug development facilities, the need to overcome the narrow-minded paradigm that flavonoids will never be as efficacious as "true" cancer therapies, and possibly most substantial, the indifference expressed by drug companies in advancing development of natural products. This last problem is generally thought to be due to the lack of patent space for most polyphenols. It is increasingly important for scientists, particularly ones working with natural products, to be familiar with ways to make their work patentable in order to bring it to fruition. Some possible avenues for opening patent space include unique NP encapsulations or formulations of flavonoid combinations. Most importantly, the goal of effective clinical use of flavonoids as therapeutic and chemopreventive agents will require a combined collaborative effort by the entire scientific community, with a redirected emphasis toward moving forward and addressing the problems rather than lying stagnant and rediscovering more of the same.

REFERENCES

Ahmad, Iftekhar U., Jeffrey D. Forman, Fazlul H. Sarkar, Gilda G. Hillman, Elisabeth Heath, Ulka Vaishampayan, Michael L. Cher, Fundagul Andic, Peter J. Rossi, and Omer Kucuk. 2010. Soy isoflavones in conjunction with radiation therapy in patients with prostate cancer. *Nutrition and Cancer* 62:996–1000.

Akiyama, T., J. Ishida, S. Nakagawa, H. Ogawara, S. Watanabe, N. Itoh, M. Shibuya, and Y. Fukami. 1987. Genistein, a specific inhibitor of tyrosine-specific protein kinases. *Journal of Biological Chemistry* 262:5592–5595.

Albanes, Demetrius. 1996. Alpha-tocopherol and beta-carotene supplements and lung cancer incidence in the alpha-tocopherol, beta-carotene cancer prevention study: effects of base-line characteristics and study compliance. *Journal of the National Cancer Institute* 88:1560–1570.

Albanes, Demetrius, Olli P. Heinonen, Philip R. Taylor, Jussi K. Huttunen et al. 1996. Alpha-tocopherol and beta-carotene supplements and lung cancer incidence in the alpha-tocopherol, beta-carotene cancer prevention study: effects of base-line characteristics and study compliance. *Journal of the National Cancer Institute* 88:1560–1570.

Bansal, Shyam S., Mehak Goel, Farrukh Aqil, Manicka V. Vadhanam, and Ramesh C. Gupta. 2011. Advanced drug-delivery systems of curcumin for cancer chemoprevention. *Cancer Prevention Research* 4: 1158–1171.

Basaria, A. Wisniewski, K. Dupree, T. Bruno, M. Y. Song, F. Yao, A. Ojumu, M. John, and A. S. Dobs. 2009. Effect of high-dose isoflavones on cognition, quality of life, androgens, and lipoprotein in post-menopausal women. *Journal of Endocrinological Investigation* 32:150–155.

Belguise, Karine, Shangqin Guo, and Gail E. Sonenshein. 2007. Activation of FOXO3a by the green tea polyphenol epigallocatechin-3-gallate induces estrogen receptor α expression reversing invasive phenotype of breast cancer cells. *Cancer Research* 67:5763–5770.

Bettuzzi, Saverio, Maurizio Brausi, Federica Rizzi, Giovanni Castagnetti, Giancarlo Peracchia, and Arnaldo Corti. 2006. Chemoprevention of human prostate cancer by oral administration of green tea catechins in volunteers with high-grade prostate intraepithelial neoplasia: a preliminary report from a one-year proof-of-principle study. *Cancer Research* 66:1234–1240.

Bigelow, Rebecca L. and J. A. Cardelli. 2006. The green tea catechins, (–)-Epigallocatechin-3-gallate (EGCG) and (–)-Epicatechin-3-gallate (ECG), inhibit HGF//Met signaling in immortalized and tumorigenic breast epithelial cells. *Oncogene* 25:1922–1930.

Bigelow, Rebecca L. and James A. Cardelli. In press. Effect of green tea catechins on intracellular signaling in breast tissue: implications for cancer. In *Tea in Health and Disease Prevention*, edited by V. R. Preedy: Elsevier Watham, MA. 1145–1159.

Bolca, Selin, Mireia Urpi-Sarda, Phillip Blondeel, Nathalie Roche, Lynn Vanhaecke, Sam Possemiers, Nawaf Al-Maharik, Nigel Botting, Denis De Keukeleire, Marc Bracke, Arne Heyerick, Claudine Manach, and Herman Depypere. 2010. Disposition of soy isoflavones in normal human breast tissue. *The American Journal of Clinical Nutrition* 91:976–984.

Boyd, Norman F., Helen Guo, Lisa J. Martin, Limei Sun, Jennifer Stone, Eve Fishell, Roberta A. Jong, Greg Hislop, Anna Chiarelli, Salomon Minkin, and Martin J. Yaffe. 2007. Mammographic density and the risk and detection of breast cancer. *New England Journal of Medicine* 356:227–236.

Boyd, Norman F., G. A. Lockwood, J. W. Byng, D. L. Tritchler, and M. J. Yaffe. 1998. Mammographic densities and breast cancer risk. *Cancer Epidemiology Biomarkers & Prevention* 7:1133–1144.

Boyd, Norman F., J. W. Byng, R. A. Jong, E. K. Fishell, L. E. Little, A. B. Miller, G. A. Lockwood, D. L. Tritchler, and M. J. Yaffe. 1995. Quantitative classification of mammographic densities and breast cancer risk: results from the Canadian National Breast Screening Study. *Journal of the National Cancer Institute* 87:670–675.

Brausi, Maurizio, Federica Rizzi, and Saverio Bettuzzi. 2008. Chemoprevention of human prostate cancer by green tea catechins: two years later. A follow-up update. *European Urology* 54:472–473.

Brink, Elizabeth, Veronique Coxam, Simon Robins, Kristiina Wahala, Aedin Cassidy, Francesco Branca, and on behalf of the PHYTOS Investigators. 2008. Long-term consumption of isoflavone-enriched foods does not affect bone mineral density, bone metabolism, or hormonal status in early postmenopausal women: a randomized, double-blind, placebo controlled study. *The American Journal of Clinical Nutrition* 87:761–770.

Brisson, Jacques, Benoit Brisson, Gary Cote, Elizabeth Maunsell, Sylvie Berube, and Jean Robert. 2000. Tamoxifen and mammographic breast densities. *Cancer Epidemiology Biomarkers & Prevention* 9:911–915.

Brusselmans, Koen, Ruth Vrolix, Guido Verhoeven, and Johannes V. Swinnen. 2005. Induction of cancer cell apoptosis by flavonoids is associated with their ability to inhibit fatty acid synthase activity. *Journal of Biological Chemistry* 280:5636–5645.

Brusselmans, Koen, Ellen De Schrijver, Walter Heyns, Guido Verhoeven, and Johannes V. Swinnen. 2003. Epigallocatechin-3-gallate is a potent natural inhibitor of fatty acid synthase in intact cells and selectively induces apoptosis in prostate cancer cells. *International Journal of Cancer* 106:856–862.

Bundred, Nigel J., E. Anderson, R. I. Nicholson, M. Dowsett, M. Dixon, and J. F. Robertson. 2002. Fulvestrant, an estrogen receptor downregulator, reduces cell turnover index more effectively than tamoxifen. *Anticancer Research* 22:2317–2319.

Campbell, Julie S., J. A. Cardelli, and Jerry McLarty. 2010. Effects of presurgical administration of an oral green tea extract in women with operable breast cancer. Paper read at American Association for Cancer Research, Frontiers in Cancer Prevention, at Philadelphia, PA.

Cao, Feng, T. Y. Jin, and Y. F. Zhou. 2006. Inhibitory effect of isoflavones on prostate cancer cells and PTEN gene. *Biomedical and Environmental Science* 19:35–41.

Chang, Polly Y., Jon Mirsalis, Edward S. Riccio, James P. Bakke, Pamela S. Lee, Julie Shimon, Sandra Phillips, David Fairchild, Yukihiko Hara, and James A. Crowell. 2003. Genotoxicity and toxicity of the potential cancer-preventive agent polyphenon E. *Environmental and Molecular Mutagenesis* 41:43–54.

Chen, Zong Ping, John B Schell, Chi-Tang Ho, and Kuang Yu Chen. 1998. Green tea epigallocatechin gallate shows a pronounced growth inhibitory effect on cancerous cells but not on their normal counterparts. *Cancer Letters* 129:173–179.

Chiu, Feng-Lan, and Jen-Kun Lin. 2008. Downregulation of androgen receptor expression by luteolin causes inhibition of cell proliferation and induction of apoptosis in human prostate cancer cells and xenografts. *The Prostate* 68:61–71.

Choan, E., Roanne Segal, Derek Jonker, Shawn Malone, Neil Reaume, Libni Eapen, and Victor Gallant. 2005. A prospective clinical trial of green tea for hormone refractory prostate cancer: an evaluation of the complementary/alternative therapy approach. *Urologic Oncology: Seminars and Original Investigations* 23:108–113.

Chow, Catherine K., David Venzon, Elizabeth C. Jones, Ahalya Premkumar, Joyce O'Shaughnessy, and JoAnne Zujewski. 2000. Effect of tamoxifen on mammographic density. *Cancer Epidemiology Biomarkers & Prevention* 9:917–921.

Chow, H.-H. Sherry, Yan Cai, David S. Alberts, Iman Hakim, Robert Dorr, Farah Shahi, James A. Crowell, Chung S. Yang, and Yukihiko Hara. 2001 Phase I pharmacokinetic study of tea polyphenols following single-dose administration of epigallocatechin gallate and polyphenon E. *Cancer Epidemiology Biomarkers & Prevention* 1053–1058.

Chow, H.-H. Sherry, Yan Cai, Iman A. Hakim, James A. Crowell, Farah Shahi, Chris A. Brooks, Robert T. Dorr, Yukihiko Hara, and David S. Alberts. 2003. Pharmacokinetics and safety of green tea polyphenols after multiple-dose administration of epigallocatechin gallate and polyphenon E in healthy individuals: *Clinical Cancer Research* 9:3312–3319.

Cole, Bernard F., J. A. Baron, R. S. Sandler, R. W. Haile, D. J. Ahnen, R. S. Bresalier, G. McKeown-Eyssen, R. W. Summers, R. I. Rothstein, C. A. Burke, D. C. Snover, T. R. Church, J. I. Allen, D. J. Robertson, G. J. Beck, J. H. Bond, T. Byers, J. S. Mandel, L. A. Mott, L. H. Pearson, E. L. Barry, J. R. Rees, N. Marcon, F. Saibil, P. M. Ueland, and E. R. Greenberg. 2007. Folic acid for the prevention of colorectal adenomas: a randomized clinical trial. *JAMA* 297:2351–2359.

Coleman, David T., Rebecca Bigelow, and James A. Cardelli. 2009. Inhibition of fatty acid synthase by luteolin post-transcriptionally down-regulates c-Met expression independent of proteosomal/lysosomal degradation. *Molecular Cancer Therapeutics* 8:214–224.

Constantinou, Andreas I., Daniel Lantvit, Michael Hawthorne, Xiaoying Xu, Richard B. van Breemen, and John M. Pezzuto. 2001. Chemopreventive effects of soy protein and purified soy isoflavones on DMBA-induced mammary tumors in female Sprague-Dawley rats. *Nutrition and Cancer* 41:75–81.

Crew, Katherine D., P. H. Brown, and H. Greenlee. 2011. Phase IB randomized, double-blinded, placebo-controlled, dose escalation study of Polyphenon E in women with a history of hormone receptor-negative breast cancer. Paper read at American Association for Cancer Research, Frontiers in Cancer Prevention, at Boston, MA.

Cuzick, Jack, Jane Warwick, Elizabeth Pinney, Stephen W. Duffy, Simon Cawthorn, Anthony Howell, John F. Forbes, and Ruth M. L. Warren. 2011. Tamoxifen-induced reduction in mammographic density and breast cancer risk reduction: a nested case-control study. *Journal of the National Cancer Institute* 103:744–752.

Cuzick, Jack, Jane Warwick, Elizabeth Pinney, Ruth M. L. Warren, and Stephen W. Duffy. 2004. Tamoxifen and breast density in women at increased risk of breast cancer. *Journal of the National Cancer Institute* 96:621–628.

Dalais, Fabien S., Andreanyta Meliala, Naiyana Wattanapenpaiboon, Mark Frydenberg, David A. I. Suter, William K. Thomson, and Mark L. Wahlqvist. 2004. Effects of a diet rich in phytoestrogens on prostate-specific antigen and sex hormones in men diagnosed with prostate cancer. *Urology* 64:510–515.

Davis, Joanne N., N. Muqim, M. Bhuiyan, O. Kucuk, K. J. Pienta, and F. H. Sarkar. 2000. Inhibition of prostate specific antigen expression by genistein in prostate cancer cells. *International Journal of Oncology* 16:1091–1097.

Dayyani, Farshid, Gary E. Gallick, Christopher J. Logothetis, and Paul G. Corn. 2011. Novel therapies for metastatic castrate-resistant prostate cancer. *Journal of the National Cancer Institute* 103:1665–1675.

deVere White, Ralph W., Alexander Tsodikov, Eschelle C. Stapp, Stephanie E. Soares, Hajime Fujii, and Robert M. Hackman. 2010. Effects of a high dose, aglycone-rich soy extract on prostate-specific antigen and serum isoflavone concentrations in men with localized prostate cancer. *Nutrition and Cancer* 62:1036–1043.

deVere White, Ralph W., Robert M. Hackman, Stephanie E. Soares, Laurel A. Beckett, Yueju Li, and Buxiang Sun. 2004. Effects of a genistein-rich extract on PSA levels in men with a history of prostate cancer. *Urology* 63:259–263.

Dillingham, Barbara L., Brianne L. McVeigh, Johanna W. Lampe, and Alison M. Duncan. 2005. Soy protein isolates of varying isoflavone content exert minor effects on serum reproductive hormones in healthy young men. *The Journal of Nutrition* 135:584–591.

Dowsett, Mitch, I. E. Smith, S. R. Ebbs, J. M. Dixon, A. Skene, R. A'Hern, J. Salter, S. Detre, M. Hills, and G. Walsh. 2007. Prognostic value of Ki67 expression after short-term presurgical endocrine therapy for primary breast cancer. *Journal of the National Cancer Institute* 99:167–170.

Dowsett, Mitch, Nigel J. Bundred, Andrea Decensi, Richard C. Sainsbury, Yili Lu, Margaret J. Hills, Fredric J. Cohen, Paolo Veronesi, Mary E. R. O'Brien, Teri Scott, and Douglas B. Muchmore. 2001. Effect of raloxifene on breast cancer cell Ki67 and apoptosis. *Cancer Epidemiology Biomarkers & Prevention* 10:961–966.

Dowsett, Mitch, J. Michael Dixon, Kieran Horgan, Janine Salter, Margaret Hills, and Eileen Harvey. 2000. Antiproliferative effects of idoxifene in a placebo-controlled trial in primary human breast cancer. *Clinical Cancer Research* 6:2260–2267.

Du, Mengyuan, Xujuan Yang, James A. Hartman, Paul S. Cooke, Daniel R. Doerge, Young H. Ju, and William G. Helferich. 2012. Low-dose dietary genistein negates the therapeutic effect of tamoxifen in athymic nude mice. *Carcinogenesis* 33:895–901.

Duhon, Damian, Rebecca L. H. Bigelow, David T. Coleman, Joshua J. Steffan, Chris Yu, Will Langston, Christopher G. Kevil, and James A. Cardelli. 2010. The polyphenol epigallocatechin-3-gallate affects lipid rafts to block activation of the c-Met receptor in prostate cancer cells. *Molecular Carcinogenesis* 49:739–749.

Duo, J., G. G. Ying, G. W. Wang, and L. Zhang. 2012. Quercetin inhibits human breast cancer cell proliferation and induces apoptosis via Bcl-2 and Bax regulation. *Molecular Medicine Reports* 5:1453–1456.

Eddy, Sean F., Susan E. Kane, and Gail E. Sonenshein. 2007. Trastuzumab-resistant HER2-driven breast cancer cells are sensitive to epigallocatechin-3 gallate. *Cancer Research* 67:9018–9023.

Fan, S., Q. Meng, K. Auborn, T. Carter, and E. M. Rosen. 2006. BRCA1 and BRCA2 as molecular targets for phytochemicals indole-3-carbinol and genistein in breast and prostate cancer cells. *British Journal of Cancer* 94:407–426.

Fang, Jing, Qiong Zhou, Xiang-lin Shi, and Bing-hua Jiang. 2006. Luteolin inhibits insulin-like growth factor 1 receptor signaling in prostate cancer cells. *Carcinogenesis* 28:713–723.

Farabegoli, F., A. Papi, and M. Orlandi. 2011. (–)-Epigallocatechin-3-gallate down-regulates EGFR, MMP-2, MMP-9 and EMMPRIN and inhibits the invasion of MCF-7 tamoxifen-resistant cells. *Bioscience Reports* 31:99–108.

Faure, ED., P. Chantre, and P Mares. 2002. Effects of a standardized soy extract on hot flushes: a multicenter, double-blind, randomized, placebo-controlled study. *Menopause* 9.

Fischer, Leslie, Chrysa Mahoney, A. Robert Jeffcoat, Matthew A. Koch, Brian F. Thomas, John L. Valentine, Thomas Stinchcombe, Jarol Boan, James A. Crowell, and Steven H. Zeisel. 2004. Clinical characteristics and pharmacokinetics of purified soy isoflavones: multiple-dose administration to men with prostate neoplasia. *Nutrition and Cancer* 48:160–170.

Fox, Stephen, Daniele Generali, and Adrian Harris. 2007. Breast tumour angiogenesis. *Breast Cancer Research* 9:216.

Franzen, Carrie A., Evangeline Amargo, Viktor Todorović, Bhushan V. Desai, Sabil Huda, Salida Mirzoeva, Karen Chiu, Bartosz A. Grzybowski, Teng-Leong Chew, Kathleen J. Green, and Jill C. Pelling. 2009. The chemopreventive bioflavonoid apigenin inhibits prostate cancer cell motility through the focal adhesion kinase/Src signaling mechanism. *Cancer Prevention Research* 2:830–841.

Gann, Peter H., Ralph Kazer, Robert Chatterton, Susan Gapstur, Kim Thedford, Irene Helenowski, Sue Giovanazzi, and Linda Van Horn. 2005. Sequential, randomized trial of a low-fat, high-fiber diet and soy supplementation: effects on circulating IGF-I and its binding proteins in premenopausal women. *International Journal of Cancer* 116:297–303.

Gardner, Christopher D., Beibei Oelrich, Jenny P. Liu, David Feldman, Adrian A. Franke, and James D. Brooks. 2009. Prostatic soy isoflavone concentrations exceed serum levels after dietary supplementation. *The Prostate* 69:719–726.

Gastaldi, Stefania, Paolo Comoglio, and Livio Trusolino. 2010. The Met oncogene and basal-like breast cancer: another culprit to watch out for? *Breast Cancer Research* 12:208.

Goel, Ajay, Sonia Jhurani, and Bharat B. Aggarwal. 2008. Multi-targeted therapy by curcumin: how spicy is it? *Molecular Nutrition & Food Research* 52:1010–1030.

Golden, Encouse B., Philip Y. Lam, Adel Kardosh, Kevin J. Gaffney, Enrique Cadenas, Stan G. Louie, Nicos A. Petasis, Thomas C. Chen, and Axel H. Schanthal. 2009. Green tea polyphenols block the anticancer effects of bortezomib and other boronic acid based proteasome inhibitors. *Blood* 113:5927–5937.

Gonzalez-Angulo, Ana M., Jaime Ferrer-Lozano, Katherine Stemke-Hale, Aysegul Sahin, Shuying Liu, Juan A. Barrera, Octavio Burgues, Ana M. Lluch, Huiqin Chen, Gabriel N. Hortobagyi, Gordon B. Mills, and Funda Meric-Bernstam. 2011. PI3K pathway mutations and PTEN levels in primary and metastatic breast cancer. *Molecular Cancer Therapeutics* 10:1093–1101.

Grainger, Elizabeth M., Steven J. Schwartz, Shihua Wang, Nuray Z. Unlu, Thomas W.-M. Boileau, Amy K. Ferketich, J. Paul Monk, Michael C. Gong, Robert R. Bahnson, Valerie L. DeGroff, and Steven K. Clinton. 2008. A combination of tomato and soy products for men with recurring prostate cancer and rising prostate specific antigen. *Nutrition and Cancer* 60:145–154.

Group. 1994. The effect of vitamin E and beta carotene on the incidence of lung cancer and other cancers in male smokers. *New England Journal of Medicine* 330:1029–1035.

Guo, Yanping, Shihua Wang, Dahlys R. Hoot, and Steven K. Clinton. 2007. Suppression of VEGF-mediated autocrine and paracrine interactions between prostate cancer cells and vascular endothelial cells by soy isoflavones. *The Journal of Nutritional Biochemistry* 18:408–417.

Gupta, Subash, Ji Kim, Sahdeo Prasad, and Bharat Aggarwal. 2010. Regulation of survival, proliferation, invasion, angiogenesis, and metastasis of tumor cells through modulation of inflammatory pathways by nutraceuticals. In *Cancer and Metastasis Reviews*: Springer, Netherlands.

Gupta, Sanjay, F. Afaq, and H. Mukhtar. 2002. Involvement of nuclear factor-kappa B, Bax and Bcl-2 in induction of cell cycle arrest and apoptosis by apigenin in human prostate carcinoma cells. *Oncogene* 21:3727–3738.

Guy, Laurent, Nicolas Vedrine, Mireia Urpi-Sarda, Angel Gil-Izquierdo, Nawaf Al-Maharik, Jean-Paul Boiteux, Augustin Scalbert, Christian Remesy, Nigel P. Botting, and Claudine Manach. 2008. Orally administered isoflavones are present as glucuronides in the human prostate. *Nutrition and Cancer* 60:461–468.

Hamilton-Reeves, Jill M., Salome A. Rebello, Will Thomas, Mindy S. Kurzer, and Joel W. Slaton. 2007a. Effects of soy protein isolate consumption on prostate cancer biomarkers in men with HGPIN, ASAP, and low-grade prostate cancer. *Nutrition and Cancer* 60:7–13.

Hamilton-Reeves, Jill M., Salome A. Rebello, William Thomas, Joel W. Slaton, and Mindy S. Kurzer. 2007b. Isoflavone-rich soy protein isolate suppresses androgen receptor expression without altering estrogen receptor-β expression or serum hormonal profiles in men at high risk of prostate cancer. *The Journal of Nutrition* 137:1769–1775.

Hargreaves, Danielle F., Christopher S. Potten, Claudia Harding, Lesley E. Shaw, Michael S. Morton, Stephen A. Roberts, Anthony Howell, and Nigel J. Bundred. 1999. Two-week dietary soy supplementation has an estrogenic effect on normal premenopausal breast. *Journal of Clinical Endocrinology & Metabolism* 84:4017–4024.

Henning, Susanne M., William Aronson, Yantao Niu, Francisco Conde, Nicolas H. Lee, Navindra P. Seeram, Ru-Po Lee, Jinxiu Lu, Diane M. Harris, Aune Moro, Jenny Hong, Leung Pak-Shan, R. James Barnard, Hossein G. Ziaee, George Csathy, Vay L. W. Go, Hejing Wang, and David Heber. 2006. Tea polyphenols and theaflavins are present in prostate tissue of humans and mice after green and black tea consumption. *The Journal of Nutrition* 136:1839–1843.

Hooper, Lee, J. J. Ryder, M. S. Kurzer, J.W. Lampe, M. J. Messina, W. R. Phipps, and A. Cassidy. 2009. Effects of soy protein and isoflavones on circulating hormone concentrations in pre- and post-menopausal women: a systematic review and meta-analysis. *Human Reproduction Update* 15:423–440.

Hooper, Lee, Giri Madhavan, Jeffrey A. Tice, Sam J. Leinster, and Aeden Cassidy. 2010. Effects of isoflavones on breast density in pre- and post-menopausal women: a systematic review and meta-analysis of randomized controlled trials. *Human Reproduction Update* 16:745–760.

Hsieh, Ching-Yi, Ross C. Santell, Sandra Z. Haslam, and William G. Helferich. 1998. Estrogenic effects of genistein on the growth of estrogen receptor-positive human breast cancer (MCF-7) cells in vitro and in vivo. *Cancer Research* 58:3833–3838

Hsieh, Tze-Chen, and Joseph M. Wu. 2009. Targeting CWR22Rv1 prostate cancer cell proliferation and gene expression by combinations of the phytochemicals EGCG, genistein and quercetin. *Anticancer Research* 29:4025–4032.

Huang, Hsiu-Chen, Tzong-Der Way, Chih-Li Lin, and Jen-Kun Lin. 2008. EGCG Stabilizes p27kip1 in E2-stimulated MCF-7 cells through down-regulation of the Skp2 protein. *Endocrinology* 149:5972–5983.

Huang, Ying-Tang, Lung-Ta Lee, Ping-Ping H. Lee, Yung-Sheng Lin, and Ming-Ting Lee. 2005. Targeting of focal adhesion kinase by flavonoids and small-interfering RNAs reduces tumor cell migration ability. *Anticancer Research* 25:2017–2025.

Ide, Hisamitsu, Shino Tokiwa, Kentaro Sakamaki, Koujiro Nishio, Shuji Isotani, Satoru Muto, Takanori Hama, Hiroko Masuda, and Shigeo Horie. 2010. Combined inhibitory effects of soy isoflavones and curcumin on the production of prostate-specific antigen. *The Prostate* 70:1127–1133.

Iwasaki, Motoki, M. Inoue, S. Sasazuki, T. Miura, N. Sawada, T. Yamaji, T. Shimazu, W. C. Willett, and S. Tsugane. 2010. Plasma tea polyphenol levels and subsequent risk of breast cancer among Japanese women: a nested case-control study. *Breast Cancer Research and Treatment* 124:827–834.

Jarred, Renea A., Mohammad Keikha, Caroline Dowling, Stephen J. McPherson, Anne M. Clare, Alan J. Husband, John S. Pedersen, Mark Frydenberg, and Gail P. Risbridger. 2002 Induction of apoptosis in low to moderate-grade human prostate carcinoma by red clover-derived dietary isoflavones. *Cancer Epidemiology Biomarkers & Prevention* 11:1689–1696

Jatoi, Aminah, Neil Ellison, Patrick A. Burch, Jeff A. Sloan, Shaker R. Dakhil, Paul Novotny, Winston Tan, Tom R. Fitch, Kendrith M. Rowland, Charles Y. F. Young, and Patrick J. Flynn. 2003. A phase II trial of green tea in the treatment of patients with androgen independent metastatic prostate carcinoma. *Cancer* 97:1442–1446.

Johnson, Jeremy J., H. H. Bailey, and H. Mukhtar. 2010. Green tea polyphenols for prostate cancer chemoprevention: a translational perspective. *Phytomedicine* 17:3–13.

Joniau, Steven, L. Goeman, T. Roskams, E. Lerut, R. Oyen, and H. Van Poppel. 2007. Effect of nutritional supplement challenge in patients with isolated high-grade prostatic intraepithelial neoplasia. *Urology* 69:1102–1106.

Kang, Nam Joo, Seung Ho Shin, Hyong Joo Lee, and Ki Won Lee. 2011. Polyphenols as small molecular inhibitors of signaling cascades in carcinogenesis. *Pharmacology & Therapeutics* 130:310–324.

Kaur, Parminder, Sanjeev Shukla, and Sanjay Gupta. 2008. Plant flavonoid apigenin inactivates Akt to trigger apoptosis in human prostate cancer: an in vitro and in vivo study. *Carcinogenesis* 29:2210–2217.

Khan, Naghma, Vaqar Mustafa Adhami, and Hasan Mukhtar. 2009. Review: green tea polyphenols in chemo-prevention of prostate cancer: preclinical and clinical studies. *Nutrition and Cancer* 61:836–841.

Khan, Seema A., Robert T. Chatterton, Nancy Michel, Michelle Bryk, Oukseub Lee, David Ivancic, Richard Heinz, Carola M. Zalles, Irene B. Helenowski, Borko D. Jovanovic, Adrian A. Franke, Maarten C. Bosland, Jun Wang, Nora M. Hansen, Kevin P. Bethke, Alexander Dew, Margerie Coomes, and Raymond C. Bergan. 2012. Soy isoflavone supplementation for breast cancer risk reduction: a randomized phase II trial. *Cancer Prevention Research* 5:309–319.

Khan, Shabana, Jianping Zhao, Ikhlas Khan, Larry Walker, and Asok Dasmahapatra. 2011. Potential utility of natural products as regulators of breast cancer-associated aromatase promoters. *Reproductive Biology and Endocrinology* 9:91. doi:10.1186/1477-7827-9-91.

Kinjo, Junei, R. Tsuchihashi, K. Morito, T. Hirose, T. Aomori, T. Nagao, H. Okabe, T. Nohara, and Y. Masamune. 2004. Interactions of phytoestrogens with estrogen receptors alpha and beta (III). Estrogenic activities of soy isoflavone aglycones and their metabolites isolated from human urine. *Biological and Pharmaceutic Bulletin* 27:185–188.

Klein, Eric A., I. M. Thompson, Jr., C. M. Tangen, J. J. Crowley, M. S. Lucia, P. J. Goodman, L. M. Minasian, L. G. Ford, H. L. Parnes, J. M. Gaziano, D. D. Karp, M. M. Lieber, P. J. Walther, L. Klotz, J. K. Parsons, J. L. Chin, A. K. Darke, S. M. Lippman, G. E. Goodman, F. L. Meyskens, Jr., and L. H. Baker. 2011. Vitamin E and the risk of prostate cancer: the Selenium and Vitamin E Cancer Prevention Trial (SELECT). *JAMA* 306:1549–1556.

Kridel, Steven J., Fumiko Axelrod, Natasha Rozenkrantz, and Jeffrey W. Smith. 2004. Orlistat is a novel inhibitor of fatty acid synthase with antitumor activity. *Cancer Research* 64:2070–2075.

Kuiper, George G. J. M., Josephine G. Lemmen, Bo Carlsson, J. Christopher Corton, Stephen H. Safe, Paul T. van der Saag, Bart van der Burg, and Jan-Ake Gustafsson. 1998. Interaction of estrogenic chemicals and phytoestrogens with estrogen receptor. *Endocrinology* 139:4252–4263.

Kumar, Nagi B., Jeffrey P. Krischer, Kathy Allen, Diane Riccardi, Karen Besterman-Dahan, Raoul Salup, Lovellen Kang, Ping Xu, and Julio Pow-Sang. 2007. A phase II randomized, placebo-controlled clinical trial of purified isoflavones in modulating steroid hormones in men diagnosed with localized prostate cancer. *Nutrition and Cancer* 59:163–168.

Kumar, Nagi B., Alan Cantor, Kathy Allen, Diane Riccardi, Karen Besterman-Dahan, John Seigne, Mohamad Helal, Raoul Salup, and Julio Pow-Sang. 2004. The specific role of isoflavones in reducing prostate cancer risk. *The Prostate* 59:141–147.

Kwan, Winkle, Graeme Duncan, Cheri Van Patten, Mitchell Liu, and Jan Lim. 2010. A phase II trial of a soy beverage for subjects without clinical disease with rising prostate-specific antigen after radical radiation for prostate cancer. *Nutrition and Cancer* 62:198–207.

Lamy, Sylvie, Valerie Bedard, David Labbe, Herve Sartelet, Chantal Barthomeuf, Denis Gingras, and Richard Beliveau. 2008. The dietary flavones apigenin and luteolin impair smooth muscle cell migration and VEGF expression through inhibition of PDGFR-β phosphorylation. *Cancer Prevention Research* 1:452–459.

Lazarevic, Bato, C. Hammarstrom, J. Yang, H. Ramberg, L. M. Diep, S. J. Karlsen, O. Kucuk, F. Saatcioglu, K. A. Tasken, and A. Svindland. 2012. The effects of short-term genistein intervention on prostate biomarker expression in patients with localised prostate cancer before radical prostatectomy. *British Journal of Nutrition* 1–10.

Lazarevic, Bato, Gro Boezelijn, Lien My Diep, Kristin Kvernrod, Olov Ogren, Hakon Ramberg, Anders Moen, Nicolai Wessel, R. Egil Berg, Wolfgang Egge-Jacobsen, Clara Hammarstrom, Aud Svindland, Omer Kucuk, Fahri Saatcioglu, Kristin A. Taskèn, and Steinar J. Karlsen. 2011. Efficacy and safety of short-term genistein intervention in patients with localized prostate cancer prior to radical prostatectomy: a randomized, placebo-controlled, double-blind phase 2 clinical trial. *Nutrition and Cancer* 63:889–898.

Lee, Lung-Ta, Ying-Tang Huang, Jiuan-Jiuan Hwang, Amy Y.-L. Lee, Ferng-Chun Ke, Chang-Jen Huang, Chithan Kandaswami, Ping-Ping H. Lee, and Ming-Ting Lee. 2004. Transinactivation of the epidermal growth factor receptor tyrosine kinase and focal adhesion kinase phosphorylation by dietary flavonoids: effect on invasive potential of human carcinoma cells. *Biochemical Pharmacology* 67:2103–2114.

Lee, Wei-Jiunn, Wen-Kang Chen, Chau-Jong Wang, Wea-Lung Lin, and Tsui-Hwa Tseng. 2008. Apigenin inhibits HGF-promoted invasive growth and metastasis involving blocking PI3K/Akt pathway and [beta]4 integrin function in MDA-MB-231 breast cancer cells. *Toxicology and Applied Pharmacology* 226:178–191.

Li, Ming, Zhiwei He, Svetlana Ermakova, Duo Zheng, Faqing Tang, Yong-Yeon Cho, Feng Zhu, Wei-Ya Ma, Yuk Sham, Evgeny A. Rogozin, Ann M. Bode, Ya Cao, and Zigang Dong. 2007. Direct inhibition of insulin-like growth factor-I receptor kinase activity by epigallocatechin-3-gallate regulates cell transformation. *Cancer Epidemiology Biomarkers & Prevention* 16:598–605.

Li, Yiwei, Fakhara Ahmed, Shadan Ali, Philip A. Philip, Omer Kucuk, and Fazlul H. Sarkar. 2005. Inactivation of nuclear factor kB by soy isoflavone genistein contributes to increased apoptosis induced by chemotherapeutic agents in human cancer cells. *Cancer Research* 65:6934–6942.

Liang, Yu-Chih, Shoei-Yn Lin-Shiau, Chieh-Fu Chen, and Jen-Kun Lin. 1999. Inhibition of cyclin-dependent kinases 2 and 4 activities as well as induction of cdk inhibitors p21 and p27 during growth arrest of human breast carcinoma cells by (–)-epigallocatechin-3-gallate. *Journal of Cellular Biochemistry* 75:1–12.

Lin, Cheng-Wei, Wen-Chi Hou, Shing-Chuan Shen, Shu-Hui Juan, Ching-Huai Ko, Ling-Mei Wang, and Yen-Chou Chen. 2008. Quercetin inhibition of tumor invasion via suppressing PKC/ERK/AP-1-dependent matrix metalloproteinase-9 activation in breast carcinoma cells. *Carcinogenesis* 29:1807–1815.

Liu, Kuo-Ching, Chun-Yi Yen, Rick Sai-Chuen Wu, Jai-Sing Yang, Hsu-Feng Lu, Kung-Wen Lu, Chyi Lo, Hung-Yi Chen, Nou-Ying Tang, Chih-Chung Wu, and Jing-Gung Chung. 2012. The roles of endoplasmic reticulum stress and mitochondrial apoptotic signaling pathway in quercetin-mediated cell death of human prostate cancer PC-3 cells. *Environmental Toxicology* doi:10.1002/tox.21769.

Long, Xinghua, Meiyun Fan, Robert M. Bigsby, and Kenneth P. Nephew. 2008. Apigenin inhibits antiestrogen-resistant breast cancer cell growth through estrogen receptor-α-dependent and estrogen receptor-α-independent mechanisms. *Molecular Cancer Therapeutics* 7:2096–2108.

Lukaczer, Dan, G. Darland, M. Tripp, D. Liska, R. H. Lerman, B. Schiltz, and J. S. Bland. 2005. Clinical effects of a proprietary combination isoflavone nutritional supplement in menopausal women: a pilot trial. *Aternative Therapies in Health and Medicine* 11:60–65.

MacGregor, Charles A., P. A. Canney, G. Patterson, R. McDonald, and J. Paul. 2005. A randomised double-blind controlled trial of oral soy supplements versus placebo for treatment of menopausal symptoms in patients with early breast cancer. *European Journal of Cancer* 41:708–714.

Mafuvadze, Benford, I. Benakanakere, and S. M. Hyder. 2010. Apigenin blocks induction of vascular endothelial growth factor mRNA and protein in progestin-treated human breast cancer cells. *Menopause* 17:1055–1063.

Mai, Zhiming, George L. Blackburn, and Jin-Rong Zhou. 2007. Genistein sensitizes inhibitory effect of tamoxifen on the growth of estrogen receptor-positive and HER2-overexpressing human breast cancer cells. *Molecular Carcinogenesis* 46:534–542.

Manach, Claudine, Gary Williamson, Christine Morand, Augustin Scalbert, and Christian Remesy. 2005. Bioavailability and bioefficacy of polyphenols in humans. I. Review of 97 bioavailability studies. *The American Journal of Clinical Nutrition* 81:230S–242S.

Marini, Herbert, Alessandra Bitto, Domenica Altavilla, Bruce P. Burnett, Francesca Polito, Vincenzo Di Stefano, Letteria Minutoli, Marco Atteritano, Robert M. Levy, Rosario D'Anna, Nicola Frisina, Susanna Mazzaferro, Francesco Cancellieri, Maria Letizia Cannata, Francesco Corrado, Alessia Frisina, Vincenzo Adamo, Carla Lubrano, Carlo Sansotta, Rolando Marini, Elena Bianca Adamo, and Francesco Squadrito. 2008. Breast safety and efficacy of genistein aglycone for postmenopausal bone loss: a follow-up study. *Journal of Clinical Endocrinology & Metabolism* 93:4787–4796.

Markaverich, Barry M., Mary Vijjeswarapu, Kevin Shoulars, and Mary Rodriguez. 2010. Luteolin and gefitinib regulation of EGF signaling pathway and cell cycle pathway genes in PC-3 human prostate cancer cells. *The Journal of Steroid Biochemistry and Molecular Biology* 122:219–231.

Maskarinec, Gertraud, Nicholas J. Ollberding, Shannon M. Conroy, Yukiko Morimoto, Ian S. Pagano, Adrian A. Franke, Elisabet Gentzschein, and Frank Z. Stanczyk. 2011. Estrogen levels in nipple aspirate fluid and serum during a randomized soy trial. *Cancer Epidemiology Biomarkers & Prevention* 20:1815–1821.

Maskarinec, Gertraud, Jana Steude, Adrian Franke, and Robert Cooney. 2009. Inflammatory markers in a 2-year soy intervention among premenopausal women. *Journal of Inflammation* 6:9.

Maskarinec, Gertraud, Y. Morimoto, S. Hebshi, S. Sharma, A. A. Franke, and F. Z. Stanczyk. 2006. Serum prostate-specific antigen but not testosterone levels decrease in a randomized soy intervention among men. *European Journal of Clinical Nutrition* 60:1423–1429.

Maskarinec, Gertraud, Y. Takata, S. P. Murphy, A. A. Franke, and R. Kaaks. 2005. Insulin-like growth factor-1 and binding protein-3 in a 2-year soya intervention among premenopausal women. *British Journal of Nutrition* 94:362–367.

Masuda, Muneyuki, Masumi Suzui, Jin T. E. Lim, and I. Bernard Weinstein. 2003 Epigallocatechin-3-gallate inhibits activation of HER-2/neu and downstream signaling pathways in human head and neck and breast carcinoma cells. *Clinical Cancer Research* 9:3486–3491.

Maubach, Julie, H. T. Depypere, J. Goeman, J. Van der Eycken, A. Heyerick, M. E. Bracke, P. Blondeel, and D. De Keukeleire. 2004. Distribution of soy-derived phytoestrogens in human breast tissue and biological fluids. *Obstetrics & Gynecology* 103:892–898.

McCormack, Valerie A., and Isabel dos Santos Silva. 2006. Breast density and parenchymal patterns as markers of breast cancer risk: a meta-analysis. *Cancer Epidemiology Biomarkers & Prevention* 15:1159–1169.

McLarty, Jerry, Rebecca L. H. Bigelow, Mylinh Smith, Don Elmajian, Murali Ankem, and James A. Cardelli. 2009. Tea polyphenols decrease serum levels of prostate-specific antigen, hepatocyte growth factor, and vascular endothelial growth factor in prostate cancer patients and inhibit production of hepatocyte growth factor and vascular endothelial growth factor in vitro. *Cancer Prevention Research* 2:673–682.

McLaughlin, John M., Susan Olivo-Marston, Mara Z. Vitolins, Marisa Bittoni, Katherine W. Reeves, Cecilia R. Degraffinreid, Steven J. Schwartz, Steven K. Clinton, and Electra D. Paskett. 2011. Effects of tomato- and soy-rich diets on the IGF-I hormonal network: a crossover study of postmenopausal women at high risk for breast cancer. *Cancer Prevention Research* 4:702–710.

Menendez, Javier A., and Ruth Lupu. 2007. Fatty acid synthase and the lipogenic phenotype in cancer pathogenesis. *Nature Reviews Cancer* 7:763–777.

Menendez, Javier A., L. Vellon, and R. Lupu. 2005. Antitumoral actions of the anti-obesity drug orlistat in breast cancer cells: blockade of cell cycle progression, promotion of apoptotic cell death and PEA3-mediated transcriptional repression of Her2/neu (erbB-2) oncogene. *Annals of Oncology* 16:1253–1267.

Micalizzi, Douglas, Susan Farabaugh, and Heide Ford. 2010. Epithelial-mesenchymal transition in cancer: parallels between normal development and tumor progression. In *Journal of Mammary Gland Biology and Neoplasia*: Springer, Netherlands.

Milligan, Shawn A., Patrick Burke, David T. Coleman, Rebecca L. Bigelow, Joshua J. Steffan, Jennifer L. Carroll, Briana Jill Williams, and James A. Cardelli. 2009. The green tea polyphenol EGCG potentiates the antiproliferative activity of c-Met and epidermal growth factor receptor inhibitors in non-small cell lung cancer cells. *Clinical Cancer Research* 15:4885–4894.

Mirzoeva, Salida, Nam Deuk Kim, Karen Chiu, Carrie A. Franzen, Raymond C. Bergan, and Jill C. Pelling. 2008. Inhibition of HIF-1 alpha and VEGF expression by the chemopreventive bioflavonoid apigenin is accompanied by Akt inhibition in human prostate carcinoma PC3-M cells. *Molecular Carcinogenesis* 47:686–700.

Mittal, Anshu, M. S. Pate, R. C. Wylie, T. O. Tollefsbol, and S. K. Katiyar. 2004. EGCG down-regulates telomerase in human breast carcinoma MCF-7 cells, leading to suppression of cell viability and induction of apoptosis. *International Journal of Oncology* 24:703–710.

Miyanaga, Naoto, Hideyuki Akaza, Shiro Hinotsu, Tomoaki Fujioka, Seiji Naito, Mikio Namiki, Satoru Takahashi, Yoshihiko Hirao, Shigeo Horie, Taiji Tsukamoto, Mitsuru Mori, and Hirokazu Tsuji. 2012. Prostate cancer chemoprevention study: an investigative randomized control study using purified isoflavones in men with rising prostate-specific antigen. *Cancer Science* 103:125–130.

Montales, Maria Theresa E., Omar M. Rahal, Jie Kang, Theodore J. Rogers, Ronald L. Prior, Xianli Wu, and Rosalia C. M. Simmen. 2012. Repression of mammosphere formation of human breast cancer cells by soy isoflavone genistein and blueberry polyphenolic acids suggests diet-mediated targeting of cancer stem-like/progenitor cells. *Carcinogenesis* 33:652–660.

Morimoto, Yukiko, Shannon M. Conroy, Ian S. Pagano, Marissa Isaki, Adrian A. Franke, Frank J. Nordt, and Gertraud Maskarinec. 2012. Urinary estrogen metabolites during a randomized soy trial. *Nutrition and Cancer* 64:307–314.

Musgrove, Elizabeth A., and Robert L. Sutherland. 2009. Biological determinants of endocrine resistance in breast cancer. *Nature Reviews Cancer* 9:631–643.

Nair, Hareesh B., Bokyung Sung, Vivek R. Yadav, Ramaswamy Kannappan, Madan M. Chaturvedi, and Bharat B. Aggarwal. 2010. Delivery of antiinflammatory nutraceuticals by nanoparticles for the prevention and treatment of cancer. *Biochemical Pharmacology* 80:1833–1843.

Nakamura, H., Y. Wang, T. Kurita, H. Adomat, and G. R. Cunha. 2011. Genistein increases epidermal growth factor receptor signaling and promotes tumor progression in advanced human prostate cancer. *PLoS One* 6:e20034.

Nguyen, Mike M., Frederick R. Ahmann, Raymond B. Nagle, Chiu-Hsieh Hsu, Joseph A. Tangrea, Howard L. Parnes, Mitchell H. Sokoloff, Matthew B. Gretzer, and H.-H. Sherry Chow. 2012. Randomized, double-blind, placebo-controlled trial of polyphenon e in prostate cancer patients before prostatectomy: evaluation of potential chemopreventive activities. *Cancer Prevention Research* 5:290–298.

Nhan, Sukwan, Karl E. Anderson, Manubai Nagamani, James J. Grady, and Lee-Jane W. Lu. 2005. Effect of a soymilk supplement containing isoflavones on urinary F2 isoprostane levels in premenopausal women. *Nutrition and Cancer* 53:73–81.

Nikander, Eini, Merja Metsä-Heikkilä, Olavi Ylikorkala, and Aila Tiitinen. 2004a. Effects of phytoestrogens on bone turnover in postmenopausal women with a history of breast cancer. *Journal of Clinical Endocrinology & Metabolism* 89:1207–1212.

Nikander, Eini, Aila Tiitinen, Kalevi Laitinen, Matti Tikkanen, and Olavi Ylikorkala. 2004b. Effects of isolated isoflavonoids on lipids, lipoproteins, insulin sensitivity, and ghrelin in postmenopausal women. *Journal of Clinical Endocrinology & Metabolism* 89:3567–3572.

Nikander, Eini, A. Kilkkinen, M. Metsä-Heikkilä, H. Adlercreutz, P. Pietinen, A. Tiitinen, and O. Ylikorkala. 2003. A randomized placebo-controlled crossover trial with phytoestrogens in treatment of menopause in breast cancer patients. *Obstetrics & Gynecology* 101:1213–1220.

Noori-Daloii, Mohammad, Majid Momeny, Mehdi Yousefi, Forough Shirazi, Mehdi Yaseri, Nasrin Motamed, Nazanin Kazemialiakbar, and Saeed Hashemi. 2011. Multifaceted preventive effects of single agent quercetin on a human prostate adenocarcinoma cell line (PC-3): implications for nutritional transcriptomics and multi-target therapy. In *Medical Oncology*: Humana Press Inc, New York City.

Omenn, Gilbert S., Gary Goodman, Mark Thornquist, James Grizzle, Linda Rosenstock, Scott Barnhart, John Balmes, Martin G. Cherniack, Mark R. Cullen, Andrew Glass, James Keogh, Frank Meyskens, Barbara Valanis, and James Williams. 1994. The beta-carotene and retinol efficacy trial (CARET) for chemoprevention of lung cancer in high risk populations: smokers and asbestos-exposed workers. *Cancer Research* 54:2038s–2043s.

Pandey, Mitali, Parminder Kaur, Sanjeev Shukla, Ata Abbas, Pingfu Fu, and Sanjay Gupta. 2011. Plant flavone apigenin inhibits HDAC and remodels chromatin to induce growth arrest and apoptosis in human prostate cancer cells: in vitro and in vivo study. *Molecular Carcinogenesis* 51:952–962.

Park, Chang E., H. Yun, E. B. Lee, B. I. Min, H. Bae, W. Choe, I. Kang, S. S. Kim, and J. Ha. 2010. The antioxidant effects of genistein are associated with AMP-activated protein kinase activation and PTEN induction in prostate cancer cells. *Journal of Medicinal Food* 13:815–20.

Pendleton, John, Winston Tan, Satoshi Anai, Myron Chang, Wei Hou, Kathleen Shiverick, and Charles Rosser. 2008. Phase II trial of isoflavone in prostate-specific antigen recurrent prostate cancer after previous local therapy. *BMC Cancer* 8:132.

Pianetti, Stefania, Shangqin Guo, Kathryn T. Kavanagh, and Gail E. Sonenshein. 2002. Green tea polyphenol epigallocatechin-3 gallate inhibits Her-2/Neu signaling, proliferation, and transformed phenotype of breast cancer cells. *Cancer Research* 62:652–655

Qin, Wenyi, Weizhu Zhu, Huidong Shi, John E. Hewett, Rachel L. Ruhlen, Ruth S. MacDonald, George E. Rottinghaus, Yin-Chieh Chen, and Edward R. Sauter. 2009. Soy isoflavones have an antiestrogenic effect and alter mammary promoter hypermethylation in healthy premenopausal women. *Nutrition and Cancer* 61:238–244.

Quella, Susan K., Charles L. Loprinzi, Debra L. Barton, James A. Knost, Jeff A. Sloan, Beth I. LaVasseur, Debra Swan, Kenneth R. Krupp, Kathy D. Miller, and Paul J. Novotny. 2000 Evaluation of soy phytoestrogens for the treatment of hot flashes in breast cancer survivors: A North Central Cancer Treatment Group Trial. *Journal of Clinical Oncology* 18:1068.

Rannikko, Antti, Anssi Petas, Sakari Rannikko, and Herman Adlercreutz. 2006. Plasma and prostate phytoestrogen concentrations in prostate cancer patients after oral phytoestrogen supplementation. *The Prostate* 66:82–87.

Rich, Rebecca L., Lise R. Hoth, Kieran F. Geoghegan, Thomas A. Brown, Peter K. LeMotte, Samuel P. Simons, Preston Hensley, and David G. Myszka. 2002. Kinetic analysis of estrogen receptor/ligand interactions. *Proceedings of the National Academy of Sciences* 99:8562–8567.

Rocha, Sandra, Roman Generalov, Maria do Carmo Pereira, Ivone Peres, Petras Juzenas, and Manuel A. N. Coelho. 2010. Epigallocatechin gallate-loaded polysaccharide nanoparticles for prostate cancer chemoprevention. *Nanomedicine* 6:79–87.

Roy, Anshu M., M. S. Baliga, and S. K. Katiyar. 2005. Epigallocatechin-3-gallate induces apoptosis in estrogen receptor-negative human breast carcinoma cells via modulation in protein expression of p53 and Bax and caspase-3 activation. *Molecular Cancer Therapeutics* 4:81–90.

Sanna, Vanna, Gianfranco Pintus, Anna Maria Roggio, Stefania Punzoni, Anna Maria Posadino, Alessandro Arca, Salvatore Marceddu, Pasquale Bandiera, Sergio Uzzau, and Mario Sechi. 2011. Targeted biocompatible nanoparticles for the delivery of epigallocatechin 3-gallate to prostate cancer cells. *Journal of Medicinal Chemistry* 54:1321–1332.

Sartippour, Maryam R., Zhi-Ming Shao, David Heber, Perrin Beatty, Liping Zhang, Canhui Liu, Lee Ellis, Wen Liu, Vay Liang Go, and Mai N. Brooks. 2002. Green tea inhibits vascular endothelial growth factor (VEGF) induction in human breast cancer cells. *The Journal of Nutrition* 132:2307–2311

Satoh, Haruna, K. Nishikawa, K. Suzuki, R. Asano, N. Virgona, T. Ichikawa, K. Hagiwara, and T. Yano. 2003. Genistein, a soy isoflavone, enhances necrotic-like cell death in a breast cancer cell treated with a chemotherapeutic agent. *Research Communications in Molecular Pathology and Pharmacology* 113–114:149–158.

Scalbert, Augustin, Claudine Manach, Christine Morand, Christian Ramsey, and Liliana Jimanez. 2005. Dietary polyphenols and the prevention of diseases. *Critical Reviews in Food Science and Nutrition* 45:287–306.

Schwartz, Janice A., Gouzhen Liu, and Sam C. Brooks. 1998. Genistein-mediated attenuation of tamoxifen-induced antagonism from estrogen receptor-regulated genes. *Biochemical and Biophysical Research Communications* 253:38–43.

Sebastian, Sinto, Jeffrey Settleman, Stephan J. Reshkin, Amalia Azzariti, Antonia Bellizzi, and Angelo Paradiso. 2006. The complexity of targeting EGFR signalling in cancer: from expression to turnover. *Biochimica et Biophysica Acta (BBA)—Reviews on Cancer* 1766:120–139.

Seely, Dugald, Edward J. Mills, Ping Wu, Shailendra Verma, and Gordon H. Guyatt. 2005. The effects of green tea consumption on incidence of breast cancer and recurrence of breast cancer: a systematic review and meta-analysis. *Integrative Cancer Therapies* 4:144–155.

Sen, Cherisse, Yukiko Morimoto, Sreang Heak, Robert V. Cooney, Adrian A. Franke, and Gertraud Maskarinec. 2012. Soy foods and urinary isoprostanes: results from a randomized study in premenopausal women. *Food & Function* 3:517–521.

Sen, Triparna, Anindita Dutta, and Amitava Chatterjee. 2010. Epigallocatechin-3-gallate (EGCG) downregulates gelatinase-B (MMP-9) by involvement of FAK/ERK/NF[kappa]B and AP-1 in the human breast cancer cell line MDA-MB-231. *Anti-Cancer Drugs* 21.

Senthilkumar, Kalimuthu, Ramachandran Arunkumar, Perumal Elumalai, Govindaraj Sharmila, Dharmalingam Nandhagopal Gunadharini, Sivanantham Banudevi, Gunasekar Krishnamoorthy, Chellakan Selvanesan Benson, and Jagadeesan Arunakaran. 2011. Quercetin inhibits invasion, migration and signalling molecules involved in cell survival and proliferation of prostate cancer cell line (PC-3). *Cell Biochemistry and Function* 29:87–95.

Senthilkumar, Kalimuthu, Perumal Elumalai, Ramachandran Arunkumar, Sivanantham Banudevi, Nandagopal Gunadharini, Govindaraj Sharmila, Kandaswamy Selvakumar, and Jagadeesan Arunakaran. 2010. Quercetin regulates insulin like growth factor signaling and induces intrinsic and extrinsic pathway mediated apoptosis in androgen independent prostate cancer cells (PC-3). In *Molecular and Cellular Biochemistry*: Springer, Netherlands.

Seo, Hye-Sook, David DeNardo, Yves Jacquot, Ioanna Laïos, Doris Vidal, Carmen Zambrana, Guy Leclercq, and Powel Brown. 2006. Stimulatory effect of genistein and apigenin on the growth of breast cancer cells correlates with their ability to activate ER alpha. In *Breast Cancer Research and Treatment*: Springer, Netherlands.

Seo, Young Jin, Bum Soo Kim, So Young Chun, Yoon Kyu Park, Ku Seong Kang, and Tae Gyun Kwon. 2011. Apoptotic effects of genistein, biochanin-A and apigenin on LNCaP and PC-3 cells by p21 through transcriptional inhibition of polo-like kinase-1. *Journal of Korean Medical Science* 26:1489–1494.

Setchell, Kenneth D. R., Nadine M. Brown, Pankaj Desai, Linda Zimmer-Nechemias, Brian E. Wolfe, Wayne T. Brashear, Abby S. Kirschner, Aedin Cassidy, and James E. Heubi. 2001 Bioavailability of pure isoflavones in healthy humans and analysis of commercial soy isoflavone supplements. *The Journal of Nutrition* 131:1362S–1375S.

Sharma, Preetika, Amy Wisniewski, Milena Braga-Basaria, Xiaoqiang Xu, Mary Yep, Samuel Denmeade, Adrian S. Dobs, Theodore DeWeese, Michael Carducci, and Shehzad Basaria. 2009. Lack of an effect of high dose isoflavones in men with prostate cancer undergoing androgen deprivation therapy. *The Journal of Urology* 182:2265–2273.

Shehzad, Adeeb, Fazli Wahid, and Young Sup Lee. 2010. Curcumin in cancer chemoprevention: molecular targets, pharmacokinetics, bioavailability, and clinical trials. *Archiv der Pharmazie* 343:489–499.

Shukla., Sanjeev, and Sanjay Gupta. 2009. Apigenin suppresses insulin-like growth factor I receptor signaling in human prostate cancer: An in vitro and in vivo study. Vol. 48, *Molecular Carcinogenesis*: Wiley Subscription Services, Inc., A Wiley Company Hoboken, NJ.

Shukla, Sanjeev, and Sanjay Gupta. 2004. Molecular mechanisms for apigenin-induced cell-cycle arrest and apoptosis of hormone refractory human prostate carcinoma DU145 cells. *Molecular Carcinogenesis* 39:114–126.

Shukla, Sanjeev, Gregory MacLennan, Pingfu Fu, and Sanjay Gupta. 2012. Apigenin attenuates insulin-like growth factor-I signaling in an autochthonous mouse prostate cancer model. In *Pharmaceutical Research*: Springer, Netherlands.

Shukla, Sanjeev, Gregory T. MacLennan, Chris A. Flask, Pingfu Fu, Anil Mishra, Martin I. Resnick, and Sanjay Gupta. 2007. Blockade of beta-catenin signaling by plant flavonoid apigenin suppresses prostate carcinogenesis in TRAMP mice. *Cancer Research* 67:6925–6935.

Shutava, Tatsiana G., Shantanu S. Balkundi, Pranitha Vangala, Joshua J. Steffan, Rebecca L. Bigelow, James A. Cardelli, D. Patrick O'Neal, and Yuri M. Lvov. 2009. Layer-by-layer-coated gelatin nanoparticles as a vehicle for delivery of natural polyphenols. *ACS Nano* 3:1877–1885.

Siddiqui, Imtiaz, and Hasan Mukhtar. 2010. Nanochemoprevention by bioactive food components: a Perspective. In *Pharmaceutical Research*: Springer, Netherlands.

Siddiqui, Imtiaz A., Mohammad Asim, Bilal B. Hafeez, Vaqar M. Adhami, Rohinton S. Tarapore, and Hasan Mukhtar. 2011. Green tea polyphenol EGCG blunts androgen receptor function in prostate cancer. *The FASEB Journal* 25:1198–1207.

Siddiqui, Imtiaz A., Vaqar M. Adhami, Dhruba J. Bharali, Bilal B. Hafeez, Mohammad Asim, Sabih I. Khwaja, Nihal Ahmad, Huadong Cui, Shaker A. Mousa, and Hasan Mukhtar. 2009. Introducing nanochemoprevention as a novel approach for cancer control: proof of principle with green tea polyphenol epigallocatechin-3-gallate. *Cancer Research* 69:1712–1716.

Singh, Bhupendra, Sarah M. Mense, Nimee K. Bhat, Sandeep Putty, William A. Guthiel, Fabrizio Remotti, and Hari K. Bhat. 2010. Dietary quercetin exacerbates the development of estrogen-induced breast tumors in female ACI rats. *Toxicology and Applied Pharmacology* 247:83–90.

Singh-Gupta, Vinita, Hao Zhang, Sanjeev Banerjee, Dejuan Kong, Julian J. Raffoul, Fazlul H. Sarkar, and Gilda G. Hillman. 2009. Radiation-induced HIF-1a cell survival pathway is inhibited by soy isoflavones in prostate cancer cells. *International Journal of Cancer* 124:1675–1684.

Slusarz, Anna, Nader S. Shenouda, Mary S. Sakla, Sara K. Drenkhahn, Acharan S. Narula, Ruth S. MacDonald, Cynthia L. Besch-Williford, and Dennis B. Lubahn. 2010. Common botanical compounds inhibit the hedgehog signaling pathway in prostate cancer. *Cancer Research* 70:3382–3390.

Staedler, Davide, Elita Idrizi, Blanka Kenzaoui, and Lucienne Juillerat-Jeanneret. 2011. Drug combinations with quercetin: doxorubicin plus quercetin in human breast cancer cells. In *Cancer Chemotherapy and Pharmacology*: Springer Berlin/Heidelberg. 68:1161–1172.

Stearns, Mark E., and M. Wang. 2011. Synergistic effects of the green tea extract epigallocatechin-3-gallate and taxane in eradication of malignant human prostate tumors. *Translational Oncology* 4:147–156.

Stearns, Mark E., Michael D. Amatangelo, Devika Varma, Chris Sell, and Shaun M. Goodyear. 2010. Combination therapy with epigallocatechin-3-gallate and doxorubicin in human prostate tumor modeling studies: inhibition of metastatic tumor growth in severe combined immunodeficiency mice. *The American Journal of Pathology* 177:3169–3179.

Stendell-Hollis, Nicole R., C. A. Thomson, P. A. Thompson, J. W. Bea, E. C. Cussler, and I. A. Hakim. 2010. Green tea improves metabolic biomarkers, not weight or body composition: a pilot study in overweight breast cancer survivors. *Journal of Human Nutrition and Dietetics* 23:590–600.

Suganuma, Masami, Achinto Saha, and Hirota Fujiki. 2011. New cancer treatment strategy using combination of green tea catechins and anticancer drugs. *Cancer Science* 102:317–323.

Sun, Can-Lan, Jian-Min Yuan, Woon-Puay Koh, and Mimi C. Yu. 2006. Green tea, black tea and breast cancer risk: a meta-analysis of epidemiological studies. *Carcinogenesis* 27:1310–1315.

Surh, Young-Joon. 2003. Cancer chemoprevention with dietary phytochemicals. *Nature Reviews Cancer* 3:768–780.

Swami, Srilatha, Aruna V. Krishnan, Jacqueline Moreno, Rumi S. Bhattacharyya, Christopher Gardner, James D. Brooks, Donna M. Peehl, and David Feldman. 2009. Inhibition of prostaglandin synthesis and actions by genistein in human prostate cancer cells and by soy isoflavones in prostate cancer patients. *International Journal of Cancer* 124:2050–2059.

Tang, Su-Ni, Chandan Singh, Dara Nall, Daniel Meeker, Sharmila Shankar, and Rakesh Srivastava. 2010. The dietary bioflavonoid quercetin synergizes with epigallocathechin gallate (EGCG) to inhibit prostate cancer stem cell characteristics, invasion, migration and epithelial-mesenchymal transition. *Journal of Molecular Signaling* 5:14.

Tarahovsky, Yury, Evgueny Muzafarov, and Yuri Kim. 2008. Rafts making and rafts braking: how plant flavonoids may control membrane heterogeneity. In *Molecular and Cellular Biochemistry*: Springer, Netherlands.

Teas, Jane, Mohammad R. Irhimeh, Susan Druker, Thomas G. Hurley, James R. Hébert, Todd M. Savarese, and Mindy S. Kurzer. 2011. Serum IGF-1 concentrations change with soy and seaweed supplements in healthy postmenopausal American women. *Nutrition and Cancer* 63:743–748.

Teillet, Florence, Ahcene Boumendjel, Jean Boutonnat, and Xavier Ronot. 2008. Flavonoids as RTK inhibitors and potential anticancer agents. *Medicinal Research Reviews* 28:715–745.

Thangapazham, Rajesh L., Anoop K. Singh, Anuj Sharma, James Warren, Jaya P. Gaddipati, and Radha K. Maheshwari. 2007. Green tea polyphenols and its constituent epigallocatechin gallate inhibits proliferation of human breast cancer cells in vitro and in vivo. *Cancer Letters* 245:232–241.

Thomas, Francis, Jeff M. P. Holly, Rajendra Persad, Amit Bahl, and Claire M. Perks. 2011. Green tea extract (epigallocatechin-3-gallate) reduces efficacy of radiotherapy on prostate cancer cells. *Urology* 78:475.e15–475.e21.

Urban, Donald, W. Irwin, M. Kirk, M. A. Markiewicz, R. Myers, M. Smith, H. Weiss, W. E. Grizzle, and S. Barnes. 2001. The effect of isolated soy protein on plasma biomarkers in elderly men with elevated serum prostate specific antigen. *The Journal of Urology* 165:294–300.

Vaishampayan, Ulka, Maha Hussain, Mousumi Banerjee, Soley Seren, Fazlul H. Sarkar, Joseph Fontana, Jeffrey D. Forman, Michael L. Cher, Isaac Powell, J. Edson Pontes, and Omer Kucuk. 2007. Lycopene and soy isoflavones in the treatment of prostate cancer. *Nutrition and Cancer* 59:1–7.

van Leenders, G. J., R. Sookhlall, W. J. Teubel, C. M. de Ridder, S. Reneman, A. Sacchetti, K. J. Vissers, W. van Weerden, and G. Jenster. 2011. Activation of c-MET induces a stem-like phenotype in human prostate cancer. *PLoS One* 6:e26753.

Van Patten, Cheri L., Ivo A. Olivotto, G. Keith Chambers, Karen A. Gelmon, T. Gregory Hislop, Edith Templeton, Angela Wattie, and Jerilynn C. Prior. 2002. Effect of soy phytoestrogens on hot flashes in postmenopausal women with breast cancer: a randomized, controlled clinical trial. *Journal of Clinical Oncology* 20:1449–1455.

Varkaris, Andreas, Paul G. Corn, Sanchaika Gaur, Farshid Dayyani, Christopher J. Logothetis, and Gary E. Gallick. 2011. The role of HGF/c-Met signaling in prostate cancer progression and c-Met inhibitors in clinical trials. *Expert Opinion on Investigational Drugs* 20:1677–1684.

Wang, Piwen, William J. Aronson, Min Huang, Yanjun Zhang, Ru-Po Lee, David Heber, and Susanne M. Henning. 2010. Green tea polyphenols and metabolites in prostatectomy tissue: implications for cancer prevention. *Cancer Prevention Research* 3:985–993.

Way, Tzong-Der, Ming-Ching Kao, and Jen-Kun Lin. 2004. Apigenin induces apoptosis through proteasomal degradation of HER2/neu in HER2/neu-overexpressing breast cancer cells via the phosphatidylinositol 3-kinase/Akt-dependent pathway. *Journal of Biological Chemistry* 279:4479–4489.

Weatherman, Ross V., R. J. Fletterick, and T. S. Scanlan. 1999. Nuclear-receptor ligands and ligand-binding domains. *Annual Review of Biochemistry* 68:559–581.

Williams, Robert J., Jeremy P. E. Spencer, and Catherine Rice-Evans. 2004. Flavonoids: antioxidants or signalling molecules? *Free Radical Biology and Medicine* 36:838–849.

Wolfe, J. N. 1976. Breast patterns as an index of risk for developing breast cancer *American Journal of Roentgenology* 126:1130–1137.

Wong, Man-Yi, and Gigi N. C. Chiu. 2011. Liposome formulation of co-encapsulated vincristine and quercetin enhanced antitumor activity in a trastuzumab-insensitive breast tumor xenograft model. *Nanomedicine: Nanotechnology, Biology and Medicine* 7:834–840.

Wong, William C., E. L. Wong, H. Li, J. H. You, S. Ho, J. Woo, and E. Hui. 2012. Isoflavones in treating watchful waiting benign prostate hyperplasia: a double-blinded, randomized controlled trial. *Journal of Alternative and Complement Medicine* 18:54–60.

Wu, Anna H., Darcy Spicer, Frank Z. Stanczyk, Chiu-Chen Tseng, Chung S. Yang, and Malcolm C. Pike. 2012. Effect of 2-month controlled green tea intervention on lipoprotein cholesterol, glucose, and hormone levels in healthy postmenopausal women. *Cancer Prevention Research* 5:393–402.

Wu, Anna H., Chiu-Chen Tseng, David Van Den Berg, and Mimi C. Yu. 2003. Tea intake, COMT genotype, and breast cancer in Asian-American women. *Cancer Research* 63:7526–7529.

Xing, Nianzeng, Yi Chen, Susan H. Mitchell, and Charles Y. F. Young. 2001. Quercetin inhibits the expression and function of the androgen receptor in LNCaP prostate cancer cells. *Carcinogenesis* 22:409–414.

Yang, Chung S. 1997. Inhibition of carcinogenesis by tea. *Nature* 389:134–135.

Yang, Chung S., and Zhi-Yuan Wang. 1993. Tea and cancer. *Journal of the National Cancer Institute* 85:1038–1049.

Yuan, Huiqing, Charles Young, Yuanyuan Tian, Zhifang Liu, Mengye Zhang, and Hongxiang Lou. 2010. Suppression of the androgen receptor function by quercetin through protein-protein interactions of Sp1, c-Jun, and the androgen receptor in human prostate cancer cells. In *Molecular and Cellular Biochemistry*: Springer, Netherlands.

Yuan, Huiqing, Aiyu Gong, and Charles Y. Young. 2005. Involvement of transcription factor Sp1 in quercetin-mediated inhibitory effect on the androgen receptor in human prostate cancer cells. *Carcinogenesis* 26:793–801.

Yuan, Huiqing, Yunqian Pan, and Charles Y. F. Young. 2004. Overexpression of c-Jun induced by quercetin and resverol inhibits the expression and function of the androgen receptor in human prostate cancer cells. *Cancer Letters* 213:155–163.

Yunos, Nurhanan M., P. Beale, J. Q. Yu, and F. Huq. 2011. Synergism from sequenced combinations of curcumin and epigallocatechin-3-gallate with cisplatin in the killing of human ovarian cancer cells. *Anticancer Research* 31:1131–1140.

Zhang, Yimin, Guoge Han, Biao Fan, Yunfeng Zhou, Xuan Zhou, Lei Wei, and Jingwei Zhang. 2009. Green tea epigallocatechin-3-gallate down-regulates VASP expression and inhibits breast cancer cell migration and invasion by attenuating Rac1 activity. *European Journal of Pharmacology* 606:172–179.

Zhou, Qiong, Bing Yan, Xiaowen Hu, Xue-Bing Li, Jie Zhang, and Jing Fang. 2009. Luteolin inhibits invasion of prostate cancer PC3 cells through E-cadherin. *Molecular Cancer Therapeutics* 8:1684–1691.

Zhou, Weibo, P. Jeanette Simpson, Jill M. McFadden, Craig A. Townsend, Susan M. Medghalchi, Aravinda Vadlamudi, Michael L. Pinn, Gabriele V. Ronnett, and Francis P. Kuhajda. 2003. Fatty acid synthase inhibition triggers apoptosis during S phase in human cancer cells. *Cancer Research* 63:7330–7337

20 Cancer Prevention by Isoflavone

Yiwei Li, Dejuan Kong, Aamir Ahmad,
Bin Bao, and Fazlul H. Sarkar

CONTENTS

20.1 INTRODUCTION

Despite significant efforts made in the field of cancer research, cancer is still the second most common cause of death in the United States, exceeded only by heart disease, with an estimated 1,638,910 new cases and 577,190 deaths in 2012 (Siegel et al. 2012). In the world, the World Health Organization's (WHO's) World Cancer Report, the most comprehensive global examination of cancer, estimated that cancer incidence could increase by 50% to 15 million new cases in 2020, suggesting the epidemic nature of cancer in the world. So far, there is no effective treatment for a complete cure of cancer; therefore, cancer prevention has become an important strategy to fight against cancers. It is generally accepted that one-third of cancers could be prevented by maintaining healthy lifestyles and diets. In addition, it is known that inflammation and oxidative stress are important biological mechanisms by which carcinogenesis occurs. Therefore, antioxidant and anti-inflammatory effects of novel agents are important for preventing, suppressing, or reversing the development of carcinogenesis. Importantly, many natural agents from plant-based diet have shown their anti-inflammation and anticarcinogen activities without systemic toxicity. Therefore, these natural agents have recently received much attention in the fields of cancer chemoprevention and chemotherapy. The in vitro and in vivo studies have demonstrated that natural agents could inhibit the development of cancer from premalignant lesions by the suppression of inflammation and carcinogenesis. Moreover, these chemopreventive agents also exert anticancer effects by inhibiting cancer cell growth, invasion, and metastasis. Because of their antitumor effect and nontoxic feature, these natural agents have been used in combination treatment with conventional chemotherapeutics or radiotherapy (Banerjee et al. 2005; Bava et al. 2005; Chan et al. 2003; Li et al. 2005, 2006) for better treatment outcome. Recently, more clinical trials using natural agents in combination with conventional cancer therapy are being conducted to evaluate these novel therapeutic strategies in the clinic. Therefore, using natural agents has opened a newer avenue toward winning the war against cancers.

It is well known that there are wide geographic variations in the incidence of different types of cancer. The most common cancer in the United States is prostate cancer in men and breast cancer in women. However, the incidences of prostate and breast cancers are much lower in Asian countries compared to the United States. It is believed that isoflavone-rich food in the Asian diet partly contributes to this difference. Intakes of 39.4 to 47.4 mg soy isoflavone per day from diets in the Asian populations have been reported, whereas the dietary consumption of soy isoflavones is less than 1 mg/day in the American population (Arai et al. 2000; Chen et al. 1999; Setchell and Cassidy 1999). Soybean is the most common source of isoflavones in Asian food. The major isoflavone in soybean is genistein. A plasma concentration of genistein in the range of 1.4 ± 0.7 to 4.09 ± 0.94 µM was measured in people consuming foods rich in isoflavones, while plasma concentration of genistein in the nanomolar range was reported in Americans and Europeans (Adlercreutz et al. 1993, 1994; King and Bursill 1998; Morton et al. 1994; Xu et al. 2000), consistent with the differences in isoflavone intake and incidence of prostate and breast cancer. More importantly, epidemiological studies have shown that high consumption of soybean is inversely associated with the risk of prostate and breast cancers (Adlercreutz et al. 1995; Jacobsen et al. 1998; Lee et al. 1991), suggesting the protective effects of isoflavone on cancer prevention. However, it is important to note that the beneficial effect is due to the consumption of food that provides isoflavone and not just pure genistein.

Isoflavone is an antioxidant and has also been found to suppress inflammation and induce apoptotic cell death in vivo and in vitro. Isoflavone genistein is identified as a protein tyrosine kinase (PTK) inhibitor. PTKs are known to play key roles in carcinogenesis and cell growth; therefore, inhibition of PTK is one of the mechanisms for isoflavone-mediated suppression of carcinogenesis. In recent years, growing evidence from xenograft animal models and in vitro studies has demonstrated that isoflavone could inhibit the development and progression of cancers, suggesting that isoflavone could be a promising agent for cancer prevention and/or treatment through exerting its antioxidant, anti-inflammatory, and proapoptotic effects. In addition, studies have shown that up to 27.46 ± 15.38 µM of genistein in human plasma could be achieved after receiving an isoflavone supplement at a dose of 16.0 mg/kg (Busby et al. 2002), suggesting the bioavailability of isoflavone genistein from the supplement for cancer prevention. In this chapter, we will summarize the known effects of isoflavone and the molecular mechanisms underlying cancer chemoprevention by isoflavone.

20.2 INFLAMMATION AND CANCER

Inflammation occurs when external pathogens (such as bacteria) enter into the human body or if intrinsic factors (such as autoimmunogen) exist in a body. It is a very common event in humans, and such a process gets resolved within a short period of time and maintains the normal physiological homeostasis. However, chronic inflammation could promote tumorigenesis through the sustained production of reactive oxygen species (ROS), leading to DNA damage, cell proliferation, apoptosis evasion, and angiogenesis. It is known that inflammations produce ROS and reactive nitrogen species (RNS), which subsequently lead to oxidative damage and DNA base nitration. If DNA repair is malfunctioning at that time, damaged DNA will not be repaired. Thus, the genome will suffer from DNA mutation, which will eventually lead to tumorigenesis.

During the process of chronic inflammation, leukocytes and other inflammatory cells at the location of inflammation secrete inflammatory factors. These inflammatory factors include cytokines, growth factors, and angiogenic regulators, which interact with immune, stromal, endothelial, and epithelial cells. These inflammatory factors are required for proper cell and tissue repair. They stimulate epithelial cell proliferation to repair wounds caused by pathogens or inflammation itself. All these events are inflammatory responses. If inflammation functions properly, the inflammatory response is self-limiting. However, if an excessive response exists, the cell proliferation will be uncontrolled, and the regenerated tissues will grow uncontrollably, leading to the development of cancers. Moreover, the inflammatory mediators such as cytokines, prostaglandins, and growth factors, which are regulated by nuclear factor kappaB (NF-κB), can induce genetic and epigenetic changes including mutations in tumor suppressor genes, DNA methylation, and posttranslational modifications, leading to the development and progression of cancer (Hussain and Harris 2007). The well-known pieces of evidence in supporting the relationship between inflammation and cancer are high risk of colorectal cancer in patients with chronic inflammatory bowel disease, high incidence of gastric cancer in patients with chronic gastritis resulting from *Heliobacter pylori* infection, and about a 10-fold increase in the risk of liver cancer in patients with chronic hepatitis B infection.

It is well known that inflammation-induced ROS can activate NF-κB, which is one of the most important regulators of inflammatory response. In addition, excessive innate immunity activation could lead to the deregulation of inhibitor of NF-κB, alpha (IκBα), leading to the activation of NF-κB. The activation of NF-κB has been found in human inflammatory diseases such as rheumatoid arthritis (Simmonds and Foxwell 2008), atherosclerosis (Hajra et al. 2000), gastritis (Isomoto et al. 2000), and inflammatory bowel disease (Schreiber et al. 1998). Importantly, NF-κB has been described as a major culprit in cancer because constitutively activated NF-κB has been found in most human cancers (Karin 2006), suggesting the relationship between inflammation and cancer. It has been reported that NF-κB is activated in Hodgkin's tumor (Bargou et al. 1997); multiple myeloma cells (Hideshima et al. 2002); and head and neck (Allen et al. 2007), breast (Nakshatri et al. 1997), prostate (Shukla et al. 2004), pancreatic (Li et al. 2004; Holcomb et al. 2008), and gastric (Levidou et al. 2007) cancer cells. In cancer cells, NF-κB is activated through constitutive activation of IκB kinase (IKK) followed by the phosphorylation and degradation of IκBα.

Moreover, the activation of NF-κB also contributes to cancer progression, invasion, and metastasis. Inhibition of constitutive NF-κB activity by a mutant IκBα (S32A, S36A) completely suppressed the liver metastasis of pancreatic cancer cells (Fujioka et al. 2003a). The downregulation of NF-κB activity also inhibited the tumorigenic phenotype of nonmetastatic pancreatic cancer cells (Fujioka et al. 2003b). Constitutively activated NF-κB also upregulated the expression of its downstream genes, plasminogen activator, urokinase (uPA) and matrix metallopeptidase 9 (MMP-9), both of which are the critical proteases involved in cancer invasion and metastasis (Wang et al. 1999). These findings demonstrate that NF-κB plays important roles in cancer progression, invasion, and metastasis.

Furthermore, NF-κB is involved in de novo and acquired resistance to chemotherapeutic agents. It has been found that chemotherapeutic agents can activate NF-κB in cancer cells, resulting in the resistance of cancer cells to chemotherapy (Chuang et al. 2002; Li et al. 2005; Yeh et al. 2002). In addition, interleukin 1 (IL-1) and E3-ubiquitin ligase receptor could also induce the activation of NF-κB, leading to increased chemoresistance in human cancer cells (Arlt et al. 2002; Muerkoster et al. 2005). These reports suggest that the activation of NF-κB contributes to the development of chemoresistance in cancers. Therefore, inhibition of NF-κB activity is likely to function as a potent therapeutic strategy for the treatment of chemoresistant cancers.

Nonsteroidal anti-inflammatory drugs have been widely used for the treatment of inflammatory disease. It has been found that these drugs could inhibit the inflammatory response through the downregulation of NF-κB activity (Yamamoto and Gaynor 2001). However, it is now becoming clear that the inhibition of NF-κB activity is desirable not only for the treatment of inflammation but also for cancer therapy (Bharti and Aggarwal 2002). Many anti-inflammatory drugs and antioxidants can inhibit NF-κB activity, reduce oxidative stress, and induce apoptosis; therefore, they could also be potent agents for the treatment of cancers as documented in the following sections.

20.3 ANTI-INFLAMMATORY EFFECTS OF ISOFLAVONE

It is known that isoflavone can regulate inflammatory pathways, especially NF-κB pathway. In an animal study, isoflavone genistein was found to inhibit NF-κB activation during acute lung injury induced by lipopolysaccharide (LPS) in rats (Kang et al. 2001). Intratracheal treatment of rats with LPS resulted in lung injury and inflammatory response with upregulation of NF-κB in lung tissue. However, pretreatment with genistein inhibited the LPS-induced injury, inflammation, and NF-κB activation. In another study of human cystic fibrosis bronchial tissues, isoflavones showed an anti-inflammatory response (Tabary et al. 1999). Treatment of cystic fibrosis gland cells with isoflavone genistein resulted in decreased IL-8 production. Isoflavone genistein also reversed the effects of LPS-induced nuclear translocation of NF-κB by increasing IκBα protein levels in cystic fibrosis gland cells (Tabary et al. 2001). The isoflavone daidzein has also been shown to suppress NF-κB and signal transducer and activator of transcription 1 (STAT1), which are important transcription factors for inducible nitric oxide synthase (iNOS) expression involved in inflammation (Hamalainen et al. 2007), suggesting the inhibitory effect of daidzein on inflammation. These results collectively suggest that both genistein and daidzein, which are the main constituents of isoflavone, are important agents for controlling inflammation and oxidative stress.

It is known that wound healing occurs in sequential periods including hemostasis, inflammation, proliferation, and remodeling. Among these periods, inflammation is a critical period for wound healing. A recent study has shown that genistein could modulate the wound healing process by altering the inflammatory response through an antioxidant effect (Park et al. 2011). In an animal study, the wound closure in mice fed with genistein was much faster than that in the control group. Genistein also modulated NF-κB and tumor necrosis factor (TNF) expression during the early stage of wound healing. These results suggest that genistein could inhibit oxidative stress by enhancing antioxidant capacity and regulating proinflammatory cytokine expression during wound healing.

In diabetic patients, treatment-mediated complications remain a substantial challenge because of the oxidative and inflammatory status that exists in the patients with diabetes. A recent study has shown that isoflavone genistein reverted the proinflammatory cytokine and ROS overproduction and restored the nerve growth factor (NGF) content in the diabetic sciatic nerve (Valsecchi et al. 2011), suggesting that isoflavone genistein has anti-inflammatory effects and could be useful for the treatment of diabetes complications.

It is known that chronic inflammation in the prostate can promote prostate carcinogenesis. Because an elevated level of prostate-specific antigen (PSA) also reflects the presence of inflammation in the prostate, the strategies to lower PSA value could potentially have beneficial effects for the inhibition of inflammation and prevention of prostate cancer development. It has been found that isoflavones combined with curcumin had anti-inflammatory and antioxidant properties and that the production of PSA was decreased by the combined treatment in an experimental study and clinical trials (Ide et al. 2010), suggesting the inhibitory effects of isoflavone on inflammation and cancer development. However, a further novel clinical trial is required to confirm these early findings.

20.4 ANTICANCER EFFECTS OF ISOFLAVONE

20.4.1 Inhibition of Cancer Development by Isoflavone

It is well known that lifestyles, including diets and environmental factors, play important roles in the development of cancer. These dietary and environmental factors can exert their effects through the modulation of inflammation. Epidemiological studies have revealed that there is a significant difference in the incidence of cancers among different ethnic groups, which could be partly attributed to dietary habits. The incidences of hormone-related cancers are much higher in the US and European countries compared to Asian countries. One of the major differences in diet between these populations is the consumption of a diet high in soy products; therefore, soy isoflavone has received much attention as a dietary component in reducing the incidence of hormone-related cancers (Adlercreutz et al. 1995; Hebert et al. 1998).

The epidemiological studies on geographical differences in the incidence of breast cancer showed that dietary habits could elicit preventive effects of soy products on breast carcinogenesis. A high incidence of breast cancer has been found in Western countries and the United States as indicated earlier, while Asian women have a very low rate of breast cancer. A much higher level of isoflavones in plasma has been reported in Asian women with low breast cancer incidence (Adlercreutz et al. 1995), suggesting a protective role of soy-derived substances against breast cancer. It was reported that Asian women who immigrated to the United States and adopted Western lifestyles had increasing breast cancer incidence (Deapen et al. 2002; Ziegler et al. 1993), suggesting that consumption of soy-rich food in their native countries may have played a role in reducing the risk of breast cancer. Experimental studies have shown that isoflavones could bind to estrogen receptors because of their structural similarity with estrogens. After binding, isoflavones initiate only a weak response; however, they block the binding of more potent estrogens at the same time, leading to the prevention of breast cancer.

Similar to the effect of isoflavone on breast cancer, soy-rich foods also have a protective role against prostate cancer. Prostate cancer is the most common male cancer in the United States and Europe. In contrast, the incidence of prostate cancer in Asia is much lower than that in the United States and Europe. This difference has been believed to be partly due to the consumption of a diet that provides complex dietary factors found in soy-rich food. The lower risk of prostate cancer has been linked with consumption of soy foods and isoflavones in China (Lee et al. 2003; Yan and Spitznagel 2009). High intake of soy milk was associated with lower risk of prostate cancer in the United States (Jacobsen et al. 1998). These findings suggest that isoflavones may be potent agents for prostate cancer chemoprevention.

In addition to breast and prostate cancer cells, isoflavones also showed inhibitory effects on other hormone-related cancers, including endometrial and ovarian. Isoflavone consumption has been inversely associated with the risk of endometrial cancer (Horn-Ross et al. 2003). Epidemiological studies also showed that the intake of soy and isoflavones was associated with reduced risk of ovarian cancer (Zhang et al. 2004). Moreover, it has been found that soy consumptions not only decreased the risk of hormone-related cancers but also prevented hormone-independent cancers including lymphoma, lung, and colorectal cancer in humans (Yang et al. 2011; Chihara et al. 2012; Yan et al. 2010). In addition, animal experiments showed that isoflavone genistein could inhibit the growth of human leukemia cells transplanted into mice (Uckun et al. 1995). Dietary soy isoflavones also protected ovarectomized ERαKO and wild-type mice from carcinogen-induced colon cancer (Guo et al. 2004). Furthermore, dietary soy isoflavone inhibited metastasis of melanoma and pancreatic cancer cells and significantly improved survival of mice (Li et al. 1999; Buchler et al. 2003), suggesting the anticarcinogenesis and anti-metastatic effects of isoflavone.

20.4.2 Inhibition of Cancer Progression by Isoflavone

Recently, emerging evidence has suggested that isoflavones not only prevent cancer development but also could inhibit cancer progression and sensitize cancer cells to conventional chemotherapy. To enhance the antitumor activity of conventional chemotherapeutics, isoflavone and isoflavone analogs have been used in experiments and in clinical trials. We have reported that isoflavone genistein in vitro and in vivo could enhance growth inhibition and apoptotic cell death caused by chemotherapeutic agents including cisplatin, docetaxel, doxorubicin, and gemcitabine in prostate, breast, pancreas, and lung cancers (El-Rayes et al. 2006; Banerjee et al. 2005; Li et al. 2004, 2006). It has been found that pretreatment of cancer cells with isoflavone genistein prior to treatment with lower doses of chemotherapeutic agents caused a significantly greater degree of growth inhibition and apoptosis, suggesting that increased anticancer activities of chemotherapeutic agents with lower toxicity to normal cells could be achieved by a combination treatment with isoflavone genistein and conventional chemotherapeutics. Moreover, animal studies have shown that dietary isoflavone genistein could enhance the antitumor activities of gemcitabine and docetaxel in an animal tumor model, leading to greater apoptotic cell death and tumor growth inhibition (Banerjee et al. 2005;

Li et al. 2005). In addition to solid tumors, isoflavone genistein also sensitized diffuse large-cell lymphoma to cyclophosphamide, doxorubicin, vincristine, and prednisone (CHOP) chemotherapy, leading to a greater inhibition of lymphoma cell growth (Mohammad et al. 2003). Furthermore, in a study on a prostate bone metastasis animal model, isoflavone genistein enhanced the antitumor, anti-invasion, and antimetastatic activities of docetaxel through the inhibition of osteoclastic bone resorption and prostate cancer bone metastasis (Li et al. 2006). These findings suggest that iso-flavone genistein could be useful for combination therapy with conventional chemotherapeutics for the inhibition of cancer progression. Moreover, it is our opinion that isoflavone could be given chronically to cancer patients as an adjuvant therapy for the prevention of tumor recurrence, and thus, cancer could be viewed as a chronic disease and should be treated as such where isoflavone could be important.

Several isoflavone analogs have been synthesized for cancer treatment. It has been reported that isoflavone analogs can inhibit cancer cell growth in vitro with low half maximal inhibitory concentration (IC_{50}). Importantly, these synthetic isoflavones at low concentrations could also enhance the anticancer activity of clinically available chemotherapeutic agents, suggesting their potent effects as adjuncts to conventional therapeutics. Phenoxodiol is one of the isoflavone analogs and has shown a promising anticancer effect. One of the major benefits of phenoxodiol is its ability to sensitize cancer cells to the antitumor effects of conventional chemotherapeutics (Alvero et al. 2006). Moreover, in cancer cells that became resistant to the effects of conventional chemotherapeutics, phenoxodiol restored chemosensitivity (Kamsteeg et al. 2003; Sapi et al. 2004). By treatment of chemoresistant cancer cells with phenoxodiol first, drug resistance was removed, making cancer cells susceptible once again to standard chemotherapeutics such as cisplatin, carboplatin, taxanes, and gemcitabine. Phenoxodiol is currently undergoing clinical studies in phase II/III trials for assessing its efficacy in combination with carboplatin, docetaxel, cisplatin, or paclitaxel in patients with ovarian, fallopian tube, or primary peritoneal cavity cancers.

The in vitro and in vivo experimental studies have also shown that the efficacy of radiotherapy could be enhanced by isoflavones (Hillman and Singh-Gupta 2011). In an animal study, isoflavone genistein treatment combined with radiation led to a greater inhibition of tumor growth and metastasis to lymph nodes compared to either genistein or radiation alone (Hillman et al. 2004), suggesting that isoflavone genistein could enhance the radiosensitivity of cancer cells. The in vitro study also showed that isoflavone genistein treatment combined with radiation led to a greater inhibition in the colony formation with enhanced cancer cell death compared to either genistein or radiation alone. Mechanistic studies revealed that enhanced anticancer effects by isoflavone genistein and radiation were mediated via upregulation of p21[WAF1/Cip1] (cyclin-dependent kinase inhibitor 1A) and downregulation of NF-κB, apurinic/apyrimidinic endonuclease 1/redox factor-1 (APE-1), and cyclin B, leading to the G_2/M arrest and increased radio-sensitivity (Raffoul et al. 2006, 2007; Singh-Gupta et al. 2011). These findings demonstrate that the combination treatment with isoflavone and radiotherapy could be an important and novel strategy for the treatment of cancers.

Most importantly, isoflavone genistein also showed its ability to reduce the angiogenic, invasive, and metastatic potentials of cancers. We have found that in breast cancer cells, isoflavone genistein could inhibit the expression of c-erb-B2 (v-erb-b2 erythroblastic leukemia viral oncogene homolog 2), MMP-2, and MMP-9 proteins, which are highly associated with cancer invasion and metastasis (Y. Li et al. 1999). From gene expression profiling, we also found that isoflavone genistein downreg-ulated the expression of protease M, vascular endothelial growth factor (VEGF), neuropilin, throm-bospondin (TSP), and transforming growth factor beta (TGF-β) (Li and Sarkar 2002a), all of which are related to angiogenesis and metastasis. Moreover, we found that isoflavone genistein inhibited prostate cancer cell metastasis to the bone through regulation of osteoprotegerin (OPG)/receptor activator of NF-κB (RANK)/receptor activator of NF-κB ligand (RANKL)/MMP-9 signaling (Li et al. 2006). Furthermore, isoflavone was found to induce drug sensitivity and caused reversal of epithelial–mesenchymal transition (EMT) phenotype in pancreatic cancers (Li et al. 2009), sug-gesting its potent inhibitory effects on drug resistance and metastasis of pancreatic cancer.

20.4.3 CELL SIGNALING ALTERED BY ISOFLAVONE

Because cellular signaling in a living cell is a complex signal network with positive or negative feedback loops, it is important to note that deregulation of multiple cellular signaling pathways including NF-κB, Akt (v-akt murine thymoma viral oncogene homolog), Wnt (wingless-type mouse mammary tumor virus (MMTV) integration site family), Notch, androgen receptor (AR), and so forth is involved in cancer development and progression. Importantly, isoflavone has been found to have the capacity to regulate multiple cellular signaling pathways. Therefore, targeting multiple signaling (multitargeting) by natural compound isoflavone combined with conventional therapy could open newer avenues for cancer therapy.

As described in the previous section that isoflavone can inhibit inflammation through down-regulation of NF-κB, isoflavone can also inhibit the activation of NF-κB in cancer cells. It is well known that NF-κB, which is activated in most cancers, inhibits apoptosis. We found that isoflavone significantly inhibited the DNA-binding activity of NF-κB and induced apoptosis in various cancer cells (Davis et al. 1999; Li and Sarkar 2002b). Moreover, isoflavone pretreatment abrogated the activation of NF-κB stimulated by TNFα (Davis et al. 2001). Recent studies showed that the induction of apoptosis and inhibition of cell proliferation by isoflavones, genistein, and biochanin-A were regulated by NF-κB–dependent and –independent pathways (Lee and Park 2013; Kole et al. 2011), suggesting the complexities of the biological activity of isoflavones. All of these findings suggest that isoflavone has an inhibitory effect on NF-κB activation in humans, suggesting that soy isoflavone could exert its cancer chemopreventive activity through the inhibition of NF-κB signaling and induction of apoptosis (Figure 20.1).

Isoflavone-mediated inhibition of cancer cell growth could also be regulated by Akt signaling, another important signaling pathway involved in cancer development and progression. We have previously investigated the effects of isoflavone on Akt signaling (Li and Sarkar 2002b). We found that isoflavone did not alter the level of total Akt protein; however, the phosphorylated Akt protein at Ser473 and the corresponding Akt kinase activity were decreased after isoflavone treatment. Isoflavone pretreatment also abrogated the activation of Akt by epidermal growth factor (EGF). Furthermore, isoflavone genistein could exert its inhibitory effects on the NF-κB pathway through the Akt pathway, leading to the inhibition of cell growth and induction of apoptosis. In addition, Akt could also inhibit apoptosis through the inhibition of glycogen synthase kinase-3 beta (GSK-3β) and forkhead box O3a (FOXO3a). We found that isoflavone could upregulate the expression of GSK-3β

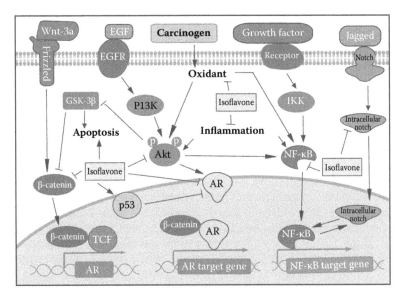

FIGURE 20.1 Cellular signaling pathways altered by isoflavone.

and inhibit the phosphorylation of Akt and FOXO3a, leading to increased apoptosis and decreased cell growth (Li et al. 2008). Isoflavone also abrogated the phosphorylation of Akt and FOXO3a stimulated by insulin-like growth factor-I (IGF-I) (Li et al. 2008). It is also reported that genistein can induce apoptosis via the regulation of Akt, NF-κB, and p21^{WAF1} (Ma et al. 2011; Privat et al. 2010). All of these findings suggest that the regulation of the Akt pathway by isoflavone contributes to the chemopreventive and chemotherapeutic effects of isoflavone (Figure 20.1).

In addition to the cross talk between NF-κB and Akt, Wnt signaling also interacts with Akt signaling, promoting cancer cell proliferation and preventing cancer cells from apoptosis. We found that isoflavone could increase the expression of GSK-3β, promote GSK-3β binding to β-catenin, induce phosphorylation of β-catenin, and eventually lead to the induction of apoptotic cell death, suggesting that isoflavone could inhibit both Akt and Wnt signaling to induce apoptosis and inhibit cancer cell proliferation (Li et al. 2008). Other investigators also reported that genistein could inhibit basal and Wnt-induced growth and downregulate the expression of Wnt targets, c-Myc (v-*myc* myelocytomatosis viral oncogene homolog), and cyclin D1 (Su and Simmen 2009). It has also been reported that isoflavone could downregulate the expression of Wnt-5a (Su et al. 2007) and Wnt-7a (Wagner and Lehmann 2006). Animal experiments coupled with microarray gene expression analysis showed that isoflavone could downregulate Wnt signaling in the tumor tissues of animals and that isoflavone treatment resulted in decreased expression of Wnt target gene cyclin D1, which is a regulator of apoptosis (Su et al. 2007). These findings collectively suggest that isoflavone could induce apoptosis and inhibit cancer cell growth through the downregulation of Wnt signaling (Figure 20.1).

Notch is another important signaling molecule involved in cancer development and progression. The inhibitory effects of isoflavone on Notch signaling have been reported. We found that isoflavone could downregulate Notch signaling, which caused the downregulation of NF-κB activity, leading to the induction of apoptosis and the inhibition of cell proliferation in pancreatic cancer cells (Wang et al. 2006). Other investigators also reported that genistein could inhibit the expression of Notch1 and Notch2 (Su et al. 2007; Janardhanan et al. 2009), which is consistent with our findings. All of these results suggest that isoflavone could inhibit cancer cell growth and induce apoptosis through the downregulation of Notch signaling pathways, which is known to cross talk with the NF-κB signaling pathway (Figure 20.1).

In prostate cancer cells, Akt could also cross talk with AR and activate AR signaling in a ligand-independent manner, leading to hormone-independent prostate cancer growth (Figure 20.1). We and other investigators have reported that isoflavone genistein could inhibit AR expression, decrease nuclear AR binding to androgen-responsive elements, and thereby downregulate the expression of the AR downstream target PSA in androgen-sensitive LNCaP cells, resulting in the induction of apoptosis and the inhibition of cancer cell growth (Davis et al. 2002; Tepper et al. 2007). Furthermore, isoflavone-induced inhibition of cell proliferation and induction of apoptosis were also mediated via the regulation of the Akt/FOXO3a/GSK-3β/AR signaling network (Li et al. 2008). An animal study also showed that dietary genistein inhibited AR expression in the rat prostate at the concentrations found in humans on a soy diet (Fritz et al. 2002). Therefore, the downregulation of AR expression by isoflavone could be an important strategy for the prevention and/or treatment of prostate cancer.

Recently, emerging evidence has shown that microRNAs (miRNAs) play an important role in cancer development and progression. We have examined the effects of isoflavone on miRNAs in pancreatic cancer cells that are gemcitabine resistant and have the typical EMT phenotype. We found that isoflavone treatment could upregulate the expression of microRNA (miR)-200, leading to the downregulation of zinc finger E-box binding homeobox 1 (ZEB1) and vimentin and the reversal of EMT (Li et al. 2009). Importantly, we found that isoflavone treatment or miR-200 reexpression enhanced sensitivity of gemcitabine-resistant pancreatic cells to gemcitabine, causing increased pancreatic cancer cell death induced by gemcitabine (Li et al. 2009). These results demonstrate that isoflavone treatment could enhance the sensitivity of gemcitabine-resistant cells to gemcitabine through miR-200–mediated reversal of EMT status. Other investigators also showed that genistein could downregulate miR-221/222, resulting in the upregulation of the ras homolog gene family, member I (ARHI), one of the tumor suppressors, and the induction of apoptosis (Chen et al. 2011). Therefore, targeting miRNAs by isoflavone could be another molecular mechanism by which isoflavone could inhibit the development and progression of cancer. Thus, isoflavone could become an effective agent for the prevention and/or treatment of human malignancies.

20.5 CLINICAL TRIALS USING ISOFLAVONE IN CANCER CLINIC

Since several in vitro experiments and in vivo animal studies have shown the preventive and therapeutic effects of isoflavone on cancers, isoflavone has been tested in clinical trials for assessing its effects on cancer patients, especially prostate cancer. Several phase I clinical trials have been conducted to investigate the toxicity and effects of isoflavones in patients with prostate cancer (Busby et al. 2002; Fischer et al. 2004; Kumar et al. 2004; Takimoto et al. 2003). The results have demonstrated that isoflavone genistein could be administrated safely with minimal side effects and that the plasma genistein concentration achieved was comparable to the concentrations used in most in vitro experiments. Importantly, supplementing early-stage prostate cancer patients with soy isoflavones decreased markers of cancer cell proliferation such as serum PSA and free testosterone, suggesting the beneficial effects of isoflavone on early-stage prostate cancer (Kumar et al. 2004). We have conducted a phase II clinical trial to investigate the modulation in serum PSA levels in patients with prostate cancer by soy isoflavone supplementation. We found a decrease in the rate of rise of serum PSA upon soy isoflavone intervention (Hussain et al. 2003). Other investigators also reported similar results in a phase II clinical trial evaluating the efficacy of isoflavone in patients with PSA recurrent prostate cancer after prior therapy (Pendleton et al. 2008). They found that dietary isoflavone decreased the slope of rising PSA, providing evidence in support of the use of isoflavone supplements against prostate cancer (Pendleton et al. 2008). Another clinical trial has been conducted to determine the biological effects of soy protein isolate (SPI) consumption on AR expression patterns in men at high risk of developing advanced prostate cancer. It was found that the consumption of SPI significantly suppressed AR expression, suggesting that isoflavone could be beneficial in preventing prostate cancer by inhibition of AR activation and PSA expression (Hamilton-Reeves et al. 2007). In a prospective follow-up study, the effects of a dietary supplementation including isoflavone were tested in men with high-grade prostatic intraepithelial neoplasia (HGPIN). It was found that 67.6% of patients showed a stable or decreasing PSA level and had a lower risk (25.5%) of prostate cancer after isoflavone supplementation, suggesting that the supplements could decrease the level of PSA, thereby decreasing the risk of prostate cancer (Joniau et al. 2007). All the results from these clinical studies have demonstrated that soy isoflavone could decrease the rate of rise in serum PSA levels without any toxicity in prostate cancer patients. Because of the anti-AR/PSA effects of soy isoflavone with no significant side effects, soy isoflavone supplementation could become an ideal strategy for prostate cancer prevention and treatment.

A pilot clinical study has been conducted to investigate the effects of soy isoflavone on acute and subacute toxicity of external beam radiation therapy in patients with localized prostate cancer (Ahmad et al. 2010). It was found that isoflavone-treated patients had less urinary incontinence, less urgency, and better erectile function as compared to the placebo group, suggesting that soy isoflavone combination with radiation therapy could reduce the urinary, intestinal, and sexual adverse effects in patients with prostate cancer.

Recently, more phase II and III clinical trials using isoflavone are being conducted to test the effects of isoflavone in the prevention and treatment of prostate, breast, head and neck, bladder, and endometrial cancers. Because numerous in vitro experiments and in vivo animal studies have demonstrated that isoflavone could enhance the antitumor activity of other chemotherapeutic agents, several clinical trials are being conducted using isoflavone genistein or isoflavone analogs in combination with IL-2, docetaxel, cisplatin, paclitaxel, or other natural agents such as lycopene and vitamin D in the treatment of melanoma and kidney and ovarian cancers. Moreover, several clinical trials are being conducted to test the effects of isoflavone treatment combined with radiotherapy in patients with prostate cancer. We believe that the results from these clinical trials will further demonstrate the beneficial value of isoflavone in cancer prevention and treatment.

20.6 CONCLUSION AND PERSPECTIVES

In conclusion, the results from epidemiological studies, in vitro experiments, and in vivo human and animal studies clearly demonstrate that isoflavone exerts its inhibitory effects on carcinogenesis and cancer progression. It is known that the inhibition of cancer development and progression by isoflavone is mediated through the regulation of multiple cellular signaling pathways including NF-κB, Akt, Wnt, Notch, AR, and miRNA-regulated signaling pathways. Importantly, in vitro and in vivo studies have further demonstrated that isoflavone could enhance the antitumor activity of chemotherapy and radiotherapy mediated by targeting multiple signaling pathways. Based on many preclinical findings as to the benefit of isoflavone, multiple clinical trials are being conducted in order to fully evaluate the effects of isoflavone and its analogs in the inhibition of development and progression of various cancer types. We believe that further in-depth mechanistic studies in vitro together with results from relevant animal model studies in vivo and the outcome of existing clinical trials will lead to an appreciation of the clinical value of isoflavone for the prevention of tumor development and progression. Moreover, our vision is that isoflavone could become an adjuvant therapy for the treatment of cancer, assuming that cancer is a chronic disease.

ACKNOWLEDGMENTS

The authors' work cited in this review article was funded by grants from the National Cancer Institute, National Institutes of Health (5R01CA083695, 5R01CA108535, 5R01CA132794, 5R01CA131151, and 1R01CA154321 awarded to FHS). We also thank the Puschelberg and Guido foundations for their generous contribution to support our research.

REFERENCES

Adlercreutz, C.H., B.R. Goldin, S.L. Gorbach et al. 1995. Soybean phytoestrogen intake and cancer risk. *J Nutr* 125:757S–70S.

Adlercreutz, H., T. Fotsis, S. Watanabe et al. 1994. Determination of lignans and isoflavonoids in plasma by isotope dilution gas chromatography-mass spectrometry. *Cancer Detect Prev* 18:259–71.

Adlercreutz, H., T. Fotsis, J. Lampe et al. 1993. Quantitative determination of lignans and isoflavonoids in plasma of omnivorous and vegetarian women by isotope dilution gas chromatography-mass spectrometry. *Scand J Clin Lab Invest Suppl* 215:5–18.

Ahmad, I.U., J.D. Forman, F.H. Sarkar et al. 2010. Soy isoflavones in conjunction with radiation therapy in patients with prostate cancer. *Nutr Cancer* 62:996–1000.

Allen, C.T., J.L. Ricker, Z. Chen, and W.C. Van. 2007. Role of activated nuclear factor-kappaB in the pathogenesis and therapy of squamous cell carcinoma of the head and neck. *Head Neck* 29:959–71.

Alvero, A.B., D. O'Malley, D. Brown et al. 2006. Molecular mechanism of phenoxodiol-induced apoptosis in ovarian carcinoma cells. *Cancer* 106:599–608.

Arai, Y., M. Uehara, Y. Sato et al. 2000. Comparison of isoflavones among dietary intake, plasma concentration and urinary excretion for accurate estimation of phytoestrogen intake. *J Epidemiol* 10:127–35.

Arlt, A., J. Vorndamm, S. Muerkoster et al. 2002. Autocrine production of interleukin 1beta confers constitutive nuclear factor kappaB activity and chemoresistance in pancreatic carcinoma cell lines. *Cancer Res* 62:910–6.

Banerjee, S., Y. Zhang, S. Ali et al. 2005. Molecular evidence for increased antitumor activity of gemcitabine by genistein in vitro and in vivo using an orthotopic model of pancreatic cancer. *Cancer Res* 65:9064–72.

Bargou, R.C., F. Emmerich, D. Krappmann et al. 1997. Constitutive nuclear factor-kappaB-RelA activation is required for proliferation and survival of Hodgkin's disease tumor cells. *J Clin Invest* 100:2961–9.

Bava, S.V., V.T. Puliappadamba, A. Deepti, A. Nair, D. Karunagaran, and R.J. Anto. 2005. Sensitization of taxol-induced apoptosis by curcumin involves down-regulation of nuclear factor-kappaB and the serine/threonine kinase Akt and is independent of tubulin polymerization. *J Biol Chem* 280:6301–8.

Bharti, A.C. and B.B. Aggarwal. 2002. Nuclear factor-kappa B and cancer: its role in prevention and therapy. *Biochem Pharmacol* 64:883–8.

Buchler, P., A.S. Gukovskaya, M. Mouria et al. 2003. Prevention of metastatic pancreatic cancer growth in vivo by induction of apoptosis with genistein, a naturally occurring isoflavonoid. *Pancreas* 26:264–73.

Busby, M.G., A.R. Jeffcoat, L.T. Bloedon et al. 2002. Clinical characteristics and pharmacokinetics of purified soy isoflavones: single-dose administration to healthy men. *Am J Clin Nutr* 75:126–36.

Chan, M.M., D. Fong, K.J. Soprano, W.F. Holmes, and H. Heverling. 2003. Inhibition of growth and sensitization to cisplatin-mediated killing of ovarian cancer cells by polyphenolic chemopreventive agents. *J Cell Physiol* 194:63–70.

Chen, Y., M.S. Zaman, G. Deng et al. 2011. MicroRNAs 221/222 and genistein-mediated regulation of ARHI tumor suppressor gene in prostate cancer. *Cancer Prev Res (Phila)* 4:76–86.

Chen, Z., W. Zheng, L.J. Custer et al. 1999. Usual dietary consumption of soy foods and its correlation with the excretion rate of isoflavonoids in overnight urine samples among Chinese women in Shanghai. *Nutr Cancer* 33:82–7.

Chihara, D., K. Matsuo, J. Kanda et al. 2012. Inverse association between soy intake and non-Hodgkin lymphoma risk among women: a case-control study in Japan. *Ann Oncol* 23:1061–6.

Chuang, S.E., P.Y. Yeh, Y.S. Lu et al. 2002. Basal levels and patterns of anticancer drug-induced activation of nuclear factor-kappaB (NF-kappaB), and its attenuation by tamoxifen, dexamethasone, and curcumin in carcinoma cells. *Biochem Pharmacol* 63:1709–16.

Davis, J.N., O. Kucuk, and F.H. Sarkar. 2002. Expression of prostate-specific antigen is transcriptionally regulated by genistein in prostate cancer cells. *Mol Carcinog* 34:91–101.

Davis, J.N., O. Kucuk, Z. Djuric, and F.H. Sarkar. 2001. Soy isoflavone supplementation in healthy men prevents NF-kappa B activation by TNF-alpha in blood lymphocytes. *Free Radic Biol Med* 30:1293–302.

Davis, J.N., O. Kucuk, and F.H. Sarkar. 1999. Genistein inhibits NF-kappa B activation in prostate cancer cells. *Nutr Cancer* 35:167–74.

Deapen, D., L. Liu, C. Perkins, L. Bernstein, and R.K. Ross. 2002. Rapidly rising breast cancer incidence rates among Asian-American women. *Int J Cancer* 99:747–50.

El-Rayes, B.F., S. Ali, I.F. Ali, P.A. Philip, J. Abbruzzese, and F.H. Sarkar. 2006. Potentiation of the effect of erlotinib by genistein in pancreatic cancer: the role of Akt and nuclear factor-kappaB. *Cancer Res* 66:10553–9.

Fischer, L., C. Mahoney, A.R. Jeffcoat et al. 2004. Clinical characteristics and pharmacokinetics of purified soy isoflavones: multiple-dose administration to men with prostate neoplasia. *Nutr Cancer* 48:160–70.

Fritz, W.A., J. Wang, I.E. Eltoum, and C.A. Lamartiniere. 2002. Dietary genistein down-regulates androgen and estrogen receptor expression in the rat prostate. *Mol Cell Endocrinol* 186:89–99.

Fujioka, S., G.M. Sclabas, C. Schmidt et al. 2003a. Function of nuclear factor kappaB in pancreatic cancer metastasis. *Clin Cancer Res* 9:346–54.

Fujioka, S., G.M. Sclabas, C. Schmidt et al. 2003b. Inhibition of constitutive NF-kappa B activity by I kappa B alpha M suppresses tumorigenesis. *Oncogene* 22:1365–70.

Guo, J.Y., X. Li, J.D. Browning, Jr. et al. 2004. Dietary soy isoflavones and estrone protect ovariectomized ERalphaKO and wild-type mice from carcinogen-induced colon cancer. *J Nutr* 134:179–82.

Hajra, L., A.I. Evans, M. Chen, S.J. Hyduk, T. Collins, and M.I. Cybulsky. 2000. The NF-kappa B signal transduction pathway in aortic endothelial cells is primed for activation in regions predisposed to atherosclerotic lesion formation. *Proc Natl Acad Sci U S A* 97:9052–7.

Hamalainen, M., R. Nieminen, P. Vuorela, M. Heinonen, and E. Moilanen. 2007. Anti-inflammatory effects of flavonoids: genistein, kaempferol, quercetin, and daidzein inhibit STAT-1 and NF-kappaB activations, whereas flavone, isorhamnetin, naringenin, and pelargonidin inhibit only NF-kappaB activation along with their inhibitory effect on iNOS expression and NO production in activated macrophages. *Mediators Inflamm* 2007:45673.

Hamilton-Reeves, J.M., S.A. Rebello, W. Thomas, J.W. Slaton, and M.S. Kurzer. 2007. Isoflavone-rich soy protein isolate suppresses androgen receptor expression without altering estrogen receptor-beta expression or serum hormonal profiles in men at high risk of prostate cancer. *J Nutr* 137:1769–75.

Hebert, J.R., T.G. Hurley, B.C. Olendzki, J. Teas, Y. Ma, and J.S. Hampl. 1998. Nutritional and socioeconomic factors in relation to prostate cancer mortality: a cross-national study. *J Natl Cancer Inst* 90:1637–47.

Hideshima, T., D. Chauhan, P. Richardson et al. 2002. NF-kappaB as a therapeutic target in multiple myeloma. *J Biol Chem* 277:16639–47.

Hillman, G.G. and V. Singh-Gupta. 2011. Soy isoflavones sensitize cancer cells to radiotherapy. *Free Radic Biol Med* 51:289–98.

Hillman, G.G., Y. Wang, O. Kucuk et al. 2004. Genistein potentiates inhibition of tumor growth by radiation in a prostate cancer orthotopic model. *Mol Cancer Ther* 3:1271–9.

Holcomb, B., M. Yip-Schneider, and C.M. Schmidt. 2008. The role of nuclear factor kappaB in pancreatic cancer and the clinical applications of targeted therapy. *Pancreas* 36:225–35.

Horn-Ross, P.L., E.M. John, A.J. Canchola, S.L. Stewart, and M.M. Lee. 2003. Phytoestrogen intake and endometrial cancer risk. *J Natl Cancer Inst* 95:1158–64.

Hussain, M., M. Banerjee, F.H. Sarkar et al. 2003. Soy isoflavones in the treatment of prostate cancer. *Nutr Cancer* 47:111–7.

Hussain, S.P. and C.C. Harris. 2007. Inflammation and cancer: an ancient link with novel potentials. *Int J Cancer* 121:2373–80.

Ide, H., S. Tokiwa, K. Sakamaki et al. 2010. Combined inhibitory effects of soy isoflavones and curcumin on the production of prostate-specific antigen. *Prostate* 70:1127–33.

Isomoto, H., Y. Mizuta, M. Miyazaki et al. 2000. Implication of NF-kappaB in Helicobacter pylori-associated gastritis. *Am J Gastroenterol* 95:2768–76.

Jacobsen, B.K., S.F. Knutsen, and G.E. Fraser. 1998. Does high soy milk intake reduce prostate cancer incidence? The Adventist Health Study (United States). *Cancer Causes Control* 9:553–7.

Janardhanan, R., N.L. Banik, and S.K. Ray. 2009. N-Myc down regulation induced differentiation, early cell cycle exit, and apoptosis in human malignant neuroblastoma cells having wild type or mutant p53. *Biochem Pharmacol* 78:1105–14.

Joniau, S., L. Goeman, T. Roskams, E. Lerut, R. Oyen, and P.H. Van. 2007. Effect of nutritional supplement challenge in patients with isolated high-grade prostatic intraepithelial neoplasia. *Urology* 69:1102–6.

Kamsteeg, M., T. Rutherford, E. Sapi et al. 2003. Phenoxodiol—an isoflavone analog—induces apoptosis in chemoresistant ovarian cancer cells. *Oncogene* 22:2611–20.

Kang, J.L., H.W. Lee, H.S. Lee et al. 2001. Genistein prevents nuclear factor-kappa B activation and acute lung injury induced by lipopolysaccharide. *Am J Respir Crit Care Med* 164:2206–12.

Karin, M. 2006. Nuclear factor-kappaB in cancer development and progression. *Nature* 441:431–6.

King, R.A. and D.B. Bursill. 1998. Plasma and urinary kinetics of the isoflavones daidzein and genistein after a single soy meal in humans. *Am J Clin Nutr* 67:867–72.

Kole, L., B. Giri, S.K. Manna, B. Pal, and S. Ghosh. 2011. Biochanin-A, an isoflavon, showed anti-proliferative and anti-inflammatory activities through the inhibition of iNOS expression, p38-MAPK and ATF-2 phosphorylation and blocking NFkappaB nuclear translocation. *Eur J Pharmacol* 653:8–15.

Kumar, N.B., A. Cantor, K. Allen et al. 2004. The specific role of isoflavones in reducing prostate cancer risk. *Prostate* 59:141–7.

Lee, H.P., L. Gourley, S.W. Duffy, J. Esteve, J. Lee, and N.E. Day. 1991. Dietary effects on breast-cancer risk in Singapore. *Lancet* 337:1197–200.

Lee, M.M., S.L. Gomez, J.S. Chang, M. Wey, R.T. Wang, and A.W. Hsing. 2003. Soy and isoflavone consumption in relation to prostate cancer risk in China. *Cancer Epidemiol Biomarkers Prev* 12:665–8.

Lee, Y.K. and O.J. Park. 2013. Soybean isoflavone genistein regulates apoptosis through NF-kappaB dependent and independent pathways. *Exp Toxicol Pathol* 65(1–2):1–6.

Levidou, G., P. Korkolopoulou, N. Nikiteas et al. 2007. Expression of nuclear factor kappaB in human gastric carcinoma: relationship with I kappaB a and prognostic significance. *Virchows Arch* 450:519–27.

Li, D., J.A. Yee, M.H. McGuire, P.A. Murphy, and L. Yan. 1999. Soybean isoflavones reduce experimental metastasis in mice. *J Nutr* 129:1075–8.

Li, L., B.B. Aggarwal, S. Shishodia, J. Abbruzzese, and R. Kurzrock. 2004. Nuclear factor-kappaB and IkappaB kinase are constitutively active in human pancreatic cells, and their down-regulation by curcumin (diferuloylmethane) is associated with the suppression of proliferation and the induction of apoptosis. *Cancer* 101:2351–62.

Li, Y. and F.H. Sarkar. 2002a. Down-regulation of invasion and angiogenesis-related genes identified by cDNA microarray analysis of PC3 prostate cancer cells treated with genistein. *Cancer Lett* 186:157–64.

Li, Y. and F.H. Sarkar. 2002b. Inhibition of nuclear factor kappaB activation in PC3 cells by genistein is mediated via Akt signaling pathway. *Clin Cancer Res* 8:2369–77.

Li, Y., T.G. VandenBoom, D. Kong et al. 2009. Up-regulation of miR-200 and let-7 by natural agents leads to the reversal of epithelial-to-mesenchymal transition in gemcitabine-resistant pancreatic cancer cells. *Cancer Res* 69:6704–12.

Li, Y., Z. Wang, D. Kong, R. Li, S.H. Sarkar, and F.H. Sarkar. 2008. Regulation of Akt/FOXO3a/GSK-3beta/ AR signaling network by isoflavone in prostate cancer cells. *J Biol Chem* 283:27707–16.

Li, Y., O. Kucuk, M. Hussain, J. Abrams, M.L. Cher, and F.H. Sarkar. 2006. Antitumor and antimetastatic activities of docetaxel are enhanced by genistein through regulation of osteoprotegerin/receptor activator of nuclear factor-kappaB (RANK)/RANK ligand/MMP-9 signaling in prostate cancer. *Cancer Res* 66:4816–25.

Li, Y., F. Ahmed, S. Ali, P.A. Philip, O. Kucuk, and F.H. Sarkar. 2005. Inactivation of nuclear factor kappaB by soy isoflavone genistein contributes to increased apoptosis induced by chemotherapeutic agents in human cancer cells. *Cancer Res* 65:6934–42.

Li, Y., K.L. Ellis, S. Ali et al. 2004. Apoptosis-inducing effect of chemotherapeutic agents is potentiated by soy isoflavone genistein, a natural inhibitor of NF-kappaB in BxPC-3 pancreatic cancer cell line. *Pancreas* 28:e90–e95.

Li, Y., M. Bhuiyan, and F.H. Sarkar. 1999. Induction of apoptosis and inhibition of c-erbB-2 in MDA-MB-435 cells by genistein. *Int J Oncol* 15:525–33.

Ma, Y., J. Wang, L. Liu et al. 2011. Genistein potentiates the effect of arsenic trioxide against human hepatocellular carcinoma: role of Akt and nuclear factor-kappaB. *Cancer Lett* 301:75–84.

Mohammad, R.M., A. Al-Katib, A. Aboukameel, D.R. Doerge, F. Sarkar, and O. Kucuk. 2003. Genistein sensitizes diffuse large cell lymphoma to CHOP (cyclophosphamide, doxorubicin, vincristine, prednisone) chemotherapy. *Mol Cancer Ther* 2:1361–8.

Morton, M.S., G. Wilcox, M.L. Wahlqvist, and K. Griffiths. 1994. Determination of lignans and isoflavonoids in human female plasma following dietary supplementation. *J Endocrinol* 142:251–9.

Muerkoster, S., A. Arlt, B. Sipos et al. 2005. Increased expression of the E3-ubiquitin ligase receptor subunit betaTRCP1 relates to constitutive nuclear factor-kappaB activation and chemoresistance in pancreatic carcinoma cells. *Cancer Res* 65:1316–24.

Nakshatri, H., P. Bhat-Nakshatri, D.A. Martin, R.J. Goulet, Jr., and G.W. Sledge, Jr. 1997. Constitutive activation of NF-kappaB during progression of breast cancer to hormone-independent growth. *Mol Cell Biol* 17:3629–39.

Park, E., S.M. Lee, I.K. Jung, Y. Lim, and J.H. Kim. 2011. Effects of genistein on early-stage cutaneous wound healing. *Biochem Biophys Res Commun* 410:514–9.

Pendleton, J.M., W.W. Tan, S. Anai et al. 2008. Phase II trial of isoflavone in prostate-specific antigen recurrent prostate cancer after previous local therapy. *BMC Cancer* 8:132.

Privat, M., C. Aubel, S. Arnould, Y. Communal, M. Ferrara, and Y.J. Bignon. 2010. AKT and p21 WAF1/CIP1 as potential genistein targets in BRCA1-mutant human breast cancer cell lines. *Anticancer Res* 30:2049–54.

Raffoul, J.J., S. Banerjee, V. Singh-Gupta et al. 2007. Down-regulation of apurinic/apyrimidinic endonuclease 1/redox factor-1 expression by soy isoflavones enhances prostate cancer radiotherapy in vitro and in vivo. *Cancer Res* 67:2141–9.

Raffoul, J.J., Y. Wang, O. Kucuk, J.D. Forman, F.H. Sarkar, and G.G. Hillman. 2006. Genistein inhibits radiation-induced activation of NF-kappaB in prostate cancer cells promoting apoptosis and G2/M cell cycle arrest. *BMC Cancer* 6:107.

Sapi, E., A.B. Alvero, W. Chen et al. 2004. Resistance of ovarian carcinoma cells to docetaxel is XIAP dependent and reversible by phenoxodiol. *Oncol Res* 14:567–78.

Schreiber, S., S. Nikolaus, and J. Hampe. 1998. Activation of nuclear factor kappa B inflammatory bowel disease. *Gut* 42:477–84.

Setchell, K.D. and A. Cassidy. 1999. Dietary isoflavones: biological effects and relevance to human health. *J Nutr* 129:758S–67S.

Shukla, S., G.T. MacLennan, P. Fu et al. 2004. Nuclear factor-kappaB/p65 (Rel A) is constitutively activated in human prostate adenocarcinoma and correlates with disease progression. *Neoplasia* 6:390–400.

Siegel, R., D. Naishadham, and A. Jemal. 2012. Cancer statistics, 2012. *CA Cancer J Clin* 62:10–29.

Simmonds, R.E. and B.M. Foxwell. 2008. Signalling, inflammation and arthritis: NF-kappaB and its relevance to arthritis and inflammation. *Rheumatology (Oxford)* 47:584–90.

Singh-Gupta, V., M.C. Joiner, L. Runyan et al. 2011. Soy isoflavones augment radiation effect by inhibiting APE1/Ref-1 DNA repair activity in non-small cell lung cancer. *J Thorac Oncol* 6:688–98.

Su, Y. and R.C. Simmen. 2009. Soy isoflavone genistein up-regulates epithelial adhesion molecule e-cadherin expression and attenuates {beta}-catenin signaling in mammary epithelial cells. *Carcinogenesis* 30(2):331–9.

Su, Y., F.A. Simmen, R. Xiao, and R.C. Simmen. 2007. Expression profiling of rat mammary epithelial cells reveals candidate signaling pathways in dietary protection from mammary tumors. *Physiol Genomics* 30:8–16.

Tabary, O., S. Escotte, J.P. Couetil et al. 2001. Relationship between IkappaBalpha deficiency, NFkappaB activity and interleukin-8 production in CF human airway epithelial cells. *Pflugers Arch* 443 Suppl 1:S40–S44.

Tabary, O., S. Escotte, J.P. Couetil et al. 1999. Genistein inhibits constitutive and inducible NFkappaB activation and decreases IL-8 production by human cystic fibrosis bronchial gland cells. *Am J Pathol* 155:473–81.

Takimoto, C.H., K. Glover, X. Huang et al. 2003. Phase I pharmacokinetic and pharmacodynamic analysis of unconjugated soy isoflavones administered to individuals with cancer. *Cancer Epidemiol Biomarkers Prev* 12:1213–21.

Tepper, C.G., R.L. Vinall, C.B. Wee et al. 2007. GCP-mediated growth inhibition and apoptosis of prostate cancer cells via androgen receptor-dependent and -independent mechanisms. *Prostate* 67:521–35.

Uckun, F.M., W.E. Evans, C.J. Forsyth et al. 1995. Biotherapy of B-cell precursor leukemia by targeting genistein to CD19-associated tyrosine kinases. *Science* 267:886–91.

Valsecchi, A.E., S. Franchi, A.E. Panerai, A. Rossi, P. Sacerdote, and M. Colleoni. 2011. The soy isoflavone genistein reverses oxidative and inflammatory state, neuropathic pain, neurotrophic and vasculature deficits in diabetes mouse model. *Eur J Pharmacol* 650:694–702.

Wagner, J. and L. Lehmann. 2006. Estrogens modulate the gene expression of Wnt-7a in cultured endometrial adenocarcinoma cells. *Mol Nutr Food Res* 50:368–72.

Wang, W., J.L. Abbruzzese, D.B. Evans, and P.J. Chiao. 1999. Overexpression of urokinase-type plasminogen activator in pancreatic adenocarcinoma is regulated by constitutively activated RelA. *Oncogene* 18:4554–63.

Wang, Z., Y. Zhang, Y. Li, S. Banerjee, J. Liao, and F.H. Sarkar. 2006. Down-regulation of Notch-1 contributes to cell growth inhibition and apoptosis in pancreatic cancer cells. *Mol Cancer Ther* 5:483–93.

Xu, X., H.J. Wang, P.A. Murphy, and S. Hendrich. 2000. Neither background diet nor type of soy food affects short-term isoflavone bioavailability in women. *J Nutr* 130:798–801.

Yamamoto, Y. and R.B. Gaynor. 2001. Therapeutic potential of inhibition of the NF-kappaB pathway in the treatment of inflammation and cancer. *J Clin Invest* 107:135–42.

Yan, L. and E.L. Spitznagel. 2009. Soy consumption and prostate cancer risk in men: a revisit of a meta-analysis. *Am J Clin Nutr* 89:1155–63.

Yan, L., E.L. Spitznagel, and M.C. Bosland. 2010. Soy consumption and colorectal cancer risk in humans: a meta-analysis. *Cancer Epidemiol Biomarkers Prev* 19:148–58.

Yang, W.S., P. Va, M.Y. Wong, H.L. Zhang, and Y.B. Xiang. 2011. Soy intake is associated with lower lung cancer risk: results from a meta-analysis of epidemiologic studies. *Am J Clin Nutr* 94:1575–83.

Yeh, P.Y., S.E. Chuang, K.H. Yeh, Y.C. Song, C.K. Ea, and A.L. Cheng. 2002. Increase of the resistance of human cervical carcinoma cells to cisplatin by inhibition of the MEK to ERK signaling pathway partly via enhancement of anticancer drug-induced NF kappa B activation. *Biochem Pharmacol* 63:1423–30.

Zhang, M., X. Xie, A.H. Lee, and C.W. Binns. 2004. Soy and isoflavone intake are associated with reduced risk of ovarian cancer in southeast china. *Nutr Cancer* 49:125–30.

Ziegler, R.G., R.N. Hoover, M.C. Pike et al. 1993. Migration patterns and breast cancer risk in Asian-American women. *J Natl Cancer Inst* 85:1819–27.

21 Anti-Inflammatory Efficacy of Silibinin
Role in Cancer Chemoprevention

Alpna Tyagi, Gagan Deep, and Rajesh Agarwal

CONTENTS

21.1 INFLAMMATION AND CANCER

21.1.1 INFLAMMATION AND ITS ROLE IN NEOPLASTIC DEVELOPMENT

Inflammation is a physiological response of the body to infection, irritation, and injury. At the site of the infection, inflammation is one of the initial responses to the presence of pathogens and triggers immune action by recruiting phagocytes, which then attack and eradicate the invading pathogens and also interact with the adaptive immune system to generate a long-term response (Porta et al. 2011a; Balkwill and Mantovani 2001; Coussens and Werb 2002). In response to tissue injury, a series of events begin and continue for months and years to restore the afflicted tissue (Coussens and Werb 2002; Stadelmann et al. 1998). Repairing of tissue injury/wound healing is a complex and dynamic process and can be divided into three distinct phases, namely, the inflammatory phase, the proliferative phase, and the remodeling phase (Coussens and Werb 2002; Stadelmann et al. 1998). The inflammatory phase involves activation and directional movement of leukocytes (neutrophils, monocytes, eosinophils, etc.) from the venous system to the sites of injury (Coussens and Werb 2002; Koh and DiPietro 2011). Neutrophils initiate wound healing by releasing early-response proinflammatory cytokines such as tumor necrosis factor α (TNFα), interleukin 1α (IL-1α), and IL-1β (Costin et al. 2012). These proinflammatory cytokines facilitate leukocyte adherence to the

401

vascular endothelium, thus targeting and restricting leukocytes to the area of tissue repair, and initiate repair by inducing the expression of matrix metalloproteinase (MMP) and keratinocyte/fibroblast growth factor (KGF/FGF) by fibroblasts (Chedid et al. 1994). Circulating monocytes are also guided to migrate from the venous system to the site of tissue injury by these proinflammatory cytokines (Balkwill and Mantovani 2001; Mantovani et al. 1992). The neutrophil number declines as the deployment of monocytes to the site of injury begins (Osusky et al. 1997; Coussens and Werb 2002). Monocytes, at the injury spot, are differentiated into macrophages and are the main source for cytokines and growth factors (transforming growth factor beta 1 [TGF-β1], TGF-α, insulin-like growth factor-I [IGF-I] and IGF-II, basic FGF [bFGF], TNFα, and IL-1) that control the tissue repair process (Porta et al. 2011b). Macrophages also regulate tissue remodeling by stimulating the production of proteolytic enzymes (MMPs, urokinase-type plasminogen activator [uPA]), inducing extracellular matrix (ECM) components, modulating angiogenesis, and eliminating apoptotic and necrotic cells (Koh and DiPietro 2011; DiPietro 1995; Fritsch et al. 1997). At the site of injury, ECM forms a platform upon which fibroblast and endothelial cells proliferate and migrate and provide a niche for the reconstitution of a normal microenvironment (DiPietro 1995; Koh and DiPietro 2011; Lu et al. 2012; Porta et al. 2011b). In general, the acute inflammation works as a defensive mechanism to protect the body; however, the chronic inflammation could predispose to the development of various types of diseases such as Alzheimer's, cardiovascular problems, asthma, and cancer (Mantovani et al. 2008; Aggarwal et al. 2006).

The concept of functional association between inflammation and cancer is not new. In 1863, Virchow noted the presence of leukocytes in neoplastic tissue and hypothesized a connection between chronic inflammation and cancer (Balkwill and Mantovani 2001). The presence of certain irritants together with inflammation at the site of the tissue injury promotes cell proliferation (Balkwill and Mantovani 2001). Although cell proliferation alone is not enough to develop cancer, persistent cell proliferation is required in an environment loaded with inflammatory cells, activated stroma, growth factors, and DNA damage–promoting agents to potentiate and/or promote cancer development. A microenvironment rich in inflammatory cells and growth factors supports the continuous growth of proliferating cells together with sustained DNA damage and or/mutagenic assault (Coussens and Werb 2002). Cell proliferation is also boosted during the tissue regeneration process at the site of wound healing; however, proliferation and inflammation start subsiding after the removal of assaulting agents or the completion of tissue repair (Coussens and Werb 2002). Conversely, in the case of neoplastic initiation/progression, both inflammation and cell proliferation continue at the affected site; in another sense, tumors are a kind of wound that fails to heal (Dvorak 1986). There are several instances where inflammatory lesions precede cancer development. For example, chronic reflux esophagitis and ulcerative colitis are associated with enhanced risk of developing esophageal and colorectal cancer, respectively. Furthermore, several infectious diseases causing chronic inflammation have also been linked with cancer development such as *Helicobacter pylori* infection with gastric cancer, human papillomavirus (HPV) infection with cervical, hepatitis C with hepatic cancer, and the urinary form of schistosomiasis with bladder cancer. Therefore, inflammation is closely associated with neoplastic development.

21.1.2 INFLAMMATORY COMPONENTS IN TUMOR MICROENVIRONMENT

Tumors reside in a complex inflammatory microenvironment, which is characterized by the presence of several types of immune cells, such as macrophages, dendritic cells, mast cells, neutrophils, eosinophils, lymphocytes, and so forth. These cells produce a variety of cytokines and cytotoxic mediators including reactive oxygen species (ROS), serine/cysteine proteases, growth factors, and MMPs in the tumor vicinity (Kuper et al. 2000; Wahl and Kleinman 1998; Erreni et al. 2011). Here, we have briefly described the important inflammatory cells as well as soluble mediators present in a tumor inflammatory microenvironment.

Macrophages are derived from the circulating monocyte precursors and are recruited into the tumor microenvironment by chemokines such as monocyte chemotactic protein (MCP). Macrophages are generally the most abundant immune population in the tumor microenvironment (Biswas et al. 2008; Gordon and Taylor 2005; Gordon 2003). Few previously published studies have shown that tumor-associated macrophages (TAMs) have a dual role in neoplasm. TAMs can kill tumor cells following activation by IL-12 and interferon (IFN) (Duluc et al. 2009; Erreni et al. 2011). However, now it is widely accepted that TAMs have mostly protumoral functions (Erreni et al. 2011). TAMs produce numerous potent angiogenic factors, cytokines, growth factors, as well as proteases, thereby stimulating tumor cell proliferation, angiogenesis, migration, invasion, and metastasis and potentiating overall neoplastic progression (Schoppmann et al. 2002; Mantovani et al. 1992).

Dendritic cells are derived from hematopoietic stem cells in the bone marrow and are the key antigen-presenting cells (APCs) for initiating immune response (Ho et al. 2001; Pinzon-Charry et al. 2005). Under physiological conditions, progenitors differentiate into immature dendritic cells, which then circulate in the blood and are delivered to peripheral tissues to sample antigens of assorted origin and act as sentinels for immune monitoring (Pinzon-Charry et al. 2005; Ho et al. 2001). Dendritic cells play an important part in both the activation of antigen-specific immunity and the maintenance of tolerance, providing a link between innate and adaptive immunity. Following an encounter with a tumor antigen or danger signals, immature dendritic cells initiate their maturation process and move to regional lymph nodes, where they activate effector cells for the clearance of the tumor (Pinzon-Charry et al. 2005). However, tumor-associated dendritic cells (TADCs) generally contain an immature phenotype with defective ability to stimulate T cells (Allavena et al. 2000) and provide to the cancer cells one of the critical mechanisms to escape immune surveillance (Pinzon-Charry et al. 2005). In recent years, several lines of evidence have indicated that tumor cells interrupt dendritic cells' maturation and differentiation process, which could be responsible for the failure of effective antitumor response by the host (Pinzon-Charry et al. 2005).

Mast cells are derived from the bone marrow and are important regulators of immune response. These cells depart the bone marrow as committed progenitors before trafficking through the circulation to their target tissues, where they stay as sentinel cells and respond to a challenge by undergoing terminal differentiation (Gurish and Austen 2001; Gurish et al. 1995; Galli 1990). The highest numbers of mast cell progenitors are in the skin, airway, and digestive tract, where they perform as a first line of defense against infiltrating pathogens and parasites (Grimbaldeston et al. 2006; Galli 1990). Mast cells are the first among the innate immune cells responding to tumor initiation, as reported in an inducible mouse model of polyposis (Gounaris et al. 2007). However, in the tumor microenvironment, these cells also contribute to neoplastic progression by releasing extracellular proteases, proangiogenic factors, and chemokines and recruiting macrophages, neutrophils, and eosinophils (Kuper et al. 2000; Di Carlo et al. 2001).

Natural killer (NK) cells, bone marrow–derived lymphocytes, patrol the body and interact with many types of cells. NK cells have been shown to lyse tumor targets in both *in vivo* and *in vitro* models and are also considered proficient in eliminating metastatic cells in the circulation (Zamai et al. 2007; van den Broek et al. 1995). Protective actions of NK cells are associated with cytotoxicity and cytokine production. NK cells mediate cytotoxicity by perforin and proteases or death ligand interactions (FasL and TNF-related apoptosis-inducing ligand [TRAIL]) (Zamai et al. 2007; van den Broek et al. 1995), all of which play an important role in innate immunity. NK cells also produce large numbers of cytokines such as IFN, TNF, and colony-stimulating factor (CSF). Overall, NK cells are the essential component of the immune response that consistently protects a person from serious infections (van den Broek et al. 1995; Takeda et al. 2001; Smyth et al. 2001).

Cytokines are a large group of proteins, peptides, or glycoproteins that are released by specific cells of the immune system throughout the body, which mediate and regulate immunity, inflammation, and hematopoiesis (Mocellin et al. 2001). IFNγ is a proinflammatory cytokine as it augments proinflammatory activity of TNF and also induces nitric oxide (NO) production. IL-1 production also aids in the development of metastasis as IL-1 receptor antagonist significantly decreases tumor development in a mouse model of metastasis (Balkwill and Mantovani 2001). IL-1β–deficient mice are also resistant to the development of experimental metastases (Vidal-Vanaclocha et al. 2000). Moreover, inflammatory cytokines, namely, IL-1, IL-4, IL-6, and IL-8, also influence tumor growth by controlling cancer stem cell populations (Korkaya et al. 2011). Blocking IL-4 signaling in colon cancer cells sensitizes cancer stem cells to apoptotic death and increases the efficacy of conventional cytotoxic therapy (Francipane et al. 2008). However, a cytokine can have opposite roles depending upon its concentration or the microenvironment conditions. For example, TNF, the most important mediator of inflammation, has roles in both tissue destruction (proinflammatory role) and wound healing (anti-inflammatory role). TNF could raze blood vessels but could also induce the expression of several proangiogenic factors (Kollias et al. 1999). Likewise, a high dose of TNF could eliminate or shrink blood vessels selectively in tumor cells, but chronically produced TNF acts as an endogenous tumor promoter, contributing to the tissue remodeling and stromal development required for tumor growth (Balkwill and Mantovani 2001).

Chemokines, chemotactic cytokines, are defined functionally as soluble and small-molecular-weight (8-14 kDa) proteins that bind their cognate G-protein–coupled receptors (GPCRs) to elicit a cellular response (Rossi and Zlotnik 2000). The foremost task of chemokines is to act as a chemoattractant to direct the migration of cells. Cells that are attracted by chemokines follow a path of increasing concentration toward the source of the chemokine (Rossi and Zlotnik 2000). Chemokines are classified into four groups based on the positioning of the conserved two N-terminal cysteine residues, namely, CXC, CC, CX3C, and C chemokines (Zlotnik and Yoshie 2000; Baggiolini et al. 1997; Luster 1998; Rossi and Zlotnik 2000). CXC chemokines are active on lymphocytes and neutrophils, whereas CC chemokines act on monocytes, eosinophils, dendritic cells, lymphocytes, and NK cells but not on neutrophils. CXC and CC are the two major groups of chemokines that are produced by most tumor cells. These chemokines facilitate tumor growth, angiogenesis, and/or metastasis (Zaja-Milatovic and Richmond 2008; Raman et al. 2007). Melanoma, breast, lung, prostate, colorectal, pancreatic, head and neck, and ovarian cancers are the examples where chemokines have been shown to exert autocrine control over neoplastic cell proliferation (Raman et al. 2007).

21.1.3 KEY MOLECULAR MEDIATORS LINKING INFLAMMATION TO CANCER

There are several mediators and mechanisms involved in both extrinsic and intrinsic inflammation pathways that contribute to cancer progression (Mantovani et al. 2008). In the extrinsic pathway, chronic inflammation and/or infection are the driving force that increases the risk for cancer development. In the intrinsic pathway, genetic alterations are the primary cause of cancer development; and mutated tumor cells produce inflammatory mediators and recruit inflammatory cells in their microenvironment (Figure 21.1) (Mantovani et al. 2008; Colotta et al. 2009). The key inflammatory molecular mediators that have been implicated in the development of cancer include several transcription factors (nuclear factor kappaB [NF-κB], signal transducer and activator of transcription 3 [STAT3], hypoxia inducible factor-1 alpha [HIF-1α], activator protein 1 [AP-1], etc.) and proinflammatory enzymes (cyclooxygenase 2 [COX2], inducible NO synthase [iNOS], MMPs, etc.) (Figure 21.1) (Mantovani 2010; Aggarwal et al. 2006; Balkwill 2009; Balkwill and Mantovani 2001; Greten et al. 2004; Karin 2006; Lee et al. 2009; Danese and Mantovani 2010).

NF-κB is activated by inflammatory signals, including TNFα, IL-1, viruses, toll-like receptors (TLRs), and nucleotide-binding oligomerization domain (NODs) and antigen receptors, and regulates expression of multiple proinflammatory genes (Yoshimura 2006; Karin 2006). NF-κB is constitutively activated in most cancers (Shen and Tergaonkar 2009). Under normal cellular conditions, NF-κB remains in a complex form with inhibitor of NF-κB (IκB) in the cytoplasm. However, following an inflammatory stimulus, IκB gets phosphorylated, ubiquitinated, and degraded, and that allows NF-κB to translocate to the nucleus, where it activates the transcription of proinflammatory cytokines (IL-1, IL-6, TNFα, IL-4, IL-8, macrophage inflammatory protein-1α, MCP-1,

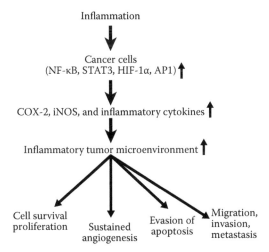

Inflammation

Cancer cells
(NF-κB, STAT3, HIF-1α, AP1) ↑

COX-2, iNOS, and inflammatory cytokines ↑

Inflammatory tumor microenvironment ↑

Cell survival
proliferation   Sustained   Evasion of   Migration,
                   angiogenesis   apoptosis   invasion,
                                                  metastasis

FIGURE 21.1 Molecular pathways linking inflammation and cancer. Inflammation in the tumor micro-environment activates several transcriptional factors (NF-κB, STAT3, HIF-1α, AP-1, etc.) in cancer cells. These transcriptional factors enhance the production of several inflammatory mediators such as cytokines and enzymes. The inflammatory tumor microenvironment contributes to tumor development via promoting cell proliferation, angiogenesis, and metastasis and evading apoptosis.

etc.); antiapoptotic proteins (B-cell lymphoma2 [Bcl2], Bcl-xL, and cellular inhibitor of apoptosis [cIAP]); proangiogenic factors (vascular endothelial growth factor [VEGF], adhesion molecules, and E-selectin); and enzymes (iNOS, COX2, and MMPs). NF-κB activation promotes cell proliferation, angiogenesis, and metastasis and renders cancer cells more resistant to necrosis and apoptotic death (Helbig et al. 2003). NF-κB also plays a critical role in leukocyte adhesion and migration through regulating the adhesion molecules, namely, E-selectin, vascular cell adhesion molecule 1, and intercellular adhesion molecule 1 (Chen et al. 1995).

STAT3 signaling is a major intrinsic pathway for cancer inflammation due to its frequent activation in malignant cells and plays a key role in regulating several genes that are decisive for inflammation in the tumor microenvironment. Constitutive activation of STAT3 has been observed in many types of tumors such as prostate, ovarian, breast, and head and neck, and it is predominantly activated by several cytokines including IFNγ, IL-6, and IL-4 (Haura et al. 2005; Hodge et al. 2005; O'Shea et al. 2002). For example, IL-6 is reported to be involved in the progression of colon cancer through activating STAT3 (Bromberg and Wang 2009), and the IL-6–Janus kinase (JAK)–STAT3 pathway is reported to play an important role in linking the inflammatory microenvironment and cancer progression (Hodge et al. 2005; Lu et al. 2006). STAT3 also promotes cell proliferation, survival, angiogenesis, and metastasis and thus functions as an oncogene (Bromberg and Wang 2009; Johnston and Grandis 2011; Hodge et al. 2005).

HIF-1α activates a wide range of hypoxia-responsive molecules, such as iNOS, VEGF, glucose transporter 1, and many glycolytic enzymes (Lu et al. 2006; Semenza 1999). A hypoxic condition is a common feature at the site of inflammation resulting from the metabolic shift in the injured cells (Kong et al. 2004). Thus, HIF-1α expression is increased at the site of inflammation and promotes chronic inflammation by preventing apoptosis in hypoxic neutrophils and lymphocytes (Walmsley et al. 2005; Lu et al. 2006; Makino et al. 2003). Hypoxic conditions at the site of inflammation also cause HIF-1α–dependent NF-κB activation (Zhou et al. 2003; Jung et al. 2003a,b; Walmsley et al. 2005). Under normoxic conditions, HIF-1α is induced by proinflammatory cytokines such as TNFα, IFNγ, and IL-1β in an NF-κB–dependent manner (Jung et al. 2003a,b; Zhou et al. 2003). For example, IL-1β–induced COX2 mediates HIF-1α expression through its product prostaglandin E2 (PGE$_2$) (Jung et al. 2003; Lu et al. 2006). Also, HIF-1α directly binds to the COX2 promoter region and regulates COX2 expression in colorectal carcinoma cell lines (Lu et al. 2006). Overexpressed HIF-1α facilitates the aggressive phenotype of cancer cells with enhanced glycolytic activity and angiogenesis through increased VEGF expression, a potent angiogenic factor that is essential for tumor growth and metastasis (Jain 2002).

AP-1 is another transcriptional factor that plays a critical role in both inflammation and cancer. It is constitutively active in many cancers such as head and neck, cervical, prostate, and breast. AP-1 amplifies the production of proinflammatory cytokines (IL-6, TNFα, IFNβ, etc.) (Fennewald et al. 2007). Blockade of AP-1 activation downregulates IL-6 expression and leads to the inhibition of STAT3 phosphorylation (Zerbini et al. 2003). Several inflammatory cytokines also have been known to activate the mitogen-activated protein kinase (MAPK) cascade (extracellular signal–regulated kinases 1 and 2 [ERK1/2], c-Jun amino-terminal kinases 1 and 2 [JNK1/2], and p38) that further induces Jun (cJun, JunB, and JunD) and Fos (cFos, FosB, Fra-1, and Fra-2) family members, which form the AP-1 transcription factor (Kaminska 2005; Yoshimura 2006; Chittezhath et al. 2008). The Jun members either homodimerize or heterodimerize with different Fos members, whereas Fos members heterodimerize only with Jun family members; therefore, Jun is the essential partner to form AP-1 complexes. In a nutshell, AP-1 is the key regulator of a wide range of cellular process including cell proliferation, cell death, cell differentiation, inflammation, and innate immune responses (Adcock 1997).

Apart from NF-κB, STAT3, HIF-1α, and AP-1, there are other transcription factors such as Nrf2 and nuclear factor of activated T cells (NFATs) that have been reported to regulate inflammation and cancer progression (Lu et al. 2006). COX2 and NO induce Nrf2 expression, which leads to the reduced susceptibility of cancer cells toward apoptotic signals (Lu et al. 2006). NFAT plays an important role in the inflammatory responses by regulating the expression of a broad range of proinflammatory cytokines, such as IL-2, IL-3, IL-4, IL-5, IL-13, and TNFα (Rao et al. 1997; Crabtree 1999; Kiani et al. 2000). In both T cells and colon carcinoma cells COX2 expression is regulated by NFAT activation (Duque et al. 2005; Jimenez et al. 2004).

COX2, an enzyme required for the production of PG, is the key mediator in inflammation and inflammation-associated cancers (Nathan 2002; Steele et al. 2003). COX2 expression is induced by a broad range of stimuli such as proinflammatory cytokines (IL-1 and TNFα), growth factors (epidermal growth factor receptor [EGFR] and VEGF), and transcription factors (NF-κB, STATs, and HIF-1α). High expression of COX2 has been observed in nearly all types of tumors and has an important role in tumor initiation and maintenance by cellular proliferation, antiapoptotic activity, angiogenesis, and metastasis (Hida et al. 1998).

NO synthase (NOS) includes three isoforms: neuronal (nNOS or NOS-1), cytokine-inducible (iNOS or NOS-2), and endothelial (eNOS or NOS-3). nNOS and eNOS produce low levels of NO, whereas iNOS produces higher levels of NO as a response to inflammatory stimuli. NO is a highly reactive molecule and is an important molecular regulator of both inflammation and cancer development (Kim et al. 2005; Lu et al. 2006). iNOS could be induced by various factors including NF-κB, HIF-1α, STAT3, inflammatory cytokines, and wingless-type MMTV integration family-signaling or microbial endotoxins (Kim et al. 2005; Lu et al. 2006). Induction of iNOS expression in monocytes, macrophages, and neutrophils leads to the production of NO, and its high levels in both the tumor cells and the tumor microenvironment contribute to cancer progression (Schetter et al. 2009; Kanwar et al. 2009). iNOS signaling also induces COX2 expression, which is a promising link between inflammation and cancer (Rao 2004).

21.1.4 Inflammation: Cancer-Preventive and Therapeutic Opportunities

The critical role of inflammation in cancer is evident from studies where researchers observed lower cancer risk among long-term users of nonsteroidal anti-inflammatory drugs (NSAIDs) (Baron and Sandler 2000; Garcia-Rodriguez and Huerta-Alvarez 2001). The use of these anti-inflammatory drugs has been reported to reduce colon cancer risk by 40%–50% and is also considered preventive

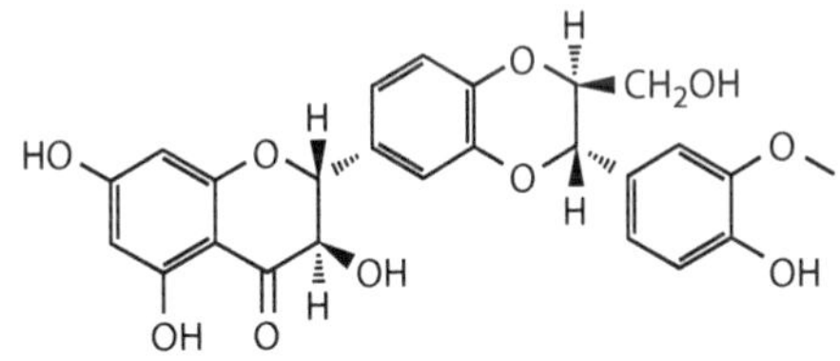

FIGURE 21.2 Chemical structure of silibinin.

against the development of lung, esophagus, breast, prostate, and stomach cancers (Baron and Sandler 2000; Garcia-Rodriguez and Huerta-Alvarez 2001). However, the chronic use of NSAIDs also causes serious gastrointestinal complications, and specific COX2 inhibitor use could enhance the risk of cardiovascular diseases. Therefore, alternative efforts are required to target the inflammatory component in the tumor microenvironment. Several nontoxic natural cancer chemopreventive agents (silibinin, curcumin, isothiocyanate, green tea, etc.) have shown remarkable efficacy in targeting the transcriptional factors (NF-κB, STAT3, HIFα, AP-1, etc.) as well as enzymes (COX2, iNOS, MMPs, etc.) regulating inflammation and have also shown immunomodulatory properties (Sen et al. 2011; Tyagi et al. 2009; Raina et al. 2013). Here, we have discussed the anti-inflammatory effects of one such cancer chemopreventive agent, that is, silibinin (Figure 21.2).

21.2 SILIBININ

21.2.1 SILIBININ SOURCE AND TRADITIONAL USES IN HUMAN HEALTH AND TOXICITY

Silibinin ($C_{25}H_{22}O_{10}$, molecular weight 482.44) is isolated from the seeds of the milk thistle plant (*Silybum marianum*, family Asteraceae). Milk thistle extract (also known as silymarin) has been used for centuries to treat a wide range of ailments related to the liver, kidney, and gall bladder. Milk thistle extract is now employed against liver cirrhosis, chronic hepatitis, and toxin-induced liver damage, including the severe liver damage from *Amanita phalloides* ("death cap" mushroom poisoning). Milk thistle extract or silibinin is sold as a dietary supplement and is one of the most frequently sold herbal products in the United States. Silibinin use is extremely safe, and its formulations have not shown toxicity or adverse effects in several toxicity tests (Hoh et al. 2006; Flaig et al. 2007; Singh et al. 2002). For example, in oral toxicity studies in rats, a dose of 2000 mg/kg per day of Siliphos for 26 weeks did not adversely affect the body/liver weight and liver enzymes (aspartate transaminase [AST], alanine aminotransferase [ALT]), suggesting the nontoxic nature of this compound (Kidd and Head 2005). In a recent 2-year feed study, there was no toxicity observed in B6C3F1 mice exposed to 12,500, 25,000, or 50,000 ppm milk thistle extract (toxicology and carcinogenesis studies of milk thistle extract in F344/N rats and B6C3F1 mice 2011). *In vivo* studies performed by our group have also shown that both silymarin and silibinin are well tolerated and have no toxicity in mouse models (Zhao and Agarwal 1999; Singh et al. 2002; Flaig et al. 2007). In recently conducted clinical trials, it was shown that 13 g/day of silibinin in the form of phytosome (Siliphos) is well tolerated in advanced prostate cancer patients (Flaig et al. 2007, 2010; Hoh et al. 2006). In general, silibinin consumption in humans is safe and has several health benefits (Flaig et al. 2007).

21.2.2 SILIBININ METABOLISM AND BIOAVAILABILITY

Silibinin, depending upon the formulation, constitutes about 50%–60% of silymarin (Davis-Searles et al. 2005). Pharmacokinetic analyses have shown that flavonoids present in silymarin are rapidly metabolized to their conjugates, such as sulfates and glucuronides, and could be detected in the human plasma; compared to free silibinin, conjugated silibinin metabolites have slower elimination from the system (Wen et al. 2008). Due to its large multiring structure, which makes its absorption difficult by simple diffusion, silibinin bioavailability is usually low (Silybin-phosphatidylcholine complex. Monograph 2009). Also, silibinin has poor miscibility with oils and other lipids that limits its ability to cross the lipid-rich outer membrane of the enterocytes of the intestine (Silybin-phosphatidylcholine complex. Monograph 2009). Thus, to achieve enhanced bioavailability of silibinin, it is combined with phosphatidylcholine, and this formulation is known as silipide (trade name Siliphos) (Kidd 2009; Wang et al. 2010; Yanyu et al. 2006). In completed pharmacokinetic studies, a higher amount of silibinin was absorbed in the plasma and liver when healthy subjects were fed with Siliphos as compared to conventional silibinin (Kidd and Head 2005; Kidd 2009; Yanyu et al. 2006; Wang et al. 2010). Furthermore, prostate and colon cancer patients fed with Siliphos showed high plasma bioavailability of silibinin (Flaig et al. 2007, 2010; Hoh et al. 2006); however, colon tissue showed more bioavailability of silibinin as compared to prostate tissue (Flaig et al. 2007, 2010; Hoh et al. 2006; Fennewald et al. 2007), suggesting the organ-specific differences in silibinin's bioavailability following oral administration. Recently, efforts have been made to further enhance silibinin's bioavailability by formulating silibinin nanosuspensions (Wang et al. 2010).

21.2.3 Silibinin: Cancer Chemopreventive Efficacy

In the last two decades, several reports have been published regarding the chemopreventive and anticancer efficacy of silibinin against cancer of different organs (Tyagi et al. 2009; Raina et al. 2008; Rajamanickam et al. 2009; Ramasamy et al. 2011; Roy et al. 2012; Singh et al. 2004; Tyagi et al. 2007; Deep et al. 2011). Silibinin's anticancer efficacy is through targeting pleiotropic biological processes such as cell proliferation, apoptosis, autophagy, angiogenesis, invasion, migration, and metabolism (Deep et al. 2011; Dhanalakshmi et al. 2005; Kaur et al. 2010; Ramasamy et al. 2011; Tyagi et al. 2004; Raina et al. 2009). Molecular efficacy studies have shown multiple signaling molecules as silibinin's targets, including p53, ataxia telangiectasia mutated (ATM), EGFR, MAPKs, AP-1, NF-κB, STATs, cyclins, cyclin-dependent kinases (CDKs), CDK inhibitors, β-catenin, androgen receptor, VEGF, VEGF receptor, and so forth (Deep et al. 2011; Tyagi et al. 2006, 2011; Roy et al. 2007; Raina et al. 2009; Singh et al. 2008). Recently, we have reported the strong antimetastatic potential of silibinin in transgenic adenocarcinoma of mouse prostate (TRAMP)–mice via inhibiting Snail-1, vimentin, β-catenin, and several proteases (Singh et al. 2008; Raina et al. 2008). In another study, it was shown that silibinin delays the development of spontaneous mammary tumors and reduces the mammary tumor masses in Her-2/neu transgenic mice (Provinciali et al. 2007). Silibinin has also been tested in prostate and colon cancer patients for its efficacy, and currently, its usefulness is being evaluated clinically against other diseases such as mushroom poisoning, diabetic nephropathy, asthma, hepatitis, and so forth (Hoh et al. 2006; Flaig et al. 2007, 2010). Overall, silibinin possess broad-spectrum chemopreventive efficacy against cancer.

21.3 ANTI-INFLAMMATORY EFFICACY OF SILIBININ AGAINST VARIOUS CANCERS

Several studies in the past have shown that silibinin possesses strong anti-inflammatory efficacy against cancer through modulating transcriptional factors, inflammatory enzymes, cytokines, and immune cells; these studies, along with mechanistic details in various cancers, are discussed below.

21.3.1 Colon Cancer

Chronic inflammation is one of the primary causes for colorectal cancer (CRC) development. Therefore, inflammatory bowel diseases (IBDs) such as ulcerative colitis and Crohn's disease increase the risk of developing CRC (Coussens and Werb 2002; Elwood et al. 2009). CRC exhibits increased expression of proinflammatory cytokines and enzymes (iNOS and COX2) and constitutive activation of transcription factors (NF-κB, STAT3, and HIF-1α). Silibinin has been reported to target several molecular mediators of inflammation in CRC. For example, silibinin efficacy has been reported against human CRC cells via inhibiting the TNFα-induced activation of inflammatory mediator NF-κB (Raina et al. 2013). Silibinin also decreased the protein levels of Bcl2, iNOS, COX2, MMP-9, and VEGF, which are upregulated via TNFα-induced NF-κB activation (Raina et al. 2013). Silibinin has been shown to inhibit the growth of SW480 and LoVo tumors in nude mice accompanied with strong NF-κB inhibition in the tumor tissues (Raina et al. 2013). Silibinin also inhibited the iNOS, COX2, and VEGF expression in HT29 tumor xenografts, suggesting its anti-inflammatory potential against CRC (Singh et al. 2008). In other studies, oral feeding of silibinin inhibited the azoxymethane-induced colon tumorigenesis in A/J mice and male Fisher 344 rats and significantly decreased the azoxymethane-induced iNOS and COX2 expression in colon tissues (Velmurugan et al. 2008; Ravichandran et al. 2010). Silibinin also suppressed the spontaneous tumorigenesis in the APC$^{min/+}$ mouse, a genetically predisposed animal model of human familial adenomatous polyposis, by modulating COX2, iNOS, HIF-1α, VEGF, PGE$_2$, and β-catenin expression selectively in the small intestinal polyps (Rajamanickam et al. 2009, 2010). Esmaily et al. (2011) have reported that silibinin inhibits NF-κB activity as well as the levels of IL-1β, TNFα, thiobarbituric acid–reactive substances (TBARS), protein carbonyl, and myeloperoxidase activity in a trinitrobenzene sulfonic acid (TNBS)–induced colitis rat model. Overall, these results in multiple study models have confirmed that silibinin possesses strong anti-inflammatory efficacy, and that contributes toward its chemopreventive efficacy against CRC.

21.3.2 LUNG CANCER

Cigarette smoking is responsible for almost 90% of lung cancer risk in men and 70%–80% in women (Walser et al. 2008). Cigarette smoke contains several known carcinogens and also generates high levels of ROS, which could lead to impairment of epithelial and endothelial cell function as well as inflammation in the lung. Further, pulmonary diseases that are associated with a high risk for lung cancer are characterized by profound abnormalities in the inflammatory pathways (Reynolds et al. 2006; Smith et al. 2006; Kim et al. 2008). These pathways, including cytokines, growth factors, iNOS, PGE$_2$, NF-κB, STAT3, and macrophages, have several deleterious effects that simultaneously pave the path for tumor promotion and progression (Lee et al. 2012). Silibinin has been reported to target multiple inflammation-related pathways in lung tumors (Chittezhath et al. 2008; Tyagi et al. 2012). For example, silibinin treatment inhibited multiple cytokine-induced signaling pathways that regulate iNOS expression in human lung adenocarcinoma A549 cells (Chittezhath et al. 2008). Dietary feeding of silibinin decreased the cell proliferation and angiogenesis in urethane-induced lung tumorigenesis by inhibiting iNOS expression (Singh et al. 2004; Ramasamy et al. 2011). Silibinin has also been shown to prevent lung tumorigenesis in wild-type but not in iNOS$^{-/-}$ mice, suggesting that silibinin exerts most of its chemopreventive and antiangiogenic effects via inhibition of iNOS expression in lung tumors (Ramasamy et al. 2011). Further, silibinin inhibited the growth and caused regression of urethane-induced lung adenocarcinoma via targeting the TAMs and cytokine production and inhibiting several transcription factors (NF-κB, HIF-1α, and STAT3) (Tyagi et al. 2009). Also, silibinin inhibited cytokine mixture–induced ERK1/2, STAT1/3, and NF-κB activation as well as COX2, iNOS, MMP-2, and MMP-9 expression in mouse lung epithelial LM2 cells (Tyagi et al. 2012). Furthermore, silibinin diminished the cytokine mixture–induced migration of LM2 cells, which could be via STAT1/3 inhibition (Tyagi et al. 2012). Chen et al. (2005) have earlier reported that silibinin treatment reduces expression of MMP-2 and uPA concomitantly with significant inhibition of A549 cell invasiveness. Silibinin has also been reported to enhance the chemosensitivity of A549 tumors via targeting the NF-κB pathway (Singh et al. 2004). Together, these results have revealed that silibinin suppresses lung tumor growth and progression mainly through its anti-inflammatory activity by interfering with iNOS expression and transcriptional factor activation.

21.3.3 Skin Cancer

Chronic exposure to solar ultraviolet radiation (UVR) is an important carcinogen that leads to the development of precancerous and cancerous skin lesions, and it is considered as the most important etiologic agent in human skin cancer (Roy et al. 2012). In addition to UVR, chemical exposure has also been known to induce a cutaneous inflammatory response, which includes the infiltration of leukocytes into the dermis, production of proinflammatory enzymes (iNOS and COX2) and cytokines, and induction of transcription factors (NF-κB, STAT3, AP-1, and HIF-1α) and growth factors (VEGF and EGF) (Gu et al. 2007; Singh et al. 2006; Meeran et al. 2007; Vaid et al. 2010). Various studies have suggested that all these factors together are accountable for skin carcinogenesis (Vaid et al. 2010; Singh et al. 2006; Gu et al. 2007). We have shown that chronic exposure to a physiological dose of UVB (30 mJ/cm^2) strongly increased the expression of iNOS, COX2, and HIF-1α and activated NF-κB and STAT3 signaling in both skin and skin tumors (Gu et al. 2007), and these events were strongly suppressed by pretopical or posttopical treatment or dietary feeding of silibinin in SKH-1 hairless mice (Gu et al. 2007). Similarly, 12-O-tetradecanoylphorbol-13-acetate (TPA) exposure resulted in edema and increased levels of inflammatory cytokine (IL-1α) and COX2 activity in SENCAR mouse epidermis; silymarin treatment inhibited the TPA-induced edema and expression of IL-1α and COX2 (Zhao et al. 1999).

The arachidonic acid metabolism via lipoxygenase and COX pathways produces hydroxyeicosatetraenoic acid and PG metabolites, respectively, and has been associated with inflammation and tumor promotion (Zhao et al. 1999). Silymarin treatment strongly inhibited the tumor promoter–induced arachidonic acid metabolism accompanied by inhibition of lipoxygenase and COX activities (Zhao et al. 1999). Furthermore, silymarin inhibited the TPA-induced epidermal lipid peroxidation and myeloperoxidase activity (Zhao et al. 1999). Silibinin treatment has also shown protective effects in mouse epidermal JB6 cells by inhibiting UVB- and EGF-induced AP-1 and NF-κB signaling pathways (Singh et al. 2006). Meeran et al. (2006) have reported that silibinin and silymarin treatment inhibited the UVB-induced local and systemic immunosuppression. Silymarin also inhibited the UVB-induced immunosuppressive cytokine IL-10 and simultaneously enhanced the levels of the immunostimulatory cytokine IL-12 in the mouse skin, suggesting that silymarin's protective effect is mediated through immunostimulatory cytokine IL-12 (Meeran et al. 2006). Together, these studies clearly advocate a high protective action of silibinin against tumor promotion in mouse skin tumorigenesis models by targeting the inflammatory components.

21.3.4 Prostate, Bladder, and Breast Cancer

Findings from numerous studies have suggested that inflammation is likely to have an important role in prostate, bladder, and breast cancer carcinogenesis (De Marzo et al. 2007; Yang et al. 2008; Laoui et al. 2011). For the development of these malignancies, environmental factors are also critically involved apart from the hereditary factors (De Marzo et al. 2007; Yang et al. 2008; Laoui et al. 2011). One such potential environmental factor that has gained attention is the chronic inflammation caused by dietary factors, hormonal changes, infections, and so forth (Yang et al. 2008; Laoui et al. 2011; De Marzo et al. 2007). Metastasis is the main cause of death especially in prostate and breast cancers, and proinflammatory cytokines are known to promote motility and invasiveness of cancer cells (Deep and Agarwal 2010; Mulholland et al. 2012). The increased motility and invasiveness of tumor cells are due to decreased cell–cell adhesion, which is reminiscent of epithelial–mesenchymal transition (EMT) that occurs during embryonic development, wound healing, and metastasis (Deep and Agarwal 2010; Mulholland et al. 2012). Snail, a zinc finger transcription factor, is stabilized by the inflammatory cytokine TNFα through NF-κB activation (Wu et al. 2009) and controls EMT by repressing E-cadherin expression (Cano et al. 2000). Silibinin has been shown to decrease metastasis of prostate cancer cells to distant organs by inhibiting Snail-1 expression and enhancing E-cadherin expression in prostate tumor tissues in TRAMP mice (Raina et al. 2008; Singh et al. 2008). Wu et al. (2010) have shown that silibinin reverses EMT in metastatic prostate cancer cells by targeting NF-κB, Zinc finger E-box-binding homeobox (ZEB1), and Slug transcription factors. Silibinin also inhibited the constitutively active NF-κB, STAT3, and HIF-1α in prostate cancer cells (Agarwal et al. 2007; Dhanalakshmi et al. 2002; Jung et al. 2009). Furthermore, TNFα-induced activation of NF-κB was also inhibited by silibinin treatment in prostate cancer cells (Dhanalakshmi et al. 2002). Silibinin also suppressed growth of PC-3 orthotopic xenograft via inhibiting STAT activation (Singh et al. 2009). Therefore, silibinin has shown anticancer efficacy against prostate cancer via targeting multiple inflammatory molecules. Silymarin and silibinin treatment also inhibited NF-κB activation in N-butyl-N-(4-hydroxybutyl) nitrosamine–induced urinary bladder carcinogenesis in male ICR mice (Tyagi et al. 2007). However, more studies are needed to validate the anti-inflammatory role of silibinin in prostate and bladder cancers. In human epidermal growth factor receptor 2 (HER-2)/neu transgenic mice, which spontaneously develop mammary tumors at an early age, silibinin administration delayed the development of spontaneous mammary tumors, reduced the number and size of tumors, and diminished lung metastasis. Silibinin effects were associated with an increased infiltration of neutrophils and CD (cluster of differentiation) 4 and CD8 T cells; however, there was a slight decrease in macrophage number (Provinciali et al. 2007). Overall, these *in vivo* and *in vitro* studies have suggested that silibinin could effectively target inflammatory molecular mediators in prostate, bladder, and breast cancers.

21.4   CONCLUSIONS

For a long time, the focus to treat cancer has been entirely on growth inhibition and death induction in cancer cells. Recently, separate lines of research have pointed attention toward a potential link between inflammation and cancer development, even in cases where the underlying chronic infections are absent. Thus, inflammation in cancer represents the complementary perspective that could help to develop effective antitumor responses via targeting immune cells in the microenvironment (such as TAM recruitment and polarization); transcription factor activation (NF-κB, STATs, HIF-1α, AP-1, etc.); or the excessive production of proinflammatory cytokines/chemokines in the tumor vicinity. In this direction, prevention/intervention of cancer by using natural agents holds promise. Silibinin, a natural cancer chemopreventive agent, has shown strong anti-inflammatory efficacy against many cancers through targeting multiple signaling pathways, cytokines, growth factors, and immune cells. However, more focused studies are needed in inflammation-specific preclinical models to establish its detailed anti-inflammatory efficacy and mechanisms.

ACKNOWLEDGMENT

Original studies are supported in part by NCI RO1 grants CA102514, CA112304, and CA140368.

REFERENCES

Adcock, I.M. 1997. Transcription factors as activators of gene transcription: AP-1 and NF-kappa B. *Monaldi Arch Chest Dis* 52:178–86.

Agarwal, C., A. Tyagi, M. Kaur, and R. Agarwal. 2007. Silibinin inhibits constitutive activation of Stat3, and causes caspase activation and apoptotic death of human prostate carcinoma DU145 cells. *Carcinogenesis* 28:1463–70.

Aggarwal, B.B., S. Shishodia, S.K. Sandur, M.K. Pandey, and G. Sethi. 2006. Inflammation and cancer: How hot is the link? *Biochem Pharmacol* 72:1605–21.

Allavena, P., A. Sica, A. Vecchi, M. Locati, S. Sozzani, and A. Mantovani. 2000. The chemokine receptor switch paradigm and dendritic cell migration: its significance in tumor tissues. *Immunol Rev* 177:141–9.

Baggiolini, M., B. Dewald, and B. Moser. 1997. Human chemokines: an update. *Annu Rev Immunol* 15:675–705.

Balkwill, F. 2009. Tumour necrosis factor and cancer. *Nat Rev Cancer* 9:361–71.

Balkwill, F., and A. Mantovani. 2001. Inflammation and cancer: back to Virchow? *Lancet* 357:539–45.

Baron, J.A., and R.S. Sandler. 2000. Nonsteroidal anti-inflammatory drugs and cancer prevention. *Annu Rev Med* 51:511–23.

Biswas, S.K., A. Sica, and C.E. Lewis. 2008. Plasticity of macrophage function during tumor progression: regulation by distinct molecular mechanisms. *J Immunol* 180:2011–7.

Bromberg, J., and T.C. Wang. 2009. Inflammation and cancer: IL-6 and STAT3 complete the link. *Cancer Cell* 15:79–80.

Cano, A., M.A. Perez-Moreno, I. Rodrigo et al. 2000. The transcription factor snail controls epithelial-mesenchymal transitions by repressing E-cadherin expression. *Nat Cell Biol* 2:76–83.

Chedid, M., J.S. Rubin, K.G. Csaky, and S.A. Aaronson. 1994. Regulation of keratinocyte growth factor gene expression by interleukin 1. *J Biol Chem* 269:10753–7.

Chen, C.C., C.L. Rosenbloom, D.C. Anderson, and A.M. Manning. 1995. Selective inhibition of E-selectin, vascular cell adhesion molecule-1, and intercellular adhesion molecule-1 expression by inhibitors of I kappa B-alpha phosphorylation. *J Immunol* 155:3538–45.

Chen, P.N., Y.S. Hsieh, H.L. Chiou, and S.C. Chu. 2005. Silibinin inhibits cell invasion through inactivation of both PI3K-Akt and MAPK signaling pathways. *Chem Biol Interact* 156:141–50.

Chittezhath, M., G. Deep, R.P. Singh, C. Agarwal, and R. Agarwal. 2008. Silibinin inhibits cytokine-induced signaling cascades and down-regulates inducible nitric oxide synthase in human lung carcinoma A549 cells. *Mol Cancer Ther* 7:1817–26.

Colotta, F., P. Allavena, A. Sica, C. Garlanda, and A. Mantovani. 2009. Cancer-related inflammation, the seventh hallmark of cancer: links to genetic instability. *Carcinogenesis* 30:1073–81.

Costin, G.E., S.A. Birlea, and D.A. Norris. 2012. Trends in wound repair: cellular and molecular basis of regenerative therapy using electromagnetic fields. *Curr Mol Med* 12:14–26.

Coussens, L.M., and Z. Werb. 2002. Inflammation and cancer. *Nature* 420:860–7.

Crabtree, G.R. 1999. Generic signals and specific outcomes: signaling through Ca2+, calcineurin, and NF-AT. *Cell* 96:611–4.

Danese, S., and A. Mantovani. 2010. Inflammatory bowel disease and intestinal cancer: a paradigm of the Yin-Yang interplay between inflammation and cancer. *Oncogene* 29:3313–23.

Davis-Searles, P.R., Y. Nakanishi, N.C. Kim, et al. 2005. Milk thistle and prostate cancer: differential effects of pure flavonolignans from Silybum marianum on antiproliferative end points in human prostate carcinoma cells. *Cancer Res* 65:4448–57.

De Marzo, A.M., E.A. Platz, S. Sutcliffe et al. 2007. Inflammation in prostate carcinogenesis. *Nat Rev Cancer* 7:256–69.

Deep, G., and R. Agarwal. 2010. Antimetastatic efficacy of silibinin: molecular mechanisms and therapeutic potential against cancer. *Cancer Metastasis Rev* 29:447–63.

Deep, G., S.C. Gangar, C. Agarwal, and R. Agarwal. 2011. Role of E-cadherin in antimigratory and antiinvasive efficacy of silibinin in prostate cancer cells. *Cancer Prev Res (Phila)* 4:1222–32.

Dhanalakshmi, S., C. Agarwal, R.P. Singh, and R. Agarwal. 2005. Silibinin up-regulates DNA-protein kinase-dependent p53 activation to enhance UVB-induced apoptosis in mouse epithelial JB6 cells. *J Biol Chem* 280:20375–83.

Dhanalakshmi, S., R.P. Singh, C. Agarwal, and R. Agarwal. 2002. Silibinin inhibits constitutive and TNFalpha-induced activation of NF-kappaB and sensitizes human prostate carcinoma DU145 cells to TNFalpha-induced apoptosis. *Oncogene* 21:1759–67.

Di Carlo, E., G. Forni, P. Lollini, M.P. Colombo, A. Modesti, and P. Musiani. 2001. The intriguing role of polymorphonuclear neutrophils in antitumor reactions. *Blood* 97:339–45.

DiPietro, L.A. 1995. Wound healing: the role of the macrophage and other immune cells. *Shock* 4:233–40.

Duluc, D., M. Corvaisier, S. Blanchard et al. 2009. Interferon-gamma reverses the immunosuppressive and protumoral properties and prevents the generation of human tumor-associated macrophages. *Int J Cancer* 125:367–73.

Duque, J., M. Fresno, and M.A. Iniguez. 2005. Expression and function of the nuclear factor of activated T cells in colon carcinoma cells: involvement in the regulation of cyclooxygenase-2. *J Biol Chem* 280: 8686–93.

Dvorak, H.F. 1986. Tumors: wounds that do not heal. Similarities between tumor stroma generation and wound healing. *N Engl J Med* 315:1650–9.

Elwood, P.C., A.M. Gallagher, G.G. Duthie, L.A. Mur, and G. Morgan. 2009. Aspirin, salicylates, and cancer. *Lancet* 373:1301–9.

Erreni, M., A. Mantovani, and P. Allavena. 2011. Tumor-associated Macrophages (TAM) and Inflammation in Colorectal Cancer. *Cancer Microenviron* 4:141–54.

Esmaily, H., A. Vaziri-Bami, A.E. Miroliaee, M. Baeeri, and M. Abdollahi. 2011. The correlation between NF-kappaB inhibition and disease activity by coadministration of silibinin and ursodeoxycholic acid in experimental colitis. *Fundam Clin Pharmacol* 25:723–33.

Fennewald, S.M., E.P. Scott, L. Zhang et al. 2007. Thioaptamer decoy targeting of AP-1 proteins influences cytokine expression and the outcome of arenavirus infections. *J Gen Virol* 88:981–90.

Flaig, T.W., M. Glode, D. Gustafson et al. 2010. A study of high-dose oral silybin-phytosome followed by prostatectomy in patients with localized prostate cancer. *Prostate* 70:848–55.

Flaig, T.W., D.L. Gustafson, L.J. Su et al. 2007. A phase I and pharmacokinetic study of silybin-phytosome in prostate cancer patients. *Invest New Drugs* 25:139–46.

Francipane, M.G., M.P. Alea, Y. Lombardo, M. Todaro, J.P. Medema, and G. Stassi. 2008. Crucial role of interleukin-4 in the survival of colon cancer stem cells. *Cancer Res* 68:4022–5.

Fritsch, C., P. Simon-Assmann, M. Kedinger, and G.S. Evans. 1997. Cytokines modulate fibroblast phenotype and epithelial-stroma interactions in rat intestine. *Gastroenterology* 112:826–38.

Galli, S.J. 1990. New insights into "the riddle of the mast cells": microenvironmental regulation of mast cell development and phenotypic heterogeneity. *Lab Invest* 62:5–33.

Garcia-Rodriguez, L.A., and C. Huerta-Alvarez. 2001. Reduced risk of colorectal cancer among long-term users of aspirin and nonaspirin nonsteroidal antiinflammatory drugs. *Epidemiology* 12:88–93.

Gordon, S. 2003. Alternative activation of macrophages. *Nat Rev Immunol* 3:23–35.

Gordon, S., and P.R. Taylor. 2005. Monocyte and macrophage heterogeneity. *Nat Rev Immunol* 5:953–64.

Gounaris, E., S.E. Erdman, C. Restaino et al. 2007. Mast cells are an essential hematopoietic component for polyp development. *Proc Natl Acad Sci U S A* 104:19977–82.

Greten, F.R., L. Eckmann, T.F. Greten et al. 2004. IKKbeta links inflammation and tumorigenesis in a mouse model of colitis-associated cancer. *Cell* 118:285–96.

Grimbaldeston, M.A., M. Metz, M. Yu, M. Tsai, and S.J. Galli. 2006. Effector and potential immunoregulatory roles of mast cells in IgE-associated acquired immune responses. *Curr Opin Immunol* 18:751–60.

Gu, M., R.P. Singh, S. Dhanalakshmi, C. Agarwal, and R. Agarwal. 2007. Silibinin inhibits inflammatory and angiogenic attributes in photocarcinogenesis in SKH-1 hairless mice. *Cancer Res* 67:3483–91.

Gurish, M.F., and K.F. Austen. 2001. The diverse roles of mast cells. *J Exp Med* 194:F1–5.

Gurish, M.F., W.S. Pear, R.L. Stevens et al. 1995. Tissue-regulated differentiation and maturation of a v-abl-immortalized mast cell-committed progenitor. *Immunity* 3:175–86.

Haura, E.B., J. Turkson, and R. Jove. 2005. Mechanisms of disease: Insights into the emerging role of signal transducers and activators of transcription in cancer. *Nat Clin Pract Oncol* 2:315–24.

Helbig, G., K.W. Christopherson, 2nd, P. Bhat-Nakshatri et al. 2003. NF-kappaB promotes breast cancer cell migration and metastasis by inducing the expression of the chemokine receptor CXCR4. *J Biol Chem* 278:21631–8.

Hida, T., Y. Yatabe, H. Achiwa et al. 1998. Increased expression of cyclooxygenase 2 occurs frequently in human lung cancers, specifically in adenocarcinomas. *Cancer Res* 58:3761–4.

Ho, C.S., J.A. Lopez, S. Vuckovic, C.M. Pyke, R.L. Hockey, and D.N. Hart. 2001. Surgical and physical stress increases circulating blood dendritic cell counts independently of monocyte counts. *Blood* 98:140–5.

Hodge, D.R., E.M. Hurt, and W.L. Farrar. 2005. The role of IL-6 and STAT3 in inflammation and cancer. *Eur J Cancer* 41:2502–12.

Hoh, C., D. Boocock, T. Marczylo et al. 2006. Pilot study of oral silibinin, a putative chemopreventive agent, in colorectal cancer patients: silibinin levels in plasma, colorectum, and liver and their pharmacodynamic consequences. *Clin Cancer Res* 12:2944–50.

Jain, R.K. 2002. Tumor angiogenesis and accessibility: role of vascular endothelial growth factor. *Semin Oncol* 29:3–9.

Jimenez, J.L., M.A. Iniguez, M.A. Munoz-Fernandez, and M. Fresno. 2004. Effect of phosphodiesterase 4 inhibitors on NFAT-dependent cyclooxygenase-2 expression in human T lymphocytes. *Cell Signal* 16:1363–73.

Johnston, P.A., and J.R. Grandis. 2011. STAT3 signaling: anticancer strategies and challenges. *Mol Interv* 11:18–26.

Jung, H.J., J.W. Park, J.S. Lee et al. 2009. Silibinin inhibits expression of HIF-1alpha through suppression of protein translation in prostate cancer cells. *Biochem Biophys Res Commun* 390:71–6.

Jung, Y., J.S. Isaacs, S. Lee, J. Trepel, Z.G. Liu, and L. Neckers. 2003a. Hypoxia-inducible factor induction by tumour necrosis factor in normoxic cells requires receptor-interacting protein-dependent nuclear factor kappa B activation. *Biochem J* 370:1011–7.

Jung, Y.J., J.S. Isaacs, S. Lee, J. Trepel, and L. Neckers. 2003b. IL-1beta-mediated up-regulation of HIF-1alpha via an NFkappaB/COX-2 pathway identifies HIF-1 as a critical link between inflammation and oncogenesis. *Faseb J* 17:2115–7.

Kaminska, B. 2005. MAPK signalling pathways as molecular targets for anti-inflammatory therapy—from molecular mechanisms to therapeutic benefits. *Biochim Biophys Acta* 1754:253–62.

Kanwar, J.R., R.K. Kanwar, H. Burrow, and S. Baratchi. 2009. Recent advances on the roles of NO in cancer and chronic inflammatory disorders. *Curr Med Chem* 16:2373–94.

Karin, M. 2006. Nuclear factor-kappaB in cancer development and progression. *Nature* 441:431–6.

Kaur, M., B. Velmurugan, A. Tyagi, C. Agarwal, R.P. Singh, and R. Agarwal. 2010. Silibinin suppresses growth of human colorectal carcinoma SW480 cells in culture and xenograft through down-regulation of beta-catenin-dependent signaling. *Neoplasia* 12:415–24.

Kiani, A., A. Rao, and J. Aramburu. 2000. Manipulating immune responses with immunosuppressive agents that target NFAT. *Immunity* 12:359–72.

Kidd, P.M. 2009. Bioavailability and activity of phytosome complexes from botanical polyphenols: the silymarin, curcumin, green tea, and grape seed extracts. *Altern Med Rev* 14:226–46.

Kidd, P., and K. Head. 2005. A review of the bioavailability and clinical efficacy of milk thistle phytosome: a silybin-phosphatidylcholine complex (Siliphos). *Altern Med Rev* 10:193–203.

Kim, V., T.J. Rogers, and G.J. Criner. 2008. New concepts in the pathobiology of chronic obstructive pulmonary disease. *Proc Am Thorac Soc* 5:478–85.

Kim, Y.H., K.J. Woo, J.H. Lim et al. 2005. 8-Hydroxyquinoline inhibits iNOS expression and nitric oxide production by down-regulating LPS-induced activity of NF-kappaB and C/EBPbeta in Raw 264.7 cells. *Biochem Biophys Res Commun* 329:591–7.

Koh, T.J., and L.A. DiPietro. 2011. Inflammation and wound healing: the role of the macrophage. *Expert Rev Mol Med* 13:e23.

Kollias, G., E. Douni, G. Kassiotis, and D. Kontoyiannis. 1999. On the role of tumor necrosis factor and receptors in models of multiorgan failure, rheumatoid arthritis, multiple sclerosis and inflammatory bowel disease. *Immunol Rev* 169:175–94.

Kong, T., H.K. Eltzschig, J. Karhausen, S.P. Colgan, and C.S. Shelley. 2004. Leukocyte adhesion during hypoxia is mediated by HIF-1-dependent induction of beta2 integrin gene expression. *Proc Natl Acad Sci U S A* 101:10440–5.

Korkaya, H., S. Liu, and M.S. Wicha. 2011. Regulation of cancer stem cells by cytokine networks: attacking cancer's inflammatory roots. *Clin Cancer Res* 17:6125–9.

Kuper, H., H.O. Adami, and D. Trichopoulos. 2000. Infections as a major preventable cause of human cancer. *J Intern Med* 248:171–83.

Laoui, D., K. Movahedi, E. Van Overmeire et al. 2011. Tumor-associated macrophages in breast cancer: distinct subsets, distinct functions. *Int J Dev Biol* 55:861–7.

Lee, H., A. Herrmann, J.H. Deng et al. 2009. Persistently activated Stat3 maintains constitutive NF-kappaB activity in tumors. *Cancer Cell* 15:283–93.

Lee, J., V. Taneja, and R. Vassallo. 2012. Cigarette smoking and inflammation: cellular and molecular mechanisms. *J Dent Res* 91:142–9.

Lu, H., W. Ouyang, and C. Huang. 2006. Inflammation, a key event in cancer development. *Mol Cancer Res* 4:221–33.

Lu, P., V.M. Weaver, and Z. Werb. 2012. The extracellular matrix: a dynamic niche in cancer progression. *J Cell Biol* 196:395–406.

Luster, A.D. 1998. Chemokines—chemotactic cytokines that mediate inflammation. *N Engl J Med* 338:436–45.

Makino, Y., H. Nakamura, E. Ikeda et al. 2003. Hypoxia-inducible factor regulates survival of antigen receptor-driven T cells. *J Immunol* 171:6534–40.

Mantovani, A. 2010. Molecular pathways linking inflammation and cancer. *Curr Mol Med* 10:369–73.

Mantovani, A., P. Allavena, A. Sica, and F. Balkwill. 2008. Cancer-related inflammation. *Nature* 454:436–44.

Mantovani, A., F. Bussolino, and E. Dejana. 1992. Cytokine regulation of endothelial cell function. *Faseb J* 6:2591–9.

Meeran, S.M., S. Katiyar, C.A. Elmets, and S.K. Katiyar. 2006. Silymarin inhibits UV radiation-induced immunosuppression through augmentation of interleukin-12 in mice. *Mol Cancer Ther* 5:1660–8.

Meeran, S.M., S. Katiyar, C.A. Elmets, and S.K. Katiyar. 2007. Interleukin-12 deficiency is permissive for angiogenesis in UV radiation-induced skin tumors. *Cancer Res* 67:3785–93.

Mocellin, S., E. Wang, and F.M. Marincola. 2001. Cytokines and immune response in the tumor microenvironment. *J Immunother* 24:392–407.

Mulholland, D.J., N. Kobayashi, M. Ruscetti et al. 2012. Pten loss and RAS/MAPK activation cooperate to promote EMT and metastasis initiated from prostate cancer stem/progenitor cells. *Cancer Res* 7:1878–89.

Nathan, C. 2002. Points of control in inflammation. *Nature* 420:846–52.

O'Shea, J.J., M. Gadina, and R.D. Schreiber. 2002. Cytokine signaling in 2002: new surprises in the Jak/Stat pathway. *Cell* 109 Suppl:S121–31.

Osusky, R., P. Malik, and S.J. Ryan. 1997. Retinal pigment epithelium cells promote the maturation of monocytes to macrophages in vitro. *Ophthalmic Res* 29:31–6.

Pinzon-Charry, A., T. Maxwell, and J.A. Lopez. 2005. Dendritic cell dysfunction in cancer: a mechanism for immunosuppression. *Immunol Cell Biol* 83:451–61.

Porta, C., E. Riboldi, and A. Sica. 2011a. Mechanisms linking pathogens-associated inflammation and cancer. *Cancer Lett* 305:250–62.

Porta, C., E. Riboldi, M.G. Totaro, L. Strauss, A. Sica, and A. Mantovani. 2011b. Macrophages in cancer and infectious diseases: the 'good' and the 'bad.' *Immunotherapy* 3:1185–202.

Provinciali, M., F. Papalini, F. Orlando et al. 2007. Effect of the silybin-phosphatidylcholine complex (IdB 1016) on the development of mammary tumors in HER-2/neu transgenic mice. *Cancer Res* 67:2022–9.

Raina, K., C. Agarwal, and R. Agarwal. 2013. Effect of silibinin in human colorectal cancer cells: Targeting the activation of NF-kappaB signaling. *Mol Carcinog* 52:195–206.

Raina, K., N.J. Serkova, and R. Agarwal. 2009. Silibinin feeding alters the metabolic profile in TRAMP prostatic tumors: 1H-NMRS-based metabolomics study. *Cancer Res* 69:3731–5.

Raina, K., S. Rajamanickam, R.P. Singh, G. Deep, M. Chittezhath, and R. Agarwal. 2008. Stage-specific inhibitory effects and associated mechanisms of silibinin on tumor progression and metastasis in transgenic adenocarcinoma of the mouse prostate model. *Cancer Res* 68:6822–30.

Rajamanickam, S., M. Kaur, B. Velmurugan, R.P. Singh, and R. Agarwal. 2009. Silibinin suppresses spontaneous tumorigenesis in APC min/+ mouse model by modulating beta-catenin pathway. *Pharm Res* 26:2558–67.

Rajamanickam, S., B. Velmurugan, M. Kaur, R.P. Singh, and R. Agarwal. 2010. Chemoprevention of intestinal tumorigenesis in APCmin/+ mice by silibinin. *Cancer Res* 70:2368–78.

Raman, D., P.J. Baugher, Y.M. Thu, and A. Richmond. 2007. Role of chemokines in tumor growth. *Cancer Lett* 256:137–65.

Ramasamy, K., L.D. Dwyer-Nield, N.J. Serkova et al. 2011. Silibinin prevents lung tumorigenesis in wild-type but not in iNOS–/– mice: potential of real-time micro-CT in lung cancer chemoprevention studies. *Clin Cancer Res* 17:753–61.

Rao, A., C. Luo, and P.G. Hogan. 1997. Transcription factors of the NFAT family: regulation and function. *Annu Rev Immunol* 15:707–47.

Rao, C. V. 2004. Nitric oxide signaling in colon cancer chemoprevention. *Mutat Res* 555:107–19.

Ravichandran, K., B. Velmurugan, M. Gu, R.P. Singh, and R. Agarwal. 2010. Inhibitory effect of silibinin against azoxymethane-induced colon tumorigenesis in A/J mice. *Clin Cancer Res* 16:4595–606.

Reynolds, P.R., M.G. Cosio, and J.R. Hoidal. 2006. Cigarette smoke-induced Egr-1 upregulates proinflammatory cytokines in pulmonary epithelial cells. *Am J Respir Cell Mol Biol* 35:314–9.

Rossi, D., and A. Zlotnik. 2000. The biology of chemokines and their receptors. *Annu Rev Immunol* 18:217–42.

Roy, S., G. Deep, C. Agarwal, and R. Agarwal. 2012. Silibinin prevents ultraviolet B radiation-induced epidermal damages in JB6 cells and mouse skin in a p53-GADD45alpha-dependent manner. *Carcinogenesis* 33:629–36.

Roy, S., M. Kaur, C. Agarwal, M. Tecklenburg, R.A. Sclafani, and R. Agarwal. 2007. p21 and p27 induction by silibinin is essential for its cell cycle arrest effect in prostate carcinoma cells. *Mol Cancer Ther* 6:2696–707.

Schetter, A.J., G.H. Nguyen, E.D. Bowman et al. 2009. Association of inflammation-related and microRNA gene expression with cancer-specific mortality of colon adenocarcinoma. *Clin Cancer Res* 15:5878–87.

Schoppmann, S.F., P. Birner, J. Stockl et al. 2002. Tumor-associated macrophages express lymphatic endothelial growth factors and are related to peritumoral lymphangiogenesis. *Am J Pathol* 161:947–56.

Semenza, G.L. 1999. Regulation of mammalian O2 homeostasis by hypoxia-inducible factor 1. *Annu Rev Cell Dev Biol* 15:551–78.

Sen, G.S., S. Mohanty, D.M. Hossain et al. 2011. Curcumin enhances the efficacy of chemotherapy by tailoring p65NFkappaB-p300 cross-talk in favor of p53-p300 in breast cancer. *J Biol Chem* 286:42232–47.

Shen, H.M., and V. Tergaonkar. 2009. NFkappaB signaling in carcinogenesis and as a potential molecular target for cancer therapy. *Apoptosis* 14:348–63.

Silybin-phosphatidylcholine complex. Monograph. 2009. *Altern Med Rev* 14:385–90.

Singh, R.P., S. Dhanalakshmi, S. Mohan, C. Agarwal, and R. Agarwal. 2006. Silibinin inhibits UVB- and epidermal growth factor-induced mitogenic and cell survival signaling involving activator protein-1 and nuclear factor-kappaB in mouse epidermal JB6 cells. *Mol Cancer Ther* 5:1145–53.

Singh, R.P., S. Dhanalakshmi, A.K. Tyagi, D.C. Chan, C. Agarwal, and R. Agarwal. 2002. Dietary feeding of silibinin inhibits advance human prostate carcinoma growth in athymic nude mice and increases plasma insulin-like growth factor-binding protein-3 levels. *Cancer Res* 62:3063–9.

Singh, R.P., M. Gu, and R. Agarwal. 2008. Silibinin inhibits colorectal cancer growth by inhibiting tumor cell proliferation and angiogenesis. *Cancer Res* 68:2043–50.

Singh, R.P., G.U. Mallikarjuna, G. Sharma et al. 2004. Oral silibinin inhibits lung tumor growth in athymic nude mice and forms a novel chemocombination with doxorubicin targeting nuclear factor kappaB-mediated inducible chemoresistance. *Clin Cancer Res* 10:8641–7.

Singh, R.P., K. Raina, G. Deep, D. Chan, and R. Agarwal. 2009. Silibinin suppresses growth of human prostate carcinoma PC-3 orthotopic xenograft via activation of extracellular signal-regulated kinase 1/2 and inhibition of signal transducers and activators of transcription signaling. *Clin Cancer Res* 15:613–21.

Singh, R.P., K. Raina, G. Sharma, and R. Agarwal. 2008. Silibinin inhibits established prostate tumor growth, progression, invasion, and metastasis and suppresses tumor angiogenesis and epithelial-mesenchymal transition in transgenic adenocarcinoma of the mouse prostate model mice. *Clin Cancer Res* 14:7773–80.

Smith, C.J., T.A. Perfetti, and J.A. King. 2006. Perspectives on pulmonary inflammation and lung cancer risk in cigarette smokers. *Inhal Toxicol* 18:667–77.

Smyth, M.J., E. Cretney, K. Takeda et al. 2001. Tumor necrosis factor-related apoptosis-inducing ligand (TRAIL) contributes to interferon gamma-dependent natural killer cell protection from tumor metastasis. *J Exp Med* 193:661–70.

Stadelmann, W.K., A.G. Digenis, and G.R. Tobin. 1998. Physiology and healing dynamics of chronic cutaneous wounds. *Am J Surg* 176:26S–38S.

Steele, V.E., E.T. Hawk, J.L. Viner, and R.A. Lubet. 2003. Mechanisms and applications of non-steroidal anti-inflammatory drugs in the chemoprevention of cancer. *Mutat Res* 523–524:137–44.

Takeda, K., M.J. Smyth, E. Cretney et al. 2001. Involvement of tumor necrosis factor-related apoptosis-inducing ligand in NK cell-mediated and IFN-gamma-dependent suppression of subcutaneous tumor growth. *Cell Immunol* 214:194–200.

Toxicology and carcinogenesis studies of milk thistle extract (CAS No. 84604-20-6) in F344/N rats and B6C3F1 mice (Feed Studies). 2011. *Natl Toxicol Program Tech Rep Ser* 1–177.

Tyagi, A., C. Agarwal, L.D. Dwyer-Nield, R.P. Singh, A.M. Malkinson, and R. Agarwal. 2012. Silibinin modulates TNF-alpha and IFN-gamma mediated signaling to regulate COX2 and iNOS expression in tumorigenic mouse lung epithelial LM2 cells. *Mol Carcinog* 51:832–42.

Tyagi, A., C. Agarwal, G. Harrison, L.M. Glode, and R. Agarwal. 2004. Silibinin causes cell cycle arrest and apoptosis in human bladder transitional cell carcinoma cells by regulating CDKI-CDK-cyclin cascade, and caspase 3 and PARP cleavages. *Carcinogenesis* 25:1711–20.

Tyagi, A., K. Raina, R.P. Singh et al. 2007. Chemopreventive effects of silymarin and silibinin on N-butyl-N-(4-hydroxybutyl) nitrosamine induced urinary bladder carcinogenesis in male ICR mice. *Mol Cancer Ther* 6:3248–55.

Tyagi, A., R.P. Singh, C. Agarwal, and R. Agarwal. 2006. Silibinin activates p53-caspase 2 pathway and causes caspase-mediated cleavage of Cip1/p21 in apoptosis induction in bladder transitional-cell papilloma RT4 cells: evidence for a regulatory loop between p53 and caspase 2. *Carcinogenesis* 27:2269–80.

Tyagi, A., R.P. Singh, K. Ramasamy et al. 2009. Growth inhibition and regression of lung tumors by silibinin: modulation of angiogenesis by macrophage-associated cytokines and nuclear factor-kappaB and signal transducers and activators of transcription 3. *Cancer Prev Res (Phila)* 2:74–83.

Vaid, M., S.D. Sharma, and S.K. Katiyar. 2010. Honokiol, a phytochemical from the Magnolia plant, inhibits photocarcinogenesis by targeting UVB-induced inflammatory mediators and cell cycle regulators: development of topical formulation. *Carcinogenesis* 31:2004–11.

van den Broek, M.F., D. Kagi, R.M. Zinkernagel, and H. Hengartner. 1995. Perforin dependence of natural killer cell-mediated tumor control in vivo. *Eur J Immunol* 25:3514–6.

Velmurugan, B., R.P. Singh, A. Tyagi, and R. Agarwal. 2008. Inhibition of azoxymethane-induced colonic aberrant crypt foci formation by silibinin in male Fisher 344 rats. *Cancer Prev Res (Phila)* 1:376–84.

Vidal-Vanaclocha, F., G. Fantuzzi, L. Mendoza et al. 2000. IL-18 regulates IL-1beta-dependent hepatic melanoma metastasis via vascular cell adhesion molecule-1. *Proc Natl Acad Sci U S A* 97:734–9.

Wahl, L.M., and H.K. Kleinman. 1998. Tumor-associated macrophages as targets for cancer therapy. *J Natl Cancer Inst* 90:1583–4.

Walmsley, S.R., C. Print, N. Farahi et al. 2005. Hypoxia-induced neutrophil survival is mediated by HIF-1alpha-dependent NF-kappaB activity. *J Exp Med* 201:105–15.

Walser, T., X. Cui, J. Yanagawa et al. 2008. Smoking and lung cancer: the role of inflammation. *Proc Am Thorac Soc* 5:811–5.

Wang, Y., D. Zhang, Z. Liu et al. 2010. In vitro and in vivo evaluation of silybin nanosuspensions for oral and intravenous delivery. *Nanotechnology* 21:155104.

Wen, Z., T.E. Dumas, S.J. Schrieber, R.L. Hawke, M.W. Fried, and P.C. Smith. 2008. Pharmacokinetics and metabolic profile of free, conjugated, and total silymarin flavonolignans in human plasma after oral administration of milk thistle extract. *Drug Metab Dispos* 36:65–72.

Wu, K., J. Zeng, L. Li et al. 2010. Silibinin reverses epithelial-to-mesenchymal transition in metastatic prostate cancer cells by targeting transcription factors. *Oncol Rep* 23:1545–52.

Wu, Y., J. Deng, P.G. Rychahou, S. Qiu, B.M. Evers, and B.P. Zhou. 2009. Stabilization of snail by NF-kappaB is required for inflammation-induced cell migration and invasion. *Cancer Cell* 15:416–28.

Yang, H., J. Gu, X. Lin et al. 2008. Profiling of genetic variations in inflammation pathway genes in relation to bladder cancer predisposition. *Clin Cancer Res* 14:2236–44.

Yanyu, X., S. Yunmei, C. Zhipeng, and P. Qineng. 2006. The preparation of silybin-phospholipid complex and the study on its pharmacokinetics in rats. *Int J Pharm* 307:77–82.

Yoshimura, A. 2006. Signal transduction of inflammatory cytokines and tumor development. *Cancer Sci* 97:439–47.

Zaja-Milatovic, S., and A. Richmond. 2008. CXC chemokines and their receptors: a case for a significant biological role in cutaneous wound healing. *Histol Histopathol* 23:1399–407.

Zamai, L., C. Ponti, P. Mirandola et al. 2007. NK cells and cancer. *J Immunol* 178:4011–6.

Zerbini, L.F., Y. Wang, J.Y. Cho, and T.A. Libermann. 2003. Constitutive activation of nuclear factor kappaB p50/p65 and Fra-1 and JunD is essential for deregulated interleukin 6 expression in prostate cancer. *Cancer Res* 63:2206–15.

Zhao, J., and R. Agarwal. 1999. Tissue distribution of silibinin, the major active constituent of silymarin, in mice and its association with enhancement of phase II enzymes: implications in cancer chemoprevention. *Carcinogenesis* 20:2101–8.

Zhao, J., Y. Sharma, and R. Agarwal. 1999. Significant inhibition by the flavonoid antioxidant silymarin against 12-O-tetradecanoylphorbol 13-acetate-caused modulation of antioxidant and inflammatory enzymes, and cyclooxygenase 2 and interleukin-1alpha expression in SENCAR mouse epidermis: implications in the prevention of stage I tumor promotion. *Mol Carcinog* 26:321–33.

Zhou, J., T. Schmid, and B. Brune. 2003. Tumor necrosis factor-alpha causes accumulation of a ubiquitinated form of hypoxia inducible factor-1alpha through a nuclear factor-kappaB-dependent pathway. *Mol Biol Cell* 14:2216–25.

Zlotnik, A., and O. Yoshie. 2000. Chemokines: a new classification system and their role in immunity. *Immunity* 12:121–7.

22 Cancer Prevention by Antioxidant Compounds from Berries

Noah P. Zimmerman, Dan Peiffer, and Gary D. Stoner

CONTENTS

22.1 INTRODUCTION

22.1.1 INFLAMMATION AND CANCER

Chronic inflammation is a recognized risk factor in the development of various cancers. The link between inflammation and cancer has been suggested by epidemiological and experimental data (Grivennikov et al. 2010), and confirmed by numerous reports demonstrating that inflammatory cells can promote disease by inducing cell proliferation and invasion and supporting cancer cell survival. Chronic inflammatory states are now widely accepted as an important factor that leads to an environment fostering genomic lesions, tumor initiation, and progression. For example, epidemiological studies have identified multiple risk factors for colon cancer, with chronic inflammation thought to be the leading cause (Rizzo et al. 2011). Meta-analysis has shown that patients suffering from inflammatory bowel diseases, such as Crohn's disease and ulcerative colitis, have a relative risk of developing bowel cancers of 33.2 compared to the general population (Canavan et al. 2006). These diseases affect approximately 1 to 2 of every 1000 people in developed countries and are on the rise worldwide (Molodecky et al. 2012). Links between inflammation and cancer have been confirmed in a number of animal models, particularly in the colon (Clapper et al. 2007; Harris et al. 2001), liver (Rogers and Houghton 2009), and pancreas (pancreatitis) (Satake et al. 1986). Chronic inflammation is thought to induce DNA modifications in the intestinal epithelial cells through the release of reactive oxygen species (ROS) and reactive nitrogen species (RNS) by inflammatory cells (Meira et al. 2008; Westbrook et al. 2009) and can result in chromosomal instability as well as DNA methylation (Grady and Carethers 2008).

One mechanism through which inflammation and carcinogenesis are linked is through the production of reactive oxygen and nitrogen intermediates leading to oxidative damage of DNA, proteins, and lipids. ROS and RNS can cause DNA base changes and strand breaks and induce the expression of oncogenes or damage to tumor suppressor genes (Cerutti 1994; Wiseman and Halliwell 1996). Cancer cells exist under constant oxidative stress, which induces mutations and thereby increases their survival potential (Shinkai et al. 1986). This stress may also activate redox signaling that can lead to the inactivation of tumor suppressor genes and the activation of prosurvival proteins such as nuclear factor kappaB (NF-κB) and activator protein 1 (AP-1) (Ripple et al. 1999). As low levels of ROS can induce proliferation in cancer cells (Arora-Kuruganti et al. 1999), foods high in antioxidant phytochemicals are important for the prevention of diseases related to oxidant stress, such as cancer. This chapter presents an overview of the role for a few of the major polyphenolic antioxidant compounds in berries, that is, anthocyanins, ellagic acid (EA), and flavonols, in chemoprevention. It should be noted that more research is needed to elucidate the active constituents of berries, as the ability to assess metabolic degradation, metabolite interactions, and synergistic effects of these constituents has only recently been technologically possible.

22.1.2　Oxidative Stress and Antioxidant Defenses

Oxidative stress is a result of the disparity between ROS such as hydroxyl radicals and RNS such as nitric oxide (NO) and the ability of cells to detoxify the reactive free radicals. Free radicals are highly reactive molecules and chemical species that produce oxidative damage. Oxidative stress is generated by chemical species containing unpaired electrons as a result of cell lysis, oxidative burst, or the presence of an excess of free transition metals. These species can attack proteins, DNA, and lipid membranes, thereby disrupting cellular functions and integrity, and can lead to cell death as a result of lipid peroxidation (LPO) and DNA fragmentation (Fang et al. 2009). Extensive research has revealed multiple mechanisms by which oxidative stress is involved in diseases such as diabetes, cardiovascular diseases, ulcerative colitis, and cancer (Ferguson 2010; Hofseth et al. 2003; Hussain et al. 2003; Roessner et al. 2008; Tsutsui et al. 2011).

ROS are products of normal cellular processes, such as mitochondrial respiration (Fridovich 1978; Poyton et al. 2009). During normal cellular respiration, respiratory intermediates escape the mitochondria and interact with cellular molecules. During states of inflammation, however, leukocytes and other immune cells such as macrophages release a respiratory burst, which results in activation of a membrane-bound oxidase that catalyzes the reduction of oxygen to superoxide anion. This release of reactive oxygen intermediates not only is highly reactive by itself but also generates other oxidizing agents such as hydroxyl radicals and hydrogen peroxide, which can damage neighboring cells. The oxidative reactivity of ROS and RNS species is variable. Compounds such as H_2O_2, O_2, and NO are relatively selective in the biological molecules with which they interact, while the radical OH⁻ is highly reactive with multiple biological molecules. Furthermore, free radicals demonstrate reactivity very near the sight of production, while nonradical ROS can diffuse through tissues and expand their reactivity (Boots et al. 2008).

Antioxidant defenses are integral to survival. Enzymes such as superoxide dismutase, catalase, and glutathione peroxidase are important proteins that protect from oxidative damage through catalytic breakdown of reactive molecules such as superoxide and hydrogen peroxide. Molecules such as glutathione and flavonoids are important in scavenging, absorbing, and detoxifying reactive species. In chronic inflammatory diseases and cancer, the defenses against reactive species can be weakened and oxidant stress increased. During these times, an increased external supply of antioxidants, as can be obtained through dietary constituents, can be beneficial in reestablishing oxidative balance through multiple means such as direct absorption, increasing antioxidant enzyme activity, or inhibiting enzymes that produce ROS. The remaining portion of this chapter will include a discussion of the major antioxidant compounds in berries and their known antioxidant, anti-inflammatory, and anticarcinogenic effects.

22.2 BERRIES, ANTIOXIDANTS, AND CANCER PREVENTION

Epidemiological studies indicate that persons who consume a diet rich in vegetables and fruits have a reduced risk of cancer at multiple organ sites (Chen et al. 2012; Stoner 2009; Wang et al. 2011). Because fruits and vegetables are major sources of antioxidants (and other protective substances), it is hypothesized that these antioxidants are responsible for a significant part of their cancer-preventive effects. Indeed, experimental studies with polyphenolic antioxidants such as the catechins in green tea, curcumin in turmeric, resveratrol in red wine, and quercetin in apples have demonstrated their chemopreventive effects at multiple organ sites and correlated these effects with their ability to scavenge ROS (Stoner 2009).

Berries are richly abundant in compounds with antioxidant and chemopreventive activity. These include several structural and chemical classes including flavonoids (anthocyanins, flavanols, flavonols); condensed tannins (proanthocyanidins); phenolic acids (hydroxybenzoic and hydroxycinnamic acids); hydrolyzable tannins (ellagitannins); lignans; stilbenoids; triterpenes; and sterols (Seeram 2008). The structures of these compounds and their chemistry and biological effects have been described in detail (Seeram 2008). Among the most prevalent of these compounds are the anthocyanins, ellagitannins (EA), quercetin, and kaempferol (Figure 22.1), which are responsible for much of the antioxidant activity of berries (Borges et al. 2010). This chapter will discuss the chemopreventive effects of the anthocyanins, EA, quercetin, and kaempferol in detail. In addition to these compounds, berries also contain other constituents with potential chemopreventive effects, including minerals, such as calcium and selenium; vitamins, such as A, E, C, and folic acid; and carotenoids, such as β-carotene and lutein (Stoner 2009). The cancer-preventive effects of some of these constituents are due, at least in part, to their antioxidant capacity. Approximately 35%–50% of the dry weight of berries is fiber, and the fiber fraction also exhibits chemopreventive effects (Wang and Stoner 2008). The bioactive constituents in berry fiber have not been fully identified; however, the conversion of berry fiber to short-chain fatty acids such as butyrate by the enteric microbiota may contribute to their chemopreventive effects (Flint et al. 2008).

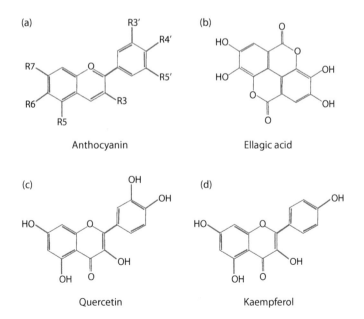

FIGURE 22.1 Chemical structures of bioactive polyphenols commonly found in berries. (a) Anthocyanin backbone. (b) EA. (c) Quercetin. (d) Kaempferol.

22.2.1 Anthocyanins

Anthocyanins occur in fruits and vegetables and, as stated above, are among the most prevalent polyphenolic compounds in berries. The daily intake of anthocyanins by US citizens is estimated to be about 200 mg or about ninefold higher than that of other dietary flavonoids (Stoner 2009). Epidemiological studies suggest that the consumption of anthocyanins lowers the risk for cardiovascular disease, diabetes, arthritis, and cancer, due, in part, to their antioxidant and anti-inflammatory activities (Seeram 2008).

The anthocyanins occur in nature as glycosides, having different sugars bound to an aglycone nucleus (Giusti et al. 1999). The chemistry and biosynthesis of the anthocyanins have been described in detail (LS Wang et al. 2012; Wang and Stoner 2008) and will be discussed only briefly here. Anthocyanins are water soluble and, depending upon pH and the presence of chelating metal ions, are intensely colored blue, purple, and red. They are responsible for the color of many foodstuffs, including multiple berry types. The stability of anthocyanins is dependent on pH, temperature, and the presence of light and oxygen (McGhie and Walton 2007). Therefore, the manner in which berries are handled postharvest can have a significant effect on their content of anthocyanins. The direct antioxidant activity of anthocyanins is a result of their phenolic structure and is due primarily to the presence of hydroxyl groups in position 3 of ring C and positions 3′, 4′, and 5′ in ring B of the molecule (Figure 22.1).

The ability of berry anthocyanins to scavenge ROS such as superoxide, peroxides, hydrogen peroxide, and hydroxyl radicals has been demonstrated in multiple cell culture systems. For example, in Caco-2 colon cancer cells, Renis et al. (2008) monitored ROS production by measuring the hydrolysis of 2′,7′-dichlorofluorescein diacetate to fluorescent 2′,7′-dichlorofluorescein in the presence of ROS. ROS production in Caco-2 cells was decreased after treatment with cyanidin-3-O-β-glucopyranoside, a common anthocyanin (Parry et al. 2006). Using a similar method, ROS production by noncancerous MCF-10F human breast cells was shown to be decreased by the anthocyanin delphinidin-3-glucoside as well as the aglycone delphinidin (Singletary et al. 2007). In rat hepatocyte clone 9 cells, several anthocyanidins and anthocyanins, including delphinidin and cyanidin-3-O-glucoside (C3G), suppressed cellular damage and oxidative stress-induced cell death (Shih et al. 2007). In a model of ultraviolet B (UVB)-mediated oxidative stress using HaCaT skin cells, the antioxidant effects of delphinidin were measured by both the Trolox assay and the LPO assay (Afaq et al. 2007). Treatment with delphinidin resulted in a protective effect from UVB-mediated apoptosis, LPO, and 8-hydroxydeoxyguanosine (8-OHdG) DNA adduct formation in HaCaT cells (Afaq et al. 2007). Beyond simple ROS scavenging activities, delphinidin also decreased levels of the proapoptotic protein Bax and increased the antiapoptotic protein B-cell lymphoma-2 (Bcl-2) (Hafeez et al. 2008).

Results from these in vitro studies provided mechanistic insights and rationale for subsequent in vivo studies in animal model systems. In a study by Cooke et al. (2006), administration of C3G in the diet of APC$^{min/+}$ mice resulted in a significant decrease in adenoma number and size, particularly interfering with the development of smaller (<1 mm) adenomas. C3G was recovered from the intestinal mucosa at submicrogram/gram tissue levels and from the urine at microgram/milliliter levels. While the authors mention they were able to recover anthocyanins from the liver and kidney, no mention is made as to the levels observed at these sites.

Stoner and coworkers conducted a series of biofractionation studies using freeze-dried black raspberries (BRBs) and demonstrated that their component anthocyanins are responsible for a significant portion of their anti-inflammatory and chemopreventive activities. The anthocyanins are the most prevalent polyphenols in BRBs, accounting for approximately 3%–5% of the dry weight of the berries. Initially, a methanol extract of BRBs was shown to inhibit benzo(a)pyrene [B(a)P]-induced transformation of Syrian hamster embryo cells in vitro (Xue et al. 2001). Subsequently, this same extract was shown to inhibit benzo(a)pyrene diol-epoxide (BPDE)-induced transactivation of AP-1 and NF-κB in cultured JB-6 mouse epidermal cells, in part by targeting the mitogen-activated protein kinase (MAPK) and phosphotidylinositol 3-kinase/Akt pathways (Hecht et al. 2006; Huang et al. 2002). These findings are potentially important in view of the roles of AP-1 and NF-κB in inflammation and carcinogenesis. Using high-performance liquid chromatography (HPLC), Hecht et al. (2006) isolated 55 fractions of the bioactive alcoholic extract of BRBs and compared each fraction in terms of its relative ability to inhibit BPDE-induced activation of AP-1 and NF-κB in JB-6 cells. The fractions with the highest inhibitory activity coincided with the three most prevalent anthocyanins in BRBs (cyanidin-3-*O*-rutinoside, cyanidin-3-*O*-xylosylrutinoside, and C3G), providing in vitro evidence of the importance of these compounds in chemoprevention. Interestingly, a pentane fraction, which did not contain anthocyanins, had no effect on cellular NF-κB or AP-1 activities. In a later report, Wang et al. (2009) compared diets containing either whole BRB powder or an anthocyanin-enriched extract of BRBs (each diet containing the same amount of anthocyanins) for their relative ability to inhibit *N*-nitrosomethylbenzylamine (NMBA)-induced tumors in the F344 rat esophagus. The anthocyanin-enriched fraction was nearly as effective as whole berries in reducing NMBA-induced esophageal tumorigenesis, providing in vivo evidence of the anticarcinogenic effects of BRB anthocyanins. In addition, both the whole berry and anthocyanin-enriched diets protectively modulated the protein expression levels of genes associated with cell proliferation (Ki-67, Erk1/2); apoptosis (Bcl-2; Bax); inflammation (cyclooxygenase 2 [COX2] and prostaglandin E2 [PGE$_2$], NF-κB, cluster determinant 45 [CD45, leukocyte common antigen]); and angiogenesis (vascular endothelial growth factor 1 [VEGF1], hypoxia-inducing factor-1 alpha [HIF-1α], and CD34) in esophageal tumors. These studies demonstrated that BRB anthocyanins influence the expression levels of genes associated with multiple cellular functions that can go awry in carcinogenesis. Figure 22.2 depicts multiple cellular functions and associated genes that are influenced by the anthocyanins in BRBs (Wang et al. 2009).

While anthocyanins exhibit great potential as cancer chemopreventive agents, it is notable that relatively low concentrations are observed in the urine and plasma after ingestion, suggesting low bioavailability. Indeed, through the use of HPLC and mass spectrometry, studies in murine models assessing the levels of anthocyanins in tissues, primarily urine and plasma, demonstrate low levels of the parent molecules as well as their conjugated metabolites (He et al. 2006; Manach et al. 2005; Talavera et al. 2004). Similarly, in healthy human subjects that were administered with freeze-dried BRB powder (45 g/day) orally in a slurry of water over a 7-day period, the levels of anthocyanins and EA in the plasma and urine after 1–4 h were found to be less than 1% of the administered dose (Stoner et al. 2005). The metabolic degradation of anthocyanins may alter their bioavailability as the type and number of glycosylations have been shown to affect the absorption of anthocyanins into plasma and urine (He et al. 2006). Deglycosylation of anthocyanins to their corresponding aglycone

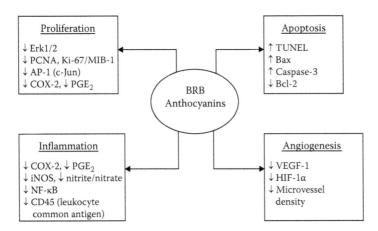

FIGURE 22.2 Scheme showing the effects of BRB anthocyanins on proliferation, apoptosis, inflammation, angiogenesis, and associated genes.

by removal of the sugar may contribute to steric hindrance and add hydroxyl groups, which could aid in cellular uptake (He et al. 2006). Deglycosylation of anthocyanins is primarily associated with the activities of two enzymes, β-glucosidase and lactase–phlorizin hydrolase (LPH), which are present in the intestinal and oral epithelium (Mallery et al. 2011). The presence of these enzymes in tissues, as well as in enteric bacteria, suggests the potential for enhancing the deglycosylation of anthocyanins and their increased bioavailability. Interestingly, a recent study in human oral tissues demonstrated the potential for processing, absorption, and release of a major metabolite of BRB anthocyanins (Mallery et al. 2011). This metabolite is protocatechuic acid (PCA), which is produced in part from the anthocyanins by oral and enteric bacteria. PCA itself has been shown to elicit anticancer effects through the induction of apoptosis by stimulation of the MAPK pathway (Yip et al. 2006). Moreover, PCA has demonstrated anti-inflammatory effects. NO production was decreased by 20% in lipopolysaccharide (LPS)-stimulated RAW 264.7 macrophages treated with PCA compared to control cells (Hidalgo et al. 2012).

The extent to which anthocyanins and anthocyanin metabolites can alter carcinogenesis is an expanding subject of research. While this review introduces the role of anthocyanins in cancer chemoprevention, more extensive discussions are provided by (LS Wang et al. 2012).

22.2.2 Ellagic Acid

EA is a polyphenol found abundantly in many plants, especially in tree bark. It is present in plants in the form of hydrolyzable tannins called ellagitannins. Ellagitannins are esters of glucose with hexahydroxydiphenic acid, and when hydrolyzed, they yield EA. EA is a very stable compound and is moderately soluble in dimethylsulfoxide, slightly soluble in other organic solvents, and relatively insoluble in water. Our laboratory and others have demonstrated its presence in a variety of berry types, including blackberries, BRBs, red raspberries, strawberries, and cranberries (Daniel and Stoner 1991; Dixit et al. 1985). It is present primarily in the seeds and pulp of the berry; there is very little in the juice. Compared to other berry types, BRBs have among the highest levels of EA, ranging from 166 to 225 mg/100 g dry weight (Mandal and Stoner 1990). In early studies, EA was shown to inhibit lung tumors in mice induced by B(a)P (Boukharta et al. 1992), BPDE (Mukhtar et al. 1984), or 4-(methylnitrosamino)-3-pyridyl-1-butanone (NNK) (Boukharta et al. 1992), and skin tumors in mice induced by 3-methylcholanthrene (MCA) (Mukhtar et al. 1984) or initiated by B(a)P or 7,12-dimethylbenz(a)anthracene (DMBA) and promoted by 12-O-tetradecanoylphorbol-13-acetate (TPA) (Chang et al. 1985). In 1990, we reported that dietary EA inhibits the formation of NMBA-induced esophageal tumors in rats (Mandal and Stoner 1990), and in 1991, it was shown to inhibit azoxymethane (AOM)-induced colon tumors in rats (Rao et al. 1991). More recently, Aiyer et al. (2008) reported the ability of dietary EA to reduce estrogen-mediated mammary tumors in ACI rats.

Several mechanisms have been described to account for the chemopreventive effects of EA. Mechanisms for its ability to inhibit tumor initiation are as follows: (1) It reduces the formation of carcinogen–DNA adducts by inhibiting the metabolic activation of carcinogens and inducing phase II enzymes involved in carcinogen detoxification. For example, in a report by Ahn et al. (1996), rats fed with EA had a decrease in P450 content in the liver by up to 25%. In contrast, in these same animals, the activities of the hepatic phase II enzymes, glutathione S-transferase (GST), nicotinamide adenine dinucleotide phosphate (NADPH):quinone reductase, and uridine diphosphate (UDP)-glucuronosyltransferase, increased 26%, 17%, and 75%, respectively, when compared to control rats. In a separate study, EA was found to detoxify carcinogens by inducing the transcription of GSTs through the antioxidant response element of the Ya gene (Barch et al. 1995). (2) It directly binds EA to the reactive metabolites of carcinogens, such as BPDE, thus inhibiting its ability to form adducts in DNA (Chang et al. 1985).

EA also affects cellular and molecular events associated with tumor promotion and progression by affecting rates of cellular proliferation and apoptosis, as well as the formation of new blood vessels (angiogenesis). In a study utilizing muscadine grape extracts, EA was shown to decrease the rate of Caco-2 intestinal cell proliferation and increase apoptosis through heightened activation of caspase-3 (Mertens-Talcott et al. 2006). EA also induced a significant decrease in the G0/G1 phase of the cell cycle, from 45% to 18%. Similar results were observed in cervical carcinoma cells (CaSki). CaSki cells treated with EA had increased DNA fragmentation indicative of apoptosis over a 24- to 72-h treatment schedule (Narayanan et al. 1999). A higher proportion of cells treated for 48 h with EA remained in G1 arrest (80%) compared to untreated cells (30%), inhibiting overall cell growth. The authors also reported an increase in the messenger RNA (mRNA) and protein levels of the cdk inhibitory protein, p21, suggesting a potential mechanism by which EA can affect cell cycle progression. A subsequent study provided further information regarding EAs ability to affect p21 using SW 480 colon cancer cells (Narayanan and Re 2001). After 48 h of treatment with micromolar concentrations of EA, insulin-like growth factor (IGF-II) was downregulated, and p21 activated. Interestingly, a low dose of EA combined with quercetin decreased proliferation and increased cytotoxicity and apoptosis in a human leukemia cell line (Narayanan and Re 2001).

EA in pomegranate juice has been shown to suppress the COX2 enzyme by 79% in human colon cancer cells (Adams et al. 2006) with a similar effect in human colonic fibroblasts (Gonzalez-Sarrias et al. 2010). The polyphenol also reduced COX2 expression in normal human monocytes without toxic effects and without affecting COX1 expression (Karlsson et al. 2010), making it a candidate for chemoprevention in normal individuals. In vivo, EA reduced COX2 expression in a rat colon carcinogenesis model (Umesalma and Sudhandiran 2010) as well as in a mouse model of Crohn's disease (Rosillo et al. 2011). These studies indicate that EA can reduce the accumulation of prostaglandins in tissues by regulating COX2, thereby positively affecting cellular events associated with prostaglandin activity including cell proliferation, inflammation, and apoptosis.

EA treatment has been shown to have an oxidant effect on a variety of cell types and organisms. One mechanism for this may be through its ability to reduce oxidative stress on cells via the regulation of inducible NO synthase (iNOS), thus reducing the presence of the oxidant NO. The activity of iNOS has shown to be regulated in mouse lymphocytes (Gerhauser et al. 2003) and human endothelial cells (Lee et al. 2010) by EA. In both studies, EA was shown to reduce iNOS expression, which correlated with reduced NO production. EA also reduced iNOS overexpression in both the rat and mouse colon in vivo. In the rat colon, EA reduced iNOS levels to that in the control group (Umesalma and Sudhandiran 2010), and similar results were observed in a mouse model of Crohn's disease, a disease associated with chronic inflammation in the colon (Rosillo et al. 2011).

EA is also capable of inhibiting VEGF-induced phosphorylation of epidermal growth factor receptor 2 (EGFR-2), leading to inhibition of the signal transduction pathway utilized in endothelial cells by these receptors (Labrecque et al. 2005). Similarly, EA inhibited VEGF2 expression in breast cancer cells, resulting in a decrease in breast cancer angiogenesis (N. Wang et al. 2012).

22.2.3 FLAVONOLS

22.2.3.1 Quercetin

Quercetin is the most abundant dietary flavonol in the plant kingdom. In BRBs, quercetin is present in concentrations between 35 and 45 mg/100 g dry weight (Yang et al. 2000) or about one-fifth the concentration of EA. The average daily intake of quercetin in the human diet is estimated to be as high as 200–500 mg/day in those who consume diets high in fruit and vegetables (Harwood et al. 2007) and between 5 and 40 mg/day in most citizens (Hertog et al. 1995). The relationship between quercetin intake and risk for cardiovascular disease and cancer has been reviewed in depth by Russo et al. (2012).

Unlike the anthocyanins and EA, pharmacokinetic studies in the rat have shown that quercetin has high bioavailability, which allows for diverse tissue distribution in the small intestine, colon, liver, and kidney. The highest concentrations were found in the lung, where levels approached 15.3 nmol/g tissue in rats consuming a diet containing 1% quercetin (de Boer et al. 2005). After absorption into tissues, quercetin is conjugated primarily to glucuronic acid as well as sulfate and methyl groups (Harwood et al. 2007) to form quercetin-3-O-glucuronide, 3'-O-methylquercetin-3-glucuronide, and quercetin-3'-O-sulfate. Metabolism of quercetin occurs not only through enzymatic activity from intestinal tissues but also through degradation by the intestinal bacteria. The primary products of quercetin degradation are hydroxyphenylacetic acids, which are excreted in urine (Aura et al. 2002).

Quercetin is among the most potent antioxidants of the polyphenols (Ratnam et al. 2006). It is an avid scavenger of H_2O_2, O_2 (Cushnie and Lamb 2005; Hanasaki et al. 1994), as well as RNS such as NO and peroxynitrite (Haenen et al. 1997; Heijnen et al. 2001). Heijnen et al. (2002) assessed the antioxidant activity of quercetin through electrochemical analysis of freshly prepared rat microsomes and found that upon methylation of the 5-OH groups, the activity was greatly reduced, suggesting that the catechol group on ring B and the OH group at position 3 of the AC ring are important for activity. The antioxidant abilities of quercetin in vivo have been determined in feeding studies. At 0.2% of the diet, quercetin inhibited LPO in rats, and the plasma had a significantly higher total antioxidant status when compared to untreated controls (Hollman et al. 1995). In another study, pretreatment of freshly isolated human leukocytes with quercetin at concentrations of 1–100 μM for 1 h protected against oxidative DNA damage induced by H_2O_2, as measured by the comet assay (Wilms et al. 2005).

Beyond direct ROS scavenging activities, quercetin affects other events that are important in carcinogenesis. Lee et al. (2008) found that quercetin inhibited mitogen activated protein kinase kinase 1 (MEK1) activity in mouse epidermal cells, thereby inhibiting TPA-induced transformation. They further showed that quercetin causes mild inhibitory effects on Raf1, resulting in a decrease in AP-1 and NF-κB signaling. An additional target in the NF-κB pathway was identified by Peet and Li (1999), who observed that quercetin was able to inhibit both IkappaB kinases (IKKα and IKKβ), consistent with its known abilities to inhibit tumor necrosis factor (TNF)-induced NF-κB activation. These results suggest that quercetin is able to interfere with the NF-κB pathway at multiple levels, thus providing a mechanistic rationale for its anti-inflammatory activities.

In animal models, quercetin has shown promise as an effective chemopreventative agent. In a recent report by Murphy et al. (2011) oral treatment of APC[min/+] mice with 0.02% quercetin for 16 weeks significantly decreased overall intestinal polyp number by 67% compared to untreated control animals. Furthermore, after 16 weeks of treatment, quercetin significantly decreased macrophage numbers in the intestinal villi of the small intestine. In the DMBA-induced hamster buccal pouch tumor model, animals treated with 25 mg/kg quercetin by gastric administration at the same time as DMBA administration over a 14-week period showed a significant decrease in development of squamous cell carcinoma compared to animals that received DMBA alone (Priyadarsini et al. 2011). In this model, quercetin increased caspase activity and decreased biomarkers of tissue invasion and angiogenesis. Quercetin at 10 mg/kg in the diet was also effective in inhibiting the growth of Walker 256 carcinoma cells in rats, decreasing tumor growth by 50% when compared to controls (Camargo et al. 2011). Furthermore, daily administration of quercetin resulted in a significant increase in survival of the rats.

Finally, through its ability to suppress heat shock protein expression, quercetin increased the cell-killing effects of hyperthermia and the chemotherapeutic agents *cis*-diaminedichloroplatinum II and etoposide for Ewing's tumor cells (Debes et al. 2003). It has also been shown to sensitize human hepatoma cells to TNF-related apoptosis-inducing ligand (TRAIL)-induced apoptosis by Sp1-mediated upregulation of the death receptor DR5 and proteasome-mediated downregulation of c-FLIP, an inhibitor of caspase-8 (Kim et al. 2008). Therefore, in addition to its role as a chemopreventive agent, quercetin may be very useful for sensitizing tumor cells to chemotherapeutic agents.

22.2.3.2 Kaempferol

Kaempferol is a natural flavonoid in many fruits and vegetables such as strawberries, broccoli, tea, and other plant sources. Kaempferol is well absorbed when administered orally. Dupont et al.

(2004) used HPLC analysis with a level of detection at 0.003 μM in plasma to determine that only about 2% of the ingested kaempferol was lost in urine over the first 24 h, while the remainder was absorbed into tissue. Kaempferol also appears to have greater stability in plasma than quercetin (DuPont et al. 2004).

Kaempferol is an effective anti-inflammatory, antioxidant, and chemopreventive agent. With respect to its effects on inflammation, in a dextran sodium sulfate (DSS)-induced model of colitis in mice, kaempferol significantly decreased the disease activity index (DAI) and levels of NO and PGE_2 (Park et al. 2012). In a study of oxidant-induced colorectal carcinoma in rats, 1,2-dimethyl-hydrazine, a strong oxidant and carcinogen, was used to induce damage to DNA, protein, and lipid membranes. Treatment with 200 mg/kg kaempferol in the diet for 16 weeks restored the activities of the antioxidants glutathione and glutathione peroxidase in the liver and colon of animals. The levels of LPO, assessed by erythrocyte lysis and thiobarbituric acid, were reduced in animals fed with kaempferol and appeared to be dose dependent (Nirmala and Ramanathan 2011).

Kaempferol exerts cytotoxic effects in multiple cancer cell types primarily through the induction of apoptosis. In a report using SW 480 colon cancer cells, Yoshida et al. (2008) demonstrated that kaempferol sensitized the cells to TRAIL-induced apoptosis. Cells treated with 10–40 μM kaempferol showed little induction of apoptosis compared to untreated control cells; however, the addition of TRAIL to cells treated with kaempferol led to a significant increase in apoptosis. This increase in apoptosis was likely due to the increase in DR4 and DR5 TRAIL receptor expression, induced by kaempferol treatment (Yoshida et al. 2008). Kaempferol was also shown to enhance the cell-killing effects of cisplatin on ovarian cancer cells by promoting apoptosis caused by downregulation of c-Myc (Luo et al. 2011). In two reports, kaempferol induced apoptosis in colon and lung cancer cells through the intrinsic pathway, as shown by its ability to induce poly(ADP-ribose) polymerase (PARP) cleavage and caspase-3 activation (Li et al. 2009; Nguyen et al. 2003). Therefore, like quercetin, kaempferol appears to be a promising sensitizing agent in the treatment of tumor cells with therapeutic drugs.

22.3 CONCLUSION AND PERSPECTIVES

Berries represent a mixture of bioactive compounds that undoubtedly work in synergy to produce antioxidant, antiproliferative, anti-inflammatory, and proapoptotic effects. Among the most active compounds in berries are the anthocyanins, ellagitannins (EA), quercetin, and kaempferol, all phenolic antioxidants. Probably the most active of these are the anthocyanins because of their relative abundance in berries and the fact that their anticancer activity in at least one animal model of esophagus cancer was nearly equal to that of whole berries. The fact that PCA is the major metabolite of the anthocyanins in some berry types, and that PCA itself is an effective chemopreventive agent, suggests that additional studies on the chemopreventive effects of PCA are warranted. At least two advantages of using PCA for chemoprevention rather than the anthocyanins are its ease of synthesis and relatively low cost. EA was the subject of intense study in the 1980s, having been shown to exhibit chemopreventive activity against carcinogen-induced cancer in the rodent skin, lung, esophagus, colon, and liver. However, interest in EA as a chemopreventive agent was reduced over time by its low solubility and minimal bioavailability. In view of the fact that other phenolic compounds with minimal bioavailability (e.g., curcumin and the green tea polyphenols) have been the subject of intense research in chemoprevention, it is possible that research with EA was abandoned too quickly. In that regard, the recent report of its ability to inhibit estrogen-induced breast cancer in rats (Aiyer et al. 2008) is intriguing and worthy of follow-up. Quercetin and kaempferol may well be worthy of additional studies as well, both for chemoprevention and as agents that sensitize tumor cells to chemotherapeutic drugs.

Studies in multiple laboratories suggest that the antioxidant effects of berry components may be responsible for a significant portion of their biological activities; however, this has not been confirmed. It may well be that the direct effects of berry compounds, including those discussed in this chapter, on gene expression at the level of gene transcription and translation may be equally or more important than their ability to scavenge ROS. Similarly, their effects on enzyme activity, such as on the dimethyltransferases involved in DNA methylation, may be of importance. It is clear that additional studies at the molecular level are required to further determine the mechanisms of action of berry bioactives.

ACKNOWLEDGMENTS

The authors' work cited in this review was funded, in part, by National Cancer Institute grant NCI R01 CA103180. We also thank Advancing a Healthier Wisconsin for their generous support of our research.

REFERENCES

Adams LS, Seeram NP, Aggarwal BB, Takada Y, Sand D, and Heber D. 2006. Pomegranate juice, total pomegranate ellagitannins, and punicalagin suppress inflammatory cell signaling in colon cancer cells. *J. Agric. Food Chem.* 54 (3): 980–985.

Afaq F, Syed DN, Malik A et al. 2007. Delphinidin, an anthocyanidin in pigmented fruits and vegetables, protects human HaCaT keratinocytes and mouse skin against UVB-mediated oxidative stress and apoptosis. *J. Invest. Dermatol.* 127 (1): 222–232.

Ahn D, Putt D, Kresty L, Stoner GD, Fromm D, and Hollenberg PF. 1996. The effects of dietary ellagic acid on rat hepatic and esophageal mucosal cytochromes P450 and phase II enzymes. *Carcinogenesis* 17 (4): 821–828.

Aiyer HS, Srinivasan C, and Gupta RC. 2008. Dietary berries and ellagic acid diminish estrogen-mediated mammary tumorigenesis in ACI rats. *Nutr. Cancer* 60 (2): 227–234.

Arora-Kuruganti P, Lucchesi PA, and Wurster RD. 1999. Proliferation of cultured human astrocytoma cells in response to an oxidant and antioxidant. *J. Neurooncol.* 44 (3): 213–221.

Aura AM, O'Leary KA, Williamson G et al. 2002. Quercetin derivatives are deconjugated and converted to hydroxyphenylacetic acids but not methylated by human fecal flora in vitro. *J. Agric. Food Chem.* 50 (6): 1725–1730.

Barch DH, Rundhaugen LM, and Pillay NS. 1995. Ellagic acid induces transcription of the rat glutathione S-transferase-Ya gene. *Carcinogenesis* 16 (3): 665–668.

Boots AW, Haenen GR, and Bast A. 2008. Health effects of quercetin: from antioxidant to nutraceutical. *Eur. J. Pharmacol.* 585 (2–3): 325–337.

Borges G, Degeneve A, Mullen W, and Crozier A. 2010. Identification of flavonoid and phenolic antioxidants in black currants, blueberries, raspberries, red currants, and cranberries. *J. Agric. Food Chem.* 58 (7): 3901–3909.

Boukharta M, Jalbert G, and Castonguay A. 1992. Biodistribution of ellagic acid and dose-related inhibition of lung tumorigenesis in A/J mice. *Nutr. Cancer* 18 (2): 181–189.

Camargo CA, da Silva ME, da Silva RA, Justo GZ, Gomes-Marcondes MC, and Aoyama H. 2011. Inhibition of tumor growth by quercetin with increase of survival and prevention of cachexia in Walker 256 tumor-bearing rats. *Biochem. Biophys. Res. Commun.* 406 (4): 638–642.

Canavan C, Abrams KR, and Mayberry J. 2006. Meta-analysis: colorectal and small bowel cancer risk in patients with Crohn's disease. *Aliment. Pharmacol. Ther.* 23 (8): 1097–1104.

Cerutti PA. 1994. Oxy-radicals and cancer. *Lancet* 344 (8926): 862–863.

Chang RL, Huang MT, Wood AW et al. 1985. Effect of ellagic acid and hydroxylated flavonoids on the tumorigenicity of benzo[a]pyrene and (+/-)-7 beta, 8 alpha-dihydroxy-9 alpha, 10 alpha-epoxy-7,8,9,10-tetrahydrobenzo[a]pyrene on mouse skin and in the newborn mouse. *Carcinogenesis* 6 (8): 1127–1133.

Chen T, Yan F, Qian J et al. 2012. Randomized phase II trial of lyophilized strawberries in patients with dysplastic precancerous lesions of the esophagus. *Cancer Prev. Res. (Phila)* 5 (1): 41–50.

Clapper ML, Cooper HS, and Chang WC. 2007. Dextran sulfate sodium-induced colitis-associated neoplasia: a promising model for the development of chemopreventive interventions. *Acta Pharmacol. Sin.* 28 (9): 1450–1459.

Cooke D, Schwarz M, Boocock D et al. 2006. Effect of cyanidin-3-glucoside and an anthocyanin mixture from bilberry on adenoma development in the ApcMin mouse model of intestinal carcinogenesis—relationship with tissue anthocyanin levels. *Int. J. Cancer* 119 (9): 2213–2220.

Cushnie TP, and Lamb AJ. 2005. Antimicrobial activity of flavonoids. *Int. J. Antimicrob. Agents* 26 (5): 343–356.

Daniel EM, and Stoner GD. 1991. The effects of ellagic acid and 13-cis-retinoic acid on N-nitrosobenzyl-methylamine-induced esophageal tumorigenesis in rats. *Cancer Lett.* 56 (2): 117–124.

de Boer VC, Dihal AA, van der Woude H et al. 2005. Tissue distribution of quercetin in rats and pigs. *J. Nutr.* 135 (7): 1718–1725.

Debes A, Oerding M, Willers R, Gobel U, and Wessalowski R. 2003. Sensitization of human Ewing's tumor cells to chemotherapy and heat treatment by the bioflavonoid quercetin. *Anticancer Res.* 23 (4): 3359–3366.

Dixit R, Teel RW, Daniel FB, and Stoner GD. 1985. Inhibition of benzo(a)pyrene and benzo(a)pyrene-trans-7,8-diol metabolism and DNA binding in mouse lung explants by ellagic acid. *Cancer Res.* 45 (7): 2951–2956.

DuPont MS, Day AJ, Bennett RN, Mellon FA, and Kroon PA. 2004. Absorption of kaempferol from endive, a source of kaempferol-3-glucuronide, in humans. *Eur. J. Clin. Nutr.* 58 (6): 947–954.

Fang J, Seki T, and Maeda H. 2009. Therapeutic strategies by modulating oxygen stress in cancer and inflammation. *Adv. Drug Deliv. Rev.* 61 (4): 290–302.

Ferguson LR. 2010. Chronic inflammation and mutagenesis. *Mutat. Res.* 690 (1–2): 3–11.

Flint HJ, Bayer EA, Rincon MT, Lamed R, and White BA. 2008. Polysaccharide utilization by gut bacteria: potential for new insights from genomic analysis. *Nat. Rev. Microbiol.* 6 (2): 121–131.

Fridovich I. 1978. The biology of oxygen radicals. *Science (New York, N. Y.)* 201 (4359): 875–880.

Gerhauser C, Klimo K, Heiss E et al. 2003. Mechanism-based in vitro screening of potential cancer chemopreventive agents. *Mutat. Res.* 523–524: 163–172.

Giusti MM, Rodriguez-Saona LE, and Wrolstad RE. 1999. Molar absorptivity and color characteristics of acylated and non-acylated pelargonidin-based anthocyanins. *J. Agric. Food Chem.* 47 (11): 4631–4637.

Gonzalez-Sarrias A, Larrosa M, Tomas-Barberan FA, Dolara P, and Espin JC. 2010. NF-kappaB-dependent anti-inflammatory activity of urolithins, gut microbiota ellagic acid-derived metabolites, in human colonic fibroblasts. *Br. J. Nutr.* 104 (4): 503–512.

Grady WM, and Carethers JM. 2008. Genomic and epigenetic instability in colorectal cancer pathogenesis. *Gastroenterology* 135 (4): 1079–1099.

Grivennikov SI, Greten FR, and Karin M. 2010. Immunity, inflammation, and cancer. *Cell* 140 (6): 883–899.

Haenen GR, Paquay JB, Korthouwer RE, and Bast A. 1997. Peroxynitrite scavenging by flavonoids. *Biochem. Biophys. Res. Commun.* 236 (3): 591–593.

Hafeez BB, Siddiqui IA, Asim M et al. 2008. A dietary anthocyanidin delphinidin induces apoptosis of human prostate cancer PC3 cells in vitro and in vivo: involvement of nuclear factor-kappaB signaling. *Cancer Res.* 68 (20): 8564–8572.

Hanasaki Y, Ogawa S, and Fukui S. 1994. The correlation between active oxygens scavenging and antioxidative effects of flavonoids. *Free Radic. Biol. Med.* 16 (6): 845–850.

Harris GK, Gupta A, Nines RG et al. 2001. Effects of lyophilized black raspberries on azoxymethane-induced colon cancer and 8-hydroxy-2′-deoxyguanosine levels in the Fischer 344 rat. *Nutr. Cancer* 40 (2): 125–133.

Harwood M, Danielewska-Nikiel B, Borzelleca JF, Flamm GW, Williams GM, and Lines TC. 2007. A critical review of the data related to the safety of quercetin and lack of evidence of in vivo toxicity, including lack of genotoxic/carcinogenic properties. *Food Chem. Toxicol.* 45 (11): 2179–2205.

He J, Magnuson BA, Lala G, Tian Q, Schwartz SJ, and Giusti MM. 2006. Intact anthocyanins and metabolites in rat urine and plasma after 3 months of anthocyanin supplementation. *Nutr. Cancer* 54 (1): 3–12.

Hecht SS, Huang C, Stoner GD et al. 2006. Identification of cyanidin glycosides as constituents of freeze-dried black raspberries which inhibit anti-benzo[a]pyrene-7,8-diol-9,10-epoxide induced NFkappaB and AP-1 activity. *Carcinogenesis* 27 (8): 1617–1626.

Heijnen CG, Haenen GR, Oostveen RM, Stalpers EM, and Bast A. 2002. Protection of flavonoids against lipid peroxidation: the structure activity relationship revisited. *Free Radic. Res.* 36 (5): 575–581.

Heijnen CG, Haenen GR, van Acker FA, van der Vijgh WJ, and Bast A. 2001. Flavonoids as peroxynitrite scavengers: the role of the hydroxyl groups. *Toxicol. in Vitro* 15 (1): 3–6.

Hertog MG, Kromhout D, Aravanis C et al. 1995. Flavonoid intake and long-term risk of coronary heart disease and cancer in the seven countries study. *Arch. Intern. Med.* 155 (4): 381–386.

Hidalgo M, Martin-Santamaria S, Recio I et al. 2012. Potential anti-inflammatory, anti-adhesive, anti/estrogenic, and angiotensin-converting enzyme inhibitory activities of anthocyanins and their gut metabolites. *Genes Nutr.* 7 (2): 295–306.

Hofseth LJ, Hussain SP, Wogan GN, and Harris CC. 2003. Nitric oxide in cancer and chemoprevention. *Free Radic. Biol. Med.* 34 (8): 955–968.

Hollman PC, de Vries JH, van Leeuwen SD, Mengelers MJ, and Katan MB. 1995. Absorption of dietary quercetin glycosides and quercetin in healthy ileostomy volunteers. *Am. J. Clin. Nutr.* 62 (6): 1276–1282.

Huang C, Huang Y, Li J, Hu W et al. 2002. Inhibition of benzo(a)pyrene diol-epoxide-induced transactivation of activated protein 1 and nuclear factor kappaB by black raspberry extracts. *Cancer Res.* 62 (23): 6857–6863.

Hussain SP, Hofseth LJ, and Harris CC. 2003. Radical causes of cancer. *Nat. Rev. Cancer* 3 (4): 276–285.

Karlsson S, Nanberg E, Fjaeraa C, and Wijkander J. 2010. Ellagic acid inhibits lipopolysaccharide-induced expression of enzymes involved in the synthesis of prostaglandin E2 in human monocytes. *Br. J. Nutr.* 103 (8): 1102–1109.

Kim JY, Kim EH, Park SS, Lim JH, Kwon TK, and Choi KS. 2008. Quercetin sensitizes human hepatoma cells to TRAIL-induced apoptosis via Sp1-mediated DR5 up-regulation and proteasome-mediated c-FLIPS down-regulation. *J. Cell Biochem.* 105 (6): 1386–1398.

Labrecque L, Lamy S, Chapus A et al. 2005. Combined inhibition of PDGF and VEGF receptors by ellagic acid, a dietary-derived phenolic compound. *Carcinogenesis* 26 (4): 821–826.

Lee KW, Kang NJ, Heo YS et al. 2008. Raf and MEK protein kinases are direct molecular targets for the chemopreventive effect of quercetin, a major flavonol in red wine. *Cancer Res.* 68 (3): 946–955.

Lee WJ, Ou HC, Hsu WC et al. 2010. Ellagic acid inhibits oxidized LDL-mediated LOX-1 expression, ROS generation, and inflammation in human endothelial cells. *J. Vasc. Surg.* 52 (5): 1290–1300.

Li W, Du B, Wang T, Wang S, and Zhang J. 2009. Kaempferol induces apoptosis in human HCT116 colon cancer cells via the ataxia-telangiectasia mutated-p53 pathway with the involvement of p53 upregulated modulator of apoptosis. *Chem. Biol. Interact.* 177 (2): 121–127.

Luo H, Rankin GO, Li Z, Depriest L, and Chen YC. 2011. Kaempferol induces apoptosis in ovarian cancer cells through activating p53 in the intrinsic pathway. *Food Chem.* 128 (2): 513–519.

Mallery SR, Budendorf DE, Larsen MP et al. 2011. Effects of human oral mucosal tissue, saliva, and oral microflora on intraoral metabolism and bioactivation of black raspberry anthocyanins. *Cancer Prev. Res. (Phila)* 4 (8): 1209–1221.

Manach C, Williamson G, Morand C, Scalbert A, and Remesy C. 2005. Bioavailability and bioefficacy of polyphenols in humans. I. Review of 97 bioavailability studies. *Am. J. Clin. Nutr.* 81 (1 Suppl): 230S–242S.

Mandal S, and Stoner GD. 1990. Inhibition of N-nitrosobenzylmethylamine-induced esophageal tumorigenesis in rats by ellagic acid. *Carcinogenesis* 11 (1): 55–61.

McGhie TK, and Walton MC. 2007. The bioavailability and absorption of anthocyanins: towards a better understanding. *Mol. Nutr. Food Res.* 51 (6): 702–713.

Meira LB, Bugni JM, Green SL et al. 2008. DNA damage induced by chronic inflammation contributes to colon carcinogenesis in mice. *J. Clin. Invest* 118 (7): 2516–2525.

Mertens-Talcott SU, Lee JH, Percival SS, and Talcott ST. 2006. Induction of cell death in Caco-2 human colon carcinoma cells by ellagic acid rich fractions from muscadine grapes (Vitis rotundifolia). *J. Agric. Food Chem.* 54 (15): 5336–5343.

Molodecky NA, Soon IS, Rabi DM et al. 2012. Increasing incidence and prevalence of the inflammatory bowel diseases with time, based on systematic review. *Gastroenterology* 142 (1): 46–54.

Mukhtar H, Das M, Del Tito BJJ, and Bickers DR. 1984. Protection against 3-methylcholanthrene-induced skin tumorigenesis in Balb/C mice by ellagic acid. *Biochem. Biophys. Res. Commun.* 119 (2): 751–757.

Murphy EA, Davis JM, McClellan JL, and Carmichael MD. 2011. Quercetin's effects on intestinal polyp multiplicity and macrophage number in the Apc(Min/+) mouse. *Nutr. Cancer* 63 (3): 421–426.

Narayanan BA, Geoffroy O, Willingham MC, Re GG, and Nixon DW. 1999. p53/p21(WAF1/CIP1) expression and its possible role in G1 arrest and apoptosis in ellagic acid treated cancer cells. *Cancer Lett.* 136 (2): 215–221.

Narayanan BA, and Re GG. 2001. IGF-II down regulation associated cell cycle arrest in colon cancer cells exposed to phenolic antioxidant ellagic acid. *Anticancer Res.* 21 (1A): 359–364.

Nguyen TT, Tran E, Ong CK et al. 2003. Kaempferol-induced growth inhibition and apoptosis in A549 lung cancer cells is mediated by activation of MEK-MAPK. *J. Cell Physiol* 197 (1): 110–121.

Nirmala P, and Ramanathan M. 2011. Effect of kaempferol on lipid peroxidation and antioxidant status in 1,2-dimethyl hydrazine induced colorectal carcinoma in rats. *Eur. J. Pharmacol.* 654 (1): 75–79.

Park MY, Ji GE, and Sung MK. 2012. Dietary kaempferol suppresses inflammation of dextran sulfate sodium-induced colitis in mice. *Dig. Dis. Sci.* 57 (2): 355–363.

Parry J, Su L, Moore J et al. 2006. Chemical compositions, antioxidant capacities, and antiproliferative activities of selected fruit seed flours. *J. Agric. Food Chem.* 54 (11): 3773–3778.

Peet GW, and Li J. 1999. IkappaB kinases alpha and beta show a random sequential kinetic mechanism and are inhibited by staurosporine and quercetin. *J. Biol. Chem.* 274 (46): 32655–32661.

Poyton RO, Ball KA, and Castello PR. 2009. Mitochondrial generation of free radicals and hypoxic signaling. *Trends Endocrinol. Metab* 20 (7): 332–340.

Priyadarsini RV, Vinothini G, Murugan RS, Manikandan P, and Nagini S. 2011. The flavonoid quercetin modulates the hallmark capabilities of hamster buccal pouch tumors. *Nutr. Cancer* 63 (2): 218–226.

Rao CV, Tokumo K, Rigotty J, Zang E, Kelloff G, and Reddy BS. 1991. Chemoprevention of colon carcinogenesis by dietary administration of piroxicam, alpha-difluoromethylornithine, 16 alpha-fluoro-5-androsten-17-one, and ellagic acid individually and in combination. *Cancer Res.* 51 (17): 4528–4534.

Ratnam DV, Ankola DD, Bhardwaj V, Sahana DK, and Kumar MN. 2006. Role of antioxidants in prophylaxis and therapy: A pharmaceutical perspective. *J. Control Release* 113 (3): 189–207.

Renis M, Calandra L, Scifo C et al. 2008. Response of cell cycle/stress-related protein expression and DNA damage upon treatment of CaCo2 cells with anthocyanins. *Br. J. Nutr.* 100 (1): 27–35.

Ripple MO, Henry WF, Schwarze SR, Wilding G, and Weindruch R. 1999. Effect of antioxidants on androgen-induced AP-1 and NF-kappaB DNA-binding activity in prostate carcinoma cells. *J. Natl. Cancer Inst.* 91 (14): 1227–1232.

Rizzo A, Pallone F, Monteleone G, and Fantini MC. 2011. Intestinal inflammation and colorectal cancer: a double-edged sword? *World J. Gastroenterol.* 17 (26): 3092–3100.

Roessner A, Kuester D, Malfertheiner P, and Schneider-Stock R. 2008. Oxidative stress in ulcerative colitis-associated carcinogenesis. *Pathol. Res. Pract.* 204 (7): 511–524.

Rogers AB, and Houghton J. 2009. Helicobacter-based mouse models of digestive system carcinogenesis. *Methods Mol. Biol.* 511: 267–295.

Rosillo MA, Sanchez-Hidalgo M, Cardeno A, and de la Lastra CA. 2011. Protective effect of ellagic acid, a natural polyphenolic compound, in a murine model of Crohn's disease. *Biochem. Pharmacol.* 82 (7): 737–745.

Russo M, Spagnuolo C, Tedesco I, Bilotto S, and Russo GL. 2012. The flavonoid quercetin in disease prevention and therapy: facts and fancies. *Biochem. Pharmacol.* 83 (1): 6–15.

Satake K, Mukai R, Kato Y, and Umeyama K. 1986. Effects of cerulein on the normal pancreas and on experimental pancreatic carcinoma in the Syrian golden hamster. *Pancreas* 1 (3): 246–253.

Seeram NP. 2008. Berry fruits for cancer prevention: current status and future prospects. *J. Agric. Food Chem.* 56 (3): 630–635.

Shih PH, Yeh CT, and Yen GC. 2007. Anthocyanins induce the activation of phase II enzymes through the antioxidant response element pathway against oxidative stress-induced apoptosis. *J. Agric. Food Chem.* 55 (23): 9427–9435.

Shinkai K, Mukai M, and Akedo H. 1986. Superoxide radical potentiates invasive capacity of rat ascites hepatoma cells in vitro. *Cancer Lett.* 32 (1): 7–13.

Singletary KW, Jung KJ, and Giusti M. 2007. Anthocyanin-rich grape extract blocks breast cell DNA damage. *J. Med. Food* 10 (2): 244–251.

Stoner GD. 2009. Foodstuffs for preventing cancer: the preclinical and clinical development of berries. *Cancer Prev. Res. (Phila)* 2 (3): 187–194.

Stoner GD, Sardo C, Apseloff G et al. 2005. Pharmacokinetics of anthocyanins and ellagic acid in healthy volunteers fed freeze-dried black raspberries daily for 7 days. *J. Clin. Pharmacol.* 45 (10): 1153–1164.

Talavera S, Felgines C, Texier O et al. 2004. Anthocyanins are efficiently absorbed from the small intestine in rats. *J. Nutr.* 134 (9): 2275–2279.

Tsutsui H, Kinugawa S, and Matsushima S. 2011. Oxidative stress and heart failure. *Am. J. Physiol Heart Circ. Physiol* 301 (6): H2181–H2190.

Umesalma S, and Sudhandiran G. 2010. Differential inhibitory effects of the polyphenol ellagic acid on inflammatory mediators NF-kappaB, iNOS, COX-2, TNF-alpha, and IL-6 in 1,2-dimethylhydrazine-induced rat colon carcinogenesis. *Basic Clin. Pharmacol. Toxicol.* 107 (2): 650–655.

Wang LS, Arnold M, Huang YW et al. 2011. Modulation of genetic and epigenetic biomarkers of colorectal cancer in humans by black raspberries: a phase I pilot study. *Clin. Cancer Res.* 17 (3): 598–610.

Wang LS, Carmella S, Keyes R et al. 2012. Anthocyanins and Cancer Prevention. In *Nutraceuticals and Cancer*, ed. Fazlul H. Sarkar, 201–229. Springer, New York.

Wang LS, Hecht SS, Carmella SG et al. 2009. Anthocyanins in black raspberries prevent esophageal tumors in rats. *Cancer Prev. Res. (Phila)* 2 (1): 84–93.

Wang LS, and Stoner GD. 2008. Anthocyanins and their role in cancer prevention. *Cancer Lett.* 269 (2): 281–290.

Wang N, Wang ZY, Mo SL et al. 2012. Ellagic acid, a phenolic compound, exerts anti-angiogenesis effects via VEGFR-2 signaling pathway in breast cancer. *Breast Cancer Res. Treat* 134 (3): 943–55.

Westbrook AM, Wei B, Braun J, and Schiestl RH. 2009. Intestinal mucosal inflammation leads to systemic genotoxicity in mice. *Cancer Res.* 69 (11): 4827–4834.

Wilms LC, Hollman PC, Boots AW, and Kleinjans JC. 2005. Protection by quercetin and quercetin-rich fruit juice against induction of oxidative DNA damage and formation of BPDE-DNA adducts in human lymphocytes. *Mutat. Res.* 582 (1-2): 155–162.

Wiseman H, and Halliwell B. 1996. Damage to DNA by reactive oxygen and nitrogen species: role in inflammatory disease and progression to cancer. *Biochem. J.* 313 (Pt 1): 17–29.

Xue H, Aziz RM, Sun N et al. 2001. Inhibition of cellular transformation by berry extracts. *Carcinogenesis* 22 (2): 351–356.

Yang K, Lamprecht SA, Liu Y et al. 2000. Chemoprevention studies of the flavonoids quercetin and rutin in normal and azoxymethane-treated mouse colon. *Carcinogenesis* 21 (9): 1655–1660.

Yip EC, Chan AS, Pang H, Tam YK, and Wong YH. 2006. Protocatechuic acid induces cell death in HepG2 hepatocellular carcinoma cells through a c-Jun N-terminal kinase-dependent mechanism. *Cell Biol. Toxicol.* 22 (4): 293–302.

Yoshida T, Konishi M, Horinaka M et al. 2008. Kaempferol sensitizes colon cancer cells to TRAIL-induced apoptosis. *Biochem. Biophys. Res. Commun.* 375 (1): 129–133.

Section VII

Garlic Organosulfur Compounds and Crucifer Glucusinolates

23 Garlic and Cancer Prevention

Chi Chen

CONTENTS

23.1 INTRODUCTION

Garlic (*Allium sativum*) belongs to the genus *allium*, which includes over 800 bulbous plant species such as leek, shallot, chive, scallion, and onions (Li, Zhou et al. 2010). Besides being consumed as an important flavoring component in the human diet, garlic has been extensively used as a medicine for many centuries, and its positive effects on human health have been observed throughout this long-term usage (Dausch and Nixon 1990). In fact, garlic preparations are the most widely used dietary supplements in US households (Timbo, Ross et al. 2006). Many claims on the health-promoting effects of garlic in traditions and cultures have been confirmed by clinical and preclinical research in the past decades, while controversies or disapproval also occurred to some folklore beliefs on garlic (Butt, Sultan et al. 2009). The biological responses associated with garlic and its preparations are very diverse, including alteration of lipid metabolism, modulation of the immune system, induction of the detoxifying and antioxidant system, regulation of signal transduction pathways, and selective cytotoxicity. Observations of these health-related bioactivities imply the value of garlic in antimicrobial treatment and the prevention of cardiovascular diseases and cancers.

23.2 CHEMISTRY OF BIOACTIVE GARLIC COMPOUNDS

The distinctive and complex chemistry of garlic is the foundation of its dietary and biomedical applications (Block 1985). For garlic itself, the existence of diverse chemical species in garlic cloves mainly serves the purposes of nutrient deposit and defense against microbes and pests (Amagase, Petesch et al. 2001). During the preparation of garlic products and/or through the interaction with the biological system after garlic consumption, this diversity in chemistry is further expanded through both enzymatic and nonenzymatic reactions on garlic compounds. Structurally, chemical components of garlic can be simply classified as either sulfur-containing compounds or non–sulfur-containing compounds. Sulfur-containing compounds are the most important bioactive components in garlic, including over 30 different organosulfur compounds (OSCs), while non–sulfur-containing compounds include nutrients (fructans, free amino acids, and fibers) and bioactive phytochemicals (saponins and phytoalexins).

23.2.1 Organosulfur Compounds

As a multivalent element, sulfur in nature exists in various forms, ranging from electron-rich status (–2 valence) to electron-deficient status (+6 valence). One prominent feature of garlic is that OSCs in garlic not only exist in high abundance but also mainly contain sulfur in the reduced status. This distinctive character of garlic OSCs has a major influence on the reactivity and bioactivity of garlic and its preparations, such as antioxidant activity and the interaction with signaling pathways. The primary sulfur-containing constituents in intact garlic cloves are γ-glutamylcysteine and its derivatives (Lancaster and Shaw 1989). Through the reactions mediated by γ-glutamyltranspeptidase and other enzymes, alliin is formed as the main precursor of many OSCs in stored garlic cloves. The fates of γ-glutamylcysteine and alliin are largely determined by the processing and extraction procedures, especially by the catalysis of alliinase. In the intact garlic clove, alliinase and its substrate (alliin) are located in two separate subcellular spaces, that is, the vacuole and cytosol, respectively. When crushing and cutting of a garlic clove ruptures the vacuole, alliinase is released to catalyze the formation of allicin, an essential intermediate for forming many OSCs in subsequent extraction processes (Figure 23.1). Garlic oil, prepared by steam distillation, contains a variety of volatile sulfides with a strong garlic smell, such as diallyl sulfide (DAS), diallyl disulfide (DADS), and diallyl

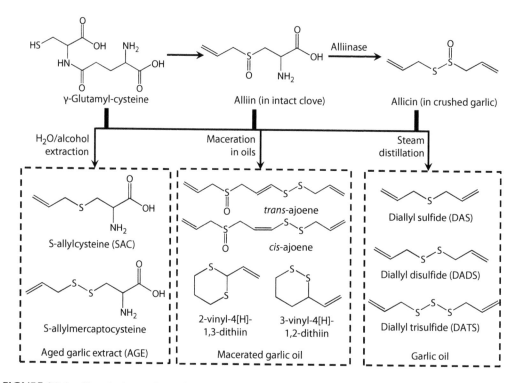

FIGURE 23.1 Chemical transformation of bioactive garlic compounds. Unprocessed garlic cloves contain abundant γ-glutamylcysteines, while chopping and crushing produce allicin through alliinase-mediated reactions. Extraction processes, including long-term water extraction, maceration in oil, and steam distillation, further affect the chemical components of commonly consumed garlic preparations.

trisulfide (DATS), while the decomposed products of allicin, such as ajoenes and dithiins, are the major OSCs in the oil macerate of garlic. Compared to these oil preparations of garlic, aged garlic extract (AGE), which is prepared by soaking garlic in aqueous media (water or diluted alcohol), contains mainly water-soluble OSCs, including S-allylcysteine (SAC) and S-allylmercaptocysteine (SAMC) (Figure 23.1). As sulfur atom and functional groups in OSCs largely determine the bioactivities of these molecules, garlic preparations containing different composition of OSCs show different effects in disease prevention and cytotoxicity.

23.2.2 Non–Sulfur-Containing Compounds

Even though the most prominent bioactive components in garlic are OSCs, a considerable amount of non–sulfur-containing nutrients and phytochemicals also exists in garlic, including saccharides (fructan and pectin); lipids (fatty acids, glycolipids, phospholipids, and prostaglandins); amino acids; vitamins; flavonoids; phenolics; and anthocyanins (Fenwick and Hanley 1985; Ryu, Ide et al. 2001). Among them, several phytoalexins and saponins have shown distinctive activities against microbes, oxidative stress, and carcinogenesis (Matsuura 2001; Kodera, Ichikawa et al. 2002).

23.2.3 In Vivo Metabolism of Garlic Compounds

The chemical complexity of bioactive garlic compounds is further increased after intake since the majority of them go through extensive biotransformation inside the body. For example, allicin and its derivatives (diallyl sulfides, ajoenes, and vinyldithiins) are not detectable in human blood, urine, or stool after consuming a significant amount of fresh garlic or pure allicin (Lawson, Ransom et al. 1992; Lawson, Bauer et al. 1998), even though the bioavailability of both allicin and vinyldithiin is quite high (>60% and >70%, respectively) (Lachmann, Lorenz et al. 1994). Instead, allyl methyl sulfide (AMS) and acetone in the breath have been identified as the degradation products of allicin and its derivatives in humans (Lawson and Wang 2005). Besides AMS, allyl methyl sulfoxide (AMSO) and allyl methyl sulfone (AMSO$_2$) have been identified as the metabolites of DADS in rats. Among them, AMSO$_2$ is the most abundant metabolite (Germain, Auger et al. 2002). Furthermore, the in vivo metabolism of γ-glutamylallylcysteine, the major OSC in fresh garlic cloves, resembles its metabolic fate within garlic, which is the hydrolysis by γ-glutamyltranspeptidase to form SAC and then the acetylation by N-acetyltransferase to generate SAMC in the kidney (Verhagen, Hageman et al. 2001). Based on its consistent appearance in the urine of garlic consumers, SAMC may function as an exposure biomarker of intact garlic.

23.3 CHEMOPREVENTIVE ACTIVITIES OF GARLIC

Chemoprevention aims to impede, arrest, or reverse the carcinogenic process using pharmacological or dietary agents (Sporn and Suh 2002). Feasibility and efficacy of chemopreventive compounds against different types of cancer have been demonstrated in many animal experiments and several clinical trials (Sporn and Suh 2000). Transformation of a normal cell to a malignant tumor is a multiple-stage process, including initiation, promotion, and progression. During this transformation, the disruption, dysfunction, and dysregulation of biological entities (such as metabolites, proteins, RNA, DNA, cytoskeleton) and biological pathways (such as metabolism, signal transduction, hormone release) occur in each stage of carcinogenesis (Kreeger and Lauffenburger 2010), leading to the changes in metabolome, proteome, transcriptome, and genome and affecting the fundamental cell processes such as death, proliferation, differentiation, and migration (Figure 23.2). The chronic process of carcinogenesis as well as the complexity of carcinogenesis-induced changes in the biological system provides numerous opportunities for chemoprevention. In fact, current strategies applied in the chemoprevention field are evolved from the knowledge on various aspects of carcinogenesis (Chen and Kong 2005). According to the end points and targets of chemopreventive

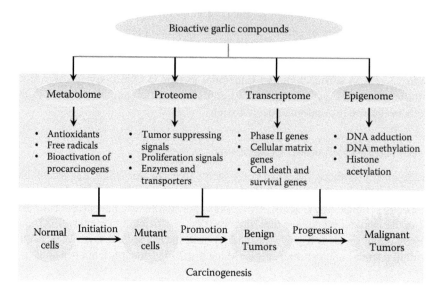

FIGURE 23.2 Carcinogenesis is a multiple-stage pathogenic event, comprising numerous molecular and cellular processes that are targets for intervention and interference. Bioactive garlic compounds can affect these processes through their effects on small-molecule metabolites, proteins, gene expression, and DNA structure, resulting in diverse antitumorigenic activities.

treatments, the majority of chemopreventive compounds can be broadly classified as either blocking agents or suppressing agents (1999). Blocking agents, which aim to prevent the occurrence of DNA mutation caused by carcinogens, encompass groups of mechanistically diversified compounds, such as substances that reduce the formation of reactive species in the body; chemicals that inhibit the metabolic activation of procarcinogens or enhance their detoxification; antioxidants that scavenge free radicals; and chemicals that trap ultimate carcinogens, preventing their interactions with DNA. Different from blocking agents, suppressing agents mostly interfere with the promotion and progression stages of carcinogenesis. Generally, the chemopreventive activity of suppressing agents is attributed to their influence on cell proliferation, differentiation, senescence, and apoptosis (Manson, Gescher et al. 2000). It should be noted that many chemopreventive compounds, including garlic compounds, can function as both blocking and suppressing agents in different stages of carcinogenesis since they can affect multiple targets and pathways in this process.

Dietary compounds are highly desirable for developing as chemopreventive agents because of their safety, low toxicity, and general acceptance as dietary supplements. Among many identified dietary chemopreventive compounds, garlic compounds, especially OSCs, possess distinctive chemical and biological properties to make them potent agents to intervene in many important events in carcinogenesis.

23.3.1 EPIDEMIOLOGICAL AND PRECLINICAL EVIDENCE

An inverse relationship between garlic intake and cancer incidence has been observed in many epidemiological studies (Milner 2006; Rivlin 2009). Results from these studies indicated that garlic alone or together with other nutrients can decrease the incidence of prostate (Hsing, Chokkalingam et al. 2002), colon (Steinmetz, Kushi et al. 1994), laryngeal (Zheng, Blot et al. 1992), breast (Challier, Perarnau et al. 1998), and gastric cancers (Buiatti, Palli et al. 1989; You, Blot et al. 1989). However, a recent evidence-based review on the relation between garlic and cancer has suggested that currently available information from dietary surveys or dietary interventions in humans is not yet sufficient to support strong cancer-preventive effects of garlic or to make relevant claims in the Food and Drug Administration (FDA)–regulated garlic products due to the deficiencies in some of these epidemiological studies, such as the lack of control samples or stringent statistical analysis, or the insufficient validation of dietary assessment method or surrogate biomarkers of cancer risk (Kim and Kwon 2009). In contrast to the ambivalence related to the health effects of garlic in humans, the chemopreventive effects of garlic have been consistently observed in numerous animal studies. Administration of garlic extract and compounds has been shown to inhibit tumorigenesis in multiple organs and tissues, including the liver (Haber-Mignard, Suschetet et al. 1996), skin (Sadhana, Rao et al. 1988), cervix (Hussain, Jannu et al. 1990), colon (Sumiyoshi and Wargovich 1990), and breast (Gued, Thomas et al. 2003), in various carcinogenesis animal models. In addition, together with in vitro analysis using cells, subcellular fractions, and enzymes, these animal studies revealed the molecular mechanisms that potentially underlie the cancer-preventive effects of garlic, that is, direct antioxidant function (Section 23.3.2), regulation of bioactivation and detoxifying enzymes (Section 23.3.3), antiproliferation and induction of apoptosis (Section 23.3.4), and immunoregulation (Section 23.3.5) (Figure 23.2).

23.3.2 DIRECT ANTIOXIDANT FUNCTION

Oxidative stress has been defined as an important contributor in carcinogenesis and many chronic diseases (Reuter, Gupta et al. 2010). Production of reactive oxygen species (ROS) from both endogenous processes and exogenous exposures causes unwanted oxidation and damage to DNA and other macromolecules, which can become the source of carcinogenic lesions. In addition, proinflammatory responses can be triggered by oxidative damages, further raising the level of oxidative stress. Reduced sulfur structures in the body, including glutathione (GSH), *N*-acetylcysteine (NAC), and thioredoxin, are an important part of the endogenous antioxidant system for removing ROS, while garlic is one of a few dietary sources that can directly supply sulfur-containing compounds as exogenous antioxidants (Yin and Cheng 1998). Chemical analysis has defined that the antioxidant activity of allicin, the precursor of many OSCs, is mainly attributed to its sulfenic acid moiety (Vaidya, Ingold et al. 2009). Furthermore, other non–sulfur-containing compounds in garlic, such as flavonoids and organoselenium compounds, also possess antioxidant activity (Cai, Uden et al. 1994; Dong, Lisk et al. 2001). It should be noted that not all garlic compounds function as antioxidants. Instead, the prooxidant properties of some OSCs, such as DATS (Antosiewicz, Herman-Antosiewicz et al. 2006), contribute to their chemopreventive activity through upregulating detoxifying enzymes, inhibiting the cell cycle, or triggering cell death (detailed in Sections 23.3.3 and 23.3.4).

23.3.3 REGULATION OF BIOACTIVATION AND DETOXIFYING ENZYMES

The final fate of carcinogens, whether from exogenous or endogenous sources, largely depends on their interaction with the metabolic system in the body. Alteration of gene expression and enzymatic activity related to the biotransformation of carcinogens can significantly affect the consequences of chemically initiated carcinogenesis. Based on their influence on the carcinogens, metabolizing enzymes can be categorized as bioactivation enzymes or detoxifying enzymes. The majority of bioactivation reactions are mediated by cytochrome P450 enzymes (P450s), though sulfation and acetylation reactions catalyzed by sulfotransferases and *N*-acetyltransferases can also contribute to the bioactivation of procarcinogens, especially some heterocyclic amines (Malfatti, Buonarati et al. 1994; Glatt 1997). The production of reactive metabolites from these bioactivation reactions results in the formation of adducts with DNA and proteins. Direct consequences from these interactions are mutations and/or disruption of intracellular and intercellular signaling pathways (Guengerich and Liebler 1985). In contrast, the detoxifying/defense system in the body includes a wide spectrum of phase I and phase II metabolizing enzymes, such as aldehyde–ketone reductase (AKR), glutathione reductase (GR), epoxide hydrolase (EH), glutathione S-transferase (GST), NAD(P)H quinone oxidoreductase (NQO), and UDP-glucuronosyltransferase (UGT). These can compete with the bioactivation enzymes by eliminating reactive metabolites via the reduction reactions or the conjugation reactions (GSH conjugation, glucuronidation, or sulfation) to render them less reactive and more water soluble, and therefore to facilitate their excretion from the cell and ultimately from the body (Jakoby and Ziegler 1990). The physiological balance between bioactivation enzymes and detoxifying enzymes, to some extent, may determine the risk of chemically induced carcinogenesis (Kensler 1997).

The chemopreventive activities of bioactive garlic compounds, especially OSCs, are closely related to their influences on xenobiotic metabolism system. In fact, the subtle structural differences among OSCs have a major impact on their effects on bioactivation and detoxifying enzymes (Yang, Chhabra et al. 2001). The influences of OSCs on P450 enzymes are diverse. It has been shown that DAS, DADS, and AMS competitively inhibited cytochrome P450 2E1 (CYP2E1), the P450 enzyme mainly responsible for the bioactivation of several small-molecule carcinogens, such as benzene, 1,2-dimethylhydrazine, and azoxymethane (Brady, Ishizaki et al. 1991; Davenport and Wargovich 2005; Wargovich 2006), but they also robustly increased the transcriptional levels of CYP1A1, 2B1, and 3A1 in the rat liver (Brady, Ishizaki et al. 1991; Wu, Sheen et al. 2002). Therefore, the role of garlic OSCs in the P450-mediated bioactivation or deactivation of carcinogens may be substrate specific. As for the influence on phase II detoxifying enzymes, the positive effects of OSCs, especially DADS and DATS, on GST (Hatono, Jimenez et al. 1996), GR (Wu, Sheen et al. 2001), NQO (Singh, Pan et al. 1998), as well as H- and L-ferritin (Thomas, Zhang et al. 2002), were consistently observed in animal and cell models. The consequences of inhibiting bioactivation and promoting detoxification by garlic OSCs have been examined in many chemical-induced carcinogenesis models. The results indicated that garlic OSCs, especially allyl sulfides (DAS, DADS, DATS), are effective in inhibiting 1,2-dimethylhydrazine–induced and azoxymethane-induced colon cancer, benzopyrene-induced and nitrosodiethylamine-induced forestomach cancer, and N-nitrosomethylbenzylamine-induced esophageal cancer, as well as renal and liver cancers in animal models (Wargovich 1987; Sparnins, Barany et al. 1988; Wargovich, Woods et al. 1988; Wattenberg, Sparnins et al. 1989; Takahashi, Hakoi et al. 1992; Reddy, Rao et al. 1993).

Mechanisms underlying the regulatory effects of garlic OSCs on xenobiotics metabolizing enzymes have been also characterized. The inhibitory effect of DAS on CYP2E1 is actually mediated by the enzyme itself since diallyl sulfoxide (DASO) and diallyl sulfone (DASO$_2$), two DAS metabolites formed by CYP2E1, are better competitive inhibitors of CYP2E1 than DAS (Yang, Chhabra et al. 2001). Different from the direct interaction that occurs in the garlic OSC–mediated enzyme inhibition, the upregulation of xenobiotics metabolizing enzymes is mainly controlled by transcriptional activities. Constitutive androstane receptor (CAR), a nuclear receptor, has been shown to be activated by DAS, potentially through an indirect interaction, leading to the induction of CYP2B enzymes (Fisher, Augustine et al. 2007), while nuclear factor E2–related factor 2 (Nrf2) is mainly responsible for the induction of many detoxifying enzymes by garlic OSCs, including allyl sulfides and ajoene (Kay, Won Yang et al. 2010; Chen, Pung et al. 2004). In contrast to the antioxidant activity of some OSCs (detailed in Section 23.3.2), the induction of detoxifying enzymes is generally initiated by the prooxidant activity of these OSCs, such as the production of hydrogen peroxide (Jin and Baillie 1997; Munday, Munday et al. 2003). In fact, the antioxidants GSH and NAC can abrogate the inducing effects of allyl sulfides on the detoxifying enzyme (Chen, Pung et al. 2004). Mechanistically, disruption of redox balance by garlic OSCs triggers the dissociation of Nrf2 from its anchoring protein Keap1 in the cytoplasm and promotes the migration of Nrf2 into the nucleus. Subsequently, the binding of Nrf2 to the antioxidant response element (ARE), an enhancer sequence in the promoter region of many detoxifying enzyme genes, results in the increased gene expression and enzyme activity (Chen and Kong 2004). Interestingly, even though the final consequence of consuming garlic OSCs is the elevation of intracellular GSH level, the GSH concentration in primary rat hepatocytes was decreased dramatically in the early hours of OSC exposure (Sheen, Lii et al. 1996). Overall, upregulation of the detoxification system through Nrf2 and ARE is a reflection of the adaptation response to the stress signals from garlic OSCs. Among the three most abundant allyl sulfides in garlic oil, DATS is the most potent inducer of gene expression (Chen, Pung et al. 2004). Since DATS comprises as much as 50% of garlic volatile fraction (Yu, Wu et al. 1989), it is likely that DATS, not DAS and DADS, is the major effective component in garlic essential oil preparations responsible for the upregulation of the detoxification system.

23.3.4 Antiproliferation and Induction of Apoptosis

While the inhibition of bioactivation enzymes and the induction of detoxifying system are mainly intended to prevent the initiation of carcinogenesis, the antiproliferative and proapoptotic activities of chemopreventive agents aim to halt and reverse the carcinogenic process (Manson 2003). The antiproliferation can be achieved by cell cycle arrest and/or the inhibition of differentiation and angiogenesis (Knowles and Milner 2001). In both cell culture and animal models, several garlic OSCs have been shown to decrease the growth of neoplastic cells through blocking the cell cycle and induction of G2/M phase arrest (Frantz, Hughes et al. 2000; Li, Ciu et al. 2002). Suppression of p34^{cdc2} kinase activity, responsible for the progression of the cells from the G2 phase to the M phase, has been revealed as a contributing mechanism of garlic-induced antiproliferative activities (Knowles and Milner 2000). In addition, the induction of histone acetylation and the inhibition of telomerase activity also account for the antiproliferative effects of garlic OSCs since these down-regulatory events could suppress the transcriptional activities important in cell division and growth (Druesne-Pecollo and Latino-Martel 2011; Ye, Yang et al. 2005).

Apoptosis or programmed cell death is an orchestrated process, represented by membrane blebbing, cell shrinkage, protein degradation, chromatin condensation, and DNA fragmentation. The induction of apoptosis not only is a goal of chemotherapy for cancer but also represents a protective strategy against the neoplastic transformation of genetically damaged cells and the development of the tumor. It has been shown that bioactive garlic compounds, including DAS, DADS, DATS, SAC, SAMC, allicin, and ajoene, are among the phytochemical chemopreventive agents that can induce apoptosis in adenoma and carcinoma cells (Nagini 2008), and the induction of apoptosis by these agents is at least partially responsible for their chemopreventive activities (Kong, Yu et al. 2001). The main factor determining whether the cytotoxic effects of garlic OSCs to preneoplastic or neoplastic cells are antiproliferative or proapoptotic is the dose of exposure during the treatment. As the doses of garlic OSCs increase, the effects of chemopreventive treatments progress from the decrease in cell proliferation to the induction of apoptosis. Indeed, many signaling pathways involved in the antiproliferation also contribute to the garlic OSC-induced apoptosis. In addition, the proapoptotic signaling and degradation events have been identified in the garlic OSC-treated cells, including the activation of mitogen-activated protein kinases (MAPKs:c-Jun amino-terminal kinase [JNK], p38, and extracellular signal–regulated kinases 1 and 2 [ERK1/2]); upregulation of Bax and downregulation of Bcl-2 protein; release of cytochrome c; activation of caspases-3, -8, and -9; cleavage of poly(ADP-ribose) polymerase (PARP); and microtubule depolymerization (Nagini 2008). The potency of garlic OSCs to induce apoptosis is correlated to the capacity to induce oxidative stress, suggesting that, similar to the induction of detoxifying enzymes, the redox imbalance is also the triggering factor in garlic OSC-induced cell death. Besides antiproliferation and apoptosis, recent studies have shown that several garlic OSCs, including DAS, DADS, and DATS, can suppress the invasion and migration abilities of carcinoma cells through inhibiting the expression of matrix metalloproteinases (Lai, Hsu et al. 2011; Meyer, Ueberham et al. 2004).

23.3.5 Immunoregulation

Immune response has a very significant role in carcinogenesis. Inflammation, especially chronic inflammation, contributes to the development of three stages of carcinogenesis (initiation, promotion, and progression) through altering the signaling events and microenvironment of preneoplastic and neoplastic cells (Coussens and Werb 2002). On the other hand, stimulating the recognition of tumor antigens by immune cells can facilitate the immunosurveillance and removal of cancerous cells (Finn 2008). Correlating to the dual functional roles of the immune system in carcinogenesis, garlic OSCs have both immunostimulating and immunosuppressing functions according to the treatments and subjects. AGE has been shown to inhibit histamine release and suppress immunoglobulin E (IgE)–mediated antigen-specific skin reactions (Kyo, Uda et al. 2001). The potential chemopreventive effects of allicin on colon cancer have been partially attributed to the attenuation of intestinal inflammation by inhibiting the expression and secretion of proinflammatory cytokines, such as interleukin 1β (IL-1β) and IL-8 (Lang, Lahav et al. 2004). In addition, DATS has been shown to inhibit the phorbol ester–induced expression of cyclooxygenase 2 (COX2), which is responsible for synthesizing prostaglandins (Shrotriya, Kundu et al. 2010). On the other hand, the immunostimulating effects of garlic are represented by the increase in the total white blood cell count (Kuttan 2000), alliin-enhanced engulfing capacity of phagocytes (Salman, Bergman et al. 1999), and stimulated synthesis of tumor necrosis factor (TNFα) and nitric oxide (NO) from primary human lymphocytes or macrophages (Purev, Chung et al. 2012; Bhattacharyya, Girish et al. 2007).

23.4 PERSPECTIVES ON GARLIC-ELICITED CHEMOPREVENTIVE ACTIVITIES

Even though epidemiological studies have not provided a definite conclusion on the role of garlic in human health (potentially due to insufficient garlic intake or inadequate survey population), the data from animal experiments and cell cultures have vindicated that garlic and its bioactive compounds and preparations have the inhibitory activities on all stages of carcinogenesis. Based on our current understanding on the mechanisms, it is clear that the chemopreventive activities of garlic are the consequences of combinatorial effects of bioactive garlic compounds on multiple targets in carcinogenesis, including the inhibition of carcinogen bioactivation, the facilitation of carcinogen detoxification and elimination, the suppression of proliferation, the induction of apoptosis, as well as the modulation of immune responses. However, the efficacy and application of garlic in cancer prevention are still hampered by some issues that are more or less specific to garlic and are caused by the lack of information and the limitation of experimental approaches. First, there is a great uncertainty on the chemical composition of garlic preparations since it is dramatically affected by enzyme exposure and physical and chemical conditions (such as temperature and extraction solvent) during the preparation process. As the garlic compounds with high bioactivity and good safety from chemoprevention are not clearly defined, it is difficult to define and establish a correlation between the content of OSCs in these preparations and the efficacy of cancer prevention. Potential coexistence of chemicals with opposite bioactivities (antioxidant vs. prooxidant, immunostimulant vs. immunosuppressor) may further complicate the application of these garlic preparations. Second, because of their chemical reactivity, all garlic OSCs are extensively metabolized in vivo, and the parent compounds are hardly detectable or exist in very minor amounts in the body. Therefore, the active compounds in the target sites of chemoprevention are not likely the same compounds consumed by experimental animals or humans. The direct implication of this phenomenon is that the mechanism behind the observed chemopreventive activities of garlic compounds and preparations might be different from the mechanism revealed by an in vitro cell culture model, which might be deficient in biotransformation capacity. Lastly, besides the mechanisms discussed in this review, other effects of garlic consumption, such as the modulation of the vascular system and lipid metabolism, could also contribute to garlic-induced chemoprevention since all these events are interconnected with the transformation, proliferation, and apoptosis of cells as well as immune responses. To resolve these issues, more mechanistic and comprehensive investigations on various aspects of garlic-elicited bioactivities are required. As the influence of bioactive garlic compounds on a biological system occurs at multiple sites and multiple levels (Figure 23.2), systems biology approaches, including metabolomics, proteomics, transcriptomics, and genomics, will provide more insights on the value and mechanism of garlic in cancer prevention.

ACKNOWLEDGMENT

Research on diet and health in C. Chen's lab is partially supported by a United States Department of Agriculture Experimental Station project (MIN-18-082).

REFERENCES

(1999). "Prevention of cancer in the next millennium: Report of the Chemoprevention Working Group to the American Association for Cancer Research." *Cancer Res* 59(19): 4743–58.

Amagase, H., B. L. Petesch et al. (2001). "Intake of garlic and its bioactive components." *J Nutr* 131(3s): 955S–62S.

Antosiewicz, J., A. Herman-Antosiewicz et al. (2006). "c-Jun NH(2)-terminal kinase signaling axis regulates diallyl trisulfide-induced generation of reactive oxygen species and cell cycle arrest in human prostate cancer cells." *Cancer Res* 66(10): 5379–86.

Bhattacharyya, M., G. V. Girish et al. (2007). "Systemic production of IFN-alpha by garlic (Allium sativum) in humans." *J Interferon Cytokine Res* 27(5): 377–82.

Block, E. (1985). "The chemistry of garlic and onions." *Sci Am* 252(3): 114–9.

Brady, J. F., H. Ishizaki et al. (1991). "Inhibition of cytochrome P-450 2E1 by diallyl sulfide and its metabolites." *Chem Res Toxicol* 4(6): 642–7.

Buiatti, E., D. Palli et al. (1989). "A case-control study of gastric cancer and diet in Italy." *Int J Cancer* 44(4): 611–6.

Butt, M. S., M. T. Sultan et al. (2009). "Garlic: nature's protection against physiological threats." *Crit Rev Food Sci Nutr* 49(6): 538–51.

Cai, X. J., P. C. Uden et al. (1994). "Allium chemistry—identification of natural-abundance organoselenium volatiles from garlic, elephant garlic, onion, and Chinese chive using headspace gas-chromatography with atomic-emission detection." *J Agric Food Chem* 42(10): 2081–4.

Challier, B., J. M. Perarnau et al. (1998). "Garlic, onion and cereal fibre as protective factors for breast cancer: a French case-control study." *Eur J Epidemiol* 14(8): 737–47.

Chen, C. and A. N. Kong (2004). "Dietary chemopreventive compounds and ARE/EpRE signaling." *Free Radic Biol Med* 36(12): 1505–16.

Chen, C. and A. N. Kong (2005). "Dietary cancer-chemopreventive compounds: from signaling and gene expression to pharmacological effects." *Trends Pharmacol Sci* 26(6): 318–26.

Chen, C., D. Pung et al. (2004). "Induction of detoxifying enzymes by garlic organosulfur compounds through transcription factor Nrf2: effect of chemical structure and stress signals." *Free Radic Biol Med* 37(10): 1578–90.

Coussens, L. M. and Z. Werb (2002). "Inflammation and cancer." *Nature* 420(6917): 860–7.

Dausch, J. G. and D. W. Nixon (1990). "Garlic: a review of its relationship to malignant disease." *Prev Med* 19(3): 346–61.

Davenport, D. M. and M. J. Wargovich (2005). "Modulation of cytochrome P450 enzymes by organosulfur compounds from garlic." *Food Chem Toxicol* 43(12): 1753–62.

Dong, Y., D. Lisk et al. (2001). "Characterization of the biological activity of gamma-glutamyl-Se-methylseleno-cysteine: a novel, naturally occurring anticancer agent from garlic." *Cancer Res* 61(7): 2923–8.

Druesne-Pecollo, N. and P. Latino-Martel (2011). "Modulation of histone acetylation by garlic sulfur compounds." *Anticancer Agents Med Chem* 11(3): 254–9.

Fenwick, G. R. and A. B. Hanley (1985). "The genus Allium. Part 2." *Crit Rev Food Sci Nutr* 22(4): 273–377.

Finn, O. J. (2008). "Cancer immunology." *N Engl J Med* 358(25): 2704–15.

Fisher, C. D., L. M. Augustine et al. (2007). "Induction of drug-metabolizing enzymes by garlic and allyl sulfide compounds via activation of constitutive androstane receptor and nuclear factor E2-related factor 2." *Drug Metab Dispos* 35(6): 995–1000.

Frantz, D. J., B. G. Hughes et al. (2000). "Cell cycle arrest and differential gene expression in HT-29 cells exposed to an aqueous garlic extract." *Nutr Cancer* 38(2): 255–64.

Germain, E., J. Auger et al. (2002). "In vivo metabolism of diallyl disulphide in the rat: identification of two new metabolites." *Xenobiotica* 32(12): 1127–38.

Glatt, H. (1997). "Sulfation and sulfotransferases 4: bioactivation of mutagens via sulfation." *FASEB J* 11(5): 314–21.

Gued, L. R., R. D. Thomas et al. (2003). "Diallyl sulfide inhibits diethylstilbestrol-induced lipid peroxidation in breast tissue of female ACI rats: Implications in breast cancer prevention." *Oncol Rep* 10(3): 739–43.

Guengerich, F. P. and D. C. Liebler (1985). "Enzymatic activation of chemicals to toxic metabolites." *Crit Rev Toxicol* 14(3): 259–307.

Haber-Mignard, D., M. Suschetet et al. (1996). "Inhibition of aflatoxin B1- and N-nitrosodiethylamine-induced liver preneoplastic foci in rats fed naturally occurring allyl sulfides." *Nutr Cancer* 25(1): 61–70.

Hatono, S., A. Jimenez et al. (1996). "Chemopreventive effect of S-allylcysteine and its relationship to the detoxification enzyme glutathione S-transferase." *Carcinogenesis* 17(5): 1041–4.

Hsing, A. W., A. P. Chokkalingam et al. (2002). "Allium vegetables and risk of prostate cancer: a population-based study." *J Natl Cancer Inst* 94(21): 1648–51.

Hussain, S. P., L. N. Jannu et al. (1990). "Chemopreventive action of garlic on methylcholanthrene-induced carcinogenesis in the uterine cervix of mice." *Cancer Lett* 49(2): 175–80.

Jakoby, W. B. and D. M. Ziegler (1990). "The enzymes of detoxication." *J Biol Chem* 265(34): 20715–8.

Jin, L. and T. A. Baillie (1997). "Metabolism of the chemoprotective agent diallyl sulfide to glutathione conjugates in rats." *Chem Res Toxicol* 10(3): 318–27.

Kay, H. Y., J. Won Yang et al. (2010). "Ajoene, a stable garlic by-product, has an antioxidant effect through Nrf2-mediated glutamate-cysteine ligase induction in HepG2 cells and primary hepatocytes." *J Nutr* 140(7): 1211–9.

Kensler, T. W. (1997). "Chemoprevention by inducers of carcinogen detoxication enzymes." *Environ Health Perspect* 105 (Suppl 4): 965–70.

Kim, J. Y. and O. Kwon (2009). "Garlic intake and cancer risk: an analysis using the Food and Drug Administration's evidence-based review system for the scientific evaluation of health claims." *Am J Clin Nutr* 89(1): 257–64.

Knowles, L. M. and J. A. Milner (2000). "Diallyl disulfide inhibits p34(cdc2) kinase activity through changes in complex formation and phosphorylation." *Carcinogenesis* 21(6): 1129–34.

Knowles, L. M. and J. A. Milner (2001). "Possible mechanism by which allyl sulfides suppress neoplastic cell proliferation." *J Nutr* 131(3s): 1061S–6S.

Kodera, Y., M. Ichikawa et al. (2002). "Pharmacokinetic study of allixin, a phytoalexin produced by garlic." *Chem Pharm Bull (Tokyo)* 50(3): 354–63.

Kong, A. N., R. Yu et al. (2001). "Signal transduction events elicited by cancer prevention compounds." *Mutat Res* 480–481: 231–41.

Kreeger, P. K. and D. A. Lauffenburger (2010). "Cancer systems biology: a network modeling perspective." *Carcinogenesis* 31(1): 2–8.

Kuttan, G. (2000). "Immunomodulatory effect of some naturally occurring sulphur-containing compounds." *J Ethnopharmacol* 72(1-2): 93–9.

Kyo, E., N. Uda et al. (2001). "Immunomodulatory effects of aged garlic extract." *J Nutr* 131(3s): 1075S–9S.

Lachmann, G., D. Lorenz et al. (1994). "[The pharmacokinetics of the S35 labeled labeled garlic constituents alliin, allicin and vinyldithiine]." *Arzneimittelforschung* 44(6): 734–43.

Lai, K. C., S. C. Hsu et al. 2011. "Diallyl sulfide, diallyl disulfide, and diallyl trisulfide inhibit migration and invasion in human colon cancer colo 205 cells through the inhibition of matrix metalloproteinase-2, -7, and -9 expressions." *Environ Toxicol* doi: 10.1002/tox.20737.

Lancaster, J. E. and M. L. Shaw (1989). "Gamma-glutamyl-transferase peptides in the biosynthesis of S-Alk(En) Yl-L-cysteine sulfoxides (flavor precursors) in allium." *Phytochemistry* 28(2): 455–460.

Lang, A., M. Lahav et al. (2004). "Allicin inhibits spontaneous and TNF-alpha induced secretion of proinflammatory cytokines and chemokines from intestinal epithelial cells." *Clin Nutr* 23(5): 1199–208.

Lawson, L. D., R. Bauer et al. (1998). *Phytomedicines of Europe: Chemistry and Biological Activity.* Washington, DC: American Chemical Society.

Lawson, L. D., D. K. Ransom et al. (1992). "Inhibition of whole blood platelet-aggregation by compounds in garlic clove extracts and commercial garlic products." *Thromb Res* 65(2): 141–56.

Lawson, L. D. and Z. J. Wang (2005). "Allicin and allicin-derived garlic compounds increase breath acetone through allyl methyl sulfide: use in measuring allicin bioavailability." *J Agric Food Chem* 53(6): 1974–83.

Li, M., J. R. Ciu et al. (2002). "Antitumor activity of Z-ajoene, a natural compound purified from garlic: antimitotic and microtubule-interaction properties." *Carcinogenesis* 23(4): 573–9.

Li, Q. Q., S. D. Zhou et al. (2010). "Phylogeny and biogeography of Allium (Amaryllidaceae: Allieae) based on nuclear ribosomal internal transcribed spacer and chloroplast rps16 sequences, focusing on the inclusion of species endemic to China." *Ann Bot* 106(5): 709–33.

Malfatti, M. A., M. H. Buonarati et al. (1994). "The role of sulfation and/or acetylation in the metabolism of the cooked-food mutagen 2-amino-1-methyl-6-phenylimidazo[4,5-b]pyridine in Salmonella typhimurium and isolated rat hepatocytes." *Chem Res Toxicol* 7(2): 139–47.

Manson, M. M. (2003). "Cancer prevention—the potential for diet to modulate molecular signalling." *Trends Mol Med* 9(1): 11–8.

Manson, M. M., A. Gescher et al. (2000). "Blocking and suppressing mechanisms of chemoprevention by dietary constituents." *Toxicol Lett* 112–113: 499–505.

Matsuura, H. (2001). "Saponins in garlic as modifiers of the risk of cardiovascular disease." *J Nutr* 131(3s): 1000S–5S.

Meyer, K., E. Ueberham et al. (2004). "Influence of organosulphur compounds from garlic on the secretion of matrix metalloproteinases and their inhibitor TIMP-1 by cultured HUVEC cells." *Cell Biol Toxicol* 20(4): 253–60.

Milner, J. A. (2006). "Preclinical perspectives on garlic and cancer." *J Nutr* 136(3 Suppl): 827S–31S.

Munday, R., J. S. Munday et al. (2003). "Comparative effects of mono-, di-, tri-, and tetrasulfides derived from plants of the Allium family: redox cycling in vitro and hemolytic activity and Phase 2 enzyme induction in vivo." *Free Radic Biol Med* 34(9): 1200–11.

Nagini, S. (2008). "Cancer chemoprevention by garlic and its organosulfur compounds-panacea or promise?" *Anticancer Agents Med Chem* 8(3): 313–21.

Purev, U., M. J. Chung et al. (2012). "Individual differences on immunostimulatory activity of raw and black garlic extract in human primary immune cells." *Immunopharmacol Immunotoxicol* 34(4):651–60.

Reddy, B. S., C. V. Rao et al. (1993). "Chemoprevention of colon carcinogenesis by organosulfur compounds." *Cancer Res* 53(15): 3493–8.

Reuter, S., S. C. Gupta et al. (2010). "Oxidative stress, inflammation, and cancer: how are they linked?" *Free Radic Biol Med* 49(11): 1603–16.

Rivlin, R. S. (2009). "Can garlic reduce risk of cancer?" *Am J Clin Nutr* 89(1): 17–8.

Ryu, K., N. Ide et al. (2001). "N alpha-(1-deoxy-D-fructos-1-yl)-L-arginine, an antioxidant compound identified in aged garlic extract." *J Nutr* 131(3s): 972S–6S.

Sadhana, A. S., A. R. Rao et al. (1988). "Inhibitory action of garlic oil on the initiation of benzo[a]pyrene-induced skin carcinogenesis in mice." *Cancer Lett* 40(2): 193–7.

Salman, H., M. Bergman et al. (1999). "Effect of a garlic derivative (alliin) on peripheral blood cell immune responses." *Int J Immunopharmacol* 21(9): 589–97.

Sheen, L. Y., C. K. Lii et al. (1996). "Effect of the active principle of garlic--diallyl sulfide--on cell viability, detoxification capability and the antioxidant system of primary rat hepatocytes." *Food Chem Toxicol* 34(10): 971–8.

Shrotriya, S., J. K. Kundu et al. (2010). "Diallyl trisulfide inhibits phorbol ester-induced tumor promotion, activation of AP-1, and expression of COX-2 in mouse skin by blocking JNK and Akt signaling." *Cancer Res* 70(5): 1932–40.

Singh, S. V., S. S. Pan et al. (1998). "Differential induction of NAD(P)H:quinone oxidoreductase by anti-carcinogenic organosulfides from garlic." *Biochem Biophys Res Commun* 244(3): 917–20.

Sparnins, V. L., G. Barany et al. (1988). "Effects of organosulfur compounds from garlic and onions on benzo[a]pyrene-induced neoplasia and glutathione S-transferase activity in the mouse." *Carcinogenesis* 9(1): 131–4.

Sporn, M. B. and N. Suh (2000). "Chemoprevention of cancer." *Carcinogenesis* 21(3): 525–30.

Sporn, M. B. and N. Suh (2002). "Chemoprevention: an essential approach to controlling cancer." *Nat Rev Cancer* 2(7): 537–43.

Steinmetz, K. A., L. H. Kushi et al. (1994). "Vegetables, fruit, and colon cancer in the Iowa Women's Health Study." *Am J Epidemiol* 139(1): 1–15.

Sumiyoshi, H. and M. J. Wargovich (1990). "Chemoprevention of 1,2-dimethylhydrazine-induced colon cancer in mice by naturally occurring organosulfur compounds." *Cancer Res* 50(16): 5084–7.

Takahashi, S., K. Hakoi et al. (1992). "Enhancing effects of diallyl sulfide on hepatocarcinogenesis and inhibitory actions of the related diallyl disulfide on colon and renal carcinogenesis in rats." *Carcinogenesis* 13(9): 1513–8.

Thomas, M., P. Zhang et al. (2002). "Diallyl disulfide increases rat h-ferritin, L-ferritin and transferrin receptor genes in vitro in hepatic cells and in vivo in liver." *J Nutr* 132(12): 3638–41.

Timbo, B. B., M. P. Ross et al. (2006). "Dietary supplements in a national survey: Prevalence of use and reports of adverse events." *J Am Diet Assoc* 106(12): 1966–74.

Vaidya, V., K. U. Ingold et al. (2009). "Garlic: source of the ultimate antioxidants—sulfenic acids." *Angew Chem Int Ed Engl* 48(1): 157–160.

Verhagen, H., G. J. Hageman et al. (2001). "Biomonitoring the intake of garlic via urinary excretion of allyl mercapturic acid." *Br J Nutr* 86 Suppl 1: S111–4.

Wargovich, M. J. (1987). "Diallyl sulfide, a flavor component of garlic (Allium sativum), inhibits dimethylhydrazine-induced colon cancer." *Carcinogenesis* 8(3): 487–9.

Wargovich, M. J. (2006). "Diallylsulfide and allylmethylsulfide are uniquely effective among organosulfur compounds in inhibiting CYP2E1 protein in animal models." *J Nutr* 136(3 Suppl): 832S–4S.

Wargovich, M. J., C. Woods et al. (1988). "Chemoprevention of N-nitrosomethylbenzylamine-induced esophageal cancer in rats by the naturally occurring thioether, diallyl sulfide." *Cancer Res* 48(23): 6872–5.

Wattenberg, L. W., V. L. Sparnins et al. (1989). "Inhibition of N-nitrosodiethylamine carcinogenesis in mice by naturally occurring organosulfur compounds and monoterpenes." *Cancer Res* 49(10): 2689–92.

Wu, C. C., L. Y. Sheen et al. (2001). "Effects of organosulfur compounds from garlic oil on the antioxidation system in rat liver and red blood cells." *Food Chem Toxicol* 39(6): 563–9.

Wu, C. C., L. Y. Sheen et al. (2002). "Differential effects of garlic oil and its three major organosulfur components on the hepatic detoxification system in rats." *J Agric Food Chem* 50(2): 378–83.

Yang, C. S., S. K. Chhabra et al. (2001). "Mechanisms of inhibition of chemical toxicity and carcinogenesis by diallyl sulfide (DAS) and related compounds from garlic." *J Nutr* 131(3s): 1041S–5S.

Ye, Y., H. Y. Yang et al. (2005). "[Z-ajoene causes cell cycle arrest at G2/M and decrease of telomerase activity in HL-60 cells]." *Zhonghua Zhong Liu Za Zhi* 27(9): 516–20.

Yin, M. C. and W. S. Cheng (1998). "Antioxidant activity of several Allium members." *J Agric Food Chem* 46(10): 4097–101.

You, W. C., W. J. Blot et al. (1989). "Allium vegetables and reduced risk of stomach cancer." *J Natl Cancer Inst* 81(2): 162–4.

Yu, T. H., C. M. Wu et al. (1989). "Volatile compounds from garlic." *J Agric Food Chem* 37(3): 725–30.

Zheng, W., W. J. Blot et al. (1992). "Diet and other risk factors for laryngeal cancer in Shanghai, China." *Am J Epidemiol* 136(2): 178–91.

24 Molecular Mechanisms of Cancer Chemoprevention with Benzyl Isothiocyanate

Anuradha Sehrawat and Shivendra V. Singh

CONTENTS

24.1 INTRODUCTION

A diet rich in fruits and vegetables is considered protective against cancer, and this association is quite persuasive for cruciferous vegetables. Common edible cruciferous vegetables include broccoli, watercress, kale, cabbage, bok choy, collard greens, and horseradish. Initial evidence for the protective effect of cruciferous vegetables against cancer emerged from population-based case-control studies. An inverse association between dietary intake of cruciferous vegetables and cancer risk has been noted for different types of malignancies, including those of the stomach (Chyou et al. 1990), ovary (Pan et al. 2004), lung (Steinmetz et al. 1993), prostate (Kolonel et al. 2000), bladder (Michaud et al. 1999), and colon, to cite a few (Moy et al. 2008). The anticarcinogenic effect of cruciferous vegetables is partly attributed to chemicals with an isothiocyanate (ITC; $-N = C = S$) functional group (Hecht 2000; Conaway et al. 2002; Keum et al. 2004). Bioavailability, safety, efficacy, and ability to target multiple oncogenic pathways are desired attributes for a clinically useful cancer chemopreventive agent. The ITCs meet all of these criteria substantiated by laboratory research over the past three decades. ITCs are not only orally bioavailable but also effective inhibitors of cancer development in rodents (Warin et al. 2009; Singh et al. 2009; Powolny et al. 2011). Efficacy of ITCs for prevention of cancer has now been established in rodent models of chemically induced and oncogene-driven cancers (Hecht 2000; Conaway et al. 2002; Keum et al. 2004; Warin et al. 2009; Wu et al. 2009; Cavell et al. 2011). The ITCs are stored as glucosinolate precursors (β-thioglucoside N-hydroxysulfates) in cruciferous plants. The ITCs are produced upon plant cell wall damage (e.g., cutting or chewing) due to enzymatic hydrolysis of corresponding glucosinolates in a reaction catalyzed by myrosinase (a thioglucoside glucohydrolase). The glucosinolates can also be degraded to the corresponding ITCs by the intestinal microflora, although the extent of such degradation is still unresolved (Getahun and Chung 1999). The absorption and excretion of ITCs are substantially lower from cooked than from raw cruciferous vegetables (Shapiro et al. 2001).

More than 100 structurally different glucosinolate precursors of ITCs have been identified in various plants (Fahey et al. 2001). Many naturally occurring ITCs have been extensively studied for their anticancer efficacy, including benzyl ITC (BITC), phenethyl isothiocyanate (PEITC), allyl isothiocyanate, and sulforaphane. Evidence also exists to indicate that even a subtle difference in ITCs structure can translate into remarkable divergence in the mechanism of their anticancer effect (Hecht 2000). Scientific literature is mature enough to warrant a review of preclinical evidence supporting cancer chemopreventive potential of BITC, which has the ability to inhibit chemically induced as well as spontaneous cancer development in rodents (Hecht 2000; Warin et al. 2009). In vivo growth of human cancer cells implanted in athymic mice is also retarded by BITC administration (Warin et al. 2010; Boreddy et al. 2011a). In cultured cancer cells, BITC targets multiple pathways to exhibit a variety of anticancer effects, including inhibition of carcinogen-activating enzymes and induction of carcinogen-inactivating enzymes (Hecht 2000; Conaway et al. 2002), apoptosis induction and growth arrest (Xiao et al. 2006), inhibition of angiogenesis (Boreddy et al. 2011b), and inhibition of epithelial–mesenchymal transition (EMT) (Sehrawat and Singh 2011).

24.2 METABOLISM AND PHARMACOKINETICS OF BITC

Similar to other ITCs, BITC accumulates rapidly in cancer cells and conjugates with intracellular thiols including glutathione (GSH) (Zhang 2000). The GSH conjugation of BITC is catalyzed by GSH S-transferases (GSTs), but this reaction is believed to be reversible (Zhang et al. 1995). Cellular accumulation of BITC is followed by transporter-mediated export as dithiocarbamates (Callaway et al. 2004). The BITC–GSH conjugate is further metabolized to an N-acetylcysteine (NAC) conjugate (Mennicke et al. 1988). Administration of a BITC–cysteine conjugate resulted in rapid absorption and mainly urinary excretion in rats, the principal metabolite (62% of the dose) being the mercapturic acid (Brusewitz et al. 1977). Metabolism of BITC is different in dogs, with hippuric acid (i.e., the glycine conjugate) being the primary metabolite (Brusewitz et al. 1977). In guinea pigs and rabbits, a cyclic mercaptopyruvate conjugate (4-hydroxy-4-carboxy-3-benzylthiazolidin-2-thione) was the primary urinary metabolite, with only trace amounts of NAC conjugate after oral administration of BITC or its GSH and NAC conjugates (Gorler et al. 1982). After ingestion of BITC by human volunteers, the NAC conjugate was rapidly excreted in urine, representing more than 50% of the initial dose with maximum concentrations evident 2–6 h after dosing (Mennicke et al. 1988). Although the biological effects of NAC conjugates of ITCs are not fully understood, they have been reported to show a weaker cytotoxicity possibly due to the dissociative conversion into free ITCs (Bruggeman et al. 1986). Stable reaction products of ITCs with albumin and hemoglobin have been identified (Kumar and Sabbioni 2010). Oral administration of 12 μmol of BITC to tumor-bearing athymic mice resulted in approximately 6.5 μM BITC in the plasma after 1 h, with a cumulative concentration approaching 7.5 μmol/g in the tumors after 46 days of treatment (Boreddy et al. 2011a). However, detailed pharmacokinetics for BITC remains to be determined.

24.3 PRECLINICAL EVIDENCE FOR ANTICANCER EFFECT OF BITC

24.3.1 INHIBITION OF CHEMICALLY INDUCED CANCER

The ability of BITC to block chemical carcinogenesis was first recognized by Wattenberg (1977) more than 30 years ago. Since then, a number of studies from different laboratories have documented the cancer chemopreventive effect of BITC. For example, BITC was shown to be an effective inhibitor of rat mammary and mouse lung tumorigenesis induced by 7,12-dimethylbenz[a] anthracene and benzo[a]pyrene (B[a]P), respectively (Wattenberg 1977, 1981, 1987; Lin et al. 1993; Hecht et al. 2000). The BITC-mediated inhibition of B[a]P-induced lung tumorigenesis in mice was accompanied by suppression of DNA adduction (Sticha et al. 2000, 2002). When administered by gavage 15 min prior to the carcinogen challenge, BITC almost completely inhibited forestomach tumor formation resulting from diethylnitrosamine (DEN) (Wattenberg 1987). Studies have shown that the NAC conjugate of BITC retains chemopreventive activity. For example, dietary administration of a BITC–NAC conjugate during the postinitiation stage inhibited B[a]P-induced lung tumorigenesis in mice (Yang et al. 2002). The incidence and multiplicity of tumors in the small intestine and the incidence of colon tumors in female ACI/N rats induced by methylazoxymethanol acetate were reduced significantly by BITC administration (Sugie et al. 1994). The BITC treatment significantly inhibited lung tumor multiplicity in mice induced by 5-methylchrysene and dibenz[a,h]anthracene (Hecht el al. 2002). Dietary BITC administration inhibited incidence and average number of liver neoplasms in rats induced by DEN (Sugie et al. 1993). The effect of dietary BITC administration on urinary bladder carcinogenesis was examined in rats simultaneously treated with N-butyl-N-(4-hydroxybutyl)nitrosamine (Okazaki et al. 2002). Carcinogen-induced dysplasia, papilloma, and carcinoma incidences and multiplicities were dramatically decreased by simultaneous treatment with BITC in a dose-dependent manner (Okazaki et al. 2002). The feeding of male Syrian hamsters with a diet supplemented with BITC resulted in a significant decrease in pancreatic atypical hyperplasia and adenocarcinoma induced by N-nitrosobis(2-oxopropyl)amine (Kuroiwa et al. 2006). On the other hand, BITC failed to confer protection against lung cancer induced by the tobacco-specific carcinogen 4-(methylnitrosamino)-1-(3-pyridyl)-1-butanone (NNK) (Morse et al. 1989, 1990). Similarly, BITC administration was not protective against esophageal tumor induction by N-nitrosomethylbenzylamine in rats (Wilkinson et al. 1995).

It is important to point out that BITC has been shown to promote bladder carcinogenesis in rats (Hirose et al. 1998; Akagi et al. 2003; Okazaki et al. 2003). In experiments designed to determine the postinitiation effect of BITC against hepatocarcinogenesis and urinary bladder carcinogenesis, rats were pretreated with DEN and N-butyl-N-(4-hydroxybutyl)nitrosamine prior to the BITC administration in the diet at a 0.1% dose (Hirose et al. 1998). The incidence of papillary or nodular hyperplasia and carcinoma was significantly elevated in the BITC treatment group (Hirose et al. 1998). Inflammatory changes characterized by cellular infiltration, apoptosis/single cell necrosis, cytoplasmic vacuolation, erosion, and hemorrhage in the urinary bladder were observed after acute administration of 0.1% BITC in the diet within 2–3 days (Akagi et al. 2003). As noted above, BITC strongly enhanced rat urinary bladder carcinogenesis after initiation with N-butyl-N-(4-hydroxybutyl)nitrosamine, while potently inhibiting induction of these lesions when given simultaneously with the carcinogen (Okazaki et al. 2002). In a follow-up study, simultaneous treatment with BITC and a lower dose of the same carcinogen did not inhibit, but rather enhanced, rat urinary bladder carcinogenesis (Okazaki et al. 2003). The mechanism by which BITC may act as a carcinogen or bladder tumor promoter is not fully understood but may be related to the metabolism and disposition of BITC in vivo. As discussed above, BITC is primarily excreted in the urine as a mercapturic acid. Excessive exposure of the bladder epithelium to BITC metabolite as the cause of urinary bladder carcinogenesis is one of the proposed mechanisms for this effect. However, there is no evidence to indicate that BITC or any other ITC compound is a bladder carcinogen or bladder tumor promoter in humans based on epidemiological data (Michaud et al. 1999). In fact, consumption of raw cruciferous vegetables was inversely associated with bladder cancer risk in a hospital-based case-control study involving 275 individuals with incident primary bladder cancer and 825 controls (Tang et al. 2008). The same group of investigators reported later that intake of broccoli was inversely associated with bladder cancer mortality (Tang et al. 2010). It is possible that rats are unusually sensitive to bladder carcinogenesis by BITC. Notably, at least two studies have documented clastogenic effects of BITC (Musk and Johnson 1993; Musk et al. 1995). Furthermore, BITC treatment exhibited genotoxic effects in HepG2 cells, but substantially weaker effects were obtained in vivo (Kassie et al. 1999).

24.3.2 SUPPRESSION OF ONCOGENE-DRIVEN CANCER DEVELOPMENT

Dietary administration of a diet of 3 mmol BITC/kg for 25 weeks markedly suppressed the incidence and/or burden of mammary hyperplasia and carcinoma in female mouse mammary tumor virus-neu (MMTV-neu) mice without causing weight loss or affecting the neu protein level. The BITC-mediated prevention of mammary carcinogenesis was found to correlate with significant reduction in cell proliferation, increased apoptosis, T-cell infiltration, and induction of E-cadherin (Warin et al. 2009).

24.3.3 INHIBITION OF CANCER XENOGRAFT GROWTH AND METASTASIS

Intraperitoneal and oral administration of BITC inhibited growth of MDA-MB-231 human breast cancer cells subcutaneously implanted in female nude mice without any harmful side effects (Warin et al. 2010). Oral administration of BITC suppressed 4T1 mammary carcinoma xenograft growth in BALB/c mice (Kim et al. 2011). Oral administration of 12 μmol BITC resulted in growth retardation of pancreatic cancer xenografts in athymic mice (Sahu and Srivastava 2009; Batra et al. 2010; Boreddy et al. 2011a). BITC inhibited murine WEHI-3 leukemia cells in vitro and promoted phagocytosis in BALB/c mice in vivo (Tsou et al. 2009).

Pulmonary metastasis multiplicity and total pulmonary metastasis volume of 4T1 murine mammary carcinoma cells injected into the inguinal mammary fat pads of syngeneic female BALB/c mice were decreased by gavage for 4 weeks with BITC (Kim et al. 2011).

24.4 MOLECULAR MECHANISMS FOR ANTICANCER EFFECTS OF BITC

24.4.1 ALTERATION OF CARCINOGEN-METABOLIZING ENZYMES

Evidence exists to suggest that prevention of preinitiation cancer development by BITC may involve modulation of carcinogen metabolism (Smith 2001). Cytochrome P450 (CYP)–dependent monooxygenases (phase 1 enzymes) play critical roles in the activation of carcinogens (Gonzalez 1988). Inhibition of specific CYP isoforms is one mechanism underlying the chemopreventive response to many agents. BITC and the GSH conjugate of BITC were found to inhibit dealkylation of pentoxyresorufin and ethoxyresorufin in liver microsomes, reactions predominantly mediated by CYP2B1 and CYP1A1/1A2 (Conaway et al. 1996). Because CYP2B1 is one of the isozymes involved in NNK activation (Guo et al. 1991), its inhibition appears to be an important mechanism for the chemopreventive activity of BITC against NNK-induced cancer. The BITC treatment inhibited the 7-ethoxy-4-(trifluoromethyl)coumarin O-deethylation activity of purified and reconstituted CYP2E1 in a time- and concentration-dependent manner (Moreno et al. 1999). The BITC inactivated CYP2B1 in a time- and concentration-dependent manner (Goosen et al. 2000). In a follow-up study, inactivation of rat and human CYP in microsomes and the reconstituted system by BITC was investigated (Goosen et al. 2001). The BITC was shown to be a mechanism-based inactivator of rat CYP1A1, CYP1A2, CYP2B1, and CYP2E1, as well as human CYP2B6 and CYP2D6 (Goosen et al. 2001). Furthermore, BITC was unable to inactivate the CYP2E1 mutant, in which the conserved threonine at position 303 was replaced by alanine (Moreno et al. 2001). CYP2A6 and CYP2A13 are thought to be the primary human enzymes responsible for the in vivo metabolism of nicotine and NNK, respectively. BITC treatment efficiently inhibited CYP2A6- and CYP2A13-mediated coumarin 7 hydroxylation (von Weymarn et al. 2006). Furthermore, these authors demonstrated significant inhibition of CYP2A6-mediated metabolism of nicotine and CYP2A13-mediated alpha-hydroxylation of NNK by BITC (von Weymarn et al. 2006).

Induction of phase 2 enzymes [e.g., GST and NAD(P)H:quinone oxidoreductase (QR)] is another mechanism by which chemopreventive agents function to inhibit preinitiation cancer development (Talalay et al. 1990; Hayes and Pulford 1995). Administration of BITC in the diet (0.5%, w/w) for 2 weeks resulted in an increase in QR activity in the lung, kidney, urinary bladder, proximal small intestine, and colon of female CD-1 mice (Benson et al. 1986). A BITC-mediated increase in hepatic and forestomach GST activity has also been reported (Benson and Barretto 1985). Intracellular accumulation of BITC in mouse skin papilloma cells correlated with elevation of GSH content, QR activity, and GST activity (Ye and Zhang 2001). Rat liver epithelial RL34 cells were used to study the mechanism underlying GST induction by BITC (Nakamura et al. 2000). The BITC was found to significantly induce GST activity in RL34 cells by increasing levels of class-pi isozyme, which was further enhanced by GSH depletion by diethyl maleate (Nakamura et al. 2000). These data suggested the involvement of a redox-sensitive mechanism in BITC-mediated induction of GST (Nakamura et al. 2000). The BITC treatment induced the expression of CYP1A1 in LS-174 colon cancer cells, but caused an increase in the protein levels of aldo-keto reductase 1C1, QR, and gamma-glutamylcysteine synthetase heavy subunit (Bonnesen et al. 2001). Collectively, these results indicate that modulation of carcinogen metabolism by inhibition of CYP and induction of phase 2 enzymes is an important mechanism potentially contributing to suppression of cancer initiation, as summarized in Figure 24.1.

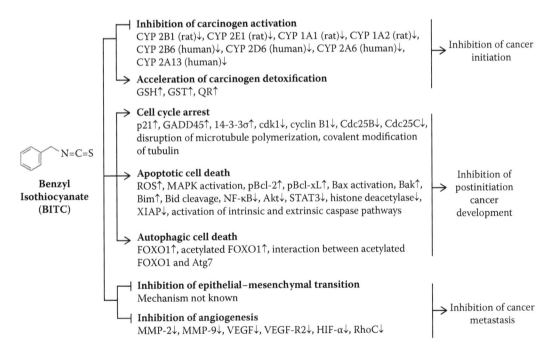

FIGURE 24.1 Molecular mechanisms underlying cancer chemopreventive response to BITC. Abbreviations: Apaf, apoptosis protease activating factor-1; XIAP, X-linked inhibitor of apoptosis; VEGF-R2, VEGF receptor; HIF-1α, hypoxia inducible factor-1 alpha.

24.4.2 CELL CYCLE ARREST

Proper cell cycle progression is ensured by checkpoints, which are often inactivated in cancer cells (Molinari 2000). Hasegawa et al. (1993) were the first to show cell cycle arrest in the G2/M phase by BITC in HeLa cells. Cell cycle arrest in cultured cancer cells after treatment with BITC has been observed in leukemia (Miyoshi et al. 2004a,b), breast cancer (Xiao et al. 2006), pancreatic cancer (Srivastava and Singh 2004; Zhang et al. 2006; Sahu et al. 2009b), lung cancer (Mi et al. 2008), multiple myeloma (Mi et al. 2011), melanoma (Huang et al. 2012), osteosarcoma (Wu et al. 2011), colon cancer (Visanji et al. 2004; Miyoshi et al. 2007; Odom et al. 2009), and bladder cancer cells (Tang and Zhang 2004; Tang et al. 2006). The G2/M phase arrest is the most frequently observed cell cycle change after treatment of cancer cells with BITC. However, a few studies have shown arrest in other phases of the cell cycle after treatment with BITC, which may be a cell line–specific phenomenon (Zhang et al. 2003; Wu et al. 2011). For example, short-term (3 h) exposure of HL-60 cells to 10 μM BITC followed by culture for 21 h in drug-free media resulted in G2/M phase cell cycle arrest, whereas 24-h continuous treatment predominantly caused arrest in the G1 phase (Zhang et al. 2003). Other investigators have observed G2/M arrest by 24-h BITC treatment in HL-60 cells (Miyoshi et al. 2004a; Jakubikova et al. 2005), which was associated with upregulation of expression of many cell cycle–related genes including p21 (Cip1/Waf1), growth arrest and DNA damage (GADD) 45, and 14-3-3sigma (Miyoshi et al. 2004a). A dose-dependent difference in the phase of cell cycle arrest by BITC treatment was observed in U2OS osteogenic sarcoma cells (Wu et al. 2011). Exposure of Jurkat T leukemia cells to 2.5 and 5 μM BITC for 15 h resulted in inhibition of G2/M progression that coincided with the apoptosis induction (Miyoshi et al. 2004b). The experiment using the phase-specific synchronized cells indicated increased sensitivity to apoptosis in G2/M phase–arrested cells upon treatment with BITC (Miyoshi et al. 2004b). The mechanism by which BITC causes cell cycle arrest is not fully understood, and most studies have relied on changes in cell cycle–related genes or proteins to explain this phenomenon (Miyoshi et al. 2004a; Srivastava and Singh 2004; Xiao et al. 2006; Zhang et al. 2006; Sahu et al. 2009b; Mi et al. 2008, 2011; Huang et al. 2012). However, a handful of studies have attempted to delineate the molecular basis for BITC-induced cell cycle arrest. For example, p38 mitogen-activated protein kinase (MAPK) inhibitor significantly attenuated the accumulation of phosphorylated (inactive) cyclin-dependent kinase 1 (cdk1) protein and the G2/M arrest in Jurkat T leukemia cells (Miyoshi et al. 2004b). The BITC-induced G2/M arrest in BxPC-3 cells was accompanied by a marked decline in the protein levels of cdk1, cyclin B1, and cell division cycle 25B (Cdc25B) (Srivastava and Singh 2004). In MDA-MB-231 and MCF-7 human breast cancer cells, BITC treatment caused a decrease in protein levels of cyclin B1, cdk1, and Cdc25C (Xiao et al. 2006); all these proteins are involved in regulation of G2/M transition (Molinari 2000). Interestingly, a normal mammary epithelial cell line (MCF-10A) was significantly more resistant to cell cycle arrest by BITC, which may partly explain the relative insensitivity of MCF-10A cells to growth suppression by this compound (Xiao et al. 2006). To the contrary, BITC was cytotoxic to MCF-12A cells, which is another human mammary epithelial cell line (Tseng et al. 2004). The molecular basis for the discrepancy in sensitivity of MCF-10A versus MCF-12A cells to cytotoxic effects of BITC is still unclear. In Capan-2 human pancreatic cancer cells, BITC treatment caused phosphorylation of histone H2A.X (H2A.X), suggesting DNA damage and permanent G2/M phase cell cycle arrest (Zhang et al. 2006). The BITC-mediated G2/M arrest in Capan-2 cells was associated with upregulation of cyclin-dependent kinase inhibitor p21 (Waf1/Cip1) and suppression of cyclin B1, cdk1, and Cdc25C protein levels, leading to inhibition of cdk1 kinase activity (Zhang et al. 2006). In a follow-up study, the same group of investigators showed that BITC-induced G2M arrest in Capan-2 cells was significantly attenuated by pretreatment with MAPK kinase (MEK-1) inhibitor but not c-Jun N-terminal kinase (JNK) or p38 MAPK–specific inhibitor (Sahu et al. 2009b). Furthermore, the BITC-mediated G2/M arrest was significantly blocked by NAC or tiron (Sahu et al. 2009b). These results implicated reactive oxygen species (ROS)–dependent activation of extracellular signal–regulated kinase (ERK) in BITC-induced G2/M arrest (Sahu et al. 2009b).

In BxPC-3 cells, pretreatment with BITC increased gamma irradiation–induced G2/M phase arrest in association with DNA damage (Sahu et al. 2009a). The BITC treatment resulted in G2 as well as mitotic arrest in A549 lung cancer cells, which was accompanied by disruption of microtubule polymerization and covalent modification of tubulin (Mi et al. 2008). Selective degradation of alpha- and beta-tubulin by BITC treatment was observed in A549 cells (Mi et al. 2009a). The BITC-induced G2/M arrest in association with inhibition of 26S and 20S proteasome was observed in multiple myeloma cells (Mi et al. 2011). Interestingly, the BITC-mediated inhibition of proteasome was shown to be independent of ROS generation or protein aggregation (Mi et al. 2011). It is reasonable to conclude that both ROS-dependent (Sahu et al. 2009b) and ROS-independent (Mi et al. 2011) mechanisms are engaged in BITC-mediated cell cycle arrest.

24.4.3 Apoptosis Induction

Apoptosis induction is a well-accepted mechanism for the postinitiation anticancer effect of BITC. BITC-induced apoptosis has been documented in cultured (Bonnesen et al. 2001; Tang and Zhang 2004, 2005; Xiao et al. 2006) as well as xenografted cancer cells (Kim et al. 2011; Boreddy et al. 2011a). However, suprapharmacological concentrations of BITC (e.g., 100 µM) may lead to necrotic cell death (Miyoshi et al. 2008). Apoptosis is an evolutionary conserved, complex, and tightly regulated mechanism of cellular suicide to eliminate unwanted cells during development as well as in many pathological conditions (Green 2000; Reed 2001). Two major pathways of apoptosis are well characterized: the mitochondria-mediated intrinsic pathway (mediated by activation of caspase-7 and caspase-9) and the death receptor–mediated extrinsic pathway through activation of caspase-8 (Green and Reed 1998; Ashkenazi and Dixit 1998; Hengartner 2000). Execution of BITC-induced apoptosis likely depends on both mitochondrial and death receptor pathways (Nakamura et al. 2002; Tang and Zhang 2005; Xiao et al. 2006; Basu and Haldar 2009; Liu et al. 2011; Huang et al. 2012). For example, BITC-mediated activation of both caspase-8 and caspase-9 was observed in human bladder (Tang and Zhang 2004) and breast cancer cells (Xiao et al. 2006). On the other hand, BITC-treated ovarian cancer cells exhibited activation of caspase-9 only (Kalkunte et al. 2006). The NAC conjugate of BITC can also trigger apoptosis, at least in bladder cancer cells (Tang et al. 2006). The mechanism by which BITC causes apoptosis has been the topic of intense research in the past decade. Mechanistic observations to explain BITC-induced apoptosis in cancer cells have been reviewed previously (Nakamura 2009). It is now clear that BITC has the ability to target multiple pathways leading to apoptosis induction. The key mechanisms upstream of caspase activation in BITC-induced apoptosis include the following: ROS production due to inhibition of mitochondrial respiration (Nakamura et al. 2002; Xiao et al. 2006, 2008; Wu et al. 2010), MAPK activation (Lui et al. 2003; Sahu et al. 2009b; Yan et al. 2011), MAPK-mediated phosphorylation of B-cell lymphoma 2 (Bcl-2) and B-cell lymphoma extra-large (Bcl-xL) (Miyoshi et al. 2004b; Tang and Zhang 2005; Basu and Haldar 2008), ROS–MAPK–dependent activation of Bax (Xiao et al. 2008), mitochondrial translocation of Bak (Tang and Zhang 2005), disruption of the association between Bcl-xL and both Bak and Bax in the mitochondrial membrane (Tang and Zhang 2005), inhibition of nuclear factor kappaB (NF-κB) (Srivastava and Singh 2004; Wu et al. 2010), inhibition of signal transducer and activator of transcription 3 (STAT3) (Sahu and Srivastava 2009; Hutzen et al. 2009), inhibition of Akt and Forkhead box protein O1 (FOXO1) (Wu et al. 2010; Boreddy et al. 2011a), inhibition of histone deacetylase (Batra et al. 2010), covalent binding to proteins (Mi and Chung 2008), Bid cleavage (Basu and Haldar 2009), selective depletion of mutant p53 but not wild-type p53 (Wang et al. 2011), release of apoptosis inducing factor and endonuclease G (Liu et al. 2011), nitric oxide production (Huang et al. 2012), down-modulation of rat sarcoma GTPase-Activating Protein/ Ras-related C3 botulinum toxin substrate 1 (Basu and Haldar 2009), and suppression of inhibitor of apoptosis–family protein expression (Kim and Singh 2010). The exact relationship between BITC-mediated molecular alterations listed above and apoptosis induction is not entirely clear because of fragmented data. A mechanistic model emerging from systematic investigation from our own laboratory using breast cancer cells predicts ROS-dependent activation of JNK leading to activation of Bax and caspases (Xiao et al. 2006, 2008). This mechanistic model also accommodates MAPK-mediated phosphorylation of Bcl-2 and Bcl-xL, which is expected to cause activation of Bax and Bak (Miyoshi et al. 2004b; Tang and Zhang 2005; Basu and Haldar 2008). On the other hand, Chung and colleagues have proposed an alternate model involving ROS-independent covalent protein binding as an early event in BITC-induced apoptosis (Mi and Chung 2008). The precise mechanism by which protein binding triggers BITC-induced apoptosis is not fully understood. Nevertheless, apoptosis induction seems an important mechanism by which BITC may not only prevent postinitiation cancer development (Warin et al. 2009) but also eliminate cancer cells (Boreddy et al. 2011a; Kim et al. 2011).

24.4.4 AUTOPHAGIC CELL DEATH

Recent studies have implicated ROS in induction of autophagy (Gibson 2010), which is an evolutionary conserved process for bulk degradation of cellular components including organelles (e.g., mitochondria) and considered a valid cancer chemotherapeutic target (Chen and Karantza 2011). We have studied autophagic response to BITC using cultured breast cancer cells (MDA-MB-231, MCF-7, MDA-MB-468, BT-474, and BRI-JM04) and MDA-MB-231 xenografts from control and BITC-treated mice as models (Xiao et al. 2012). The BITC-treated breast cancer cells and MDA-MB-231 xenografts from BITC-treated mice exhibited several features characteristic of autophagy (Xiao et al. 2012). On the other hand, the normal mammary epithelial cell line (MCF-10A) was resistant to BITC-induced autophagy (Xiao et al. 2012). Autophagy induction by BITC contributed to its cytotoxic effect (Xiao et al. 2012). The BITC-induced autophagy was associated with increased expression and acetylation of FOXO1 (Xiao et al. 2012). BITC treatment has been shown to induce formation of aggresome-like structures in HeLa cells (Mi et al. 2009b). Aggresome formation is believed to be a mechanism for removal of unwanted or misfolded proteins through mediation of the ubiquitin–proteasome system (Kopito 2000). Further studies are needed to determine the connection, if any, between BITC-induced autophagy and aggresome-like structure formation. Likewise, it remains to be determined if autophagy induction by BITC is unique to breast cancer cells.

24.4.5 INHIBITION OF ANGIOGENESIS, CELL MIGRATION, AND CELL INVASION

Because angiogenesis is critical not only for tumor growth but also for metastatic spread (Folkman 1971), the antiangiogenic effect of BITC has been examined by several investigators. In MDA-MB-231 xenografts, analysis of the vasculature in the tumors from BITC-treated mice indicated smaller vessel area compared with control tumors based on immunohistochemistry for angiogenesis marker cluster of differentiation 31 (CD31) (Warin et al. 2010). The BITC-mediated inhibition of angiogenesis in vivo correlated with downregulation of vascular endothelial growth factor (VEGF) receptor 2 protein level in the tumor (Warin et al. 2010). Oral BITC treatment reduced hemoglobin content and CD31 and VEGF expression in vivo, as well as circulating levels of VEGF (Kim et al. 2011). The BITC treatment caused a significant reduction in the levels of matrix metalloproteinase 2 (MMP-2) and MMP-9 and downregulated urokinase-type plasminogen activator and plasminogen activator inhibitor-I in breast cancer cells and xenografts (Kim et al. 2011). Inhibition of neovascularization in the rat aorta and chicken chorioallantoic membrane was also shown (Boreddy et al. 2011b).

Inhibition of cancer cell migration and invasion by BITC has been documented in various cancer cell types, including breast (Warin et al. 2010; Kim et al. 2012), colon (Lai et al. 2010), gastric (Ho et al. 2011), and pancreatic cancer cells (Boreddy et al. 2011b). For example, BITC inhibited migration and invasion of BxPC-3 and PanC-1 pancreatic cancer cells in association with suppression of VEGF and MMP-2 levels, reduction in phosphorylation of VEGF receptor (Tyr-1175), and suppression of hypoxia-inducible factor-1α and RhoC (Boreddy et al. 2011b). In another study, BITC was shown to inhibit basal as well as hepatocyte growth factor–induced migration of MDA-MB-231 and 4T1 breast cancer cells (Kim et al. 2012). We have shown recently that BITC inhibits leptin-stimulated migration of breast cancer cells (Kim et al. 2011). Collectively, these results indicate that BITC has the ability to inhibit several steps necessary for cancer metastasis including angiogenesis, cell migration, and cell invasion by affecting multiple pathways.

24.4.6 Inhibition of EMT

The BITC-mediated prevention of mammary cancer development in MMTV-neu mice was associated with a marked increase in levels of E-cadherin protein (Warin et al. 2009). Induction of E-cadherin concomitant with loss of mesenchymal marker proteins (e.g., vimentin) is a biochemical hallmark of EMT reversal (Thiery 2002; Hugo et al. 2007). The EMT is a process by which epithelial cells acquire spindle-shaped morphology, leading to reduced intercellular adhesion but increased motility (Thiery 2002; Hugo et al. 2007). Using MDA-MB-231 cells as a model, we demonstrated BITC-mediated inhibition of EMT (Sehrawat and Singh 2011). The transforming growth factor beta (TGFβ)/tumor necrosis factor alpha (TNFα)–treated MCF-10A cells display higher propensity for migration and cytoskeleton remodeling with actin reorganization. The BITC treatment was able to inhibit cytoskeletal remodeling and formation of actin stress fibers, leading to suppression of TGFβ/TNFα-stimulated cell migration (Sehrawat and Singh 2011). Moreover, the BITC-mediated inhibition of MDA-MB-231 xenograft growth in vivo was associated with a significant increase in protein levels of E-cadherin and suppression of vimentin and fibronectin protein expression (Sehrawat and Singh 2011). The mechanism by which BITC inhibits EMT is still elusive, but this response seems independent of ROS or STAT3 (Sehrawat and Singh, unpublished results). Further investigation is needed to determine if EMT inhibition by BITC is unique to breast cancer cells.

24.4.7 Effect of BITC on microRNA

The microRNA (miR) function as either oncogenes or tumor suppressors and can have multiple target genes (Croce 2009). It was shown very recently that BITC treatment altered the expression of putative miR-221 and miR-375 to switch hyperproliferative cancer cells to a hypoproliferative state in pancreatic adenocarcinoma cells (BxPC-3 and CFPAC-1) (Basu et al. 2011). miR-221 and miR-375 are known to be abnormally expressed in pancreatic cancer patients (Szafranska et al. 2007). Ectopic expression of miR-375 or enforced silencing of miR-221 in cultured pancreatic cancer cells sensitized cells to antiproliferative action of BITC (Basu et al. 2011). Additional work is needed to identify other potential miRNAs targeted by BITC.

24.4.8 Chemotherapy and Radiation Sensitization

BITC has the ability to sensitize cancer cells to chemotherapy and radiation therapy. It was shown to inhibit efflux of anticancer drugs by affecting P-glycoprotein and breast cancer resistance protein (Tseng et al. 2002; Ji and Morris 2004, 2005; Hu and Morris 2004). Pretreatment with BITC resulted in sensitization of BxPC-3 pancreatic cancer cells to gamma radiation–induced cell cycle arrest and apoptosis involving inhibition of NF-κB and activation of p38 MAPK (Sahu et al. 2009a). The BITC increased sensitivity to x-ray in MIAPaCa-2 and PANC-1 pancreatic cancer cells in association with increased apoptosis, suppression of X-linked inhibitor of apoptosis protein, and increase in apoptosis protease activating factor-1 (Ohara et al. 2011). The BITC treatment resulted in sensitization of a panel of pancreatic cancer cells to TNF-related apoptosis-inducing ligand (TRAIL)–induced apoptosis due to dual activation of extrinsic and intrinsic pathways (Wicker et al. 2010). In NCI-H596 non–small-cell lung cancer cells, BITC enhanced the efficacy of cisplatin (Di Pasqua et al. 2010). Neither cellular platinum accumulation nor DNA platination accounted for the increased cytotoxicity (Di Pasqua et al. 2010). However, the in vivo relevance of these cellular findings is still unclear.

24.4.9 SUPPRESSION OF ESTROGEN RECEPTOR α

Estrogen signaling plays an important role in mammary cancer development by increasing the rate of mammary epithelial cell proliferation and differentiation. The growth-promoting function of estrogen is mediated by estrogen receptor α (ERα). BITC treatment significantly inhibited estrogen-stimulated cell growth and suppressed ERα expression in MCF-7 and T-47D breast cancer cells in a dose- and time-dependent manner (Kang et al. 2009). Antiestrogenic activity of BITC is appealing for mammary cancer prevention considering successful clinical application of selective estrogen receptor modulators such as tamoxifen and raloxifene (Fisher et al. 1998; Cauley et al. 2001).

24.5 CONCLUDING REMARKS AND FUTURE DIRECTIONS

Research over the past three decades has provided not only preclinical evidence for the efficacy of BITC for prevention of cancer but also valuable insights into the mechanism of its anticancer effects. Clinical development of BITC as a chemopreventive agent against cancer seems more plausible today mainly because of the knowledge acquired over the past few decades. At the same time, there are a few hurdles in the clinical development of BITC. First, a formulation of pure BITC suitable for clinical investigation is not yet available. Second, pharmacokinetic data for BITC are still lacking. Third, suitable biomarker(s) predictive of response are needed for pilot clinical trials to justify clinical investigations with cancer incidence as the primary end point, which are too expensive, requiring substantial resources and thousands of subjects. Finally, the question of whether BITC-mediated promotion of bladder cancer is unique to rats requires further investigation because this may turn out to be a major impediment in long-term usage of BITC necessary for cancer prevention in high-risk subjects.

ACKNOWLEDGMENT

Work cited from our laboratory was supported by grant CA129347, awarded by the National Cancer Institute.

REFERENCES

Akagi, K., M. Sano, K. Ogawa, M. Hirose, H. Goshima, and T. Shirai. 2003. Involvement of toxicity as an early event in urinary bladder carcinogenesis induced by phenethyl isothiocyanate, benzyl isothiocyanate, and analogues in F344 rats. *Toxicol Pathol* 31:388–96.

Ashkenazi, A., and V.M. Dixit. 1998. Death receptors: signaling and modulation. *Science* 281:1305–8.

Basu, A., and S. Haldar. 2008. Dietary isothiocyanate mediated apoptosis of human cancer cells is associated with Bcl-xL phosphorylation. *Int J Oncol* 33:657–63.

Basu, A., and S. Haldar. 2009. Anti-proliferative and proapoptotic effects of benzyl isothiocyanate on human pancreatic cancer cells is linked to death receptor activation and RasGAP/Rac1 down-modulation. *Int J Oncol* 35:593–9.

Basu, A., H. Alder, A. Khiyami, P. Leahy, C.M. Croce, and S. Haldar. 2011. MicroRNA-375 and MicroRNA-221: Potential noncoding RNAs associated with antiproliferative activity of benzyl isothiocyanate in pancreatic cancer. *Genes Cancer* 2:108–19.

Batra, S., R.P. Sahu, P.K. Kandala, and S.K. Srivastava. 2010. Benzyl isothiocyanate-mediated inhibition of histone deacetylase leads to NF-κB turnoff in human pancreatic carcinoma cells. *Mol Cancer Ther* 9:1596–608.

Benson, A.M., and P.B. Barretto. 1985. Effects of disulfiram, diethyldithiocarbamate, bisethylxanthogen, and benzyl isothiocyanate on glutathione transferase activities in mouse organs. *Cancer Res* 45:4219–23.

Benson, A.M., P.B. Barretto, J.S. Stanley. 1986. Induction of DT-diaphorase by anticarcinogenic sulfur compounds in mice. *J Natl Cancer Inst* 76:467–73.

Bonnesen, C., I.M. Eggleston, J.D. Hayes. 2001. Dietary indoles and isothiocyanates that are generated from cruciferous vegetables can both stimulate apoptosis and confer protection against DNA damage in human colon cell lines. *Cancer Res* 61:6120–30.

Boreddy, S.R., K.C. Pramanik, S.K. Srivastava. 2011a. Pancreatic tumor suppression by benzyl isothiocyanate is associated with inhibition of PI3K/AKT/FOXO pathway. *Clin Cancer Res* 17:1784–95.

Boreddy, S.R., R.P. Sahu, S.K. Srivastava. 2011b. Benzyl isothiocyanate suppresses pancreatic tumor angiogenesis and invasion by inhibiting HIF-α/VEGF/Rho-GTPases: pivotal role of STAT-3. *PLoS ONE* 6:e25799.

Bruggeman, I.M., J.H. Temmink, P.J. van Bladeren. 1986. Glutathione- and cysteine- mediated cytotoxicity of allyl and benzyl isothiocyanate. *Toxicol Appl Pharmacol* 83:349–59.

Brusewitz, G., B.D. Cameron, L.F. Chasseaud et al. 1977. The metabolism of benzyl isothiocyanate and its cysteine conjugate. *Biochem J* 162:99–107.

Callaway, E.C., Y. Zhang, W. Chew, and H. Chow. 2004. Cellular accumulation of dietary anticarcinogenic isothiocyanates is followed by transporter-mediated export as dithiocarbamates. *Cancer Lett* 204:23–31.

Cauley, J.A., L. Norton, M.E. Lippman et al. 2001. Continued breast cancer risk reduction in postmenopausal women treated with raloxifene: 4-year results from the MORE trial. *Breast Cancer Res Treat* 65:125–34.

Cavell, B.E., S.S. Syed Alwi, A. Donlevy, and G. Packham. 2011. Anti-angiogenic effects of dietary isothiocyanates: mechanisms of action and implications for human health. *Biochem Pharmacol* 81:327–36.

Chen, N., and V. Karantza. 2011. Autophagy as a therapeutic target in cancer. *Cancer Biol Ther* 11:157–68.

Chyou, P.H., A.M. Nomura, J.H. Hankin, and G.N. Stemmermann. 1990. A case-cohort study of diet and stomach cancer. *Cancer Res* 50:7501–4.

Conaway, C.C., D. Jiao, and F.L. Chung. 1996. Inhibition of rat liver cytochrome P450 isozymes by isothiocyanates and their conjugates: a structure-activity relationship study. *Carcinogenesis* 17:2423–7.

Conaway, C.C., Y.M. Yang, and F.L. Chung. 2002. Isothiocyanates as cancer chemopreventive agents: their biological activities and metabolism in rodents and humans. *Curr Drug Metab* 3:233–55.

Croce, C.M. 2009. Causes and consequences of microRNA dysregulation in cancer. *Nat Rev Genet* 10:704–14.

Di Pasqua, A.J., C. Hong, M.Y. Wu et al. 2010. Sensitization of non-small cell lung cancer cells to cisplatin by naturally occurring isothiocyanates. *Chem Res Toxicol* 23:1307–9.

Fahey, J.W., A.T. Zalcmann, and P. Talalay. 2001 The chemical diversity and distribution of glucosinolates and isothiocyanates among plants. *Phytochem* 56:5–51.

Fisher, B., J.P. Costantino, D.L. Wickerham et al. 1998. Tamoxifen for prevention of breast cancer: report of the National Surgical Adjuvant Breast and Bowel project P-1 study. *J Natl Cancer Inst* 90:1371–88.

Folkman, J. 1971. Tumor angiogenesis: therapeutic implications. *N Engl J Med* 285:1182–6.

Getahun, S.M., and F.L. Chung. 1999. Conversion of glucosinolates to isothiocyanates in humans after ingestion of cooked watercress. *Cancer Epidemiol Biomarkers Prev* 8:447–51.

Gibson, S.B. 2010. A matter of balance between life and death: targeting reactive oxygen species (ROS)-induced autophagy for cancer therapy. *Autophagy* 6:835–7.

Gonzalez, F.J. 1988. The molecular biology of cytochrome P450s. *Pharmacol Rev* 40:243–88.

Goosen, T.C., D.E. Mills, and P.F. Hollenberg. 2001. Effects of benzyl isothiocyanate on rat and human cytochromes P450: identification of metabolites formed by P450 2B1. *J Pharmacol Exp Ther* 296:198–206.

Goosen, T.C., U.M. Kent, L. Brand, and P.F. Hollenberg. 2000. Inactivation of cytochrome P450 2B1 by benzyl isothiocyanate, a chemopreventative agent from cruciferous vegetables. *Chem Res Toxicol* 13:1349–59.

Gorler, K., G. Krumbiegel, W.H. Mennicke, and H.U. Siehl. 1982. The metabolism of benzyl isothiocyanate and its cysteine conjugate in guinea-pigs and rabbits. *Xenobiotica* 12:535–42.

Green, D.R. 2000. Apoptotic pathways: paper wraps stone blunts scissors. *Cell* 102:1–4.

Green, D.R., and J.C. Reed. 1998. Mitochondria and apoptosis. *Science* 281:1309–12.

Guo, Z., T.J. Smith, H. Ishizaki, and C.S. Yang. 1991. Metabolism of 4-(methylnitrosamino)-1-(3-pyridyl)-1-butanone (NNK) by cytochrome P450IIB1 in a reconstituted system. *Carcinogenesis* 12:2277–82.

Hasegawa, T.H., Nishino, and A. Iwashima. 1993. Isothiocyanates inhibit cell cycle progression of HeLa cells at G2/M phase. *Anticancer Drugs* 4:273–9.

Hayes, J.D., and D.J. Pulford. 1995. The glutathione *S*-transferase supergene family: regulation of GST* and the contribution of the isoenzymes to cancer chemoprotection and drug resistance. *Crit Rev Biochem Mol Biol* 30:445–600.

Hecht, S.S. 2000. Inhibition of carcinogenesis by isothiocyanates. *Drug Metab Rev* 32:395–411.

Hecht, S.S., P.M. Kenney, M. Wang, and P. Upadhyaya. 2002. Benzyl isothiocyanate: an effective inhibitor of polycyclic aromatic hydrocarbon tumorigenesis in A/J mouse lung. *Cancer Lett* 187:87–94.

Hecht, S.S., P.M. Kenney, M. Wang, N. Trushin, and P. Upadhyaya. 2000. Effects of phenethyl isothiocyanate and benzyl isothiocyanate, individually and in combination, on lung tumorigenesis induced in A/J mice by benzo[a]pyrene and 4-(methylnitrosamino)-1-(3-pyridyl)-1-butanone. *Cancer Lett* 150:49–56.

Hengartner, M.O. 2000. The biochemistry of apoptosis. *Nature* 407:770–6.

Hirose, M., T. Yamaguchi, N. Kimoto et al. 1998. Strong promoting activity of phenylethyl isothiocyanate and benzyl isothiocyanate on urinary bladder carcinogenesis in F344 male rats. *Int J Cancer* 77:773–7.

Ho, C.C., K.C. Lai, S.C. Hsu et al. 2011. Benzyl isothiocyanate (BITC) inhibits migration and invasion of human gastric cancer AGS cells via suppressing ERK signal pathways. *Hum Exp Toxicol* 30:296–306.

Hu, K., and M.E. Morris. 2004. Effects of benzyl-, phenethyl-, and alpha-naphthyl isothiocyanates on P-glycoprotein- and MRP1-mediated transport. *J Pharm Sci* 93:1901–11.

Huang, S.H., L.W. Wu, A.C. Huang et al. 2012. Benzyl isothiocyanate (BITC) induces G$_2$/M phase arrest and apoptosis in human melanoma A375.S2 cells through ROS and both mitochondria-dependent and death receptor-mediated multiple signaling pathways. *J Agric Food Chem* 60:665–75.

Hugo, H., M.L. Ackland, T. Blick et al. 2007. Epithelial-mesenchymal and mesenchymal-epithelial transitions in carcinoma progression. *J Cell Physiol* 213:374–83.

Hutzen, B., W. Willis, S. Jones et al. 2009. Dietary agent, benzyl isothiocyanate inhibits signal transducer and activator of transcription 3 phosphorylation and collaborates with sulforaphane in the growth suppression of PANC-1 cancer cells. *Cancer Cell Int* 9:24.

Jakubikova, J., Y. Bao, and J. Sedlak. 2005. Isothiocyanates induce cell cycle arrest, apoptosis and mitochondrial potential depolarization in HL-60 and multidrug-resistant cell lines. *Anticancer Res* 25:3375–86.

Ji, Y., and M.E. Morris. 2005. Membrane transport of dietary phenethyl isothiocyanate by ABCG2 (breast cancer resistance protein). *Mol Pharm* 2:414–9.

Ji, Y., and M.E. Morris. 2004. Effect of organic isothiocyanates on breast cancer resistance protein (ABCG2)-mediated transport. *Pharm Res* 21:2261–9.

Kalkunte, S., N. Swamy, D.S. Dizon, and L. Brard. 2006. Benzyl isothiocyanate (BITC) induces apoptosis in ovarian cancer cells in vitro. *J Exp Ther Oncol* 5:287–300.

Kang, L., L. Ding, and Z.Y. Wang. 2009. Isothiocyanates repress estrogen receptor alpha expression in breast cancer cells. *Oncol Rep* 21:185–92.

Kassie, F., B. Pool-Zobel, W. Parzefall, and S. Knasmüller. 1999. Genotoxic effects of benzyl isothiocyanate, a natural chemopreventive agent. *Mutagenesis* 14:595–604.

Keum, Y.S., W.S. Jeong, and A.N. Kong. 2004. Chemoprevention by isothiocyanates and their underlying molecular signaling mechanisms. *Mutat Res* 555:191–202.

Kim, E.J., S.J. Eom, J.E. Hong, J.Y. Lee, M.S. Choi, and J.H. Park. 2012. Benzyl isothiocyanate inhibits basal and hepatocyte growth factor-stimulated migration of breast cancer cells. *Mol Cell Biochem* 359:431–40.

Kim, E.J., J.E. Hong, S.J. Eom, J.Y. Lee, and J.H. Park. 2011. Oral administration of benzyl- isothiocyanate inhibits solid tumor growth and lung metastasis of 4T1 murine mammary carcinoma cells in BALB/c mice. *Breast Cancer Res Treat* 130:61–71.

Kim, S.H., and S.V. Singh. 2010. p53-Independent apoptosis by benzyl isothiocyanate in human breast cancer cells is mediated by suppression of XIAP expression. *Cancer Prev Res* 3:718–26.

Kim, S.H., A. Nagalingam, N.K. Saxena, S.V. Singh, and D. Sharma. 2011. Benzyl isothiocyanate inhibits oncogenic actions of leptin in human breast cancer cells by suppressing activation of signal transducer and activator of transcription 3. *Carcinogenesis* 32:359–67.

Kolonel, L.N., J.H. Hankin, A.S. Whittemore et al. 2000. Vegetables, fruits, legumes and prostate cancer: a multiethnic case-control study. *Cancer Epidemiol Biomarkers Prev* 9:795–804.

Kopito, R.R. 2000. Aggresomes, inclusion bodies and protein aggregation. *Trends Cell Biol* 10:524–30.

Kumar, A., and G. Sabbioni. 2010. New biomarkers for monitoring the levels of isothiocyanates in humans. *Chem Res Toxicol* 23:756–65.

Kuroiwa, Y., A. Nishikawa, Y. Kitamura et al. 2006. Protective effects of benzyl isothiocyanate and sulforaphane but not resveratrol against initiation of pancreatic carcinogenesis in hamsters. *Cancer Lett* 241:275–80.

Lai, K.C., A.C. Huang, S.C. Hsu et al. 2010. Benzyl isothiocyanate (BITC) inhibits migration and invasion of human colon cancer HT29 cells by inhibiting matrix metalloproteinase-2/-9 and urokinase plasminogen (uPA) through PKC and MAPK signaling pathway. *J Agric Food Chem* 58:2935–42.

Lin, J.M., S. Amin, N. Trushin, and S.S. Hecht. 1993. Effects of isothiocyanates on tumorigenesis by benzo[a] pyrene in murine tumor models. *Cancer Lett* 74:151–9.

Liu, K.C., Y.T. Huang, P.P. Wu et al. 2011. The roles of AIF and Endo G in the apoptotic effects of benzyl isothiocyanate on DU 145 human prostate cancer cells via the mitochondrial signaling pathway. *Int J Oncol* 38:787–96.

Lui, V.W., A.L. Wentzel, D. Xiao, K.L. Lew, S.V. Singh, and J.R. Grandis. 2003. Requirement of a carbon spacer in benzyl isothiocyanate-mediated cytotoxicity and MAPK activation in head and neck squamous cell carcinoma. *Carcinogenesis* 24:1705–12.

Mennicke, W.H., K. Gorler, G. Krumbiegel, D. Lorenz, and N. Rittman. 1988. Studies on the metabolism and excretion of benzyl isothiocyanate in man. *Xenobiotica* 18:441–7.

Mi, L., and F.L. Chung. 2008. Binding to protein by isothiocyanates: a potential mechanism for apoptosis induction in human non-small lung cancer cells. *Nutr Cancer* 60(suppl.)1:12–20.

Mi, L., N. Gan, and F.L. Chung. 2011. Isothiocyanates inhibit proteasome activity and proliferation of multiple myeloma cells. *Carcinogenesis* 32:216–23.

Mi, L., N. Gan, A. Cheema et al. 2009a. Cancer preventive isothiocyanates induce selective degradation of cellular alpha- and beta-tubulins by proteasomes. *J Biol Chem* 284:17039–51.

Mi, L., N. Gan, and F.L. Chung. 2009b. Aggresome-like structure induced by isothiocyanates is novel proteasome-dependent degradation machinery. *Biochem Biophys Res Commun* 388:456–62.

Mi, L., Z. Xiao, B.L. Hood et al. 2008. Covalent binding to tubulin by isothiocyanates. A mechanism of cell growth arrest and apoptosis. *J Biol Chem* 283:22136–46.

Michaud D.S., D. Spiegelman, S.K. Clinton, E.B. Rimm, W.C. Willett, and E.L. Giovannucci. 1999. Fruit and vegetable intake and incidence of bladder cancer in a male prospective cohort. *J Natl Cancer Inst* 91:605–13.

Miyoshi, N., E. Watanabe, T. Osawa et al. 2008. ATP depletion alters the mode of cell death induced by benzyl isothiocyanate. *Biochim Biophys Acta* 1782:566–73.

Miyoshi, N., K. Uchida, T. Osawa, and Y. Nakamura. 2007. Selective cytotoxicity of benzyl isothiocyanate in the proliferating fibroblastoid cells. *Int J Cancer* 120:484–92.

Miyoshi, N., K. Uchida, T. Osawa, and Y. Nakamura. 2004a. Benzyl isothiocyanate modifies expression of the G_2/M arrest-related genes. *Biofactors* 21:23–6.

Miyoshi, N., K. Uchida, T. Osawa, and Y. Nakamura. 2004b. A link between benzyl isothiocyanate-induced cell cycle arrest and apoptosis: involvement of mitogen-activated protein kinases in the Bcl-2 phosphorylation. *Cancer Res* 64:2134–42.

Molinari, M. 2000. Cell cycle checkpoints and their inactivation in human cancer. *Cell Prolif* 33:261–74.

Moreno, R.L., T. Goosen, U.M. Kent, F.L. Chung, and P.F. Hollenberg. 2001. Differential effects of naturally occurring isothiocyanates on the activities of cytochrome P450 2E1 and the mutant P450 2E1 T303A. *Arch Biochem Biophys* 391:99–110.

Moreno, R.L., U.M. Kent, K. Hodge, and P.F. Hollenberg. 1999. Inactivation of cytochrome P450 2E1 by benzyl isothiocyanate. *Chem Res Toxicol* 12:582–7.

Morse, M.A., J.C. Reinhardt, S.G, Amin, S.S. Hecht, G.D. Stoner, and F.L. Chung. 1990. Effect of dietary aromatic isothiocyanates fed subsequent to the administration of 4- (methylnitrosamino)-1-(3-pyridyl)-1-butanone on lung tumorigenicity in mice. *Cancer Lett* 49:225–30.

Morse, M.A., S.G. Amin, S.S. Hecht, and F.L. Chung. 1989. Effects of aromatic isothiocyanates on tumorigenicity, O6-methylguanine formation, and metabolism of the tobacco-specific nitrosamine 4-(methylnitrosamino)-1-(3-pyridyl)-1-butanone in A/J mouse lung. *Cancer Res* 49:2894–7.

Moy, K.A., J.M. Yuan, F.L. Chung et al. 2008 Urinary total isothiocyanates and colorectal cancer: a prospective study of men in Shanghai, China. *Cancer Epidemiol Biomarkers Prev* 17:1354–59.

Musk, S.R., and I.T. Johnson. 1993. The clastogenic effects of isothiocyanates. *Mutat Res* 300:111–7.

Musk, S.R., S.B. Astley, S.M. Edwards, P. Stephenson, R.B. Hubert, and I.T. Johnson. 1995. Cytotoxic and clastogenic effects of benzyl isothiocyanate towards cultured mammalian cells. *Food Chem Toxicol* 33:31–7.

Nakamura, Y. 2009. Chemoprevention by isothiocyanates: molecular basis of apoptosis induction. *Forum Nutr* 61:170–81.

Nakamura, Y., H. Ohigashi, S. Masuda et al. 2000. Redox regulation of glutathione S-transferase induction by benzyl isothiocyanate: correlation of enzyme induction with the formation of reactive oxygen intermediates. *Cancer Res* 60:219–25.

Nakamura, Y., M. Kawakami, A. Yoshihiro et al. 2002. Involvement of the mitochondrial death pathway in chemopreventive benzyl isothiocyanate-induced apoptosis. *J Biol Chem* 277:8492–9.

Odom, R.Y., M.Y. Dansby, M.A. Rollins-Hairston, K.M. Jackson, and W.G. Kirlin. 2009. Phytochemical induction of cell cycle arrest by glutathione oxidation and reversal by N-acetylcysteine in human colon carcinoma cells. *Nutr Cancer* 61:332–9.

Ohara, M., S. Kimura, A. Tanaka, K. Ohnishi, R. Okayasu, and N. Kubota. 2011. Benzyl isothiocyanate sensitizes human pancreatic cancer cells to radiation by inducing apoptosis. *Int J Mol Med* 28:1043–7.

Okazaki, K., T. Umemura, T. Imazawa, A. Nishikawa, T. Masegi, and M. Hirose. 2003. Enhancement of urinary bladder carcinogenesis by combined treatment with benzyl isothiocyanate and N-butyl-N-(4-hydroxybutyl)nitrosamine in rats after initiation. *Cancer Sci* 94:948–52.

Okazaki, K., M. Yamagishi, H.Y. Son et al. 2002. Simultaneous treatment with benzyl isothiocyanate, a strong bladder promoter, inhibits rat urinary bladder carcinogenesis by N-butyl-N-(4-hydroxybutyl)nitrosamine. *Nutr Cancer* 42:211–6.

Pan, S.Y., A.M. Ugnat, Y. Mao et al. 2004. A case-control study of diet and the risk of ovarian cancer. *Cancer Epidemiol Biomarkers Prev* 13:1521–7.

Powolny, A.A., A. Bommareddy, E.R. Hahm et al. 2011. Chemopreventative potential of the cruciferous vegetable constituent phenethyl isothiocyanate in a mouse model of prostate cancer. *J Natl Cancer Inst* 103:571–84.

Reed, J.C. 2001. Apoptosis-regulating proteins as targets for drug discovery. *Trends Mol Med* 7:314–9.

Sahu, R.P., and S.K. Srivastava. 2009. The role of STAT-3 in the induction of apoptosis in pancreatic cancer cells by benzyl isothiocyanate. *J Natl Cancer Inst* 101:176–93.

Sahu, R.P., M.W. Epperly, and S.K. Srivastava. 2009a. Benzyl isothiocyanate sensitizes human pancreatic cancer cells to radiation therapy. *Front Biosci* 1:568–76.

Sahu, R.P., R. Zhang, S. Batra, Y. Shi, and S.K. Srivastava. 2009b. Benzyl isothiocyanate-mediated generation of reactive oxygen species causes cell cycle arrest and induces apoptosis via activation of MAPK in human pancreatic cancer cells. *Carcinogenesis* 30:1744–53.

Sehrawat, A., and S.V. Singh. 2011. Benzyl isothiocyanate inhibits epithelial-mesenchymal transition in cultured and xenografted human breast cancer cells. *Cancer Prev Res* 4:1107–17.

Shapiro, T.A., J.W. Fahey, K.L. Wade, K.K. Stephenson, and P. Talalay. 2001. Chemoprotective glucosinolates and isothiocyanates of broccoli sprouts: metabolism and excretion in humans. *Cancer Epidemiol Biomarkers Prev* 10:501–8.

Singh, S.V., R. Warin, D. Xiao et al. 2009. Sulforaphane inhibits prostate carcinogenesis and pulmonary metastasis in TRAMP mice in association with increased cytotoxicity of natural killer cells. *Cancer Res* 69:2117–25.

Smith, T.J. 2001. Mechanisms of carcinogenesis inhibition by isothiocyanates. *Expert Opin Investig Drugs* 10:2167–74.

Srivastava, S.K., and S.V. Singh. 2004. Cell cycle arrest, apoptosis induction and inhibition of nuclear factor kappa B activation in anti-proliferative activity of benzyl isothiocyanate against human pancreatic cancer cells. *Carcinogenesis* 25:1701–9.

Steinmetz, K.A., J.D. Potter, and A.R. Folsom. 1993. Vegetables, fruit, and lung cancer in the Iowa Women's Health Study. *Cancer Res* 53:536–43.

Sticha, K.R., P.M. Kenney, G. Boysen et al. 2002. Effects of benzyl isothiocyanate and phenethyl isothiocyanate on DNA adduct formation by a mixture of benzo[a]pyrene and 4- (methylnitrosamino)-1-(3-pyridyl)-1-butanone in A/J mouse lung. *Carcinogenesis* 23:1433–9.

Sticha, K.R., M.E. Staretz, M. Wang, H. Liang, P.M. Kenney, and S.S. Hecht. 2000. Effects of benzyl isothiocyanate and phenethyl isothiocyanate on benzo[a]pyrene metabolism and DNA adduct formation in the A/J mouse. *Carcinogenesis* 21:1711–9.

Sugie, S., K. Okamoto, A. Okumura, T. Tanaka, and H. Mori. 1994. Inhibitory effects of benzyl thiocyanate and benzyl isothiocyanate on methylazoxymethanol acetate-induced intestinal carcinogenesis in rats. *Carcinogenesis* 15:1555–60.

Sugie, S., A. Okumura, T. Tanaka, and H. Mori. 1993. Inhibitory effects of benzyl isothiocyanate and benzyl thiocyanate on diethylnitrosamine-induced hepatocarcinogenesis in rats. *Jpn J Cancer Res* 84:865–70.

Szafranska, A.E., T.S. Davison, J. John et al. 2007. MicroRNA expression alterations are linked to tumorigenesis and non-neoplastic processes in pancreatic ductal adenocarcinoma. *Oncogene* 26:4442–52.

Talalay, P., H.J. Prochaska, and S.R. Spencer. 1990. Regulation of enzymes that detoxify the electrophilic forms of chemical carcinogens. *Princess Takamatsu Symp* 21:177–87.

Tang, L., and Y. Zhang. 2005. Mitochondria are the primary target in isothiocyanate-induced apoptosis in human bladder cancer cells. *Mol Cancer Ther* 4:1250–9.

Tang, L., and Y. Zhang. 2004. Dietary isothiocyanates inhibit the growth of human bladder carcinoma cells. *J Nutr* 134:2004–10.

Tang, L., G.R. Zirpoli, K. Guru et al. 2010. Intake of cruciferous vegetables modifies bladder cancer survival. *Cancer Epidemiol Biomarkers Prev* 19:1806–11.

Tang, L., G.R. Zirpoli, K. Guru et al. 2008. Consumption of raw cruciferous vegetables is inversely associated with bladder cancer risk. *Cancer Epidemiol Biomarkers Prev* 17:938–44.

Tang, L., G. Li, L. Song, and Y. Zhang. 2006. The principal urinary metabolites of dietary isothiocyanates, N-acetylcysteine conjugates, elicit the same anti-proliferative response as their parent compounds in human bladder cancer cells. *Anticancer Drugs* 17:297–305.

Thiery, J.P. 2002. Epithelial-mesenchymal transitions in tumour progression. *Nat Rev Cancer* 2:442–54.

Tseng, E., E.A. Scott-Ramsay, and M.E. Morris. 2004. Dietary organic isothiocyanates are cytotoxic in human breast cancer MCF-7 and mammary epithelial MCF-12A cell lines. *Exp Biol Med* 229:835–42.

Tseng, E., A. Kamath, and M.E. Morris. 2002. Effect of organic isothiocyanates on the P-glycoprotein- and MRP1-mediated transport of daunomycin and vinblastine. *Pharm Res* 19:1509–15.

Tsou, M.F., C.T. Peng, M.C. Shih et al. 2009. Benzyl isothiocyanate inhibits murine WEHI-3 leukemia cells in vitro and promotes phagocytosis in BALB/c mice *in vivo. Leukemia Res* 33:1505–11.

Visanji, J.M., S.J. Duthie, L. Pirie, D.G. Thompson, and P.J. Padfield. 2004. Dietary isothiocyanates inhibit Caco-2 cell proliferation and induce G2/M phase cell cycle arrest, DNA damage, and G_2/M checkpoint activation. *J Nutr* 134:3121–6.

von Weymarn, L.B., J.A. Chun, and P.F. Hollenberg. 2006. Effects of benzyl and phenethyl isothiocyanate on P450s 2A6 and 2A13: potential for chemoprevention in smokers. *Carcinogenesis* 27:782–90.

Wang, X., A.J. Di Pasqua, S. Govind et al. 2011. Selective depletion of mutant p53 by cancer chemopreventive isothiocyanates and their structure-activity relationships. *J Med Chem* 54:809–16.

Warin, R., D. Xiao, J.A. Arlotti, A. Bommareddy, and S.V. Singh. 2010. Inhibition of human breast cancer xenograft growth by cruciferous vegetable constituent benzyl isothiocyanate. *Mol Carcinog* 49:500–7.

Warin, R., W.H. Chambers, D.M. Potter, and S.V. Singh. 2009. Prevention of mammary carcinogenesis in MMTV-neu mice by cruciferous vegetable constituent benzyl isothiocyanate. *Cancer Res* 69:9473–80.

Wattenberg, L.W. 1987. Inhibitory effects of benzyl isothiocyanate administered shortly before diethylnitrosamine or benzo[a]pyrene on pulmonary and forestomach neoplasia in A/J mice. *Carcinogenesis* 8:1971–3.

Wattenberg, L.W. 1981. Inhibition of carcinogen-induced neoplasia by sodium cyanate, tert-butyl isocyanate, and benzyl isothiocyanate administered subsequent to carcinogen exposure. *Cancer Res* 41:2991–4.

Wattenberg, L.W. 1977. Inhibition of carcinogenic effects of polycyclic hydrocarbons by benzyl isothiocyanate and related compounds. *J Natl Cancer Inst* 58:395–8.

Wicker, C.A., R.P. Sahu, K. Kulkarni-Datar, S.K. Srivastava, and T.L. Brown. 2010. BITC sensitizes pancreatic adenocarcinomas to TRAIL-induced apoptosis. *Cancer Growth Metastasis* 2009(2):45–55.

Wilkinson, J.T., M.A. Morse, L.A. Kresty, and G.D. Stoner. 1995. Effect of alkyl chain length on inhibition of N-nitrosomethylbenzylamine-induced esophageal tumorigenesis and DNA methylation by isothiocyanates. *Carcinogenesis* 16:1011–5.

Wu, C.L., A.C. Huang, J.S. Yang et al. 2011. Benzyl isothiocyanate (BITC) and phenethyl isothiocyanate (PEITC)-mediated generation of reactive oxygen species causes cell cycle arrest and induces apoptosis via activation of caspase-3, mitochondria dysfunction and nitric oxide (NO) in human osteogenic sarcoma U-2 OS cells. *J Orthop Res* 29:1199–209.

Wu, X., Q.H. Zhou, and K. Xu. 2009. Are isothiocyanates potential anti-cancer drugs? *Acta Pharmacol Sin* 30:501–12.

Wu, X., Y. Zhu, H. Yan et al. 2010. Isothiocyanates induce oxidative stress and suppress the metastasis potential of human non-small cell lung cancer cells. *BMC Cancer* 10:269.

Xiao, D., A. Bommareddy, S.H. Kim et al. 2012. Benzyl isothiocyanate causes FOXO1-mediated autophagic death in human breast cancer cells. *PLoS ONE* 7:e32597.

Xiao, D., A.A. Powolny, and S.V. Singh. 2008. Benzyl isothiocyanate targets mitochondrial respiratory chain to trigger reactive oxygen species-dependent apoptosis in human breast cancer cells. *J Biol Chem* 283:30151–63.

Xiao, D., V. Vogel, and S.V. Singh. 2006. Benzyl isothiocyanate-induced apoptosis in human breast cancer cells is initiated by reactive oxygen species and regulated by Bax and Bak. *Mol Cancer Ther* 5:2931–45.

Yan, H., Y. Zhu, B. Liu et al. 2011. Mitogen-activated protein kinase mediates the apoptosis of highly metastatic human non-small cell lung cancer cells induced by isothiocyanates. *Br J Nutr* 106:1779–91.

Yang, Y.M., C.C. Conaway, J.W. Chiao et al. 2002. Inhibition of benzo(a)pyrene-induced lung tumorigenesis in A/J mice by dietary N-acetylcysteine conjugates of benzyl and phenethyl isothiocyanates during the postinitiation phase is associated with activation of mitogen- activated protein kinases and p53 activity and induction of apoptosis. *Cancer Res* 62:2–7.

Ye, L., and Y. Zhang. 2001. Total intracellular accumulation levels of dietary isothiocyanates determine their activity in elevation of cellular glutathione and induction of Phase 2 detoxification enzymes. *Carcinogenesis* 22:1987–92.

Zhang, R., S. Loganathan, I. Humphreys, and S.K. Srivastava. 2006. Benzyl isothiocyanate-induced DNA damage causes G_2/M cell cycle arrest and apoptosis in human pancreatic cancer cells. *J Nutr* 136: 2728–34.

Zhang, Y. 2000. Role of glutathione in the accumulation of anticarcinogenic isothiocyanates and their glutathione conjugates by murine hepatoma cells. *Carcinogenesis* 21:1175–82.

Zhang, Y., L. Tang, and V. Gonzalez. 2003. Selected isothiocyanates rapidly induce growth inhibition of cancer cells. *Mol Cancer Ther* 2:1045–52.

Zhang, Y., R.H. Kolm, B. Mannervik, and P. Talalay. 1995. Reversible conjugation of isothiocyanates with glutathione catalyzed by human glutathione transferases. *Biochem Biophys Res Commun* 206:748–55.

25 Suppression of Prostate Carcinogenesis by Dietary Isothiocyanates

Young-Sam Keum

CONTENTS

25.1 INTRODUCTION

Prostate cancer represents the most commonly diagnosed types of cancer and provides a major clinical and public health challenge (Stokes et al. 2010). In 2010, approximately 217,730 men are expected to be diagnosed with prostate cancer, and 32,050 prostate cancer-related deaths are predicted to occur in the United States (Jemal et al. 2009). Currently, prostate cancer is the second-leading cause of cancer-related mortality in American males, next only to lung cancer (Jemal et al. 2009). However, it should be noted that prostate cancer is a preventable disease. This belief is based on the facts that (1) prostate carcinogenesis is composed of three distinct stages (initiation, promotion, and progression), some of which can be halted or even reversed by maintaining a healthy lifestyle or conducting appropriate medical treatments, and (2) prostate tumor formation takes a considerable time to occur, which is well supported by many clinical observations that prostate cancer is hardly found in men under age 50, but the prostatic intraepithelial neoplasia (PIN) lesion, a predictive biomarker of prostate cancers, is often found at autopsy in men under age 30. Chemoprevention is a clinical strategy to inhibit, delay, or reverse carcinogenesis, using naturally occurring or synthetic chemical agents. Indeed, it is estimated that formation of most types of cancers in humans, including prostate cancer, is attributable to environmental risk factors, such as noxious chemicals, occupational irradiations, and tumor-causing viruses. The notion that formation of human cancers is affected by environmental factors, combined with genetic susceptibility, offers great optimism for chemoprevention, since most cancer-causing substances are produced and introduced into the environment by human activities. Therefore, eliminating carcinogens or at least avoiding them in the environment can reduce the incidence of cancer.

On the other hand, an alternative and more proactive way of chemoprevention is to find out the chemical agents that can suppress or halt the carcinogenic processes. Because of the expected safety due to long-term administration, our diet has been considered as a great source of chemopreventive agents. Accumulating evidence indicates that consumption of fruits or vegetables gives significant protection against formation and progression of various types of cancer. In particular, the vegetables of the Cruciferase family, also known as cruciferous vegetables, are abundant in local supermarkets and have garnered scientific interest as a source of potential chemopreventive agents. Good examples of natural cruciferous vegetables include broccoli, watercress, brussels sprouts, cabbage, and cauliflower. The bioactive food compounds in dietary cruciferous vegetables to provide protection against prostate carcinogenesis have been identified as isothiocyanates (ITCs). Glucosinolates (also known by the trivial names sinigrin and sinalbin) are chemical precursors of ITCs in cruciferous vegetables. To date, more than 100 structurally distinct glucosinolates have been identified predominantly, but not exclusively, from a variety of cruciferous vegetables (Fahey et al. 2001). However, the types of popular edible cruciferous vegetables are limited, and therefore, chemopreventive activities of selected natural ITCs have been evaluated in the experimental settings thus far. Good examples of such ITCs include allyl isothiocyanate (AITC) from cabbage, mustard, and horseradish; benzyl isothiocyanate (BITC) and phenethyl isothiocyanate (PEITC) from watercress; sulforaphane from broccoli and broccoli sprouts; erucin from daikon; and so forth.

25.2 INDUCTION OF Nrf2 PROTEIN AND PHASE II CYTOPROTECTIVE ENZYMES BY DIETARY ITCs

Normal cells are transformed after repeated exposure to carcinogens and ultimately assume carcinogenic properties, a process referred to as transformation. In fact, tumor cells are regarded as a collection of neoplastic cells that were transformed after a series of critical somatic mutations and then clonally expanded. Therefore, it is conceivable that an induction of phase II cytoprotective enzymes, such as glutathione S-transferase (GST), NAD[P]H:quinone reductase (NQO1), γ-glutamylcysteine synthetase (γ-GCS), and hemoxygenase 1 (HO-1), will play a significant role in protecting normal cells against the toxic and carcinogenic effects of detrimental electrophiles and oxidants. Biochemical studies have confirmed that transcriptional regulation of these enzymes is coordinated, in large part, by the antioxidant response element (ARE), a common nucleotide motif sequence that is found in the 5′-upstream promoter region of phase II cytoprotective enzymes (Kensler et al. 2007). NF-E2-related factor 2 (Nrf2) is a transcription factor that is sequestered in the cytosol. In response to extracellular stresses, however, it translocates into the nucleus and induces a battery of phase II cytoprotective enzymes by binding to ARE sequences in association with other coactivators or corepressor proteins (Itoh et al. 1997). Nrf2 is a basic leucine zipper protein and contains a Cap'n'Collar (CNC) structure, which is defined by the presence of a conserved 43–amino acid motif (Sykiotis and Bohmann 2010). While most CNC transcription factors are transcriptional activators, some can behave as transcriptional suppressors when naturally truncated or cleaved by caspases (Motohashi et al. 2002; Ohtsubo et al. 1999).

Domain analysis has revealed that the Nrf2 protein is composed of six highly conserved domains, so called Nrf2-ECH homology (Neh) domains (Figure 25.1, upper panel). The Neh1 domain contains

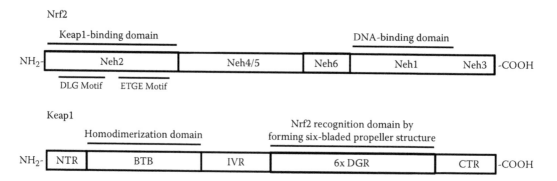

FIGURE 25.1 Domain architecture of Nrf2 and Keap1 proteins.

a basic leucine zipper (bZIP) motif and is responsible for binding to the DNA. The Neh3 domain, located mostly in the C-terminal region, plays a permissive role of transactivation of Nrf2, and the tandem of Neh4 and Neh5 domains is essential for Nrf2 transactivation. The Neh6 domain is necessary for Nrf2 protein degradation. On the other hand, the Neh2 domain, located mostly in the N-terminal region, acts as a negative regulatory domain. By using a Gal4–Neh2 fusion protein as bait in a yeast two-hybrid assay, Itoh et al. (1999) have identified multiple clones for a single protein. A close inspection of this newly identified cDNA illustrated the presence of two unusual protein interaction motifs: a broad-complex, tramtrack, and bric-a-brac (BTB) domain and a double glycine repeat (DGR). A database search for proteins harboring both motifs has revealed that it is the characteristic of the *Drosophila* cytoskeleton-binding protein, Kelch, and this newly identified protein was thus named Kelch-like ECH-associated protein 1 (Keap1). Keap1 consists of five different domains: an amino-terminal region (NTR); a broad complex, tramtrack, and BTB; an intervening region (IVR); six Kelch/ DGRs; and a carboxyl terminal region (CTR) (Figure 25.1, lower panel). Keap1 is a cytosolic protein, and its subcellular location seems to be mediated, at least in part, by binding to a cytoplasmic actin or myosin VIIa through the DGR domain (Kang et al. 2004). Now, it is well established that Keap1 is a key cytosolic anchor protein that sequesters Nrf2 in the cytoplasm and releases it in the cytoplasm, when the induction of phase II cytoprotective enzymes is necessary in response to electrophiles or oxidants.

Consumption of ITCs inhibits carcinogenesis in vivo through a variety of biochemical mechanisms of action (Clarke et al. 2008). In particular, ITCs are strong chemical inducers of phase II cytoprotective enzymes. A coordinated induction of phase II cytoprotective enzymes by ITCs is very rapid and transcriptionally regulated by Nrf2 protein (Thimmulappa et al. 2002). There exist numerous in vivo animal studies showing that Nrf2 is an essential transcription factor for the induction of phase II cytoprotective enzymes. Mice lacking the *Nrf2* gene exhibit greater susceptibility to oxidant and electrophile stresses (Ramos-Gomez et al. 2001). Homozygous disruption of *Nrf2* in mice also abrogated the inducible expression of GST and NQO1 by butylated hydroxyanisole (BHA) in the liver and intestine (Itoh et al. 1997). Likewise, primary Nrf2 (–/–) mouse embryonic fibroblasts (MEFs) failed to exhibit an induction of HO-1 protein, a phase II cytoprotective enzyme, in response to treatment with various ITCs (Keum et al. 2006; Prawan et al. 2008). Together, these facts suggest that the chemopreventive activities of ITCs could be mediated, in large part, by the induction of phase II cytoprotective enzymes through transcriptional activation of Nrf2. Accumulating evidence indicates that the regulation of Nrf2 expression in cells is not transcriptionally regulated but achieved by an elegant posttranslational modification, for example, polyubiquitination (McMahon et al. 2003). Follow-up studies have identified that Keap1 serves as a substrate linker protein for interaction of Cul3-based E3 ligase complex with Nrf2, resulting in a continuous polyubiquitination and its degradation of Nrf2. Therefore, the current biochemical model depicting Keap1–Nrf2 interactions is as follows. Nrf2 protein is constantly polyubiquitinated and degraded in the cytoplasm under basal conditions. In response to treatment with ITCs, degradation of Nrf2 protein is halted, which makes it stable and free to translocate into the nucleus, thereby activating target genes by binding to ARE. So far, the Keap1–Nrf2 pathway seems to regulate more than 100 genes, including phase II cytoprotective genes and antioxidant systems that can balance high levels of reactive oxygen species (ROS) (Kensler et al. 2007).

Biophysical analyses have indicated that the in vitro binding ratio between Keap1 and Nrf2 proteins is 2:1. As such, two Keap1 proteins employ individual DGR regions to recognize two primary sequences, for example, the ETGE and DLG motifs, located in the Neh2 domain of a single Nrf2 protein, by forming a six-bladed propeller structure. The Keap1 proteins seem to homodimerize each other via the BTB domain that enables two Keap1 proteins to simultaneously bind to a single Nrf2 protein (Tong et al. 2006). The isothermal calorimetric assay has revealed that the overlapping ETGE and DLG motifs in the Neh2 domain bind to the DGR region of Keap1 with a highly differential affinity, in which the binding affinity of the ETGE motif ($Ka = 20 \times 10^7$/M) is much stronger than that of the DLG motif ($Ka = 0.1 \times 10^7$/M) to Keap1 protein. Therefore, the so-called hinge and latch model was proposed to account for the mode of Nrf2 regulation by Keap1 (Tong et al. 2007). According to this model, the "hinge" depicts a strong-affinity interaction between the ETGE motif and Keap1, and this interaction is unaffected by stress inducers. On the other hand, the "latch" depicts a weak interaction between the DLG motif and Keap1, and a displacement of the Nrf2 DLG motif from Keap1 occurs in response to treatment with stress inducers. While this model is currently considered as a primary mechanism that explains the mode of Nrf2/Keap1 interaction, an alternative mechanism that explains the regulation of Nrf2 by Keap1 has been proposed (Li and Kong 2009). For example, Li et al. (2005) have found that a redox-sensitive nuclear exporting signal (NES) motif exists in the Neh5 domain of Nrf2, and Cys183, which is embedded in this NES motif, seems to mediate the redox sensitivity of Nrf2. Accordingly, a site-directed mutagenesis of Nrf2 (Nrf2C183A) showed that this mutant Nrf2 protein exhibited remarkably reduced nuclear transloca-tion kinetics (Li et al. 2005).

Unlike many other chemopreventive agents, ITCs are not strong antioxidants, and therefore, they do not possess the ability to directly combat environmental oxidants or electrophiles. Rather, they promote the generation of intracellular ROS and activate the two major signaling kinase cascades, that is, mitogen-activated protein kinase (MAPK) and phosphatidylinositol 3'-kinase (PI3-K), to increase the expression of Nrf2 and phase II cytoprotective enzymes in cells (Keum et al. 2004). This view is supported by the fact that pretreatment with antioxidants, for example, reduced glu-tathione (GSH) or N-acetylcysteine (NAC), can suppress ARE-dependent gene expression and an induction of phase II cytoprotective enzymes, elicited by treatment with ITCs (data not shown). Also, activation of these signaling pathways contributes not only to the activation of ARE-dependent gene expression but also to the induction of an apoptotic pathway in prostate cancer cells, such as DNA fragmentation or caspase activation (Antosiewicz et al. 2008). Therefore, potential chemopreven-tive mechanisms of ITCs seem to be different from those of other conventional chemopreventive polyphenolic antioxidants, such as curcumin, resveratrol, epigallocatechin gallate (EGCG), and so forth. Although we are aware that ROS play critical roles in the intracellular signal transduction and induction of phase II cytoprotective enzymes, the detailed biochemical mechanisms by which ROS contribute to eliciting ARE-dependent gene expression and increasing the cellular expression of Nrf2 protein and phase II cytoprotective enzymes are still unknown.

25.3 DIRECT MODIFICATIONS OF CELLULAR PROTEINS BY DIETARY ITCs

It is possible to speculate that there would be other routes for ITCs to switch on ARE-dependent gene expression aside from the generation of intracellular ROS. Dinkova-Kostova et al. (2002) have initially examined the possibility that treatment with ITCs might induce Nrf2 expression by directly modifying Keap1 cysteine (Cys) residues. Keap1 protein is a cysteine-rich protein (a total of 27 in human Keap1). Individual Cys residues are proposed as differential sensors in response to expo-sure to diverse electrophiles, and this led to a conceptual classification of ARE inducers into six classes, so-called cysteine code (Kobayashi et al. 2009). Indeed, selected Cys residues in Keap1 play an important role in Nrf2-mediated ARE transactivation. Zhang and Hannink (2003) have demonstrated that mutation of certain Cys (C) into Ser (S) residues in Keap1 perturbed Keap1-mediated repression of Nrf2 under basal conditions (C273S or C288S) or the activity of Nrf2 to escape from Keap1-mediated repression (C151S). In the same study, they showed that sulforaphane-mediated ARE–luciferase was also hampered when HA-Keap1-C151S plasmid, but not HA-Keap1-C273S or HA-Keap1-C288S plasmids, was introduced. In an attempt to find out the Cys residue(s) in Keap1 protein that sulforaphane can directly bind to, Hong et al. (2005) have mixed sulforaphane with a recombinant Keap1 protein in a test tube and observed that sulforaphane formed a direct adduct with Cys residues in recombinant Keap1 protein, depending on the workup conditions or the concentration of sulforaphane used in the experiment. Also, Hu et al. (2011) made an observa-tion that sulforaphane can form a labile but covalent adduct with a recombinant Keap1 protein at Cys151, if iodoacetamide was omitted and sample preparation time was shortened. It suggests that sulforaphane indeed serves as an electrophile that can bind to and modifies Cys residues of Keap1 in vitro. Yet, it can be surmised that not all Cys residues in Keap1 would be reactive with ITCs, because the reactivity of individual Cys residues would depend on its propensity to undergo a protonation state that is affected by several aspects, such as pKa, electrostatic interactions, and hydrophilicity of adjacent residues. In addition, there exist no reports yet, demonstrating a stable adduct formation of any of Cys residue(s) in Keap1 protein by natural ITCs in cells, and therefore, there still exist great debates, regarding whether endogenous Keap1 protein is a genuine direct target of chemopreventive ITCs.

Identification of the protein targets of ITCs is an important step to understand the molecular mechanisms by which ITCs exert their anticarcinogenic activities, and it is likely to provide us with the knowledge and tools for the future design and screening of more efficacious chemopreventive compounds. Several studies have been conducted to find out the direct targets (e.g., cellular DNA, RNA or proteins) of ITCs in cells. In particular, Mi et al. (2008) have exposed cells to radiolabeled ITCs (^{14}C-PEITC and ^{14}C-sulforaphane) and observed that no discernable adduct formation of ^{14}C-labeled ITCs with nucleotides (DNA and RNA) occurred. Hence, it is unlikely that nucleotides are direct targets of ITCs. Next, they have attempted to identify the proteins that ^{14}C-PEITC or ^{14}C-sulforaphane directly binds to, using proteomic approaches and two-dimensional electrophoresis, and observed that only a small number of protein spots contained radioactivity (Mi et al. 2008), suggesting that the number of protein targets to which ITCs can directly bind is fewer than initially expected. Undoubtedly, the primary cellular target of ITCs is a cellular reduced GSH. GSH is a cellular antioxidant tripeptide that consists of glycine (Gly), cysteine (Cys), and glutamic acid (Glu) residues. The thiol group of Cys in GSH acts as a cellular reducing agent and is important for combating against ROS, such as free radicals and peroxides, by undergoing a conjugation reaction of disulfide bonds between GSHs. In this process, GSH is converted to its oxidized form, oxidized GSH or glutathione disulfide (GSSG). Oxidized GSH can be reduced back by GSH reductase, using NADPH as an electron donor, and the ratio between reduced GSH and oxidized GSH is often considered as an indication of cellular toxicity within cells. Metabolism of glucosinolates is now well defined and closely associated with GSH. Upon consumption of cruciferous vegetables, ITCs are formed from glucosinolates and rapidly conjugated to cellular GSH. Cellular ITCs and ITC–GSH conjugates establish a constant equilibrium state by repeating conjugation and deconjugation cycles, depending on pH and the amount of available cellular ITCs and thiols. Binding of ITCs with GSH causes a depletion of cellular GSH, and depletion of intracellular GSH is believed to be responsible for ROS generation and apoptotic induction in tumor cells by ITCs. Due to the lack of a clear correlation between the depletion level of intracellular GSH and the potency of apoptosis by several ITCs, however, some still question depletion of GSH as a primary chemopreventive mechanism of natural ITCs (Mi et al. 2011).

Tubulins were identified as another direct target protein of ITCs (Mi et al. 2008). A dimer of α- and β-tubulin contributes to the formation of microtubules in cells. The dynamic equilibrium between tubulin dimers and microtubules is essential for various cellular functions, such as mitosis, cytokinesis, intracellular movement of organelles, and vesicular transport. In addition, currently valid targets of several chemotherapeutic agents are tubulin-binding chemicals (colchicine, vinblastine, and taxol, for example). Different ITCs exhibited differential binding affinities to tubulins, and in particular, the protein residues to which ITCs directly bind were shown to be Cys347 in α-tubulin and Cys308 in β-tubulin (Mi et al. 2008). Also, exposure of N-methyl phenethylamine, a structural analog of PEITC without an ITC functional group, did not exhibit binding affinity toward tubulin, indicating that ITC is indeed a functional group that interacts with tubulins. Further, circular dichroism (CD) analysis illustrated that direct binding of BITC induced a conformation change in tubulin protein structure. Conformational change of tubulin created protein misfolding and degradation of tubulins, resulting in the induction of apoptosis in tumor cells (Mi et al. 2009). Therefore, it appears that binding of ITCs to tubulins contributes to a novel chemotherapeutic mechanism. In addition to forming thiocarbamates with cysteines, it is possible that ITCs can react with amine groups, for example, existing in α-amino groups of the N-terminal residues or in ε-carbon in lysines by forming thiourea through an alkylation reaction (Mi et al. 2008). Alkylation is an irreversible reaction, but it proceeds much slower, compared with a thiocarbamation reaction. Two recent studies have demonstrated for the first time that ITCs can directly react with the N-terminal proline of macrophage migration inhibitory factor (MIF) (Cross et al. 2009; Ouertatani-Sakouhi et al. 2009). MIF is a proinflammatory and protumorigenic cytokine and a direct modification. Hence, inhibition of MIF activity by ITCs is believed to constitute another novel mechanism by which dietary ITCs inhibit carcinogenesis. Interestingly, the proline residue was found to be the only binding site in MIF protein by ITCs, although it contains three conserved cysteine residues, that is, Cys57, Cys60, and Cys81. Finally, the binding of ITCs to hydroxyl groups in protein residues is theoretically possible in addition to thiocarbamation and alkylation reactions. However, this reaction can proceed only at nonphysiological pH and creates the unstable hydroxyl conjugates, which can be easily deconjugated by switching to a physiological pH. By far, the conjugation of ITCs to hydroxyl groups in protein residues has not been observed in vivo.

25.4 PROSTATE CANCER PREVENTION BY DIETARY ITCs IN PRECLINICAL AND CLINICAL SETTINGS

Glucosinolates exist as inactive N-hydrosulfate with the sulfur linked to the β-glucose in cruciferous vegetables. When tissues in vegetables are broken by chewing or food preparation, the plant-specific myrosinase enzyme is released and comes in contact with glucosinolates, resulting in the production of chemopreventive ITCs. ITCs are characterized by the $-N = C = S$ functional group, in which the central carbon is highly electrophilic. As mentioned earlier, cellular GSH is a primary target of ITCs and responsible for further metabolism of ITCs in the body, in which conjugated ITC–GSH (dithiocarbamate) is serially metabolized into the ITC–NAC conjugate, that is, mercapturic acid, and excreted into the urine. The metabolic conversion of glucosinolates into mercapturic acid is referred to as the mercapturic acid pathway (Keum 2011). Facile and accurate quantification of ITCs in human samples is necessary for pharmacokinetic and epidemiological studies. Initially, determination of ITC concentrations in the sample was conducted by a simple high-performance liquid chromatography (HPLC)-based assay, so called the cyclocondensation assay (Figure 25.2). This assay is based on the chemical principle that ITCs can undergo successive nucleophilic additions with dithiols to produce a five-membered cyclic thiocarbonyl product. 1,2-Benzenedithiole was selected as a reactant, in which cellular or plasma ITCs are converted into 1,3-benzodithiole-2-thione in the

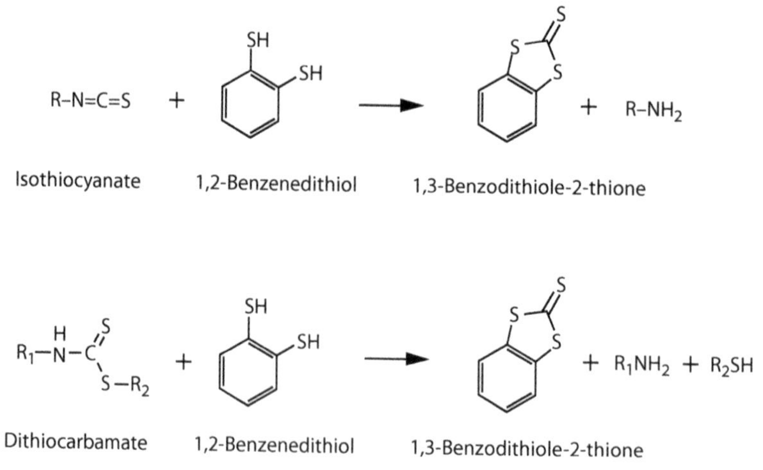

FIGURE 25.2 Chemical reaction basis for cyclocondensation assay.

presence of excessive 1,2-benzenedithiole that is, in turn, quantified by two-step hexane extractions and HPLC analysis, using ultraviolet (UV) detection at 365 nm. However, the cyclocondensation assay has a weakness: this assay does not discriminate between ITCs and dithiocarbamates (Figure 25.2). This problem can be overcome by the introduction of the liquid chromatography-tandem mass spectrometry (LC–MS–MS). In fact, LC–MS–MS exhibited a superior selectivity and sensitivity in quantifying the amount of ITCs (Ji et al. 2005).

Earlier studies have demonstrated that administration of natural ITCs in rodents exhibited significant cancer-preventive effects. Potential in vivo chemopreventive mechanisms of ITCs include (1) inhibition of cytochrome P450 enzymes, (2) induction of phase II cytoprotective enzymes, (3) induction of cell cycle arrest and apoptosis, and (4) suppression of proinflammatory genes, all of which might involve direct and/or indirect interactions of ITCs with cellular components (Cheung and Kong 2010). The first evidence of chemoprotective effects of ITCs was observed by feeding Wistar rats with α-naphthyl–ITC less than five decades ago (Sidransky et al. 1966). Since then, quite a number of naturally occurring ITCs have been demonstrated to exhibit significant inhibitory effects against carcinogen-induced tumor formation in many experimental animal models (Conaway et al. 2002). PEITC has received much attention as a potential chemopreventive agent. Using a PC-3 cell subcutaneous xenograft model, Khor et al. (2006) have demonstrated that intraperitoneal injection of PEITC, ahead of implantation of PC-3 prostate cancer cells, significantly suppressed the growth of PC-3 xenografts in nude mice. The growth-suppressive effect of PEITC was more pronounced when PEITC was coinjected with curcumin, another potential chemopreventive agent that is abundant in turmeric. However, the growth-suppressive effect of PEITC alone or in combination with curcumin was not observable when PC-3 xenografts were fully established in mice. This fact suggests that the growth-inhibitory effect of PEITC would be evident in the early phases, but not in late phases, of carcinogenesis. In addition, the potential growth-inhibitory mechanisms of PC-3 xenografts mediated by administration of PEITC in mice included apoptosis induction and suppression of the nuclear factor kappaB (NF-κB) pathway. Moreover, administration of other naturally occurring ITCs, such as sulforaphane and AITC, have been shown to exhibit significant inhibitory effects on the growth of prostate tumor xenografts in nude mice (Singh et al. 2004; Srivastava et al. 2003). Therefore, it seems that the growth-inhibitory effects of ITCs on prostate tumor xenografts in vivo seem to be a general event exerted by ITC-class natural compounds. Among many other experimental animal models, the transgenic adenocarcinoma of the mouse prostate (TRAMP) mouse model has been serving as a useful system to examine the potential chemopreventive activities of natural compounds because exogenous carcinogens or hormones are not required to induce prostate cancer in this model. Another advantage of this model lies in the fact that prostate tumor formation in TRAMP mice arises from normal cells in their natural tissue microenvironment and progresses through multiple stages, which faithfully recapitulates the human multistage carcinogenesis in terms of pathological features and lethality. Furthermore, TRAMP mice reproducibly produce PIN before prostate cancer formation and, more importantly, not only develop primary prostate tumors, but also, tumors in TRAMP mice metastasize in other organs, such as the liver, lung, and lymph node. In order to examine the chemopreventive activities of sulforaphane in TRAMP mice, Kong and colleagues have utilized broccoli sprouts as a source of sulforaphane because young broccoli sprouts are an exceptionally rich source of glucoraphanin, the glucosinolate precursor of sulforaphane, which is present in broccoli sprouts in amounts 20–50 times higher than that in mature market-stage vegetables (Fahey et al. 1997). As a result, they observed that oral administration of broccoli sprouts significantly suppressed the growth of prostate tumors and the Akt/mammalian target of rapamycin (mTOR) pathway activity but induced an apoptotic pathway in the prostate of TRAMP mice (Keum et al. 2009). More interestingly, a significant induction of Nrf2 and HO-1 proteins was also observed in the prostate of TRAMP mice when they were fed with broccoli sprouts for 16 weeks. This result shows that administration of ITCs can increase the expression of Nrf2 and phase II cytoprotective enzymes in the prostate of mice and suggests a possibility that activation of the Nrf2 signaling cascade can serve as a valid target of prostate chemoprevention in vivo.

Using a cyclocondensation assay, Ye et al. (2002) have conducted a simple pharmacokinetic analysis to study the bioavailability of ITCs in humans. They fed four healthy male volunteers with single dose of broccoli sprout preparations, which contain 200 μmol of ITCs that have been hydrolyzed by myrosinase over a period of time. Blood and urine samples were collected, and the amount of excreted ITCs was analyzed by the cyclocondensation assay. It was observed that a significant amount of ITCs was recovered from the urinary sample (77.9 ± 6.4% after 48 h), implying that ITCs are not irreversibly conjugated in the plasma or tissues. Analysis of plasma samples also showed that ITCs appear as early as 15 min after dosing and were maximally detected after 1 h, suggesting that conversion of glucosinolates into ITCs is a rapid event in the body. In order to study whether plant-specific enzyme(s) is responsible for conversion of glucosinolates into ITCs, Getahun and Chung (1999) recruited nine healthy male volunteers, fed them with 350 g boiled watercress, and collected their urinary samples. After a week, they administered an equal amount of raw watercress into the same subjects and measured the efficiency of urinary conversion of glucosinolates into ITCs. As expected, they found that a significant amount of ITCs was discovered in the urine (17.2%–77.7%) when the subjects were fed with raw watercress. However, the conversion efficiency was significantly reduced (1.2%–7.3%) when the subjects were fed with boiled watercress, implying that boiling watercress destroyed the integrity of myrosinase and impaired enzymatic conversion of glucosinolates into ITCs. In addition, Shapiro et al. (1998) have observed that incubation of watercress juice with fresh human feces converted some glucosinolates into ITCs (~18%), suggesting that, although conversion efficiency is lower than myrosinase, unidentified microflora existing in the feces might exhibit myrosinase activities. The existence of possible microflora that can mediate conversion of glucosinolates into ITCs is supported by another observation that conversion of glucosinolates is significantly lower in subjects whose microflora was possibly reduced by mechanical cleansing or oral antibiotics (Getahun and Chung 1999). Together, these observations support the idea that the functional myrosinase activity of vegetables and the presence of gut microflora that can catalyze hydrolysis of glucosinolates are important factors in increasing the bioavailability of natural ITCs and suggest that consumption of raw vegetables would be desirable to warrant chemopreventive activities of cruciferous vegetables in humans. However, as noted above, there is a wide variation in the urinary levels of ITC metabolites among individuals, and it means that only selected individuals would receive the beneficial chemopreventive activities by consuming cruciferous vegetables. Therefore, it seems necessary at present to understand which genotype(s) would be responsible for modulating the bioavailability of ITCs in humans.

Previously, Kensler and colleagues conducted a small-scale clinical study to examine the potential anticarcinogenic activities of broccoli sprouts. They recruited 200 healthy individuals in Qidong, People's Republic of China, and administered them with hot-water extracts of broccoli sprouts. As a result, they found that consumption of hot extracts of broccoli sprouts significantly suppressed the formation of aflatoxin–DNA adducts and antiphenanthrene in urine, both of which serve as useful biomarkers of carcinogen metabolites. This implies that broccoli sprouts possess antimutagenic activities in humans, possibly by accelerating the rate of detoxification and elimination of chemical carcinogens. An inverse relationship between a high intake of cruciferous vegetables and risk of most types of cancer has been observed in many case-controlled epidemiological studies as well. However, the results of some case-controlled studies obtained from patients with selected types of cancer, including prostate cancer, yielded confounding results (Kristal and Lampe 2002). The underlying reason is unclear at present, but it is interesting to note that these organs are located in the body, where any metabolites, including ITCs, are difficult to reach. While there are no solid cohort studies demonstrating prostate chemopreventive effects of ITCs, it seems that genetic polymorphism of human GST isozymes contributes, at least in part, to the potential chemopreventive effects of ITCs in humans. For example, Lin et al. (1998) have demonstrated that the inverse relationship between the risk for colorectal adenoma and an intake of broccoli was evident only in the subjects with GSTM1-null genotypes. Zhao et al. (2001) have also demonstrated that intake of ITCs reduced the risk of lung cancer to a greater extent among subjects with homozygous deletion of GSTM1 or GSTT1. London et al. (2000) have observed more significant associations between urinary level of ITCs and reduced lung cancer risks among men with homozygous deletion of GSTM1 and GSTT1. Based on our knowledge that ITCs, formed in the cells, are conjugated to cellular GSH by GST enzymes and further metabolized into the mercapturic acids, it appears that a lack of GST genotypes seems to contribute to the bioavailability of ITCs, possibly by delaying metabolism and elimination of ITC–GSH conjugates in humans. Therefore, it would be interesting to study whether consumption of cruciferous vegetables can indeed prevent prostate carcinogenesis in humans and, if so, whether men with null GST genotypes would receive more chemopreventive advantages of cruciferous vegetables in preventing prostate cancer, compared with those with functional GST genotypes.

ACKNOWLEDGMENT

This research was supported by the Basic Research Program through the National Research Foundation of Korea (NRF) funded by the Ministry of Education, Science and Technology (2011-0013733).

REFERENCES

Antosiewicz, J., Ziolkowski, W., Kar, S., Powolny, A. A. and Singh, S. V. (2008). Role of reactive oxygen intermediates in cellular responses to dietary cancer chemopreventive agents. *Planta Med* 74, 1570–1579.

Cheung, K. L. and Kong, A. N. (2010). Molecular targets of dietary phenethyl isothiocyanate and sulforaphane for cancer chemoprevention. *AAPS J* 12, 87–97.

Clarke, J. D., Dashwood, R. H. and Ho, E. (2008). Multi-targeted prevention of cancer by sulforaphane. *Cancer Lett* 269, 291–304.

Conaway, C. C., Yang, Y. M. and Chung, F. L. (2002). Isothiocyanates as cancer chemopreventive agents: their biological activities and metabolism in rodents and humans. *Curr Drug Metab* 3, 233–255.

Cross, J. V., Rady, J. M., Foss, F. W., Lyons, C. E., Macdonald, T. L. and Templeton, D. J. (2009). Nutrient isothiocyanates covalently modify and inhibit the inflammatory cytokine macrophage migration inhibitory factor (MIF). *Biochem J* 423, 315–321.

Dinkova-Kostova, A. T., Holtzclaw, W. D., Cole, R. N., Itoh, K., Wakabayashi, N., Katoh, Y., Yamamoto, M. and Talalay, P. (2002). Direct evidence that sulfhydryl groups of Keap1 are the sensors regulating induction of phase 2 enzymes that protect against carcinogens and oxidants. *Proc Natl Acad Sci U S A* 99, 11908–11913.

Fahey, J. W., Zalcmann, A. T. and Talalay, P. (2001). The chemical diversity and distribution of glucosinolates and isothiocyanates among plants. *Phytochemistry* 56, 5–51.

Fahey, J. W., Zhang, Y. and Talalay, P. (1997). Broccoli sprouts: an exceptionally rich source of inducers of enzymes that protect against chemical carcinogens. *Proc Natl Acad Sci U S A* 94, 10367–10372.

Getahun, S. M. and Chung, F. L. (1999). Conversion of glucosinolates to isothiocyanates in humans after ingestion of cooked watercress. *Cancer Epidemiol Biomarkers Prev* 8, 447–451.

Hong, F., Freeman, M. L. and Liebler, D. C. (2005). Identification of sensor cysteines in human Keap1 modified by the cancer chemopreventive agent sulforaphane. *Chem Res Toxicol* 18, 1917–1926.

Hu, C., Eggler, A. L., Mesecar, A. D. and van Breemen, R. B. (2011). Modification of keap1 cysteine residues by sulforaphane. *Chem Res Toxicol* 24, 515–521.

Itoh, K., Chiba, T., Takahashi, S., Ishii, T., Igarashi, K., Katoh, Y., Oyake, T., Hayashi, N., Satoh, K., Hatayama, I., Yamamoto, M. and Nabeshima, Y. (1997). An Nrf2/small Maf heterodimer mediates the induction of phase II detoxifying enzyme genes through antioxidant response elements. *Biochem Biophys Res Commun* 236, 313–322.

Itoh, K., Wakabayashi, N., Katoh, Y., Ishii, T., Igarashi, K., Engel, J. D. and Yamamoto, M. (1999). Keap1 represses nuclear activation of antioxidant responsive elements by Nrf2 through binding to the amino-terminal Neh2 domain. *Genes Dev* 13, 76–86.

Jemal, A., Siegel, R., Ward, E., Hao, Y., Xu, J. and Thun, M. J. (2009). Cancer statistics, 2009. *CA Cancer J Clin* 59, 225–249.

Ji, Y., Kuo, Y. and Morris, M. E. (2005). Pharmacokinetics of dietary phenethyl isothiocyanate in rats. *Pharm Res* 22, 1658–1666.

Kang, M. I., Kobayashi, A., Wakabayashi, N., Kim, S. G. and Yamamoto, M. (2004). Scaffolding of Keap1 to the actin cytoskeleton controls the function of Nrf2 as key regulator of cytoprotective phase 2 genes. *Proc Natl Acad Sci U S A* 101, 2046–2051.

Kensler, T. W., Wakabayashi, N. and Biswal, S. (2007). Cell survival responses to environmental stresses via the Keap1-Nrf2-ARE pathway. *Annu Rev Pharmacol Toxicol* 47, 89–116.

Keum, Y. S. (2011). Regulation of the Keap1/Nrf2 system by chemopreventive sulforaphane: implications of posttranslational modifications. *Ann N Y Acad Sci* 1229, 184–189.

Keum, Y. S., Jeong, W. S. and Kong, A. N. (2004). Chemoprevention by isothiocyanates and their underlying molecular signaling mechanisms. *Mutat Res* 555, 191–202.

Keum, Y. S., Khor, T. O., Lin, W., Shen, G., Kwon, K. H., Barve, A., Li, W. and Kong, A. N. (2009). Pharmacokinetics and pharmacodynamics of broccoli sprouts on the suppression of prostate cancer in transgenic adenocarcinoma of mouse prostate (TRAMP) mice: implication of induction of Nrf2, HO-1 and apoptosis and the suppression of Akt-dependent kinase pathway. *Pharm Res* 26, 2324–2331.

Keum, Y. S., Yu, S., Chang, P. P., Yuan, X., Kim, J. H., Xu, C., Han, J., Agarwal, A. and Kong, A. N. (2006). Mechanism of action of sulforaphane: inhibition of p38 mitogen-activated protein kinase isoforms contributing to the induction of antioxidant response element-mediated heme oxygenase-1 in human hepatoma HepG2 cells. *Cancer Res* 66, 8804–8813.

Khor, T. O., Keum, Y. S., Lin, W., Kim, J. H., Hu, R., Shen, G., Xu, C., Gopalakrishnan, A., Reddy, B., Zheng, X., Conney, A. H. and Kong, A. N. (2006). Combined inhibitory effects of curcumin and phenethyl isothiocyanate on the growth of human PC-3 prostate xenografts in immunodeficient mice. *Cancer Res* 66, 613–621.

Kobayashi, M., Li, L., Iwamoto, N., Nakajima-Takagi, Y., Kaneko, H., Nakayama, Y., Eguchi, M., Wada, Y., Kumagai, Y. and Yamamoto, M. (2009). The antioxidant defense system Keap1-Nrf2 comprises a multiple sensing mechanism for responding to a wide range of chemical compounds. *Mol Cell Biol* 29, 493–502.

Kristal, A. R. and Lampe, J. W. (2002). Brassica vegetables and prostate cancer risk: a review of the epidemiological evidence. *Nutr Cancer* 42, 1–9.

Li, W., Jain, M. R., Chen, C., Yue, X., Hebbar, V., Zhou, R. and Kong, A. N. (2005). Nrf2 Possesses a redox-insensitive nuclear export signal overlapping with the leucine zipper motif. *J Biol Chem* 280, 28430–28438.

Li, W. and Kong, A. N. (2009). Molecular mechanisms of Nrf2-mediated antioxidant response. *Mol Carcinog* 48, 91–104.

Lin, H. J., Probst-Hensch, N. M., Louie, A. D., Kau, I. H., Witte, J. S., Ingles, S. A., Frankl, H. D., Lee, E. R. and Haile, R. W. (1998). Glutathione transferase null genotype, broccoli, and lower prevalence of colorectal adenomas. *Cancer Epidemiol Biomarkers Prev* 7, 647–652.

London, S. J., Yuan, J. M., Chung, F. L., Gao, Y. T., Coetzee, G. A., Ross, R. K. and Yu, M. C. (2000). Isothiocyanates, glutathione S-transferase M1 and T1 polymorphisms, and lung-cancer risk: a prospective study of men in Shanghai, China. *Lancet* 356, 724–729.

McMahon, M., Itoh, K., Yamamoto, M. and Hayes, J. D. (2003). Keap1-dependent proteasomal degradation of transcription factor Nrf2 contributes to the negative regulation of antioxidant response element-driven gene expression. *J Biol Chem* 278, 21592–21600.

Mi, L., Di Pasqua, A. J. and Chung, F. L. (2011). Proteins as binding targets of isothiocyanates in cancer prevention. *Carcinogenesis* 32, 1405–1413.

Mi, L., Gan, N., Cheema, A., Dakshanamurthy, S., Wang, X., Yang, D. C. and Chung, F. L. (2009). Cancer preventive isothiocyanates induce selective degradation of cellular alpha- and beta-tubulins by proteasomes. *J Biol Chem* 284, 17039–17051.

Mi, L., Xiao, Z., Hood, B. L., Dakshanamurthy, S., Wang, X., Govind, S., Conrads, T. P., Veenstra, T. D. and Chung, F. L. (2008). Covalent binding to tubulin by isothiocyanates. A mechanism of cell growth arrest and apoptosis. *J Biol Chem* 283, 22136–22146.

Motohashi, H., O'Connor, T., Katsuoka, F., Engel, J. D. and Yamamoto, M. (2002). Integration and diversity of the regulatory network composed of Maf and CNC families of transcription factors. *Gene* 294, 1–12.

Ohtsubo, T., Kamada, S., Mikami, T., Murakami, H. and Tsujimoto, Y. (1999). Identification of NRF2, a member of the NF-E2 family of transcription factors, as a substrate for caspase-3(-like) proteases. *Cell Death Differ* 6, 865–872.

Ouertatani-Sakouhi, H., El-Turk, F., Fauvet, B., Roger, T., Le Roy, D., Karpinar, D. P., Leng, L., Bucala, R., Zweckstetter, M., Calandra, T. and Lashuel, H. A. (2009). A new class of isothiocyanate-based irreversible inhibitors of macrophage migration inhibitory factor. *Biochemistry* 48, 9858–9870.

Prawan, A., Keum, Y. S., Khor, T. O., Yu, S., Nair, S., Li, W., Hu, L. and Kong, A. N. (2008). Structural influence of isothiocyanates on the antioxidant response element (ARE)-mediated heme oxygenase-1 (HO-1) expression. *Pharm Res* 25, 836–844.

Ramos-Gomez, M., Kwak, M. K., Dolan, P. M., Itoh, K., Yamamoto, M., Talalay, P. and Kensler, T. W. (2001). Sensitivity to carcinogenesis is increased and chemoprotective efficacy of enzyme inducers is lost in nrf2 transcription factor-deficient mice. *Proc Natl Acad Sci U S A* 98, 3410–3415.

Shapiro, T. A., Fahey, J. W., Wade, K. L., Stephenson, K. K. and Talalay, P. (1998). Human metabolism and excretion of cancer chemoprotective glucosinolates and isothiocyanates of cruciferous vegetables. *Cancer Epidemiol Biomarkers Prev* 7, 1091–1100.

Sidransky, H., Ito, N. and Verney, E. (1966). Influence of alpha-naphthyl-isothiocyanate on liver tumorigenesis in rats ingesting ethionine and N-2-fluorenylacetamide. *J Natl Cancer Inst* 37, 677–686.

Singh, A. V., Xiao, D., Lew, K. L., Dhir, R. and Singh, S. V. (2004). Sulforaphane induces caspase-mediated apoptosis in cultured PC-3 human prostate cancer cells and retards growth of PC-3 xenografts in vivo. *Carcinogenesis* 25, 83–90.

Srivastava, S. K., Xiao, D., Lew, K. L., Hershberger, P., Kokkinakis, D. M., Johnson, C. S., Trump, D. L. and Singh, S. V. (2003). Allyl isothiocyanate, a constituent of cruciferous vegetables, inhibits growth of PC-3 human prostate cancer xenografts in vivo. *Carcinogenesis* 24, 1665–1670.

Stokes, M. E., Black, L., Benedict, A., Roehrborn, C. G. and Albertsen, P. (2010). Long-term medical-care costs related to prostate cancer: estimates from linked SEER-Medicare data. *Prostate Cancer Prostatic Dis* 13, 278–284.

Sykiotis, G. P. and Bohmann, D. (2010). Stress-activated cap'n'collar transcription factors in aging and human disease. *Sci Signal* 3, re3.

Thimmulappa, R. K., Mai, K. H., Srisuma, S., Kensler, T. W., Yamamoto, M. and Biswal, S. (2002). Identification of Nrf2-regulated genes induced by the chemopreventive agent sulforaphane by oligonucleotide microarray. *Cancer Res* 62, 5196–5203.

Tong, K. I., Kobayashi, A., Katsuoka, F. and Yamamoto, M. (2006). Two-site substrate recognition model for the Keap1-Nrf2 system: a hinge and latch mechanism. *Biol Chem* 387, 1311–1320.

Tong, K. I., Padmanabhan, B., Kobayashi, A., Shang, C., Hirotsu, Y., Yokoyama, S. and Yamamoto, M. (2007). Different electrostatic potentials define ETGE and DLG motifs as hinge and latch in oxidative stress response. *Mol Cell Biol* 27, 7511–7521.

Ye, L., Dinkova-Kostova, A. T., Wade, K. L., Zhang, Y., Shapiro, T. A. and Talalay, P. (2002). Quantitative determination of dithiocarbamates in human plasma, serum, erythrocytes and urine: pharmacokinetics of broccoli sprout isothiocyanates in humans. *Clin Chim Acta* 316, 43–53.

Zhang, D. D. and Hannink, M. (2003). Distinct cysteine residues in Keap1 are required for Keap1-dependent ubiquitination of Nrf2 and for stabilization of Nrf2 by chemopreventive agents and oxidative stress. *Mol Cell Biol* 23, 8137–8151.

Zhao, B., Seow, A., Lee, E. J., Poh, W. T., Teh, M., Eng, P., Wang, Y. T., Tan, W. C., Yu, M. C. and Lee, H. P. (2001). Dietary isothiocyanates, glutathione S-transferase -M1, -T1 polymorphisms and lung cancer risk among Chinese women in Singapore. *Cancer Epidemiol Biomarkers Prev* 10, 1063–1067.

Section VIII

Selenium, Herbal Medicines,
Alpha Lipoic Acid, and
Cancer Prevention

26 Cancer Prevention with Selenium

Costly Lessons and Difficult but Bright Future Prospects

Junxuan Lü, Cheng Jiang, and Jinhui Zhang

CONTENTS

26.1 INTRODUCTION

Chemoprevention of carcinogenesis is recognized as a plausible and essential approach to win the war on cancer (Klein 2005; Bode and Dong 2009). "Success stories" include the Food and Drug Administration (FDA)–approved antiestrogen tamoxifen for the prevention of estrogen receptor–positive breast cancer (Fisher et al. 1998, 2005) and raloxifene (marketed as Evista by Eli Lilly and Company), which is an oral selective estrogen receptor modulator (SERM) that has estrogenic actions on bone and antiestrogenic actions on the uterus and breast, for the prevention of osteoporosis and invasive breast cancer in postmenopausal women (Vogel et al. 2006). A major adverse effect of tamoxifen is uterine cancer; raloxifene was associated with fewer uterine cancers. Tamoxifen increased the risk of cataracts, but raloxifene did not. Both groups had more blood clots in veins and the lungs, but that side effect was more common with tamoxifen than raloxifene (Vogel et al. 2006). For prostate cancer, the controversial 5α-reductase II inhibitor drug finasteride that blocks the intraprostatic generation of the active androgen dihydrotestosterone has been shown to decrease cancer incidence by 24.8%, but with significant sexual side effects and questionable survival benefit

(Lucia et al. 2007; Thompson et al. 2003, 2008), and is not approved by FDA for prevention use. The classical single-target approach has a mixed record for developing chemopreventive agents due to complexity and the multistep and multimutation etiology nature of carcinogenesis.

Previous human studies have suggested that supplementation of selenium (Se) in the form of selenized yeast may modify the risk of and prevent human cancers in China and the United States (see next section) (Clark et al. 1996, 1998; Li et al. 2004; Brooks et al. 2001; Yu et al. 1989, 1997). However, the National Cancer Institute stopped the Selenium and Vitamin E Cancer Prevention Trial (SELECT) in October 2008, several years ahead of schedule, because of the failure to demonstrate efficacy of selenomethionine (SeMet) for prostate cancer prevention in North American men (Lippman et al. 2009). To the credit of the clinical investigators, that trial was well designed (e.g., double blinded, randomized, placebo controlled) and well executed (e.g., abiding by subject selection criteria at enrollment, supplementation compliance, and Se status monitoring) and was indeed sensitive to detect adverse effects such as a nonstatistically significant increase in type 2 diabetes risk for subjects taking the SeMet supplement and increased prostate cancer risk by vitamin E in the form of α-tocopheryl acetate (Lippman et al. 2009; Klein et al. 2011). The recently concluded Southwest Oncology Group (SWOG) trial (S9917) in men with advanced high-grade intraprostatic neoplasia (HGPIN) for the assessment of efficacy of SeMet to prevent their conversion to prostate cancer has also failed to show any risk reduction (Marshall et al. 2011). A similar fate awaited the clinical trial for Se-yeast (the major Se form is SeMet) for the "prevention" of a second primary lung cancer (Karp 2005), where Se-yeast was found to be not preventive (Karp et al. 2010).

While these well-designed and well-executed trials were costly in financial terms, their negative impacts on the credibility and reputation of the field of cancer chemoprevention research as a whole, and Se in particular, are probably far greater. Their failures to show preventive efficacy of SeMet/Se-yeast have cast doubts in the minds of many researchers and the lay public alike about the merit of Se for cancer prevention. Many would have concluded that there is no hope for using Se to prevent cancer.

Given the metabolic and biochemical differences that have been well documented between SeMet and other Se forms by us and others (Lu and Jiang 2005; Ip 1998) (Figure 26.1), we argued that the failure of SeMet in SELECT should and cannot be equated to all Se forms as ineffective for cancer prevention (Wang et al. 2009). This postulate, in the wake of the negative results of the other well-conducted trials with SeMet and Se-yeast, stands to gain greater footing based on the vast knowledge base of their cellular and molecular effects (for comprehensive reviews, see the recent publications by Lu and Jiang 2005; Lu et al. 2009) and the growing body of preclinical efficacy data in prostate and other organ sites, especially mammary carcinogenesis (Ip 1998), for Se forms other than SeMet, with desirable attributes of multiple targeting of carcinogenesis and progression. It would be a shame to "throw the baby out with the bathwater," that is, to abandon research on these newer Se agents due to the failure of SeMet or Se-yeast. There is, nevertheless, an urgent need for an objective and critical analysis of what went wrong with these well-designed and well-conducted double-blinded, randomized, and placebo-controlled trials (the gold standard for evidence-based medicine). What needs to be done to rehabilitate and revitalize the field of Se cancer prevention research toward the realization of the full health benefits of Se for mankind?

Whereas possible reasons for failure to demonstrate SeMet efficacy have been discussed in the original Lippman paper (Lippman et al. 2009) and reviewed by El-Bayoumi and others, including Se status of subjects, Se dosage, and chemical forms (El-Bayoumi 2009; Hatfield and Gladyshev 2009), we posit that the two major culprits are (1) wrong choice of subjects and patient populations for testing the antioxidant hypothesis and (2) wrong choice of Se forms for cancer chemoprevention in Se-adequate populations. The major focus of this chapter is to elaborate on these postulates. We will also provide an updated analysis of progress on newer Se forms for consideration for future translation studies, especially from a preclinical efficacy and in vivo mechanism perspective.

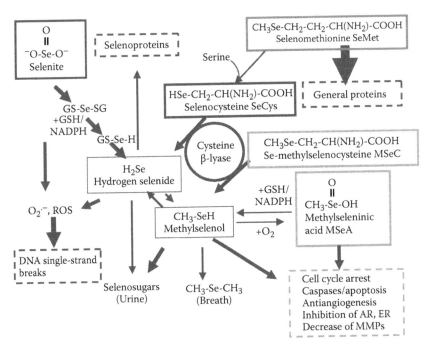

FIGURE 26.1 Structures and possible metabolic pathways for methylseleninic acid, selenoamino acids, and inorganic selenite in a chemoprevention context. For selenoamino acids, tissue cysteine β-lyases release hydrogen selenide and methylselenol from selenocysteine and methylselenocysteine, respectively. Methylselenol pool may be selectively enriched by precursor compounds or functional foods such as Se-garlic, bypassing the hydrogen selenide pool. SeMet leads to massive tissue accumulation of Se due to its nonspecific incorporation into general proteins in place of Met. Selenite can cause DNA damage, likely through reactive oxygen species.

26.2 SE NUTRITIONAL PREVENTION OF CANCER TRIAL REVISITED

Cancer preventive effects on liver cancer risk of a Se-yeast supplement were initially reported in a small-scale trial (226 subjects) with hepatitis B patients in Qi-Dong County, China, where Se intake was deficient (Whanger 2004; Yu et al. 1989, 1997), providing an important rationale and support for the "landmark" Nutritional Prevention of Cancer (NPC) trial in the United States, led by the late Dr. Larry Clark and his then Cornell University colleague Dr. Gerald Combs, Jr. (also known as [aka] the Clark study). The original report of the NPC trial results and subsequent updates of the extended data collection based on the total number of patients enrolled ($n = 1312$) (Clark et al. 1996, 1998; Duffield-Lillico et al. 2002, 2003a,b; Reid et al. 2002) suggested the possibility that a dietary Se supplement, in the form of Se-yeast, might be an effective preventive agent against solid cancers in multiple organ sites, particularly in the prostate, colon, and lung, in secondary end point analyses. Subjects in the treatment arm were given once-daily 200 μg Se (~4× the recommended daily value of 55 μg/day) as selenized brewer's yeast, which consists predominantly of SeMet (Bird et al. 1997; Ip et al. 2000), for a mean of 4.5 years, and the subjects were followed for a mean of 6.5 years. Subjects who received the Se-yeast supplement showed significantly lower incidences of cancers of the prostate (relative risk [RR] = 0.37, $P = .002$); colon (RR = 0.42, $P = .03$); and lung (RR = 0.54, $P = .04$) than the placebo group. Total cancer-related mortality was also significantly decreased by 41%. However, there was a Se-yeast associated increase in the risk of secondary nonmelanoma skin cancers (NMSC) (RR = 1.10), which were the primary end points of the trial (Clark et al. 1996; Duffield-Lillico et al. 2003b). The protective effects of Se supplementation persisted upon longer follow-up for a mean of 7.8 years for prostate cancer (RR = 0.51, $P = .009$) and colon cancer (RR = 0.46, $P = .055$) (Duffield-Lillico et al. 2002).

It is particularly noteworthy that the subjects with baseline plasma Se in the lowest tertile (<~105 ng/mL or 1.33 µM) showed the most reduction of prostate and lung cancer and total non-NMSC upon Se-yeast intervention in the NPC trial (Duffield-Lillico et al. 2002, 2003a,b; Lu and Jiang 2005). Subjects entering the trial with higher baseline Se did not show a reduction of risk for these cancers with the Se-yeast supplement. Same as in the original report (Clark et al. 1996), a small yet statistically significant increase in the occurrence of secondary NMSC due to the Se-yeast supplement persisted with longer follow-up (RR = 1.27, $P = .001$) (Duffield-Lillico et al. 2003b). It is worthy of note that the increase in secondary NMSC incidence was observed in subjects entering the trial within the second (105–123 ng/mL) and third tertiles (123 ng/mL or 1.58 µM) of baseline Se concentration. These results suggested organ site specificities of Se-yeast at a dose of 200 µg/day for the prevention of several solid cancers and for Se-associated increase in NMSC risk in this male-dominated and NMSC patient cohort. The potential benefit of preventing the top two cancers (lung cancer, prostate cancer) that account for the cancer-related mortality in North America stimulated great research interests that culminated in the initiation of several clinical prevention trials in North America to validate the preventive efficacy of SeMet for prostate cancer and Se-yeast for lung cancer. Here we will analyze the three that have been published.

As a side note, a publication of a retrospective analysis of the NPC trial subjects in 2007 suggested a significant association of Se-yeast supplementation with an increased incidence of self-reported type 2 diabetes (Stranges et al. 2007). This little-noticed piece of information is relevant in light of the side effects of SeMet revealed in SELECT (see next).

26.3 CLINICAL TRIALS FAIL TO VALIDATE PREVENTIVE ACTIVITIES OF SEMET OR SE-YEAST

26.3.1 SELECT

SELECT is a randomized, prospective, double-blind study designed to determine whether Se as SeMet and vitamin E alone and in combination can reduce the risk of prostate cancer among healthy men (Lippman et al. 2009). Coordinated by the SWOG, the study was a placebo-controlled trial with 35,533 men from 427 participating sites in the United States, Canada, and Puerto Rico randomly assigned to four groups (Se, vitamin E, Se + vitamin E, and placebo) in a double-blind fashion between August 22, 2001, and June 24, 2004. Baseline eligibility included age of 50 years or older (African-American men) or 55 years or older (all other men), a serum prostate-specific antigen (PSA) level of 4 ng/mL or less, and a digital rectal examination not suspicious for prostate cancer. Oral Se (200 µg/day from L-SeMet) and matched vitamin E placebo, vitamin E (400 IU/day of all-rac-α-tocopheryl acetate) and matched Se placebo, Se + vitamin E, or placebo + placebo was given, with a planned follow-up of a minimum of 7 years and a maximum of 12 years. The National Cancer Institute stopped the trial in late October 2008, several years ahead of the scheduled completion date, due to a possible increase of diabetes risk in SeMet-supplemented subjects and a rise in prostate cancer risk in the vitamin E–supplemented subjects. Specifically, as of October 23, 2008, median overall follow-up was 5.46 years (range, 4.17–7.33 years). Hazard ratios (99% confidence intervals [CIs]) for prostate cancer were 1.13 (99% CI = 0.95–1.35, $n = 473$, $P = .06$) for vitamin E; 1.04 (99% CI = 0.87–1.24, $n = 432$) for Se; and 1.05 (99% CI = 0.88–1.25, $n = 437$) for Se + vitamin E versus 1.00 ($n = 416$) for placebo. There were no significant differences (all $P > .15$) in any other prespecified cancer end points. At that point, there was a statistically nonsignificant increased risk of type 2 diabetes mellitus in the Se group (RR, =1.07, 99% CI = 0.94–1.22, $P = .16$) but not in the Se + vitamin E group.

On further follow-up, the increase in prostate cancer risk by α-tocopheryl acetate has reached statistical significance (Klein et al. 2011). This was based on 54,464 additional person-years of follow-up and 521 additional cases of prostate cancer since the above primary report. Compared with the placebo (referent) group, in which 529 men developed prostate cancer, 620 men in the vitamin E group developed prostate cancer (hazard ratio [HR] = 1.17, 99% CI = 1.004–1.36, P = .008), as did 575 in the Se group (HR = 1.09, 99% CI = 0.93–1.27; P = .18) and 555 in the Se + vitamin E group (HR = 1.05, 99% CI = 0.89–1.22, P = .46).

26.3.2   SWOG S9917 Trial

In November 2011, the results of the phase III trial of Se to prevent prostate cancer in men with high-grade prostatic intraepithelial neoplasia (HGPIN) (SWOG S9917) were published (Marshall et al. 2011). This is a double-blind, randomized, placebo-controlled trial of Se 200 (µg/day) as SeMet in men with HGPIN. The primary end point was progression of HGPIN to prostate cancer over a 3-year period. Of 619 enrolled patients, 423 randomized men with HGPIN (212 Se and 211 placebo) were eligible (by central pathology review) and included in the primary analysis. Three-year cancer rates were 36.6% (placebo) versus 35.6% (Se; P = .73, adjusted). The majority of patients who developed cancer on trial (70.8% for Se and 75.5% for placebo) had a Gleason score of 6 or less; there were no differences in Gleason scores between the two arms. Subset analyses included the finding of a nonsignificantly reduced prostate cancer risk (RR = 0.82, 95% CI = 0.40–1.69) in Se versus placebo patients in the lowest quartile of baseline plasma Se level (<106 ng/mL). Overall, and in all other subsets defined by baseline blood Se levels, Se supplementation had no effect on prostate cancer risk. The 36% prostate cancer rate in men with HGPIN indicates the association of this lesion with an elevated prostate cancer risk. The authors suggested that future study in this setting should focus on Se-deficient populations and Se pharmacogenetics.

26.3.3   Eastern Cooperative Oncology Group Lung Cancer Trial

The Eastern Cooperative Oncology Group (ECOG-5597) led this phase III randomized chemoprevention study of Se in patients with previously resected stage I non–small-cell lung cancer (NSCLC) (Karp 2005; Karp et al. 2010). From October 2000 to November 2009, six institutions carried out this double-blind, placebo-controlled trial using 200 µg Se daily (Se-yeast) in a 2:1 randomization versus placebo for 48 months in completely resected stage I NSCLC. Participation was 6–36 months post-op and required a negative mediastinal node biopsy, no excessive vitamin intake, normal liver function, a negative chest x-ray, and no other evidence of recurrence. A planned size of 1960 participants had been designed to detect a 40% decrease in second primary lung tumors (SPTs) with 80% power. Interim analysis occurred in October 2009 after 1561 of 1772 patients reached step 2 (completion of the 4-week [step 1] run-in period requiring at least 75% of the study drug to be taken). End points included SPTs, recurrence, and toxicity. A total of 216 SPTs developed, of which 84 (38.9%) were lung cancer. SPT (lung/overall) incidence was 1.36/3.66 per 100 person-years for placebo versus 1.91/4.11 for Se (P = .150). Five-year progression-free survival was 78% for placebo versus 72% for Se. The study was stopped according to futility analysis. Grade 1 or 2 toxicity occurred in 38% of placebo and 39% of Se. Grade 3 toxicity was 3% in placebo versus <1% in Se. Compliance was excellent (>95% at 2 years). The study authors concluded that no increase in diabetes mellitus or skin cancer was detected and that Se was safe but conferred no benefit over placebo.

Overall, these trials followed the gold standard for evidence-based medicine (i.e., double-blinded, randomized, and placebo-controlled design) and were executed for definitive validation tests of the preventive efficacy of Se in the forms of SeMet and Se-yeast for prostate and lung cancers. What went wrong? What lessons can be learned?

As we have pointed out before (Lu and Jiang 2005), the Se status of the human or animal subjects, the chemical forms and dosages of Se, and the organ/tissue Se metabolic capacity and specificity will determine the fates of ingested Se and the profiles of Se metabolites and, consequently, the biochemical, molecular, and cellular responses, which are also further defined by the organ site specificities of the cancer etiology and cell signaling pathways. These pieces of information must be considered to obtain a balanced understanding of the Se literature and for the analyses of the reasons for failure of the clinical trials.

26.4 LESSON 1: ANTIOXIDANT HYPOTHESIS WAS TESTED IN WRONG SUBJECTS/PATIENT POPULATIONS

A number of hypotheses have been proposed to account for the potential cancer chemopreventive activities of Se. Prominent among these is antioxidant protection against lipid peroxide– and reactive oxygen species (ROS)–driven initiation and promotion events (Lu and Jiang 2005; Ip 1998; Combs and Gray 1998; Whanger 2004). Others include enhanced carcinogen detoxification through phase I and II enzymes, enhanced immune surveillance, inhibition of cancer cell proliferation, and selective induction of apoptosis of transformed epithelial cells, to name a few (Combs and Gray 1998; Ip 1998; Whanger 2004). We have proposed that inhibition of cancer angiogenesis by Se metabolites may also contribute to the chemopreventive activity (Lu and Jiang 2001, 2005). In terms of the Se chemical forms, the critical Se metabolite(s) hypothesis has steadily gained both in vivo and in vitro support during the past two decades (Lu and Jiang 2005; Lu et al. 2009).

The central hypothesis for SELECT was antioxidant function of Se and/or vitamin E for the prevention of prostate cancer. The best-studied biochemical function of Se in the nutritional range of intake is as an integral part of a family of antioxidant enzymes, the Se-dependent glutathione peroxidases (SeGPXs) (Arthur 2000; Brigelius-Flohe 1999). Studies in the past with Se-deficient rodent models of cancer have, in general, shown modest protection at best with nutritional Se supplements on chemically induced carcinogenesis in mammary and other organ sites (Ip 1998; Combs and Gray 1998). The interpretation of such studies, however, was complicated by how much the protective effects were exerted by improving the activities of SeGPXs, thioredoxin reductases (TRs), and other selenoproteins or by the increase in nonprotein Se metabolites per se. The development of a transgenic mouse model a decade ago with suppressed selenoprotein synthesis through the expression of an altered selenocysteine tRNA (i6A-) has made it possible to address this question with some specificity (Moustafa et al. 2001). As reported in the original study, selenoprotein suppression was in a protein- and tissue-specific manner. Cytosolic SeGPX (GPX1) and mitochondrial TR3 were the most and least affected selenoproteins, while selenoprotein expression was most and least affected in the liver and testes, respectively. The defect in selenoprotein expression occurred at translation, since selenoprotein messenger RNA (mRNA) levels were largely unaffected (Moustafa et al. 2001).

Diwadkar-Navsariwala et al. (2006) developed double-transgenic mice with reduced selenoprotein levels because i6A-transgenic expression and prostate targeted expression of the SV40 (Simian virus) large T and small t oncogenes to that organ [C3(1)/Tag]. The resulting bigenic animals (i6A-/Tag) and control wild type (WT)/Tag mice were assessed for the presence, degree, and progression of prostatic epithelial hyperplasia and nuclear atypia. The selenoprotein-deficient mice exhibited accelerated development of lesions associated with prostate cancer progression with adequate dietary Se (0.1 ppm), implicating selenoproteins in cancer risk and development and supporting the possibility that nutritional Se prevents cancer by modulating the levels of these selenoproteins.

Irons et al. (2006) examined Se homeostasis in the liver and colon of wild-type and transgenic mice fed with Se-deficient diets supplemented with 0, 0.1 (adequate for rodents), or 2.0 ppm Se (as selenite) per gram of diet. In agreement with the earlier study (Diwadkar-Navsariwala et al. 2006), they revealed that transgenic mice had reduced liver and colon SeGPX expression, but conserved TR expression compared with wild-type mice, regardless of whether the Se was at a nutritional (0.1 ppm) or chemopreventive (2 ppm) supplementation level. The transgenic mice had more Se in the nonprotein fraction of the liver and colon than wild-type mice, indicating a greater amount of low-molecular-weight Se metabolites. Compared with wild-type mice, transgenic mice had more azoxymethane-induced aberrant crypt formation (a preneoplastic lesion for colon cancer) at both 0.1 and 2 ppm levels. Supplemental Se (0.1 to 2 ppm) decreased the number of aberrant crypts and aberrant crypt foci in both wild-type and transgenic mice. These results provide evidence that a lack of selenoprotein activity (mostly SeGPX, not TR) increases colon cancer susceptibility. Independently of the selenoprotein genotype, low-molecular-weight Se metabolites exert important cancer-protective effects of Se.

To specifically assess the function of TR, Yoo et al. (2006) used RNA interference technology to decrease TR1 expression in mouse Lewis lung carcinoma (LLC1) cells. Stable transfection of LLC1 cells with a small interfering RNA (siRNA) construct that specifically targets TR1 led to a reversal in the morphology and anchorage-independent growth properties of these cancer cells toward the normal cells. Mice fed with a diet with adequate Se levels inoculated with the TR1 knockdown cells showed a dramatic reduction in tumor progression and metastasis compared with those mice inoculated with the corresponding control vector. In addition, tumors that arose from the injected TR1 knockdown cells lost the targeting construct, suggesting that TR1 is essential for LLC tumor growth in mice. Since these data show that lowering the TR1 level in lung cancer cells is antitumorigenic in the presence of adequate dietary Se, the reverse implication is that improving TR1 activity by an Se nutritional supplement may promote this lung cancer model.

These in vivo studies together suggest that the reduction of SeGPXs (Irons et al. 2006) or TR1 (Yoo et al. 2006) have opposite consequences for cancer risk. The overall balance of the activities between TR and SeGPX could therefore be a crucial factor for determining the cancer risk in the nutritional range of Se supplementation. Such mechanistic insights are instructive for the "postmortem" analyses and syntheses of reasons for failure of the human clinical trials.

The Se status of individuals residing in the United States has been considered "nutritionally" adequate judging by their Se intake data and serum Se content. According to the Third National Health and Nutrition Examination Survey (NHANES III), the mean intake of all ages was 103 µg (Ervin et al. 2004), nearly twice the National Research Council's recommended daily allowance of 55 µg (Food and Nutrition Board 2000). From the 18,597 persons for whom serum Se values were available in NHANES III (Ford et al. 2003; Niskar et al. 2003), the mean concentration was 1.58 µM, and the median concentration was 1.56 µM. This is much higher than the 1 µM or 80 ng/mL that was found to be the upper limit for SeGPX responses to supplemental Se in healthy adults (Neve 1995). This was also supported by the Clark study in which the placebo group had a baseline plasma Se level of 114 ng Se/mL (1.4 µM) (Clark et al. 1996; Duffield-Lillico et al. 2002). In that trial, the average plasma Se level in the supplemented group was increased by some 67% to 190 ng/mL or 2.4 µM. Only two subjects (1.5%) had Se levels below 80 ng/mL (Duffield-Lillico et al. 2002). In spite of an increase in the plasma total Se level, the plasma SeGPX activity of selected subjects before and after Se supplementation was not increased (Combs et al. 2001).

In SELECT (Lippman et al. 2009), baseline medium Se was 136 ng/mL (i.e., 1.72 µM), and SeMet supplementation increased to 223, 232, 228, and 251 ng/mL in the subsequent years (2.82–3.17 µM). Such levels are therefore more than nutritionally adequate.

26.5 LESSON 2: CHOICE OF SE FORMS IN VIOLATION OF DRUG DEVELOPMENT PARADIGM

The discussion section by Lippman et al. (2009) for possible rationale for SeMet noted: "In designing SELECT, we carefully evaluated the choice of l-selenomethionine vs high-Se yeast (and other formulations) and our rationale for selecting l-selenomethionine included the following considerations: selenomethionine was the major component of apparently active high-Se yeast; evidence indicated substantial batch-to-batch variations in specific organoselenium compounds in samples of NPC yeast, making it unlikely that we could duplicate the Se yeast formulation used in the NPC study; potential genotoxicity of highly active inorganic Se compounds, such as selenite, made them potentially unsuitable for long-term prevention; lowering (vs. selenomethionine) of overall body Se stores with selenite, which is neither absorbed nor retained well; practical and safety concerns over newer Se compounds, such as monomethylated forms (eg, lacking availability, investigational new drug certification, and clinical data)." As discussed below, cell culture and animal studies did not support the anticancer efficacy of SeMet or Se-yeast.

In cell culture models, SeMet exposure levels of two orders of magnitude higher than serum total Se level were needed to show modest growth-inhibitory effects in cancer cell lines. For example, SeMet exposure inhibited the growth of A549 lung cancer cells, with IC_{50} of 65 μM, and HT29 colon cancer cells, with IC_{50} of 130 μM (Redman et al. 1997). In prostate cancer cells, 100–500 μM SeMet was needed to induce growth suppression effects and apoptosis (Menter et al. 2000). SeMet treatment of the lung and colon cancer cell lines increased the number of cells in metaphase (Redman et al. 1997). In colon and prostate cancer cells, such high levels of SeMet were required to induce G2/M arrest. Two additional studies with colon cancer cell lines reported cell cycle arrests with SeMet above 100 μM (Chigbrow and Nelson 2001; Goel et al. 2006). Whether colonic luminal SeMet concentrations can reach such high levels should be evaluated to assess the relevance of these observed effects. For non-alimentary tract cancers, the only likely route of exposure to SeMet is through vascular delivery. It would be very unlikely for such extreme high levels to be achievable through an oral SeMet supplement, as shown in a recent phase I trial with 11-fold higher daily intake of SeMet than the Clark study (Fakih et al. 2006).

A few studies, conducted in the late 1990s before SELECT was initiated, did not find any efficacy of SeMet, α-tocopheryl acetate, each alone or combination, or Se-yeast on chemically induced prostate carcinogenesis models in rats. The negative results were initially communicated as meeting proceedings, and the full results have now been published (Ozten et al. 2010; McCormick et al. 2010). In one study, the Bosland group examined the potential of SeMet and α-tocopheryl acetate to modulate prostate cancer development in the testosterone + estradiol–treated NBL rat, a model that does involve sex hormone–induced oxidative stress mechanisms and prostatic inflammation (Ozten et al. 2010). One week following the implantation with hormone-filled silastic implants, rats were fed with diets containing L-SeMet (1.5 or 3.0 mg/kg), DL-α-tocopheryl acetate (2000 or 4000 mg/ kg), or a natural-ingredient control diet (NIH-07). The development of prostate carcinomas was not affected by dietary treatment with either agent. Food intake, body weight, and mortality were also not affected. In the other study, McCormick et al. (2010) stimulated prostate epithelial cell proliferation by a sequential regimen of cyproterone acetate followed by testosterone propionate; male Wistar-Unilever rats received a single i.v. injection of N-methyl-N-nitrosourea (MNU) followed by chronic androgen stimulation via subcutaneous implantation of testosterone pellets. At 1 week post-MNU, groups of carcinogen-treated rats (39–44 per group) were fed with either a basal diet or a basal diet supplemented with SeMet (3 or 1.5 mg/kg diet, study 1); DL-α-tocopheryl acetate (vitamin E, 4000 or 2000 mg/kg diet, study 2); SeMet + vitamin E (3 + 2000 mg/kg diet or 3 + 500 mg/kg diet, study 3); or Se-yeast (target Se levels of 9 or 3 mg/kg diet, study 4). Each chemoprevention study was terminated at 13 months post-MNU, and prostate cancer incidence was determined by histopathologic evaluation. No statistically significant reductions in prostate cancer incidence were identified in any group receiving dietary supplementation with Se and/or vitamin E. Collectively, the findings from both studies suggest that SeMet and α-tocopherol supplementation does not prevent prostate cancer in rats fed with diets with nutritionally adequate levels of Se and vitamin E. Importantly, the results of these animal studies were predictive of the negative outcome of SELECT.

Experiments since SELECT was initiated, including our study with xenograft models, did not support any in vivo anticancer activity of SeMet (Corcoran et al. 2004; Li et al. 2008). In a study with orthotopic PC-3 tumors in the prostates of 6-week-old male nude mice fed with a baseline Se-replete diet (0.07 ppm), supplementing intake with different Se forms (sodium selenate, SeMet, methylselenocysteine, and Se-yeast) at two different concentrations (0.3 and 3 ppm) in drinking water, only sodium selenate significantly retarded the growth of primary prostatic tumors and the development of retroperitoneal lymph node metastases, which was associated with a decrease in angiogenesis (Corcoran et al. 2004).

Our group evaluated the growth-inhibitory effects of SeMet and selenite in comparison to two presumed methylselenol precursors, methylseleninic acid (MSeA) and Se-methylselenocysteine

(MSeC), in DU145 and PC-3 human prostate cancer xenografts in athymic nude mice (Li et al. 2008). Each Se type was given by a daily single oral-dose regimen starting the day after the subcutaneous inoculation of cancer cells. We analyzed serum, liver, and tumor Se content to confirm supplementation status and apoptosis indices and tumor microvessel density for association with antitumor efficacy. Furthermore, we analyzed lymphocyte DNA integrity to detect the genotoxic effect of Se treatments. The data show that SeMet did not have any inhibitory effect in spite of Se retention an order of magnitude higher in the liver and tumors of the SeMet-treated mice than in those from mice treated with selenite or MSeA and MSeC in either DU145 or PC-3 models. MSeA and MSeC exerted a dose-dependent inhibition of DU145 xenograft growth. Selenite treatment increased DNA single-strand breaks (SSBs) in peripheral lymphocytes, whereas the other Se forms did not. In the PC-3 xenograft model, only MSeA was growth inhibitory at a dose of 3 mg/kg body weight. In summary, our data demonstrated superior in vivo growth-inhibitory efficacy of MSeA over SeMet and selenite, against two human prostate cancer xenograft models, without the genotoxic property of selenite.

26.6 NONSELENOPROTEIN SE METABOLITES AND METHYLSELENOL HYPOTHESIS

Because Se deficiency is not a health concern in the United States, most animal models and in vitro cell culture studies since the mid-1980s have dealt with chemopreventive levels of Se and have focused on the cancerous epithelial cells as the targets of its anticancer effects. Most animal models have shown cancer chemopreventive activity of Se intake that is 20–50× greater than the nutritional requirement (Ip 1998). Based on a large body of data from these studies, it has been articulated that cancer chemoprevention by Se in the nutritionally adequate subject is independent of the antioxidant activity of plasma or tissue SeGPX (Combs and Gray 1998; Ip 1998). This paradigm was based on the observation that the dietary level of Se (2 ppm or greater as selenite) needed to achieve a significant cancer preventive activity in rodent animal models far exceeded that required (i.e., 0.1 ppm) to support maximal SeGPX in the blood (GPX3) or the target tissues from which experimental cancers arise. This view has been extended to the other selenoproteins identified subsequently in the last decade, including phospholipid glutathione peroxidase (Ph-SeGPX, aka GPX4), selenoprotein P (Sel-P), selenoprotein W (Sel-W), thyroxine deiodinases (TDIs), and TRs (Lu et al. 2009). The studies with transgenic suppression of selenoproteins (increased prostate and colon cancer risk with decreased SeGPXs in the presence of adequate dietary Se) and the TR1 knockdown transfectant cells (decreased lung cancer growth with knocked down TR1) cited above indicate likely contradicting roles of these proteins as regulators of cancer risk in the nutritional range of Se intake.

Excess Se beyond the need for selenoprotein synthesis (hydrogen selenide is cotranslationally incorporated into the SeCys-containing selenoproteins) is methylated into methylselenol, which is further methylated and excreted as dimethylselenide (volatile through breath) and trimethylselenonium (urine) or converted into selenosugars (Figure 26.1). It should be pointed out that SeMet is either incorporated into general proteins in place of Met (nonspecific substitution) or metabolized to SeCys through a transselenation pathway similar to the transsulfuration pathway for Met → cysteine conversion. The efficiency of the latter pathway will be dependent on the metabolic capacity of the cell types and organs. The liver and hepatocytes are expected to be well equipped with the metabolic enzymes, whereas, in general, nonhepatic tumor cells in culture would be expected to be limited in this ability.

Ip (1998) and Ganther (1999) led efforts to identify the putative in vivo Se metabolite pool using a mammary chemical carcinogenesis model. They proposed that the active anticancer Se metabolites were likely monomethylated Se species (presumably methylselenol) and that the chemopreventive efficacy of a given Se compound might depend on the rate of its metabolic conversion to the active Se form(s) (Ip 1998; Ganther 1999). Strong supporting evidence was obtained by comparing the cancer chemopreventive efficacy of forms of Se that fed into different Se metabolite pools with precursors of methylselenol displaying greater preventive efficacy than those for hydrogen selenide or dimethylselenide in the chemically induced rodent mammary carcinogenesis model (Ip and Ganther 1990;

Ip et al. 1991). In addition, they used arsenic as an inhibitor of the Se methylation steps, and the data showed that blocking the conversion of hydrogen selenide to methylselenol decreased the anticancer activity, whereas inhibiting the further methylation of methylselenol increased the efficacy. Extending on the methylselenol structure–activity theme, subsequent work had shown that the alkyl selenol and allyl selenol precursor compounds were more active against mammary carcinogenesis than methylselenol precursors on an equal molar basis of dietary Se intake (Ip et al. 1995, 1999). However, these structure–activity studies have not been extended beyond the mammary carcinogenesis model for assessing the general applicability of the methylselenol hypothesis in other organ sites, due, in part, to the NPC outcome of two breast cancer cases in the placebo group versus six cases in the Se-yeast group in the few women enrolled in that trial (Clark et al. 1996).

In analyzing the Se literature, it will be important to keep in mind the chemical form of Se used, the levels of Se exposure, and the serum levels in the cell culture media (e.g., 10% fetal bovine serum usually provides 100 nM Se in the final medium). In general, cell culture models using the inorganic sodium selenite salt as the source of Se have shown biphasic responses of cancer cell proliferation to incremental Se supplementation: a modest stimulatory effect in the nanomolar to sub-micromolar range and a strong suppression effect at higher Se concentrations. While the small growth stimulatory response is likely related to the nutritional actions of Se through changing the balance of SeGPXs, TRs, and other selenoproteins to achieve the optimal redox tone for growth in cell culture, studies by us and others focusing on the higher levels of Se exposure have shown that monomethyl Se compounds that are putative precursors to the methylselenol pool induce numerous cellular, biochemical, and gene expression responses that are distinct from those induced by the forms of Se that enter the hydrogen selenide pool (Lu and Jiang 2005; Ip 1998; Lu et al. 2009). These major cellular and biochemical effects are schematically summarized in Figure 26.1 and detailed in earlier reviews (Lu and Jiang 2005; Lu et al. 2009).

26.6.1 Hydrogen Selenide Pool

Sodium selenite and sodium selenide, which feed into the hydrogen selenide (H_2Se) pool, rapidly (within minutes to a few hours of Se exposure) induce DNA SSBs and S phase or G2/M cell cycle arrest and lead to subsequent cell death by apoptosis and necrosis (Lu and Jiang 2005). Sodium selenide and SeCys could recapitulate the DNA SSB induction and the apoptosis effects of selenite in the model system (Lu et al. 1995). A superoxide dismutase mimetic compound, copper dipropylsalicylate, blocked DNA SSBs and apoptosis, indicating that selenite per se did not trigger these events (Lu 2001). Recent studies have provided further support for ROS (superoxide generation) as intermediates for activating p53 Ser phosphorylation in apoptosis induced by selenite in an LNCaP prostate cancer cell model (Zhao et al. 2006; Hu et al. 2006).

However, little is known of whether the hydrogen selenide pool could reach the pharmacological levels used in these in vitro studies to affect DNA integrity (genotoxicity) in vivo. Our published data indicate that selenite given by daily oral dosage of 3 mg/kg body weight to tumor-bearing nude mice increased DNA SSBs in peripheral lymphocytes, whereas the same dosage of MSeA or MSeC lacked this effect (Li et al. 2008). Further studies in animal models and in humans are necessary to confirm the in vivo genotoxicity of selenite.

26.6.2 Methylselenol Pool

We and others have shown that putative methylselenol precursors such as methylselenocyanate (MSeCN) and MSeC induced apoptosis of mammary tumor epithelial cells and leukemia cells without the induction of DNA SSBs (Lu et al. 1995, 1996; Kaeck et al. 1997). Furthermore, we and others have reported that methyl Se–induced cancer cell apoptosis was caspase dependent, whereas selenite-induced cell death was independent of these death proteases in prostate cancer and leukemia cells lacking functional p53 (Jiang et al. 2001; Kim et al. 2001). The methyl Se or methylselenol led to G1 arrest (Lu et al. 1996; Kaeck et al. 1997; Jiang et al. 2002; Wang et al. 2001, 2002; Zhu et al. 2002). Inhibitory effects on cyclin-dependent kinases (Zhu et al. 2002; Sinha and Medina 1997) and protein kinase C (Sinha et al. 1999) have been attributed to the methyl Se pool. In terms of genotoxicity implications, our data show that at a daily oral dosage of 3 mg/kg body weight, MSeA and MSeC significantly suppressed human DU145 xenograft growth without increasing DNA SSBs in the peripheral lymphocytes of the host mice, whereas the same dosage of selenite caused increased DNA SSBs and was ineffective for suppressing xenograft growth (Li et al. 2008).

In addition to these cellular effects, methylselenol precursors exert a rapid inhibitory effect on the expression of key molecules involved in angiogenesis regulation. For example, we have shown that subapoptotic doses of MSeA inhibited the expression and secretion of the angiogenic factor vascular endothelial growth factor (VEGF) in several cancer cell lines (Jiang et al. 2000). Methyl Se also inhibited the expression of matrix metalloproteinase 2 (MMP-2) in the vascular endothelial cells (Jiang et al. 1999, 2000). These effects plus a potent inhibitory effect on the cell cycle progression of vascular endothelial cells (Wang et al. 2001, 2002) indicate that methylselenol can be a key inhibitor of angiogenic switch regulation in early lesions and in tumors (Lu and Jiang 2005). Furthermore, we and others have recently shown that MSeA and methylselenol released by methioninase from SeMet inhibit androgen receptor expression and its signaling to PSA (Cho et al. 2004; Dong et al. 2004; Zhao et al. 2004) as well as PSA stability (Cho et al. 2004). MSeA has been also shown to inhibit estrogen receptor signaling in breast and endometrial cancer cells (Lee et al. 2005; Shah et al. 2005a,b; Lu et al. 2009).

26.7   EFFICACY AND MOLECULAR TARGETS OF MONOMETHYLATED SE IN PROSTATE CANCER MODELS

As noted above, we have shown that orally administered MSeA and MSeC dose-dependently (1 and 3 mg Se/kg) inhibit the in vivo growth of DU145 human prostate cancer xenografts in athymic nude mice, whereas selenite and SeMet are not active (Li et al. 2008). MSeA is more active than MSeC against PC-3 xenograft growth. In terms of tolerability, all four Se compounds at the tested doses of 3 mg/kg or lower did not adversely affect the body weight of the mice. Measurement of tissue Se content showed that SeMet treatment led to 9.1-fold more liver Se retention, approximately 3.6 times higher than mice treated with an equal dose of methyl Se, despite the least potency of SeMet to affect DU145 or PC-3 xenograft growth. The observed massive tissue Se accumulation (nonspecific incorporation in place of Met into proteins) and the lack of anticancer potency agreed well with earlier work with SeMet in conventional rodent models (Ip and Hayes 1989; Ip et al. 1991).

26.7.1   MSeA or MSeC Inhibits Primary Prostate Carcinogenesis in the TRAMP Model

We used the transgenic adenocarcinoma of mouse prostate (TRAMP) model to establish the efficacy of MSeA and MSeC against prostate carcinogenesis and to characterize potential mechanisms (Wang et al. 2009). Eight-week-old male TRAMP mice (C57B/6 background) were given a daily oral dose of water, MSeA, or MSeC at 3 mg Se/kg body weight and were euthanized at either 18 or 26 weeks of age. By 18 weeks of age, the genitourinary tract and dorsolateral prostate weights for the MSeA- and MSeC-treated groups were lower than for the control ($P < .01$). At 26 weeks, 4 of 10 control mice had genitourinary weight >2 g, and only 1 of 10 in each of the Se groups did. The efficacy was accompanied by delayed lesion progression, increased apoptosis, and decreased proliferation without appreciable changes of T-antigen expression in the dorsolateral prostate of Se-treated mice and decreased serum insulin-like growth factor I when compared with control mice. In another experiment, giving MSeA to TRAMP mice from 10 or 16 weeks of age increased their survival to 50 weeks of age and delayed death due to synaptophysin-positive neuroendocrine carcinomas, synaptophysin-negative prostate lesions, and seminal vesicle hypertrophy. Wild-type mice receiving MSeA from 10 weeks did not exhibit decreased body weight or genitourinary weight or increased serum alanine aminotransferase compared with the control mice. Therefore, these Se compounds were effective at inhibiting this model of prostate carcinogenesis.

26.7.2 Proteomic Profiling Data Challenge the Methylselenol Paradigm

We applied the isobaric tag for relative and absolute quantization (iTRAQ, Applied Biosystems) proteomic approach to profile protein changes of the TRAMP prostate and to characterize their modulation by MSeA and MSeC to identify their potential molecular targets (Zhang et al. 2010). Dorsolateral prostates from wild-type mice at 18 weeks of age and TRAMP mice treated with water (control), MSeA, or MSeC (3 mg Se/kg) from 8 to 18 weeks of age were pooled (9–10 mice per group) and subjected to protein extraction, followed by protein denaturation, reduction, and alkylation. After tryptic digestion, the peptides were labeled with iTRAQ reagents, mixed together, and analyzed by two-dimensional liquid chromatography/tandem mass spectrometry. Of 342 proteins identified with >95% confidence, the expression of 75 proteins was significantly different between TRAMP and wild-type mice. MSeA mainly affected proteins related to prostate functional differentiation, androgen receptor signaling, protein (mis)folding, and endoplasmic reticulum stress responses (e.g., [GRP78] 78 kDa glucose-regulated protein), whereas MSeC affected proteins involved in phase II detoxification (e.g., glutathione S-transferase GSTM1) or cytoprotection and in stromal cells. Although MSeA and MSeC are presumed precursors of methylselenol and were equally effective against the TRAMP model, their distinct affected protein profiles suggest that biological differences in their molecular targets outweigh the similarities.

Furthermore, we analyzed the prostate proteome signatures of mice treated with MSeA, MSeC, SeMet, and selenite for hypothesis generation concerning their potential in vivo molecular targets and cancer risk modification (Zhang et al. 2011). Nude mice bearing subcutaneous PC-3 xenografts were treated daily with each Se form (3 mg Se/kg) orally for 45 days. Five prostates were pooled from each group. Their proteomes were profiled by (LC-MS/MS) liquid chromatography coupled with tandem mass spectrometry with iTRAQ labeling. Of the 1088 proteins identified, 72 were significantly modulated by one or more Se forms. MSeA and MSeC each induced separate sets of tumor suppressor proteins and suppressed different oncoproteins. Proteins induced by selenite and shared with MSeC were

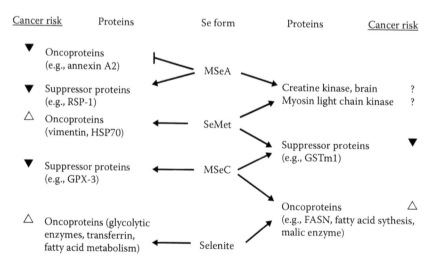

FIGURE 26.2 Representative proteins affected by different forms of Se in the noncarcinogenic prostate of nude mice given oral Se treatment (3 mg/kg) for 5 weeks. Proteins were detected by iTRAQ proteomics and most were verified by Western blot. (Reprinted from Zhang, J. et al., *Nutr Cancer* 63, 5, 778–789, 2011.)

related to energy metabolism (e.g., fatty-acid synthase), and those induced by SeMet included vimentin and heat shock protein-70, favoring cancer growth. While proteome changes induced by MSeA were associated with prostate cancer risk reduction, desirable risk-reducing signatures induced by MSeC (e.g., inducing GSTM1 and increasing GPX-3) were counterbalanced by risk-promoting patterns shared with selenite and SeMet (e.g., inducing fatty acid synthase [FASN], an oncoprotein for prostate cancer). We hypothesized that the balance of oncogenic versus suppressor protein patterns in the prostate might impact the direction of prostate cancer risk modification by a given Se (Figure 26.2).

While methylselenol has been assumed an in vivo active anticancer metabolite pool (Ip 1998; Lu and Jiang 2005), the proteomic data question the validity of the methylselenol paradigm and suggest unique potential molecular targets for each of these chemoprevention-active Se forms with little "protein target" overlap between MSeA and MSeC. Together, the proteomic data suggest that MSeA and MSeC are not interchangeable and that there is a possible adverse prostate cancer risk profile for MSeC through oncoproteins such as FASN. Whether such findings are present in mammary and other tissues should be examined to assess the generalizability to other organ sites.

26.8 CONCLUSIONS AND PERSPECTIVES

The outcomes of the three clinical trials with SeMet or Se-yeast for prostate and lung cancer prevention have been disappointing to many and devastating to the field of cancer chemoprevention as a whole and Se cancer research field in particular. We elaborated on two factors that, in our opinion, were the major culprits for the failure of these studies to detect preventive efficacy of SeMet or Se-yeast, namely, inappropriate subject/patient populations to test the antioxidant hypothesis and ineffective forms of Se in cell culture and animal models chosen for human clinical trials. The mechanistic studies reviewed above have indicated that the Se forms are critical for chemoprevention, depending on their entry into two distinct Se metabolite pools that exert diverse and differential effects on signaling pathways, leading to cell cycle arrests and cell death/apoptosis. In cell culture models, the methylselenol "precursors" have many desirable attributes of cancer chemoprevention and therapy, including targeting key signaling pathways and angiogenic switch regulators in general cancers as well as sex hormone signaling in gender-specific cancers. The hydrogen selenide pool in excess of selenoprotein synthesis can lead to DNA SSBs and genotoxicity to normal cells. Accumulating data support MSeC and MSeA as more meritorious candidates than SeMet or selenite for future clinical investigations of cancer preventive efficacy. Proteomic profiling has uncovered more differences than similarities for the proteome affected by these Se forms. Based on lessons of the concluded trials, it will be essential and necessary that efficacy validation and chronic safety evaluations (such as diabetes risk) and molecular targets and cellular pathways be thoroughly investigated in relevant preclinical animal models with respect to each of these effective Se forms to provide scientific rationale for future translational studies in humans. Mechanism-driven smaller-scale phase I/II trials must be carried out with these newer Se agents to guide future decisions for definitive chemoprevention efficacy validation trials on the SELECT scale.

ACKNOWLEDGMENT

This work was supported in part by the US National Cancer Institute (CA R01 126880). We regret the inability to cite many worthy papers due to space limitations.

REFERENCES

Arthur, J. R. "The Glutathione Peroxidases." *Cell Mol Life Sci* 57, no. 13–14 (2000): 1825–35.
Bird, S. M., P. C. Uden, J. F. Tyson, E. Block, and Denoyer, E. "Speciation of Selenoaminoacids and Organoselenium Compounds in Selenium-Enriched Yeast Using High-Performance Liquid Chromatography-Inductively Coupled Plasma Mass Spectrometry." *J Anal Atom Spectrom* 12 (1997): 785–88.

Bode, A. M., and Z. Dong. "Cancer Prevention Research—Then and Now." *Nat Rev Cancer* 9, no. 7 (2009): 508–16.

Brigelius-Flohe, R. "Tissue-Specific Functions of Individual Glutathione Peroxidases." *Free Radic Biol Med* 27, no. 9–10 (1999): 951–65.

Brooks, J. D., E. J. Metter, D. W. Chan, L. J. Sokoll, P. Landis, W. G. Nelson, D. Muller, R. Andres, and H. B. Carter. "Plasma Selenium Level before Diagnosis and the Risk of Prostate Cancer Development." *J Urol* 166, no. 6 (2001): 2034–8.

Chigbrow, M., and M. Nelson. "Inhibition of Mitotic Cyclin B and Cdc2 Kinase Activity by Selenomethionine in Synchronized Colon Cancer Cells." *Anticancer Drugs* 12, no. 1 (2001): 43–50.

Cho, S. D., C. Jiang, B. Malewicz, Y. Dong, C. Y. Young, K. S. Kang, Y. S. Lee, C. Ip, and J. Lu. "Methyl Selenium Metabolites Decrease Prostate-Specific Antigen Expression by Inducing Protein Degradation and Suppressing Androgen-Stimulated Transcription." *Mol Cancer Ther* 3, no. 5 (2004): 605–11.

Clark, L. C., G. F. Combs, Jr., B. W. Turnbull, E. H. Slate, D. K. Chalker, J. Chow, L. S. Davis, R. A. Glover, G. F. Graham, E. G. Gross, A. Krongrad, J. L. Lesher, Jr., H. K. Park, B. B. Sanders, Jr., C. L. Smith, and J. R. Taylor. "Effects of Selenium Supplementation for Cancer Prevention in Patients with Carcinoma of the Skin. A Randomized Controlled Trial. Nutritional Prevention of Cancer Study Group." *JAMA* 276, no. 24 (1996): 1957–63.

Clark, L. C., B. Dalkin, A. Krongrad, G. F. Combs, Jr., B. W. Turnbull, E. H. Slate, R. Witherington, J. H. Herlong, E. Janosko, D. Carpenter, C. Borosso, S. Falk, and J. Rounder. "Decreased Incidence of Prostate Cancer with Selenium Supplementation: Results of a Double-Blind Cancer Prevention Trial." *Br J Urol* 81, no. 5 (1998): 730–4.

Combs, G. F., Jr., L. C. Clark, and B. W. Turnbull. "An Analysis of Cancer Prevention by Selenium." *Biofactors* 14, no. 1–4 (2001): 153–9.

Combs, G. F., Jr., and W. P. Gray. "Chemopreventive Agents: Selenium." *Pharmacol Ther* 79, no. 3 (1998): 179–92.

Corcoran, N. M., M. Najdovska, and A. J. Costello. "Inorganic Selenium Retards Progression of Experimental Hormone Refractory Prostate Cancer." *J Urol* 171, no. 2 Pt 1 (2004): 907–10.

Diwadkar-Navsariwala, V., G. S. Prins, S. M. Swanson, L. A. Birch, V. H. Ray, S. Hedayat, D. L. Lantvit, and A. M. Diamond. "Selenoprotein Deficiency Accelerates Prostate Carcinogenesis in a Transgenic Model." *Proc Natl Acad Sci U S A* 103, no. 21 (2006): 8179–84.

Dong, Y., S. O. Lee, H. Zhang, J. Marshall, A. C. Gao, and C. Ip. "Prostate Specific Antigen Expression Is Down-Regulated by Selenium through Disruption of Androgen Receptor Signaling." *Cancer Res* 64, no. 1 (2004): 19–22.

Duffield-Lillico, A. J., B. L. Dalkin, M. E. Reid, B. W. Turnbull, E. H. Slate, E. T. Jacobs, J. R. Marshall, and L. C. Clark. "Selenium Supplementation, Baseline Plasma Selenium Status and Incidence of Prostate Cancer: An Analysis of the Complete Treatment Period of the Nutritional Prevention of Cancer Trial." *BJU Int* 91, no. 7 (2003a): 608–12.

Duffield-Lillico, A. J., M. E. Reid, B. W. Turnbull, G. F. Combs, Jr., E. H. Slate, L. A. Fischbach, J. R. Marshall, and L. C. Clark. "Baseline Characteristics and the Effect of Selenium Supplementation on Cancer Incidence in a Randomized Clinical Trial: A Summary Report of the Nutritional Prevention of Cancer Trial." *Cancer Epidemiol Biomarkers Prev* 11, no. 7 (2002): 630–9.

Duffield-Lillico, A. J., E. H. Slate, M. E. Reid, B. W. Turnbull, P. A. Wilkins, G. F. Combs, Jr., H. K. Park, E. G. Gross, G. F. Graham, M. S. Stratton, J. R. Marshall, and L. C. Clark. "Selenium Supplementation and Secondary Prevention of Nonmelanoma Skin Cancer in a Randomized Trial." *J Natl Cancer Inst* 95, no. 19 (2003b): 1477–81.

El-Bayoumy, K. "The Negative Results of the Select Study Do Not Necessarily Discredit the Selenium-Cancer Prevention Hypothesis." *Nutr Cancer* 61, no. 3 (2009): 285–6.

Ervin, R. B., C. Y. Wang, J. D. Wright, and J. Kennedy-Stephenson. "Dietary Intake of Selected Minerals for the United States Population: 1999–2000." *Adv Data*, no. 341 (2004): 1–5.

Fakih, M. G., L. Pendyala, P. F. Smith, P. J. Creaven, M. E. Reid, V. Badmaev, R. G. Azrak, J. D. Prey, D. Lawrence, and Y. M. Rustum. "A Phase I and Pharmacokinetic Study of Fixed-Dose Selenomethionine and Irinotecan in Solid Tumors." *Clin Cancer Res* 12, no. 4 (2006): 1237–44.

Fisher, B., J. P. Costantino, D. L. Wickerham, R. S. Cecchini, W. M. Cronin, A. Robidoux, T. B. Bevers, M. T. Kavanah, J. N. Atkins, R. G. Margolese, C. D. Runowicz, J. M. James, L. G. Ford, and N. Wolmark. "Tamoxifen for the Prevention of Breast Cancer: Current Status of the National Surgical Adjuvant Breast and Bowel Project P-1 Study." *J Natl Cancer Inst* 97, no. 22 (2005): 1652–62.

Fisher, B., J. P. Costantino, D. L. Wickerham, C. K. Redmond, M. Kavanah, W. M. Cronin, V. Vogel, A. Robidoux, N. Dimitrov, J. Atkins, M. Daly, S. Wieand, E. Tan-Chiu, L. Ford, and N. Wolmark. "Tamoxifen for Prevention of Breast Cancer: Report of the National Surgical Adjuvant Breast and Bowel Project P-1 Study." *J Natl Cancer Inst* 90, no. 18 (1998): 1371–88.

Food and Nutrition Board, Institute of Medicine. *Selenium. Dietary References Intakes for Vitamin C, Vitamin E, Selenium and Carotenoids*. Washington, DC: National Academy Press, 2000.

Ford, E. S., A. H. Mokdad, W. H. Giles, and D. W. Brown. "The Metabolic Syndrome and Antioxidant Concentrations: Findings from the Third National Health and Nutrition Examination Survey." *Diabetes* 52, no. 9 (2003): 2346–52.

Ganther, H. E. "Selenium Metabolism, Selenoproteins and Mechanisms of Cancer Prevention: Complexities with Thioredoxin Reductase." *Carcinogenesis* 20, no. 9 (1999): 1657–66.

Goel, A., F. Fuerst, E. Hotchkiss, and C. R. Boland. "Selenomethionine Induces P53 Mediated Cell Cycle Arrest and Apoptosis in Human Colon Cancer Cells." *Cancer Biol Ther* 5, no. 5 (2006): 529–35.

Hatfield, D. L., and V. N. Gladyshev. "The Outcome of Selenium and Vitamin E Cancer Prevention Trial (Select) Reveals the Need for Better Understanding of Selenium Biology." *Mol Interv* 9, no. 1 (2009): 18–21.

Hu, H., C. Jiang, T. Schuster, G. X. Li, P. T. Daniel, and J. Lu. "Inorganic Selenium Sensitizes Prostate Cancer Cells to Trail-Induced Apoptosis through Superoxide/P53/Bax-Mediated Activation of Mitochondrial Pathway." *Mol Cancer Ther* 5, no. 7 (2006): 1873–82.

Ip, C. "Lessons from Basic Research in Selenium and Cancer Prevention." *J Nutr* 128, no. 11 (1998): 1845–54.

Ip, C., M. Birringer, E. Block, M. Kotrebai, J. F. Tyson, P. C. Uden, and D. J. Lisk. "Chemical Speciation Influences Comparative Activity of Selenium-Enriched Garlic and Yeast in Mammary Cancer Prevention." *J Agric Food Chem* 48, no. 9 (2000): 4452.

Ip, C., and H. E. Ganther. "Activity of Methylated Forms of Selenium in Cancer Prevention." *Cancer Res* 50, no. 4 (1990): 1206–11.

Ip, C., and C. Hayes. "Tissue Selenium Levels in Selenium-Supplemented Rats and Their Relevance in Mammary Cancer Protection." *Carcinogenesis* 10, no. 5 (1989): 921–5.

Ip, C., C. Hayes, R. M. Budnick, and H. E. Ganther. "Chemical Form of Selenium, Critical Metabolites, and Cancer Prevention." *Cancer Res* 51, no. 2 (1991): 595–600.

Ip, C., S. Vadhanavikit, and H. Ganther. "Cancer Chemoprevention by Aliphatic Selenocyanates: Effect of Chain Length on Inhibition of Mammary Tumors and Dmba Adducts." *Carcinogenesis* 16, no. 1 (1995): 35–8.

Ip, C., Z. Zhu, H. J. Thompson, D. Lisk, and H. E. Ganther. "Chemoprevention of Mammary Cancer with Se-Allylselenocysteine and Other Selenoamino Acids in the Rat." *Anticancer Res* 19, no. 4B (1999): 2875–80.

Irons, R., B. A. Carlson, D. L. Hatfield, and C. D. Davis. "Both Selenoproteins and Low Molecular Weight Selenocompounds Reduce Colon Cancer Risk in Mice with Genetically Impaired Selenoprotein Expression." *J Nutr* 136, no. 5 (2006): 1311–7.

Jiang, C., H. Ganther, and J. Lu. "Monomethyl Selenium—Specific Inhibition of Mmp-2 and Vegf Expression: Implications for Angiogenic Switch Regulation." *Mol Carcinog* 29, no. 4 (2000): 236–50.

Jiang, C., W. Jiang, C. Ip, H. Ganther, and J. Lu. "Selenium-Induced Inhibition of Angiogenesis in Mammary Cancer at Chemopreventive Levels of Intake." *Mol Carcinog* 26, no. 4 (1999): 213–25.

Jiang, C., Z. Wang, H. Ganther, and J. Lu. "Caspases as Key Executors of Methyl Selenium-Induced Apoptosis (Anoikis) of Du-145 Prostate Cancer Cells." *Cancer Res* 61, no. 7 (2001): 3062–70.

Jiang, C., Z. Wang, H. Ganther, and J. Lu. "Distinct Effects of Methylseleninic Acid Versus Selenite on Apoptosis, Cell Cycle, and Protein Kinase Pathways in Du145 Human Prostate Cancer Cells." *Mol Cancer Ther* 1, no. 12 (2002): 1059–66.

Kaeck, M., J. Lu, R. Strange, C. Ip, H. E. Ganther, and H. J. Thompson. "Differential Induction of Growth Arrest Inducible Genes by Selenium Compounds." *Biochem Pharmacol* 53, no. 7 (1997): 921–6.

Karp, D. D. "Ecog 5597: Phase Iii Chemoprevention Trial of Selenium Supplementation in Persons with Resected Stage I Non-Small-Cell Lung Cancer." *Clin Adv Hematol Oncol* 3, no. 4 (2005): 313–5.

Karp, D. D., S. J. Lee, G. L. Shaw-Wright, D. H. Johnson, M. R. Johnston, G. E. Goodman, G. H. Clamon, G. S. Okawara, R. Marks, and J. C. Ruckdeschel. *J. Clin Oncol* 28, no. 18S (2010): supplement; abstract CRA 7004.

Kim, T., U. Jung, D. Y. Cho, and A. S. Chung. "Se-Methylselenocysteine Induces Apoptosis through Caspase Activation in Hl-60 Cells." *Carcinogenesis* 22, no. 4 (2001): 559–65.

Klein, E. A. "Can Prostate Cancer Be Prevented?" *Nat Clin Pract Urol* 2, no. 1 (2005): 24–31.

Klein, E. A., I. M. Thompson, Jr., C. M. Tangen, J. J. Crowley, M. S. Lucia, P. J. Goodman, L. M. Minasian, L. G. Ford, H. L. Parnes, J. M. Gaziano, D. D. Karp, M. M. Lieber, P. J. Walther, L. Klotz, J. K. Parsons, J. L. Chin, A. K. Darke, S. M. Lippman, G. E. Goodman, F. L. Meyskens, Jr., and L. H. Baker. "Vitamin E and the Risk of Prostate Cancer: The Selenium and Vitamin E Cancer Prevention Trial (Select)." *JAMA* 306, no. 14 (2011): 1549–56.

Lee, S. O., N. Nadiminty, X. X. Wu, W. Lou, Y. Dong, C. Ip, S. A. Onate, and A. C. Gao. "Selenium Disrupts Estrogen Signaling by Altering Estrogen Receptor Expression and Ligand Binding in Human Breast Cancer Cells." *Cancer Res* 65, no. 8 (2005): 3487–92.

Li, G. X., H. J. Lee, Z. Wang, H. Hu, J. D. Liao, J. C. Watts, G. F. Combs, Jr., and J. Lu. "Superior in vivo Inhibitory Efficacy of Methylseleninic Acid against Human Prostate Cancer over Selenomethionine or Selenite." *Carcinogenesis* 29, no. 5 (2008): 1005–12.

Li, H., M. J. Stampfer, E. L. Giovannucci, J. S. Morris, W. C. Willett, J. M. Gaziano, and J. Ma. "A Prospective Study of Plasma Selenium Levels and Prostate Cancer Risk." *J Natl Cancer Inst* 96, no. 9 (2004): 696–703.

Lippman, S. M., E. A. Klein, P. J. Goodman, M. S. Lucia, I. M. Thompson, L. G. Ford, H. L. Parnes, L. M. Minasian, J. M. Gaziano, J. A. Hartline, J. K. Parsons, J. D. Bearden, 3rd, E. D. Crawford, G. E. Goodman, J. Claudio, E. Winquist, E. D. Cook, D. D. Karp, P. Walther, M. M. Lieber, A. R. Kristal, A. K. Darke, K. B. Arnold, P. A. Ganz, R. M. Santella, D. Albanes, P. R. Taylor, J. L. Probstfield, T. J. Jagpal, J. J. Crowley, F. L. Meyskens, Jr., L. H. Baker, and C. A. Coltman, Jr. "Effect of Selenium and Vitamin E on Risk of Prostate Cancer and Other Cancers: The Selenium and Vitamin E Cancer Prevention Trial (Select)." *JAMA* 301, no. 1 (2009): 39–51.

Lu, J. "Apoptosis and Angiogenesis in Cancer Prevention by Selenium." *Adv Exp Med Biol* 492 (2001): 131–45.

Lu, J., H. Hu, and C. Jiang. "Regulation of Signaling Pathways by Selenium in Cancer." In *Dietary Modulation of Cell Signaling Pathways*, edited by Y. J. Surh, Z. Dong, E. Cadenas and L. Packer, 273–314. Boca Raton, FL: CRC Press, 2009.

Lu, J., and C. Jiang. "Antiangiogenic Activity of Selenium in Cancer Chemoprevention: Metabolite-Specific Effects." *Nutr Cancer* 40, no. 1 (2001): 64–73.

Lu, J., and C. Jiang. "Selenium and Cancer Chemoprevention: Hypotheses Integrating the Actions of Selenoproteins and Selenium Metabolites in Epithelial and Non-Epithelial Target Cells." *Antioxid Redox Signal* 7, no. 11–12 (2005): 1715–27.

Lu, J., C. Jiang, M. Kaeck, H. Ganther, S. Vadhanavikit, C. Ip, and H. Thompson. "Dissociation of the Genotoxic and Growth Inhibitory Effects of Selenium." *Biochem Pharmacol* 50, no. 2 (1995): 213–9.

Lu, J., H. Pei, C. Ip, D. J. Lisk, H. Ganther, and H. J. Thompson. "Effect on an Aqueous Extract of Selenium-Enriched Garlic on in vitro Markers and in vivo Efficacy in Cancer Prevention." *Carcinogenesis* 17, no. 9 (1996): 1903–7.

Lucia, M. S., J. I. Epstein, P. J. Goodman, A. K. Darke, V. E. Reuter, F. Civantos, C. M. Tangen, H. L. Parnes, S. M. Lippman, F. G. La Rosa, M. W. Kattan, E. D. Crawford, L. G. Ford, C. A. Coltman, Jr., and I. M. Thompson. "Finasteride and High-Grade Prostate Cancer in the Prostate Cancer Prevention Trial." *J Natl Cancer Inst* 99, no. 18 (2007): 1375–83.

Marshall, J. R., C. M. Tangen, W. A. Sakr, D. P. Wood, Jr., D. L. Berry, E. A. Klein, S. M. Lippman, H. L. Parnes, D. S. Alberts, D. F. Jarrard, W. R. Lee, J. M. Gaziano, E. D. Crawford, B. Ely, M. Ray, W. Davis, L. M. Minasian, and I. M. Thompson, Jr. "Phase III Trial of Selenium to Prevent Prostate Cancer in Men with High-Grade Prostatic Intraepithelial Neoplasia: Swog S9917." *Cancer Prev Res (Phila)* 4, no. 11 (2011): 1761–9.

McCormick, D. L., K. V. Rao, W. D. Johnson, M. C. Bosland, R. A. Lubet, and V. E. Steele. "Null Activity of Selenium and Vitamin E as Cancer Chemopreventive Agents in the Rat Prostate." *Cancer Prev Res (Phila)* 3, no. 3 (2010): 381–92.

Menter, D. G., A. L. Sabichi, and S. M. Lippman. "Selenium Effects on Prostate Cell Growth." *Cancer Epidemiol Biomarkers Prev* 9, no. 11 (2000): 1171–82.

Moustafa, M. E., B. A. Carlson, M. A. El-Saadani, G. V. Kryukov, Q. A. Sun, J. W. Harney, K. E. Hill, G. F. Combs, L. Feigenbaum, D. B. Mansur, R. F. Burk, M. J. Berry, A. M. Diamond, B. J. Lee, V. N. Gladyshev, and D. L. Hatfield. "Selective Inhibition of Selenocysteine Trna Maturation and Selenoprotein Synthesis in Transgenic Mice Expressing Isopentenyladenosine-Deficient Selenocysteine tRNA." *Mol Cell Biol* 21, no. 11 (2001): 3840–52.

Neve, J. "Human Selenium Supplementation as Assessed by Changes in Blood Selenium Concentration and Glutathione Peroxidase Activity." *J Trace Elem Med Biol* 9, no. 2 (1995): 65–73.

Niskar, A. S., D. C. Paschal, S. M. Kieszak, K. M. Flegal, B. Bowman, E. W. Gunter, J. L. Pirkle, C. Rubin, E. J. Sampson, and M. McGeehin. "Serum Selenium Levels in the Us Population: Third National Health and Nutrition Examination Survey, 1988–1994." *Biol Trace Elem Res* 91, no. 1 (2003): 1–10.

Ozten, N., L. Horton, S. Lasano, and M. C. Bosland. "Selenomethionine and Alpha-Tocopherol Do Not Inhibit Prostate Carcinogenesis in the Testosterone Plus Estradiol-Treated Nbl Rat Model." *Cancer Prev Res (Phila)* 3, no. 3 (2010): 371–80.

Redman, C., M. J. Xu, Y. M. Peng, J. A. Scott, C. Payne, L. C. Clark, and M. A. Nelson. "Involvement of Polyamines in Selenomethionine Induced Apoptosis and Mitotic Alterations in Human Tumor Cells." *Carcinogenesis* 18, no. 6 (1997): 1195–202.

Reid, M. E., A. J. Duffield-Lillico, L. Garland, B. W. Turnbull, L. C. Clark, and J. R. Marshall. "Selenium Supplementation and Lung Cancer Incidence: An Update of the Nutritional Prevention of Cancer Trial." *Cancer Epidemiol Biomarkers Prev* 11, no. 11 (2002): 1285–91.

Shah, Y. M., M. Al-Dhaheri, Y. Dong, C. Ip, F. E. Jones, and B. G. Rowan. "Selenium Disrupts Estrogen Receptor (Alpha) Signaling and Potentiates Tamoxifen Antagonism in Endometrial Cancer Cells and Tamoxifen-Resistant Breast Cancer Cells." *Mol Cancer Ther* 4, no. 8 (2005a): 1239–49.

Shah, Y. M., A. Kaul, Y. Dong, C. Ip, and B. G. Rowan. "Attenuation of Estrogen Receptor Alpha (Eralpha) Signaling by Selenium in Breast Cancer Cells Via Downregulation of Eralpha Gene Expression." *Breast Cancer Res Treat* 92, no. 3 (2005b): 239–50.

Sinha, R., S. C. Kiley, J. X. Lu, H. J. Thompson, R. Moraes, S. Jaken, and D. Medina. "Effects of Methylselenocysteine on Pkc Activity, Cdk2 Phosphorylation and Gadd Gene Expression in Synchronized Mouse Mammary Epithelial Tumor Cells." *Cancer Lett* 146, no. 2 (1999): 135–45.

Sinha, R., and D. Medina. "Inhibition of Cdk2 Kinase Activity by Methylselenocysteine in Synchronized Mouse Mammary Epithelial Tumor Cells." *Carcinogenesis* 18, no. 8 (1997): 1541–7.

Stranges, S., J. R. Marshall, R. Natarajan, R. P. Donahue, M. Trevisan, G. F. Combs, F. P. Cappuccio, A. Ceriello, and M. E. Reid. "Effects of Long-Term Selenium Supplementation on the Incidence of Type 2 Diabetes: A Randomized Trial." *Ann Intern Med* 147, no. 4 (2007): 217–23.

Thompson, I. M., P. J. Goodman, C. M. Tangen, M. S. Lucia, G. J. Miller, L. G. Ford, M. M. Lieber, R. D. Cespedes, J. N. Atkins, S. M. Lippman, S. M. Carlin, A. Ryan, C. M. Szczepanek, J. J. Crowley, and C. A. Coltman, Jr. "The Influence of Finasteride on the Development of Prostate Cancer." *N Engl J Med* 349, no. 3 (2003): 215–24.

Thompson, I. M., C. M. Tangen, H. L. Parnes, S. M. Lippman, and C. A. Coltman, Jr. "Does the Level of Prostate Cancer Risk Affect Cancer Prevention with Finasteride?" *Urology* 71, no. 5 (2008): 854–7.

Vogel, V. G., J. P. Costantino, D. L. Wickerham, W. M. Cronin, R. S. Cecchini, J. N. Atkins, T. B. Bevers, L. Fehrenbacher, E. R. Pajon, Jr., J. L. Wade, 3rd, A. Robidoux, R. G. Margolese, J. James, S. M. Lippman, C. D. Runowicz, P. A. Ganz, S. E. Reis, W. McCaskill-Stevens, L. G. Ford, V. C. Jordan, and N. Wolmark. "Effects of Tamoxifen Vs Raloxifene on the Risk of Developing Invasive Breast Cancer and Other Disease Outcomes: The Nsabp Study of Tamoxifen and Raloxifene (Star) P-2 Trial." *JAMA* 295, no. 23 (2006): 2727–41.

Wang, L., M. J. Bonorden, G. X. Li, H. J. Lee, H. Hu, Y. Zhang, J. D. Liao, M. P. Cleary, and J. Lu. "Methyl-Selenium Compounds Inhibit Prostate Carcinogenesis in the Transgenic Adenocarcinoma of Mouse Prostate Model with Survival Benefit." *Cancer Prev Res (Phila)* 2, no. 5 (2009): 484–95.

Wang, Z., C. Jiang, H. Ganther, and J. Lu. "Antimitogenic and Proapoptotic Activities of Methylseleninic Acid in Vascular Endothelial Cells and Associated Effects on Pi3k-Akt, Erk, Jnk and P38 Mapk Signaling." *Cancer Res* 61, no. 19 (2001): 7171–8.

Wang, Z., C. Jiang, and J. Lu. "Induction of Caspase-Mediated Apoptosis and Cell-Cycle G1 Arrest by Selenium Metabolite Methylselenol." *Mol Carcinog* 34, no. 3 (2002): 113–20.

Whanger, P. D. "Selenium and Its Relationship to Cancer: An Update Dagger." *Br J Nutr* 91, no. 1 (2004): 11–28.

Yoo, M. H., X. M. Xu, B. A. Carlson, V. N. Gladyshev, and D. L. Hatfield. "Thioredoxin Reductase 1 Deficiency Reverses Tumor Phenotype and Tumorigenicity of Lung Carcinoma Cells." *J Biol Chem* 281, no. 19 (2006): 13005–8.

Yu, S. Y., W. G. Li, Y. J. Zhu, W. P. Yu, and C. Hou. "Chemoprevention Trial of Human Hepatitis with Selenium Supplementation in China." *Biol Trace Elem Res* 20, no. 1–2 (1989): 15–22.

Yu, S. Y., Y. J. Zhu, and W. G. Li. "Protective Role of Selenium against Hepatitis B Virus and Primary Liver Cancer in Qidong." *Biol Trace Elem Res* 56, no. 1 (1997): 117–24.

Zhang, J., L. Wang, L. B. Anderson, B. Witthuhn, Y. Xu, and J. Lu. "Proteomic Profiling of Potential Molecular Targets of Methyl-Selenium Compounds in the Transgenic Adenocarcinoma of Mouse Prostate Model." *Cancer Prev Res (Phila)* 3, no. 8 (2010): 994–1006.

Zhang, J., L. Wang, G. Li, L. B. Anderson, Y. Xu, B. Witthuhn, and J. Lu. "Mouse Prostate Proteomes Are Differentially Altered by Supranutritional Intake of Four Selenium Compounds." *Nutr Cancer* 63, no. 5 (2011): 778–89.

Zhao, H., M. L. Whitfield, T. Xu, D. Botstein, and J. D. Brooks. "Diverse Effects of Methylseleninic Acid on the Transcriptional Program of Human Prostate Cancer Cells." *Mol Biol Cell* 15, no. 2 (2004): 506–19.

Zhao, R., N. Xiang, F. E. Domann, and W. Zhong. "Expression of P53 Enhances Selenite-Induced Superoxide Production and Apoptosis in Human Prostate Cancer Cells." *Cancer Res* 66, no. 4 (2006): 2296–304.

Zhu, Z., W. Jiang, H. E. Ganther, and H. J. Thompson. "Mechanisms of Cell Cycle Arrest by Methylseleninic Acid." *Cancer Res* 62, no. 1 (2002): 156–64.

27 Chemoprevention of Lung Cancer by Ginseng

Michael S. You, Lucina C. Rouggly, Ming Hu,
Zhen Yang, Ming You, and Yian Wang

CONTENTS

27.1 INTRODUCTION

Ginseng is a traditional herbal medicine widely used in China and other Asian countries for hundreds of years. Among Chinese herbs, ginseng has been considered a tonic, used to improve physical condition and to prolong life, presumably by preventing or delaying the onset of various chronic diseases such as cancer and diabetes (Yun 2003). Epidemiological studies suggest that ginseng is a chemopreventive agent against a variety of cancer types, including cancer of the lip, oral cavity/pharynx, esophagus, stomach, colon, liver, pancreas, laryngis, lung, and ovary (Yun 2003). Users of ginseng had decreased cancer risk compared to nonusers, and the decrease greatly depended on the frequency of ginseng intake (Yun and Choi 1990). A large cohort study with 4634 adults (2362 men, 2272 women) over 40 years of age showed that ginseng users had a decreased cancer risk (relative risk [RR] = 0.40, 95% confidence interval [CI]: 0.28–0.56) compared with nonusers (Yun and Choi 1998; Yun 2001). The general conclusion from these studies is that ginseng has nontoxic and non–organ-specific preventive effects against several types of cancer, including lung cancer.

There are numerous reports on the mechanisms of ginseng's chemopreventive activity. Possible mechanisms include antioxidation, antitumor promotion, inhibition of cell proliferation, and induction of apoptosis (Hofseth and Wargovich 2007; Helms 2004). Ginseng has been shown to attenuate lipid peroxidation in rat brain homogenates and is also capable of scavenging superoxide generated by xanthine oxidase or by 12-*O*-tetradecanoylphorbol-13-acetate (TPA) in differentiated human promyelocytic leukemia HL-60 cells (Keum et al. 2000). Topical application of ginseng extract suppressed TPA-induced skin tumor promotion in ICR mice. Moreover, topical application of ginsenoside Rg3 inhibited TPA-induced mouse epidermal ornithine decarboxylase activity and skin tumor promotion. In a more recent study, ginsenoside Rg3 inhibited TPA-stimulated activation of nuclear factor kappaB (NF-κB) and extracellular signal–regulated kinase (ERK), one of the mitogen-activated protein kinases (MAPKs) in mouse skin as well as cultured human breast epithelial cells (Surh et al. 2001).

Several reports have shown that ginseng or ginsenosides (components isolated from ginseng, such as Rh1 and Rh2) suppressed the growth of various cancer cells (Ota et al. 1991; Liu et al. 2000). Ginseng can induce expression of the p21 tumor suppressor in human breast cancer cells (MCF-7 and MDA-MB-231) (Duda et al. 2001). Transfection of p21 reporter constructs in breast cancer cells demonstrated p53-independent activation of the p21 promoter (Duda et al. 2001). Polyacetylenic compounds from ginseng roots inhibited growth of human melanoma cells through induction of G1 cell cycle arrest and p27 function (Moon et al. 2000). An intestinal bacterial metabolite of ginseng, protopanaxadiol saponin Rb1 (M1), and a metabolic derivative from three mixtures (Rb1, Rb2, and Rc)—IH-901—induced apoptosis in tumor cells (Lee et al. 2000; Wakabayashi et al. 1998). Further studies suggest that the proapoptotic effect of IH-901 involves a mitochondria-mediated pathway and its downstream caspase-8 activation and Bid cleavage (Oh and Lee 2004). Interestingly, ginseng can also inhibit radiation-induced apoptosis in intestinal crypt cells and has a radioprotective effect (Kim et al. 2003a). Similarly, ginseng has protective effects against 1-methyl-4-phenylpyridinium–induced apoptosis in rat pheochromocytoma PC12 cells (Kim et al. 2003b). Inhibition of the ras signal transduction pathway, such as ERK, was reported (Surh et al. 2001) and further supported by experiments that found that ginseng or ginsenosides inhibit activator protein 1 (AP-1) activation (Choi et al. 2003; Keum et al. 2003). Ginsenoside Rd was found to inhibit Jun B and Fra-1 protein levels and AP-1 activation induced by lipopolysaccharide (LPS) plus tumor necrosis factor α (TNFα) (Choi et al. 2003). Ginsenoside Rg3 elicits a potent inhibitory effect on the activation of AP-1 that is responsible for c-jun and c-fos oncogenic transactivation in TPA-treated mouse skin (Keum et al. 2003). In the same study, Rg3 also inhibited TPA-induced activation of NF-κB (Keum et al. 2003). These results suggest that the chemopreventive effect of ginseng may be mediated through downregulation of NF-κB and AP-1 transcription factors.

27.2 EPIDEMIOLOGY

Table 27.1 summarized epidemiological studies on the chemoprevention of lung cancer by ginseng. Yun and Choi (1990) reported a case–control study on the effect of ginseng consumption and cancer risk. Among the 905 pairs of cases and controls, 62% of the cases (562 of 905 cases) had a history of ginseng intake compared to 75% of the controls (674 of 905 controls). They found that the odds ratio (OR) of cancer in relation to ginseng intake was 0.56, with a 95% CI of 0.45–0.69. A trend test showed a significant decrease in the proportion of cancer cases with increasing frequency of intake for males ($P < .00001$) as well as for females ($P < .05$). Chi-square homogeneity tests also confirmed significant differences between cases and controls for both sexes ($P < .001$). Another large ($n = 1987$) case–control study was reported by the same group (Yun and Choi 1995) and found a decrease in the risk of several cancer types (head and neck, esophagus, stomach, colorectal, liver, pancreas, lung, and ovary). The decrease in cancer risk was associated with the frequency, duration, and dose of ginseng intake. Interestingly, in cancers of the lung, lip, oral cavity and pharynx, and liver, smokers with ginseng intake had decreased ORs compared with smokers with no ginseng intake. However, there was no relationship between ginseng intake and cancers of the breast, cervix,

TABLE 27.1
Epidemiological Studies on the Chemoprevention of Lung Cancer by Ginseng

Agent	Population	Cancer	Results	Reference/PMID #
Ginseng	Patients at Korean Cancer Center ($n = 905$)	Multiple cancers	Decreased risk	Yun and Choi (1990)/ 2084014
Combined treatment[a]	SCLC patients in General Hospital of PLA, Beijing ($n = 54$)	SCLC	Raised survival rate	Cha et al. (1994)/ 7867442
Fresh, white, and red *Panax* ginseng extract and powder	Patients at Korean Cancer Center ($n = 1987$)	Multiple cancers	Decreased risk	Yun and Choi (1995b)/ 7655337
Fresh, white, and red *Panax* ginseng	Kangwha-eup, Korea ($n = 4634$)	Multiple cancers	Decreased risk	Yun and Choi (1998)/ 9698120
Ginseng	Medline database (1983–1998)	Multiple cancers	Not conclusive	Shin et al. (2000) review/10880039
Fresh, white, and red *Panax* ginseng extract and powder	Patients at the Korean Cancer Center	Multiple cancers	Decreased risk	Yun (2001) review/11905620
Red ginseng powder	Patients with stage III gastric cancer ($n = 42$)	Gastric cancer	Inhibits recurrence	Suh et al. (2002)/ 12568276
Fresh, white, and red *Panax* ginseng	Patients at Korean Cancer Center ($n = ?$)	Multiple cancers	Decreased risk	Yun (2003) review/12628504
Ginseng	Women from Shanghai, China ($n = 74,942$)	Gastric cancer	No effect	Kamangar et al. (2007)/ 17372265
Ginseng	African- or European-American women from Philadelphia and New Jersey ($n = 949$ patients; $n = 1524$ controls)	Breast cancer	No effect	Rebbeck et al. (2007)/ 17205521
Ginseng product: Shenqi	Cancer patients in China ($n = 60$)	Esophageal cancer	Improved cellular immunity	Wang et al. (2007)/ 17626759
Ginseng	General Korean population (55 years of age or older, $n = 6282$)		↓ All-cause mortality in men but not in women	Yi et al. (2009)/ 19678784
Ginseng	Males from western Washington State ($n = 35,239$)	Prostate cancer	No effect	Brasky et al. (2011)/ 21598177

[a] Combined treatment modalities of chemotherapy, radiotherapy, immunotherapy, and traditional Chinese medicine (including ginseng).

bladder, and thyroid gland. These findings suggest that ginseng users have a decreased risk for certain types of cancers compared with nonusers (Yun and Choi 1995). A prospective cohort study evaluated the preventive effects of ginseng against cancer in a population residing in a ginseng cultivation area based on the results from previous case–control studies (Yun and Choi 1998). The study interviewed 4634 people 40 years or older and collected data on ginseng intake, age at initial intake, frequency and duration of intake, and the types of ginseng. Multiple logistic regression calculation was used to estimate RR when controlling simultaneously for covariates. Ginseng users were found to have a decreased risk ($RR = 0.40$, 95% $CI = 0.28$–0.56) compared with nonusers. They also found decreased risks for gastric and lung cancer (Yun and Choi 1998). These data from epidemiological studies support a positive association between ginseng intake and decreased lung cancer risk.

27.3 GINSENG PREPARATIONS

In the past two decades, both *Panax* ginseng (Asian ginseng) and *Panax quinquefolius* L. (American ginseng [AG]) have attracted many scientists' and physicians' interest due to their potent pharmacological effects (Qi et al. 2010). Based on different preparation methods, *Panax* ginseng is classified into three types in the traditional herbal market: fresh ginseng, white ginseng, and red ginseng (Yun 2001). White ginseng is prepared from fresh ginseng after sun drying, with the water content usually less than 14% (Kim 2008). Red ginseng is manufactured by steaming fresh ginseng at 95°C–100°C for 2–3 h and then drying (Zhang et al. 2012).

Both white ginseng and red ginseng exhibit chemoprevention and anticancer activity (Kim 2008). The heat processing can hydrolyze and degrade most primary ginsenosides, including Rb1, Rb2, and Rc, to secondary ginsenosides by cleavage of sugar moieties (Christensen 2009). The same principle also applies to AG in that, after steam treatment (100°C–120°C), the antiproliferative effect of AG is significantly enhanced (Wang et al. 2007a). The enhanced anticancer activity is correlated with steaming time in that the activity of ginseng extract steamed for 2 h is greater than that of roots steamed for 1 h (Wang et al. 2007a). In addition, the quantity of seven ginsenosides decreased, whereas five other ginsenosides increased after heat processing.

There are many different formulations of ginseng on the market as anticancer drugs. ShenYi capsule, which contains 95% ginsenoside Rg3, has been used in China for treating non–small-cell lung cancer (NSCLC) and esophageal cancer since 2006 (Lu et al. 2008; Huang et al. 2009). The combination of ShenYi capsule with chemotherapy produces significantly enhanced therapeutic effects compared with chemotherapy alone in terms of 1-year survival time and quality of life. This may be due to improved immune function and antiangiogenic effects (Lu et al. 2008). Another ginseng preparation, "Shenmai" injection, which is composed of red ginseng and *Ophiopogon* (a genus of herbaceous perennial plants), has been used to treat cardiomyopathy, myocardial infarction, and hypertension in China (Xiaohui et al. 2006; Yang et al. 2009; Xia et al. 2010). Its major components are ginsenosides Rb1, Rb2, Rb3, Re, Rc, Rh1, Rg1, and Rg2 (Xiaohui et al. 2006). Also, Xuesaitong, administered as tablets or by injection, and Danshen tablets are the commercial formulations of *Panax notoginseng*. These ginseng formulations are used in China for treating various diseases including high blood pressure, depression, and inflammation (Song et al. 2010b; Feng et al. 2011). Many other raw ginseng and finished products (tablet, capsule matrixes) are available as dietary supplements (Harkey et al. 2001; Brown 2011).

27.4 CHEMISTRY, PHARMACOKINETICS, AND PHARMACOLOGY OF GINSENG

27.4.1 CHEMISTRY OF GINSENG

Ginsenosides, the dammarane-type triterpene saponins, have been found to be the major components responsible for ginseng's pharmacological activity, especially in the chemoprevention of lung cancer (Hasegawa 2004; Gu et al. 2009; Qi et al. 2011a). More than 150 ginsenosides have been identified so far, and Rb1, Rb2, Rc, Re, and Rg1 are the main naturally occurring constituents, representing 80% of ginsenosides (Li et al. 2004; Kim et al. 2005; Christensen 2009). There are four major groups of ginsenosides, including protopanaxadiol (PPD), protopanaxatriol (PPT), type C, and type D (Haijiang et al. 2003). Rb1, Rb2, and Rc represent quantitatively the main components of the PPD ginsenosides, whereas Rg1 and Re are the main components of PPT ginsenosides (Chang et al. 2002). Rk1, Rg5, Rk2, and Rh3 are the major dehydration metabolites of Rg3 and Rh2, the active anticancer components among ginsenosides (Qi et al. 2010). Some minor ginsenosides, like F0, F11, 25-OH-PPT, and 25-OH-PPT, do not belong to any of these four groups and therefore are considered as "other ginsenosides." PPD-series ginsenosides have sugar moieties attached to the β-OH at the C-3 and/or C-20 position, whereas PPT-series ginsenosides possess sugar moieties attached to the α-OH at C-6 and/or β-OH at C-20; type C and type D series are the dehydrogenated derivatives of PPT and PPD, with a double bond in the aliphatic side chain (Lu et al. 2009) (Figure 27.1).

PPD series

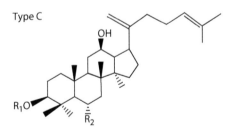

PPD series	R1	R2
Rb1	Glu^2-Glu	Glu^6-Glu
Rb2	Glu^2-Glu	Glu^2-Arap
Rb3	Glu^2-Glu	Glu^2-Xyl
Rc	Glu^2-Glu	Glu^6-Araf
Rd	Glu^2-Glu	H
Rg3	Glu^2-Glu	H
Rh2	Glu	H
F2	Glu	Glu
CK	H	Glu
PPD	H	H

PPT series

PPT series	R1	R2
Rh1	Glu	H
Rg1	Glu	Glu
Re	Glu^2-Rha	Glu
F1	H	Glu
R1	Glu^2-Xyl	Glu
Rg2	Glu^2-Rha	H
R2	H	Glu^2-Xyl
PPT	H	H

Type C

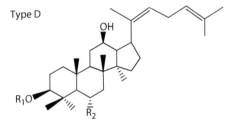

Type C	R1	R2
Rg5	Glc^2-Glc	H
Rh3	Glc	H

Type D

Type D	R1	R2
Rk1	Glc^2-Glc	H
Rk2	Glc	H

FIGURE 27.1 Chemical structures of ginsenosides including PPD series, PPT series, type C, and type D. Arap = α-L-arabinose (pyranose); Araf = α-L-arabinose (furanose); Glu = β-D-glucose; Rha = α-L-rhamnose; Xyl = β-D-xylose.

27.4.2 Pharmacokinetics of Ginsenosides

Ginsenosides have been shown to exhibit chemopreventive and anticancer activities, especially in lung cancer (Lee et al. 1999; Yun 2003). However, their low oral bioavailability (generally <5%) is the major factor leading to ambiguous results in clinical trials and represents a major obstacle for developing ginseng or ginsenosides as effective chemopreventive/chemotherapeutic agents (Table 27.2). Gu et al. (2009) reported that oral bioavailability of ginsenoside Rh2 is 5% in the rat after oral administration at 1, 3, and 9 mg/kg. The oral bioavailability of Rg3 is 0.5% in dogs after 2 mg/kg (Li et al. 2005) and was not detectable in rat plasma after oral administration at 100 mg/kg (Qian et al. 2005b). In humans, the plasma level of ginsenoside Rg3 (the approved anticancer drug in China) is below the quantification limit (2.5 ng/mL), at 0.8 mg/kg, and C_{max} is only 15.6 ng/mL at 3.2 mg/kg (Wang et al. 1999; Pang et al. 2001). Ginsenoside Re has very low oral bioavailability, ranging from 0.19% to 0.28% after oral administration of 50 mg/kg in mice (Joo et al. 2010). The ginsenoside aglycone PPD exhibits relatively high oral bioavailability at 20%–22% after using oil and emulsion formulations at 25 mg/kg (Han et al. 2010).

Many factors are responsible for the low bioavailability of ginsenosides, including low aqueous solubility, poor permeability, good substrate for efflux transporters, instability in gastrointestinal (GI) fluid, enzymatic degradation by glucosidases, and extensive metabolism (Qian et al. 2005a; Gu et al. 2009; Li et al. 2009a; Li et al. 2011b; Hao et al. 2010). Evaluation of presystemic stability of ginsenoside in the GI tract is important as some reports indicate that ginsenosides in vivo can be deglycosylated by intestinal bacteria via stepwise cleavage of the sugar moieties (Bae et al. 2004; Hasegawa 2004; Qi et al. 2011b). In vivo metabolism of ginsenosides should be considered since some ginsenosides, especially the potent ginsenosides with less sugar moieties, are very hydrophobic and may be metabolized and eliminated in vivo (Hao et al. 2010). Yang et al. (2011, 2012) found that ginsenoside Rh2 and compound K (CK) are good substrates of P-glycoprotein (P-gp) and that

TABLE 27.2

Oral Bioavailability of Various Ginsenosides in Rodents after Oral Administration at Different Doses

In Rat	Oral Bioavailability (%)	Dose (mg/kg)	Reference
Rh2	4.7	1, 3, 9	(Gu et al. 2009)
Rh2	N/A (<LOQ)	100	(Qian et al. 2005a)
	<1	5	
	<1	20	
Rg3(r)	N/A (<LOQ)	100	(Qian et al. 2005b)
Rg3	2.63	10	(Xie et al. 2005)
CK	3.52–6.57	30	(Lee et al. 2006)
	1.8	5	
	4.3	10	
	35.0	20	(Paek et al. 2006)
Re	0.16–0.28	1	(Joo et al. 2010)
Rb1	4.35	10	(Xu et al. 2003)
Rd	2.36	10	(Li et al. 2007)
Rg1	1.33	100	(Sun et al. 2005)
PPD	36.8	2	(Ren et al. 2008)
	20.7	25	
	22.4	25	(Han et al. 2010)

Note: LOQ, limit of quantitation.

inhibition of P-gp can significantly increase ginsenoside Rh2's oral bioavailability from 1% to 30% in A/J mice. Similarly, many other ginsenosides were found to be the substrates of ATP-binding cassette (ABC) transporters (Liu et al. 2009; Gu et al. 2010).

27.4.3 Pharmacology of Ginseng

Epidemiological data from a case–control study of 1987 pairs of Korean subjects showed that the long-term consumption of ginseng is associated with a significant reduction in many different types of malignancies including lung cancer (Yun 2003). The chemoprevention and anticancer mechanisms of ginsenosides include mitigation of DNA damage, induction of apoptosis, antiangiogenesis, and inhibition of proliferation as well as positive immunomodulation (Helms 2004). CK is one of the extensively investigated ginsenosides. CK displayed potent chemoprevention and anticancer activities in various cancer cell lines, and the mechanisms of action include induction of apoptosis (Cho et al. 2009; Jeong et al. 2010), suppression of NF-κB pathway activation (Ming et al. 2010), and inhibition of mutagenicity (Lee et al. 1998). Although CK has low abundance in raw ginseng or ginseng extract, previous studies indicated that it could be the major metabolite of ginsenosides after oral administration to rats (Akao et al. 1998), suggesting possible biotransformation of primary ginsenosides to secondary ginsenosides in vivo. Lee et al. (1999) also showed that the mean IC_{50} value of CK against four other human cancer cell lines was 32.9 μM, whereas the primary ginsenoside Rb1 (ginsenoside present in abundance in nature), the precursor of CK, produced no cytotoxic effects on any of the four cancer cell lines. These results are consistent with several structure–activity relationship studies indicating that the anticancer activity of ginsenoside is inversely correlated with the number of sugars, suggesting that the hydrolysis products have stronger anticancer activities than the precursor ginsenosides (Li et al. 2009b; Musende et al. 2009).

Ginsenoside Rh2s are another frequently studied ginsenoside that displays potent anticancer activity, especially in lung cancer cell lines (Cheng et al. 2006; Wang et al. 2006). A 9-week animal study showed that Rh2s have a tendency to decrease lung tumor incidence in mice after oral consumption (Yun 2003). Ginsenoside Rh2 has been shown to induce G1 phase arrest, followed by progression to apoptosis, in many human cancer cell lines (Cheng et al. 2005; Kim et al. 2011a; Li et al. 2011a). Ginsenosides Rg3 and Rg5 produce a statistically significant reduction in lung tumor incidence, and Rh2 had a tendency to decrease the incidence (Yun 2003). Rg3 can induce apoptosis by interfering with several signaling pathways, including modulating the AMP-activated protein kinase (AMPK) and transient receptor potential melastatin 7 channels (Yuan et al. 2010; Kim et al. 2011a). Ginsenoside 20(S)-protopanaxadiol inhibits the proliferation and invasion of human fibrosarcoma HT-1080 cells through apoptosis (Li et al. 2006). The chemoprevention of Rb1 and Re showed protective effects on DNA damage and in inducing DNA repair (Zhang et al. 2008; Cai et al. 2009). Rg5 ameliorates lung inflammation, possibly by inhibiting the binding of LPS to toll-like receptor 4 (TLR4) on macrophages (Kim et al. 2011b).

27.5 ANIMAL MODELS

Ginseng contains at least 150 different ginsenosides of PPD, PPT, or oleanane categories (Li et al. 2004; Kim et al. 2005; Christensen 2009; Yun 1999). These ginsenosides appear to have various biological activities including antioxidation, anti–tumor promotion, induction of p21 or p27, activation of NF-κB, activation of ERK, inhibition of cell proliferation, and induction of apoptosis. As mentioned earlier, ginseng is a potent inhibitor of carcinogenesis in many rodent models including lung, skin, liver, mammary gland, uterine cervix, brain, and colon and inhibits tumor cell growth in xenograft models (Tables 27.3 and 27.4).

TABLE 27.3

Inhibitory Effect of Ginseng or Ginseng Products in Xenograft Tumor Models

Ginseng Product	Cancer Cell Line	Xenograft Tumor	Reference/PMID #
25-OCH3-PPD	A549	Lung cancer—adenocarcinoma	Wang et al. (2009a)/19131140
CK	NCI-H460	Lung cancer—large cell	Chae et al. (2009)/19526988
Lipid-soluble red ginseng extract	NCI-H460	Lung cancer—large cell	Lee et al. (2010a)/20136429
Ginsenoside-Rb2	B16-BL6	Metastasis to lung—melanoma	Sato et al. (1994)/7522731
20(R)- and 20(S)-ginsenoside-Rg3	B16-BL6	Metastasis to lung—melanoma	Mochizuki et al. (1995)/8845804
20(R)- and 20(S)-ginsenoside-Rg3	26-M3.1	Metastasis to lung—colon cancer	Mochizuki et al. (1995)/8845804
Ginsenoside Rp1	B16-F10	Metastasis to lung—melanoma	Park et al. (2008)/18758081
Ginsenoside Rh2	MCF-7, MDA-MB-231	Breast cancer	Choi et al. (2011)/21080338
Apozem	H22	Liver cancer	Li et al. (2008)/18652353
Panax notoginseng	Hep3B	Liver cancer	Lin et al. (2010)/20681639
D-Rh(2)	H22	Liver cancer	Wei et al. (2011)/22196118
Red ginseng extract A and B	B16	Melanoma	Xiaoguang et al. (1998)/9533434
M4	B16-BL6	Melanoma	Hasegawa et al. (2002)/12132658
Ethanol extracts of *Panax notoginseng*	B16	Melanoma	Chen et al. (2006) 16965745
Ginsenoside Rh2	HRA	Ovarian cancer	Tode (1993a)/8258727
Ginsenoside Rh2	HRA	Ovarian cancer	Tode et al. (1993b)/8270603
Ginsenoside Rg3 cyclophosphamide	SKOV-3	Ovarian cancer	Xu et al. (2007)/17442207
Ginsenoside Rg3	SKOV-3	Ovarian cancer	Xu et al. (2008)/18959116
TBS-101	PC-3	Prostate cancer	Evans et al. (2009)/19846929
KG-135 (sun ginseng)	DU145	Prostate cancer	Yoo et al. (2010)/19765891
Red ginseng extract A and B	S180	Sarcoma	Xiaoguang et al. (1998)/9533434

27.5.1 XENOGRAFT TUMOR MODELS

Table 27.3 summarized efficacy results of ginseng xenograft tumor models. Multiple studies have been conducted using mouse cancer xenograft models to test the effects of ginseng on cancer development. Established human cancer cell lines (approximately 2×10^6 per injection) were inoculated subcutaneously into the backs of immunocompromised mice. Ginseng treatment was initiated either ~2 weeks before or ~2 weeks after cancer cell injection. (Wang et al. 2009a) have studied a newly identified natural product from *Panax notoginseng*, 20(S)-25-methoxyl-dammarane-3beta, 12beta, 20-triol [25-OCH(3)-PPD], for its activity against cancer cell growth. They reported that this compound decreased survival, inhibited proliferation, and induced apoptosis and G1 cell cycle arrest in human lung cancer cell lines (A549, H358, and H838). These abilities of 25-OCH(3)-PPD were also observed in xenografts produced by A549 lung cancer cells. At the same time, 25-OCH(3)-PPD exhibited low toxicity to noncancer cells, and no observable toxicity was seen when the compound was administered to animals (Wang et al. 2009a).

Chae et al. (2009) reported that NCI-H460 human large lung cancer cells are more susceptible to gamma-ray radiation–induced cell death when pretreated with CK (prepared by the incubation of PPD-type ginsenosides with *Bacteroides* JY-6, a human intestinal bacterium). The increased apoptosis induced by the combined treatment (gamma-ray radiation plus CK) was apparent by the presence of nuclear fragmentation, loss of mitochondrial membrane potential, and activation of caspase-3. Furthermore, CK enhances gamma–ray radiation-induced regression of NCI-H460 tumor xenografts in nude mice (Chae et al. 2009).

Lee et al. (2010a) prepared lipid-soluble ginseng extract (LSGE) by *n*-hexane extraction of red ginseng. They administrated the LSGE orally to BALB/c-nu mice with established xenograft tumors produced by human lung cancer (NCI-H460) cells. The extract produced a dose-dependent tumor inhibitory effect without any apparent toxicity (Lee et al. 2010a).

Ginseng products have also been found to inhibit the growth of xenograft tumors in mice derived from the liver (Li et al. 2008; Lin et al. 2010; Wei et al. 2011); melanoma (Xiaoguang et al. 1998; Hasegawa et al. 2002; Chen et al. 2006); sarcoma (Xiaoguang et al. 1998); ovarian cancer (Tode et al. 1993a,b; Xu et al. 2007, 2008); and prostate cancer cell lines (Evans et al. 2009; Yoo et al. 2010). Although the growth of HRA cells (derived from ascites of a patient with serous cystadenocarcinoma of the ovary) transplanted into nude mice was not significantly inhibited by Rh2 (a ginsenoside isolated from red ginseng) alone, survival of the mice was prolonged when cisplatin was administered with Rh2, suggesting a synergistic effect between cisplatin and Rh2 (Tode et al. 1992).

Li et al. (2008) transplanted H22 liver cancer cells to mice. The tumor weight, body weight, spleen index and thymus gland index, natural killer (NK) cell activity, proliferation of T lymphocytes, and interleukin 2 (IL-2) level were measured. Growth of H22 xenograft tumors was markedly inhibited by ginseng–Chinese date–licorice root along with an improved immune function in tumor-bearing mice (Li et al. 2008). Lin et al. (2010) have tested *Panax notoginseng* (fermented ginseng broth) for its antiproliferative activity against hepatoma Hep3B cells xenografted in severe combined immunodeficient (SCID) mice. They found that both tumor volume and tumor weight were reduced by approximately 60%. High-performance liquid chromatography (HPLC) analyses showed that saponins in *Panax notoginseng*, including notoginsenoside R1 and ginsenosides Rg1, Rb1, Rd, and Rh4, decreased but ginsenosides Rh1 and Rg3 increased during fermentation. Liquid chromatography–tandem mass spectrometry (LC–MS/MS) revealed that the minor saponins ginsenoside F(1), PPT, and notoginseng R2 also exist in the fermentation product. It appears that ginsenoside Rg3, ginsenoside Rh1, and PPT are responsible for the enhanced antihepatocarcinoma activity of *Panax notoginseng* fermentation broth (Lin et al. 2010). Ginsenoside Rh2 is one of the most important ginsenosides with anticancer properties in red ginseng. Cytotoxicity tests with the human hepatocyte cell line, QSG-7701 (IC$_{50}$, 37.3 μM), indicated that Rh2 might be strongly cytotoxic to normal liver cells. In order to decrease the toxicity, Wei et al. (2011) structurally modified ginsenoside Rh2 by reacting with octanoyl chloride to add dioctanoyl ester onto Rh2, and they named it D-Rh2. They then showed by MTT assay that the cytotoxicity of D-Rh2 toward human hepatocyte cells (IC$_{50}$, 80.5 μM) was significantly lower than that of Rh2 (IC$_{50}$, 37.3 μM). At the same time, the antitumor activity of D-Rh2 remained the same as that of Rh2 in xenograft tumors of mice bearing H22 liver cancer cells (Wei et al. 2011).

Sato et al. (1994) studied the effect of ginsenoside-Rb2 extracted from *Panax* ginseng on angiogenesis and metastasis produced by B16-BL6 melanoma cells in syngeneic mice. Intravenous (i.v.) administration of ginsenoside-Rb2 on days 1, 3, or 7 after tumor inoculation achieved a remarkable reduction in the number of vessels oriented toward the tumor mass but did not cause a significant inhibition of tumor growth. Intratumoral or oral administration of ginsenoside-Rb2 caused a marked inhibition of both neovascularization and tumor growth. Interestingly, they found that multiple administrations of ginsenoside-Rb2 after i.v. inoculation of B16-BL6 melanoma cells resulted in a significant inhibition of lung metastasis, and an inhibition of tumor-associated angiogenesis by ginsenoside-Rb2 may partly contribute to the inhibition of lung tumor metastasis (Sato et al. 1994). A year later, Mochizuki et al. (1995) (from the same group at Hokkaido University,

TABLE 27.4
Inhibitory Effect of Ginseng or Ginseng Products on Carcinogen-Induced Tumors in Rodents

Ginseng Product	Carcinogen	Tumor	Rodent	Inhibition Effect	Reference/PMID #
Korean red ginseng	DMBA	Lung adenoma	ICR mice	Yes	Yun et al. (1983)/6420059
Korean red ginseng	Urethane	Lung adenoma	ICR mice	Yes	Yun et al. (1983)/6420059
Korean red ginseng	Aflatoxin B1	Lung adenoma	ICR mice	Yes	Yun et al. (1983)/6420059
Red ginseng extract	B(a)P	Lung adenoma	A/J mice	Yes	Yun (1995)/7645968
Fr.3	B(a)P	Lung adenoma	N:GP(S) mice	Yes	Yun et al. (1993)/ 8302951
Red ginseng extract	B(a)P	Lung adenoma	N:GP(S) mice	Yes	Yun (1995)/7645968
Red ginseng	B(a)P	Lung adenoma	A/J mice	Yes	Yan et al. (2006)/16533426
EFLA400	B(a)P	Lung adenoma	Swiss albino mice	Yes	Panwar et al. (2005)/16272690
Fresh ginseng	B(a)P	Lung adenoma	N:GP(S) mice	No	Yun (1995)/7645968
Bioginseng	ENU	Brain and spinal cord	Rats	Yes	Bespalov et al. (2001)/11748376
250 ppm ginseng	AOM + WD	Colon tumor	A/J mice	Yes	Dougherty et al. (2011)/22070864
White ginseng	DEN	Colon tumor	F344/DuCrj rats	Yes	Ichihara et al. (2002)/12718582
Red and white ginseng	DEN	GST-P–positive foci in liver	F344/DuCrj rats	No	Ichihara et al. (2002)/12718582
Ginseng powder	AOM	Colon/ACF	Rats	Yes	Volate et al. (2005)/15831530
Korean red ginseng	AOM	Colon/ACF	F344 rats	Yes	Wargovich (2001)/11748382
Red ginseng	DMH	Colon/ACF	F344 rats	Yes	Li et al. (2000)/10798218
Ginseng	None	Fibrosarcoma of mammary	F344/N rats	Yes	NTP/21921964
MR2	DEN/BP (phenobarbital)	Hepatic tumor	Mice	Yes	Konoshima et al. (1999b)/10660083
Korean red ginseng	Aflatoxin B1	Hepatoma	ICR mice	Yes	Yun et al. (1983)/6420059
Pfaffia paniculata	None	Leukemia	AKR/J mice	Yes	Watanabe et al. (2000)/10917139
Ginseng	DEN	Liver	Rats	Yes	Wu and Zhu (1990)/2255002

Red ginseng extracts	None	Liver	C3H/He mice	Yes	Nishino et al. (2001)/11748379
Bioginseng	MNU	Mammary	Rats	Yes	Bespalov et al. (2001)/11748376
American ginseng	DMBA	Mammary tumors	SENCAR mice	No	Wurz et al. (2006)/17476970
Pfaffia paniculata root	DEN	Preneoplastic hepatic lesions	BALB/c mice	Yes	da Silva et al. (2005)/16039950
WKRG	Testosterone	Prostate hyperplasia	Rats	Yes	Bae et al. (2012)/22101440
Bioginseng	DMBA	SCC of uterus, cervix, vagina	Mice	Yes	Bespalov et al. (1993a)/8312554
Red ginseng extract A/B	DMBA/croton oil	Skin papilloma	Mice	Yes	Xiaoguang et al. (1998)/9533434
Red ginseng extract A/B	DMBA/croton oil	Skin papilloma	Mice	Yes	Xiaoguang et al. (1998)/9533434
EFLA400	DMBA	Skin papilloma	Swiss albino	Yes	Panwar et al. (2005)/15799001
Ginsenoside Rg3	TPA and DMBA	Skin tumor	ICR mice	Yes	Keum et al. (2003)/12628505
RSYRT	DMBA and ATP	Skin tumor	CD-1 mice	Yes	Nishino et al. (2001)/11748379
MR2	NOR-1 and TPA	Skin tumor	Mice	Yes	Konoshima et al. (1999b)/10660083
MR2	Peroxynitrite/TPA	Skin tumor	Mice	Yes	Konoshima et al. (1999b)/10660083
Araliaceae	DMBA and Fumonisin B1	Skin tumor	Mice	Yes	Konoshima et al. (1999a)/10549877
Araliaceae	NOR-1 and TPA	Skin tumor	Mice	Yes	Konoshima et al. (1999a)/10549877
MR2	DMBA and TPA	Skin tumor	Mice	Yes	Konoshima et al. (1998)/9743252
American ginseng	AOM/dextran sulfate sodium	Ulcerative colitis	Mice	Yes	Cui et al. (2010)/20729391
IH-901	DMBA and TPA	Skin papilloma	Mice	Yes	Lee et al. (2005)/15498788
Bioginseng	DMBA	Uterine/cervical/vaginal tumor	Mice	Yes	Bespalov et al. (2001)/11748376

Note: NOR-1, nitric oxide donor, (+/−)-(E)-methyl-2-[(E)-hydroxyimino]-5-nitro-6-methoxy-3-hexen amide; SCC, squamous cell carcinoma.

Japan) reported their studies of the inhibitory effects of two saponin preparations from red ginseng, 20(R)-ginsenoside-Rg3 [20(R)-Rg3] and 20(S)-ginsenoside-Rg3 [20(S)-Rg3], on B16-BL6 melanoma and colon 26-M3.1 carcinoma metastasis to the lungs of syngeneic mice. In an experimental metastasis model using B16-BL6 melanoma, consecutive i.v. administrations of 10 and 100 μg per mouse of 20(R)- or 20(S)-Rg3 1, 2, 3, and 4 days after tumor inoculation led to a significant decrease in lung metastasis. The oral administration of both saponins (100–1000 μg per mouse) induced a significant decrease in lung metastasis of B16-BL6 melanoma. Also, both ginseng saponins were effective at inhibiting lung metastasis produced by colon 26-M3.1 carcinoma cells. Their study also indicated that both ginseng saponins, 20(R)- and 20(S)-Rg3, possess an ability to inhibit lung metastasis of tumor cells, and the mechanism of their antimetastatic effects is related to inhibition of the adhesion and invasion of tumor cells and also to antiangiogenesis activity (Mochizuki et al. 1995).

27.5.2 Primary Tumor Models

As shown in Table 27.4, the chemopreventive efficacy of ginseng has been demonstrated in an ICR mouse lung tumor model using 7,12-dimethylbenz(a)anthracene (DMBA), urethane, and aflatoxin B1 as carcinogens (Yun et al. 1983), and in N:GP(S) and A/J mice using benzo(a)pyrene [B(a)P] as the carcinogen (Yun et al. 1995a; Yan et al. 2006). Similar results were reported by a group of scientists in India (Panwar et al. 2005) on B(a)P-induced lung adenomas in Swiss albino mice. Furthermore, two specific ginsenosides, Rg3 and Rg5, caused statistically significant reductions in lung tumor incidence in mice (Yun et al. 2001a). In one of our studies, red ginseng was evaluated in A/J mice treated with the tobacco-specific carcinogen B(a)P for its ability to inhibit pulmonary adenoma formation and growth. Administration of red ginseng in drinking water decreased tumor multiplicity by 36% and tumor load (sum of tumor volume per lung) by 70% in a tumor progression protocol (Yan et al. 2006).

In a two-stage mouse skin model with DMBA and TPA, ginseng exhibits an inhibitory effect against the development of skin papillomas in a dose-dependent manner (Xiaoguang et al. 1998). When ginseng was given in the diet, it suppressed aberrant crypt foci (ACF) induced by 1,2-dimethylhydrazine or azoxymethane in Fisher 344 rats (Li et al. 2000). More significantly, ginseng appears to be more effective against ACF development at the postinitiation stage of colon carcinogenesis (Wargovich 2001). Oral administration of red ginseng extract (RGE) caused significant suppression of spontaneous liver tumor formation in C3H/He male mice, the development of diethylnitrosamine-induced liver cancer in rats, methyl-N-nitrosourea–induced mammary adenocarcinoma in rats, N-ethyl-N-nitrosourea–induced brain and spinal cord tumors in rats, and DMBA-induced mammary, uterine, cervix, and vaginal tumors in mice (Wu and Zhu 1990; Bespalov et al. 1993a,b, 2001). White ginseng was found to decrease the incidence of adenocarcinomas in the small intestine and colon in a medium-term multiorgan carcinogenesis model without any effect on the number of ACF (Ichihara et al. 2002).

27.6 CLINICAL STUDIES

Table 27.5 summarizes clinical studies on ginseng's effect against cancer. Among these studies, only one was focused on cancer prevention in high-risk populations: a randomized, double-blinded, placebo-controlled trial involving 643 chronic atrophic gastritis patients in four hospitals in Zhejiang Province, China (Yun et al. 2010). Effects of long-term use of Korean RGE on the incidence of human primary cancers in a non–organ-specific manner were evaluated. One gram of RGE was administered orally to each patient per week for 3 years, and follow-up was made for 8 years. The development of various cancers (including cancers of the lung, stomach, liver, colon, esophagus, and prostate) was monitored, and they found that the relative cancer risk (95% CI) was highly decreased in male patients (Yun et al. 2010).

Cha et al. (1994) reported their findings on the nonsurgical treatment of small-cell lung cancer (SCLC) with chemotherapy (vincristine, cyclophosphamide, methotrexate, and carmustine) plus a ginseng formula made of the leaf of Asiatic ginseng and the root of *Astragalus membranaceus* Bge, among other components. Although the cohort was small (54 SCLC patients), they reported a complete response of 59.2%, a partial response of 38.9%, and an overall response of 98.1%. The survival of these patients was prolonged when they were treated long term (especially more than 2 years or 10 courses), combined with chemotherapy, radiotherapy, and adjuvants such as traditional Chinese medicine and immunotherapy (Cha et al. 1994).

Additional studies have shown an enhancing effect of ginseng on chemotherapy (Navelbine and cisplatin or vinorelbine and cisplatin) in NSCLC patients (Chen et al. 2009; Sun et al. 2006). Chen et al. (2009) reported their findings of combined Chinese drugs and chemotherapy in treating advanced NSCLC. Sixty-three stage IIIB and IV NSCLC patients were enrolled, and all 63 patients were treated with Navelbine and cisplatin. These patients were assigned to two groups randomly. One group received Shengmai injection (i.v. dripping) and Gujin Granule (oral intake). The response rate, median survival time, 1-year survival rate, and median time to progression (TTP) were recorded. Sixty-one patients (33 from the treatment group and 28 from the control group) completed the trial. Based on their calculations, combined Navelbine and cisplatin and Chinese drugs can enhance the short-term therapeutic efficacy in the treatment of NSCLC and prolong patients' median survival time but show no evident impact on TTP (Chen et al. 2009). Subsequently, Sun et al. (2006) performed a randomized, prospective, multicenter clinical trial of (vinorelbine and cisplatin) plus ginseng Rg3 (an active component isolated from ginseng) in the treatment of stage III–IV NSCLC patients. One hundred and fifteen patients were enrolled into the trial, and 106 patients were evaluated for clinical efficacy. The results indicated slight improvements in response rate and survival time (median and mean) in the Rg3 arm compared with the placebo arm. The authors suggested that these results should be confirmed in future clinical trials (Sun et al. 2006).

27.7 MECHANISMS

Ginseng has been shown to inhibit cancer cell proliferation and tumor growth. There are several major molecular mechanisms involving ginseng's anticancer properties: antioxidation, induction of apoptosis, induction of cell cycle arrest, and anti-invasion/metastasis. Table 27.6 summarizes the major molecular mechanisms of ginseng on cell growth and apoptosis.

27.7.1 GINSENG AND CELL CYCLE ARREST

Ginseng and its related products can induce cell cycle arrest as demonstrated in several cancer cell lines, including breast, colon, laryngeal, cervical, and prostate cancer and melanoma. These effects associated with ginseng treatment are predominantly related to inducing G1 phase arrest. Oh et al. (1999) studied the antiproliferating effect of ginsenoside Rh2 on MCF-7 human breast cancer cells. They found that Rh2 significantly inhibited cell growth in a concentration-dependent manner through G1 cell cycle arrest. This effect was reversible upon removal of Rh2 from the medium. Rh2 treatment downregulated the protein level of cyclin D3 and upregulated the expression of cyclin-dependent kinase (CDK) inhibitor p21$^{WAF1/CIP1}$. Increased levels of p21 were associated with increased binding of p21 and CDK2 concomitant with a marked decrease in CDK2 and cyclin E–dependent kinase activities, with no changes in the expression of CDK2 or cyclin E. Rh2 markedly reduced p-Rb–enhanced association of unphosphorylated Rb and of transcription factor E2F-1. These data suggest that Rh2 inhibits the growth of MCF-7 cells by inducing protein expression of p21 and reducing the protein levels of cyclin D, resulting in downregulation of the activity of cyclin/CDK complex kinase, decreased phosphorylation of Rb, and inhibition of E2F release (Oh et al. 1999). This study was supported by the findings of Duda et al. (2001). The p21 protein functions as a universal cell cycle inhibitor by binding to cyclin/CDK complexes. In another human breast

TABLE 27.5
Clinical Findings on Ginseng Use[a]

Ginseng	Cohort	Study	Findings	Institution	Reference/PMID #
Shenmai (GP)	63 stomach cancer	Patients were randomly divided into two groups	Shenmai might improve immune function; Shenmai might facilitate chemotherapy	Zhejiang Provincial Hospital, China	Lin et al. (1995)/8580688
RT + GSP	131 nasopharyngeal carcinoma	Patients were randomly divided into two groups	GSP improves immune function effect in patients during RT; GSP eliminates adverse reaction to RT	Cancer Center of Sun Yat-Sen University, China	Xie et al. (2001)/12577414
Red ginseng	42 stage III gastric cancer		Inhibits recurrence; Positive immunomodulatory activities	Korea University College of Medicine, Korea	Suh et al. (2002)/12568276
Ginseng	233 breast cancer	Questionnaires/risk calculations	Could potentially increase the risk of breast cancer; Potentially interacts with tamoxifen or aromatase inhibitor	Lund University Hospital, Sweden	Malekzadeh et al. (2005)/16329453
Ginseng	1455 breast cancer (Shanghai Breast Cancer Study)	Questionnaires/risk calculations	Reduced risk of death in regular users; Improves quality of life in regular users	Vanderbilt University, USA	Cui et al. (2006)/16484447
Sun ginseng (SG)	28 gynecologic cancer; 13 liver cancer; 12 other cancers	Randomized, double-blind, placebo-controlled pilot trial	Improves some aspects of mental and physical functioning	Gachon Medical School, Korea	Kim et al. (2006)/16882101
Rg3	115 stage III–IV NSCLC—all treated with vinorelbine and cisplatin	Patients were randomly divided into control and trial groups	Improves response rate and survival time	Cancer Hospital/Institute, Chinese Academy of Medical Sciences, China	Sun et al. (2006)/21172156

Shenqi (GP)	60 esophageal carcinoma, received two-field dissection	Patients were randomly divided into control and trial groups	Improves cellular immunity of patients after modern two-field dissection		Skate Key Lab of Oncology in South China, China	Wang et al. (2007b)/ 17626759
Shengmai (GP) and Gujin granule (CAM)	63 stage IIIB and IV NSCLC—all treated with Navelbine and cisplatin	Patients were randomly divided into two groups	Combination chemotherapy can enhance short-term therapeutic efficacy	Combined chemotherapy can prolong patients' median survival		Chen et al. (2009)/ 20082245
AG	290 all cancer	Randomized in a double-blind manner	Some activity on cancer-related fatigue	Tolerable toxicity	Mayo Clinic, USA	Barton et al. (2010)/ 19415341
RGE	643 chronic atrophic gastritis	Randomized, double-blinded, placebo-controlled trial	Lowers the incidence of non–organ-specific cancers in males		Korea Institute of Cancer Chemoprevention, Korea	Yun et al. (2010)/ 20521975
CVT-E002 (GP)	293 early-stage, untreated CML	Double-blind, placebo-controlled, randomized trial	It did not reduce the number of ARI days or antibiotic use	With a trend toward reduced rates of ARI and significantly less sore throat	Wake Forest University School of Medicine, USA	High et al. (2012)/ 22266154

Note: GSP, ginseng polysaccharide: RT, radiotherapy.

[a] Case reports were not listed.

TABLE 27.6

Major Molecular Mechanisms of Ginseng on Cell Growth and Apoptosis

Ginseng	Effect	Modulated Target(s)	Cell Line	Original Cancer	Reference/PMID
AGBE	Antiproliferation	Synergistic with 5-FU; G2/M phase arrest	SW-480; HCT-116; HT-29	Human colon cancer	Li et al. (2009c)/19724877
Panax ginseng	Antiproliferation	Inhibited HCC in rats; prolonged survival time	DEN-induced HCC *in vivo*	Rat liver cancer	Li (1991)/1816418
Ginsenoside Rb1, Rg1	Antiproliferation	Antiproliferation	HuH-7	Human hepatoma	Okita et al. (1993)/7681712
Panax pseudo-ginseng	Antiproliferation	Suppresses growth	LNCaP	Human prostate cancer	Hsieh and Wu (2002)/11836572
Ginsenoside Rg1	Antiproliferation	Inhibits TNFα-enhanced proliferation; ↓ G-protein receptor kinase, PKC, N-ras	VSMC	Vascular smooth muscle	Ma et al. (2006)/16867250
White ginseng (WG)	Antiproliferation	Inhibits proliferation in a dose-dependent manner; Expression of p21	HCT-116	Human colon cancer	Fishbein et al. (2009)/19407967
G-Rh2	Cell cycle regulation	Inhibits cell growth; G1 arrest; ↓ cyclin D3; p21	MCF-7	Human breast cancer	Oh et al. (1999)/10200336
Panaxydol	Cell cycle regulation	Antiproliferation; decreases cell number; Inhibits G(1)-S transition; ↓ CDK2; p27 KiP1	SK-MEL-1	Human melanoma	Moon et al. (2000)/10704940
AG	Cell cycle regulation	Inhibits human breast cancer cell growth; AG induced p21 mRNA expression; Independent of p53	MDA-MB-231; MCF-7	Human breast cancer	Duda et al. (2001)/11748377
Ginseng saponin IH-901	Cell cycle regulation	Antiproliferation; Cell cycle arrests in the G0/G1 phase; ↓ VEGF and bFGF; CC3 and CC9	ECV304	Endothelial cells	Ming et al. (2009)/20055170
KG-135	Cell cycle regulation	Induces cell growth arrest; Arrests cells at the G1 phase of cell cycle; ↓ activity of cyclins D1 and B1	HeLa	Human cervix adenocarcinoma	Lee et al. (2009c)/19148524
Rh2	Cell cycle regulation	Inhibited viability; Causes G(0)/G(1) phase arrest; Inhibited G(1)-S CDKs/cyclin activity	MDA-MB-231; MCF-7	Human breast cancer	Choi et al. (2009)/19629651

Compound	Pathway	Effect	Mechanism	Molecular targets	Cell line	Cancer type	Reference
GE	Cell cycle regulation	Cell cycle arrest in p21wt cells; cell death in p21-/-	G0/G1 arrest	p53; p21; ↓ p-MEK	HCT-116	Human colon cancer	King and Murphy (2010)/19674880
KG-135	Cell cycle regulation	Growth inhibition	G1 arrest; p21	↓ PCNA	DU145; PC-3	Human prostate cancer	Yoo et al. (2010)/19765891
Ginseng pectin	Cell cycle regulation	Antiproliferation; induces apoptosis	Induced CC arrest in the G2/M phase		HT-29	Human colon cancer	Cheng et al. (2011)/20165990
GE	MAPK pathway	Inhibits proliferation of MCF-7	↓ p-MEK1/2; ↓ p-ERK1/2; p-Raf-1	mRNA and protein expression of RKIP	MCF-7 cells	Human breast cancer	King and Murphy (2007)/17407973
PND	MAPK pathway	Inhibits proliferation; induces differentiation	Changes differentiation markers	Intracellular cAMP; p21 and p-ERK1/2	SMMC-7721	Human liver carcinoma	Wang et al. (2011)/21628989
Ginsenoside Rd	MAPK pathway	Inhibited migration, invasion, and metastasis	↓ expression of MMPs; blocks MAPK signaling	↓ AP-1; focal adhesion formation	HepG2	Human HCC	Yoon et al. (2011)/21982435
Ginsenoside Rg3	Wnt/β-catenin pathway	Inhibits growth of colon tumor cell growth	Blocking translocation of ß-catenin	Decreases PCNA expression	HCT-116	Colorectal tumor	He et al. (2011)/21152855
RG	Differentiation	Inhibits proliferation; synergistic with 5-FU	Induces G1 arrest		HCT-116	Human colon cancer	Fishbein (2009)/19407967
M1	Apoptosis	Induce apoptosis in tumor cells	$p27^{Kip1}$	↓ c-Myc; ↓cyclin D1	B16-BL6	Mouse melanoma	Wakabayashi et al. (1998)/9618279
Ginsenoside Rg3	Apoptosis	↓ cell growth via a CC3-mediated apoptosis	p21 and p27; G1 phase arrest	↓ PSA, androgen receptor, and PCNA	LNCaP	Human prostate carcinoma	Liu et al. (2000)/10972198
IH-901	Apoptosis	Via cytochrome c–mediated caspase-3	Proteolytic cleavage of PARP	Independent of Bcl-2 modulation	HL-60	Human myeloid leukemia	Lee et al. (2000)/10927026
Ginsenoside Rh2	Apoptosis	Inhibited growth	Via caspase-3 and -8 pathway		A375-S2	Human melanoma	Fei et al. (2002)/11931705
MGG	Apoptosis	Nitric oxide in mouse peritoneal macrophage	↓ caspase-8; and –caspase-3	↓ TNFα secretion	HL-60	Human leukemia	Koo et al. (2007)/17265560
Panaxydol	Apoptosis	Inhibited proliferation; induction of apoptosis	↓ Expression of bcl-2	Levels of Bax and caspase-3	C6	Rat glioma	Hai et al. (2007)/17320424
Ginsenoside Rk1	Apoptosis	Antitumor activity	↓ telomerase; ↓ cell growth; ↓ hTERT	Caspases-8 and -3; ↓ FADD and c-Myc	HepG2	Human HCC	Kim et al. (2008)/18451501

(continued)

TABLE 27.6 (Continued)
Major Molecular Mechanisms of Ginseng on Cell Growth and Apoptosis

Ginseng	Effect		Modulated Target(s)	Cell Line	Original Cancer	Reference/PMID
Saponins of *Panax* ginseng	Apoptosis	Induces apoptosis in HL-60 cells	Expression of Bax mRNA, ↓ expression of bcl-xl mRNA	HL-60		Fang et al. (2008)/ 18718060
Korean RGE	Apoptosis	↓ telomerase activity; activation of caspase 3	↓ antiapoptotic Bcl-2, Bcl-X(L), ↓ COX2, iNOS, hTERT, and c-Myc	U937	Human leukemia	Park et al. (2009)/ 19041934
Ginsenoside Rg3	Apoptosis	↓ cell growth	Causes G0/G1 arrest, ↓ HIF-1α during hypoxia	Hep-2	Human laryngeal cancer	Wang et al. (2009b)/ 19445134
Ginsenoside Rg3	Apoptosis	Antiproliferative; induces apoptosis	↓ Rho GDP dissociation inhibitor, Tropomyosin 1 and annexin 5	HT29	Colon cancer	Lee et al. (2009a)/ 19352032
Compound K	Apoptosis	Induces mitochondria-dependent apoptosis	Modulates Bax and Bcl-2 expression, Activation of caspase-9 and -3	HT29	Human colon cancer	Lee et al. (2010b)/ 21614182
KG-135	Apoptosis	Synergistic with etoposide	Stabilizes p53, Stimulates Bax/ p21-mediated pathways	HeLa		Lee et al. (2010c)/ 20226587
Ethyl acetate extract of PGP	Apoptosis	Antiproliferation	Differentiation, Apoptosis via p53, p21, caspase-8	B16F10	Melanoma	Park et al. (2010)/ 20691773
Compound K	Apoptosis	Inhibited HCC cell growth; attenuates metastasis	Via Bid-mediated mitochondrial pathway		HCC	Song et al. (2010b)/ 21121651
Lipid-soluble GE	Apoptosis	Antiproliferation	Caspase-8, -9, -3, G0/G1 arrest; ↓ S phase cells	NCI-H460	Human lung cancer	Kang et al. (2011)/ 21611769
Panaxynol and panaxydol	Apoptosis	Inhibited proliferation of HL-60	Caspase-3 activation, Proteolytic activation of PKCδ	HL-60	Human leukemia	Yan et al. (2011)/ 21716177
Rd and Rg3	Inflammatory response	Antiproliferative effect		HCT-116	Human colon cancer	Fishbein (2009)/ 19407967
G-Rh2	Inflammatory response	Inhibits proliferation		SMMC-7721	HCC	Zeng et al. (2004)/ 15301707
Ginseng	Inflammatory response	Anticarcinogenic effect	↓ natural killer activity		B(a)P-induced lung adenoma in mice	Yun et al. (1987)/ 3480057

Ginsenan S-IIA	Inflammatory response	Induces cytokine (IL-8) production	IL-8 mRNA expression	THP-1	Human monocytic cell line	Sonoda (1998)/9506829
Withania somnifera	Inflammatory response	Nitric oxide production		J774	Macrophage	Luvone (2003)/12551750
BST204	Inflammatory response	No effect on COX2 in unstimulated RAW 264.7		RAW 264.7	Mouse macrophage	Seo et al. (2005)/15778128
BST204	Inflammatory response	↓ CO-2, ↓ PGE in LPS-stimulated RAW 264.7	↓ p70 S6 kinase activation	RAW 264.7	Mouse macrophage	Seo et al. (2005)/15778128
PN-F	Inflammatory response	Anti-inflammatory	↓ nitric oxide, PGE_2, TNFα, and IL-1β	Blocking NF-κB pathway in ∅	RAW 264.7	Mouse macrophage (∅)	Jung et al. (2009)/19162159
LEAG	Inflammatory response	Antiproliferation	↓ COX2	↓ p-NF-κB p65	MDA-MB-231; MCF7	Human breast cancer	Peralta et al. (2009)/19815237
GRd	Inflammatory response	Attenuates the inflammatory response	Reduces accumulation of leukocytes	↓ TNFα, IL-1β, and IL-6	Rat in vivo	TNBS-induced relapsing colitis	Yang et al. (2012)/22227208
Ginsenoside Rg1	PPAR-γ	Modulating pathology in Alzheimer's disease	Rg1 may be a PPAR-γ agonist	Attenuates Aβ generation	N2a-APP695 cells		Chen (2012)/22166376
Ginsenoside Rg3	Metastasis	Inhibitory effect of tumor metastasis	↓ adhesion and invasion of tumor cells	Antiangiogenesis	Lung metastasis	Melanoma, colon carcinoma	Mochizuki et al. (1995)/8845804
Ginsenoside Rg3	Metastasis	Inhibits ovarian cancer metastasis	Inhibition of tumor-induced angiogenesis	Decreases MMP-9 expression	Lung metastasis	Ovarian cancer	Xu et al. (2008)/18959116

Note: Aβ, β-amyloid; COX2, cyclooxygenase 2; GRd, ginsenoside Rd; PGE, prostaglandin E; PPAR-γ, peroxisome proliferator–activated receptor-gamma; RG, red ginseng; WG, white ginseng.

cancer model, Duda et al. (2001) found that AG transcriptionally activates p21 messenger RNA (mRNA) in hormone-sensitive (MCF-7) and -insensitive (MDA-MB-231) breast cancer cell lines. Their results suggest that AG inhibits breast cancer cell growth through transcriptional activation of the p21 gene, independent of p53 (Duda et al. 2001). Studies by Choi et al. (2009) have shown that ginsenoside Rh2 (Rh2) significantly inhibits the viability of both MCF-7 and MDA-MB-231 breast cancer cells in a dose-dependent manner. This inhibition was correlated with G0/G1 phase cell cycle arrest, accompanied by downregulation of CDK and cyclins. This led to decreased interactions between cyclin D1 and CDK4/CDK6 and increased recruitment of p15^{Ink4B} and p27^{Kip1} to cyclin D1/CDK4 and cyclin D1/CDK6 complexes. Rh2 markedly reduced the levels of p-Rb and decreased the transcriptional activity of E2F1 in a luciferase reporter assay. Rh2-induced cell cycle arrest was significantly attenuated by knockdown of p15^{Ink4B} and/or p27^{Kip1} proteins. Rh2-mediated cell cycle arrest in human breast cancer cells is caused by p15^{Ink4B}- and p27^{Kip1}-dependent inhibition of kinase activities associated with G1–S–specific CDK/cyclin complexes (Choi et al. 2009). Recently, Choi et al. (2011) undertook a study to determine the molecular mechanisms of ginsenoside Rh2 (Rh2)–induced cell death in human breast cancer cell lines as well as in in vivo xenografts. Female nude mice (6–8 weeks old) were gavaged orally with either 0.1 mL vehicle or vehicle containing 2 or 5 mg Rh2/kg body weight thrice per week for 2 weeks before tumor cell implantation. After 2 weeks of pretreatment, exponentially growing MDA-MB-231 cells were injected subcutaneously onto the back of each mouse. Tumors were allowed to grow for 90 days. Oral gavage of 5 mg Rh2/kg body weight caused significant apoptosis of MDA-MB-231 xenografts. Increases in Bax and Bak and decreases in Bcl-2 and Bcl-xL protein transcript levels were observed in the tumors. Tumors from Rh2-treated mice had markedly higher counts of apoptotic bodies and reduced proliferation indices when compared with control tumors (Choi et al. 2011). However, the change in tumor burden was not mentioned (Choi et al. 2011).

Moon et al. (2000) have shown that panaxydol (PND), a series of cytotoxic polyacetylenic compounds from *Panax* ginseng, markedly reduced proliferation of human melanoma cell line, SK-MEL-1. Cell cycle analysis revealed that PND inhibited cell cycle progression at the G1–S transition phase by increasing the protein expression of p27^{KIP} and decreasing CDK2 activity in a dose-dependent manner. Protein levels of p21^{WAF1}, p16^{INK4a}, p53, p-Rb, and E2F-1 were not changed. These results indicate that PND induces G1 cell cycle arrest by decreasing CDK2 activity and upregulating p27^{KIP1} protein expression (Moon et al. 2000).

Lee et al. (2009c) reported that a ginseng preparation called KG-135, containing ginsenosides Rk1, Rg3, and Rg5, was able to arrest the cell cycle of HeLa cells (human cervical cancer). KG-135 arrests cells in the G1 phase of the cell cycle with an IC$_{50}$ value of 69 µg/mL. G1 phase arrest is associated with downregulation of cyclin D1/CDK4 and cyclin B1/Cdc2 activities. Downregulation of G1 CDK activities is kinetically well related to decreased intracellular protein levels of these kinases. In addition, decreases in the levels of cyclin D1/CDK4 and cyclin B1, but not of Cdc2, were prevented by cotreatment with MG-132, a potent proteasome inhibitor. Thus, KG-135–induced arrest of the cell cycle at the G1 phase in HeLa cells represents a novel mechanism that involves proteasome-mediated degradation of the cyclins (cyclin D1 and B1) and CDK4 proteins (Lee et al. 2009c). Recently, similar observations of KG-135 on cell cycle regulation have been reported by Yoo et al. (2010) using human prostate cancer cells. Wang et al. (2009b) reported that Rg3 significantly inhibited the growth of human laryngeal cancer Hep-2 cells and arrested them in the G0/G1 phase during normoxia and hypoxia. The mRNA and protein expression of hypoxia-inducible factor-1 alpha (HIF-1α) was also downregulated (Wang et al. 2009b). King and Murphy (2010) found that p21$^{+/+}$ HCT-116 human colon cancer cells treated with water-extracted AG (*Panax quinquefolius*) were arrested in the G0/G1 phase of the cell cycle, the expression of p53 and p21 proteins was increased, and phospho-MAPK kinase (MEK) levels were decreased. In contrast, cells deficient in p21 (p21$^{-/-}$) displayed reduced cell viability, an elevated number of dead cells, and increased expression of Bax and cleaved caspase-3 proteins. This study suggests that the ginseng extract causes cell cycle arrest in p21 wild-type cells, while it leads p21-deficient cells to undergo cell death (King and

Murphy 2010). The regulatory effects of ginseng on cell cycle arrest were demonstrated by using another human colon cancer cell line, HT-29 (Cheng et al. 2011).

There is one report on G2/M phase arrest induced by AG berry extract (AGBE). Li et al. (2009c) reported that AGBE, which contains major ginsenosides as its active components, enhanced the chemopreventive effect of 5-fluorouracil (5-FU) on human colorectal cancer cells (SW-480, HCT-116, and HT-29). AGBE (0.1–1.0 mg/mL) significantly inhibited SW-480, HCT-116, and HT-29 cell growth in a concentration-dependent manner. Cell growth decreased more with the combined treatment with 5-FU and AGBE than with 5-FU or AGBE alone. Enhancement of S and G2/M cell cycle arrest, rather than stimulation of apoptosis, appears to be the principal mechanism for the effects of AGBE on 5-FU chemotherapy (Li et al. 2009c).

27.7.2 EFFECTS OF GINSENG ON MAPK PATHWAY

King and Murphy (2007) have shown antiproliferative effects of hot water–extracted AG on MCF-7 human breast cancer cells. By using an antibody microarray, they found several key cell survival proteins altered in ginseng treated cells, including members of the MAPK family. Hot water–extracted AG decreased phospho-MEK1/2 and phospho-ERK1/2 levels and increased phospho-Raf-1. The expression of Raf-1 kinase inhibitor protein (RKIP) was transiently, yet significantly, upregulated following cell treatment. These results suggest that AG may act to inhibit breast cancer cell proliferation by increasing the expression of RKIP, resulting in inhibition of the MAPK pathway (King and Murphy 2007). PND is one of the main nonpeptidyl small molecules isolated from lipophilic fractions of *Panax notoginseng*. Wang et al. (2011) indicated that changes in differentiation markers in SMMC-7721 cells by PND can be reversed by either the ERK kinase 1/2 (MEK1/2) inhibitor, U0126, or sorafenib, and they suggested that PND might be of value for further exploration as a potential anticancer agent via cAMP- and MAPK-dependent mechanisms. Using a different approach, Yoon et al. (2011) investigated the effects of ginsenoside Rd on tumor invasion and metastasis in human liver cancer cells (HepG2) and its possible mechanism(s) of action. HepG2 cells treated with ginsenoside Rd at different concentrations exhibited decreased migration and invasiveness using scratch-wound and Boyden chamber assays. They also used reverse transcription polymerase chain reaction (RT-PCR), Western blot analysis, gelatin zymography, promoter assays, and treatment with inhibitors of MAPK signaling to study the molecular mechanisms by which ginsenoside Rd inhibits the invasion and migration of HepG2 cells. They found that treatment with ginsenoside Rd dose- and time-dependently inhibited the migration and invasion of HepG2 cells by (1) reducing the expression of matrix metalloproteinase 1 (MMP-1), MMP-2, and MMP-7; (2) blocking MAPK signaling by inhibiting the phosphorylation of ERK and p38 MAPK; (3) inhibiting AP-1 activation; and (4) inducing focal adhesion formation and modulating vinculin localization and expression. Treatment of HepG2 cells with ginsenoside Rd significantly inhibited metastasis, most likely by blocking MMP activation and MAPK signaling pathways involved in cancer cell migration (Yoon et al. 2011).

27.7.3 EFFECTS OF GINSENG ON WNT/β-CATENIN PATHWAY

Most colorectal cancers are associated with aberrant activation of the Wnt/ß-catenin signaling pathway. He et al. (2011) investigated the anticancer activity of Rg3 on colorectal cancer cells and its underlying molecular mechanism(s) of action. They found that Rg3 inhibited cancer cell proliferation and viability in vitro. The inhibitory effect is mediated at least in part by blocking nuclear translocation of the ß-catenin protein and hence inhibiting ß-catenin/Tcf transcriptional activity. Allelic deletion of the oncogenic ß-catenin in HCT-116 cells renders the cells more sensitive to Rg3-induced growth inhibition. Using the xenograft tumor model of human colorectal cancer, they demonstrated that Rg3 effectively inhibited the growth of tumors derived from the human colorectal cancer cell line HCT-116. Rg3 inhibited cell proliferation, decreased proliferating cell nuclear antigen (PCNA) expression, and diminished nuclear staining intensity of ß-catenin. They emphasized that the anticancer activity of Rg3 may, in part, be caused by blocking the nuclear translocation of ß-catenin in colon cancer cells.

27.7.4 GINSENG AND APOPTOSIS

Numerous studies have demonstrated the proapoptotic effects of ginseng. Antiapoptotic proteins such as BCL-2, BCL-XL, and MCL-1 bind with proapoptotic proteins to induce apoptosis. BCL-2– family proteins are key regulators of apoptosis.

Lee et al. (2000) investigated the antiproliferative and proapoptotic effects of IH-901 (20-O-[beta-D-glucopyranosyl]-20(S)-protopanaxadiol) on HL-60 cells (a human promyelocytic leukemia cell line). They found that IH-901 is significantly cytotoxic toward HL-60 cells, with an IC_{50} at 24.3 μM following a 96 h incubation. Treatment of HL-60 cells with IH-901 resulted in apoptosis caused by the activation of caspase-3 protease and subsequent proteolytic cleavage of poly(ADP-ribose) polymerase (PARP). The induced apoptosis occurred via mitochondrial cytochrome c release independently of Bcl-2 modulation (Lee et al. 2000). Sansam, a wild ginseng grown deep in the mountains (also known as mountain-grown ginseng [MGG]), belongs to Araliaceae and *Panax*. Koo et al. (2007) have investigated the effects of MGG on HL-60 cells. They found that MGG is a potent inducer of apoptosis, inhibiting the activities of caspase-3 and -8 (Koo et al. 2007). Fang et al. (2008) reported that total saponins of *Panax* ginseng (TSPG) increase the percentage of apoptotic HL-60 cells in a dose-dependent manner, while the expression of BAX mRNA increased and bcl-xl expression decreased gradually. The effect on upregulation of BAX mRNA and downregulation of bcl-xl mRNA probably plays an important role in apoptosis of HL-60 cells induced by TSPG (Fang et al. 2008). Similar results of ginseng were reported by Park et al. (2009) on leukemia cells. They found that treatment of human leukemia cells (U937) with Korean red ginseng (KRG, *Panax* ginseng C.A. Meyer Radix Rubra) extract resulted in growth inhibition and induction of apoptosis in a dose-dependent manner. The increase in apoptosis was associated with downregulation of antiapoptotic Bcl-2, Bcl-X(L), an inhibitor of apoptosis (IAP) family members, and the activation of caspase-3 (Park et al. 2009). Panaxynol and PND are naturally occurring polyacetylenes, isolated from the lipophilic fractions of *Panax notoginseng*, which exerts antiproliferative effects against malignant cells. Yan et al. (2011) examined the antiproliferation and proapoptotic effects of panaxynol and PND on human promyelocytic leukemia HL60 cells and investigated their mechanism of action. They found that panaxynol and PND markedly inhibited the proliferation of HL60 cells via an apoptotic pathway. Western blot analysis revealed proteolytic activation of protein kinase Cδ, caspase-3 activation, and cleavage of PARP in HL60 cells treated by panaxynol and PND (Yan et al. 2011).

Wakabayashi et al. (1998) investigated inhibitory mechanisms of a metabolic component of ginseng protopanaxadiol saponins, called M1, on the growth of tumor cells. They found that M1 inhibited the proliferation of B16-BL6 mouse melanoma cells in a time- and dose-dependent manner. At 40 μM, M1 induced apoptotic cell death within 24 h. M1 rapidly upregulates p27^{Kip1} and downregulates the expression of c-Myc and cyclin D1. They suggested that the regulation of apoptosis-related proteins by M1 is responsible for the induction of apoptotic cell death, and this probably leads to antimetastatic activity in vivo (Wakabayashi et al. 1998). Rh2 suppresses the growth of human melanoma A375-S2 cells in vitro by inducing apoptosis, which is partially dependent on caspase-8 and caspase-3 pathways (Fei et al. 2002).

In human prostate carcinoma LNCaP cells, Rg3 activated the expression of CDK inhibitors p21 and p27. It also caused cell cycle arrest at the G1 phase and subsequently inhibited cell growth through a caspase-3–mediated apoptosis by interfering with the expression of apoptosis-related genes, bcl-2 and caspase-3 (Liu et al. 2000).

PND is a naturally occurring nonpeptidyl small molecule isolated from the lipophilic fractions of *Panax notoginseng*. PND inhibited the growth of various kinds of malignant cell lines, including glioma cells (Hai et al. 2007). PND markedly inhibited proliferation of rat C6 glioma cells in a dose-dependent manner, with an ID_{50} of 40 μM. Cell apoptosis was observed at 48 h in the presence of PND. Western blot analysis showed decreased expression of bcl-2 and increased levels of Bax and caspase-3 in C6 cells treated by PND, suggesting profound effects of PND on the growth and apoptosis of glioma cells (Hai et al. 2007).

Rk1 is one of the major components of heat-processed *Panax* ginseng C.A. Meyer, sun ginseng (SG). Kim et al. (2008) investigated the mechanisms underlying the antitumor activity of Rk1 in human liver cancer HepG2 cells in vitro. They found that Rk1 markedly inhibited telomerase activity and cell growth; obviously decreased expression levels of telomerase reverse transcriptase (hTERT) and c-Myc mRNA; and decreased expression of Fas-associated death domain (FADD). They also found that Rk1 induced apoptosis through activation of caspase-8 and -3. They suggested that the antitumor activity of Rk1 involves coordination between inhibition of telomerase activity and induction of apoptosis (Kim et al. 2008).

CK, a metabolite of ginseng saponin, induced mitochondrial-dependent and caspase-dependent apoptosis in HT-29 human colon cancer cells via generation of reactive oxygen species (ROS) (I.K. Lee et al. 2010b). CK induced apoptosis via the activation of c-Jun amino-terminal kinase (JNK) and p38 MAPK (Lee et al. 2010c). CK exhibits anticancer activity in the liver. Song et al. (2010b) reported a novel mechanism of CK-induced apoptosis of liver cancer cells via the Bid-mediated mitochondrial pathway. Bid expression in subcutaneous liver tumor tissues and in liver metastasis decreased dramatically with CK treatment (Song et al. 2010b).

KG-135 (a quality-controlled red ginseng–specific formulation containing nearly equal amounts of three major ginsenosides: Rk1, Rg3, and Rg5) potentiates cytotoxicity of etoposide by modulating apoptotic signaling in HeLa cells through a mechanism that involves stabilization of p53 and stimulation of Bax- and p21-mediated apoptotic signaling pathways. These results suggest that KG-135 represents a useful candidate adjuvant for cancer treatment that could potentially minimize the adverse effects of current clinical chemotherapeutics (Lee et al. 2010c).

Recently, Kang et al. (2011) investigated the effects of an LSGE on the NCI-H460 human lung cancer cells. LSGE inhibited the proliferation of NCI-H460 cells in a dose-dependent manner and caused cell cycle arrest at the G0/G1 phase. The expression levels of CDK2, CDK4, CDK6, cyclin D3, and cyclin E related to G0/G1 cell cycle progression was altered by LSGE. LSGE induced cell death through stimulating apoptosis, which was accompanied by increased activity of caspase, including caspase-8, caspase-9, and caspase-3. Along with enhancement of caspase activity, LSGE increased protein levels of cleaved caspase-3, caspase-8, caspase-9, and PARP (cleaved PARP is used as a marker of cell apoptosis). In summary, their findings indicate that LSGE inhibits human lung cancer cell growth by causing cell cycle arrest at the G0/G1 phase and by inducing caspase-mediated apoptosis (Kang et al. 2011). Also, the PGP ethyl acetate fraction (EtOAc, containing ginsenosides Rd, Rg3, Rb2, Rg1, and Rb1) of LSGE increases the sub-G1 cell population of B16F10 melanoma cells through inducing p53/p21 and activating caspase-8 (Park et al. 2010).

20(S)-Rg3 inhibits cell proliferation by inhibiting mitosis, DNA replication and repair, and growth factor signaling. The cytotoxic effects of 20(S)-Rg3 in colorectal cancer (CRC) are also associated with its ability to induce apoptosis. Lee et al. (2009a) investigated the mechanisms of the antiproliferative effect of 20(S)-Rg3 at the protein level in HT-29 colon cancer cells and identified altered expressions of apoptosis-associated proteins, downregulation of Rho GDP dissociation inhibitor, and upregulation of tropomyosin 1, annexin 5, and glutathione *S*-transferase p1 (Lee et al. 2009b).

27.7.5 Effects of Ginseng on Cancer Metastasis

Mochizuki et al. (1995) examined the inhibitory effect of two saponin preparations from red ginseng, 20(R)-ginsenoside-Rg3 [20(R)-Rg3] and 20(S)-ginsenoside-Rg3 [20(S)-Rg3], in comparison with that of ginsenoside-Rb2, on lung metastasis produced by two highly metastatic tumor cell lines, B16-BL6 melanoma and colon 26-M3.1 carcinoma, in syngeneic mice. In an in vitro analysis, both saponin preparations significantly inhibited the adhesion of B16-BL6 melanoma cells to fibronectin (FN) and laminin (LM). Similarly, they inhibited the invasion of B16-BL6 cells into reconstituted basement membrane (Matrigel)/FN in a dose-dependent manner. In an experimental metastasis model using B16-BL6 melanoma, consecutive i.v. administrations of 100 µg per mouse of 20(R)- or 20(S)-Rg3 1, 2, 3, and 4 days after tumor inoculation led to significant decreases in lung metastasis. The inhibitory effects of i.v. administration of both ginseng saponins on the tumor metastasis of B16-BL6 melanoma were also observed at the low dose of 10 µg per mouse. Oral administration (p.o.) of both saponins (100–1000 µg per mouse) induced a significant decrease in lung metastasis of B16-BL6 melanoma. Moreover, both ginseng saponins were effective in inhibiting lung metastasis produced by colon 26-M3.1 carcinoma cells. When 20(R)- or 20(S)-Rg3 was orally administered consecutively after tumor inoculation in a spontaneous metastasis model using B16-BL6 melanoma, both significantly inhibited lung metastasis. In an experiment involving neovascularization by tumor cells in vivo, both saponin preparations decreased the number of blood vessels oriented toward the tumor mass, with no repression of tumor size. These findings suggest that both 20(R)- and 20(S)-Rg3 possess an ability to inhibit lung metastasis of tumor cells, and the mechanism of their antimetastatic effect is related to inhibition of the adhesion and invasion of tumor cells, and also to antiangiogenic activity (Mochizuki et al. 1995). Xu et al. (2008) investigated the effect of ginsenoside Rg3 on human ovarian cancer cell (SKOV-3) metastasis to the mouse lung using a tumor-induced angiogenesis assay. The effect of Rg3 on invasive ability of SKOV-3 cells in vitro was evaluated in Boyden chambers, and immunofluorescence staining was used to determine the expression of MMP-9 in SKOV-3 cells. Rg3 significantly inhibited the metastasis of ovarian cancer. The inhibitory effect was partially due to inhibition of tumor-induced angiogenesis and a decrease in invasive ability and MMP-9 expression of SKOV-3 cells (Xu et al. 2008). An early study by Mochizuki et al. (1995) suggested that ginseng saponins, 20(R)- and 20(S)-Rg3, possessed the ability to inhibit cancer cell lung metastasis, and the antimetastatic effect is related to inhibition of cell adhesion and tumor cell invasion as well as antiangiogenesis activity.

27.7.6 ANTIOXIDANT EFFECT OF GINSENG

Kim et al. (2011c) investigated the antioxidant effects of *Panax* ginseng C.A. Meyer on healthy volunteers. In a double-blind randomized controlled design, they divided 82 healthy participants (21 men and 61 women) into three groups: control group and two ginseng groups (1 or 2 g/day) for 4 weeks. The following were measured before and after the trial: serum levels of ROS and malondialdehyde (MDA); total antioxidant capacity (TAC); the activities of catalase, superoxide dismutase (SOD), glutathione reductase (GSH-Rd), and glutathione peroxidase (GSH-Px); and total glutathione content. They found that 4 weeks of ginseng use led to significant decreases in serum levels of ROS and MDA. Notably, the total glutathione content and GSH-Rd activity considerably improved in the groups that received 2 g of ginseng. No significant alterations were observed in TAC and catalase, SOD, and GSH-Px activities. They concluded that ginseng has antioxidant properties (Kim et al. 2011c).

27.8 SUMMARY AND FUTURE PERSPECTIVES

Ginseng has long been used in traditional medicine in Asia to improve physical condition and to prolong life (Yun 2003). Ginseng appears to accomplish this by preventing or delaying the onset of various diseases such as cancer and diabetes (Yun 2003). Epidemiological studies suggest that ginseng is chemopreventive against a variety of cancer types (cancer of the lip, oral cavity, pharynx, esophagus, stomach, colon, liver, pancreas, laryngis, lung, and ovary) (Yun 2003). It contains at least 150 different ginsenosides of PPD, PPT, or oleanane categories (Li et al. 2004; Kim et al. 2005; Christensen 2009; Yun 2001). Ginseng is a potent inhibitor of carcinogenesis in many rodent models including the lung, skin, liver, mammary gland, uterine cervix, brain, and colon (Yun 2003). Furthermore, two specific ginsenosides, Rg3 and Rg5, caused statistically significant reductions in lung tumor incidence in mice (Yun et al. 2001a,b). The chemopreventive activity of ginseng is related to antioxidation, anti–tumor promotion, inhibition of cell proliferation, and induction of apoptosis (Hofseth and Wargovich 2007; Helms 2004). Inhibition of ras gene–activated signal transduction pathways such as ERK has been reported (Surh et al. 2001), and this is supported by experiments showing that ginseng or ginsenosides inhibit AP-1 activation (Choi et al. 2003; Keum et al. 2003). These results indicate that ginseng has multiple chemopreventive effects in various in vitro and in vivo systems (Helms 2004; Hofseth and Wargovich 2007; Panwar et al. 2005; Yan et al. 2006). Future studies should include systematic characterization of the efficacy of ginseng in both mouse lung adenocarcinoma and squamous cell carcinoma models, the identification of key active components of ginseng via in vitro activity–guided fractionation, pharmacokinetic and biopharmaceutical characterizations of ginseng, and chemoprevention clinical trials of ginseng against lung cancer in humans.

ACKNOWLEDGMENTS

This work was supported by a National Institutes of Health (NIH) grant (R01 AT005522). We would like to thank Dr. Gary D. Stoner, Dr. Jay Tichelaar, Dr. Jing Pan, Dr. Qi Zhang, and Ms. Marleen Janson for reading this manuscript.

ABBREVIATIONS AND DEFINITIONS

25-OCH3-PPD: 20(S)-25-methoxyl-dammarane-3beta, 12beta, 20-triol
5-FU: 5-fluorouracil
ACF: aberrant crypt foci
AG: American ginseng
AGBE: American ginseng berry extract
Araliaceae: extract of the roots of *Panax notoginseng*
ARI: acute respiratory illness
B(a)P: tobacco-specific carcinogen benzo(a)pyrene
bioginseng: produced from a tissue culture of ginseng root cultured on standard medium, whereas panaxel and panaxel-5 were produced from ginseng tissue root cultures using standard mediums enriched with 2-carboxyethylgermanium sesquioxide and 1-hydroxygermatran-monohydrate, respectively;
BST204: a fermented ginseng extract
CAM: complementary alternative medicine
CC3: cleave caspase-3
CK: compound K, an intestinal bacterial metabolite of ginseng saponin
CML: chronic lymphocytic leukaemia
DEN: *N*-nitrosodiethylamine
DMBA: 7,12-dimethylbenz[a]anthracene
D-Rh(2): structural modification of ginsenoside Rh(2) by reacting with octanoyl chloride to give a dioctanoyl ester of Rh(2)
EFLA400: a standardized *Panax* ginseng extract
ENU: *N*-ethyl-*N*-nitrosourea
FADD: Fas-associated death domain
Fr.3: the ethanol-insoluble fraction of ginseng fraction 3
GE: ginseng extract
ginsan: purified from Panax ginseng C.A. Meyer (Araliaceae), with a molecular weight of 150,000 and devoid of lectin properties
G-Rh2: ginsenoside Rh2
GST-P: glutathione *S*-transferase placental form

HCC: hepatocellular carcinoma

hTERT: telomerase reverse transcriptase

IH-901: one of the novel intestinal bacterial metabolites, 20-O-(beta-D-glucopyranosyl)-20(S)-protopanaxadiol, of ginseng protopanaxadiol saponins

KG-135: a quality-controlled standardized ginsenoside of red ginseng, specific formulation containing ~equal amounts of three major ginsenosides (Rk1, Rg3, and Rg5)

LEAG: lyophilized aqueous extract of American ginseng

LPS: lipopolysaccharide

LSGE: lipid-soluble ginseng extract

M1: intestinal bacterial metabolite of ginseng protopanaxadiol saponins

M4: 20(S)-protopanaxatriol, the main bacterial metabolite of protopanaxatriol-type ginsenosides

MGG: mountain-grown ginseng

MNU: N-methyl-N-nitrosourea

MR2: majonoside-R2, obtained from the rhizome and root of Panax vietnamensis (Vietnamese ginseng)

∅: macrophage

PARP: poly(ADP-ribose) polymerase

PGP: Phellinus linteus grown on *Panax ginseng*

PN-F: Panax notoginseng flower

Rg2: ginseng saponin ginsenoside Rh2

RGE: red ginseng extract

RKIP: Raf-1 kinase inhibitor protein

RSYRT: extracts of Ren-Shen-Yang-Rong-Tang, a white ginseng–containing Chinese medicinal prescription

TNBS: 2,4,6-trinitrobenzenesulfonic acid

TPA: 12-O-tetradecanoylphorbol-13-acetate

WD: Western diet containing 20% fat

WKRG: water extract of Korean red ginseng (daily intraperitoneal injection)

REFERENCES

Akao, T., M. Kanaoka, and K. Kobashi. 1998. Appearance of compound K, a major metabolite of ginsenoside Rb1 by intestinal bacteria, in rat plasma after oral administration—measurement of compound K by enzyme immunoassay. *Biol Pharm Bull* 21:245–9.

Bae, E.A., M.J. Han, E.J. Kim, and D.H. Kim. 2004. Transformation of ginseng saponins to ginsenoside Rh2 by acids and human intestinal bacteria and biological activities of their transformants. *Arch Pharm Res* 27:61–7.

Bae, J.S., H.S. Park, J.W. Park, S.H. Li, and Y.S. Chun. 2012. Red ginseng and 20(S)-Rg3 control testosterone-induced prostate hyperplasia by deregulating androgen receptor signaling. *J Nat Med* 66:476–85.

Barton, D.L., G.S. Soori, B.A. Bauer et al. 2010. Pilot study of Panax quinquefolius (American ginseng) to improve cancer-related fatigue: a randomized, double-blind, dose-finding evaluation: NCCTG trial N03CA. *Support Care Cancer* 18:179–87.

Bespalov, V.G., V.V. Davydov, A.I. Limarenko, L.I. Slepian, and V.A. Aleksandrov. 1993a. [The inhibition of the development of experimental tumors of the cervix uteri and vagina by using tinctures of the cultured-cell biomass of the ginseng root and its germanium-selective stocks]. *Biull Eksp Biol Med* 116:534–6. Russian.

Bespalov, V.G., V.A. Aleksandrov, and M.I. Lidak. 1993b. [An experimental study of the possibilities of using pentoxifylline for the prevention of cancer at different sites]. *Eksp Klin Farmakol* 56:35–7. Russian.

Bespalov, V.G., V.A. Alexandrov, A.Y. Limarenko et al. 2001. Chemoprevention of mammary, cervix and nervous system carcinogenesis in animals using cultured Panax ginseng drugs and preliminary clinical trials in patients with precancerous lesions of the esophagus and endometrium. *J Korean Med Sci* 16 Suppl:S42–53.

Brasky, T.M., A.R. Kristal, S.L. Navarro et al. 2011. Specialty supplements and prostate cancer risk in the VITamins and Lifestyle (VITAL) cohort. *Nutr Cancer* 63:573–82.

Brown, P.N. 2011. Determination of ginsenoside content in Asian and North American ginseng raw materials and finished products by high-performance liquid chromatography: single-laboratory validation. *J AOAC Int* 94:1391–9.

Cai, B.X., S.L. Jin, D. Luo, X.F. Lin, and J. Gao. 2009. Ginsenoside Rb1 suppresses ultraviolet radiation-induced apoptosis by inducing DNA repair. *Biol Pharm Bull* 32:837–41.

Cha, R.J., D.W. Zeng, and Q.S. Chang. 1994. [Non-surgical treatment of small cell lung cancer with chemo-radio-immunotherapy and traditional Chinese medicine]. *Zhonghua Nei Ke Za Zhi* 33:462–6. Chinese.

Chae, S., K.A. Kang, W.Y. Chang et al. 2009. Effect of compound K, a metabolite of ginseng saponin, combined with gamma-ray radiation in human lung cancer cells in vitro and in vivo. *J Agric Food Chem* 57:5777–82.

Chang, T.K., J. Chen, and S.A. Benetton. 2002. In vitro effect of standardized ginseng extracts and individual ginsenosides on the catalytic activity of human CYP1A1, CYP1A2, and CYP1B1. *Drug Metab Dispos* 30:378–84.

Chen, L.M., Z.Y. Lin, Y.G. Zhu et al. 2012. Ginsenoside Rg1 attenuates β-amyloid generation via suppressing PPARγ-regulated BACE1 activity in N2a-APP695 cells. *Eur J Pharmacol* 675:15–21.

Chen, P.F., L.M. Liu, Z. Chen et al. 2006. [Effects of ethanol extracts of Panax notoginseng on liver metastasis of B16 melanoma grafted in mice]. *Zhong Xi Yi Jie He Xue Bao* 4:500–3.

Chen, Y.Z., Z.D. Li, F. Gao et al. 2009. Effects of combined Chinese drugs and chemotherapy in treating advanced non-small cell lung cancer. *Chin J Integr Med* 15:415–9.

Cheung, L.W., K.W. Leung, C.K. Wong, R.N. Wong, and A.S. Wong. 2011. Ginsenoside-Rg1 induces angiogenesis via non-genomic crosstalk of glucocorticoid receptor and fibroblast growth factor receptor-1. *Cardiovasc Res* 89:419–25.

Cho, S.H., K.S. Chung, J.H. Choi, D.H. Kim, and K.T. Lee. 2009. Compound K, a metabolite of ginseng saponin, induces apoptosis via caspase-8-dependent pathway in HL-60 human leukemia cells. *BMC Cancer* 9:449.

Choi, S.S., J.K. Lee, E.J. Han et al. 2003. Effect of ginsenoside Rd on nitric oxide system induced by lipopolysaccharide plus TNF-alpha in C6 rat glioma cells. *Arch Pharm Res* 26:375–82.

Choi, S., T.W. Kim, and S.V. Singh. 2009. Ginsenoside Rh2-mediated G1 phase cell cycle arrest in human breast cancer cells is caused by p15 Ink4B and p27 Kip1-dependent inhibition of cyclin-dependent kinases. *Pharm Res* 26:2280–8.

Choi, S., J.Y. Oh, and S.J. Kim. 2011. Ginsenoside Rh2 induces Bcl-2 family proteins-mediated apoptosis in vitro and in xenografts in vivo models. *J Cell Biochem* 112:330–40.

Christensen, L.P. 2009. Ginsenosides chemistry, biosynthesis, analysis, and potential health effects. *Adv Food Nutr Res* 55:1–99

Cui, Y., X.O. Shu, Y.T. Gao et al. 2006. Association of ginseng use with survival and quality of life among breast cancer patients. *Am J Epidemiol* 163:645–53.

Cui, X., Y. Jin, D. Poudyal et al. 2010. Mechanistic insight into the ability of American ginseng to suppress colon cancer associated with colitis. *Carcinogenesis* 31:1734–41.

da Silva, T.C., A. Paula da Silva, G. Akisue et al. 2005. Inhibitory effects of Pfaffia paniculata (Brazilian ginseng) on preneoplastic and neoplastic lesions in a mouse hepatocarcinogenesis model. *Cancer Lett* 226:107–13.

Dougherty, U., R. Mustafi, Y. Wang et al. 2011. American ginseng suppresses Western diet-promoted tumorigenesis in model of inflammation-associated colon cancer: role of EGFR. *BMC Complement Altern Med* 11:111.

Duda, R.B., S.S. Kang, S.Y. Archer, S. Meng, and R.A. Hodin. 2001. American ginseng transcriptionally activates p21 mRNA in breast cancer cell lines. *J Korean Med Sci* 16 Suppl:S54–60.

Evans, S., N. Dizeyi, P.A. Abrahamsson, and J. Persson. 2009. The effect of a novel botanical agent TBS-101 on invasive prostate cancer in animal models. *Anticancer Res* 29:3917–24.

Fang, X.M., Y. Li, J.C. Qian, H.X. Zhou, and J.X. Wang. 2008. [Effect of total saponins of Panaxginseng on bax and bcl-xl gene expression in HL-60 cells]. *Zhongguo Shi Yan Xue Ye Xue Za Zhi* 16:781–4.

Feng, H., W. Chen, and C. Zhu. 2011. Pharmacokinetics study of bio-adhesive tablet of Panax notoginseng saponins. *Int Arch Med* 4:18.

Fei, X.F., B.X. Wang, S. Tashiro et al. 2002. Apoptotic effects of ginsenoside Rh2 on human malignant melanoma A375-S2 cells. *Acta Pharmacol Sin* 23:315–22.

Fishbein, A.B., C.Z. Wang, X.L. Li et al. 2009. Asian ginseng enhances the anti-proliferative effect of 5-fluorouracil on human colorectal cancer: comparison between white and red ginseng. *Arch Pharm Res* 32:505–13.

Gu, Y., G.J. Wang, J.G. Sun et al. 2009. Pharmacokinetic characterization of ginsenoside Rh2, an anticancer nutrient from ginseng, in rats and dogs. *Food Chem Toxicol* 47:2257–68.

Gu, Y., G.J. Wang, X.L. Wu et al. 2010. Intestinal absorption mechanisms of ginsenoside Rh2: stereoselectivity and involvement of ABC transporters. *Xenobiotica* 40:602–12.

Hai, J., Q. Lin, Y. Lu, H. Zhang, and J. Yi. 2007. Induction of apoptosis in rat C6 glioma cells by panaxydol. *Cell Biol Int* 31:711–5.

Haijiang, Z., W. Yongjiang, and C. Yiyu. 2003. Analysis of 'SHENMAI' injection by HPLC/MS/MS. *J Pharm Biomed Anal* 31:175–83.

Han, M., J. Chen, S. Chen, and X. Wang. 2010. Development of a UPLC-ESI-MS/MS assay for 20(S)-protopanaxadiol and pharmacokinetic application of its two formulations in rats. *Anal Sci* 26: 749–53.

Hao, H., L. Lai, C. Zheng et al. 2010. Microsomal cytochrome p450-mediated metabolism of protopanaxa-triol ginsenosides: metabolite profile, reaction phenotyping, and structure-metabolism relationship. *Drug Metab Dispos* 38:1731–9.

Harkey, M.R., G.L. Henderson, M.E. Gershwin, J.S. Stern, and R.M. Hackman. 2001. Variability in commer-cial ginseng products: an analysis of 25 preparations. *Am J Clin Nutr* 73:1101–6.

Hasegawa, H. 2004. Proof of the mysterious efficacy of ginseng: basic and clinical trials: metabolic activation of ginsenoside: deglycosylation by intestinal bacteria and esterification with fatty acid. *J Pharmacol Sci* 95:153–7.

Hasegawa, H., R. Suzuki, T. Nagaoka et al. 2002. Prevention of growth and metastasis of murine melanoma through enhanced natural-killer cytotoxicity by fatty acid-conjugate of protopanaxatriol. *Biol Pharm Bull* 25:861–6.

He, B.C., J.L. Gao, X. Luo et al. 2011. Ginsenoside Rg3 inhibits colorectal tumor growth through the down-regulation of Wnt/ß-catenin signaling. *Int J Oncol* 38:437–45.

Helms, S. 2004. Cancer prevention and therapeutics: Panax ginseng. *Altern Med Rev* 9:259–274.

High, K.P., D. Case, D. Hurd et al. 2012. A randomized, controlled trial of Panax quinquefolius extract (CVT-E002) to reduce respiratory infection in patients with chronic lymphocytic leukemia. *J Support Oncol* Jan 20. PMID: 22266154

Hofseth, L.J., and M.J. Wargovich. 2007. Inflammation, cancer, and targets of ginseng. *J Nutr* 137(1 Suppl):183S–5S. Review.

Hsieh, T.C., and J.M. Wu. 2002. Mechanism of action of herbal supplement PC-SPES: elucidation of effects of individual herbs of PC-SPES on proliferation and prostate specific gene expression in androgen-dependent LNCaP cells. *Int J Oncol* 20:583–8.

Huang, J.Y., Y. Sun, Q.X. Fan, and Y.Q. Zhang. 2009. [Efficacy of Shenyi Capsule combined with gemcitabine plus cisplatin in treatment of advanced esophageal cancer: a randomized controlled trial]. *Zhong Xi Yi Jie He Xue Bao* 7:1047–51.

Ichihara, T., H. Wanibuchi, S. Iwai et al. 2002. White, but not red, ginseng inhibits progression of intestinal carcinogenesis in rats. *Asian Pac J Cancer Prev* 3:243–50.

Iuvone, T., G. Esposito, F. Capasso, A.A. Izzo. 2003. Induction of nitric oxide synthase expression by *Withania somnifera* in macrophages. *Life Sci.* 72:1617–25.

Jeong, A., H.J. Lee, S.J. Jeong et al. 2010. Compound K inhibits basic fibroblast growth factor-induced angio-genesis via regulation of p38 mitogen activated protein kinase and AKT in human umbilical vein endo-thelial cells. *Biol Pharm Bull* 33:945–50.

Joo, K.M., J.K. Lee, H.Y. Jeon et al. 2010. Pharmacokinetic study of ginsenoside Re with pure ginsenoside Re and ginseng berry extracts in mouse using ultra performance liquid chromatography/mass spectrometric method. *J Pharm Biomed Anal* 51:278–83.

Jung, H.W., U.K. Seo, J.K. Kim, K.H. Leem, and Y.K. Park. 2009. Flower extract of Panax notoginseng attenu-ates lipopolysaccharide-induced inflammatory response via blocking of NF-kappaB signaling pathway in murine macrophages. *J Ethnopharmacol* 122:313–9.

Kamangar, F., Y.T. Gao, X.O. Shu et al. 2007. Ginseng intake and gastric cancer risk in the Shanghai Women's Health Study cohort. *Cancer Epidemiol Biomarkers Prev* 16:629–30.

Kang, M.R., H.M. Kim, J.S. Kang et al. 2011. Lipid-soluble ginseng extract induces apoptosis and G0/G1 cell cycle arrest in NCI-H460 human lung cancer cells. *Plant Foods Hum Nutr* 66:101–6.

Keum, Y.S., K.K. Park, J.M. Lee et al. 2000. Antioxidant and anti-tumor promoting activities of the methanol extract of heat-processed ginseng. *Cancer Lett* 150:41–8.

Keum, Y.S., S.S. Han, K.S. Chun et al. 2003. Inhibitory effects of the ginsenoside Rg3 on phorbol ester-induced cyclo-oxygenase-2 expression, NF-kappaB activation and tumor promotion. *Mutat Res* 523–524:75–85.

Kim, B.J., S.Y. Nah, J.H. Jeon, I. So, and S.J. Kim. 2011a. Transient receptor potential melastatin 7 channels are involved in ginsenoside Rg3-induced apoptosis in gastric cancer cells. *Basic Clin Pharmacol Toxicol* 109:233–9.

Kim, E.H., M.H. Jang, M.C. Shin, M.S. Shin, and C.J. Kim. 2003b. Protective effect of aqueous extract of Ginseng radix against 1-methyl-4-phenylpyridinium-induced apoptosis in PC12 cells. *Biol Pharm Bull* 26:1668–73.

Kim, H.G., S.R. Yoo, H.J. Park et al. 2011c. Antioxidant effects of Panax ginseng C.A. Meyer in healthy subjects: a randomized, placebo-controlled clinical trial. *Food Chem Toxicol* 49:2229–35.

Kim, J. 2008. Protective effects of Asian dietary items on cancers—soy and ginseng. *Asian Pac J Cancer Prev* 9:543–8.

Kim, J.H., C.Y. Park, and S.J. Lee. 2006. Effects of sun ginseng on subjective quality of life in cancer patients: a double-blind, placebo-controlled pilot trial. *J Clin Pharm Ther* 31:331–4.

Kim, M.K., J.W. Lee, K.Y. Lee, and D.C. Yang. 2005. Microbial conversion of major ginsenoside rb(1) to pharmaceutically active minor ginsenoside rd. *J Microbiol* 43:456–62.

Kim, S.R., S.K. Jo, and S.H. Kim. 2003a. Modification of radiation response in mice by ginsenosides, active components of Panax ginseng. *In Vivo* 17:77–81.

Kim, T.W., E.H. Joh, B. Kim, and D.H. Kim. 2011b. Ginsenoside Rg5 ameliorates lung inflammation in mice by inhibiting the binding of LPS to toll-like receptor-4 on macrophages. *Int Immunopharmacol* 12:110–6.

Kim, Y.J., H.C. Kwon, H. Ko et al. 2008. Anti-tumor activity of the ginsenoside Rk1 in human hepatocellular carcinoma cells through inhibition of telomerase activity and induction of apoptosis. *Biol Pharm Bull* 31:826–30.

King, M.L., and L.L. Murphy. 2007. American ginseng (*Panax quinquefolius* L.) extract alters mitogen-activated protein kinase cell signaling and inhibits proliferation of MCF-7 cells. *J Exp Ther Oncol* 6:147–55.

King, M.L., and L.L. Murphy. 2010. Role of cyclin inhibitor protein p21 in the inhibition of HCT116 human colon cancer cell proliferation by American ginseng (*Panax quinquefolius*) and its constituents. *Phytomedicine* 17:261–8.

Konoshima, T., M. Takasaki, H. Tokuda et al. 1998. Anti-tumor-promoting activity of majonoside-R2 from Vietnamese ginseng, Panax vietnamensis Ha et Grushv. (I). *Biol Pharm Bull* 21:834–8.

Konoshima, T., M. Takasaki, and H. Tokuda. 1999a. Anti-carcinogenic activity of the roots of Panax notoginseng. II. *Biol Pharm Bull* 22:1150–2.

Konoshima, T., M. Takasaki, E. Ichiishi et al. 1999b. Cancer chemopreventive activity of majonoside-R2 from Vietnamese ginseng, Panax vietnamensis. *Cancer Lett* 147:11–6.

Koo, H.N., H.J. Jeong, I.Y. Choi et al. 2007. Mountain grown ginseng induces apoptosis in HL-60 cells and its mechanism have little relation with TNF-alpha production. *Am J Chin Med* 35:169–82.

Lee, B.H., S.J. Lee, J.H. Hur et al. 1998. In vitro antigenotoxic activity of novel ginseng saponin metabolites formed by intestinal bacteria. *Planta Med* 1998;64:500–3.

Lee, I.K., K.A. Kang, C.M. Lim et al. 2010b. Compound K, a metabolite of ginseng saponin, induces mitochondria-dependent and caspase-dependent apoptosis via the generation of reactive oxygen species in human colon cancer cells. *Int J Mol Sci* 11:4916–31.

Lee, J.Y., J.W. Shin, K.S. Chun et al. 2005. Antitumor promotional effects of a novel intestinal bacterial metabolite (IH-901) derived from the protopanaxadiol-type ginsenosides in mouse skin. *Carcinogenesis* 26:359–67.

Lee, P.S., T.W. Song, J.H. Sung et al. 2006. Pharmacokinetic characteristics and hepatic distribution of IH-901, a novel intestinal metabolite of ginseng saponin, in rats. *Planta Med* 72:204–10.

Lee, S.D., S.K. Park, E.S. Lee et al. 2010a. A lipid-soluble red ginseng extract inhibits the growth of human lung tumor xenografts in nude mice. *J Med Food* 13:1–5.

Lee, S.J., J.H. Sung, C.K. Moon, and B.H. Lee. 1999. Antitumor activity of a novel ginseng saponin metabolite in human pulmonary adenocarcinoma cells resistant to cisplatin. *Cancer Lett* 144:39–43.

Lee, S.J., W.G. Ko, J.H. Kim et al. 2000. Induction of apoptosis by a novel intestinal metabolite of ginseng saponin via cytochrome c-mediated activation of caspase-3 protease. *Biochem Pharmacol* 60:677–85.

Lee, S.Y., G.T. Kim, S.H. Roh et al. 2009a. Proteomic analysis of the anti-cancer effect of 20S-ginsenoside Rg3 in human colon cancer cell lines. *Biosci Biotechnol Biochem* 73:811–6.

Lee, S.Y., G.T. Kim, S.H. Roh et al. 2009b. Proteome changes related to the anti-cancer activity of HT29 cells by the treatment of ginsenoside Rd. *Pharmazie* 64:242–7.

Lee, W.H., J.S. Choi, H.Y. Kim et al. 2009c. Heat-processed neoginseng, KG-135, down-regulates G1 Cyclin-dependent kinase through the proteasome-mediated pathway in HeLa cells. *Oncol Rep* 21:467–74.

Lee, W.H., J.S. Choi, H.Y. Kim et al. 2010c. Potentiation of etoposide-induced apoptosis in HeLa cells by co-treatment with KG-135, a quality-controlled standardized ginsenoside formulation. *Cancer Lett* 294:74–81.

Li, B., J. Zhao, C.Z. Wang et al. 2011a. Ginsenoside Rh2 induces apoptosis and paraptosis-like cell death in colorectal cancer cells through activation of p53. *Cancer Lett* 301:185–92.

Li, G., Z. Wang, Y. Sun, and K. Liu. 2006. Ginsenoside 20(S)-protopanaxadiol inhibits the proliferation and invasion of human fibrosarcoma HT1080 cells. *Basic Clin Pharmacol Toxicol* 98:588–92.

Li, H., M. Ye, H. Guo et al. 2009a. Biotransformation of 20(S)-protopanaxadiol by Mucor spinosus. *Phytochemistry* 70:1416–20.

Li, J., M. Xie, and Y. Gan. 2008. [Effect of Xiaochaihu decoction and different herbal formulation of component on inhibiting H22 liver cancer in mice and enhancing immune function]. *Zhongguo Zhong Yao Za Zhi* 33:1039–44. Chinese.

Li, K., X. Chen, J. Xu, X. Li, and D. Zhong. 2005. Liquid chromatography/tandem mass spectrometry for pharmacokinetic studies of 20(R)-ginsenoside Rg3 in dog. *Rapid Commun Mass Spectrom* 19:813–7.

Li, L., X. Chen, D. Li, and D. Zhong. 2011b. Identification of 20(S)-protopanaxadiol metabolites in human liver microsomes and human hepatocytes. *Drug Metab Dispos* 39:472–83.

Li, L., J.L. Zhang, Y.X. Sheng et al. 2004. Liquid chromatographic method for determination of four active saponins from Panax notoginseng in rat urine using solid-phase extraction. *J Chromatogr B Analyt Technol Biomed Life Sci* 808:177–83.

Li, W., H. Wanibuchi, E.I. Salim et al. 2000. Inhibition by ginseng of 1,2-dimethylhydrazine induction of aberrant crypt foci in the rat colon. *Nutr Cancer* 36:66–73.

Li, W., Y. Liu, J.W. Zhang et al. 2009b. Anti-androgen-independent prostate cancer effects of ginsenoside metabolites in vitro: mechanism and possible structure-activity relationship investigation. *Arch Pharm Res* 32:49–57.

Li, X., G. Wang, J. Sun et al. 2007. Pharmacokinetic and absolute bioavailability study of total panax notoginsenoside, a typical multiple constituent traditional Chinese medicine (TCM) in rats. *Biol Pharm Bull* 30:847–51.

Li, X.L., C.Z. Wang, S. Sun et al. 2009c. American ginseng berry enhances chemopreventive effect of 5-FU on human colorectal cancer cells. *Oncol Rep* 22:943–52.

Li, X., X.G. Wu. 1991. Effects of ginseng on hepatocellular carcinoma in rats induced by diethylnitrosamine—a further study. *J Tongji Med Univ* 11:73–80.

Lin, S.Y., L.M. Liu, and L.C. Wu. 1995. [Effects of Shenmai injection on immune function in stomach cancer patients after chemotherapy]. *Zhongguo Zhong Xi Yi Jie He Za Zhi* 15:451–3. Chinese.

Lin, Y.W., Y.C. Mou, C.C. Su, and B.H. Chiang. 2010. Antihepatocarcinoma activity of lactic acid bacteria fermented Panax notoginseng. *J Agric Food Chem* 58:8528–34.

Liu, H., J. Yang, F. Du et al. 2009. Absorption and disposition of ginsenosides after oral administration of Panax notoginseng extract to rats. *Drug Metab Dispos* 37:2290–8.

Liu, W.K., S.X. Xu, and C.T. Che. 2000. Anti-proliferative effect of ginseng saponins on human prostate cancer cell line. *Life Sci* 67:1297–306.

Lu, J.M., Q. Yao, and C. Chen. 2009. Ginseng compounds: an update on their molecular mechanisms and medical applications. *Curr Vasc Pharmacol* 7:293–302.

Lu, P., W. Su, Z.H. Miao et al. 2008. Effect and mechanism of ginsenoside Rg3 on postoperative life span of patients with non-small cell lung cancer. *Chin J Integr Med* 14:33–6.

Ma, Z.C., Y. Gao, Y.G. Wang et al. 2006. Ginsenoside Rg1 inhibits proliferation of vascular smooth muscle cells stimulated by tumor necrosis factor-alpha. *Acta Pharmacol Sin* 27:1000–6.

Malekzadeh, F., C. Ros, C. Ingvar, and H. Jernström. 2005. [Natural remedies and hormone preparations—potential risk for breast cancer patients. A study surveys the use of agents which possibly counteract with the treatment]. *Lakartidningen* 102:3226–8, 3230–1. Swedish.

Ming, Y.L., Z.Y. Chen, L.H. Chen et al. 2009. [Inhibitory effect of ginseng saponin IH901 on proliferation and metastasis of ECV304 cell line and its molecular mechanism]. *Yao Xue Xue Bao* 44:967–72. Chinese.

Ming, Y., Z. Chen, L. Chen et al. 2010. Ginsenoside compound K attenuates metastatic growth of hepatocellular carcinoma, which is associated with the translocation of nuclear factor-kappaB p65 and reduction of matrix metalloproteinase-2/9. *Planta Med* 77:428–33.

Mochizuki, M., Y.C. Yoo, K. Matsuzawa et al. 1995. Inhibitory effect of tumor metastasis in mice by saponins, ginsenoside-Rb2, 20(R)- and 20(S)-ginsenoside-Rg3, of red ginseng. *Biol Pharm Bull* 18:1197–202.

Moon, J., S.J. Yu, H.S. Kim, and J. Sohn. 2000. Induction of G(1) cell cycle arrest and p27(KIP1) increase by panaxydol isolated from Panax ginseng. *Biochem Pharmacol* 59:1109–16.

Musende, A.G., A. Eberding, C. Wood et al. 2009. Pre-clinical evaluation of Rh2 in PC-3 human xenograft model for prostate cancer in vivo: formulation, pharmacokinetics, biodistribution and efficacy. *Cancer Chemother Pharmacol* 64:1085–95.

Nishino, H., H. Tokuda, T. Ii et al. 2001. Cancer chemoprevention by ginseng in mouse liver and other organs. *J Korean Med Sci* 16 Suppl:S66–9.

Oh, M., Y.H. Choi, S. Choi et al. 1999. Anti-proliferating effects of ginsenoside Rh2 on MCF-7 human breast cancer cells. *Int J Oncol* 14:869–75.

Oh, S.H., and B.H. Lee. 2004. A ginseng saponin metabolite-induced apoptosis in HepG2 cells involves a mitochondria-mediated pathway and its downstream caspase-8 activation and Bid cleavage. *Toxicol Appl Pharmacol* 194:221–9.

Okita, K., Q. Li, T. Murakamio, and M. Takahashi. 1993. Anti-growth effects with components of Sho-saiko-to (TJ-9) on cultured human hepatoma cells. *Eur J Cancer Prev* 2:169–75.

Ota, T., M. Maeda, and S. Odashima. 1991. Mechanism of action of ginsenoside Rh2: uptake and metabolism of ginsenoside Rh2 by cultured B16 melanoma cells. *J Pharm Sci* 80:1141–6.

Paek, I.B., Y. Moon, J. Kim et al. 2006. Pharmacokinetics of a ginseng saponin metabolite compound K in rats. *Biopharm Drug Dispos* 27:39–45.

Pang, H., H.J. Wang, L. Fu, and C.Y. Su. 2001. [Pharmacokinetic studies of 20(R)-ginsenoside RG3 in human volunteers]. *Yao Xue Xue Bao* 36:170–3.

Panwar, M., R. Samarth, M. Kumar, W.J. Yoon, and A. Kumar. 2005. Inhibition of benzo(a)pyrene induced lung adenoma by panax ginseng extract, EFLA400, in Swiss albino mice. *Biol Pharm Bull* 28:2063–7.

Park, H.J., E.S. Han, and D.K. Park. 2010. The ethyl acetate extract of PGP (Phellinus linteus grown on Panax ginseng) suppresses B16F10 melanoma cell proliferation through inducing cellular differentiation and apoptosis. *J Ethnopharmacol* 132:115–21.

Park, S.E., C. Park, S.H. Kim et al. 2009. Korean red ginseng extract induces apoptosis and decreases telomerase activity in human leukemia cells. *J Ethnopharmacol* 121:304–12.

Park, T.Y., M.H. Park, W.C. Shin et al. 2008. Anti-metastatic potential of ginsenoside Rp1, a novel ginsenoside derivative. *Biol Pharm Bull* 31:1802–5.

Peralta, E.A., L.L. Murphy, J. Minnis, S. Louis, and G.L. Dunnington. 2009. American Ginseng inhibits induced COX-2 and NFKB activation in breast cancer cells. *J Surg Res* 157:261–7.

Qi, L.W., C.Z. Wang, and C.S. Yuan. 2010. American ginseng: potential structure-function relationship in cancer chemoprevention. *Biochem Pharmacol* 80:947–54.

Qi, L.W., C.Z. Wang, and C.S. Yuan. 2011a. Ginsenosides from American ginseng: chemical and pharmacological diversity. *Phytochemistry* 72:689–99.

Qi, L.W., C.Z. Wang, and C.S. Yuan. 2011b. Isolation and analysis of ginseng: advances and challenges. *Nat Prod Rep* 28:467–95.

Qian, T., Z. Cai, R.N. Wong, and Z.H. Jiang. 2005a. Liquid chromatography/mass spectrometric analysis of rat samples for in vivo metabolism and pharmacokinetic studies of ginsenoside Rh2. *Rapid Commun Mass Spectrom* 19:3549–54.

Qian, T., Z. Cai, R.N. Wong, N.K. Mak, and Z.H. Jiang. 2005b. In vivo rat metabolism and pharmacokinetic studies of ginsenoside Rg3. *J Chromatogr B Analyt Technol Biomed Life Sci* 816:223–32.

Rebbeck, T.R., A.B. Troxel, S. Norman et al. 2007. A retrospective case-control study of the use of hormone-related supplements and association with breast cancer. *Int J Cancer* 120:1523–8.

Ren, H.C., J.G. Sun, G.J. Wang et al. 2008. Sensitive determination of 20(S)-protopanaxadiol in rat plasma using HPLC-APCI-MS: application of pharmacokinetic study in rats. *J Pharm Biomed Anal* 48:1476–80.

Sato, K., M. Mochizuki, I. Saiki et al. 1994. Inhibition of tumor angiogenesis and metastasis by a saponin of Panax ginseng, ginsenoside-Rb2. *Biol Pharm Bull* 17:635–9.

Seo, J.Y., J.H. Lee, N.W. Kim et al. 2005. Effect of a fermented ginseng extract, BST204, on the expression of cyclooxygenase-2 in murine macrophages. *Int Immunopharmacol* 5:929–36.

Shin, H.R., J.Y. Kim, T.K. Yun, G. Morgan, and H. Vainio. 2000. The cancer-preventive potential of Panax ginseng: a review of human and experimental evidence. *Cancer Causes Control* 11:565–76. Review.

Song, G., S. Guo, W. Wang et al. 2010b. Intestinal metabolite compound K of ginseng saponin potently attenuates metastatic growth of hepatocellular carcinoma by augmenting apoptosis via a Bid-mediated mitochondrial pathway. *J Agric Food Chem* 58:12753–60.

Song, M., S. Zhang, X. Xu, T. Hang, and L. Jia. 2010a. Simultaneous determination of three Panax notoginseng saponins at sub-nanograms by LC-MS/MS in dog plasma for pharmacokinetics of compound Danshen tablets. *J Chromatogr B Analyt Technol Biomed Life Sci* 878:3331–7.

Sonoda, Y., T. Kasahara, N. Mukaida et al. 1998. Stimulation of interleukin-8 production by acidic polysaccharides from the root of Panax ginseng. *Immunopharmacology* 38:287–94.

Suh, S.O., M. Kroh, N.R. Kim, Y.G. Joh, and M.Y. Cho. 2002. Effects of red ginseng upon postoperative immunity and survival in patients with stage III gastric cancer. *Am J Chin Med* 30:483–94.

Sun, J., G. Wang, X. Haitang, L. Hao, P. Guoyu, and T. Tucker. 2005. Simultaneous rapid quantification of ginsenoside Rg1 and its secondary glycoside Rh1 and aglycone protopanaxatriol in rat plasma by liquid chromatography-mass spectrometry after solid-phase extraction. *J Pharm Biomed Anal* 38:126–32.

Sun, Y., H. Lin, Y. Zhu et al. 2006. [A randomized, prospective, multi-centre clinical trial of NP regimen (vinorelbine+cisplatin) plus Gensing Rg3 in the treatment of advanced non-small cell lung cancer patients.] *Zhongguo Fei Ai Za Zhi* 9:254–8. Chinese.

Surh, Y.J., H.K. Na, J.Y. Lee, and Y.S. Keum. 2001. Molecular mechanisms underlying anti-tumor promoting activities of heat-processed Panax ginseng C.A. Meyer. *J Korean Med Sci* 16 Suppl:S38–41. Review.

Tode, T., Y. Kikuchi, H. Sasa et al. 1992. [In vitro and in vivo effects of ginsenoside Rh2 on the proliferation of serous cystadenocarcinoma of the human ovary]. *Nihon Sanka Fujinka Gakkai Zasshi* 44:589–94. Japanese.

Tode, T., Y. Kikuchi, J. Hirata et al. 1993a. [Inhibitory effects of oral administration of ginsenoside Rh2 on tumor growth in nude mice bearing serous cyst adenocarcinoma of the human ovary]. *Nihon Sanka Fujinka Gakkai Zasshi* 45:1275–82. Japanese.

Tode, T., Y. Kikuchi, T. Kita et al. 1993b. Inhibitory effects by oral administration of ginsenoside Rh2 on the growth of human ovarian cancer cells in nude mice. *J Cancer Res Clin Oncol* 120:24–6.

Volate, S.R., D.M. Davenport, S.J. Muga, and M.J. Wargovich. 2005. Modulation of aberrant crypt foci and apoptosis by dietary herbal supplements (quercetin, curcumin, silymarin, ginseng and rutin). *Carcinogenesis* 26:1450–6.

Wakabayashi, C., K. Murakami, H. Hasegawa, J. Murata, and I. Saiki. 1998. An intestinal bacterial metabolite of ginseng protopanaxadiol saponins has the ability to induce apoptosis in tumor cells. *Biochem Biophys Res Commun* 246:725–30.

Wang, B.S., L.S. Zhang, D.M. Song, J.H. Zhang, and Y.M. Liu. 2009b. [Effect of ginsenoside Rg3 on apoptosis of Hep-2 and expression of HIF-1alpha in human laryngeal cancer cell line under anoxic conditions]. *Zhong Yao Cai* 32:102–6. Chinese.

Wang, C.Z., H.H. Aung, M. Ni et al. 2007a. Red American ginseng: ginsenoside constituents and antiproliferative activities of heat-processed Panax quinquefolius roots. *Planta Med* 73:669–74.

Wang, H., H. Zou, L. Kong et al. 1999. Determination of ginsenoside Rg3 in plasma by solid-phase extraction and high-performance liquid chromatography for pharmacokinetic study. *J Chromatogr B Biomed Sci Appl* 731:403–9.

Wang, J.Y., G.W. Ma, S.Q. Dai et al. 2007b. [Effect of cellular immune supportive treatment on immunity of esophageal carcinoma patients after modern two-field lymph node dissection]. *Ai Zheng* 26:778–81. Chinese.

Wang, W., E.R. Rayburn, J. Hang et al. 2009a. Anti-lung cancer effects of novel ginsenoside 25-OCH(3)-PPD. *Lung Cancer* 65:306–11.

Wang, Z., Q. Zheng, K. Liu, G. Li, and R. Zheng. 2006. Ginsenoside Rh(2) enhances antitumour activity and decreases genotoxic effect of cyclophosphamide. *Basic Clin Pharmacol Toxicol* 98:411–5.

Wang, Z.J., L. Song, L.C. Guo, M. Yin, and Y.N. Sun. 2011. Induction of differentiation by panaxydol in human hepatocarcinoma SMMC-7721 cells via cAMP and MAP kinase dependent mechanism. *Yakugaku Zasshi* 131:993–1000.

Wargovich, M.J. 2001. Colon cancer chemoprevention with ginseng and other botanicals. *J Korean Med Sci* 16 Suppl:S81–6. Review.

Watanabe, T., M. Watanabe, Y. Watanabe, and C. Hotta. 2000. Effects of oral administration of Pfaffia paniculata (Brazilian ginseng) on incidence of spontaneous leukemia in AKR/J mice. *Cancer Detect Prev* 24:173–8.

Wei, G.Q., Y.N. Zheng, W. Li et al. 2011. Structural modification of ginsenoside Rh(2) by fatty acid esterification and its detoxification property in antitumor. *Bioorg Med Chem Lett* 22:1082–5.

Wu, X.G., and D.H. Zhu. 1990. Influence of ginseng upon the development of liver cancer induced by diethyl-nitrosamine in rats. *J Tongji Med Univ* 10:141–5, 133.

Wurz, G.T., C. Marchisano-Karpman, and M.W. DeGregorio. 2006. Ineffectiveness of American ginseng in the prevention of dimethylbenzanthracene-induced mammary tumors in mice. *Oncol Res* 16:251–60.

Xia, C.H., J.G. Sun, G.J. Wang et al. 2010. Herb-drug interactions: in vivo and in vitro effect of Shenmai injection, a herbal preparation, on the metabolic activities of hepatic cytochrome P450 3A1/2, 2C6, 1A2, and 2E1 in rats. *Planta Med* 76:245–50.

Xiaoguang, C., L. Hongyan, L. Xiaohong et al. 1998. Cancer chemopreventive and therapeutic activities of red ginseng. *J Ethnopharmacol* 60:71–8.

Xiaohui, F., W. Yi, and C. Yiyu. 2006. LC/MS fingerprinting of Shenmai injection: a novel approach to quality control of herbal medicines. *J Pharm Biomed Anal* 40:591–7.

Xie, F.Y., Z.F. Zeng, and H.Y. Huang. 2001. [Clinical observation on nasopharyngeal carcinoma treated with combined therapy of radiotherapy and ginseng polysaccharide injection]. *Zhongguo Zhong Xi Yi Jie He Za Zhi* 21:332–4. Chinese.

Xie, H.T., G.J. Wang, J.G. Sun et al. 2005. High performance liquid chromatographic-mass spectrometric determination of ginsenoside Rg3 and its metabolites in rat plasma using solid-phase extraction for pharmacokinetic studies. *J Chromatogr B Analyt Technol Biomed Life Sci* 818:167–73.

Xu, Q.F., X.L. Fang, and D.F. Chen. 2003. Pharmacokinetics and bioavailability of ginsenoside Rb1 and Rg1 from Panax notoginseng in rats. *J Ethnopharmacol* 84:187–92.

Xu, T.M., Y. Xin, M.H. Cui, X. Jiang, and L.P. Gu. 2007. Inhibitory effect of ginsenoside Rg3 combined with cyclophosphamide on growth and angiogenesis of ovarian cancer. *Chin Med J* (Engl) 120:584–8.

Xu, T.M., M.H. Cui, Y. Xin et al. 2008. Inhibitory effect of ginsenoside Rg3 on ovarian cancer metastasis. *Chin Med J* (Engl) 121:1394–7.

Yan, Y., Y. Wang, Q. Tan et al. 2006. Efficacy of polyphenon E, red ginseng, and rapamycin on benzo(a)pyrene-induced lung tumorigenesis in A/J mice. *Neoplasia* 8:52–8.

Yan, Z., R. Yang, Y. Jiang et al. 2011. Induction of apoptosis in human promyelocytic leukemia HL60 cells by panaxynol and panaxydol. *Molecules* 16:5561–73.

Yang, L., S.J. Xu, Z.F. Wu, Y.M. Liu, and X. Zeng. 2009. Determination of ginsenoside-Rg(1) in human plasma and its application to pharmacokinetic studies following intravenous administration of 'Shenmai' injection. *Phytother Res* 23:65–71.

Yang, X.L., T.K. Guo, Y.H. Wang et al. 2012. Ginsenoside Rd attenuates the inflammatory response via modulating p38 and JNK signaling pathways in rats with TNBS-induced relapsing colitis. *Int Immunopharmacol* 2012 Jan 5. PMID: 22227208

Yang, Z., S. Gao, J. Wang et al. 2011. Enhancement of oral bioavailability of 20(S)-ginsenoside Rh2 through improved understanding of its absorption and efflux mechanisms. *Drug Metab Dispos* 39:1866–72.

Yang, Z., J.R. Wang, T. Niu, S. Gao, T. Yin, Z.H. Jiang, M. You, and M. Hu. 2012. Inhibition of P-glycoprotein leads to improved oral bioavailability of compound K, an anti-cancer metabolite of red ginseng extract produced by gut microflora. *Drug Metab Dispos* 40:1538–44.

Yi, S.W., J.W. Sull, J.S. Hong, J.A. Linton, and H. Ohrr. 2009. Association between ginseng intake and mortality: Kangwha cohort study. *J Altern Complement Med* 15:921–8.

Yoo, J.H., H.C. Kwon, Y.J. Kim, J.H. Park, and H.O. Yang. 2010. KG-135, enriched with selected ginsenosides, inhibits the proliferation of human prostate cancer cells in culture and inhibits xenograft growth in athymic mice. *Cancer Lett* 289:99–110.

Yoon, J.H., Y.J. Choi, S.W. Cha, and S.G. Lee. 2011. Anti-metastatic effects of ginsenoside Rd via inactivation of MAPK signaling and induction of focal adhesion formation. *Phytomedicine* 19:284–92.

Yuan, H.D., H.Y. Quan, Y. Zhang, S.H. Kim, and S.H. Chung. 2010. 20(S)-Ginsenoside Rg3-induced apoptosis in HT-29 colon cancer cells is associated with AMPK signaling pathway. *Mol Med Report* 3:825–31.

Yun, T.K. 1999. Update from Asia. Asian studies on cancer chemoprevention. *Ann N Y Acad Sci.* 889:157–92. Review.

Yun, T.K. 2001. Panax ginseng—a non-organ-specific cancer preventive? *Lancet Oncol* 2:49–55. Review.

Yun, T.K. 2003. Experimental and epidemiological evidence on non-organ specific cancer preventive effect of Korean ginseng and identification of active compounds. *Mutat Res* 523-524:63–74. Review.

Yun, T.K., and S.Y. Choi. 1990. A case-control study of ginseng intake and cancer. *Int J Epidemiol* 19:871–6.

Yun, T.K., and Y.S. Choi. 1995. Preventive effect of ginseng intake against various human cancers: a case-control study on 1987 pairs. *Cancer Epidemiol Biomarkers Prev* 4:401–8.

Yun, T.K., and Y.S. Choi. 1998. Non-organ specific cancer prevention of ginseng: a prospective study in Korea. *Int J Epidemiol* 27:359–64.

Yun, T.K., Y.S. Yun, and I.W. Han. 1983. Anticarcinogenic effect of long-term oral administration of red ginseng on newborn mice exposed to various chemical carcinogens. *Cancer Detect Prev* 6:515–25.

Yun, T.K., S.H. Kim, and Y.S. Lee. 1995. Trial of a new medium-term model using benzo(a)pyrene induced lung tumor in newborn mice. *Anticancer Res* 15:839–45.

Yun, T.K., Y.S. Lee, Y.H. Lee, S.I. Kim, and H.Y. Yun. 2001a. Anticarcinogenic effect of Panax ginseng C.A. Meyer and identification of active compounds. *J Korean Med Sci* 16 Suppl:S6–18. Review.

Yun, T.K., Y.S. Lee, Y.H. Lee, S.I. Kim, and H.Y. Yun. 2001b. Anticarcinogenic effect of Panax ginseng C.A. Meyer and identification of active compounds. *J Korean Med Sci* 16 Suppl:S6–18.

Yun, T.K., S. Zheng, S.Y. Choi et al. 2010. Non-organ-specific preventive effect of long-term administration of Korean red ginseng extract on incidence of human cancers. *J Med Food* 13:489–94.

Yun, Y.S., H.S. Moon, Y.R. Oh et al. 1987. Effect of red ginseng on natural killer cell activity in mice with lung adenoma induced by urethan and benzo(a)pyrene. *Cancer Detect Prev* Suppl 1:301–9.

Yun, Y.S., Y.S. Lee, S.K. Jo, and I.S. Jung. 1993. Inhibition of autochthonous tumor by ethanol insoluble fraction from Panax ginseng as an immunomodulator. *Planta Med* 59:521–4.

Zeng, X.L., and Z.G. Tu. 2004. [Induction of differentiation by ginsenoside Rh2 in hepatocarcinoma cell SMMC-7721]. *Ai Zheng* 23:879–84. Chinese.

Zhang, H.M., S.L. Li, H. Zhang et al. 2012. Holistic quality evaluation of commercial white and red ginseng using a UPLC-QTOF-MS/MS-based metabolomics approach. *J Pharm Biomed Anal* 62:258–73.

Zhang, Q.H., C.F. Wu, L. Duan, J.Y. Yang. 2008. Protective effects of ginsenoside Rg(3) against cyclophosphamide-induced DNA damage and cell apoptosis in mice. *Arch Toxicol* 82:117–23.

28 Anti-Inflammatory Botanical Dietary Supplements for Women's Health
Role in Breast Cancer Prevention?

Birgit M. Dietz and Judy L. Bolton

CONTENTS

28.1 INTRODUCTION: BREAST CANCER RISK AND BOTANICAL ALTERNATIVES FOR HORMONE REPLACEMENT THERAPY

Breast cancer is the second most common malignancy among women and also the second leading cause of cancer death for women (DeSantis et al. 2011). Experimental and epidemiological data strongly associate excessive estrogen exposure, such as in hormone replacement therapy (HRT), with the development of breast cancer (Bolton 2011; Chen et al. 2008). The release of the initial results from the Women's Health Initiative (WHI) Study in July 2002 highlighted the increased risk of breast cancer due to HRT (Rossouw et al. 2002). A recent analysis of data from the National

Cancer Institute's Surveillance, Epidemiology, and End Results (SEER) registries has shown that age-adjusted incidence rate of breast cancer fell sharply in 2003 and has been sustained through 2005, which seemed to be related to the drop in the use of HRT (Ravdin et al. 2007; Chlebowski et al. 2009).

Besides estrogen, accumulating evidence suggests that chronic inflammation is associated with estrogen carcinogenesis in the breast (Howe 2007; Frasor et al. 2009; Aggarwal and Sung 2011). Upregulation of the inducible isoform cyclooxygenase 2 (COX2), which plays an important role in inflammatory activities, has been identified in many human cancers and precancerous lesions (Howe 2007). COX2 overexpression has been detected in approximately 40% of cases of human breast carcinoma as well as in preinvasive ductal carcinoma in situ (DCIS) lesions. Epidemiologic analyses and several experimental studies have shown that nonsteroidal anti-inflammatory drugs and selective COX2 inhibitors can suppress breast cancer (Howe 2007). Also, breast cancer recurrence has been associated with an increase in inflammatory markers (Pierce et al. 2009).

Because of the troubling findings of the WHI studies, many women seeking safer alternatives to traditional HRT for the alleviation of menopausal symptoms are turning to botanical dietary supplements (Cheema et al. 2007; Kupferer et al. 2009; Mahady et al. 2003; Rees 2009). The efficacy of these botanical dietary supplements for the alleviation of menopausal symptoms has not been established (North American Menopause Society 2004, 2011). In fact, most placebo-controlled clinical trials looking at menopausal symptom relief show no efficacy compared to placebo (Geller et al. 2009; Nelson et al. 2006; Piersen et al. 2004; Palacio et al. 2009). However, there is a large placebo effect, which might explain the popularity of these botanicals. There could be other beneficial health effects for these botanical dietary supplements, including chemoprevention of cancer (Mandlekar et al. 2006). Observational studies have suggested that a diet consisting of fruits and vegetables can prevent cancer (Bradlow and Sepkovic 2002), and recent data suggest that many botanicals used for women's health have cytoprotective potential (Dijsselbloem et al. 2004; Hemachandra et al. 2012; Dietz et al. 2005, 2008; Bolton 2011; Einbond et al. 2007; Mense et al. 2008). In particular, many anti-inflammatory properties have been described for these botanicals (Surh 2003; Luqman and Pezzuto 2010). It is the focus of this review to discuss the anti-inflammatory properties of botanical dietary supplements used for women's health and their potential role in breast cancer prevention.

28.2 MECHANISMS OF ESTROGEN CARCINOGENESIS

The molecular mechanisms of estrogen carcinogenesis are still not well understood (Yager and Davidson 2006; Cavalieri et al. 2006; Russo et al. 2000; Russo and Russo 2006). Malignant phenotypes arise as a result of a series of mutations, most likely in genes associated with tumor suppressor, oncogene, DNA repair, or endocrine functions (Henderson and Feigelson 2000). Three major pathways (Figure 28.1) are considered to be important in estrogen carcinogenesis of the breast, including (1) the hormonal pathway leading to stimulation of tissue growth; (2) the chemical pathway involving estrogen metabolism to reactive intermediates that damage DNA (Bolton 2011; Yager and Davidson 2006); and (3) the inflammatory pathway, which leads to promotion, proliferation, and metastasis of malignant cells (Howe 2007; Frasor et al. 2009; Aggarwal and Sung 2011; Pierce et al. 2009).

28.2.1 HORMONAL PATHWAY

Estrogen stimulates cell proliferation through estrogen receptor (ER)–mediated signaling pathways, resulting in an increased risk of genomic mutations during DNA replication (Figure 28.1, Hormonal) (Henderson and Feigelson 2000; Revankar et al. 2005; Song et al. 2006). Phytoestrogens in botanical extracts can mimic or antagonize the action of estradiol at the ERs (Piersen 2003). In postmenopausal women, estradiol is produced by aromatization of androgens in extragonadal sites, such as the breast tissue (Simpson et al. 1999). Therefore, estradiol levels in breast tissue of postmenopausal

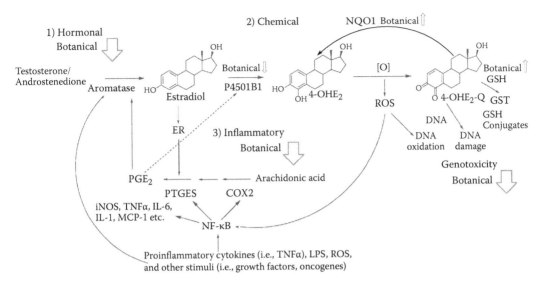

FIGURE 28.1 Multitargeted modulation of breast carcinogenesis by botanicals. Postulated pathways of estrogen carcinogenesis and potential mechanisms of botanicals to prevent estrogen carcinogenesis in the breast.

women may be relatively high. In fact, it has been demonstrated that aromatase activity is highest in or near breast tumor sites (Brueggemeier et al. 2003). Thus, local regulation of aromatase by both endogenous factors as well as botanicals could influence the levels of estrogen in the breast tissue.

28.2.2 CHEMICAL PATHWAY

The chemical pathway involves estrogen metabolism, mediated by cytochrome P450s that generate reactive electrophilic estrogen o-quinones and reactive oxygen species (ROS) through redox cycling of these o-quinones (Bolton and Thatcher 2008; Bolton 2011; Cavalieri and Rogan 2011) (Figure 28.1, Chemical). P4501B1 metabolism could be particularly significant, since only the 4-hydroxylated metabolites of estrone/estradiol have shown significant carcinogenic properties in contrast to the 2-hydroxylated metabolites in various animal studies (Liehr et al. 1986; Newbold and Liehr 2000). In addition, P4501B1 messenger RNA (mRNA) levels had higher expression in breast tissue of women with breast cancer, whereas expression of protective enzymes such as NAD(P)H:quinone oxidoreductase 1 (NQO1) was lower (Singh et al. 2005). Finally, epidemiological studies have suggested a link between genetic polymorphism in estrogen 4-hydroxylases and a risk for developing breast cancer (Zheng et al. 2000; Kisselev et al. 2005). These data suggest that estrogen metabolites are obligate contributors to the development of cancer. Reduction of CYP4501B1 through botanicals would therefore decrease the tumorigenic potential of estrogens. Estrogen quinones can be eliminated by reduction with NQO1 or conjugation with glutathione S-transferase (GST) to facilitate their excretion. Therefore, it is one chemopreventive strategy to increase detoxification enzymes, such as NQO1 and GST, by natural agents (Hong and Sporn 1997; Kensler 1997; Chen and Tony Kong 2004).

28.2.3 INFLAMMATORY PATHWAY

Chronic inflammation has been shown to increase tumor promotion and progression in various tumors (Figure 28.1, Inflammatory) (Aggarwal and Sung 2011). Recent data suggest a direct link between chronic inflammation and breast cancer (DeNardo and Coussens 2007; Calogero et al. 2007; Howe 2007; Frasor et al. 2008). It has been demonstrated that estrogen shows proinflammatory behavior in breast tissue (Frasor et al. 2008). Estrogen regulates genes that encode inflammatory mediators, such as microsomal prostaglandin E synthase-1 (PTGES) (Frasor et al. 2003). This gene and COX2 transform arachidonic acid into prostaglandin E2 (PGE_2) (Park et al. 2006). PGE_2 is a key protumorigenic prostanoid and plays an important role in breast cancer (Howe 2007). For example, PGE_2 leads to an increase in invasiveness and metastasis (Timoshenko et al. 2003; Ma et al. 2006). In addition, PGE_2 can upregulate aromatase expression, leading to an enhanced local production of estrogens within the breast (Richards and Brueggemeier 2003). Interestingly, it has been shown that PTGES is synergistically upregulated by estradiol and proinflammatory cytokines such as tumor necrosis factor α (TNFα) (Frasor et al. 2008), leading to a positive feedback loop that can contribute to estrogen-dependent breast cancer (Frasor et al. 2009). Furthermore, it has been shown that PGE_2 upregulates CYP1B1 in the breast adenocarcinoma cell line of the Michigan Cancer Foundation (MCF-7), thus increasing estrogen metabolism to genotoxic metabolites (Han et al. 2010).

The other enzyme that is responsible for the production of PGE_2 is the inducible isoform COX2 (Park et al. 2006). COX2 is undetectable in normal breast tissue, but it is overexpressed in about 40% of human breast carcinomas (Howe 2007), which correlates with several parameters that are characteristic of aggressive breast cancer, such as large tumor size and high proliferation. Furthermore, epidemiologic and experimental evidence suggests a protective effect of COX-inhibitory drugs in breast cancer (Howe 2007).

PTGES, COX2, and other inflammatory enzymes, such as inducible nitric oxide synthase (iNOS), interleukin 6 (IL-6), and TNFα, are regulated by the transcription factor nuclear factor kappa-light-chain-enhancer of activated B cells (NF-κB) (Aggarwal et al. 2006). NF-κB has been found to be constitutively activated in most cancers (Aggarwal et al. 2009). NF-κB is activated by proinflammatory cytokines, ultraviolet (UV) radiation, lipopolysaccharide (LPS), and ROS (Aggarwal 2004). ROS overproduction during redox cycling of 4-hydroxyestradiol may increase nuclear translocation of NF-κB and contributes to transformation of MCF-10A cells (Park et al. 2009). Various feedback loops exist between the hormonal and chemical estrogen carcinogenesis pathways and inflammatory responses (Figure 28.1). One strategy of cancer prevention is the inhibition of inflammatory enzymes such as COX2, PTGES, and iNOS and inhibition of PGE_2 receptors. Inhibition of NF-κB in particular may be a very promising potential chemopreventive approach, since NF-κB regulates several inflammatory enzymes (Surh 2003; Aggarwal et al. 2009).

28.3 BOTANICAL MODULATION OF ESTROGEN CARCINOGENESIS

Recent literature data suggest that botanical dietary supplements for women's health issues might have chemopreventive properties that could modulate estrogen-dependent cancers (Mandlekar et al. 2006; Surh 2003). What follows is a summary of three of the most common botanicals (black cohosh, red clover, hops) used for postmenopausal women's health and their potential to modulate estrogen carcinogenesis.

28.3.1 BLACK COHOSH

Black cohosh (*Cimicifuga racemosa*) has been traditionally used by Native Americans and is currently a popular alternative to HRT (Mahady et al. 2003). Black cohosh contains triterpene glycosides and aromatic acids as the main active compound classes (Figure 28.2) (Fabricant 2005). Commercially available extracts are often standardized to the main triterpenes, 23-epi-26-deoxyactein and actein (Figure 28.2) (Fabricant and Farnsworth 2005). The efficacy of black cohosh preparations to ameliorate hot flashes is controversial (Osmers et al. 2005; Liske et al. 2002; Fabricant and Farnsworth 2005; Liebermann 1998; Geller et al. 2009). No estrogenic effects have been demonstrated for black cohosh in endometrial or breast tissue (Seidlova-Wuttke et al. 2003; Liske et al. 2002), and black cohosh extracts had no proliferative effect on hormone-sensitive tissues (endometrium, mammary) in several animal studies (Freudenstein et al. 2002; Kretzschmar

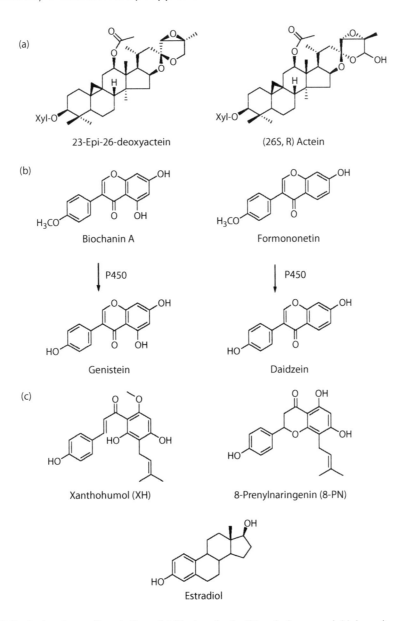

FIGURE 28.2 Isolated constituents from (a) black cohosh, (b) red clover, and (c) hops in comparison to estradiol.

et al. 2005; Burdette et al. 2003; Bodinet and Freudenstein 2002; Walji et al. 2007). Serotonergic, opioidic, and/or dopaminergic activities have been reported for black cohosh extracts in vitro, suggesting alternative mechanisms for possible menopausal symptom relief (Burdette et al. 2003; Rhyu et al. 2006; Jarry et al. 2003).

28.3.1.1 Hormonal Pathway

Several antiproliferative properties are described for black cohosh in breast cancer cells, mainly through ER-independent mechanisms (Einbond et al. 2004; Hostanska et al. 2004a). Black cohosh's antiproliferative effects on breast cancer cells are reported to be mediated through induction of apoptosis and through modulation of cell cycle proteins leading to cell cycle arrest (Hostanska et al. 2004a,b;

Einbond et al. 2004). In vitro and in vivo studies showed that black cohosh downregulates the expression of cell cycle regulator protein cyclin D1 and cell growth regulator (ID3), with actein representing the most active compound (Einbond et al. 2007, 2012). In addition, black cohosh extract as well as actein may induce mitochondrial damage. One in vitro study using a black cohosh extract describes inhibition of estradiol-induced cell proliferation and estradiol-induced genes (Zierau et al. 2002), but a direct antiestrogenic activity of black cohosh could not be determined (Overk et al. 2005).

28.3.1.2 Chemical Pathway

Antioxidant effects have been described for black cohosh (Booth et al. 2006; Burdette et al. 2002). A methanol extract of black cohosh has been shown to protect DNA from menadione-induced single-strand breaks and oxidative damage (Burdette et al. 2002). Bioassay-directed fractionation of the extract revealed that the polyphenolic acids methyl caffeate, caffeic acid, ferulic acid, cimiracemate A, cimiracemate B, and fukinolic acid exhibit antioxidative activities and reduce menadione-induced DNA damage. These data suggest that black cohosh can protect against cellular DNA damage caused by ROS. Recently, black cohosh and hop extracts were analyzed for their potential to inhibit 4-hydroxylation of estradiol (Hemachandra et al. 2012). While the hop extract significantly inhibited the formation of 4-hydroxyestradiol in MCF-10 cells, the black cohosh extract did not influence estrogen metabolism.

28.3.1.3 Inflammatory Pathway

Literature reports demonstrate moderate anti-inflammatory activities for black cohosh (Schmid et al. 2009). Aqueous *C. racemosa* extracts (0–6 mg/mL) inhibited nitric oxide (NO) production in LPS-stimulated macrophages by reduction of iNOS expression without affecting iNOS activity. Also, incubation with the extract was associated with a concentration-dependent reduction of interferon beta and interferon regulatory factor 1 mRNA. Among the triterpene glycosides, 23-epi-26-deoxyactein was identified as the active principle. The triterpene inhibited NO production in LPS-activated murine macrophages (RAW 264.7 cells) by around 44% at a concentration of 20 μg/mL. Since *C. racemosa* did not affect nuclear translocation of NF-κB (p65 subunit) protein, the mechanism of action still needs to be elucidated (Schmid et al. 2009). Yang et al. (2009) reported that based on bioassay-guided fractionation using LPS-induced primary blood macrophages, cimiracemate A was identified as an active compound. At a concentration of 140 μM, cimiracemate A reduced LPS-induced TNFα production by 47%. Analysis of the mechanistic pathway revealed that cimiracemate A inhibited LPS-induced translocation of the subunit p65 into the nucleus and LPS-induced extracellular signal–regulated kinase (ERK) phosphorylation.

In vivo studies in Sprague-Dawley rats demonstrated that after one dose of black cohosh extract (35.7 mg/kg bodyweight [BW]), inflammatory response genes were upregulated, while genes that regulate DNA replication, apoptosis inhibitory proteins, and regulation of cell growth were downregulated (Einbond et al. 2012). Interestingly, in a retrospective case–control study with breast cancer survivors, black cohosh treatment was associated with breast cancer protection (Rebbeck et al. 2007).

Overall, these studies suggest that black cohosh might modulate breast carcinogenesis mainly through antiproliferative pathways. Anti-inflammatory activities for black cohosh have also been reported, although high concentrations were used (Schmid et al. 2009; Yang et al. 2009). Studies in animal models and in women at physiologically relevant levels are necessary to determine whether these extracts show any anti-inflammatory activity in the prevention of breast cancer.

28.3.2 Red Clover

Red clover (*Trifolium pratense*) is an herbaceous plant used traditionally by Native Americans for the treatment of lung, nervous system, and reproductive system ailments (Booth and Piersen 2005; Booth et al. 2006). Red clover has a high content of estrogenic isoflavones, making it a popular botanical dietary supplement for the alleviation of menopausal symptoms (Piersen et al. 2004).

Previous studies have shown that red clover extracts have estrogenic properties in vitro (Burdette et al. 2002; Liu et al. 2001; Overk et al. 2005); however, the clinical efficacy of red clover extracts to alleviate menopausal hot flashes is controversial (Geller et al. 2009; Piersen et al. 2004; Booth and Piersen 2005; Tice et al. 2003). There are stronger epidemiological data suggesting that the isoflavones in red clover and soy are chemopreventive for breast and endometrial cancer (North American Menopause Society 2011) and may contribute to the lower incidence of breast cancer in Japanese women (Yamamoto et al. 2003; Adlercreutz 2002; Seibel et al. 2009).

28.3.2.1 Hormonal Pathway

The main compounds responsible for the estrogenic activity in red clover are the isoflavones genistein and daidzein (Figure 28.2) (Overk et al. 2005; Booth et al. 2006). In vivo, two other isoflavones, biochanin A and formononetin, that are contained in the extract in higher quantities are metabolized to genistein and daidzein (Overk et al. 2005). Van Meeuwen et al. (2007) evaluated the aromatase inhibiting activity of genistein and biochanin A in primary mammary fibroblast culture. The results revealed that genistein and biochanin A inhibited aromatase, with IC_{50} values of 3.6 and 25 µM, respectively.

Isoflavones have structural similarities to estradiol (Figure 28.2) and can compete with endogenous estrogens for binding to both ERα and ERβ. The binding affinity and the transcriptional pathway induced by genistein have been reported to be distinct from estradiol (An et al. 2001). At low concentrations (6 nM), genistein shows a predominant activation of ERβ-mediated activities (Kuiper et al. 1998; An et al. 2001; Overk et al. 2005; Chang et al. 2008), suggesting that genistein at these concentrations does not result in proliferation of breast cancer cells (Table 28.1) (Chang et al. 2008; Koehler et al. 2005). At higher concentrations (300 nM), however, genistein behaves very similarly to estradiol and can lead to proliferation of breast cancer cells (Chang et al. 2008; Harris et al. 2005; van Meeuwen et al. 2007). Micromolar concentrations (>1 µM) of genistein have been described to have antiproliferative properties, for example, in human epidermal growth factor receptor 2 (HER2) overexpressing breast cancer cells, partially through inhibition of tyrosine kinases (Sakla et al. 2007). Moreover, genistein (30 µM) induced apoptosis in the ER-negative breast cancer cell line, M.D. Anderson - metastatic breast-231 (MDA-MB-231), probably through inactivation of NF-κB (Sarkar et al. 2006). These investigations illustrate that genistein exerts distinct activities at different concentrations in ER-positive cells (Table 28.1). This might explain some of the conflicting results obtained in ER-positive breast cancer cells or in animal experiments studying estrogen-sensitive tissues.

Several animal and clinical studies analyzed the effect of isoflavones, in particular, genistein, on endometrial and mammary tissue, with controversial outcomes (Beck et al. 2005; Adlercreutz 2002; Burdette et al. 2002; Diel et al. 2001, 2004; Garcia-Perez et al. 2006; Mehmood et al. 2000;

TABLE 28.1

Proposed Targets and Resulting Biological Activities of Genistein as a Function of Dose in Breast Cells

Biological Effect	Antiproliferative function in ERβ-positive breast cells (Koehler et al. 2005; Chang et al. 2008)	Proliferation of ERα positive breast cells (Chang et al. 2008)	Antiproliferative, cell death (Sakla et al. 2007; Sarkar et al. 2006)
Target	ERβ	ERα	Tyrosine kinase
[Genistein]	≈6 nM	≈300 nM	≈10–50 µM

Sources: Koehler, K. F. et al., *Endocr. Rev.*, 26, 465–478, 2005; Chang, E. C. et al., *Mol. Endocrinol.*, 22, 1032–1043, 2008; Sakla, M. S. et al., *Endocrine*, 32, 69–78, 2007; Sarkar, F. H. et al., *Mini Rev. Med. Chem.*, 6, 401–407, 2006.

Rachon et al. 2007; Unfer et al. 2004; Wuttke et al. 2007). Some studies suggest that genistein suppresses mammary carcinogenesis (Sahin et al. 2011; Constantinou et al. 2001); however, many recent in vivo investigations have found that it promotes carcinogenesis in breast tissue (Ju et al. 2006; Allred et al. 2004; Toxicology and Carcinogenesis Studies of Genistein (CAS No. 446-72-0) in Sprague-Dawley Rats (Feed Study) 2008). For example, one animal study demonstrated that genistein stimulates mammary gland growth and enhances the growth of breast cancer cells (MCF-7) in ovariectomized rats (Hsieh et al. 1998). In another study, genistein potentiated the growth of ER-positive xenografts in nude mice and stimulated the growth of estrogen-dependent tumors in Sprague-Dawley rats (Ju et al. 2006; Allred et al. 2004).

Recently, a 6-month intervention study using a preparation of mixed soy isoflavones containing 150 mg genistein, 74 mg daidzein, and 11 mg glycitein was performed in healthy, high-risk adult Western women to examine the effect of these isoflavones on breast epithelial proliferation and other biomarkers in the healthy high-risk breast (Khan et al. 2012). The results revealed that the isoflavones did not reduce breast epithelial proliferation as measured by Ki-67 labeling, suggesting a lack of efficacy for breast cancer prevention. However, among treated premenopausal women, there was a statistically significant increase in the postintervention Ki-67 labeling index following soy supplementation. Gene expression studies demonstrated a mixed pattern, with more genes increasing, that suggests estrogenic activity rather than antiestrogenic activity in the isoflavone supplementation group.

These reports show that isoflavones of red clover have the potential to reduce and/or enhance the hormonal-related carcinogenic effects of endogenous estrogens. The activity of the whole complex red clover extract might be distinct from that of the isolated isoflavones. For example, uterotrophic activities have been described for genistein (Diel et al. 2004) but not for the red clover extract (Overk et al. 2008a). Indeed, a placebo-controlled clinical trial using a red clover extract in postmenopausal women revealed that it reduced bone loss but did not increase breast density (Powles 2004). Similarly, a standardized red clover extract did not influence breast density and endometrial thickness in healthy women with a family history of breast cancer (Powles et al. 2007).

Overall, whether isoflavones in red clover extracts show estrogenic and proliferative activities or apoptotic activities may be highly concentration dependent (Table 28.1). Further in vivo studies with different concentrations are warranted to obtain a better picture of the chemopreventive potential of isoflavones and the whole red clover extract.

28.3.2.2 Chemical Pathway

Genistein might modulate estrogen metabolism, which would enhance estrogen carcinogenesis (Mense et al. 2008). For example, genistein inhibited the expression of the detoxification enzyme NQO1, which might lead to an increase in estrogen-induced DNA damage (Wagner et al. 2008). In contrast, Bianco et al. (2005) report that biochanin A and genistein upregulate NQO1 in ER-negative MDA-MB-231 cells transfected with ERβ. Their investigations show that biochanin A, but not genistein, could significantly protect against estrogen-induced oxidative DNA damage in breast cancer cells. Red clover has also been demonstrated to induce UDP-glucuronosyltransferase (Pfeiffer et al. 2005), an enzyme that is directly involved in the detoxification of genotoxic compounds and of estradiol. In addition, radical scavenging effects have been described for red clover (Booth et al. 2006).

28.3.2.3 Anti-Inflammatory Pathway

Anti-inflammatory activities have been described for red clover extracts and for the isolated isoflavones, in particular, for genistein (Seibel et al. 2009; Banerjee et al. 2008; Kim et al. 2007). Many studies evaluated the influence of red clover extract and its isoflavones on proinflammatory cytokines (Mueller et al. 2010; Kole et al. 2011). For example, the effect of red clover and its isolated isoflavones on the proinflammatory cytokines, IL-6 and TNFα, was analyzed in LPS-induced macrophages (Mueller et al. 2010). A standardized red clover extract (40% isoflavones) significantly reduced the secretion of IL-6 and TNFα, with IC_{50} values of 65 and 252 μg/mL, respectively. Biochanin A exhibited the strongest TNFα inhibition (IC_{50}, 6 nM), followed by genistein (IC_{50}, 40 nM). Genistein, daidzein, and biochanin A also inhibited IL-6 secretion at nanomolar concentrations. However, the red clover extract, genistein, and biochanin A significantly reduced the concentration of the anti-inflammatory cytokine IL-10 (Mueller et al. 2010). The red clover extract (0.5 μg/mL), biochanin A (100 nM), and genistein (100 nM) also significantly reduced the expression of iNOS and NF-κB; however, only the red clover extract and biochanin A downregulated COX2 at this concentration. Different research groups demonstrated the ability of genistein and biochanin A to reduce NF-κB reporter activity (Davis et al. 1999; Kole et al. 2011; Gong et al. 2003). Davis et al. (1999) demonstrated that genistein (50 μM) decreased NF-κB DNA binding and abrogated NF-κB activation in prostate cancer cells, which were induced by various stimuli. Mechanism-of-action studies revealed that genistein reduces phosphorylation of NF-κ-B inhibitor α (IκBα), likely through inhibition of the kinase activity of mitogen-activated protein kinase kinase kinase 1 (MEKK1), thus blocking the nuclear translocation of NF-κB and preventing NF-κB activation. Kole et al. (2011) demonstrated that biochanin A dose-dependently inhibited LPS-induced NO, IL-6, IL-1β, and TNFα production in macrophages. Mechanism-of-action studies revealed that biochanin A (25 μM) exerts its anti-inflammatory activities likely through prevention of phosphorylation and degradation of IκBα, thus preventing activation of NF-κB reporter activity (Kole et al. 2011). In another investigation, genistein (30–50 μM) exhibited antiapoptotic and NF-κB downregulating activities, in part mediated by inactivation of AKT signaling in ER-negative breast cancer cells (MDA-MB-231) (Gong et al. 2003).

Various in vitro and in vivo studies analyzed the ability of genistein and other isoflavones to repress or inhibit COX2 activity (Mueller et al. 2010; Mutoh et al. 2000; Lam et al. 2004; Horia and Watkins 2007). For example, genistein has been shown to significantly repress COX2 promoter activity in human colon adenocarcinoma cells (Mutoh et al. 2000). Genistein (40 μM) reduced TGFα-induced COX2 promoter activity by around 79% (Mutoh et al. 2000). The ability of the four isoflavones to inhibit COX2 activity was analyzed in murine macrophages and in human monocytes (Lam et al. 2004). Genistein showed the highest inhibitory potential and, at 1 μM, significantly inhibited LPS-induced PGE_2 synthesis in murine macrophages by 62%. Formononetin and biochanin A demonstrated significant inhibition at 10 μM and daidzein at 40 μM. In human monocytes, only genistein (100 μM) inhibited LPS-stimulated PGE_2 synthesis significantly. Interestingly, it has been shown that genistein (1 μM) significantly inhibited 12-O-tetradecanoylphorbol-13-acetate (TPA)–induced PGE_2 synthesis in ER-negative breast cancer cells (MDA-MB-231) (Horia and Watkins 2007). Also, at 10 μM, it significantly reduced the invasion capacity of this cell line by 40% compared to the vehicle control, suggesting a chemopreventive potential of genistein in ER-negative breast cancer cells. COX2 expression was not reduced by genistein at concentrations ranging from 0.1 to 2.5 μM. In vivo studies confirmed that genistein downregulates COX2. In a rat model of 2,4,6-trinitrobenzenesulfonic acid (TNBS)–induced colitis, a phytoestrogen-rich diet or genistein (100 mg/kg BW) reduced COX2 mRNA and protein levels in the colon (Seibel et al. 2008, 2009). Since COX2 is also reported to be upregulated in breast cancer and since epidemiologic analyses suggest a protective effect of COX-inhibitory drugs with respect to both colon and breast cancer (Howe 2007), red clover and its isoflavones are predicted to modulate COX2 in the breast tissue.

In conclusion, numerous studies have shown that red clover and its isoflavones might modulate estrogen carcinogenesis through the hormonal, chemical, as well as inflammatory pathways. The data analyzing the influence of red clover or isoflavones on cell proliferation (hormonal) and on estrogen metabolism enzymes (chemical) reveal conflicting results, suggesting that red clover might enhance or decrease estrogen carcinogenesis through the hormonal and chemical pathways. The concentrations and cell type may play an important role in terms of whether isoflavones reduce or increase estrogen carcinogenesis. There is clear evidence that red clover and the isoflavones, in particular, genistein, have anti-inflammatory properties in the micromolar range, which might decrease estrogen carcinogenesis in the breast. Future animal and clinical studies have to determine whether red clover extracts have the ability to elicit chemopreventive properties in breast tissue at clinically relevant concentrations.

28.3.3 Hops

The strobiles of hops (*Humulus lupulus* L.) have a long tradition as dietary supplements for mood and sleep disturbances (Zanoli and Zavatti 2008). Various studies have shown estrogenic properties in vitro and in vivo for the prenylated flavonoid, 8-prenylnaringenin (8-PN) (Figure 28.2). Therefore, hop extracts have gained interest as botanical alternatives to HRT for the relief of menopausal symptoms (Bolca et al. 2007; Erkkola et al. 2010; Heyerick et al. 2006). In addition, chemopreventive properties have been described for hop extracts and its major compound, the prenylated chalcone, xanthohumol (XH) (Figure 28.2) (Chadwick et al. 2004; Plazar et al. 2007, 2008; Lamy et al. 2007). XH exhibits multiple biological activities, such as detoxification of carcinogens through induction of NQO1 (Dietz et al. 2005), induction of apoptosis (Pan et al. 2005; Strathmann et al. 2010), and anti-inflammatory activities (Harikumar et al. 2009; Dorn et al. 2010a). In vitro and in vivo studies suggest that hop extracts might influence all three pathways of estrogen carcinogenesis.

28.3.3.1 Hormonal Pathway

Several bioassays have shown that 8-PN in nanomolar or low micromolar concentrations mimics the hormonal activity of estradiol (Rong et al. 2001; Overk et al. 2005, 2008a). On the other hand, higher concentrations of 8-PN and micromolar concentrations of XH exhibit antiproliferative properties (Monteiro et al. 2007; Brunelli et al. 2009). The hop extract did show estrogenic activities in vitro; however, in vivo studies did not reveal estrogenic activities for the whole extract, suggesting that it may contain various counteracting phytoconstituents such as natural progestins (Overk et al. 2008a). Also, aromatase inhibiting activities have been reported for 8-PN and XH. 8-PN inhibited aromatase activity in the nanomolar range (300 nM) in microsomes of human placental tissue or fibroblasts from healthy human mammary tissue (van Meeuwen et al. 2008). In breast cancer cells, 8-PN showed the highest aromatase inhibiting activity, with an IC_{50} of 0.08 µM (Monteiro et al. 2007). XH also inhibited aromatase, with an IC_{50} of 3.2 µM.

28.3.3.2 Chemical Pathway

Recently, it has been shown that a hop extract (5 µg/mL) and 8-PN (50 nM), but not XH, inhibit 4-hydroxylation of estradiol in an ERα-negative, nontumorigenic, immortalized human breast epithelial cell line (MCF-10A) (Hemachandra et al. 2012). Mechanism-of-action studies showed that the hop extract reduced estradiol-induced P4501B1 expression. Interestingly, the hop extract and 8-PN inhibited estrogen-induced malignant cell transformation of MCF-10A cells. These experiments suggest that hops possess cancer chemopreventive activity through attenuation of estrogen metabolism mediated by 8-PN. Also, hop extracts and XH (1.7 µM) have been demonstrated to induce NQO1 activity in murine hepatoma cells (Dietz et al. 2005). The experiments showed that XH-inhibited menadione induced DNA damage due to an increase in NQO1 activity. Since reactive estrogen quinones are detoxified by NQO1 (Figure 28.1), an increase in NQO1 by hop extracts might reduce estrogen carcinogenesis through detoxification of reactive estrogen intermediates.

28.3.3.3 Anti-Inflammatory Activity

Various in vitro and in vivo reports describe anti-inflammatory activities for hop extracts, XH, and hop bitter acids (Dorn et al. 2012; Hougee et al. 2006; Saugspier et al. 2011). For example, XH and hop bitter acids inhibited the activation of the transcription factor NF-κB and expression of NF-κB–dependent proinflammatory genes in hepatic stellate cells (Dorn et al. 2010a; Saugspier et al. 2011). Lupinacci et al. (2009) reported that a hop extract (0.1 µg/mL) significantly inhibited the production of monocyte chemoattractant protein-1 (MCP-1) in LPS-activated RAW 264.7 mouse macrophages. Bioassay-guided fractionation of the extract revealed XH (2.5 µg/mL) as the major anti-inflammatory compound in RAW 264.7 mouse macrophages and human monocytes, while the bitter acids showed moderate anti-inflammatory activity (Lupinacci et al. 2009). XH inhibited IL-12 production and inhibited NF-κB binding activity to the κB site in the nucleus in LPS-stimulated macrophages (Cho et al. 2010). Lee et al. (2011) demonstrated that XH inhibited LPS-stimulated inflammatory mediators NO, IL-1β, and TNFα as well as the activation of NF-κB signaling in the murine microglial cell line, BV-2. The anti-inflammatory response of XH was attenuated by transfection with nuclear factor (erythroid-derived 2)-like 2 (Nrf2) small interfering RNA (siRNA) and in the presence of the heme oxygenase 1 inhibitor, ZnPP, suggesting that XH exerts its anti-inflammatory activity, at least in part, by upregulation of Nrf2 and heme oxygenase 1 induction (Lee et al. 2011). Harikumar et al. (2009) showed downregulation of TNF-induced NF-κB activation by XH (50 μM) in various cell lines including breast cancer cells (MCF-7). Mechanism-of-action studies showed that XH inhibits TNF-induced IκBα phosphorylation and degradation, likely through interacting with cysteine residues of IκB kinase (IKK) and p65, thus leading to suppression of nuclear translocation of p65 and inhibition of NF-κB pathways. Anti-inflammatory activity has also been determined in in vivo studies. In an oxazolone-induced chronic dermatitis model in the mouse ear, topical XH treatment reduced the degree of ear thickening induced by oxazolone, suggesting that XH reduces skin inflammation (Cho et al. 2010). In a murine model of nonalcoholic steatohepatitis and in an animal model of acute carbon tetrachloride (CCl_4)-mediated liver injury, feeding with XH reduced mRNA levels of hepatic inflammatory markers (TNFα, IL-1α, MCP-1) and IL-1α (Dorn et al. 2010a, 2012). Since phospho-p65 of NF-κB was reduced in the XH group, the authors report that the mechanism is, at least in part, through a decrease in NF-κB activity (Dorn et al. 2012). Interestingly, oral administration of XH (100 μM) to nude mice inoculated with MCF-7 cells resulted in central necrosis within tumors, reduced inflammatory cell number, as well as a significant decrease in NF-κB activity, increased percentage of apoptotic cells, and decreased microvessel density (Monteiro et al. 2008).

COX2 inhibition has also been demonstrated for a hop extract, XH, as well as the bitter acid humulone (Lee et al. 2007; Hougee et al. 2006). A CO_2 extract of hops inhibited PGE_2 production in LPS-stimulated peripheryl blood monocytes, with an IC_{50} of 3.6 μg/mL (Hougee et al. 2006). Analysis of PGE_2 production revealed that the hop extract reduced PGE_2 production through inhibition of COX2, with an IC_{50} value of 20.4 μg/mL. Mice treated with hop extract showed 24% less production of PGE_2 in ex vivo LPS-stimulated blood cells of mice with zymosan-induced acute arthritis; however, the extract did not reduce joint swelling.

In general, these studies suggest that hop extracts might have promise as a chemopreventive agent for breast carcinogenesis. 8-PN elicits estrogenic and proliferative activities; however, other phytoconstituents in hops might counteract the proliferative activity. The data analyzing the chemical pathway indicate that hops attenuate estrogen metabolism, and recent reports reveal anti-inflammatory activities for hop extracts, in particular, for XH. Future studies have to evaluate whether clinical doses of XH, 8-PN, alpha acids, and other beneficial phytoconstituents in hop botanical dietary supplements are high enough to achieve a chemopreventive potential in vivo.

28.4 CONCLUSION AND PERSPECTIVES

Anti-inflammatory activities of red clover and hops could potentially play a role in modulation of estrogen carcinogenesis in the breast. In addition, there are several other botanicals used for post-menopausal women's health with reported anti-inflammatory activity, including licorice, dang gui, and *Vitex* (Chen et al. 2010; H. Wang et al. 2006; Ahmad et al. 2010; Pandey et al. 2012; C.Y. Wang et al. 2011; Chandrasekaran et al. 2011; Wu et al. 2011). Good evidence suggests that the three licorice species, *Glycyrrhiza uralensis*, *Glycyrrhiza glabra*, and *Glycyrrhiza inflata*, exhibit anti-inflammatory activity (C.Y. Wang et al. 2011; Chandrasekaran et al. 2011; Wu et al. 2011). For example, *G. glabra* inhibited LPS-induced PGE_2 production in murine macrophages (Chandrasekaran et al. 2011). The constituents, glabridin and isoliquiritigenin, were, at least in part, responsible for COX inhibition. Another investigation analyzed the anti-inflammatory activities of an ethanol extract from *G. inflata*. The extract suppressed LPS-induced inflammatory responses in murine macrophages (Kim et al. 2006). *G. uralensis* extracts inhibited NF-κB–mediated inflammatory responses as well as strong activation of the Nrf2–ARE (antioxidant response element) antioxidative stress signaling pathways (Wu et al. 2011). C.Y. Wang et al. (2011) reported that two constituents, glycyrrhizic acid and 18β-glycyrrhetinic acid, isolated from *G. uralensis* are, at least in part, responsible for this activity. Both compounds attenuated the generation of NO, PGE_2, and ROS by suppressing the expression of proinflammatory genes via inhibition of NF-κB and phosphoinositide 3-kinase (PI3K) activity (C.Y. Wang et al. 2011). There are a limited number of studies describing the anti-inflammatory activities of dang gui (*Angelica sinensis*) and its phytoconstituent, ferulic acid (Chen et al. 2010; H. Wang et al. 2006). An aqueous extract of dang gui suppressed LPS-induced release of TNFα and NO (H. Wang et al. 2006). Ferulic acid decreased hydrogen peroxide–induced IL-1β and TNFα mRNA in porcine chondrocytes (Chen et al. 2010). Moderate anti-inflammatory activities have been described for different compounds contained in chasteberry (*Vitex agnus-castus*), such as iridoide, agnuside, and pterocarpan (Ahmad et al. 2010; Pandey et al. 2012). Regardless of questionable efficacy for menopausal symptom relief, the literature supporting the anti-inflammatory properties of red clover, hops, and licorice is strong. Future in vivo and clinical studies are warranted to analyze the effect of these botanicals on estrogen carcinogenesis in more detail.

ACKNOWLEDGMENTS

Support for this work was provided by P50 AT00155, provided to the University of Illinois at Chicago/ National Institute of Health (UIC/NIH) Center for Botanical Dietary Supplements Research in Women's Health by the Office of Dietary Supplements and the National Center for Complementary and Alternative Medicine, and by CA135237, provided to Birgit Dietz from the National Cancer Institute.

REFERENCES

Adlercreutz, H. 2002. Phyto-Oestrogens and Cancer. *Lancet Oncol.* 3: 364–73.
Aggarwal, B. B. 2004. Nuclear Factor-Kappab: The Enemy Within. *Cancer Cell* 6: 203–8.
Aggarwal, B. B., S. Shishodia, S. K. Sandur, M. K. Pandey, and G. Sethi. 2006. Inflammation and Cancer: How Hot Is the Link? *Biochem. Pharmacol.* 72: 1605–21.
Aggarwal, B. B., and B. Sung. 2011. The Relationship between Inflammation and Cancer Is Analogous to That between Fuel and Fire. *Oncology* 25: 414–8.
Aggarwal, B. B., R. V. Vijayalekshmi, and B. Sung. 2009. Targeting Inflammatory Pathways for Prevention and Therapy of Cancer: Short-Term Friend, Long-Term Foe. *Clin. Cancer Res.* 15: 425–30.
Ahmad, B., S. Azam, S. Bashir, I. Khan, A. Adhikari, and M. I. Choudhary. 2010. Anti-Inflammatory and Enzyme Inhibitory Activities of a Crude Extract and a Pterocarpan Isolated from the Aerial Parts of Vitex Agnus-Castus. *Biotechnol J* 5: 1207–15.
Allred, C. D., K. F. Allred, Y. H. Ju, L. M. Clausen, D. R. Doerge, S. L. Schantz, D. L. Korol, M. A. Wallig, and W. G. Helferich. 2004. Dietary Genistein Results in Larger Mnu-Induced, Estrogen-Dependent Mammary Tumors Following Ovariectomy of Sprague-Dawley Rats. *Carcinogenesis* 25: 211–8.
An, J., C. Tzagarakis-Foster, T. C. Scharschmidt, N. Lomri, and D. C. Leitman. 2001. Estrogen Receptor Beta-Selective Transcriptional Activity and Recruitment of Coregulators by Phytoestrogens. *J. Biol. Chem.* 276: 17808–14.
Banerjee, S., Y. Li, Z. Wang, and F. H. Sarkar. 2008. Multi-Targeted Therapy of Cancer by Genistein. *Cancer Lett.* 269: 226–42.
Beck, V., U. Rohr, and A. Jungbauer. 2005. Phytoestrogens Derived from Red Clover: An Alternative to Estrogen Replacement Therapy? *J. Steroid Biochem. Mol. Biol.* 94: 499–518.
Bianco, N. R., L. J. Chaplin, and M. M. Montano. 2005. Differential Induction of Quinone Reductase by Phytoestrogens and Protection against Oestrogen-Induced DNA Damage. *Biochem. J.* 385: 279–87.
Bodinet, C., and J. Freudenstein. 2002. Influence of Cimicifuga Racemosa on the Proliferation of Estrogen Receptor-Positive Human Breast Cancer Cells. *Breast Cancer Res. Treat.* 76: 1–10.

Bolca, S., S. Possemiers, V. Maervoet, I. Huybrechts, A. Heyerick, S. Vervarcke, H. Depypere, D. De Keukeleire, M. Bracke, S. De Henauw, W. Verstraete, and T. Van de Wiele. 2007. Microbial and Dietary Factors Associated with the 8-Prenylnaringenin Producer Phenotype: A Dietary Intervention Trial with Fifty Healthy Post-Menopausal Caucasian Women. *Br. J. Nutr.* 98: 950–9.

Bolton, J. L. Mechanisms of Estrogen Carcinogenesis: Modulation by Botanical Natural Products. In *Chemical Carcinogenesis*, edited by Penning T.M., pp. 74–94. New York: Springer, 2011.

Bolton, J. L., and G. R. Thatcher. 2008. Potential Mechanisms of Estrogen Quinone Carcinogenesis. *Chem. Res. Toxicol.* 21: 93–101.

Booth, N. L., C. R. Overk, P. Yao, J. E. Burdette, D. Nikolic, S. N. Chen, J. L. Bolton, R. B. van Breemen, G. F. Pauli, and N. R. Farnsworth. 2006. The Chemical and Biologic Profile of a Red Clover (Trifolium Pratense L.) Phase II Clinical Extract. *J. Altern. Complement. Med.* 12: 133–9.

Booth, N. L., and C. E. Piersen. "Red Clover (Trifolium Pratense)." In *Encyclopedia of Dietary Supplements*, edited by P.M. Coates, pp. 587–602. New York: Marcel Dekker, 2005.

Booth, N. L., C. E. Piersen, S. Banuvar, S. E. Geller, L. P. Shulman, and N. R. Farnsworth. 2006. Clinical Studies of Red Clover (Trifolium Pratense) Dietary Supplements in Menopause: A Literature Review. *Menopause* 13: 251–64.

Bradlow, H. L., and D. W. Sepkovic. 2002. Diet and Breast Cancer. *Ann. N. Y. Acad. Sci.* 963: 247–67.

Brueggemeier, R. W., J. A. Richards, and T. A. Petrel. 2003. Aromatase and Cyclooxygenases: Enzymes in Breast Cancer. *J. Steroid Biochem. Mol. Biol.* 86: 501–7.

Brunelli, E., G. Pinton, F. Chianale, A. Graziani, G. Appendino, and L. Moro. 2009. 8-Prenylnaringenin Inhibits Epidermal Growth Factor-Induced Mcf-7 Breast Cancer Cell Proliferation by Targeting Phosphatidylinositol-3-Oh Kinase Activity. *J. Steroid Biochem. Mol. Biol.* 113: 163–70.

Burdette, J. E., S. N. Chen, Z. Z. Lu, H. Xu, B. E. White, D. S. Fabricant, J. Liu, H. H. Fong, N. R. Farnsworth, A. I. Constantinou, R. B. Van Breemen, J. M. Pezzuto, and J. L. Bolton. 2002. Black Cohosh (Cimicifuga Racemosa L.) Protects against Menadione-Induced DNA Damage through Scavenging of Reactive Oxygen Species: Bioassay-Directed Isolation and Characterization of Active Principles. *J. Agric. Food Chem.* 50: 7022–8.

Burdette, J. E., J. Liu, S. N. Chen, D. S. Fabricant, C. E. Piersen, E. L. Barker, J. M. Pezzuto, A. Mesecar, R. B. Van Breemen, N. R. Farnsworth, and J. L. Bolton. 2003. Black Cohosh Acts as a Mixed Competitive Ligand and Partial Agonist of the Serotonin Receptor. *J. Agric. Food Chem.* 51: 5661–70.

Burdette, J. E., J. Liu, D. Lantvit, E. Lim, N. Booth, K. P. Bhat, S. Hedayat, R. B. Van Breemen, A. I. Constantinou, J. M. Pezzuto, N. R. Farnsworth, and J. L. Bolton. 2002. Trifolium Pratense (Red Clover) Exhibits Estrogenic Effects *in vivo* in Ovariectomized Sprague-Dawley Rats. *J. Nutr.* 132: 27–30.

Calogero, R. A., F. Cordero, G. Forni, and F. Cavallo. 2007. Inflammation and Breast Cancer. Inflammatory Component of Mammary Carcinogenesis in Erbb2 Transgenic Mice. *Breast Cancer Res.* 9: 211.

Cavalieri, E., D. Chakravarti, J. B. Guttenplan, E. Hart, J. Ingle, R. Jankowiak, P. Muti, E. Rogan, J. Russo, R. Santen, and T. Sutter. 2006. Catechol Estrogen Quinones as Initiators of Breast and Other Human Cancers: Implications for Biomarkers of Susceptibility and Cancer Prevention. *Biochim. Biophys. Acta* 1766: 63–78.

Cavalieri, E. L., and E. G. Rogan. 2011. Unbalanced Metabolism of Endogenous Estrogens in the Etiology and Prevention of Human Cancer. *J. Steroid Biochem. Mol. Biol.* 125: 169–80.

Chadwick, L. R., D. Nikolic, J. E. Burdette, C. R. Overk, J. L. Bolton, R. B. van Breemen, R. Froehlich, H. H. Fong, N. R. Farnsworth, and G. F. Pauli. 2004. Estrogens and Congeners from Spent Hops (*Humulus lupulus* L.). *J. Nat. Prod.* 67: 2024–32.

Chandrasekaran, C. V., H. B. Deepak, P. Thiyagarajan, S. Kathiresan, G. K. Sangli, M. Deepak, and A. Agarwal. 2011. Dual Inhibitory Effect of Glycyrrhiza Glabra (Gutgard) on Cox and Lox Products. *Phytomedicine: Int. J. Phytother. Phytopharmacol.* 18: 278–84.

Chang, E. C., T. H. Charn, S. H. Park, W. G. Helferich, B. Komm, J. A. Katzenellenbogen, and B. S. Katzenellenbogen. 2008. Estrogen Receptors Alpha and Beta as Determinants of Gene Expression: Influence of Ligand, Dose, and Chromatin Binding. *Mol. Endocrinol.* 22: 1032–43.

Cheema, D., A. Coomarasamy, and T. El-Toukhy. 2007. Non-Hormonal Therapy of Post-Menopausal Vasomotor Symptoms: A Structured Evidence-Based Review. *Arch. Gynecol. Obstet.* 276: 463–9.

Chen, C., and A. N. Tony Kong. 2004. Dietary Chemopreventive Compounds and Are/Epre Signaling. *Free Radic. Biol. Med.* 36: 1505–16.

Chen, J. Q., T. R. Brown, and J. D. Yager. 2008. Mechanisms of Hormone Carcinogenesis: Evolution of Views, Role of Mitochondria. *Adv. Exp. Med. Biol.* 630: 1–18.

Chen, M. P., S. H. Yang, C. H. Chou, K. C. Yang, C. C. Wu, Y. H. Cheng, and F. H. Lin. 2010. The Chondroprotective Effects of Ferulic Acid on Hydrogen Peroxide-Stimulated Chondrocytes: Inhibition of Hydrogen Peroxide-Induced Pro-Inflammatory Cytokines and Metalloproteinase Gene Expression at the Mrna Level. *Inflammation Res.* 59: 587–95.

Chlebowski, R. T., L. H. Kuller, R. L. Prentice, M. L. Stefanick, J. E. Manson, M. Gass, A. K. Aragaki, J. K. Ockene, D. S. Lane, G. E. Sarto, A. Rajkovic, R. Schenken, S. L. Hendrix, P. M. Ravdin, T. E. Rohan, S. Yasmeen, and G. Anderson. 2009. Breast Cancer after Use of Estrogen Plus Progestin in Postmenopausal Women. *N. Engl. J. Med.* 360: 573–87.

Cho, Y. C., S. K. You, H. J. Kim, C. W. Cho, I. S. Lee, and B. Y. Kang. 2010. Xanthohumol Inhibits Il-12 Production and Reduces Chronic Allergic Contact Dermatitis. *Int. Immunopharmacol.* 10: 556–61.

Constantinou, A. I., D. Lantvit, M. Hawthorne, X. Xu, R. B. van Breemen, and J. M. Pezzuto. 2001. Chemopreventive Effects of Soy Protein and Purified Soy Isoflavones on Dmba-Induced Mammary Tumors in Female Sprague-Dawley Rats. *Nutr. Cancer* 41: 75–81.

Davis, J. N., O. Kucuk, and F. H. Sarkar. 1999. Genistein Inhibits Nf-Kappa B Activation in Prostate Cancer Cells. *Nutr. Cancer* 35: 167–74.

DeNardo, D. G., and L. M. Coussens. 2007. Inflammation and Breast Cancer. Balancing Immune Response: Crosstalk between Adaptive and Innate Immune Cells During Breast Cancer Progression. *Breast Cancer Res.* 9: 212.

DeSantis, C., R. Siegel, P. Bandi, and A. Jemal. 2011. Breast Cancer Statistics, 2011. *CA. Cancer J. Clin.* 61: 409–18.

Diel, P., R. B. Geis, A. Caldarelli, S. Schmidt, U. L. Leschowsky, A. Voss, and G. Vollmer. 2004. The Differential Ability of the Phytoestrogen Genistein and of Estradiol to Induce Uterine Weight and Proliferation in the Rat Is Associated with a Substance Specific Modulation of Uterine Gene Expression. *Mol. Cell. Endocrinol.* 221: 21–32.

Diel, P., K. Smolnikar, T. Schulz, U. Laudenbach-Leschowski, H. Michna, and G. Vollmer. 2001. Phytoestrogens and Carcinogenesis-Differential Effects of Genistein in Experimental Models of Normal and Malignant Rat Endometrium. *Hum. Reprod.* 16: 997–1006.

Dietz, B. M., Y. H. Kang, G. Liu, A. L. Eggler, P. Yao, L. R. Chadwick, G. F. Pauli, N. R. Farnsworth, A. D. Mesecar, R. B. van Breemen, and J. L. Bolton. 2005. Xanthohumol Isolated from Humulus Lupulus Inhibits Menadione-Induced DNA Damage through Induction of Quinone Reductase. *Chem. Res. Toxicol.* 18: 1296–305.

Dietz, B. M., D. Liu, G. K. Hagos, P. Yao, A. Schinkovitz, S. M. Pro, S. Deng, N. R. Farnsworth, G. F. Pauli, R. B. van Breemen, and J. L. Bolton. 2008. Angelica Sinensis and Its Alkylphthalides Induce the Detoxification Enzyme Nad(P)H: Quinone Oxidoreductase 1 by Alkylating Keap1. *Chem. Res. Toxicol.* 21: 1939–48.

Dijsselbloem, N., W. Vanden Berghe, A. De Naeyer, and G. Haegeman. 2004. Soy Isoflavone Phyto-Pharmaceuticals in Interleukin-6 Affections. Multi-Purpose Nutraceuticals at the Crossroad of Hormone Replacement, Anti-Cancer and Anti-Inflammatory Therapy. *Biochem. Pharmacol.* 68: 1171–85.

Dorn, C., J. Heilmann, and C. Hellerbrand. 2012. Protective Effect of Xanthohumol on Toxin-Induced Liver Inflammation and Fibrosis. *International journal of clinical and experimental pathology* 5: 29–36.

Dorn, C., B. Kraus, M. Motyl, T. S. Weiss, M. Gehrig, J. Scholmerich, J. Heilmann, and C. Hellerbrand. 2010a. Xanthohumol, a Chalcon Derived from Hops, Inhibits Hepatic Inflammation and Fibrosis. *Mol. Nutr. Food Res.* 54 (Suppl 2): S205–13.

Dorn, C., T. S. Weiss, J. Heilmann, and C. Hellerbrand. 2010b. Xanthohumol, a Prenylated Chalcone Derived from Hops, Inhibits Proliferation, Migration and Interleukin-8 Expression of Hepatocellular Carcinoma Cells. *Int. J. Oncol.* 36: 435–41.

Einbond, L. S., M. Shimizu, D. Xiao, P. Nuntanakorn, J. T. Lim, M. Suzui, C. Seter, T. Pertel, E. J. Kennelly, F. Kronenberg, and I. B. Weinstein. 2004. Growth Inhibitory Activity of Extracts and Purified Components of Black Cohosh on Human Breast Cancer Cells. *Breast Cancer Res. Treat.* 83: 221–31.

Einbond, L. S., M. Soffritti, D. D. Esposti, H. A. Wu, E. Tibaldi, M. Lauriola, K. He, T. Park, T. Su, L. Huggins, X. Wang, M. Roller, and R. Brennan. 2012. Pharmacological Mechanisms of Black Cohosh in Sprague-Dawley Rats. *Fitoterapia* 83: 461–8.

Einbond, L. S., T. Su, H. A. Wu, R. Friedman, X. Wang, B. Jiang, T. Hagan, E. J. Kennelly, F. Kronenberg, and I. B. Weinstein. 2007. Gene Expression Analysis of the Mechanisms Whereby Black Cohosh Inhibits Human Breast Cancer Cell Growth. *Anticancer Res.* 27: 697–712.

Erkkola, R., S. Vervarcke, S. Vansteelandt, P. Rompotti, D. De Keukeleire, and A. Heyerick. 2010. A Randomized, Double-Blind, Placebo-Controlled, Cross-over Pilot Study on the Use of a Standardized Hop Extract to Alleviate Menopausal Discomforts. *Phytomedicine* 17: 389–96.

Fabricant, D. S. "Pharmacognostic Investigation of Black Cohosh (*Cimicifuga racemosa* (L.) Nutt.)." University of Illinois at Chicago, 2005.

Fabricant, D. S., and N. R. Farnsworth. "Black Cohosh (Cimicifuga Racemosa)." In *Encyclopedia of Dietary Supplements*, edited by P. M. Coates, pp. 41–54. New York: Marcel Dekker, 2005.

Frasor, J., J. M. Danes, B. Komm, K. C. Chang, C. R. Lyttle, and B. S. Katzenellenbogen. 2003. Profiling of Estrogen Up- and Down-Regulated Gene Expression in Human Breast Cancer Cells: Insights into Gene Networks and Pathways Underlying Estrogenic Control of Proliferation and Cell Phenotype. *Endocrinology* 144: 4562–74.

Frasor, J., A. E. Weaver, M. Pradhan, and K. Mehta. 2008. Synergistic up-Regulation of Prostaglandin E Synthase Expression in Breast Cancer Cells by 17beta-Estradiol and Proinflammatory Cytokines. *Endocrinology* 149: 6272–9.

Frasor, J., A. Weaver, M. Pradhan, Y. Dai, L. D. Miller, C. Y. Lin, and A. Stanculescu. 2009. Positive Cross-Talk between Estrogen Receptor and Nf-Kappab in Breast Cancer. *Cancer Res.* 69: 8918–25.

Freudenstein, J., C. Dasenbrock, and T. Nisslein. 2002. Lack of Promotion of Estrogen-Dependent Mammary Gland Tumors *in vivo* by an Isopropanolic Cimicifuga Racemosa Extract. *Cancer Res.* 62: 3448–52.

Garcia-Perez, M. A., R. Noguera, R. del Val, I. Noguera, C. Hermenegildo, and A. Cano. 2006. Comparative Effects of Estradiol, Raloxifene, and Genistein on the Uterus of Ovariectomized Mice. *Fertil Steril* 86: 1003–5.

Geller, S. E., L. P. Shulman, R. B. van Breemen, S. Banuvar, Y. Zhou, G. Epstein, S. Hedayat, D. Nikolic, E. C. Krause, C. E. Piersen, J. L. Bolton, G. F. Pauli, and N. R. Farnsworth. 2009. Safety and Efficacy of Black Cohosh and Red Clover for the Management of Vasomotor Symptoms: A Randomized Controlled Trial. *Menopause* 16: 1156–66.

Gong, L., Y. Li, A. Nedeljkovic-Kurepa, and F. H. Sarkar. 2003. Inactivation of Nf-Kappab by Genistein Is Mediated Via Akt Signaling Pathway in Breast Cancer Cells. *Oncogene* 22: 4702–9.

Han, E. H., H. G. Kim, Y. P. Hwang, G. Y. Song, and H. G. Jeong. 2010. Prostaglandin E2 Induces Cyp1b1 Expression Via Ligand-Independent Activation of the Eralpha Pathway in Human Breast Cancer Cells. *Toxicol. Sci.* 114: 204–16.

Harikumar, K. B., A. B. Kunnumakkara, K. S. Ahn, P. Anand, S. Krishnan, S. Guha, and B. B. Aggarwal. 2009. Modification of the Cysteine Residues in Ikappabalpha Kinase and Nf-Kappab (P65) by Xanthohumol Leads to Suppression of Nf-Kappab-Regulated Gene Products and Potentiation of Apoptosis in Leukemia Cells. *Blood* 113: 2003–13.

Harris, D. M., E. Besselink, S. M. Henning, V. L. Go, and D. Heber. 2005. Phytoestrogens Induce Differential Estrogen Receptor Alpha- or Beta-Mediated Responses in Transfected Breast Cancer Cells. *Exp. Biol. Med.* 230: 558–68.

Hemachandra, L. P., P. Madhubhani, R. Chandrasena, P. Esala, S. N. Chen, M. Main, D. C. Lankin, R. A. Scism, B. M. Dietz, G. F. Pauli, G. R. Thatcher, and J. L. Bolton. 2012. Hops (Humulus Lupulus) Inhibits Oxidative Estrogen Metabolism and Estrogen-Induced Malignant Transformation in Human Mammary Epithelial Cells (Mcf-10a). *Cancer Prev. Res. (Phila.)* 5: 73–81.

Henderson, B. E., and H. S. Feigelson. 2000. Hormonal Carcinogenesis. *Carcinogenesis* 21: 427–33.

Heyerick, A., S. Vervarcke, H. Depypere, M. Bracke, and D. De Keukeleire. 2006. A First Prospective, Randomized, Double-Blind, Placebo-Controlled Study on the Use of a Standardized Hop Extract to Alleviate Menopausal Discomforts. *Maturitas* 54: 164–75.

Hong, W. K., and M. B. Sporn. 1997. Recent Advances in Chemoprevention of Cancer. *Science* 278: 1073–77.

Horia, E., and B. A. Watkins. 2007. Complementary Actions of Docosahexaenoic Acid and Genistein on Cox-2, Pge2 and Invasiveness in Mda-Mb-231 Breast Cancer Cells. *Carcinogenesis* 28: 809–15.

Hostanska, K., T. Nisslein, J. Freudenstein, J. Reichling, and R. Saller. 2004a. Cimicifuga Racemosa Extract Inhibits Proliferation of Estrogen Receptor-Positive and Negative Human Breast Carcinoma Cell Lines by Induction of Apoptosis. *Breast Cancer Res. Treat.* 84: 151–60.

Hostanska, K., T. Nisslein, J. Freudenstein, J. Reichling, and R. Saller. 2004b. Evaluation of Cell Death Caused by Triterpene Glycosides and Phenolic Substances from Cimicifuga Racemosa Extract in Human Mcf-7 Breast Cancer Cells. *Biol. Pharm. Bull.* 27: 1970–5.

Hougee, S., J. Faber, A. Sanders, W. B. Berg, J. Garssen, H. F. Smit, and M. A. Hoijer. 2006. Selective Inhibition of Cox-2 by a Standardized Co2 Extract of Humulus Lupulus *in vitro* and Its Activity in a Mouse Model of Zymosan-Induced Arthritis. *Planta Med.* 72: 228–33.

Howe, L. R. 2007. Inflammation and Breast Cancer. Cyclooxygenase/Prostaglandin Signaling and Breast Cancer. *Breast Cancer Res.* 9: 210.

Hsieh, C. Y., R. C. Santell, S. Z. Haslam, and W. G. Helferich. 1998. Estrogenic Effects of Genistein on the Growth of Estrogen Receptor-Positive Human Breast Cancer (Mcf-7) Cells in vitro and in Vivo. *Cancer Res.* 58: 3833–8.

Jarry, H., M. Metten, B. Spengler, V. Christoffel, and W. Wuttke. 2003. In vitro Effects of the Cimicifuga Racemosa Extract Bno 1055. *Maturitas* 44 Suppl 1: S31–8.

Ju, Y. H., K. F. Allred, C. D. Allred, and W. G. Helferich. 2006. Genistein Stimulates Growth of Human Breast Cancer Cells in a Novel, Postmenopausal Animal Model, with Low Plasma Estradiol Concentrations. *Carcinogenesis* 27: 1292–9.

Kensler, T. W. 1997. Chemoprevention by Inducers of Carcinogen Detoxication Enzymes. *Environ. Health Perspect.* 105 Suppl 4: 965–70.

Khan, S. A., R. T. Chatterton, N. Michel, M. Bryk, O. Lee, D. Ivancic, R. Heinz, C. M. Zalles, I. B. Helenowski, B. D. Jovanovic, A. A. Franke, M. C. Bosland, J. Wang, N. M. Hansen, K. P. Bethke, A. Dew, M. Coomes, and R. C. Bergan. 2012. Soy Isoflavone Supplementation for Breast Cancer Risk Reduction: A Randomized Phase Ii Trial. *Cancer Prev. Res. (Phila.)* 5: 309–19.

Kim, E. K., K. B. Kwon, M. Y. Song, S. W. Seo, S. J. Park, S. O. Ka, L. Na, K. A. Kim, D. G. Ryu, H. S. So, R. Park, J. W. Park, and B. H. Park. 2007. Genistein Protects Pancreatic Beta Cells against Cytokine-Mediated Toxicity. *Mol. Cell. Endocrinol.* 278: 18–28.

Kim, J. K., S. M. Oh, H. S. Kwon, Y. S. Oh, S. S. Lim, and H. K. Shin. 2006. Anti-Inflammatory Effect of Roasted Licorice Extracts on Lipopolysaccharide-Induced Inflammatory Responses in Murine Macrophages. *Biochem. Biophys. Res. Commun.* 345: 1215–23.

Kisselev, P., W. H. Schunck, I. Roots, and D. Schwarz. 2005. Association of Cyp1a1 Polymorphisms with Differential Metabolic Activation of 17beta-Estradiol and Estrone. *Cancer Res.* 65: 2972–8.

Koehler, K. F., L. A. Helguero, L. A. Haldosen, M. Warner, and J. A. Gustafsson. 2005. Reflections on the Discovery and Significance of Estrogen Receptor Beta. *Endocr. Rev.* 26: 465–78.

Kole, L., B. Giri, S. K. Manna, B. Pal, and S. Ghosh. 2011. Biochanin-a, an Isoflavon, Showed Anti-Proliferative and Anti-Inflammatory Activities through the Inhibition of Inos Expression, P38-Mapk and Atf-2 Phosphorylation and Blocking Nfkappab Nuclear Translocation. *Eur. J. Pharmacol.* 653: 8–15.

Kretzschmar, G., T. Nisslein, O. Zierau, and G. Vollmer. 2005. No Estrogen-Like Effects of an Isopropanolic Extract of Rhizoma Cimicifugae Racemosae on Uterus and Vena Cava of Rats after 17 Day Treatment. *J. Steroid Biochem. Mol. Biol.* 97: 271–7.

Kuiper, G. G., J. G. Lemmen, B. Carlsson, J. C. Corton, S. H. Safe, P. T. van der Saag, B. van der Burg, and J. A. Gustafsson. 1998. Interaction of Estrogenic Chemicals and Phytoestrogens with Estrogen Receptor Beta. *Endocrinology* 139: 4252–63.

Kupferer, E. M., S. L. Dormire, and H. Becker. 2009. Complementary and Alternative Medicine Use for Vasomotor Symptoms among Women Who Have Discontinued Hormone Therapy. *J. Obstet. Gynecol. Neonatal Nurs.* 38: 50–9.

Lam, A. N., M. Demasi, M. J. James, A. J. Husband, and C. Walker. 2004. Effect of Red Clover Isoflavones on Cox-2 Activity in Murine and Human Monocyte/Macrophage Cells. *Nutr. Cancer* 49: 89–93.

Lamy, V., S. Roussi, M. Chaabi, F. Gosse, N. Schall, A. Lobstein, and F. Raul. 2007. Chemopreventive Effects of Lupulone, a Hop {Beta}-Acid, on Human Colon Cancer-Derived Metastatic Sw620 Cells and in a Rat Model of Colon Carcinogenesis. *Carcinogenesis* 28: 1575–81.

Lee, I. S., J. Lim, J. Gal, J. C. Kang, H. J. Kim, B. Y. Kang, and H. J. Choi. 2011. Anti-Inflammatory Activity of Xanthohumol Involves Heme Oxygenase-1 Induction Via Nrf2-Are Signaling in Microglial Bv2 Cells. *Neurochem. Int.* 58: 153–60.

Lee, J. C., J. K. Kundu, D. M. Hwang, H. K. Na, and Y. J. Surh. 2007. Humulone Inhibits Phorbol Ester-Induced Cox-2 Expression in Mouse Skin by Blocking Activation of Nf-Kappab and Ap-1: Ikappab Kinase and C-Jun-N-Terminal Kinase as Respective Potential Upstream Targets. *Carcinogenesis* 28: 1491–8.

Liebermann, S. 1998. A Review of the Effectiveness of Cimicifuga Racemosa (Black Cohosh) for the Symptoms of Menopause. *J. Women's Health* 7: 525–9.

Liehr, J. G., W. F. Fang, D. A. Sirbasku, and A. Ari-Ulubelen. 1986. Carcinogenicity of Catechol Estrogens in Syrian Hamsters. *J. Steroid Biochem.* 24: 353–6.

Liske, E., W. Hanggi, H. H. Henneicke-von Zepelin, N. Boblitz, P. Wustenberg, and V. W. Rahlfs. 2002. Physiological Investigation of a Unique Extract of Black Cohosh (Cimicifugae Racemosae Rhizoma): A 6-Month Clinical Study Demonstrates No Systemic Estrogenic Effect. *J. Womens Health Gend. Based Med.* 11: 163–74.

Liu, J., J. E. Burdette, H. Xu, C. Gu, R. B. van Breemen, K. P. Bhat, N. Booth, A. I. Constantinou, J. M. Pezzuto, H. H. Fong, N. R. Farnsworth, and J. L. Bolton. 2001. Evaluation of Estrogenic Activity of Plant Extracts for the Potential Treatment of Menopausal Symptoms. *J. Agric. Food Chem.* 49: 2472–79.

Lupinacci, E., J. Meijerink, J. P. Vincken, B. Gabriele, H. Gruppen, and R. F. Witkamp. 2009. Xanthohumol from Hop (Humulus Lupulus L.) Is an Efficient Inhibitor of Monocyte Chemoattractant Protein-1 and

Tumor Necrosis Factor-Alpha Release in Lps-Stimulated Raw 264.7 Mouse Macrophages and U937 Human Monocytes. *J. Agric. Food Chem.* 57: 7274–81.

Luqman, S., and J. M. Pezzuto. 2010. Nfkappab: A Promising Target for Natural Products in Cancer Chemoprevention. *Phytother. Res.* 24: 949–63.

Ma, X., N. Kundu, S. Rifat, T. Walser, and A. M. Fulton. 2006. Prostaglandin E Receptor Ep4 Antagonism Inhibits Breast Cancer Metastasis. *Cancer Res.* 66: 2923–7.

Mahady, G. B., J. Parrot, C. Lee, G. S. Yun, and A. Dan. 2003. Botanical Dietary Supplement Use in Peri- and Postmenopausal Women. *Menopause* 10: 65–72.

Mandlekar, S., J. L. Hong, and A. N. Kong. 2006. Modulation of Metabolic Enzymes by Dietary Phytochemicals: A Review of Mechanisms Underlying Beneficial Versus Unfavorable Effects. *Current Drug Metabolism* 7: 661–75.

Mehmood, Z., A. G. Smith, M. J. Tucker, F. Chuzel, and N. G. Carmichael. 2000. The Development of Methods for Assessing the *in vivo* Oestrogen-Like Effects of Xenobiotics in Cd-1 Mice. *Food Chem. Toxicol.* 38: 493–501.

Mense, S. M., T. K. Hei, R. K. Ganju, and H. K. Bhat. 2008. Phytoestrogens and Breast Cancer Prevention: Possible Mechanisms of Action. *Environ. Health Perspect.* 116: 426–33.

Monteiro, R., C. Calhau, A. O. Silva, S. Pinheiro-Silva, S. Guerreiro, F. Gartner, I. Azevedo, and R. Soares. 2008. Xanthohumol Inhibits Inflammatory Factor Production and Angiogenesis in Breast Cancer Xenografts. *J. Cell Biochem.* 104: 1699–707.

Monteiro, R., A. Faria, I. Azevedo, and C. Calhau. 2007. Modulation of Breast Cancer Cell Survival by Aromatase Inhibiting Hop (Humulus Lupulus L.) Flavonoids. *J. Steroid Biochem. Mol. Biol.* 105: 124–30.

Mueller, M., S. Hobiger, and A. Jungbauer. 2010. Red Clover Extract: A Source for Substances That Activate Peroxisome Proliferator-Activated Receptor Alpha and Ameliorate the Cytokine Secretion Profile of Lipopolysaccharide-Stimulated Macrophages. *Menopause* 17: 379–87.

Mutoh, M., M. Takahashi, K. Fukuda, Y. Matsushima-Hibiya, H. Mutoh, T. Sugimura, and K. Wakabayashi. 2000. Suppression of Cyclooxygenase-2 Promoter-Dependent Transcriptional Activity in Colon Cancer Cells by Chemopreventive Agents with a Resorcin-Type Structure. *Carcinogenesis* 21: 959–63.

Nelson, H. D., K. K. Vesco, E. Haney, R. Fu, A. Nedrow, J. Miller, C. Nicolaidis, M. Walker, and L. Humphrey. 2006. Nonhormonal Therapies for Menopausal Hot Flashes: Systematic Review and Meta-Analysis. *JAMA* 295: 2057–71.

Newbold, R. R., and J. G. Liehr. 2000. Induction of Uterine Adenocarcinoma in Cd-1 Mice by Catechol Estrogens. *Cancer Res.* 60: 235–7.

North American Menopause Society. 2011. The Role of Soy Isoflavones in Menopausal Health: Report of the North American Menopause Society/Wulf H. Utian Translational Science Symposium in Chicago, Il (October 2010). *Menopause* 18: 732–53.

North American Menopause Society. 2004. Treatment of Menopause-Associated Vasomotor Symptoms: Position Statement of the North American Menopause Society. *Menopause* 11: 11–33.

Osmers, R., M. Friede, E. Liske, J. Schnitker, J. Freudenstein, and H. H. Henneicke-von Zepelin. 2005. Efficacy and Safety of Isopropanolic Black Cohosh Extract for Climacteric Symptoms. *Obstet. Gynecol.* 105: 1074–83.

Overk, C. R., J. Guo, L. R. Chadwick, D. D. Lantvit, A. Minassi, G. Appendino, S. N. Chen, D. C. Lankin, N. R. Farnsworth, G. F. Pauli, R. B. van Breemen, and J. L. Bolton. 2008a. *In vivo* Estrogenic Comparisons of Trifolium Pratense (Red Clover) Humulus Lupulus (Hops), and the Pure Compounds Isoxanthohumol and 8-Prenylnaringenin. *Chem. Biol. Interact.* 176 (1): 30–9.

Overk, C. R., P. Yao, L. R. Chadwick, D. Nikolic, Y. Sun, M. A. Cuendet, Y. Deng, A. S. Hedayat, G. F. Pauli, N. R. Farnsworth, R. B. van Breemen, and J. L. Bolton. 2005. Comparison of the *in vitro* Estrogenic Activities of Compounds from Hops (Humulus Lupulus) and Red Clover (Trifolium Pratense). *J. Agric. Food Chem.* 53: 6246–53.

Overk, C. R., P. Yao, S. Chen, S. Deng, A. Imai, M. Main, A. Schinkovitz, N. R. Farnsworth, G. F. Pauli, and J. L. Bolton. 2008b. High-Content Screening and Mechanism-Based Evaluation of Estrogenic Botanical Extracts. *Comb. Chem. High Throughput Screen.* 11: 283–93.

Palacio, C., G. Masri, and A. D. Mooradian. 2009. Black Cohosh for the Management of Menopausal Symptoms: A Systematic Review of Clinical Trials. *Drugs Aging* 26: 23–36.

Pan, L., H. Becker, and C. Gerhauser. 2005. Xanthohumol Induces Apoptosis in Cultured 40-16 Human Colon Cancer Cells by Activation of the Death Receptor- and Mitochondrial Pathway. *Mol. Nutr. Food Res.* 49: 837–43.

Pandey, A., S. Bani, N. K. Satti, B. D. Gupta, and K. A. Suri. 2012. Anti-Arthritic Activity of Agnuside Mediated through the Down-Regulation of Inflammatory Mediators and Cytokines. *Inflam. Re.* 61 (4): 293–304.

Park, J. Y., M. H. Pillinger, and S. B. Abramson. 2006. Prostaglandin E2 Synthesis and Secretion: The Role of Pge2 Synthases. *Clin. Immunol.* 119: 229–40.

Park, S. A., H. K. Na, E. H. Kim, Y. N. Cha, and Y. J. Surh. 2009. 4-Hydroxyestradiol Induces Anchorage-Independent Growth of Human Mammary Epithelial Cells Via Activation of Ikappab Kinase: Potential Role of Reactive Oxygen Species. *Cancer Res.* 69: 2416–24.

Pfeiffer, E., C. R. Treiling, S. I. Hoehle, and M. Metzler. 2005. Isoflavones Modulate the Glucuronidation of Estradiol in Human Liver Microsomes. *Carcinogenesis* 26: 2172–8.

Pierce, B. L., R. Ballard-Barbash, L. Bernstein, R. N. Baumgartner, M. L. Neuhouser, M. H. Wener, K. B. Baumgartner, F. D. Gilliland, B. E. Sorensen, A. McTiernan, and C. M. Ulrich. 2009. Elevated Biomarkers of Inflammation Are Associated with Reduced Survival among Breast Cancer Patients. *J Clin Oncol* 27: 3437–44.

Piersen, C. E. 2003. Phytoestrogens in Botanical Dietary Supplements: Implications for Cancer. *Integr. Cancer Ther.* 2: 120–38.

Piersen, C. E., N. L. Booth, Y. Sun, W. Liang, J. E. Burdette, R. B. van Breemen, S. E. Geller, C. Gu, S. Banuvar, L. P. Shulman, J. L. Bolton, and N. R. Farnsworth. 2004. Chemical and Biological Characterization and Clinical Evaluation of Botanical Dietary Supplements: A Phase I Red Clover Extract as a Model. *Curr. Med. Chem.* 11: 1361–74.

Plazar, J., M. Filipic, and G. M. Groothuis. 2008. Antigenotoxic Effect of Xanthohumol in Rat Liver Slices. *Toxicol. In Vitro* 22: 318–27.

Plazar, J., B. Zegura, T. T. Lah, and M. Filipic. 2007. Protective Effects of Xanthohumol against the Genotoxicity of Benzo(a)Pyrene (Bap), 2-Amino-3-Methylimidazo[4,5-F]Quinoline (Iq) and Tert-Butyl Hydroperoxide (T-Booh) in Hepg2 Human Hepatoma Cells. *Mutat. Res.* 632: 1–8.

Powles, T. 2004. Isoflavones and Women's Health. *Breast Cancer Res.* 6: 140–2.

Powles, T. J., S. Ashley, A. Tidy, I. E. Smith, and M. Dowsett. 2007. Twenty-Year Follow-up of the Royal Marsden Randomized, Double-Blinded Tamoxifen Breast Cancer Prevention Trial. *J. Natl. Cancer Inst.* 99: 283–90.

Rachon, D., T. Vortherms, D. Seidlova-Wuttke, and W. Wuttke. 2007. Dietary Daidzein and Puerarin Do Not Affect Pituitary Lh Expression but Exert Uterotropic Effects in Ovariectomized Rats. *Maturitas* 57: 161–70.

Ravdin, P. M., K. A. Cronin, N. Howlader, C. D. Berg, R. T. Chlebowski, E. J. Feuer, B. K. Edwards, and D. A. Berry. 2007. The Decrease in Breast-Cancer Incidence in 2003 in the United States. *N. Engl. J. Med.* 356: 1670–4.

Rebbeck, T. R., A. B. Troxel, S. Norman, G. R. Bunin, A. DeMichele, M. Baumgarten, M. Berlin, R. Schinnar, and B. L. Strom. 2007. A Retrospective Case-Control Study of the Use of Hormone-Related Supplements and Association with Breast Cancer. *Int. J. Cancer* 120: 1523–8.

Rees, M. 2009. Alternative Treatments for the Menopause. *Best Pract. Res. Clin. Obstet. Gynaecol.* 23: 151–61.

Revankar, C. M., D. F. Cimino, L. A. Sklar, J. B. Arterburn, and E. R. Prossnitz. 2005. A Transmembrane Intracellular Estrogen Receptor Mediates Rapid Cell Signaling. *Science* 307: 1625–30.

Rhyu, M. R., J. Lu, D. E. Webster, D. S. Fabricant, N. R. Farnsworth, and Z. J. Wang. 2006. Black Cohosh (Actaea Racemosa, Cimicifuga Racemosa) Behaves as a Mixed Competitive Ligand and Partial Agonist at the Human Mu Opiate Receptor. *J. Agric. Food Chem.* 54: 9852–7.

Richards, J. A., and R. W. Brueggemeier. 2003. Prostaglandin E2 Regulates Aromatase Activity and Expression in Human Adipose Stromal Cells Via Two Distinct Receptor Subtypes. *J. Clin. Endocrinol. Metab.* 88: 2810–6.

Rong, H., T. Boterberg, J. Maubach, C. Stove, H. Depypere, S. Van Slambrouck, R. Serreyn, D. De Keukeleire, M. Mareel, and M. Bracke. 2001. 8-Prenylnaringenin, the Phytoestrogen in Hops and Beer, Upregulates the Function of the E-Cadherin/Catenin Complex in Human Mammary Carcinoma Cells. *Eur. J. Cell Biol.* 80: 580–5.

Rossouw, J. E., G. L. Anderson, R. L. Prentice, A. Z. LaCroix, C. Kooperberg, M. L. Stefanick, R. D. Jackson, S. A. Beresford, B. V. Howard, K. C. Johnson, J. M. Kotchen, and J. Ockene. 2002. Risks and Benefits of Estrogen Plus Progestin in Healthy Postmenopausal Women: Principal Results from the Women's Health Initiative Randomized Controlled Trial. *JAMA* 288: 321–33.

Russo, J., Y. F. Hu, X. Yang, and I. H. Russo. 2000. Developmental, Cellular, and Molecular Basis of Human Breast Cancer. *J. Natl. Cancer Inst. Monogr.* 17–37.

Russo, J., and I. H. Russo. 2006. The Role of Estrogen in the Initiation of Breast Cancer. *J. Steroid Biochem. Mol. Biol.* 102: 89–96.

Sahin, K., M. Tuzcu, N. Sahin, F. Akdemir, I. Ozercan, S. Bayraktar, and O. Kucuk. 2011. Inhibitory Effects of Combination of Lycopene and Genistein on 7,12- Dimethyl Benz(a)Anthracene-Induced Breast Cancer in Rats. *Nutr. Cancer* 63: 1279–86.

Sakla, M. S., N. S. Shenouda, P. J. Ansell, R. S. Macdonald, and D. B. Lubahn. 2007. Genistein Affects Her2 Protein Concentration, Activation, and Promoter Regulation in Bt-474 Human Breast Cancer Cells. *Endocrine* 32: 69–78.

Sarkar, F. H., S. Adsule, S. Padhye, S. Kulkarni, and Y. Li. 2006. The Role of Genistein and Synthetic Derivatives of Isoflavone in Cancer Prevention and Therapy. *Mini Rev Med Chem* 6: 401–7.

Saugspier, M., C. Dorn, W. E. Thasler, M. Gehrig, J. Heilmann, and C. Hellerbrand. 2011. Hop Bitter Acids Exhibit Anti-Fibrogenic Effects on Hepatic Stellate Cells in Vitro. *Exp. Mol. Pathol.* 92 (2): 222–8.

Schmid, D., M. Gruber, F. Woehs, S. Prinz, B. Etzlstorfer, C. Prucker, N. Fuzzati, B. Kopp, and T. Moeslinger. 2009. Inhibition of Inducible Nitric Oxide Synthesis by Cimicifuga Racemosa (Actaea Racemosa, Black Cohosh) Extracts in Lps-Stimulated Raw 264.7 Macrophages. *J. Pharm. Pharmacol.* 61: 1089–96.

Seibel, J., A. F. Molzberger, T. Hertrampf, U. Laudenbach-Leschowski, G. H. Degen, and P. Diel. 2008. In Utero and Postnatal Exposure to a Phytoestrogen-Enriched Diet Increases Parameters of Acute Inflammation in a Rat Model of Tnbs-Induced Colitis. *Arch. Toxicol.* 82: 941–50.

Seibel, J., A. F. Molzberger, T. Hertrampf, U. Laudenbach-Leschowski, and P. Diel. 2009. Oral Treatment with Genistein Reduces the Expression of Molecular and Biochemical Markers of Inflammation in a Rat Model of Chronic Tnbs-Induced Colitis. *Eur. J. Nutr.* 48: 213–20.

Seidlova-Wuttke, D., O. Hesse, H. Jarry, V. Christoffel, B. Spengler, T. Becker, and W. Wuttke. 2003. Evidence for Selective Estrogen Receptor Modulator Activity in a Black Cohosh (Cimicifuga Racemosa) Extract: Comparison with Estradiol-17beta. *Eur. J. Endocrinol.* 149: 351–62.

Simpson, E., G. Rubin, C. Clyne, K. Robertson, L. O'Donnell, S. Davis, and M. Jones. 1999. Local Estrogen Biosynthesis in Males and Females. *Endocr.-Relat. Cancer* 6: 131–7.

Singh, S., D. Chakravarti, J. A. Edney, R. R. Hollins, P. J. Johnson, W. W. West, S. M. Higginbotham, E. L. Cavalieri, and E. G. Rogan. 2005. Relative Imbalances in the Expression of Estrogen-Metabolizing Enzymes in the Breast Tissue of Women with Breast Carcinoma. *Oncol. Rep.* 14: 1091–6.

Song, R. X., P. Fan, W. Yue, Y. Chen, and R. J. Santen. 2006. Role of Receptor Complexes in the Extranuclear Actions of Estrogen Receptor Alpha in Breast Cancer. *Endocr.-Relat. Cancer* 13 Suppl 1: S3–13.

Strathmann, J., K. Klimo, S. W. Sauer, J. G. Okun, J. H. Prehn, and C. Gerhauser. 2010. Xanthohumol-Induced Transient Superoxide Anion Radical Formation Triggers Cancer Cells into Apoptosis Via a Mitochondria-Mediated Mechanism. *FASEB J.* 24 (8): 2938–50.

Surh, Y. J. 2003. Cancer Chemoprevention with Dietary Phytochemicals. *Nat. Rev. Cancer* 3: 768–80.

Tice, J. A., B. Ettinger, K. Ensrud, R. Wallace, T. Blackwell, and S. R. Cummings. 2003. Phytoestrogen Supplements for the Treatment of Hot Flashes: The Isoflavone Clover Extract (Ice) Study: A Randomized Controlled Trial. *JAMA* 290: 207–14.

Timoshenko, A. V., G. Xu, S. Chakrabarti, P. K. Lala, and C. Chakraborty. 2003. Role of Prostaglandin E2 Receptors in Migration of Murine and Human Breast Cancer Cells. *Exp. Cell Res.* 289: 265–74.

Toxicology and Carcinogenesis Studies of Genistein (Case No. 446-72-0) in Sprague-Dawley Rats (Feed Study). 2008. *Natl. Toxicol. Prog. Tech. Rep. Ser.* 1–240.

Unfer, V., M. L. Casini, L. Costabile, M. Mignosa, S. Gerli, and G. C. Di Renzo. 2004. Endometrial Effects of Long-Term Treatment with Phytoestrogens: A Randomized, Double-Blind, Placebo-Controlled Study. *Fertil. Steril.* 82: 145–8, quiz 265.

van Meeuwen, J. A., N. Korthagen, P. C. de Jong, A. H. Piersma, and M. van den Berg. 2007. (Anti)Estrogenic Effects of Phytochemicals on Human Primary Mammary Fibroblasts, Mcf-7 Cells and Their Co-Culture. *Toxicol. Appl. Pharmacol.* 221: 372–83.

van Meeuwen, J. A., S. Nijmeijer, T. Mutarapat, S. Ruchirawat, P. C. de Jong, A. H. Piersma, and M. van den Berg. 2008. Aromatase Inhibition by Synthetic Lactones and Flavonoids in Human Placental Microsomes and Breast Fibroblasts—a Comparative Study. *Toxicol. Appl. Pharmacol.* 228: 269–76.

Wagner, J., L. Jiang, and L. Lehmann. 2008. Phytoestrogens Modulate the Expression of 17alpha-Estradiol Metabolizing Enzymes in Cultured Mcf-7 Cells. *Adv. Exp. Med. Biol.* 617: 625–32.

Walji, R., H. Boon, E. Guns, D. Oneschuk, and J. Younus. 2007. Black Cohosh (Cimicifuga Racemosa [L.] Nutt.): Safety and Efficacy for Cancer Patients. *Support. Care Cancer* 15: 913–21.

Wang, C. Y., T. C. Kao, W. H. Lo, and G. C. Yen. 2011. Glycyrrhizic Acid and 18beta-Glycyrrhetinic Acid Modulate Lipopolysaccharide-Induced Inflammatory Response by Suppression of Nf-Kappab through Pi3k P110delta and P110gamma Inhibitions. *J. Agric. Food Chem.* 59: 7726–33.

Wang, H., W. Li, J. Li, B. Rendon-Mitchell, M. Ochani, M. Ashok, L. Yang, H. Yang, K. J. Tracey, P. Wang, and A. E. Sama. 2006. The Aqueous Extract of a Popular Herbal Nutrient Supplement, Angelica Sinensis, Protects Mice against Lethal Endotoxemia and Sepsis. *J. Nutr.* 136: 360–5.

Wu, T. Y., T. O. Khor, C. L. Saw, S. C. Loh, A. I. Chen, S. S. Lim, J. H. Park, L. Cai, and A. N. Kong. 2011. Anti-Inflammatory/Anti-Oxidative Stress Activities and Differential Regulation of Nrf2-Mediated Genes by Non-Polar Fractions of Tea Chrysanthemum Zawadskii and Licorice Glycyrrhiza Uralensis. *AAPS J.* 13: 1–13.

Wuttke, W., H. Jarry, and D. Seidlova-Wuttke. 2007. Isoflavones-Safe Food Additives or Dangerous Drugs? *Ageing Res. Rev.* 6: 150–88.

Yager, J. D., and N. E. Davidson. 2006. Estrogen Carcinogenesis in Breast Cancer. *N. Engl. J. Med.* 354: 270–82.

Yamamoto, S., T. Sobue, M. Kobayashi, S. Sasaki, and S. Tsugane. 2003. Soy, Isoflavones, and Breast Cancer Risk in Japan. *J. Natl. Cancer Inst.* 95: 906–13.

Yang, C. L., S. C. Chik, J. C. Li, B. K. Cheung, and A. S. Lau. 2009. Identification of the Bioactive Constituent and Its Mechanisms of Action in Mediating the Anti-Inflammatory Effects of Black Cohosh and Related Cimicifuga Species on Human Primary Blood Macrophages. *J. Med. Chem.* 52: 6707–15.

Zanoli, P., and M. Zavatti. 2008. Pharmacognostic and Pharmacological Profile of Humulus Lupulus L. *J. Ethnopharmacol.* 116: 383–96.

Zheng, W., D. W. Xie, F. Jin, J. R. Cheng, Q. Dai, W. Q. Wen, X. O. Shu, and Y. T. Gao. 2000. Genetic Polymorphism of Cytochrome P450-1b1 and Risk of Breast Cancer. *Cancer Epidemiol. Biomarkers Prev.* 9: 147–50.

Zierau, O., C. Bodinet, S. Kolba, M. Wulf, and G. Vollmer. 2002. Antiestrogenic Activities of Cimicifuga Racemosa Extracts. *J. Steroid Biochem. Mol. Biol.* 80: 125–30.

29 PHY906, a Cancer Adjuvant Therapy, Differentially Affects Inflammation of Different Tissues

Wing Lam, Scott Bussom, Zaoli Jiang, Wei Zhang, Fulan Guan, Shwu-Huey Liu, and Yung-Chi Cheng

CONTENTS

29.1   INTRODUCTION

Cancer is the second-largest killer in the United States, killing around 571,950 Americans annually or more than 1500 people a day in 2011. It means almost one of every four deaths is due to cancer (American Cancer Society 2011). At the same time, there are over 1.5 million new diagnoses of cancer annually (American Cancer Society 2011). Despite billions of dollars being spent annually to develop new cancer therapies to treat cancer, the overall 5-year relative survival rate for all diagnosed cancers has only increased by 18% from the 1970s to the 2000s (American Cancer Society 2011). Some types of cancer, such as those of the pancreas or liver, have only 6% and 14% 5-year survival rates, respectively (American Cancer Society 2011).

Early cancer drug discovery was based on a reductionist single-target approach where an "active" compound is usually purified from an herbal mixture or synthetic chemical library and tested against a single biological target. However, the effects of single target–oriented drugs are usually crippled by tumor phenotypic heterogeneity as the result of tumor microenvironment. Moreover, genetic and epigenetic heterogeneity of tumor cells, due to tumor evolution or drug treatment, can also reduce the action of a single drug. Furthermore, the long-term use of highly potent target-oriented drugs will result in drug-induced toxicities that can reduce the quality of life of a patient. Single-agent approaches to eliminate the toxicity of chemotherapy have largely been unsatisfactory, especially for nonhematological toxicities, which include gastrointestinal ailments such as diarrhea, nausea, and vomiting, as well as hand–foot syndrome. Because of this, we searched for drugs that could reduce these multiple adverse effects without compromising the antitumor efficacy of a standard chemotherapy, and this drug should also improve the quality of life for patients and enhance the therapeutic indices of chemotherapy.

Herbal medicines have been used for several millennia, are widely claimed to help with a variety of diseases or symptoms, and are believed by the general public to cause fewer side effects or dependency. Despite the assumption of safety by consumers, there were 21 case reports in cancer patients where an herbal drug was identified as the cause of toxicity (Olaku and White 2011). In Asia, herbal medicines are most commonly used by cancer patients for relieving various symptoms and diseases. In the United States, herbal medicine use also becomes more prevalent after a diagnosis of cancer, escalating in use from 5.3% before the diagnosis of cancer to 13.9% after the diagnosis of cancer (Molassiotis et al. 2005). Many individuals try certain complementary and alternative medicine (CAM) approaches to improve therapeutic effects on the tumor in the hopes of increasing survival or improving their quality of life. While there were many case reports indicating apparent antitumor effects after taking an herbal therapy (Olaku and White 2011), there is currently no herbal medicine (oral administration) approved by the Food and Drug Administration (FDA) as a drug.

Chinese herbal medicine, among all the herbal medicine traditions, is relatively well- documented and has its own theories, which essentially use a holistic/multitarget system biology approach evolved from human experience. Little scientific evidence, however, has been accumulated in the past, and most of the concepts of Chinese medicine have not been scientifically validated. Using modern scientific and technological approaches to reinvestigate the claims of Chinese medicine could help in the discovery of new drug(s) as polychemical mixtures that target different tissues. This may offer a complementary approach to the current single-compound–single-target approach. In order to examine whether herbal medicine is useful in chemotherapy, we need to solve several important issues: quality control of herbal products, the completion of adequately designed clinical trials, understanding of the mechanisms of action of herbal products, and the interactions with commonly used conventional drugs.

29.2   FDA REGULATORY REQUIREMENTS FOR HERBAL MEDICINE

A botanical product can be sold as food, a dietary supplement, and/or a drug. The FDA issued the "Guidance for Industry: Botanical Drug Products" to explain the requirements for each category. All botanicals sold in the United States as dietary supplements are regulated under the Dietary Supplement Health and Education Act of 1994 (DSHEA). Statements that "claim to diagnose, mitigate, treat, cure, or prevent a specific disease or class of diseases" are not allowed to be shown on herbal products by the DSHEA regulations. Strict quality-control information, in addition to contamination with heavy metals, pesticides, or others, is required. For such uses, botanical products must be marketed under an approved new drug application (NDA) or via the FDA's over-the-counter (OTC) drug monograph system. Safety in human use, claimed efficacy in a disease, and consistency in batch-to-batch drug qualities are the three key criteria raised in the FDA's 2004 Guidance for botanical medicine. More details on herbal medicine regulations have been recently reviewed by Liu and Cheng (2012). Currently, there is no orally administered herbal mixtures approved in the United States.

29.3 APPROACH TO SELECTING THE RIGHT HERBAL FORMULATION TO STUDY

This laboratory has a long-term research focus on cancer and viral chemotherapy. One approach in cancer chemotherapy is to relieve side effects associated with treatment with hope for improving the quality of patients' life and allowing dosage increases in patients. We initiated our traditional Chinese medicine (TCM) study after doing a literature review on TCM since it has a relatively large amount of documentation over a long history. We decided on a few criteria for the selection of TCM to study. First, we searched the literature for simple herbal formulations that had been used for a long time and were currently being used to relieve symptoms associated with cancer chemotherapy, such as diarrhea, abdominal cramps, fever, vomiting, and nausea. Our approach was based on the assumption that a "true" therapeutic effect would survive and be passed down through a long history and that "fake" or "unreliable" therapeutic effects would not be passed down over time. Those formulations that survived may have some flexibility in the quality of the herbal materials, allowing them to show consistent efficacy. Second, to help lessen the complexity of quality control, we looked for simple herbal formulations that included, at most, six herbs. Third, to help ensure that future production could be achieved, we chose a formula that contained common and easily cultivated plants.

Based on these principles, we selected a few herbal formulations and tested whether they could reduce the toxicity and antitumor effect of irinotecan (CPT-11) using a mouse model. CPT-11 in combination with 5-fluorouracil (5-FU) and leucovorin was approved by the FDA as a first-line therapy for the treatment of metastatic colon or rectal carcinoma in 1996. In 1998, CPT-11 was approved as a second-line therapy for recurrent metastatic colon or rectum carcinoma after 5-FU–based therapy. The use of CPT-11 can be limited by serous diarrhea due to its gastrointestinal toxicity (Abigerges et al. 1994; Cunningham et al. 1998). Our herbal preparation was made following a traditional method. The herbal powder mixture was boiled in water for 30 min to prepare the decoction. This decoction was then orally administered to the tumor-bearing mice by gavage together with intraperitoneal treatment with CPT-11. Of those herbal formulations tested, "Huang Qin Tang" showed promise in decreasing toxicity caused by CPT-11. Furthermore, it increased the antitumor activity of CPT-11.

Huang Qin Tang was first described in a part of *Shang Han Lun*, a key text in the Chinese herbal medicine canon, about 1800 years ago (Hsu and Hsu 1980). Huang Qin Tang is a four-herb formula composed of *Glycyrrhiza uralensis* Fisch (G), *Paeonia lactiflora* Pall (P), *Scutelleria baicalensis* Georgi (S), and *Ziziphus jujuba* Mill (Z) (Hsu and Hsu 1980). Its main use was for the treatment of different gastrointestinal symptoms, including diarrhea, nausea, and vomiting, which are also common side effects of chemotherapy (Hsu and Hsu 1980). Since Huang Qin Tang satisfied our three criteria, we chose this for further development.

29.4 CONSISTENCY OF THE PREPARATIONS OF HUANG QIN TANG

According to rigid specifications for the raw ingredients set by PhytoCeutica Inc in the United States and Sun Ten Pharmaceuticals in Taiwan, a powder mixture comprised of spray-drying starch powder of a traditional hot-water extract of *Scutelleria baicalensis* Georgi (S), *Paeonia lactiflora* Pall (P), *Glycyrrhiza uralensis* Fisch (G), and *Ziziphus jujuba* Mill (Z) was manufactured at a ratio of 3:2:2:2, respectively, following current good manufacturing practice (cGMP) standards. We termed this powder mixture PHY906.

The first challenge in the development of PHY906 as a drug was ensuring that different batches of the herbal product could be produced with consistent quality since environmental factors and manufacturing procedures can easily affect the consistency of the final herbal product. Together with PhytoCeutica Inc, we developed a comprehensive platform for integration of the chemical and biological response fingerprints of herbal products and analysis by a novel statistical methodology. This platform is termed "Phytomics QC" (Tilton et al. 2010). Different methods can be used to obtain chemical fingerprints. The methodology of choice should give (1) information-intensive fingerprints; (2) chemical resolution at the molecular level; (3) quantitative analysis; (4) robust and integrated technology; and (5) a centralized platform with standard operating procedures (SOPs). We chose liquid chromatography–mass spectrometry (LC–MS) to determine the chemical fingerprint of PHY906 because liquid chromatography-tandem mass spectrometry (LC-MS/MS) is relatively quantitative and sensitive, and it can detect a broad spectrum of chemicals, giving details of the chemical structures in the mixture. For the biological fingerprint, we chose to study the effects of PHY906 on standard enzyme/receptor assays and also on a gene expression platform using RNA oligo-array and quantitative-reverese transcriptase-PCR (qRT-PCR) in genetically stable cell lines. We also carried out in vivo experiments in mice to access the activity of PHY906 if necessary.

Chemical and biological information was then analyzed by the phytomics similarity index (PSI) software, a bioinformatics tool developed by Professor H. Zhao at Yale and PhytoCeutica, to generate, with high sensitivity, a quantitative batch-to-batch similarity index (PSI), where a score of 0 indicates no similarity and 1.0 indicates that the batches are exactly the same (Tilton et al. 2010). With this technology we demonstrated a batch-to-batch consistency (PSI) >0.9 among different batches of PHY906, even in batches manufactured 5 to 10 years apart. Although PHY906 and Huang Qin Tang share the same herbal formulation, the consistency of PHY906 is guaranteed to reproduce the results of studies, including clinical studies, and to meet clinical standards for a clinically used drug. In contrast, commercial preparations of Huang Qin Tang have a much wider range of PSIs (from 0.6 to 0.9) as compared to PHY906, and they could have a different biological activity from PHY906.

29.5 PHY906 (ALL FOUR HERBS OF PHY906 ARE REQUIRED) ENHANCES THE THERAPEUTIC INDEX OF CPT-11 IN COLON TUMOR–BEARING MICE

Once we confirmed that PHY906 could be manufactured with consistent quality using Phytomics QC, we examined whether the use of PHY906 in reducing toxicity triggered by CPT-11 would compromise the antitumor activity of CPT-11 in colon 38–bearing mice. We found that PHY906 did not compromise, but actually enhanced the antitumor activity of CPT-11 and reduced animal body weight loss caused by CPT-11. In the TCM theory of making a formula, the four herbs of PHY906 are thought to have separate functions: imperial herb, ministerial herb, assistant herb, and servant herb. The combination of all four herbs is assumed essential to achieve the best therapeutic effect (Hsu and Hsu 1980). In order to test this assumption, we compared the effect of the full herb formulation versus one-herb-deleted formulations or single-herb preparations on antitumor activity and body weight protection activity in combination therapy with CPT-11 (Liu and Cheng 2012). Herb S was determined to play a very important role in both the enhancement of antitumor activity and in protecting against body weight loss since deletion of herb S resulted in loss of both activities. Deletion of herb P decreased the antitumor activity but not the body weight loss protection. Both herb G and herb Z were required to protect against body weight loss. Individual use of any one of the four herbs displayed minimal activities for antitumor and body weight protection. These results demonstrated that all four herbs of PHY906 are required to achieve the best therapeutic effect in combination therapy with CPT-11 (Liu and Cheng 2012). This deductive approach could also be used to test the rationales behind other herb mixture formulations since many Chinese medicine formulations were invented by Chinese physicians and are based on their personal experiences or empirical understanding of herbal properties. Many of those formulations consist of more than 10 different herbs, with little scientific-based evidence to support that all herbs are required. Reducing the number of herbs in formulations, while maintaining their therapeutic effect, could reduce the difficulty of quality control and the cost of formula and is likely to increase the consistency of the herbal products. This approach would also be useful to find new indications for herbs used in TCM.

29.6 MECHANISTIC STUDIES OF THE ACTIONS OF PHY906 ON THE INTESTINE OF CPT-11–TREATED MICE

29.6.1 PHY906 DOES NOT REDUCE THE INITIAL DAMAGE, BUT IT PROMOTES INTESTINAL RECOVERY FROM DAMAGE CAUSED BY CPT-11

As mentioned above, PHY906 protected against body weight loss of animals induced by CPT-11, which could be caused by serious intestinal damage and diarrhea. Therefore, we studied whether PHY906 can reduce the intestinal damage caused by CPT-11. We compared the effects of PHY906 (oral, twice per day [b.i.d.], 500 mg/kg, day 0–3) and loperamide (oral, b.i.d., 2 mg/kg, day 0–9) treatment on tumor growth and body weight loss after a single CPT-11 treatment (360 mg/kg, day 0, i.p.) using BDF mice bearing colon 38 allografts as an animal model (Lam et al. 2010). PHY906 alone showed no animal toxicity and no significant antitumor activity. PHY906 promoted much faster body weight rebound at day 4, while loperamide, an opioid receptor agonist employed as an adjuvant drug for relieving CPT-11–induced diarrhea (Abigerges et al. 1994; Cunningham et al. 1998), required 6 days to start body weight recovery after CPT-11 treatment. Increasing PHY906 to 1 g/kg, or lengthening the treatment duration to 8 days did not improve outcomes. Traditionally, Huang Qin Tang, the PHY906 equivalent, is suggested to be taken for no more than 4 days. We focused on PHY906 500 mg/kg [b.i.d] day 0–3, and the results from day 2 and day 4 for further detailed analysis.

Since the major toxicity of CPT-11 affects the gastrointestinal tract, we examined whether the intestine was protected by PHY906. As expected, CPT-11 alone caused destruction of the mucosal architecture of several sections of intestine: proximal jejunum, middle jejunum, distal ileum, and proximal colon (Lam et al. 2010). Intestines of the CPT-11–treated group showed enlarged cell size with less condensed nuclei, inflammatory cellular infiltration, and increased number of lysozyme vesicles in the paneth cells on day 2, and the whole intestine had progressive damage through day 4 (Lam et al. 2010). PHY906 did not reduce the damage caused by CPT-11 on day 2. However, by day 4, PHY906 helped to restore normal structure, with a composition of paneth, endocrine, and goblet cells throughout the small and large intestines in the CPT-11/PHY906 group. PHY906 clearly facilitated the regrowth of intestinal cells after the CPT-11-induced damage (Lam et al. 2010). Treatment with PHY906 alone did not affect intestinal histology within 4 days (Lam et al. 2010).

29.6.2 PHY906 DECREASES APOPTOTIC CELLS AND INCREASES PROLIFERATIVE CELLS IN THE INTESTINE AFTER CPT-11 TREATMENT

Terminal deoxynucleotidyl transferase dUTP nick end labeling (TUNEL) and cleaved caspase-3 staining confirmed that PHY906 did not prevent the initial DNA damage or apoptosis caused by CPT-11 on day 2. By day 4, however, PHY906 reduced TUNEL-positive cells and cleaved caspase-3 in the PHY906/CPT-11 group across all intestinal segments. PHY906 also increased proliferative, mitotic, and transcriptional activity, as detected by immunohistochemistry staining of proliferating cell nuclear antigen (PCNA), bromodeoxyuridine (BrdU), histone 3 (H3) Ser10 phosphorylation, H3 Lysine9 acetylation, and H3 Lys4 trimethylation, in the intestinal crypt cells on day 4 (Lam et al. 2010). BrdU pulse-chase experiments demonstrated that PHY906 promotion of intestinal epithelial cell recovery was not simply due to on-site repair of the damaged cells after CPT-11 treatment but through the replacement of new crypt-generated enterocytes from day 2 to day 4 (Lam et al. 2010).

Once CPT-11 is administered, it is converted into the active metabolite SN38 (7-ethyl-10-hydroxy-camptothecin) by hepatic and intestinal carboxyesterases. SN38 can induce severe acute diarrhea in patients. The metabolism of SN38 by hepatic UDP–glucuronyltransferase forms an inactive SN38G that is excreted into intestine via the bile (Rivory et al. 1996; Humerickhouse et al. 2000). Inside the intestine, β-glucuronidases from bacteria can remove glucuronoside from SN38G to form SN38, which can further prolong and increase the intestinal damage and result in intestinal inflammation. Because PHY906 did not reduce the initial intestinal damage caused by CPT-11, it is unlikely that the glucuronides from PHY906 competed effectively with SN38G for glucuronidases in the intestine. Our previous pharmacokinetic studies also indicated that PHY906 did not affect the pharmacokinetics of CPT-11, SN38, or SN38G in the plasma of animals (Ye et al. 2008).

29.6.3 PHY906 Promoted Repopulation of Progenitor/ Stem Cell in Crypts after CPT-11 Treatment

To examine whether the repopulated crypt cells in the CPT-11/PHY906 group were intestinal progenitor cells, we examined the protein expression or messenger RNA (mRNA) expression for several intestinal stem cell markers, CD44, Lgr5, Ascl2, Olfm4. We found that PHY906 increased CD44 staining in crypts and increased Lgr5, Olfm4, and Ascl2 mRNA after CPT-11 treatment by day 4. Since CD44, Lgr5, and Ascl2 (Van der Flier et al. 2007) are Wnt-dependent genes, and the Wnt signaling pathway is important for stem cell self-renewal and for the proliferation of progenitor cells (Fevr et al. 2007), the effect of PHY906 on mRNA expression of other components of the Wnt signaling pathway was further examined. PHY906 increased several of these, including Wnt3, Fzd5, Lrp5, Pygo2, and Axin2, after CPT-11 treatment by day 4 (Lam et al. 2010). Therefore, PHY906 may promote progenitor cell regeneration through stimulation of Wnt signaling after CPT-11 treatment.

29.6.4 β-Glucuronidase-Treated PHY906 Potentiates Wnt3a Activity in the Wnt/β-Catenin Signaling Pathway

When we tested if PHY906 could directly stimulate the Wnt/β-catenin signaling pathway, we found that PHY906 alone had no appreciable activity in potentiating Wnt3a action in HEK-293 LEF/TCF luciferase reporter cells (Lam et al. 2010). We suspected that the digestive system activates PHY906 in the intestine, so we created a method called "YungChi Cheng (YCC) treatment," which includes HCl treatment at a pH of 2 to mimic the acidic conditions of the stomach and β-glucuronidase treatment (a major enzyme produced by the bacteria in the intestinal tract) to mimic what happens to PHY906 following oral administration. After YCC treatment, we found that PHY906 could then potentiate Wnt3a and increase β-catenin–LEF/TCF–mediated transcriptional responses threefold (Lam et al. 2010). We further narrowed down the active chemical(s) for this potentiation to herb S. Subsequently, we found that β-glucuronidase treatment, but not the low pH condition, is solely responsible for enhancing the Wnt-potentiating activity of PHY906 (Lam et al. 2010). We also observed that the Wnt-potentiating activity of PHY906 could be inhibited by the overexpression of UDP-glucuronyltransferases (UDP-glucuronosyltransferase 1A1 [UGT1A1] or UGT1A9) (Lam et al. 2010). Therefore, PHY906 may have a unique effect on different tissues where β-glucuronidase/UDP–glucuronyltransferase ratios vary. In our study of the gut, this would mean the β-glucuronidase activity dominates, allowing the Wnt-potentiating activity of PHY906 to be uncovered.

29.6.5 PHY906 Inhibits CPT-11–Triggered Inflammation in the Intestine

CPT-11 alone caused pathological changes of the intestine associated with increases in infiltrating neutrophils, and macrophages, along with increased inflammatory markers including tumor necrosis factor α (TNFα) and monocyte chemotactic protein (MCP-1) in the plasma on day 4 (Lam et al. 2010). Several chemokine mRNA transcripts (CCL3, CCL4, CCL5, CXCL10, CXCL14, interleukin

18 [IL-18], IL-1B) were also examined using real-time polymerase chain reaction (PCR) but were not found to be significantly altered in middle jejunum segments after treatment with PHY906/CPT-11 versus CPT-11 alone. PHY906 effectively inhibited the detection of multiple inflammatory markers induced by CPT-11 on day 4 in the intestine and plasma.

Because of the observed inflammatory changes, we then tested the effects of PHY906 on three key mediators of inflammation, nuclear factor kappaB (NF-κB), cyclooxygenase 2 (Cox2), and inducible nitric oxide synthase (iNOS). First, PHY906, and mainly herb S, could inhibit TNFα-induced NF-κB–mediated transcriptional activity (Lam et al. 2010). YCC treatment increased the NF-κB inhibitory activity of PHY906 or herb S. Secondly, PHY906, and the individual components G, P, and S, also inhibited Cox2 in the absence of β-glucuronidase. Third, we found that PHY906 or herb S could also inhibit iNOS, and this inhibition was reduced by half after YCC treatment (Lam et al. 2010).

Based on these studies, it appears that unlike single target–oriented therapeutic agents, PHY906 hits multiple sites of action on inflammatory pathways including TNFα-induced NF-κB–mediated transcriptional activity, Cox2, and iNOS enzyme activity. Since our in vitro experiments showed that YCC treatment enhanced the anti–NF-κB activity of PHY906, this suggests that the active compounds may be aglycone flavonoids. Our LC–MS data indicated that the presence of aglycone flavonoids from PHY906 such as baicalein, chrysin, oroxylin A, and wogonin increased dramatically after YCC treatment. These flavonoids have been reported by others and confirmed by us to have anti–NF-κB activity (Chen, Yang, and Lee 2000; Chi, Cheon, and Kim 2001; Chen et al. 2001; Kang et al. 2003; Lin and Shieh 1996; Wakabayashi and Yasui 2000; Shen et al. 2003). PHY906 also inhibits two downstream targets of NF-κB, Cox2 and iNOS, which are key mediators of intestinal inflammation and diarrhea. Since YCC treatment alters the inhibitory activities of PHY906 on iNOS and Cox2, different compounds within PHY906 are likely responsible for the inhibitory activities we observed. Because PHY906 directly targets iNOS and Cox2 enzymes, PHY906 may help reduce the downstream inflammatory cascades triggered by them.

Beyond the inhibition of inflammatory mediators, PHY906 was also found to have inhibitory effects on tachykinin NK1 (Liu et al. 2004) and the opiate delta receptor, both of which are associated with diarrhea, vomiting, nausea, and pain.

In summary, PHY906 reduces CPT-11–induced intestinal damage by inhibiting multiple inflammatory mediators and by facilitating intestinal repair through promoting intestinal progenitor cell proliferation (Figure 29.1).

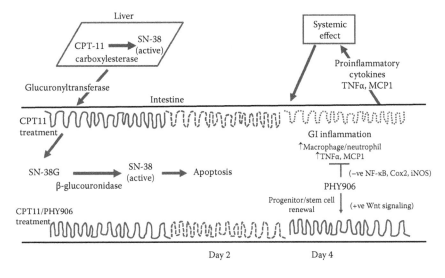

FIGURE 29.1 Summary of the mechanism of action of PHY906 in reducing gastrointestinal toxicity caused by CPT-11.

29.7   MECHANISTIC STUDIES OF ACTIONS OF PHY906 ON TUMORS AFTER CPT-11 TREATMENT

29.7.1   PHY906 INCREASES APOPTOSIS IN TUMORS AFTER CPT-11 TREATMENT

PHY906 had a completely different action on tumors than seen in the intestine after CPT-11 treatment. PHY906 monotherapy did not display any growth inhibitory effect on the colon 38 tumors. The combination of PHY906 and CPT-11 had stronger antitumor activity than CPT-11 alone. TUNEL assay and cleaved caspase-3 staining of tumor sections revealed that PHY906 increased DNA damage and apoptosis in colon 38 tumors after CPT-11 treatment from day 2 to day 4 (unpublished data).

According to pharmacokinetic studies in our animal model, PHY906 did not alter the pharmacokinetics of CPT-11, or the conversion of CPT-11 to its active metabolites, SN38, in different tissues, including plasma, tumor, liver, spleen, and kidney (Ye et al. 2008). Therefore, other reasons beyond alterations in pharmacokinetics of CPT-11 by PHY906 needed to be considered. To further explore the mechanism(s) responsible for the antitumor enhancement of CPT-11 by PHY906, we used a system biology approach that examined the differences in expression of 18,000 RNA species triggered by the four different treatments on day 3 post CPT-11 treatment in a colon 38 tumor, spleen, and liver. A few important findings were observed.

29.7.2   DIFFERENT TREATMENTS HAVE DIFFERENT EFFECTS ON mRNA/microRNA CHANGES

Each treatment had a different effect on both mRNA and microRNA (miRNA) expression in different tissues, and only a small percentage of mRNA or miRNA changes were overlapping. For example, cotreatment with CPT-11 and PHY906 had only 180 mRNA and 4 miRNA alterations that were shared by the tumor, spleen, and liver. In tumors, CPT-11/PHY906 caused 1369 unique mRNA changes and 46 unique miRNA changes (Wang et al. 2011). However, the same treatment caused 3577 mRNA/30 miRNA unique changes in the spleen and 1270 mRNA/14 miRNA unique changes in liver. It should be noted that different organs had unique transcriptional responses to different treatment. Using LC–MS, we also demonstrated that the metabolite profiles of CPT-11 and PHY906 in different tissues are also very different. These experiments clearly demonstrate tissue-specific responses to the different treatments.

29.7.3   CPT-11/PHY906 CAUSES A RELATIVE PROINFLAMMATORY AND PROAPOPTOTIC EFFECT AND MORE MACROPHAGE INFILTRATION IN TUMORS

Either PHY906 or CPT-11 alone predominantly repressed many transcripts of different signaling pathways in tumors. PHY906 alone suppressed the expression of genes in several canonical pathways related to the proinflammatory activity naturally present within the tumor (Wang et al. 2011). The observed anti-inflammatory activity of PHY906 should not impair tumor growth because the PHY906 group alone had no significant in vivo antitumor activity. CPT-11 alone selectively enhanced the expression of NF-κB–associated proapoptotic transcripts, but suppressed many NF-κB–dependent transcripts associated with innate immune responses, including interferon regulatory factor-1 (IRF-1) (Wang et al. 2011), which has proinflammatory/proapoptotic (Suk et al. 2001) and antiangiogenic properties (Lee et al. 2008). In contrast to single-agent treatment, the combination of CPT-11 with PHY906 reverted some of the anti-inflammatory effects of CPT-11 or PHY906. Ingenuity Pathway Analysis demonstrated that the overlap in the ranking of the most affected pathways were limited to proinflammatory pathways such as interferon (IFN), IL-9, and Janus kinase (JAK)/signal transducer and activator of transcription (STAT) signaling, suggesting that the combination of PHY906 and CPT-11 predominantly affected pathways associated with switching the immune response from chronic to acute in the tumor microenvironment, and this may help trigger tumor rejection (Wang et al. 2011).

Results also indicated that some important immunological regulators such as IRF-5 and IRF-9, downstream targets of INFα/β signaling, were upregulated after CPT-11/PHY906 treatment (Wang et al. 2011). IRF-5 was found to play a key role in sensitizing colon tumor cells to CPT-11 (Hu, Mancl, and Barnes 2005) or death receptor–mediated cell death (Hu and Barnes 2009). Therefore, increased expression of IRF-5 induced by CPT-11/PHY906 may explain why more apoptosis was found in the tumors from the CPT-11/PHY906 group. IRF-5 is also reported to be a potent proinflammatory transcription factor associated with immune-mediated, tissue-specific rejection (Schoenemeyer et al. 2005; Pandey et al. 2009; Ouyang et al. 2007; Krausgruber et al. 2010). Increased expression of IRF-5 in activated murine macrophages can lead to induction of several chemokines, including CCL1/I-309; CCL2/monocyte chemotactic protein 1 (MCP-1); CCL4/macrophage inflammatory protein 1b (MIP-1b); CCL5/regulated upon activation, normal T cell expressed and secreted (RANTES); and CXCL-8/IL-8 (Barnes et al. 2002). As a consequence, more inflammatory cells could be recruited to the areas of inflammation, which might increase tumor rejection. Our array and qRT-PCR results showed upregulation of CCL2/MCP-1 and CCL5/RANTES mRNA by CPT-11/PHY906. Using immunohistochemistry, we consistently found strong macrophage infiltration in tumors of the CPT-11/PHY906 treatment group (Wang et al. 2011). IRF-5 has recently been found to play an important role in polarizing macrophages toward an M1 phenotype, which is favorable toward inducing tumor rejection (Krausgruber et al. 2011). We are currently investigating whether the infiltrated macrophages display this M1 phenotype since this may provide an additional explanation for the increased antitumor activity observed in the CPT-11 + PHY906 treatment group.

In summary, PHY906 itself has a general immunosuppressive effect in tumors that does not inhibit tumor growth. When PHY906 is combined with CPT-11, PHY906 changes the gene expression profiles of a tumor toward a proinflammatory and proapoptotic one that may favor tumor rejection (Figure 29.2).

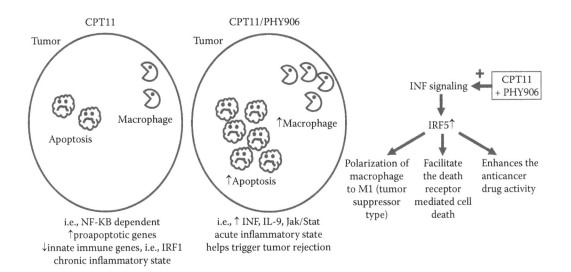

FIGURE 29.2 Summary of the mechanism of action of PHY906 in enhancing antitumor activity of CPT-11.

29.8   PHY906, WHEN COMBINED WITH DIFFERENT CHEMOTHERAPEUTIC AGENTS, ENHANCES ANTITUMOR ACTIVITY IN VIVO

Since we found that PHY906 could enhance antitumor activity when combined with CPT-11, we further tested if PHY906 can enhance the antitumor activity of other chemotherapeutic agents in different tumor models in mice. We combined PHY906 with 5-FU; capecitabine (5-FU prodrug, Xeloda); etoposide (VP-16, Etopophos, Vepesid); troxacitabine (L-OddC, Troxatyl); gemcitabine (dFdC, Gemzar); oxaliplatin (Eloxatin); sorafenib (Nexavar); sunitinib (Sutent); thalidomide; or Taxol (Liu et al. 2004). To our surprise, PHY906 increased the antitumor activities of all these agents. It is interesting to note that the above chemotherapeutic agents had different targets such as topoisomerase I/II, thymidylate synthase, ribonucleotide reductase, multiple cytoplasmic and receptor kinases, epidermal growth factor receptor (EGFR), and tubulin. These agents inhibit DNA and RNA synthesis or repair, multiple signaling transduction pathways via cell division, or tumor angiogenesis, and can induce cell death via apoptosis and autophagy. In a nude mouse HepG2 xenograft model, cotreatment with PHY906 and sorafenib triggered more cell death in tumors and increased macrophage infiltration in tumors. We are currently investigating whether PHY906 can change the immunological conditions in the tumor to favor apoptosis and tumor rejection. If confirmed, this may provide a clue to explain how PHY906 can enhance the antitumor activity of various anticancer agents. In addition, PHY906 contains multiple bioactive chemicals that could target multiple sites in the tumor or the body of an animal. Therefore, PHY906 has the potential to hit multiple signaling pathways and enhance different chemotherapeutic agents.

29.9   PHY906 CLINICAL TRIALS

As our preclinical results indicated that PHY906 reduced intestinal toxicity caused by CPT-11 and enhanced antitumor activities of different chemotherapeutic agents, clinical trials were initiated to study whether PHY906 could be of benefit to patients during treatment with chemotherapy. Currently, five clinical trials have been carried out in three different types of cancers in multiple clinical centers in both the United States and Taiwan: (1) two phase I studies on advanced colorectal cancer (CRC) in which CPT-11/5-FU/LV + PHY906 or CPT-11 + PHY906 were used; (2) one phase I/II and one phase II study on advanced hepatocellular carcinoma (HCC) in which capecitabine + PHY906 was used; and (3) one phase I/II study on advanced pancreatic cancer (APC) in which capecitabine + PHY906 was used (Farrell and Kummar 2003; Kummar et al. 2011; Saif et al. 2010, in press; Yen et al. 2009). PHY906 as oral capsules (200 mg) in various dose regimens were given to a total of 150 patients. In brief, PHY906 mitigated diarrhea and vomiting caused by CPT-11/5-FU/LV or CPT-11. In the HCC trial, capecitabine + PHY906 appeared to have less capecitabine-associated toxicity compared to other studies using similar capecitabine doses. The medium survival time was 10.9 months, which is comparable to that of sorafenib (first-line HCC therapy) US/European trials but much longer than that seen in Asian sorafenib trials, with a medium survival of 7 months. Capecitabine + PHY906 appeared to have fewer side effects than sorafenib. In the APC trial, PHY906 was suggested to increase the therapeutic index of capecitabine by reducing diarrhea and hand–foot syndrome. Details of clinical trials of PHY906 were reviewed by Liu and Cheng (2012).

29.10   DETECTION OF PHY906 CHEMICALS OR THEIR METABOLITES IN THE PLASMA OF PATIENTS FOLLOWING PHY906 TREATMENT

In order to understand what the biological active chemical(s) of PHY906 in patients could be, we established a methodology using high-performance LC–MS to detect multiple compounds in a single run. This enables us to monitor multiple chemicals from PHY906 and drugs such as CPT-11. Briefly, the chemicals from PHY906 aqueous extract, animal plasma, or patients were prepared and separated on an Agilent ZORBAX SB-C18 column and eluted with acetonitrile/0.05%

(v/v) formic acid, and final mass information was collected in a 4000 QTrap mass spectrometer (Zhang et al. 2010).

We monitored the pharmacokinetics of chemicals or their metabolites from PHY906 and CPT-11 in a phase I/ll clinical trial for advanced CRC. In this study, the pharmacokinetics of CPT-11 and its metabolites were monitored in three cohorts, with two cycles in which patients received CPT-11 (180 mg/m^2) alone in cycle 1 and received a second dose of CPT-11 (180 mg/m^2) plus different dosages of PHY906 (cohort 1, 1200 mg, b.i.d.; cohort 2, 1800 mg, b.i.d; cohort 3, 2400 mg, b.i.d.) in cycle 2 after 14 days. Results showed that in all cohorts, CPT-11 and its metabolites reached their maximum concentration, 1.5 to 5.3 μM for CPT-11, 20 to 300 nM for SN38, and 40 to 250 nM for SN38G, after about 1.5 h in the two cycles. The area under the curve (AUC) for CPT-11, SN38, and SN38G showed no significant differences among different cycles and cohorts in which a patient received CPT-11 without or with a different dosage of PHY906 (unpublished data). This indicated that PHY906 did not affect the pharmacokinetics (PKs) of CPT-11, an observation that is entirely consistent with our preclinical study results using colon 38 allograft–bearing mice. Similarly, in another clinical trial, PHY906 also did not affect the pharmacokinetics of 5-FU/CPT-11 (Zhang et al. 2010).

In contrast to a single-chemical drug, it is a great challenge to detect the multitude of chemicals in an herbal mixture such as PHY906. However, for understanding the mechanism of action of PHY906, it is critical to know the chemicals and their metabolites present in plasma after oral administration of the herbal mixture. Using LC–MS methodology, 57 compounds in the PHY906 aqueous extract were identified and tentatively assigned structures based upon their identified mass spectrometry. Different numbers of compounds were found in different herbs: 26 from G, 4 from P, 26 from S, and 1 from Z, with flavonoids constituting the major class of compounds. In total, 31 flavonoids from patients' plasma have been identified (Zhang et al. 2010). Most of the flavonoids detected are present in herb S, and some also can be found in herb G and herb P, with glucuronidation being the most common modification. This modification usually increases the aqueous solubility of flavonoids. As we mentioned above, glucuronidation may increase or decrease PHY906's activity, depending on the specific targets. Other metabolic modifications may also affect PHY906 activity; this is still under investigation.

Plasma samples from the phaseI/II clinical trial of PHY906 and CPT-11 failed to detect all the compounds from PHY906, suggesting that most of them will be subjected to metabolism or not absorbed. We detected only six parental compounds that were present in the original water extract of PHY906, but we did find 27 new metabolites (33 chemicals in total) (Zhang et al. 2010). Regarding the class of chemicals detected in the human plasma, the majority were flavonoids. Most of the chemicals from PHY906 were subjected to glucuronidation, although some were subjected to sulfonation and methylation.

Based on the pharmacokinetics results, we found two factors affecting PHY906 metabolism. The first factor is the dosage of PHY906. We determined that baicalin is a major flavonoid present in PHY906. When PHY906 is ingested orally, it is subjected to acidic conditions followed by intestinal microbial metabolism, including deglucuronidation by β-glucuronidase. As a result, most of the baicalin in the small intestine is converted to baicalein (without glucuronide). When baicalein passes through the intestine, it can be glucuronidated by different UGT isozymes to form different isomers of baicalin. The levels of baicalin and its isomers in the plasma of patients treated in cohort 2 (PHY906, 1800 mg, b.i.d.) and cohort 3 (PHY906, 2400 mg, b.i.d.) were higher than that of cohort 1 (PHY906, 1200 mg, b.i.d.). The detection of different isomers of baicalin was dose dependent. For instance, detection of baicalin in plasma required patients to ingest a total dose of 4800 mg of PHY906, but other isomers were seen with total oral doses of only 2400 mg. Increasing PHY906 from 2400 to 4800 mg did not affect the level of baicalin isomer 3; however, the optimal dosage of PHY906 for the formation of baicalin isomers 1 and 2 was 3600 mg and not 4800 mg (unpublished data).

The second factor is the individual since some metabolites varied across patients. For example, our preliminary PK analysis of oroxylin A showed that oroxylin A–(gluA)2 was detected in the plasma from patient 2, but not from patients 1 and 3 in cohort 1. In cohort 2, patient 6 had relatively high levels of both oroxylin A and oroxylin A–(gluA)2. Patients 4 and 7 had relatively low levels of oroxylin A but comparable amounts of oroxylin A–(gluA)2. Oroxylin A and oroxylin A–(gluA)2 were undetectable in patient 9 (unpublished data). With these findings, we anticipate that the different metabolite profiles of PHY906 in patients resulted from pharmacogenetic variations of key metabolizing enzymes in both normal tissue and tumor.

In humans, UGT1 and UGT2 are the most common UGTs (Owens, Basu, and Banerjee 2005). UGT1 has at least 16 isoforms and UGT2 has at least 6 (Bock 2010), and they have been reported to have different enzymatic activities and tissue distributions. Therefore, different UGT isozymes may be responsible for differences in glucuronidation of PHY906 flavonoids (Wong et al. 2009). Furthermore, individual UGT polymorphisms are also likely to affect glucuronidation reactions (Bock 2010).

Currently, we are collaborating with a bioinformatics and clinical group to study the chemical profiles of PHY906 of each patient and the response of each patient to chemotherapy. In brief, we will generate chemical profiles using clinical plasma samples from patients who received PHY906 and chemotherapy. Then the bioinformatics group will analyze and filter chemical(s) that has (have) a correlation with response to chemotherapy. We will further validate the bioactivity of the chemical(s) using in vitro assays. Results obtained will help us to predict which patients will respond better to PHY906 and to identify active compound(s) of PHY906 in patients.

29.11 SUMMARY

Through our efforts in the past 12 years, using an 1800-year-old four-herb formulation PHY906 as an example, we established new methodologies to study a polychemical-based herbal mixture while solving certain important issues in quality control. We accumulated scientifically based evidence to demonstrate that PHY906 is a multiple target–oriented herbal mixture that differentially affects inflammation of different tissues and improves therapeutic efficacy of CPT-11 in vivo. Our future challenge is how to use bioinformatics to integrate the data generated by clinical trials, animal studies, and in vitro experiments to identify active compound(s) and to predict which patients will respond better to PHY906. It is our hope that our studies can eventually form a model for the future development of "personalized medicine" and illustrate the utility of polychemical herbal medicines for treating multifactorial diseases such as cancer.

ACKNOWLEDGMENTS

We thank Sharon Lin for the critical reading of the manuscript. This work was supported by the National Cancer Institute (NCI) (1PO1CA154295-01A1) and by the National Center for Complementary and Alternative Medicine (NCCAM), National Institutes of Health (NIH), USA. Yung-Chi Cheng is a fellow of the National Foundation for Cancer Research, USA.

REFERENCES

Abigerges, D., J. P. Armand, G. G. Chabot, L. Da Costa, E. Fadel, C. Cote, P. Herait, and D. Gandia. 1994. Irinotecan (CPT-11) high-dose escalation using intensive high-dose loperamide to control diarrhea. *J Natl Cancer Inst* 86 (6):446–9.

American Cancer Society. 2011. *Cancer Facts & Figures*. Atlanta, Georgia.

Barnes, B. J., M. J. Kellum, A. E. Field, and P. M. Pitha. 2002. Multiple regulatory domains of IRF-5 control activation, cellular localization, and induction of chemokines that mediate recruitment of T lymphocytes. *Mol Cell Biol* 22 (16):5721–40.

Bock, K. W. 2010. Functions and transcriptional regulation of adult human hepatic UDP-glucuronosyltransferases (UGTs): mechanisms responsible for interindividual variation of UGT levels. *Biochem Pharmacol* 80 (6):771–7.

Chen, Y. C., S. C. Shen, L. G. Chen, T. J. Lee, and L. L. Yang. 2001. Wogonin, baicalin, and baicalein inhibition of inducible nitric oxide synthase and cyclooxygenase-2 gene expressions induced by nitric oxide synthase inhibitors and lipopolysaccharide. *Biochem Pharmacol* 61 (11):1417–27.

Chen, Y., L. Yang, and T. J. Lee. 2000. Oroxylin A inhibition of lipopolysaccharide-induced iNOS and Cox-2 gene expression via suppression of nuclear factor-kappaB activation. *Biochem Pharmacol* 59 (11):1445–57.

Chi, Y. S., B. S. Cheon, and H. P. Kim. 2001. Effect of wogonin, a plant flavone from *Scutellaria radix*, on the suppression of cyclooxygenase-2 and the induction of inducible nitric oxide synthase in lipopolysaccharide-treated RAW 264.7 cells. *Biochem Pharmacol* 61 (10):1195–203.

Cunningham, D., S. Pyrhonen, R. D. James, C. J. Punt, T. F. Hickish, R. Heikkila, T. B. Johannesen, H. Starkhammar, C. A. Topham, L. Awad, C. Jacques, and P. Herait. 1998. Randomised trial of irinotecan plus supportive care versus supportive care alone after fluorouracil failure for patients with metastatic colorectal cancer. *Lancet* 352 (9138):1413–8.

Farrell, M. P., and S. Kummar. 2003. Phase I/IIA randomized study of PHY906, a novel herbal agent, as a modulator of chemotherapy in patients with advanced colorectal cancer. *Clin Colorectal Cancer* 2 (4):253–6.

Fevr, T., S. Robine, D. Louvard, and J. Huelsken. 2007. Wnt/beta-catenin is essential for intestinal homeostasis and maintenance of intestinal stem cells. *Mol Cell Biol* 27 (21):7551–9.

Hsu, H. Y., and C. S. Hsu. 1980. *Commonly Used Chinese Herb Formulas—With Illustrations*. Long Beach, CA: Oriental Healing Art Institute.

Hu, G., and B. J. Barnes. 2009. IRF-5 is a mediator of the death receptor–induced apoptotic signaling pathway. *J Biol Chem* 284 (5):2767–77.

Hu, G., M. E. Mancl, and B. J. Barnes. 2005. Signaling through IFN regulatory factor-5 sensitizes p53-deficient tumors to DNA damage-induced apoptosis and cell death. *Cancer Res* 65 (16):7403–12.

Humerickhouse, R., K. Lohrbach, L. Li, W. F. Bosron, and M. E. Dolan. 2000. Characterization of CPT-11 hydrolysis by human liver carboxylesterase isoforms hCE-1 and hCE-2. *Cancer Res* 60 (5):1189–92.

Kang, B. Y., S. W. Chung, S. H. Kim, D. Cho, and T. S. Kim. 2003. Involvement of nuclear factor-kappaB in the inhibition of interleukin-12 production from mouse macrophages by baicalein, a flavonoid in *Scutellaria baicalensis*. *Planta Med* 69 (8):687–91.

Krausgruber, T., K. Blazek, T. Smallie, S. Alzabin, H. Lockstone, N. Sahgal, T. Hussell, M. Feldmann, and I. A. Udalova. 2011. IRF5 promotes inflammatory macrophage polarization and TH1-TH17 responses. *Nat Immunol* 12 (3):231–8.

Krausgruber, T., D. Saliba, G. Ryzhakov, A. Lanfrancotti, K. Blazek, and I. A. Udalova. 2010. IRF5 is required for late-phase TNF secretion by human dendritic cells. *Blood* 115 (22):4421–30.

Kummar, S., M. S. Copur, M. Rose, S. Wadler, J. Stephenson, M. O'Rourke, W. Brenckman, R. Tilton, S. H. Liu, Z. Jiang, T. Su, Y. C. Cheng, and E. Chu. 2011. A phase I study of the Chinese herbal medicine PHY906 as a modulator of irinotecan-based chemotherapy in patients with advanced colorectal cancer. *Clin Colorectal Cancer* 10 (2):85–96.

Lam, W., S. Bussom, F. Guan, Z. Jiang, W. Zhang, E. A. Gullen, S. H. Liu, and Y. C. Cheng. 2010. The four-herb Chinese medicine PHY906 reduces chemotherapy-induced gastrointestinal toxicity. *Sci Transl Med* 2 (45):1–8.

Lee, J. H., T. Chun, S. Y. Park, and S. B. Rho. 2008. Interferon regulatory factor-1 (IRF-1) regulates VEGF-induced angiogenesis in HUVECs. *Biochim Biophys Acta* 1783 (9):1654–62.

Lin, C. C., and D. E. Shieh. 1996. The anti-inflammatory activity of *Scutellaria rivularis* extracts and its active components, baicalin, baicalein and wogonin. *Am J Chin Med* 24 (1):31–6.

Liu, S. H., and Y. C. Cheng. 2012. Old formula, new Rx: the journey of PHY906 as cancer adjuvant therapy. *J Ethnopharmacol* 140 (3):614–23.

Liu, S.-H., Z. Jiang, T.-M. Su, W.-Y. Gao, C.-H. Leung, Y. Lee, and Y.-C. Cheng. 2004. Developing PHY906 as a broad-spectrum modulator of chemotherapeutic agents in cancer therapy. *Proc Am Assoc. Cancer Res* 45:557.

Molassiotis, A., P. Fernadez-Ortega, D. Pud, G. Ozden, J. A. Scott, V. Panteli, A. Margulies, M. Browall, M. Magri, S. Selvekerova, E. Madsen, L. Milovics, I. Bruyns, G. Gudmundsdottir, S. Hummerston, A. M. Ahmad, N. Platin, N. Kearney, and E. Patiraki. 2005. Use of complementary and alternative medicine in cancer patients: a European survey. *Ann Oncol* 16 (4):655–63.

Olaku, O., and J. D. White. 2011. Herbal therapy use by cancer patients: a literature review on case reports. *Eur J Cancer* 47 (4):508–14.

Ouyang, X., H. Negishi, R. Takeda, Y. Fujita, T. Taniguchi, and K. Honda. 2007. Cooperation between MyD88 and TRIF pathways in TLR synergy via IRF5 activation. *Biochem Biophys Res Commun* 354 (4):1045–51.

Owens, I. S., N. K. Basu, and R. Banerjee. 2005. UDP-glucuronosyltransferases: gene structures of UGT1 and UGT2 families. *Methods Enzymol* 400:1–22.

Pandey, A. K., Y. Yang, Z. Jiang, S. M. Fortune, F. Coulombe, M. A. Behr, K. A. Fitzgerald, C. M. Sassetti, and M. A. Kelliher. 2009. NOD2, RIP2 and IRF5 play a critical role in the type I interferon response to *Mycobacterium tuberculosis*. *PLoS Pathog* 5 (7):e1000500.

Rivory, L. P., M. R. Bowles, J. Robert, and S. M. Pond. 1996. Conversion of irinotecan (CPT-11) to its active metabolite, 7-ethyl-10-hydroxycamptothecin (SN-38), by human liver carboxylesterase. *Biochem Pharmacol* 52 (7):1103–11.

Saif, M. W., F. Lansigan, S. Ruta, L. Lamb, M. Mezes, K. Elligers, N. Grant, Z. L. Jiang, S. H. Liu, and Y. C. Cheng. 2010. Phase I study of the botanical formulation PHY906 with capecitabine in advanced pancreatic and other gastrointestinal malignancies. *Phytomedicine* 17 (3–4):161–9.

Saif, M. W., F. Lansigan, S. Ruta, L. Lamb, K. Elligers, M. Mezes, N. Grant, Z. Jiang, S. H. Liu, and Y. Cheng. In press. Phase I study of the botanical formulation PHY906 with capecitabine in advanced pancreatic and gastrointestinal malignancies. *Phytomedicine* 17 (3–4):161–9.

Schoenemeyer, A., B. J. Barnes, M. E. Mancl, E. Latz, N. Goutagny, P. M. Pitha, K. A. Fitzgerald, and D. T. Golenbock. 2005. The interferon regulatory factor, IRF5, is a central mediator of toll-like receptor 7 signaling. *J Biol Chem* 280 (17):17005–12.

Shen, Y. C., W. F. Chiou, Y. C. Chou, and C. F. Chen. 2003. Mechanisms in mediating the anti-inflammatory effects of baicalin and baicalein in human leukocytes. *Eur J Pharmacol* 465 (1–2):171–81.

Suk, K., I. Chang, Y. H. Kim, S. Kim, J. Y. Kim, H. Kim, and M. S. Lee. 2001. Interferon gamma (IFNgamma) and tumor necrosis factor alpha synergism in ME-180 cervical cancer cell apoptosis and necrosis. IFNgamma inhibits cytoprotective NF-kappa B through STAT1/IRF-1 pathways. *J Biol Chem* 276 (16):13153–9.

Tilton, R., A. A. Paiva, J. Q. Guan, R. Marathe, Z. Jiang, W. van Eyndhoven, J. Bjoraker, Z. Prusoff, H. Wang, S. H. Liu, and Y. C. Cheng. 2010. A comprehensive platform for quality control of botanical drugs (PhytomicsQC): a case study of Huangqin Tang (HQT) and PHY906. *Chin Med* 5:30.

Van der Flier, L. G., J. Sabates-Bellver, I. Oving, A. Haegebarth, M. De Palo, M. Anti, M. E. Van Gijn, S. Suijkerbuijk, M. Van de Wetering, G. Marra, and H. Clevers. 2007. The intestinal Wnt/TCF signature. *Gastroenterology* 132 (2):628–32.

Wakabayashi, I., and K. Yasui. 2000. Wogonin inhibits inducible prostaglandin E(2) production in macrophages. *Eur J Pharmacol* 406 (3):477–81.

Wang, E., S. Bussom, J. Chen, C. Quinn, D. Bedognetti, W. Lam, F. Guan, Z. Jiang, Y. Mark, Y. Zhao, D. F. Stroncek, J. White, F. M. Marincola, and Y. C. Cheng. 2011. Interaction of a traditional Chinese medicine (PHY906) and CPT-11 on the inflammatory process in the tumor microenvironment. *BMC Med Genomics* 4:38.

Wong, Y. C., L. Zhang, G. Lin, and Z. Zuo. 2009. Structure–activity relationships of the glucuronidation of flavonoids by human glucuronosyltransferases. *Expert Opin Drug Metab Toxicol* 5 (11):1399–419.

Ye, M., Z. Jiang, W. Lam, G. Dutschman, S. Bussom, P.-C. Chen, S.-H. Liu, and Y.-C. Cheng. 2008. A novel herb-drug interaction: irinotecan can significantly change the pharmacokinetics and pharmacodynamics of PHY906, a Chinese medicine formulation for cancer therapy. *Proc Am Assoc Cancer Res* 49:635.

Yen, Y., S. So, M. Rose, M. W. Saif, E. Chu, S. H. Liu, A. Foo, Z. Jiang, T. Su, and Y. C. Cheng. 2009. Phase I/II study of PHY906/capecitabine in advanced hepatocellular carcinoma. *Anticancer Res* 29 (10):4083–92.

Zhang, W., M. W. Saif, G. E. Dutschman, X. Li, W. Lam, S. Bussom, Z. Jiang, M. Ye, E. Chu, and Y. C. Cheng. 2010. Identification of chemicals and their metabolites from PHY906, a Chinese medicine formulation, in the plasma of a patient treated with irinotecan and PHY906 using liquid chromatography/tandem mass spectrometry (LC/MS/MS). *J Chromatogr A* 1217 (37):5785–93.

30 Lipoic Acid in the Prevention and Treatment of Inflammatory Disease and Cancer

Kate Petersen Shay, Regis F. Moreau, and Tory M. Hagen

CONTENTS

30.1 INTRODUCTION: BIOAVAILABILITY AND METABOLIC FATE OF DIETARY LIPOIC ACID

1,2-Dithiolane-3-pentanoic acid, commonly known as alpha-lipoic acid (LA), is a naturally occurring dithiol compound that is synthesized in the mitochondrion from octanoic acid. LA serves a critical role in mitochondrial energy metabolism as a necessary cofactor for mitochondrial α-ketoacid dehydrogenases, and its de novo synthesis appears to supply all of the necessary LA needed for intermediary metabolism. However, LA may also be absorbed from the diet and transiently accumulates in many tissues. Dietary sources of LA are muscle meats, heart, kidney, liver, and to a lesser degree, fruits and vegetables (Akiba et al. 1998; Packer et al. 2001; Wollin and Jones 2003). Though available in small amounts from these nutritional sources, it is not likely that appreciable quantities of LA are consumed in the typical Western diet. Rather, dietary supplements that typically range from 50 to 600 mg are the primary sources of LA, and most information as to its bioavailability and therapeutic activity comes from studies using supplements.

The potential therapeutic actions of orally supplied LA can be appreciated only with an understanding of its bioavailability, tissue accumulation, and metabolic fate. It is apparent that cells maintain active systems to transport, utilize, and excrete non–protein-bound LA. Dietary bioavailability studies show that an oral LA dose is rapidly absorbed from the gastrointestinal tract and appreciably increases plasma LA levels. Approximately 20%–40% of LA from an oral dose appears in the plasma (Bernkop-Schnurch et al. 2004; Mignini et al. 2007; Carlson et al. 2007; Teichert et al. 1998, 2003, 2005; Breithaupt-Grogler et al. 1999; Evans et al. 2002; Amenta et al. 2008). This high variability is dictated, in part, by the dose given, the food matrix involved, and whether the tablet is controlled release.

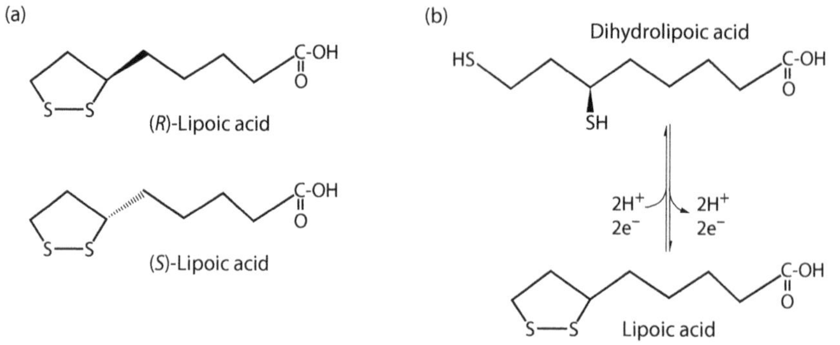

FIGURE 30.1 *R* and *S* enantiomers of lipoic acid (a); reduced and oxidized forms of lipoic acid (b).

LA has one chiral center and therefore exists in both *R*- and *S*-enantiomeric forms; however, only *R*-LA is conjugated to conserved lysine residues in an amide linkage, making this isoform essential as a cofactor in biological systems (Reed 1974) (Figure 30.1a). Most LA sold as dietary supplements is the racemic mixture. Both racemic LA and the *R* isomer are bioavailable and safe in moderate doses (Carlson et al. 2007; Mignini et al. 2007, 2011; Teichert et al. 1998, 2003; Foster 2007; Cremer et al. 2006a,b). The uptake and clearance of LA have been the focus of several studies. In one trial, volunteers were given 600 mg of the racemic mixture, and peak plasma concentrations of *R*-LA were 40%–50% higher than *S*-LA (Breithaupt-Grogler et al. 1999), the latter of which was apparently more rapidly cleared than the *R* form. This result suggests that the *R* enantiomer would be the primary form to provide as an oral supplement; however, the presence of *S*-LA in the racemic mixture may enhance bioavailability by preventing the polymerization of *R*-LA. Rapid gastrointestinal uptake of LA and appearance in the plasma is followed by an equally rapid clearance, reflecting both transport into tissues as well as glomerular filtration and renal excretion (Harrison and McCormick 1974). LA accumulates in the liver, heart, and skeletal muscle in a transient manner but can be found in other tissues as well. In a study by Panigrahi et al. (1996), an intravenous (i.v.) dose of LA (25 mg/kg body weight [b.w]) given to rats was shown to cross the blood–brain barrier and accumulated (2.14 nmol/g wet tissue) in the cerebral cortex within 60 min of administration. The level was reduced more than fourfold within 24 h after dosage but was still higher than those of controls or shams, which had no measureable LA. Another study examining the cortex and other brain regions showed lower levels of basal LA content in the brains of old rats compared to young, but a 7- to 14-day regimen of LA (intraperitoneal [i.p.], 100 mg/kg b.w.) increased its measurable levels in all regions of the brain in old rats, whereas levels in young animals were unchanged (Arivazhagan et al. 2002). A more recent study, however, did not find significant changes in brain LA content following oral gavage (50 mg/kg b.w. in rats) (Chng et al. 2009), particularly after correcting for residual blood volume. Thus, there may exist differences in brain concentrations of LA depending on mode of administration. Additionally, corrections for blood-borne LA content will be needed to resolve the extent that LA crosses the blood–brain barrier and is available for nervous tissue.

30.2 BIOCHEMICAL PROPERTIES OF LIPOIC ACID AND ITS CHEMOPROTECTIVE POTENTIAL

The oxidized (LA) and reduced (dihydrolipoic acid or DHLA) forms of lipoic acid create a potent redox couple with a standard reduction potential of −0.32 V (Figure 30.1b). Evidence shows that both LA and DHLA are capable of scavenging a variety of reactive oxygen species (Searls and Sanadi 1960; Shay et al. 2009). While neither species is active against hydrogen peroxide (Scott et al. 1994), both LA and DHLA terminate hydroxyl radicals and hypochlorous acid, while LA also eliminates singlet oxygen (Scott et al. 1994; Devasagayam et al. 1993; Suzuki et al. 1991, 1993; Yan et al. 1996; Haenen and Bast 1991). DHLA may also regenerate endogenous antioxidants, including vitamins C and E (Biewenga et al. 1997; Bast and Haenen 2003). However, it is not clear how LA as a dietary supplement augments endogenous antioxidant capacity in the long term, as it accumulates only transiently in vivo and is rapidly catabolized. It may be that the most salubrious property of the LA/DHLA redox couple is through increasing endogenous antioxidant capacity rather than directly scavenging free radicals (Shay et al. 2008). Regardless of whether LA acts as a direct scavenger of reactive oxygen species in vivo, it is clear that it exerts potent health-related benefits in pathophysiologies associated with oxidative stress (Smith et al. 2004; Scott et al. 1994; Devasagayam et al. 1993; Liu et al. 2002; Suh et al. 2004; Lodge et al. 1998; Anuradha and Varalakshmi 1999; Han et al. 1997).

The rationale for LA as a chemopreventative agent is extended from its known pharmacological properties in that, like many chemoprotectants (Mans et al. 2000), LA activates intracellular signal transduction pathways, inhibits phosphatases, and acts as a weak stressor to induce a phase II detoxification response. Thus, LA must be considered to have high chemoprotective potential against tumorigenesis. Based on the accumulation of evidence supplied below, we postulate that LA may play two very specific roles in cancer chemoprevention: as an anti-inflammatory agent and as an activator of nuclear factor erythroid 2 (NF-E2)–related factor 2 (Nrf2)–mediated stress response.

30.3 LA IN Nrf2-MEDIATED CANCER CHEMOPREVENTION

Nrf2 is a transcription factor that governs the expression of over 100 so-called phase II detoxification and antioxidant genes, which are regulated through the antioxidant response element (ARE) (Lee and Johnson 2004). While the Nrf2 gene is constitutively expressed and the protein contains a nuclear localization sequence (Jain et al. 2005), very little Nrf2 is found in the cell under quiescent conditions. This is because Nrf2 is rapidly degraded by binding to Keap1, a Kelch-like actin-binding protein that bridges Nrf2 to the Cul3 E3 ubiquitin ligase (Cullinan et al. 2004; Kobayashi et al. 2004). This system is also able to halt Nrf2 degradation under stress conditions so that the Nrf2 protein translocates to the nucleus and accumulates for binding to the ARE (Nguyen et al. 2003; Jaiswal 2004; Wakabayashi et al. 2003). It is thought that oxidation of, or electrophilic addition to, critical sulfhydryls on Keap1 may prevent Nrf2 association or else cause its release from the Keap1 complex (Zhang and Hannink 2003; Dinkova-Kostova et al. 2002; Kobayashi et al. 2006). Thus, Nrf2 is a critical surveillance protein for rapid response to xenobiotic or oxidative stress.

With regard to this particular review, not only is the Nrf2 stress response system activated by obvious environmental toxins, but several classes of nutritive compounds also induce Nrf2 nuclear accumulation under experimental conditions (Slocum and Kensler 2011). These bioactive compounds include isothiocyanates such as sulforaphane (found in broccoli); flavonoids such as quercetin (found in apples, grapes, etc.) and curcumin (found in turmeric); polyphenols such as resveratrol (found in red wine); and epigallocatechin gallate (found in green tea). Sulfur-containing compounds like the drug oltipraz and the micronutrient LA are also known activators of the Nrf2-mediated detoxification defenses. In fact, through its effect on Nrf2 activation, a small physiological dose of LA triggers upregulation of enzymes for xenobiotic detoxification (Figure 30.2a and b).

I.p. administration of LA to rodents activates Nrf2 and induces a phase II detoxification response in vivo. We previously showed that providing LA to old rats induced glutathione-synthesizing enzymes in the liver (Suh et al. 2004). Other laboratories showed that glutathione S-transferases (GSTs) (Flier et al. 2002) and/or NADPH:quinone oxidoreductase (NQO1) in either astrocytes (Flier et al. 2002) or HL-60 leukemia cells (Elangovan and Hsieh 2008) were also elevated following LA administration. Moreover, further work has clearly shown that LA-mediated gene induction appears to occur largely through initiating Nrf2 nuclear translocation and its subsequent binding to the ARE in the promoters of phase II response genes (Suh et al. 2004; Shenvi et al. 2009). Thus, LA may act in cancer chemoprevention (reviewed in Hu et al. 2010; Slocum and Kensler 2011) by increasing

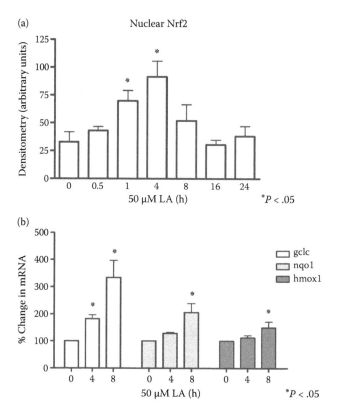

FIGURE 30.2 Lipoic acid induces nuclear accumulation of Nrf2 (a) and subsequent increase in Nrf2-dependent gene transcription (b).

transcription of enzymes that catalyze the detoxification of xenobiotics before damage to macromolecules can occur. In this way, LA would prevent procarcinogens from becoming metabolically activated into DNA-damaging agents.

30.4 INTERSECTION OF Nrf2 AND INFLAMMATION

In addition to activating an Nrf2-mediated stress response, LA may also modulate proinflammatory processes, which contributes to a multitude of pathologies including potentiation of neoplasia and tumor metastasis. This action may be both independent of and also in association with its stimulation of Nrf2-mediated gene induction. For the latter, Nrf2 knockout mice with spinal cord injury displayed more proinflammatory cytokine secretion, matrix metalloproteinase (e.g., MMP-9) activity, and nuclear factor kappaB (NF-κB) activation, compared to wild-type counterparts (Mao et al. 2010). NF-κB is a key transcription factor controlling many inflammatory responses. Its expression can inhibit Nrf2 at the transcriptional level (Liu et al. 2008).

Another study found that in astrocytes from Nrf2 knockout mice cultured with oxyhemoglobin (an inducer of cerebral vasospasm), more inflammatory markers were observed in the Nrf2$^{-/-}$ compared with wild-type astrocytes (Pan et al. 2011). Moreover, heightened expression of Nrf2-mediated genes protects against inflammation-associated damage found in spinal cord (Mao et al. 2011) and lung injury (Reddy et al. 2011) and diabetic kidney disease (Palsamy and Subramanian 2011). The mechanism through which Nrf2 influences inflammation likely has to do with the phase II enzymes that it upregulates (Kundu and Surh 2010). For instance, heme oxygenase 1 (Hmox1/HO-1) is an Nrf2-dependent gene that influences the levels of MMPs, which have normal roles in wound healing and angiogenesis but are also implicated in tumor cell invasion (Hua et al. 2011). HO-1 is induced in response to oxidative stress and hypoxia, and LA stimulates increases in both message and protein levels of HO-1 in an Nrf2-dependent manner (Ogborne et al. 2005). These and many other studies have implicated Nrf2 in inflammation prevention, and the ability of LA to transiently induce Nrf2 activity and the phase II detoxification response is a call to action for additional studies on the benefits of LA as a chemoprotectant and an anti-inflammatory agent.

30.5 LA AS A DIRECT ANTI-INFLAMMATORY AGENT

Aside from influencing the proinflammatory versus anti-inflammatory state via Nrf2, LA may directly act as an anti-inflammatory agent, especially as a means to limit chronic activation of NF-κB (Shay et al. 2009), which induces the expression of genes that lead to inflammatory cell recruitment (Van der Heiden et al. 2010). Two important studies using tumor necrosis factor alpha (TNFα)–stimulated human aortic endothelial cells and human umbilical vein endothelial cells (Zhang and Frei 2001; Ying et al. 2011) demonstrated that LA inhibits NF-κB by preventing degradation of its repressor, I-κB-α, reducing expression of intercellular adhesion molecule 1 (ICAM-1), vascular cell adhesion molecule 1 (VCAM-1), monocyte chemotactic protein-1 (MCP-1), and E-selectin. The commonly used antioxidants, N-acetyl cysteine and ascorbic acid, did not have the same effect. The aforementioned in vitro evidence for LA as an anti-inflammatory compound has now been augmented by animal studies in which 12 weeks of oral LA supplementation (20 mg/kg/day) in Watanabe hyperlipidemic rabbits inhibited NF-κB, reduced oxidative stress, and lowered atherosclerotic lesion formation (Ying et al. 2010). In human patients with renal disease, 8 weeks of oral LA supplementation (600 mg/day) significantly ($P < .05$) decreased C-reactive protein (Khabbazi et al. 2012), an important marker of inflammation. Thus, limiting chronic NF-κB–mediated expression of proinflammatory proteins and cytokines by LA may be an additional means to combat the effects of cancer-associated chronic inflammation.

In addition to this evidence, expression of the aforementioned MMPs is directly governed by NF-κB. One study found that LA inhibits MMP-9, but not MMP-2, by preventing its transcription (Bogani et al. 2007) in bovine aortic endothelial cells. However, in the breast cancer cell line MDA-MB-231, both MMP-2 and MMP-9 were decreased by LA treatment at both the messenger RNA (mRNA) and protein levels (Lee et al. 2010). MMP-9 was significantly reduced at a lower dose of LA than was MMP-2; indeed, the dose of LA required to limit MMP-2 (500–1000 μM) could be called supraphysiological, considering that its accumulation to this extent has not been measured in tissues following oral LA supplementation. However, additional studies show that a lower dose of LA (250 μM) was able to reduce cell motility in a Boyden chamber and cell invasion in Matrigel, which suggests that LA at potentially physiological levels was able to limit MMP-mediated cell migration. Both MMP-9 and MMP-2 are secreted by stromal cells, and not necessarily by cancer cells themselves, and thus may have a role in creating a microenvironment that is permissive toward cancer initiation or progression (Egeblad and Werb 2002).

In a rat model of inflammation, LA acted as both an anti-inflammatory and an antioxidant compound. LA significantly ($P < .01$) reduced carrageenan-induced paw edema, restored lost glutathione levels, and lowered lipid peroxidation (Odabasoglu et al. 2011). In this type of model, LA also lowers COX-2 mRNA and reduces nitric oxide levels (El-Shitany et al. 2010). DHLA was used as a chemoprotectant against skin tumor formation in mice, in a two-step model of initiation (7,12-dimethylbenzanthracene) and promotion (12-O-tetradecanoylphorbol-13-acetate) (Ho et al. 2007). When used prior to the initiating agent, DHLA prevented the tumors, and when used before the promoting agent, DHLA reduced the total number of tumors observed. DHLA also inhibited COX-2 activity, confirming that this compound has anti-inflammatory properties. COX-2 is upregulated at sites of inflammation and has been linked to tumorigenesis (Sethi et al. 2012), which means that lowering COX-2 with LA/DHLA may limit the permissiveness of the microenvironment toward cancer formation.

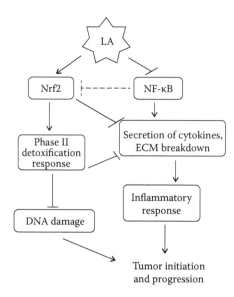

FIGURE 30.3 Cancer chemoprevention by lipoic acid: Putative mechanisms.

The anti-inflammatory properties of LA were examined in humans in the Irbesartan and Lipoic Acid in Endothelial Dysfunction (ISLAND) trial, which showed a significant ($P < .05$) decrease in serum interleukin 6 (IL-6) levels following 4 weeks of supplementation with LA (300 mg/day) (Sola et al. 2005). IL-6 is a recognized marker of inflammation and also regulates the expression of other inflammatory cytokines, such as IL-1 and TNFα (Zhang and Frei 2001). Strategies to regulate IL-6 may help combat inflammation-associated cancers (Neurath and Finotto 2011). While it remains to be seen whether experiments in culture translate to the clinical situation, it is clear that LA is able to limit chronic inflammatory processes through multiple mechanisms (Figure 30.3).

30.6 LA AS AN ADJUVANT TO CHEMOTHERAPY

LA is also being explored for its ability to reduce the proinflammatory side effects of chemotherapy that induce kidney injury (Kang et al. 2009). In a mouse model treated with cisplatin, cotreatment with LA (100 mg/kg) attenuated the drug-induced decrease in renal function through its anti-inflammatory properties. LA reduced NF-κB activity as well as expression of TNFα, ICAM-1, and MCP-1. Changes in blood urea nitrogen (BUN) and creatine levels were normalized by LA, as was the histological appearance of the tissue, which also showed reduced infiltration by CD11b-positive macrophages. The successful use of LA in this short-term model supports the suitability of more extensive studies to investigate the use of LA in countering injurious inflammation during chemotherapy regimens.

While the rationale is strong for LA as a cancer chemoprotectant to counter inflammation at the preinitiation or postinitiation stage, there is also evidence that LA may be useful as a cancer chemotherapy, especially as an adjunct with other drugs to increase tumor susceptibility. In this regard, many cancers exhibit the so-called Warburg effect, which confers on the tumor augmented growth characteristics and a competitive advantage over normal somatic tissue. Three recent studies from the same group tested the combination of LA and hydroxycitrate (METABLOC) with the aim of reducing the metabolic activities of pyruvate dehydrogenase kinase and ATP citrate lyase, respectively, in cell culture as well as in xenograft mouse models of lung and bladder carcinomas (Guais et al. 2012; Schwartz et al. 2010; Abolhassani et al. 2011). The METABLOC combination yielded synergistic cell death in T24 human bladder cancer and HT-29 human colon cancer cell lines as compared to controls or either regimen alone (Schwartz et al. 2010); moreover, its combination with cisplatin slowed tumor growth and extended median survival time over the chemotherapeutic agent alone in their model of LL/2 lung carcinoma cells in C57BL/6 mice, but it was less effective in their bladder carcinoma model. Likewise, a lung carcinoma model responded well to METABLOC combined with methotrexate (Guais et al. 2012). METABLOC combined with octreotide significantly reduced tumor growth and extended median survival time in the aforementioned lung carcinoma model as well as other models (Abolhassani et al. 2011). The combination of LA with other cancer drugs has also been extended to the clinical environment. I.v. LA used in conjunction with oral naltrexone (which inhibits opiate receptors) helped treat four cases of complex pancreatic cancer, as described in a recent report (Berkson et al. 2009). Taken together, results from this study and those using animal models suggest that there is enough evidence to support more extensive clinical trials for the use of LA in combination with other drugs to sensitize tumors for more effective chemotherapeutic action.

30.7 IS ORAL LA SAFE AND EFFECTIVE?

For consideration of LA as either a prophylactic nutrient or a chemotherapeutic compound, a thorough understanding of its safe and effective use in vivo is necessary. Actually, LA safety and potential adverse health reactions have already been studied in several clinical trials in North America and Europe. In particular, the Neurological Assessment of Thioctic Acid in Diabetic Neuropathy (NATHAN 1) trial tested the effectiveness of LA to treat diabetic distal symmetric sensorimotor polyneuropathy (DSPN) in a long-term trial. This 4-year study showed that daily oral LA supplementation (600 mg) to more than 200 patients was well tolerated, but some complications relative to a placebo group were noted (Ziegler et al. 2011). Treatment-emergent adverse events included heart rate and rhythm disorders ($P = .047$) as well as myocardial, endocardial, pericardial, and valvular disorders ($P = .088$). Urinary system disorders ($P = .071$) were also noted. However, the incidence of any of these adverse events was quite small. In fact, no significant differences in the particular cardiovascular disorders between the groups were observed. The corrected QT interval (QTc) prolongation >60 ms was significantly more frequent on placebo than that on LA ($P = .0497$). Global assessment of treatment tolerability by investigators and patients showed no differences between the LA and placebo groups. There were a greater number of serious adverse events in the LA group but more deaths in the placebo group, and none of these events reached statistical significance. Thus, long-term supplementation with LA is well tolerated, and potential adverse health reactions appear to be clinically manageable.

However, a note of caution should be sounded for the widespread use of LA as a clinical adjunct for cancer therapies in general. It must be appreciated that if Nrf2, which is induced by LA, can strengthen the defenses of healthy cells, there is also the possibility that LA treatment could make cancer cells more drug resistant via Nrf2 upregulation. Indeed, Nrf2 is upregulated in some cancers (Slocum and Kensler 2011), although in these cases, the upregulation is due to mutations in Nrf2 or Keap1. It would appear that an intact and responsive Keap1/Nrf2 axis in otherwise normal cells does not contribute to cancer formation. Instead, a dysfunction of this system appearing in precancerous or already cancerous cells is the problem. One recent report found that a Keap1 mutation is found in a small percentage of solid tumors, but none of these were coupled with Nrf2 mutations (Yoo et al. 2012).

30.8 CONCLUSIONS AND FUTURE DIRECTIONS

The well-recognized "two-hit" model for carcinogenesis postulates that DNA damage leads to mutations, which may ultimately result in unregulated mitosis and escape from the checks and balances of growth arrest and apoptosis. A permissive microenvironment and epigenetic alterations may also provide an entrée into cancer formation. Throughout this process, it is clear that the primary initiating event(s) often occurs years before manifestation of overt tumorigenesis and is aggravated by inflammation. Thus, a strong rationale has developed toward prevention of initial DNA damage, limiting the risk for progression to mutation and neoplasia. An enormous effort has ensued to define so-called chemoprotectants that can be provided via the diet that could mitigate carcinogen-induced damage. Ideally, chemoprotection would encompass anti-inflammatory as well as detoxification functions.

LA has emerged as a promising chemoprotective agent that has an array of biochemical activities. Its safety has been established through its 40+ years of use as an antidiabetic compound. Much attention has been given lately to the potential role of LA in cancer prevention. Based on the evidence presented herein, we conclude that LA elicits increased phase II detoxification and acts as a potent anti-inflammatory compound, both of which could be envisioned to limit initial damage and/or progression of neoplasia to tumorigenesis. LA may also improve age-associated pathophysiologic conditions such as cardiovascular disease and neuromuscular deficits (Smith et al. 2004; Scott et al. 1994; Devasagayam et al. 1993; Liu et al. 2002; Suh et al. 2004; Lodge et al. 1998; Anuradha and Varalakshmi 1999; Han et al. 1997). Thus, LA should be considered both as a nutritive supplement and as a pharmacotherapeutic agent. We consider this a call to action for the examination of LA in cancer chemoprevention.

However, along with this call, it should be recognized that using LA in cell culture may not reflect its mode of action in vivo. A physiologically achievable plasma concentration of LA after oral dosing is approximately 50–100 μM (reviewed in Shay et al. 2008, 2009). In our hands, cultured primary rat hepatocytes as well as human liver cancer HepG2 cells can tolerate more than 24 h of LA exposure at this low micromolar level (data not shown). However, LA kills cancer cells as well as normal cells in culture at supraphysiological concentrations. In a cell culture model, 500 μM LA caused significant HepG2 cell death after 24 h; smaller concentrations of LA took 48 h to produce significant cell death (Simbula et al. 2007). Additionally, cell culture experiments do not replicate the single-pass clearance of LA via glomerular filtration that would be found in vivo (Harrison and McCormick 1974). In cell culture models, LA is reduced to DHLA and effluxed into the media (Handelman et al. 1994), where it can be taken up again. DHLA has been shown to be more cytotoxic than LA in HL-60 cells (Yamasaki et al. 2009). Thus, caution should be used in drawing conclusions about the usefulness of LA as a cancer therapy based on in vitro data alone. Still, the studies that have emerged in the past 5 years show that LA may be a beneficial adjuvant to chemotherapy in certain human cancers by targeting metabolic pathways and apoptosis-inducing pathways or by inducing cell cycle arrest. The animal studies that have been performed to date are encouraging and suggest there is a need for more extensive studies.

ACKNOWLEDGMENTS

This work was supported by grants from the National Center for Complementary and Alternative Medicine of the National Institutes of Health under award numbers T32 AT002688 (KPS) and P01 AT002034, as well as a grant from the National Institute on Aging of the National Institutes of Health under award number R01 AG017141. The content is solely the responsibility of the authors and does not necessarily represent the official views of the National Institutes of Health.

REFERENCES

Abolhassani, M., A. Guais, E. Sanders, F. Campion, I. Fichtner, J. Bonte, G. Baronzio, G. Fiorentini, M. Israel, and L. Schwartz. 2012. Screening of well-established drugs targeting cancer metabolism: reproducibility of the efficacy of a highly effective drug combination in mice. *Invest New Drugs* 30:1331–42.

Akiba, S., S. Matsugo, L. Packer, and T. Konishi. 1998. Assay of protein-bound lipoic acid in tissues by a new enzymatic method. *Anal Biochem* 258:299–304.

Amenta, F., E. Traini, D. Tomassoni, and F. Mignini. 2008. Pharmacokinetics of different formulations of tioctic (alpha-lipoic) acid in healthy volunteers. *Clin Exp Hypertens* 30:767–75.

Anuradha, B., and P. Varalakshmi. 1999. Protective role of DL-alpha-lipoic acid against mercury-induced neural lipid peroxidation. *Pharmacol Res* 39:67–80.

Arivazhagan, P., S. Shila, S. Kumaran, and C. Panneerselvam. 2002. Effect of DL-alpha-lipoic acid on the status of lipid peroxidation and antioxidant enzymes in various brain regions of aged rats. *Exp Gerontol* 37:803–11.

Bast, A., and G. R. Haenen. 2003. Lipoic acid: a multifunctional antioxidant. *Biofactors* 17:207–13.

Berkson, B. M., D. M. Rubin, and A. J. Berkson. 2009. Revisiting the ALA/N (alpha-lipoic acid/low-dose naltrexone) protocol for people with metastatic and nonmetastatic pancreatic cancer: a report of 3 new cases. *Integr Cancer Ther* 8:416–22.

Bernkop-Schnurch, A., E. Reich-Rohrwig, M. Marschutz, H. Schuhbauer, and M. Kratzel. 2004. Development of a sustained release dosage form for alpha-lipoic acid. II. Evaluation in human volunteers. *Drug Dev Ind Pharm* 30:35–42.

Biewenga, G. P., G. R. Haenen, and A. Bast. 1997. The pharmacology of the antioxidant lipoic acid. *Gen Pharmacol* 29:315–31.

Bogani, P., M. Canavesi, T. M. Hagen, F. Visioli, and S. Bellosta. 2007. Thiol supplementation inhibits metalloproteinase activity independent of glutathione status. *Biochem Biophys Res Commun* 363:651–5.

Breithaupt-Grogler, K., G. Niebch, E. Schneider, K. Erb, R. Hermann, H. H. Blume, B. S. Schug, and G. G. Belz. 1999. Dose-proportionality of oral thioctic acid—coincidence of assessments via pooled plasma and individual data. *Eur J Pharm Sci* 8:57–65.

Carlson, D. A., A. R. Smith, S. J. Fischer, K. L. Young, and L. Packer. 2007. The plasma pharmacokinetics of R-(+)-lipoic acid administered as sodium R-(+)-lipoate to healthy human subjects. *Altern Med Rev* 12:343–51.

Chng, H. T., L. S. New, A. H. Neo, C. W. Goh, E. R. Browne, and E. C. Chan. 2009. Distribution study of orally administered lipoic acid in rat brain tissues. *Brain Res* 1251:80–6.

Cremer, D. R., R. Rabeler, A. Roberts, and B. Lynch. 2006a. Long-term safety of alpha-lipoic acid (ALA) consumption: a 2-year study. *Regul Toxicol Pharmacol* 46:193–201.

Cremer, D. R., R. Rabeler, A. Roberts, and B. Lynch. 2006b. Safety evaluation of alpha-lipoic acid (ALA). *Regul Toxicol Pharmacol* 46:29–41.

Cullinan, S. B., J. D. Gordan, J. Jin, J. W. Harper, and J. A. Diehl. 2004. The Keap1-BTB protein is an adaptor that bridges Nrf2 to a Cul3-based E3 ligase: oxidative stress sensing by a Cul3-Keap1 ligase. *Mol Cell Biol* 24:8477–86.

Devasagayam, T. P., M. Subramanian, D. S. Pradhan, and H. Sies. 1993. Prevention of singlet oxygen–induced DNA damage by lipoate. *Chem Biol Interact* 86:79–92.

Dinkova-Kostova, A. T., W. D. Holtzclaw, R. N. Cole, K. Itoh, N. Wakabayashi, Y. Katoh, M. Yamamoto, and P. Talalay. 2002. Direct evidence that sulfhydryl groups of Keap1 are the sensors regulating induction of phase 2 enzymes that protect against carcinogens and oxidants. *Proc Natl Acad Sci U S A* 99:11908–13.

Egeblad, M., and Z. Werb. 2002. New functions for the matrix metalloproteinases in cancer progression. *Nat Rev Cancer* 2:161–74.

El-Shitany, N. A., S. A. El-Masry, M. A. El-Ghareib, and K. El-Desoky. 2010. Thioctic acid protects against carrageenan-induced acute inflammation in rats by reduction in oxidative stress, downregulation of COX-2 mRNA and enhancement of IL-10 mRNA. *Fundam Clin Pharmacol* 24:91–9.

Elangovan, S., and T. C. Hsieh. 2008. Control of cellular redox status and upregulation of quinone reductase NQO1 via Nrf2 activation by alpha-lipoic acid in human leukemia HL-60 cells. *Int J Oncol* 33:833–8.

Evans, J. L., C. J. Heymann, I. D. Goldfine, and L. A. Gavin. 2002. Pharmacokinetics, tolerability, and fructosamine-lowering effect of a novel, controlled-release formulation of alpha-lipoic acid. *Endocr Pract* 8:29–35.

Flier, J., F. L. Van Muiswinkel, C. A. Jongenelen, and B. Drukarch. 2002. The neuroprotective antioxidant alpha-lipoic acid induces detoxication enzymes in cultured astroglial cells. *Free Radic Res* 36:695–9.

Foster, T. S. 2007. Efficacy and safety of alpha-lipoic acid supplementation in the treatment of symptomatic diabetic neuropathy. *Diabetes Educ* 33:111–7.

Guais, A., G. Baronzio, E. Sanders, F. Campion, C. Mainini, G. Fiorentini, F. Montagnani, M. Behzadi, L. Schwartz, and M. Abolhassani. 2012. Adding a combination of hydroxycitrate and lipoic acid (METABLOC) to chemotherapy improves effectiveness against tumor development: experimental results and case report. *Invest New Drugs* 30:200–11.

Haenen, G. R., and A. Bast. 1991. Scavenging of hypochlorous acid by lipoic acid. *Biochem Pharmacol* 42:2244–6.

Han, D., C. K. Sen, S. Roy, M. S. Kobayashi, H. J. Tritschler, and L. Packer. 1997. Protection against glutamate-induced cytotoxicity in C6 glial cells by thiol antioxidants. *Am J Physiol* 273:R1771–8.

Handelman, G. J., D. Han, H. Tritschler, and L. Packer. 1994. Alpha-lipoic acid reduction by mammalian cells to the dithiol form, and release into the culture medium. *Biochem Pharmacol* 47:1725–30.

Harrison, E. H., and D. B. McCormick. 1974. The metabolism of DL-(1,6-14C)lipoic acid in the rat. *Arch Biochem Biophys* 160:514–22.

Ho, Y. S., C. S. Lai, H. I. Liu, S. Y. Ho, C. Tai, M. H. Pan, and Y. J. Wang. 2007. Dihydrolipoic acid inhibits skin tumor promotion through anti-inflammation and anti-oxidation. *Biochem Pharmacol* 73:1786–95.

Hu, R., C. L. Saw, R. Yu, and A. N. Kong. 2010. Regulation of NF-E2–related factor 2 signaling for cancer chemoprevention: antioxidant coupled with antiinflammatory. *Antioxid Redox Signal* 13:1679–98.

Hua, H., M. Li, T. Luo, Y. Yin, and Y. Jiang. 2011. Matrix metalloproteinases in tumorigenesis: an evolving paradigm. *Cell Mol Life Sci* 68:3853–68.

Jain, A. K., D. A. Bloom, and A. K. Jaiswal. 2005. Nuclear import and export signals in control of Nrf2. *J Biol Chem* 280:29158–68.

Jaiswal, A. K. 2004. Nrf2 signaling in coordinated activation of antioxidant gene expression. *Free Radic Biol Med* 36:1199–207.

Kang, K. P., D. H. Kim, Y. J. Jung, A. S. Lee, S. Lee, S. Y. Lee, K. Y. Jang, M. J. Sung, S. K. Park, and W. Kim. 2009. Alpha-lipoic acid attenuates cisplatin-induced acute kidney injury in mice by suppressing renal inflammation. *Nephrol Dial Transplant* 24:3012–20.

Khabbazi, T., R. Mahdavi, J. Safa, and P. Pour-Abdollahi. 2012. Effects of Alpha-lipoic acid supplementation on inflammation, oxidative stress, and serum lipid profile levels in patients with end-stage renal disease on hemodialysis. *J Ren Nutr* 22:244–50.

Kobayashi, A., M. I. Kang, H. Okawa, M. Ohtsuji, Y. Zenke, T. Chiba, K. Igarashi, and M. Yamamoto. 2004. Oxidative stress sensor Keap1 functions as an adaptor for Cul3-based E3 ligase to regulate proteasomal degradation of Nrf2. *Mol Cell Biol* 24:7130–9.

Kobayashi, A., M. I. Kang, Y. Watai, K. I. Tong, T. Shibata, K. Uchida, and M. Yamamoto. 2006. Oxidative and electrophilic stresses activate Nrf2 through inhibition of ubiquitination activity of Keap1. *Mol Cell Biol* 26:221–9.

Kundu, J. K., and Y. J. Surh. 2010. Nrf2–Keap1 signaling as a potential target for chemoprevention of inflammation-associated carcinogenesis. *Pharm Res* 27:999–1013.

Lee, H. S., M. H. Na, and W. K. Kim. 2010. Alpha-lipoic acid reduces matrix metalloproteinase activity in MDA-MB-231 human breast cancer cells. *Nutr Res* 30:403–9.

Lee, J. M., and J. A. Johnson. 2004. An important role of Nrf2–ARE pathway in the cellular defense mechanism. *J Biochem Mol Biol* 37:139–43.

Liu, G. H., J. Qu, and X. Shen. 2008. NF-kappaB/p65 antagonizes Nrf2–ARE pathway by depriving CBP from Nrf2 and facilitating recruitment of HDAC3 to MafK. *Biochim Biophys Acta* 1783:713–27.

Liu, J., E. Head, A. M. Gharib, W. Yuan, R. T. Ingersoll, T. M. Hagen, C. W. Cotman, and B. N. Ames. 2002. Memory loss in old rats is associated with brain mitochondrial decay and RNA/DNA oxidation: partial reversal by feeding acetyl-L-carnitine and/or R-alpha-lipoic acid. *Proc Natl Acad Sci U S A* 99:2356–61.

Lodge, J. K., M. G. Traber, and L. Packer. 1998. Thiol chelation of Cu2+ by dihydrolipoic acid prevents human low density lipoprotein peroxidation. *Free Radic Biol Med* 25:287–97.

Mans, D. R., A. B. da Rocha, and G. Schwartsmann. 2000. Anti-cancer drug discovery and development in Brazil: targeted plant collection as a rational strategy to acquire candidate anti-cancer compounds. *Oncologist* 5:185–98.

Mao, L., H. Wang, L. Qiao, and X. Wang. 2010. Disruption of Nrf2 enhances the upregulation of nuclear factor-kappaB activity, tumor necrosis factor-alpha, and matrix metalloproteinase-9 after spinal cord injury in mice. *Mediators Inflamm* 2010:238321.

Mao, L., H. Wang, X. Wang, H. Liao, and X. Zhao. 2011. Transcription factor Nrf2 protects the spinal cord from inflammation produced by spinal cord injury. *J Surg Res* 170:e105–15.

Mignini, F., M. Capacchietti, V. Napolioni, G. Reggiardo, R. Fasani, and P. Ferrari. 2011. Single dose bioavailability and pharmacokinetic study of a innovative formulation of alpha-lipoic acid (ALA600) in healthy volunteers. *Minerva Med* 102:475–82.

Mignini, F., V. Streccioni, D. Tomassoni, E. Traini, and F. Amenta. 2007. Comparative crossover, randomized, open-label bioequivalence study on the bioequivalence of two formulations of thioctic acid in healthy volunteers. *Clin Exp Hypertens* 29:575–86.

Neurath, M. F., and S. Finotto. 2011. IL-6 signaling in autoimmunity, chronic inflammation and inflammation-associated cancer. *Cytokine Growth Factor Rev* 22:83–9.

Nguyen, T., P. J. Sherratt, H. C. Huang, C. S. Yang, and C. B. Pickett. 2003. Increased protein stability as a mechanism that enhances Nrf2-mediated transcriptional activation of the antioxidant response element. Degradation of Nrf2 by the 26 S proteasome. *J Biol Chem* 278:4536–41.

Odabasoglu, F., Z. Halici, H. Aygun, M. Halici, F. Atalay, A. Cakir, E. Cadirci, Y. Bayir, and H. Suleyman. 2011. Alpha-lipoic acid has anti-inflammatory and anti-oxidative properties: an experimental study in rats with carrageenan-induced acute and cotton pellet–induced chronic inflammations. *Br J Nutr* 105:31–43.

Ogborne, R. M., S. A. Rushworth, and M. A. O'Connell. 2005. Alpha-lipoic acid–induced heme oxygenase-1 expression is mediated by nuclear factor erythroid 2–related factor 2 and p38 mitogen-activated protein kinase in human monocytic cells. *Arterioscler Thromb Vasc Biol* 25:2100–5.

Packer, L., K. Kraemer, and G. Rimbach. 2001. Molecular aspects of lipoic acid in the prevention of diabetes complications. *Nutrition* 17:888–95.

Palsamy, P., and S. Subramanian. 2011. Resveratrol protects diabetic kidney by attenuating hyperglycemia-mediated oxidative stress and renal inflammatory cytokines via Nrf2–Keap1 signaling. *Biochim Biophys Acta* 1812:719–31.

Pan, H., H. Wang, L. Zhu, L. Mao, L. Qiao, and X. Su. 2011. Depletion of Nrf2 enhances inflammation induced by oxyhemoglobin in cultured mice astrocytes. *Neurochem Res* 36:2434–41.

Panigrahi, M., Y. Sadguna, B. R. Shivakumar, S. V. Kolluri, S. Roy, L. Packer, and V. Ravindranath. 1996. Alpha-lipoic acid protects against reperfusion injury following cerebral ischemia in rats. *Brain Res* 717:184–8.

Reddy, N. M., H. R. Potteti, T. J. Mariani, S. Biswal, and S. P. Reddy. 2011. Conditional deletion of Nrf2 in airway epithelium exacerbates acute lung injury and impairs the resolution of inflammation. *Am J Respir Cell Mol Biol* 45:1161–8.

Reed, L. J. 1974. Multienzyme complexes. *Accts Chem Res* 7:40–6.

Schwartz, L., M. Abolhassani, A. Guais, E. Sanders, J. M. Steyaert, F. Campion, and M. Israel. 2010. A combination of alpha lipoic acid and calcium hydroxycitrate is efficient against mouse cancer models: Preliminary results. *Oncol Rep* 23:1407–16.

Scott, B. C., O. I. Aruoma, P. J. Evans, C. O'Neill, A. Van der Vliet, C. E. Cross, H. Tritschler, and B. Halliwell. 1994. Lipoic and dihydrolipoic acids as antioxidants. A critical evaluation. *Free Radic Res* 20:119–33.

Searls, R. L., and D. R. Sanadi. 1960. Alpha-ketoglutaric dehydrogenase. 8. Isolation and some properties of a flavoprotein component. *J Biol Chem* 235:2485–91.

Sethi, G., M. K. Shanmugam, L. Ramachandran, A. P. Kumar, and V. Tergaonkar. 2012. Multifaceted link between cancer and inflammation. *Biosci Rep* 32:1–15.

Shay, K. P., R. F. Moreau, E. J. Smith, and T. M. Hagen. 2008. Is alpha-lipoic acid a scavenger of reactive oxygen species in vivo? Evidence for its initiation of stress signaling pathways that promote endogenous antioxidant capacity. *IUBMB Life* 60:362–7.

Shay, K. P., R. F. Moreau, E. J. Smith, A. R. Smith, and T. M. Hagen. 2009. Alpha-lipoic acid as a dietary supplement: molecular mechanisms and therapeutic potential. *Biochim Biophys Acta* 1790:1149–60.

Shenvi, S. V., E. J. Smith, and T. M. Hagen. 2009. Transcriptional regulation of rat gamma-glutamate cysteine ligase catalytic subunit gene is mediated through a distal antioxidant response element. *Pharmacol Res* 60:229–36.

Simbula, G., A. Columbano, G. M. Ledda-Columbano, L. Sanna, M. Deidda, A. Diana, and M. Pibiri. 2007. Increased ROS generation and p53 activation in alpha-lipoic acid–induced apoptosis of hepatoma cells. *Apoptosis* 12:113–23.

Slocum, S. L., and T. W. Kensler. 2011. Nrf2: control of sensitivity to carcinogens. *Arch Toxicol* 85:273–84.

Smith, A. R., S. V. Shenvi, M. Widlansky, J. H. Suh, and T. M. Hagen. 2004. Lipoic acid as a potential therapy for chronic diseases associated with oxidative stress. *Curr Med Chem* 11:1135–46.

Sola, S., M. Q. Mir, F. A. Cheema, N. Khan-Merchant, R. G. Menon, S. Parthasarathy, and B. V. Khan. 2005. Irbesartan and lipoic acid improve endothelial function and reduce markers of inflammation in the metabolic syndrome: results of the Irbesartan and Lipoic Acid in Endothelial Dysfunction (ISLAND) study. *Circulation* 111:343–8.

Suh, J. H., S. V. Shenvi, B. M. Dixon, H. Liu, A. K. Jaiswal, R. M. Liu, and T. M. Hagen. 2004. Decline in transcriptional activity of Nrf2 causes age-related loss of glutathione synthesis, which is reversible with lipoic acid. *Proc Natl Acad Sci U S A* 101:3381–6.

Suzuki, Y. J., M. Tsuchiya, and L. Packer. 1991. Thioctic acid and dihydrolipoic acid are novel antioxidants which interact with reactive oxygen species. *Free Radic Res Commun* 15:255–63.

Suzuki, Y. J., M. Tsuchiya, and L. Packer. 1993. Antioxidant activities of dihydrolipoic acid and its structural homologues. *Free Radic Res Commun* 18:115–22.

Teichert, J., R. Hermann, P. Ruus, and R. Preiss. 2003. Plasma kinetics, metabolism, and urinary excretion of alpha-lipoic acid following oral administration in healthy volunteers. *J Clin Pharmacol* 43:1257–67.

Teichert, J., J. Kern, H. J. Tritschler, H. Ulrich, and R. Preiss. 1998. Investigations on the pharmacokinetics of alpha-lipoic acid in healthy volunteers. *Int J Clin Pharmacol Ther* 36:625–8.

Teichert, J., T. Tuemmers, H. Achenbach, C. Preiss, R. Hermann, P. Ruus, and R. Preiss. 2005. Pharmacokinetics of alpha-lipoic acid in subjects with severe kidney damage and end-stage renal disease. *J Clin Pharmacol* 45:313–28.

Van der Heiden, K., S. Cuhlmann, A. Luong Le, M. Zakkar, and P. C. Evans. 2010. Role of nuclear factor kappaB in cardiovascular health and disease. *Clin Sci (Lond)* 118:593–605.

Wakabayashi, N., K. Itoh, J. Wakabayashi, H. Motohashi, S. Noda, S. Takahashi, S. Imakado, T. Kotsuji, F. Otsuka, D. R. Roop, T. Harada, J. D. Engel, and M. Yamamoto. 2003. Keap1-null mutation leads to postnatal lethality due to constitutive Nrf2 activation. *Nat Genet* 35:238–45.

Wollin, S. D., and P. J. Jones. 2003. Alpha-lipoic acid and cardiovascular disease. *J Nutr* 133:3327–30.

Yamasaki, M., A. Kawabe, K. Nishimoto, H. Madhyastha, Y. Sakakibara, M. Suiko, T. Okamoto, T. Suda, K. Uehira, and K. Nishiyama. 2009. Dihydro-alpha-lipoic acid has more potent cytotoxicity than alpha-lipoic acid. *In Vitro Cell Dev Biol Anim* 45:275–80.

Yan, L. J., M. G. Traber, H. Kobuchi, S. Matsugo, H. J. Tritschler, and L. Packer. 1996. Efficacy of hypochlorous acid scavengers in the prevention of protein carbonyl formation. *Arch Biochem Biophys* 327:330–4.

Ying, Z., T. Kampfrath, Q. Sun, S. Parthasarathy, and S. Rajagopalan. 2011. Evidence that alpha-lipoic acid inhibits NF-kappaB activation independent of its antioxidant function. *Inflamm Res* 60:219–25.

Ying, Z., N. Kherada, B. Farrar, T. Kampfrath, Y. Chung, O. Simonetti, J. Deiuliis, R. Desikan, B. Khan, F. Villamena, Q. Sun, S. Parthasarathy, and S. Rajagopalan. 2010. Lipoic acid effects on established atherosclerosis. *Life Sci* 86:95–102.

Yoo, N. J., H. R. Kim, Y. R. Kim, C. H. An, and S. H. Lee. 2012. Somatic mutations of the KEAP1 gene in common solid cancers. *Histopathology* 60:943–52.

Zhang, D. D., and M. Hannink. 2003. Distinct cysteine residues in Keap1 are required for Keap1-dependent ubiquitination of Nrf2 and for stabilization of Nrf2 by chemopreventive agents and oxidative stress. *Mol Cell Biol* 23:8137–51.

Zhang, W. J., and B. Frei. 2001. Alpha-lipoic acid inhibits TNF-alpha–induced NF-kappaB activation and adhesion molecule expression in human aortic endothelial cells. *Faseb J* 15:2423–32.

Ziegler, D., P. A. Low, W. J. Litchy, A. J. Boulton, A. I. Vinik, R. Freeman, R. Samigullin, H. Tritschler, U. Munzel, J. Maus, K. Schutte, and P. J. Dyck. 2011. Efficacy and safety of antioxidant treatment with alpha-lipoic acid over 4 years in diabetic polyneuropathy: the NATHAN 1 trial. *Diabetes Care* 34:2054–60.

Section IX

Epigenetics and Chronic Inflammation

31 Epigenetic Modifications by Dietary Phytochemicals in Cancer Prevention

Tabitha M. Hardy and Trygve O. Tollefsbol

CONTENTS

31.1 INTRODUCTION

It is now apparent that dietary phytochemicals can alter gene expression, interact with the genome and epigenome, augment protein composition, and modify epigenetic states (Subbiah and Ravi 2008; Robert 2006). While many dietary agents have been deemed harmful in excess (e.g., salt, fats, oils), several have advantageous effects. These dietary compounds are of particular interest in the prevention of diseases, including cancer, which is often thought of as both a genetic and epigenetic disease. Epigenetic alterations associated with human disease can be influenced by environmental factors and may be, at least in part, mediated by diet (Skinner and Guerrero-Bosagna 2009; Jaenisch and Bird 2003; Hardy and Tollefsbol 2011; Riley and Anderson 2011).

31.2 CANCER-RELATED EPIGENETIC MODIFICATIONS

The study of epigenetics involves heritable changes in gene expression and chromatin organization that do not include changes in the actual DNA sequence (Waddington 1942). Interestingly, epigenetic modifications are frequently reversible and are potentially important in disease prevention and therapeutics (Berger et al. 2009). DNA methylation, histone modification, and alterations to microRNA (miRNA) expression are the most common methods of epigenetic modification. Briefly, DNA methylation involves the transfer of a methyl group to the 5-carbon (C^5) of cytosine and is normally associated with a condensed chromatin state and the silencing of genes. DNA methylation

is catalyzed by DNA methyltransferases (DNMTs) that hypermethylate cytosine phosphate guanine (CpG) dinucleotides, typically promoting gene silencing and inactivation. There are four
known DNMTs: DNMT1, DNMT2, DNMT3A, and DNMT3B all of which are similar in sequence
and phylogenic analysis; however, DNMT2 appears to have very little DNA methylation activity
(Jurkowski and Jeltsch 2011). Aberrant DNA methylation and DNMT expression are often seen in
disease states. Reversing them may be the key to determining the mechanisms by which epigenetic
modifications occur.

Histone modifications, including lysine acetylation, lysine and arginine methylation, phosphorylation of serine and threonine, lysine biotinylation, lysine ubiquitination, and sumoylation, occur
at the N-terminal tails of histones (Hassan and Zempleni 2006; Feinberg, Ohlsson, and Henikoff
2006; Doi et al. 2009). The modification of histones has differential effects and may indirectly affect
chromatin function and gene regulation (Jenuwein and Allis 2001; Meeran et al. 2011). Histone
methylation can influence chromatin structure and function by adding methyl residues to lysine and
arginine amino acids. The acetylation of histones causes an open conformation of chromatin that
allows for transcription and gene expression (Kouzarides 2007). Enzymes such as histone methyltransferases (HMTs), histone acetyltransferases (HATs), histone demethylases (HDMs), and histone
deacetyltransferases (HDACs) act to catalyze histone modifications. HMTs and HATs add methyl or
acetyl groups to histones, while HDMs and HDACs remove them, respectively.

Noncoding miRNAs are composed of 18–30 RNA nucleotides that act to regulate gene expression
and are involved in chromatin remodeling and DNA methylation in cancer cells (Fabbri et al. 2007;
Friedman, Liang, and Jones 2009; Parasramka et al. 2012). miRNAs target untranslated regions of
messenger RNAs (mRNAs) and may target multiple transcripts simultaneously (Brennecke et al.
2005). Several investigations have indicated that miRNAs can operate as epigenetic modulators by
regulating *DNMTs* and other cancer-related genes (Lujambio et al. 2008; Liang et al. 2008; Yavari et
al. 2010). Additionally, miRNAs can bring about the inhibition of mRNA translation and the silencing of transcription (Ducasse and Brown 2006; Guil and Esteller 2009). A number of miRNAs are
upregulated or downregulated throughout the various stages of cancer, and global downregulation
of miRNAs has been observed in cancer cells (Taby and Issa 2010; Lu et al. 2009).

31.3 EPIGENETIC MODULATION OF CANCER BY DIETARY PHYTOCHEMICALS

Many phytochemicals from nutrients found in plants have been found to have beneficial effects on
the body when consumed. In particular, compounds from vegetables and fruits have been studied
extensively for their preventive and epigenetic effect (Weinstein 1991). Dietary phytochemicals are
vital in carrying out normal biological functions and have been of interest in the field of epigenetics.
Numerous investigations have described epigenetic alterations modified by dietary factors, focusing
on their ability to act as histone modifiers and DNMT inhibitors. This has become an important area
of study as the majority of these bioactive phytochemicals potentially play a role in cancer prevention. The chemopreventive effects of several dietary phytochemicals are thought to protect against
the development of tumors and inhibit or prevent cancer initiation and progression (Ip, Dong, and
Ganther 2002; Cheung and Kong 2010; Sarkar and Li 2002). Dietary polyphenols are also attractive therapeutic agents because of their low rate of toxicity and their ability to reverse epigenetic
modifications affecting aberrantly expressed genes (Li and Tollefsbol 2010). Also, *in vivo* and *in
vitro* investigations have demonstrated that several dietary components can inhibit cancer cell proliferation (Berletch et al. 2008; Mittal et al. 2004). Herein we will discuss the preventive properties
of several classes of dietary phytochemicals and their effects on epigenetic modifiers.

31.4 POLYPHENOLIC PHYTOCHEMICALS

Polyphenols are prevalent in fruits and vegetables. These dietary components develop from either
shikimic acid or phenylalanine and contain a hydroxyl group attached to one or more sugar residues.

TABLE 31.1
Categories of Dietary Phytochemicals

Categories of Phytochemicals	Primary Dietary Sources	Chemopreventive Epigenetic Properties
Polyphenols	Green tea, turmeric, curry, soybeans, kudzu, fava beans, grapes, red wine, peanuts, mulberry, cranberry, blueberry	DNMT, HAT, and HDAC inhibitors; modify miRNA
Organosulfur compounds	Broccoli, cabbage, kale, mushrooms, onions, watercress, garlic, Brazilian nuts, chicken, game meat, beef	DNMT and HDAC inhibitors
Carotenoids	Carrots, squash, tomatoes, corn, spinach	Induce DNA methylation and demethylation; modify histones
Alkaloids	Coffee, cocaine, nicotine, morphine, vincristine	Inhibit DNA methylation

Polyphenols make up one of the largest and most numerous categories of phytochemicals. Over 8000 dietary sources of polyphenols are believed to exist, and there are at least 10 classes of polyphenolic compounds, a number of which will be discussed (Table 31.1) (Bravo 1998).

31.4.1 GREEN TEA POLYPHENOLS

Polyphenolic compounds from teas are currently of interest because of their antioxidant, antiinflammatory, and chemopreventive properties (Relja et al. 2012; Du et al. 2009; Yang, Lambert, and Sang 2009). Catechins including (–)-epicatechin (EC), (–)-epicatechin-3-gallate (ECG), (–)-epigallocatechin (EGC), and (–)-epigallocatechin-3-gallate (EGCG) from teas have been investigated for their potential as demethylating agents (Fang, Chen, and Yang 2007; Fang et al. 2003). In addition, green tea polyphenol (GTP) treatment of cancer cells has been effective in the reactivation of silenced genes associated with tumorigenesis (Pandey, Shukla, and Gupta 2010). *In vivo* investigations involving GTPs have confirmed their effectiveness as dietary inhibitors of carcinogenesis (Tran et al. 2010; Zhang et al. 2010). The catechin EGCG comprises more than 50% of the bioactive components of green tea (Lin, Liang, and Lin-Shiau 1999). Numerous investigations have explored the chemopreventive properties of EGCG and the correlation between EGCG consumption and the inhibition of certain cancers (Chen et al. 2011; Tu et al. 2011; Kürbitz et al. 2011; Kim, Amin, and Shin 2010). The anticarcinogenic capabilities of EGCG occur through its ability to inhibit cancer cell proliferation, oxidative stress, migration, and angiogenesis (Yang, Lambert, and Sang 2009; Balasubramanian, Adhikary, and Eckert 2010; Farabegoli et al. 2007; Singh, Shankar, and Srivastava 2011). Additionally, EGCG can prompt cell cycle arrest and apoptosis as well as regulate signal transduction (Kang et al. 2010; Deng and Lin 2011).

EGCG is the most efficient of the catechins at targeting DNMTs. This compound directly inhibits DNMT activity by forming hydrogen bonds within the catalytic pocket of DNMTs, leading to demethylation and reactivation of methylation-silenced genes (Fang, Chen, and Yang 2007; Lee, Shim, and Zhu 2005; Lin, Liang, and Lin-Shiau 1999). In fact, the epigenetic modification of DNMTs by EGCG has made it a promising agent for cancer therapeutics. EGCG treatment of esophageal cells decreased DNMT activity in a time- and dose-dependent manner and reversed the hypermethylation of several tumor suppressor genes, allowing for their reactivation (Fang, Chen, and Yang 2007). Additionally, EGCG has also been found to reactivate *estrogen receptor* α (*ER-α*) in breast cancer cells and tumor suppressor proteins *p16* and *p21* in skin cancer cells (Li et al. 2010; Nandakumar, Vaid, and Katiyar 2011). In oral cancer cells, EGCG is responsible for partially reversing the hypermethylation of the reversion-inducing-cytosine-rich protein with kazal motifs (*RECK*) tumor suppressor gene (Kato et al. 2008). EGCG has also demonstrated its ability to epigenetically modify the methylation of the promoter regions of cancer-related genes including *Wnt inhibitory factor-1 (WIF-1)* and human telomerase reverse transcriptase (*hTERT*), the catalytic subunit of telomerase (Gao et al. 2009; Berletch et al. 2008). Furthermore, synthetic analogs of EGCG produced to increase efficacy and stability also reveal compelling evidence of anticarcinogenic activities (Lam et al. 2004; Meeran et al. 2011; Landis-Piwowar et al. 2007). EGCG also affects miRNA expression in hepatocellular carcinoma cells and has been identified as a HAT inhibitor (Choi et al. 2009).

31.4.2 ISOFLAVONES

Isoflavones are polyphenolic compounds found in kudzu, fava beans, and soybeans. The dietary compound genistein is perhaps the most investigated of this category. Genistein is primarily found in soybeans and functions to manipulate epigenetic events by activating and enhancing histone acetylation and HAT activity by regulating miRNA expression and by inhibiting DNMTs (Fang et al. 2005; Yu. Li et al. 2009; Barnes 1995; Yi. Li et al. 2009; Parker et al. 2009). Similar to other polyphenolic dietary compounds, genistein has anticarcinogenic properties and is believed to have chemopreventive effects on colon, prostate, esophageal, and cervical cancer cells (Barnes 1995). In prostate cancer cells, genistein treatment alters the histone and promoter methylation of *p16* and *p21* tumor suppressor genes. Additionally, genistein has been shown to inhibit DNMT activity and reactivate the expression of *p16,* O6-methylguanine-DNA methyltransferase (*MGMT*), and retinoic acid receptor β (*RARβ*) in prostate and esophageal carcinomas (Fang et al. 2005; Majid et al. 2008). Genistein also appears to inhibit the expression of *hTERT, DNMT1, DNMT3a,* and DNMT*3b* (Yu. Li et al. 2009). The estrogen-like properties of genistein have made its consumption of some concern in women who are at high risk of breast cancer and for patients with tumors sensitive to estrogen; however, low concentrations of genistein do seem to be effective and can demethylate the promoter of G1 to S phase transition 1 (*GSPT1*), which functions to protect cells from carcinogens and cytotoxins (Pandey, Shukla, and Gupta 2010). Moreover, collectively, isoflavones act in a chemopreventive manner in clinical trials. In studies conducted by Qin et al. (2009), healthy premenopausal women received either low (40 mg) or high (140 mg) doses of isoflavones daily through one menstrual cycle. Results indicate that cancer-related genes *RARβ2* and cyclin D2 (*CCND2*) were hypermethylated after treatment, possibly silencing gene activation (Qin et al. 2009).

31.4.3 RESVERATROL

Resveratrol is categorized as a stilbene and is a dietary polyphenol found most abundantly in grape skins and several other plants (Das, Mukherjee, and Ray 2010). Resveratrol can also be consumed in red wine and displays antioxidant, anti-inflammatory, and anticarcinogenic qualities. Furthermore, resveratrol has demonstrated an ability to inhibit cancer cell proliferation and inhibit cancer cell migration and metastasis *in vivo* and *in vitro* (Wu et al. 2008; Weng et al. 2010; Jang et al. 1997). Compared to other dietary compounds, resveratrol shows less DNMT inhibition than other polyphenols, including EGCG, but does inhibit DNMTs and methyl binding domain 2 (MBD2) proteins in breast cancer cells (Papoutsis et al. 2010). Moreover, resveratrol was able to prevent the silencing of tumor suppressor gene breast cancer 1, early onset (*BRCA1*) in breast cancer cells (Papoutsis et al. 2010). Although resveratrol is capable of affecting the methylation status of cancer-associated genes, its most promising feature as an epigenetic compound is its ability to augment histone acetylation and activate HDAC inhibitors *p300* and sirtuin [silent mating type informtion regulation 2 homolog 1 (*SIRT1*) Wang et al. 2008]. In fact, enhanced *p53* tumor suppressor gene acetylation is seen upon resveratrol treatment in prostate cancer cells, and *SIRT1* H3 acetylation is known to influence BRCA1 signaling in breast cancer cells (Howitz et al. 2003; Wang et al. 2008). Resveratrol-mediated activation of *SIRT1* also regulates Survivin, an antiapoptotic protein, through histone 3 lysine 9 (H3K9) deacetylation (Stünkel et al. 2007).

31.4.4 CURCUMIN

The polyphenolic dietary compound curcumin is the primary component of turmeric, a spice from the plant *Curcuma longa*. Curcumin has been used as a therapeutic compound in Indian and Chinese medicine and exhibits anti-inflammatory, antioxidant, antiangiogenic, and anticancer properties (Maheshwari et al. 2006; Goel and Aggarwal 2010). In addition, curcumin acts to modify histone activity and methylation in a number of systems. The DNMT inhibitor activity of curcumin stems from its ability to covalently block DNMT1 (Liu et al. 2009; Kuck et al. 2010). Global hypomethylation of leukemia cells and decreased global histone H3 and H4 acetylation in brain cells are seen after curcumin treatments, indicating that curcumin may also have effects on the epigenome (Liu et al. 2005; Kang, Cha, and Jeon 2006). Curcumin affects cell signaling pathways involved in apoptosis and cell cycle arrest and has shown potential as an inhibitor of *p300* activity in cancer cells (Reuter et al. 2008; Marcu et al. 2006; Balasubramanyam et al. 2004). *In vivo* studies involving curcumin allude to it as an inhibitor of both HATs and HDACs, which may make curcumin an agent of further interest in chemoprevention (Morimoto et al. 2008).

31.5 ORGANOSULFUR COMPOUNDS

Organosulfur compounds contain sulfur and are classified according to their functional groups. Common organosulfur compounds include garlic, mushrooms, cabbage, and onions, many of which are being investigated for their usage as anti-inflammatory and anticarcinogenic agents (Table 31.1). Dietary phytochemicals that are categorized as isothiocyanates contain sulfur and an additional functional group ($N = C = S$), which is typically found in cruciferous vegetables including kale, cabbage, and broccoli (Cheung and Kong 2010). In general, isothiocyanates display proapoptotic and antitumorigenic properties and exhibit inhibitory effects on cancer cell growth (Fimognari, Lenzi, and Hrelia 2008). In fact, a common isothiocyanate found in watercress, phenylethyl isothiocyanate (PEITC), has demonstrated demethylation activity and has the ability to reactivate silenced *GSTP1* genes (Wang et al. 2008). Additionally, allyl isothiocyanate (AITC), prevalent in broccoli, reportedly increases histone acetylation erythroleukemia *in vivo* (Zhang 2010; Lea et al. 2001). Histone hyperacetylation of myeloma cells has been observed after treatment with the synthetic phenylhexyl isothiocyanate (PHI). PHI also acts as an HDAC inhibitor and is involved in chromatin remodeling and *p21* activation (Lu et al. 2008). Sulforaphane (SFN), which is consumed in cruciferous vegetables like broccoli sprouts, exhibits anticarcinogenic and proapoptotic properties and is likely one of the most thoroughly investigated isothiocyanates (Higdon et al. 2007; Pledgie-Tracy, Sobolewski, and Davidson 2007; Bhamre et al. 2009). In addition, SFN also functions as an HDAC inhibitor in cancer cells and in human subjects (Myzak et al. 2007). SFN also inhibits DNMTs in breast cancer cells and inhibits the expression of *hTERT*, the catalytic subunit of telomerase, which is overexpressed in 90% of all cancers (Marcu et al. 2006; Dashwood and Ho 2008).

Allylic sulfur compounds found in garlics are also considered to be organosulfur compounds. Early investigations involving consumption of garlic and other sulfur compounds show reduced carcinogenic tumor induction in mammary, colon, skin, liver, esophageal, and stomach cells (El-Bayoumy et al. 2006). Compounds containing garlic extracts have been effective in cancer treatment and prevention *in vitro* and *in vivo* and work to induce apoptosis and inhibit the cell cycle and angiogenesis (Nian et al. 2009; Lea et al. 2001, 2010). Cancer cells treated with garlic compounds reveal the induction of histone acetylation and histone deacetylase inhibition (Alpers 2009; Nian et al. 2008). Garlic also contains a number of other compounds that may contribute to its anticancer activity, including small amounts of selenium (Se) (Morris and Levander 1970). Se is a sulfur-related nutrient found in soil and in beef, chicken, and Brazilian nuts. Se exists in various organic forms, several of which are thought to provide antioxidant effects and a protective function, particularly in carcinogenesis. In clinical trials to determine the effects of Se in nonmelanoma skin cancers, Se treatments given daily for 4.5 years show a 44% decrease in the incidence of secondary lung cancer (Clark et al. 1996). In a double-blind cancer prevention trial conducted by Clark et al. (1998), a 63% reduction in prostate cancer incidence was observed among patients given Se-enriched foods. Combination treatments of Se and genistein induce growth arrest in both hormone-dependent and hormone-independent prostate cancer cells, revealing its therapeutic potential (Kumi-Diaka et al. 2010). Se has also been shown to inhibit DNMT1 and histone deacetylase activity in prostate cancer cells, which may provide a mechanism for its chemopreventive qualities (Uthus, Yokoi, and Davis 2002).

31.6 CAROTENOIDS

Carotenoids are synthesized by plants, algae, and photosynthetic bacteria that produce hues of yellow, orange, and red found in carrots, tomatoes, corn, and many other fruits and vegetables (Table 31.1). Certain classes of carotenoids are categorized as provitamin A carotenoids that can be converted into retinol (vitamin A). Provitamin A carotenoids, including α- and β-carotenes (found in carrots, squash, spinach, etc.), along with carotenoids that are not converted to vitamin A are being investigated for their chemopreventive potential (Johanning and Piyathilake 2003). Chemopreventive studies involving carotenoids produced varied results depending on the carotenoid and the type of cancer. Investigations involving β-carotenes in human lung and prostate cancers showed very little anticancer activity but were found to reduce disease risk in breast and bladder cancers and inhibited the metastasis of melanoma cells to the lungs in C57Bl/6 mice, while lycopene, a compound found primarily in tomatoes, appears to decrease metalloproteinase and vascular endothelial growth factor (*VEGF*) levels (Pradeep and Kuttan 2003; Huang, Liao, and Hu 2008). Lycopene was effective in inhibiting metastasis in lung cancer cells in nude mice, and both lycopene and β-carotene appear to inhibit growth of hormone-independent prostate cancer cells (Yang et al. 2011).

While little is known about the effects of lycopene and epigenetic modifications, retinoic acid, an active metabolite of vitamin A, is thought to induce DNA methylation and histone modifications. Investigations by Di Croce et al. determined that retinoic acid treatment induced promoter demethylation, gene repression, and phenotype reversal in leukemia-promoting fusion proteins (Di Croce et al. 2002). Further investigations also indicate that retinoic acid reactivates the *RARβ2* tumor suppressor gene by inducing histone acetylation (Sirchia et al. 2002).

31.7 ALKALOIDS

Alkaloids are naturally occurring compounds that contain basic nitrogen atoms and are produced by both plants and animals. Caffeine, cocaine, nicotine, morphine, chemotherapeutic agents (i.e., vincristine), and other pharmacological drugs serve as examples of alkaloids (Table 31.1). Although some alkaloids are thought to be oncogenic, investigations into the anticarcinogenic properties of caffeine reveal tumor volume decreases and inhibition of metastasis in mice after caffeine is administered (André 2009; Yang et al. 2005). Furthermore, caffeic acids appear to be demethylating agents. Caffeic acid treatment of breast cancer cells shows concentration-dependent inhibition of DNA methylation and partial methylation inhibition of the *RARβ* promoter region (Lee and Zhu 2006).

31.8 CONCLUSIONS AND PERSPECTIVES

Dietary phytochemicals are of vital importance to normal physiological development. Therefore, it is not surprising that naturally occurring compounds hold significance in cancer prevention. Studies herein explore the chemopreventive properties of commonly consumed dietary factors and find that many phytochemicals display anticancer properties. Epigenetic modification of oncogenes and tumor suppressor genes by dietary factors may provide new avenues for chemotherapy. Numerous phytochemicals act as epigenetic modifiers of cancer-related genes and are becoming increasingly relevant to cancer prevention. Consumption of chemopreventive phytochemicals may serve to decrease overall cancer risk and incidence. Several studies also involved the combination of dietary compounds, which may provide a focus for future inquiries. Additionally, further investigations into the mechanism of the reversal of gene silencing and the reactivation of genes pertinent to tumor suppression and tumorigenesis by phytochemicals are needed to assess the validity of dietary agents in cancer prevention.

ACKNOWLEDGMENTS

This work was supported in part by grants from the National Cancer Institute (RO1 CA129415), the American Institute for Cancer Research, and the Norma Livingston Foundation. TMH was supported by National Institutes of Health (NIH) National Institute of General Medical Sciences (NIGMS) Institutional Research and Academic Career Development Awards (IRACDA) Program 5K12GM088010 (Dr. Bryan Noe [PI]).

REFERENCES

Alpers, David H. "Garlic and Its Potential for Prevention of Colorectal Cancer and Other Conditions." *Current Opinion in Gastroenterology* 25, no. 2 (2009): 116–21, 10.1097/MOG.0b013e32831ef221.

André, Nkondjock. "Coffee Consumption and the Risk of Cancer: An Overview." *Cancer Letters* 277, no. 2 (2009): 121–25.

Balasubramanian, Sivaprakasam, Gautam Adhikary, and Richard L. Eckert. "The Bmi-1 Polycomb Protein Antagonizes the (−)-Epigallocatechin-3-Gallate–Dependent Suppression of Skin Cancer Cell Survival." *Carcinogenesis* 31, no. 3 (2010): 496–503.

Balasubramanyam, Karanam, Radhika A. Varier, Mohammed Altaf, Venkatesh Swaminathan, Nagadenahalli B. Siddappa, Udaykumar Ranga, and Tapas K. Kundu. "Curcumin, a Novel P300/Creb-Binding Protein-Specific Inhibitor of Acetyltransferase, Represses the Acetylation of Histone/Nonhistone Proteins and Histone Acetyltransferase–Dependent Chromatin Transcription." *Journal of Biological Chemistry* 279, no. 49 (2004): 51163–71.

Barnes, Stephen. "Effect of Genistein on in Vitro and in Vivo Models of Cancer." *The Journal of Nutrition* 125, no. 3 Suppl (1995): 777S–83S.

Berger, Shelley L., Tony Kouzarides, Ramin Shiekhattar, and Ali Shilatifard. "An Operational Definition of Epigenetics." *Genes & Development* 23, no. 7 (2009): 781–83.

Berletch, Joel B., Canhui Liu, William K. Love, Lucy G. Andrews, Santosh K. Katiyar, and Trygve O. Tollefsbol. "Epigenetic and Genetic Mechanisms Contribute to Telomerase Inhibition by EGCG." *Journal of Cellular Biochemistry* 103, no. 2 (2008): 509–19.

Bhamre, Suvarna, Debashis Sahoo, Robert Tibshirani, David L. Dill, and James D. Brooks. "Temporal Changes in Gene Expression Induced by Sulforaphane in Human Prostate Cancer Cells." *The Prostate* 69, no. 2 (2009): 181–90.

Bravo, Laura. "Polyphenols: Chemistry, Dietary Sources, Metabolism, and Nutritional Significance." *Nutrition Reviews* 56, no. 11 (1998): 317–33.

Brennecke, Julius, Alexander Stark, Robert B. Russell, and Stephen M. Cohen. "Principles of MicroRNA-Target Recognition." *PLoS Biol* 3, no. 3 (2005): e85.

Chen, Pei-Ni, Shu-Chen Chu, Wu-Hsien Kuo, Ming-Yung Chou, Jen-Kun Lin, and Yih-Shou Hsieh. "Epigallocatechin-3 Gallate Inhibits Invasion, Epithelial–Mesenchymal Transition, and Tumor Growth in Oral Cancer Cells." *Journal of Agricultural and Food Chemistry* 59, no. 8 (2011): 3836–44.

Cheung, Ka, and Ah-Ng Kong. "Molecular Targets of Dietary Phenethyl Isothiocyanate and Sulforaphane for Cancer Chemoprevention." *The AAPS Journal* 12, no. 1 (2010): 87–97.

Choi, Kyung-Chul, Myung Gu Jung, Yoo-Hyun Lee, Joo Chun Yoon, Seung Hyun Kwon, Hee-Bum Kang, Mi-Jeong Kim, Jeong-Heon Cha, Young Jun Kim, Woo Jin Jun, Jae Myun Lee, and Ho-Geun Yoon. "Epigallocatechin-3-Gallate, a Histone Acetyltransferase Inhibitor, Inhibits EBV-Induced B Lymphocyte Transformation via Suppression of Rela Acetylation." *Cancer Research* 69, no. 2 (2009): 583–92.

Clark, Larry, Bruce Dalkin, Arnon Krongrad, Gerald F. Combs, Jr., Bruce W. Turnbull, Elizabeth H. Slate, Roy Witherington, James H. Herlong, Edward O. Janosko, David Carpenter, Carlos Borosso, Stephen Falk, and James Rounder. "Decreased Incidence of Prostate Cancer with Selenium Supplementation: Results of a Double-Blind Cancer Prevention Trial." *British Journal of Urology* 81, no. 5 (1998): 730–4.

Clark, Larry C., Gerald F. Combs, Bruce W. Turnbull, Elizabeth H. Slate, Dan K. Chalker, James Chow, Loretta S. Davis, Renee A. Glover, Gloria F. Graham, Earl G. Gross, Arnon Krongrad, Jack L. Lesher, H. Kim Park, Beverly B. Sanders, Cameron L. Smith, and J. Richard Taylor. "Effects of Selenium Supplementation for Cancer Prevention in Patients with Carcinoma of the Skin." *JAMA: The Journal of the American Medical Association* 276, no. 24 (1996): 1957–63.

Das, Dipak, Subhendu Mukherjee, and Diptarka Ray. "Resveratrol and Red Wine, Healthy Heart and Longevity." *Heart Failure Reviews* 15, no. 5 (2010): 467–77.

Dashwood, Roderick H., and Emily Ho. "Dietary Agents as Histone Deacetylase Inhibitors: Sulforaphane and Structurally Related Isothiocyanates." *Nutrition Reviews* 66 (2008): S36–8.

Deng, Yea-Tzy, and Jen-Kun Lin. "EGCG Inhibits the Invasion of Highly Invasive CL1-5 Lung Cancer Cells through Suppressing MMP-2 Expression Via Jnk Signaling and Induces G2/M Arrest." *Journal of Agricultural and Food Chemistry* 59 (2011): 13318–27.

Di Croce, Luciano, Veronica A. Raker, Massimo Corsaro, Francesco Fazi, Mirco Fanelli, Mario Faretta, Francois Fuks, Francesco Lo Coco, Tony Kouzarides, Clara Nervi, Saverio Minucci, and Pier Giuseppe Pelicci. "Methyltransferase Recruitment and DNA Hypermethylation of Target Promoters by an Oncogenic Transcription Factor." *Science* 295, no. 5557 (2002): 1079–82.

Doi, Akiko, In-Hyun Park, Bo Wen, Peter Murakami, Martin J. Aryee, Rafael Irizarry, Brian Herb, Christine Ladd-Acosta, Junsung Rho, Sabine Loewer, Justine Miller, Thorsten Schlaeger, George Q. Daley, and Andrew P. Feinberg. "Differential Methylation of Tissue- and Cancer-Specific CpG Island Shores Distinguishes Human Induced Pluripotent Stem Cells, Embryonic Stem Cells and Fibroblasts." *Nature Genetics* 41, no. 12 (2009): 1350–53.

Du, Yatao, Yunfei Wu, Xueli Cao, Wei Cui, Huihui Zhang, Weixi Tian, Mingjuan Ji, Arne Holmgren, and Liangwei Zhong. "Inhibition of Mammalian Thioredoxin Reductase by Black Tea and Its Constituents: Implications for Anticancer Actions." *Biochimie* 91, no. 3 (2009): 434–44.

Ducasse, Miryam, and Mark Brown. "Epigenetic Aberrations and Cancer." *Molecular Cancer* 5, no. 1 (2006): 60.

El-Bayoumy, Karam, Raghu Sinha, John T. Pinto, and Richard S. Rivlin. "Cancer Chemoprevention by Garlic and Garlic-Containing Sulfur and Selenium Compounds." *The Journal of Nutrition* 136, no. 3 (2006): 864S–9S.

Fabbri, Muller, Ramiro Garzon, Amelia Cimmino, Zhongfa Liu, Nicola Zanesi, Elisa Callegari, Shujun Liu, Hansjuerg Alder, Stefan Costinean, Cecilia Fernandez-Cymering, Stefano Volinia, Gulnur Guler, Carl D. Morrison, Kenneth K. Chan, Guido Marcucci, George A. Calin, Kay Huebner, and Carlo M. Croce. "MicroRNA-29 Family Reverts Aberrant Methylation in Lung Cancer by Targeting DNA Methyltransferases 3a and 3b." *Proceedings of the National Academy of Sciences* 104, no. 40 (2007): 15805–10.

Fang, Ming Zhu, Dapeng Chen, Yi Sun, Zhe Jin, Judith K. Christman, and Chung S. Yang. "Reversal of Hypermethylation and Reactivation of P16ink4a, Rarβ, and Mgmt Genes by Genistein and Other Isoflavones from Soy." *Clinical Cancer Research* 11, no. 19 (2005): 7033–41.

Fang, Ming Zhu, Dapeng Chen, and Chung S. Yang. "Dietary Polyphenols May Affect DNA Methylation." *The Journal of Nutrition* 137, no. 1 (2007): 223S–8S.

Fang, Ming Zhu, Yimin Wang, Ni Ai, Zhe Hou, Yi Sun, Hong Lu, William Welsh, and Chung S. Yang. "Tea Polyphenol (–)-Epigallocatechin-3-Gallate Inhibits DNA Methyltransferase and Reactivates Methylation-Silenced Genes in Cancer Cell Lines." *Cancer Research* 63, no. 22 (2003): 7563–70.

Farabegoli, Fulvia, Cristiana Barbi, Elisabetta Lambertini, and Roberta Piva. "(-)-Epigallocatechin-3-Gallate Downregulates Estrogen Receptor Alpha Function in Mcf-7 Breast Carcinoma Cells." *Cancer Detect Prev* 31 (2007): 499–504.

Feinberg, Andrew P., Rolf Ohlsson, and Steven Henikoff. "The Epigenetic Progenitor Origin of Human Cancer." *Nat Rev Genet* 7, no. 1 (2006): 21–33.

Fimognari, C., M. Lenzi, and P. Hrelia. "Chemoprevention of Cancer by Isothiocyanates and Anthocyanins: Mechanisms of Action and Structure–Activity Relationship." *Current Medicinal Chemistry* 15, no. 5 (2008): 440–7.

Friedman, Jeffrey M., Gangning Liang, and Peter A. Jones. "The Tumor Suppressor MicroRNA-101 Becomes an Epigenetic Player by Targeting the Polycomb Group Protein Ezh2 in Cancer." *Cell Cycle* 8, no. 15 (2009): 2313–14.

Gao, Zhi, Zhidong Xu, Ming-Szu Hung, Yu-Ching Lin, Tianyou Wang, Min Gong, Xiuyi Zhi, David M. Jablon, and Liang You. "Promoter Demethylation of Wif-1 by Epigallocatechin-3-Gallate in Lung Cancer Cells." *Anticancer Research* 29, no. 6 (2009): 2025–30.

Goel, Ajay, and Bharat B. Aggarwal. "Curcumin, the Golden Spice from Indian Saffron, Is a Chemosensitizer and Radiosensitizer for Tumors and Chemoprotector and Radioprotector for Normal Organs." *Nutrition and Cancer* 62, no. 7 (2010): 919–30.

Guil, Sònia, and Manel Esteller. "DNA Methylomes, Histone Codes and Mirnas: Tying It All Together." *The International Journal of Biochemistry & Cell Biology* 41, no. 1 (2009): 87–95.

Hardy, Tabitha M., and Trygve O. Tollefsbol. "Epigenetic Diet: Impact on the Epigenome and Cancer." *Epigenomics* 3, no. 4 (2011): 503–18.

Hassan, Yousef I., and Janos Zempleni. "Epigenetic Regulation of Chromatin Structure and Gene Function by Biotin." *The Journal of Nutrition* 136, no. 7 (2006): 1763–5.

Higdon, Jane V., Barbara Delage, David E. Williams, and Roderick H. Dashwood. "Cruciferous Vegetables and Human Cancer Risk: Epidemiologic Evidence and Mechanistic Basis." *Pharmacological Research* 55, no. 3 (2007): 224–36.

Howitz, Konrad T., Kevin J. Bitterman, Haim Y. Cohen, Dudley W. Lamming, Siva Lavu, Jason G. Wood, Robert E. Zipkin, Phuong Chung, Anne Kisielewski, Li-Li Zhang, Brandy Scherer, and David A. Sinclair. "Small Molecule Activators of Sirtuins Extend *Saccharomyces cerevisiae* Lifespan." *Nature* 425, no. 6954 (2003): 191–6.

Huang, Chin-Shiu, Jiunn-Wang Liao, and Miao-Lin Hu. "Lycopene Inhibits Experimental Metastasis of Human Hepatoma Sk-Hep-1 Cells in Athymic Nude Mice." *The Journal of Nutrition* 138, no. 3 (2008): 538–43.

Ip, Clement, Yan Dong, and Howard E. Ganther. "New Concepts in Selenium Chemoprevention." *Cancer and Metastasis Reviews* 21, no. 3 (2002): 281–9.

Jaenisch, Rudolf, and Adrian Bird. "Epigenetic Regulation of Gene Expression: How the Genome Integrates Intrinsic and Environmental Signals." *Nature Genetics* 33 (2003): 245–54.

Jang, Meishiang, Lining Cai, George O. Udeani, Karla V. Slowing, Cathy F. Thomas, Christopher W. W. Beecher, Harry H. S. Fong, Norman R. Farnsworth, A. Douglas Kinghorn, Rajendra G. Mehta, Richard C. Moon, and John M. Pezzuto. "Cancer Chemopreventive Activity of Resveratrol, a Natural Product Derived from Grapes." *Science* 275, no. 5297 (1997): 218–20.

Jenuwein, Thomas, and C. David Allis. "Translating the Histone Code." *Science* 293, no. 5532 (2001): 1074–80.

Johanning, Gary L., and Chandrika J. Piyathilake. "Retinoids and Epigenetic Silencing in Cancer." *Nutrition Reviews* 61, no. 8 (2003): 284–9.

Jurkowski, Tomasz P., and Albert Jeltsch. "On the Evolutionary Origin of Eukaryotic DNA Methyltransferases and Dnmt2." *PLoS ONE* 6, no. 11 (2011): e28104.

Kang, Hyung-Gyoo, Jasmine M. Jenabi, Xian Fang Liu, C. Patrick Reynolds, Timothy J. Triche, and Poul H. B. Sorensen. "Inhibition of the Insulin-Like Growth Factor I Receptor by Epigallocatechin Gallate Blocks Proliferation and Induces the Death of Ewing Tumor Cells." *Molecular Cancer Therapeutics* 9, no. 5 (2010): 1396–407.

Kang, Soo-Kyung, Seung-Heun Cha, and Hyo-Gon Jeon. "Curcumin-Induced Histone Hypoacetylation Enhances Caspase-3–Dependent Glioma Cell Death and Neurogenesis of Neural Progenitor Cells." *Stem Cells and Development* 15, no. 2 (2006): 165–74.

Kato, Keizo, Nguyen K. Long, Hiroki Makita, Mokoto Toida, Tomomi Yamashita, Daijiro Hatakeyama, Akira Hara, Hideki Mori, and Toshiyuki Shibata. "Effects of Green Tea Polyphenol on Methylation Status of Reck Gene and Cancer Cell Invasion in Oral Squamous Cell Carcinoma Cells." *The British Journal of Cancer* 99, no. 4 (2008): 647–54.

Kim, Joseph W., A. R. M. Ruhul Amin, and Dong M. Shin. "Chemoprevention of Head and Neck Cancer with Green Tea Polyphenols." *Cancer Prevention Research* 3, no. 8 (2010): 900–9.

Kouzarides, Tony. "Chromatin Modifications and Their Function." *Cell* 128, no. 4 (2007): 693–705.

Kuck, Dirk, Narender Singh, Frank Lyko, and Jose L. Medina-Franco. "Novel and Selective DNA Methyltransferase Inhibitors: Docking-Based Virtual Screening and Experimental Evaluation." *Bioorganic & Medicinal Chemistry* 18, no. 2 (2010): 822–9.

Kumi-Diaka, James, Kendra Merchant, Alberto Haces, Vanessa Hormann, and Michelle Johnson. "Genistein–Selenium Combination Induces Growth Arrest in Prostate Cancer Cells." *Journal of Medicinal Food* 13, no. 4 (2010): 842–50.

Kürbitz, Claudia, Daniel Heise, Torben Redmer, Freya Goumas, Alexander Arlt, Johannes Lemke, Gerald Rimbach, Holger Kalthoff, and Anna Trauzold. "Epicatechin Gallate and Catechin Gallate Are Superior to Epigallocatechin Gallate in Growth Suppression and Anti-Inflammatory Activities in Pancreatic Tumor Cells." *Cancer Science* 102, no. 4 (2011): 728–34.

Lam, Wai Har, Aslamuzzaman Kazi, Deborah J. Kuhn, Larry M. C. Chow, Albert S. C. Chan, Q. Ping Dou, and Tak Hang Chan. "A Potential Prodrug for a Green Tea Polyphenol Proteasome Inhibitor: Evaluation of the Peracetate Ester of (-)-Epigallocatechin Gallate [(-)-EGCG]." *Bioorganic & Medicinal Chemistry* 12, no. 21 (2004): 5587–93.

Landis-Piwowar, Kristin R., Congde Huo, Di Chen, Vesna Milacic, Guoqing Shi, Tak Hang Chan, and Q. Ping Dou. "A Novel Prodrug of the Green Tea Polyphenol (−)-Epigallocatechin-3-Gallate as a Potential Anticancer Agent." *Cancer Research* 67, no. 9 (2007): 4303–10.

Lea, Michael A., Chinwe Ibeh, Lydia Han, and Charles desBordes. "Inhibition of Growth and Induction of Differentiation Markers by Polyphenolic Molecules and Histone Deacetylase Inhibitors in Colon Cancer Cells." *Anticancer Research* 30, no. 2 (2010): 311–8.

Lea, Michael A., Verrell M. Randolph, Jennifer E. Lee, and Charles desBordes. "Induction of Histone Acetylation in Mouse Erythroleukemia Cells by Some Organosulfur Compounds Including Allyl Isothiocyanate." *International Journal of Cancer* 92, no. 6 (2001): 784–9.

Lee, Won Jun, Joong-Youn Shim, and Bao Ting Zhu. "Mechanisms for the Inhibition of DNA Methyltransferases by Tea Catechins and Bioflavonoids." *Molecular Pharmacology* 68, no. 4 (2005): 1018–30.

Lee, Won Jun, and Bao Ting Zhu. "Inhibition of DNA Methylation by Caffeic Acid and Chlorogenic Acid, Two Common Catechol-Containing Coffee Polyphenols." *Carcinogenesis* 27, no. 2 (2006): 269–77.

Li, Yiwei, Timothy G. VandenBoom, Dejuan Kong, Zhiwei Wang, Shadan Ali, Philip A. Philip, and Fazlul H. Sarkar. "Up-regulation of miR-200 and let-7 by Natural Agents Leads to the Reversal of Epithelial-to-Mesenchymal Transition in Gemcitabine-Resistant Pancreatic Cancer Cells." *Cancer Research* 69, no. 16 (2009): 6704–12.

Li, Yuanyuan, Liang Liu, Lucy G. Andrews, and Trygve O. Tollefsbol. "Genistein Depletes Telomerase Activity through Cross-Talk between Genetic and Epigenetic Mechanisms." *International Journal of Cancer* 125, no. 2 (2009): 286–96.

Li, Yuanyuan, and Trygve O. Tollefsbol. "Impact on DNA Methylation in Cancer Prevention and Therapy by Bioactive Dietary Components." *Current Medicinal Chemistry* 17 (2010): 2141–51.

Li, Yuanyuan, Yih-Ying Yuan, Syed Meeran, and Trygve Tollefsbol. "Synergistic Epigenetic Reactivation of Estrogen Receptor-Alpha (Eralpha) by Combined Green Tea Polyphenol and Histone Deacetylase Inhibitor in ERalpha-Negative Breast Cancer Cells." *Molecular Cancer* 9, no. 1 (2010): 274.

Liang, Xinhua, Xiaoqin Yang, Yaling Tang, Hao Zhou, Xian Liu, Lin Xiao, Jiarang Gao, and Zuyi Mao. "RNAi-Mediated Downregulation of Urokinase Plasminogen Activator Receptor Inhibits Proliferation, Adhesion, Migration and Invasion in Oral Cancer Cells." *Oral Oncology* 44, no. 12 (2008): 1172–80.

Lin, Jen-Kun, Yu-Chih Liang, and Shoei-Yn Lin-Shiau. "Cancer Chemoprevention by Tea Polyphenols through Mitotic Signal Transduction Blockade." *Biochemical Pharmacology* 58, no. 6 (1999): 911–5.

Liu, Hong-li, Yan Chen, Guo-hui Cui, and Jian-feng Zhou. "Curcumin, a Potent Anti-Tumor Reagent, Is a Novel Histone Deacetylase Inhibitor Regulating B-NHL Cell Line Raji Proliferation." *Acta Pharmacologica Sinica* 26, no. 5 (2005): 603–9.

Liu, Zhongfa, Zhiliang Xie, William Jones, Ryan E. Pavlovicz, Shujun Liu, Jianhua Yu, Pui-kai Li, Jiayuh Lin, Jame R. Fuchs, Guido Marcucci, Chenglong Li, and Kenneth K. Chan. "Curcumin Is a Potent DNA Hypomethylation Agent." *Bioorganic & Medicinal Chemistry Letters* 19, no. 3 (2009): 706–9.

Lu, Quanyi, Xianghua Lin, Jean Feng, Xiangmin Zhao, Ruth Gallagher, Marietta Lee, Jen-Wei Chiao, and Delong Liu. "Phenylhexyl Isothiocyanate Has Dual Function as Histone Deacetylase Inhibitor and Hypomethylating Agent and Can Inhibit Myeloma Cell Growth by Targeting Critical Pathways." *Journal of Hematology & Oncology* 1, no. 1 (2008): 6.

Lu, Tung-Ying, Cheng-Fu Kao, Chin-Tarng Lin, Dah-Yeou Huang, and Han-Chung Wu. "DNA Methylation and Histone Modification Regulate Silencing of OPG During Tumor Progression." *J Cell Biochem* 108, no. 1 (2009): 315–25.

Lujambio, Amaia, George A. Calin, Alberto Villanueva, Santiago Ropero, Montserrat Sánchez-Céspedes, David Blanco, Luis M. Montuenga, Simona Rossi, Milena S. Nicoloso, William J. Faller, William M. Gallagher, Suzanne A. Eccles, Carlo M. Croce, and Manel Esteller. "A MicroRNA DNA Methylation Signature for Human Cancer Metastasis." *Proceedings of the National Academy of Sciences* 105, no. 36 (2008): 13556–61.

Maheshwari, Radha K., Anoop K. Singh, Jaya Gaddipati, and Rikhab C. Srimal. "Multiple Biological Activities of Curcumin: A Short Review." *Life Sciences* 78, no. 18 (2006): 2081–7.

Majid, Shahana, Nobuyuki Kikuno, Jason Nelles, Emily Noonan, Yuichiro Tanaka, Ken Kawamoto, Hiroshi Hirata, Long C. Li, Hong Zhao, Steve T. Okino, Robert F. Place, Deepa Pookot, and Rajvir Dahiya. "Genistein Induces the p21WAF1/CIP1 and P16INK4a Tumor Suppressor Genes in Prostate Cancer Cells by Epigenetic Mechanisms Involving Active Chromatin Modification." *Cancer Research* 68, no. 8 (2008): 2736–44.

Marcu, Monica G., Yun-Jin Jung, Sunmin Lee, Eun-Joo Chung, Min-Jung Lee, Jane Trepel, and Len Neckers. "Curcumin Is an Inhibitor of P300 Histone Acetyltransferase." *Medical Chemistry* 2, no. 2 (2006): 169–74.

Meeran, Syed M., Shweta N. Patel, Tak-Hang Chan, and Trygve O. Tollefsbol. "A Novel Prodrug of Epigallocatechin-3-Gallate: Differential Epigenetic hTERT Repression in Human Breast Cancer Cells." *Cancer Prevention Research* 4, no. 8 (2011): 1243–54.

Mittal, Anshu, Mitchell S. Pate, Rebecca C. Wylie, Trygve O. Tollefsbol, Santosh K. Katiyar. "EGCG Down-Regulates Telomerase in Human Breast Carcinoma MCF-7 Cells, Leading to Suppression of Cell Viability and Induction of Apoptosis." *International Journal of Oncology* 24 (2004): 703–10.

Morimoto, Tatsuya, Yoichi Sunagawa, Teruhisa Kawamura, Tomohide Takaya, Hiromichi Wada, Atsushi Nagasawa, Masashi Komeda, Masatoshi Fujita, Akira Shimatsu, Toru Kita, and Koji Hasegawa. "The Dietary Compound Curcumin Inhibits p300 Histone Acetyltransferase Activity and Prevents Heart Failure in Rats." *The Journal of Clinical Investigation* 118, no. 3 (2008): 868–78.

Morris, Virginia C., and Orville A. Levander. "Selenium Content of Foods." *The Journal of Nutrition* 100, no. 12 (1970): 1383–8.

Myzak, Melinda C., Philip Tong, Wan-Mohaiza Dashwood, Roderick H. Dashwood, and Emily Ho. "Sulforaphane Retards the Growth of Human PC-3 Xenografts and Inhibits HDAC Activity in Human Subjects." *Exp. Biol. Med.* 232, no. 2 (2007): 227–34.

Nandakumar, Vijayalakshmi, Mudit Vaid, and Santosh K. Katiyar. "(–)-Epigallocatechin-3-Gallate Reactivates Silenced Tumor Suppressor Genes, Cip1/p21 and P16INK4a, by Reducing DNA Methylation and Increasing Histones Acetylation in Human Skin Cancer Cells." *Carcinogenesis*, 32, no. 4 (2011): 537–44.

Nian, Hui, Barbara Delage, Emily Ho, and Roderick H. Dashwood. "Modulation of Histone Deacetylase Activity by Dietary Isothiocyanates and Allyl Sulfides: Studies with Sulforaphane and Garlic Organosulfur Compounds." *Environmental and Molecular Mutagenesis* 50, no. 3 (2009): 213–21.

Nian, Hui, Barbara Delage, John T. Pinto, and Roderick H. Dashwood. "Allyl Mercaptan, a Garlic-Derived Organosulfur Compound, Inhibits Histone Deacetylase and Enhances Sp3 Binding on the P21WAF1 Promoter." *Carcinogenesis* 29, no. 9 (2008): 1816–24.

Pandey, Mitali, Sanjeev Shukla, and Sanjay Gupta. "Promoter Demethylation and Chromatin Remodeling by Green Tea Polyphenols Leads to Re-Expression of GSTP1 in Human Prostate Cancer Cells." *International Journal of Cancer* 126, no. 11 (2010): 2520–33.

Papoutsis, Andreas J., Sarah D. Lamore, Georg T. Wondrak, Ornella I. Selmin, and Donato F. Romagnolo. "Resveratrol Prevents Epigenetic Silencing of BRCA-1 by the Aromatic Hydrocarbon Receptor in Human Breast Cancer Cells." *The Journal of Nutrition* 140, no. 9 (2010): 1607–14.

Parasramka, Mansi A., Emily Ho, David E. Williams, and Roderick H. Dashwood. "Micrornas, Diet, and Cancer: New Mechanistic Insights on the Epigenetic Actions of Phytochemicals." *Molecular Carcinogenesis* 51, no. 3 (2012): 213–30.

Parker, Lynn P., Douglas D. Taylor, J. Kesterson, Daniel S. Metzinger, and Cicek Gercel- Taylor. "Modulation of MicroRNA Associated with Ovarian Cancer Cells by Genistein." *European Journal of Gynaecological Oncology* 30, no. 6 (2009): 616–21.

Pledgie-Tracy, Allison, Michele D. Sobolewski, and Nancy E. Davidson. "Sulforaphane Induces Cell Type–Specific Apoptosis in Human Breast Cancer Cell Lines." *Molecular Cancer Therapeutics* 6, no. 3 (2007): 1013–21.

Pradeep, Chaluvally R., and Girija Kuttan. "Effect of β-carotene on the Inhibition of Lung Metastasis in Mice." *Phytomedicine* 10, no. 2–3 (2003): 159–64.

Qin, W., W. Zhu, H. Shi, J. E. Hewett, R. L. Ruhlen, R. S. MacDonald, G. E. Rottinghaus, Y. C. Chen, and E. R. Sauter. "Soy Isoflavones Have an Antiestrogenic Effect and Alter Mammary Promoter Hypermethylation in Healthy Premenopausal Women." *Nutrition and Cancer* 61 (2009): 238–44.

Relja, Borna, Eva Töttel, Lara Breig, Dirk Henrich, Heinz Schneider, Ingo Marzi, and Mark Lehnert. "Plant Polyphenols Attenuate Hepatic Injury after Hemorrhage/Resuscitation by Inhibition of Apoptosis, Oxidative Stress, and Inflammation Via NF-KappaB in Rats." *European Journal of Nutrition* 51, no. 3 (2012): 311–21.

Reuter, Simone, Serge Eifes, Mario Dicato, Bharat B. Aggarwal, and Marc Diederich. "Modulation of Anti-Apoptotic and Survival Pathways by Curcumin as a Strategy to Induce Apoptosis in Cancer Cells." *Biochemical Pharmacology* 76, no. 11 (2008): 1340–51.

Riley, Lee B., and David W. Anderson. "Cancer Epigenetics." In *Handbook of Epigenetics: The New Molecular and Medical Genetics*, edited by T. O. Tollefsbol, 521–34. San Diego, CA: Elsevier, 2011.

Robert, Feil. "Environmental and Nutritional Effects on the Epigenetic Regulation of Genes." *Mutation Research/Fundamental and Molecular Mechanisms of Mutagenesis* 600, no. 1–2 (2006): 46–57.

Sarkar, Fazlul H., and Yiwei Li. "Mechanisms of Cancer Chemoprevention by Soy Isoflavone Genistein." *Cancer and Metastasis Reviews* 21, no. 3 (2002): 265–80.

Singh, Brahma N., Sharmila Shankar, and Rakesh K. Srivastava. "Green Tea Catechin, Epigallocatechin-3-Gallate (EGCG): Mechanisms, Perspectives and Clinical Applications." *Biochemical Pharmacology* 82, no. 12 (2011): 1807–21.

Sirchia, Silvia M., Mingqiang Ren, Roberto Pili, Elena Sironi, Giulia Somenzi, Riccardo Ghidoni, Salvatore Toma, Guido Nicolò, and Nicoletta Sacchi. "Endogenous Reactivation of the RARβ2 Tumor Suppressor Gene Epigenetically Silenced in Breast Cancer." *Cancer Research* 62, no. 9 (2002): 2455–61.

Skinner, Michael K., and Carlos Guerrero-Bosagna. "Environmental Signals and Transgenerational Epigenetics." *Epigenomics* 1, no. 1 (2009): 111–7.

Stünkel, Walter, Bee Keow Peh, Yong Cheng Tan, Vasantha M. Nayagam, Xukun Wang, Manuel Salto-Tellez, BinHui Ni, Michael Entzeroth, and Jeanette Wood. "Function of the Sirt1 Protein Deacetylase in Cancer." *Biotechnology Journal* 2, no. 11 (2007): 1360–8.

Subbiah, M. T. Ravi. "Understanding the Nutrigenomic Definitions and Concepts at the Food–Genome Junction." *OMICS: A Journal of Integrative Biology* 12, no. 4 (2008): 229–35.

Taby, Rodolphe, and Jean-Pierre J. Issa. "Cancer Epigenetics." *CA: A Cancer Journal for Clinicians* 60, no. 6 (2010): 376–92.

Tran, Phan, Soo-A Kim, Hong Choi, Jung-Hoon Yoon, and Sang-Gun Ahn. "Epigallocatechin-3-Gallate Suppresses the Expression of HSP70 and HSP90 and Exhibits Anti-Tumor Activity in Vitro and in Vivo." *BMC Cancer* 10, no. 1 (2010): 276.

Tu, Shih-Hsin, Chung-Yu Ku, Chi-Tang Ho, Ching-Shyang Chen, Ching-Shui Huang, Chia-Hwa Lee, Li-Ching Chen, Min-Hsiung Pan, Hui-Wen Chang, Chien-Hsi Chang, Yu-Jia Chang, Po-Li Wei, Chih-Hsiung Wu, and Yuan-Soon Ho. "Tea Polyphenol (−)-Epigallocatechin-3-Gallate Inhibits Nicotine- and Estrogen-Induced α9-Nicotinic Acetylcholine Receptor Upregulation in Human Breast Cancer Cells." *Molecular Nutrition & Food Research* 55, no. 3 (2011): 455–66.

Uthus, Eric O., Katsuhiko Yokoi, and Cindy D. Davis. "Selenium Deficiency in Fisher-344 Rats Decreases Plasma and Tissue Homocysteine Concentrations and Alters Plasma Homocysteine and Cysteine Redox Status." *The Journal of Nutrition* 132, no. 6 (2002): 1122–8.

Waddington, Conrad H. "The Epigenotype." *Endeavour* 1 (1942): 18–20.

Wang, Rui-Hong, Yin Zheng, Hyun-Seok Kim, Xiaoling Xu, Liu Cao, Tyler Lahusen, Mi-Hye Lee, Cuiying Xiao, Athanassios Vassilopoulos, Weiping Chen, Kevin Gardner, Yan-Gao Man, Mien-Chie Hung, Toren Finkel, and Chu-Xia Deng. "Interplay among BRCA1, SIRT1, and Survivin During BRCA1-Associated Tumorigenesis." *Molecular Cell* 32, no. 1 (2008): 11–20.

Weinstein, I. Bernard. "Cancer Prevention: Recent Progress and Future Opportunities." *Cancer Research* 51, no. 18 Suppl (1991): 5080s–5s.

Weng, Ya-Ling, Hui-Fen Liao, Anna Fen-Yau Li, Ju-Chun Chang, and Robin Y. Y. Chiou. "Oral Administration of Resveratrol in Suppression of Pulmonary Metastasis of BALB/c Mice Challenged with CT26 Colorectal Adenocarcinoma Cells." *Molecular Nutrition & Food Research* 54, no. 2 (2010): 259–67.

Wu, Hongzhong, Xin Liang, Yishi Fang, Xiaoran Qin, Yuanxing Zhang, and Jianwen Liu. "Resveratrol Inhibits Hypoxia-Induced Metastasis Potential Enhancement by Restricting Hypoxia-Induced Factor-1[Alpha] Expression in Colon Carcinoma Cells." *Biomedicine & Pharmacotherapy* 62, no. 9 (2008): 613–21.

Yang, Chih-Min, Yeu-Torng Yen, Chin-Shiu Huang, and Miao-Lin Hu. "Growth Inhibitory Efficacy of Lycopene and β-Carotene against Androgen-Independent Prostate Tumor Cells Xenografted in Nude Mice." *Molecular Nutrition & Food Research* 55, no. 4 (2011): 606–12.

Yang, Chung, Joshua Lambert, and Shengmin Sang. "Antioxidative and Anti-Carcinogenic Activities of Tea Polyphenols." *Archives of Toxicology* 83, no. 1 (2009): 11–21.

Yang, Haiyan, Jessica Rouse, Luanne Lukes, Mindy Lancaster, Timothy Veenstra, Ming Zhou, Ying Shi, Yeong-Gwan Park, and Kent Hunter. "Caffeine Suppresses Metastasis in a Transgenic Mouse Model: A Prototype Molecule for Prophylaxis of Metastasis." *Clinical and Experimental Metastasis* 21, no. 8 (2005): 719–35.

Yavari, Kamal, Mohammad Taghikhani, Mohammad Ghannadi Maragheh, Seyed Mesbah-Namin, and Mohammad Babaei. "Downregulation of IGF-IR Expression by Rnai Inhibits Proliferation and Enhances Chemosensitization of Human Colon Cancer Cells." *International Journal of Colorectal Disease* 25, no. 1 (2010): 9–16.

Zhang, Dong, Mohamed Al-Hendy, Gloria Richard-Davis, Valerie Montgomery-Rice, Chakradhari Sharan, Veera Rajaratnam, Anjali Khurana, and Ayman Al-Hendy. "Green Tea Extract Inhibits Proliferation of Uterine Leiomyoma Cells in Vitro and in Nude Mice." *American Journal of Obstetrics and Gynecology* 202, no. 3 (2010): 289.e1–e9.

Zhang, Yuesheng. "Allyl Isothiocyanate as a Cancer Chemopreventive Phytochemical." *Molecular Nutrition & Food Research* 54, no. 1 (2010): 127–35.

32 Nutritional Phytochemicals and the Management of Chronic Inflammation

Laura Marler and John M. Pezzuto

CONTENTS

32.1 INTRODUCTION

Immediate response of the innate immune systems results from wounds, infection, or other cellular damage. Immune cells are recruited, producing cytokines and activating the complement cascade. Unwanted cells or particulates are subjected to phagocytosis, and finally, T cells of the adaptive immune system are recruited. Innate immunity is a vital component of protection and early wound healing, and inflammation plays an important role in this defense (Miller and Watson 1965). Induced by cytokines secreted by the injured cells themselves, it is the first response of the body to injury or invasion and serves to create a physical barrier for pathogens (Tracey 2007). Inflammation also functions to promote early healing (Cotran et al. 1999).

Macrophages, dendritic cells, histiocytes, mastocytes, and other cells present at the site of cellular damage initiate the innate immune response by releasing inflammatory mediators (Cotran et al. 1999). These chemical signals activate and direct the migration of leukocytes such as neutrophils, eosinophils, and monocytes to the site of the injury or infection (Brigati et al. 2002). Chemotactic factors for neutrophils include complement factor 5 (C5a), leukotriene B4, kallikrein, certain bacterial products in the case of infection, and some factors released by platelets at the site (Phillipson and Kubes 2011). Aggregating platelets provide a bolus of secreted proteins such as arachidonic acid metabolites, heparin, serotonin, thrombin, fibrinogen, and albumin, as well as cell growth factors like platelet-derived growth factor (PDGF), platelet-derived angiogenesis factor, transforming growth factors (TGF-α and -β), enzymes such as heparanase and factor XIII, and protease inhibitors (plasminogen activator inhibitor-1, α2-macroglobulin, and α2-antiplasmin) (Coussens and Werb 2002). Recruitment of neutrophils occurs via a four-step process involving activation of members of the selectin family of adhesion molecules, which facilitate rolling in the vascular endothelium, triggering of signals that activate and upregulate leukocyte integrins mediated by cytokines and leukocyte-activating molecules, immobilization of neutrophils on the surface of the vascular endothelium by binding of integrins ($\alpha_4\beta_1$

and $\alpha_4\beta_7$) to endothelial vascular cell-adhesion molecule 1 (VCAM-1) and mucosal addressin cellular adhesion molecule-1 (MAdCAM-1), and transmigration of the neutrophils to sites of injury (Hartman et al. 2012; Soehnlein et al. 2009; Kobayashi 2008; Zarbock and Ley 2011). Arriving neutrophils, monocytes, and fibroblasts aid in the formation of granulation tissue and new extracellular matrix (ECM) (Coussens and Werb 2002; DiPietro 1995). Neutrophils are also responsible for the release of many early proinflammatory cytokines, including tumor necrosis factor α (TNFα), interleukin 1α (IL-1α), and IL-1β (Sadik et al. 2011; Feiken et al. 1995; Hubner et al. 1996). These cytokines not only mediate adherence of recruited leukocytes to the vascular endothelium but also induce the expression of keratinocyte growth factor (KGF/fibroblast growth factor 7 [FGF-7]) and matrix metalloproteinases (MMPs) in fibroblasts (Coussens and Werb 2002; Sadik et al. 2011). Simultaneously, mononuclear phagocytes are recruited by chemotactic factors. These include platelet factor-4 (PF-4); TGF-β; PDGF; chemokines such as monocyte chemotactic protein (MCP-1)/chemokine (C-C motif) ligand (CCL2), MCP-2/CCL8, and MCP-3/CCL7; macrophage inflammatory protein 1α and 1β (MIP-1α/CCL3 and MIP-1β/CCL4); and cytokines like IL-1β and TNFα (Weber et al. 2004). These cells can differentiate into mature macrophages, which become the major producers of growth factors and cytokines to bring about tissue repair, regulate tissue remodeling, and promote angiogenesis (through production of thrombospondin-1) (Hume 2006). Mast cells, which are important in the early stages of inflammation as well as in wound healing, also produce a variety of mediators such as heparin, heparanase, histamine, MMPs, serine proteases, and polypeptide growth factors like basic fibroblast growth factor (bFGF) and vascular endothelial growth factor (VEGF) (Collington et al. 2011).

While the process of inflammation is normally self-limiting, with the production of anti-inflammatory cytokines following closely that of proinflammatory cytokines, it is apparent that misregulation of these multiple converging factors can lead to abnormalities, which eventually result in pathogenesis. In fact, uncontrolled or chronic inflammation has been implicated in many major disease states. Diseases typically considered the result of incorrectly regulated inflammation include chronic asthma, rheumatoid arthritis, osteoarthritis, multiple sclerosis, Crohn's disease, inflammatory bowel disease, and psoriasis. Now, Alzheimer's disease, heart disease, stroke, diabetes, depression, fibromyalgia, fibrosis, pancreatitis, and cancer can be added to the list of diseases in which inflammation plays a causal role (Johnston et al. 2011; Manabe 2011; Gardner and Boles 2011; Giehl et al. 2011; Demaria et al. 2010). The association of low-grade inflammation with such a wide range of diseases has prompted questions such as that posed in a recent UC Berkeley Wellness Letter: "Is inflammation the root of all disease?" (Swartzberg 2008).

32.2 INFLAMMATION AND CANCER

The correlation of inflammation to cancer is long standing. As early as 1863, Virchow hypothesized that neoplasia originated at sites of chronic inflammation (Balkwill and Mantovani 1996). Although Virchow's theory rested on the incorrect belief that cell proliferation was the link between inflammation at sites of tissue injury and carcinogenesis, it has been seen that many of the elements of the innate immune system can work to aid the progression and continued growth of tumors (Coussens and Werb 2002). Epidemiological studies have consistently identified chronic infection or inflammation as a major risk factor for various types of cancer. It is estimated that infections and the inflammatory reactions resulting from them are linked to 15%–20% of cancer deaths (Balkwill and Mantovani 2010). Chronic inflammation is generally viewed as a promoter of the process of carcinogenesis.

In recent years, there are numerous examples of direct links between inflammation and cancer: human papillomavirus (HPV) and cervical cancer; inflammatory bowel disease and colorectal cancer; chronic pancreatitis and pancreatic cancer; and infection with *Heliobacter pylori* and stomach cancer (Schiffman et al. 2007; Itzkowitz and Yio 2004; Whitcomb 2004; Kusters et al. 2006). The continuous state of low-grade inflammation in obese individuals significantly elevates the risk of developing cancer (Chen 2011). Beyond these examples, inflammation may play a key role in tumorigenesis and progression of ovarian cancer, as well as the link between hepatitis infection and hepatocellular carcinoma (Maccia and Madeddu 2012; Di Bisceglie et al. 1991). In sum, very strong evidence supports the relationship between inflammation and cancer. But what is the nature of that link? How does this vital part of our innate immune system go so fatally awry?

In chronically inflamed tissues, cell death and/or repair mechanisms are subverted, resulting in DNA replication and proliferation of cells that have lost normal growth control (Coussens and Werb 2002). Leukocytes and other phagocytic cells produce reactive oxygen species (ROS) and reactive nitrogen species to fight infection, but these compounds can cause DNA damage in proliferating cells (Maeda and Akaike 1998). In chronic inflammatory diseases, such as rheumatoid arthritis and inflammatory bowel disease, mutations of p53 are seen at frequencies similar to those in tumors (Yamanishi et al. 2002). In addition to DNA damage caused by inflammatory cells, macrophages and T lymphocytes express macrophage migration inhibitory factor (MIF) at sites of chronic inflammation. MIF suppresses the transcriptional activity of p53, increasing the potential for accumulation of oncogenic mutations while enhancing proliferation and extending life span (Hudson et al. 1999).

The problem of DNA damage at sites of inflammation may be the mechanism for promotion, but sustained inflammation also appears to be important to tumor progression and metastasis (Vicari and Caux 2002). The chemokine receptor system can be altered dramatically in neoplastic tissue (Allavena et al. 2011). Some tumors (particularly melanoma) use chemokine factors to promote tumor growth and progression (Luan et al. 1997). Others regulate angiogenic and angiostatic factors (e.g., glutamic acid-leucine-arginine [ELR]$^+$ cysteine-X-cysteine [CXC] and ELR$^-$ CXC chemokines, potentially through the upregulation of CXCR4 by VEGF-A) (Opdenakker and Van Damme 2004; Vandercappellen et al. 2008). Further, it appears that chemokines may be involved in regulating the spectrum of metastases in diverse cancers (e.g., CXCR4 and CXCL12 in breast cancer) (Liekens et al. 2010). Indeed, inflammation appears to be a necessity for malignancy in many and possibly even all cancers. While it has been said that genetic damage is "the match that lights the fire" and inflammation is "the fuel that feeds the flames" (Balkwill and Mantovani 1996), it appears that, in causing DNA damage, inflammation serves as both the spark and the kindling for neoplasia.

32.3 ANTI-INFLAMMATORY MOLECULAR TARGETS

A number of molecular targets have been identified as potential biomarkers for inflammation (Zhu et al. 2011). These include enzymes, cytokines, G-protein–coupled receptors, nuclear hormone receptors, cell interaction molecules, or transcription factors that block the output of an inflammatory pathway when antagonized. One of the most common targets is cyclooxygenase 2 (COX2) (Seibert et al. 1995). Cyclooxygenases mediate the formation of prostaglandins, prostacyclin, and thromboxane through a double oxidation of arachidonic acid and other fatty acids to produce the precursor molecule prostaglandin H_2 (PGH_2) (Schneider and Pozzi 2011). COX1, a constitutive enzyme, functions primarily in the synthesis of prostaglandins responsible for the maintenance and protection of the gastrointestinal tract, while COX2, an inducible enzyme (Figure 32.1), is implicated in the production of prostaglandins responsible for pain and inflammation. COX2 has been found to be overexpressed in a variety of cancers, including neuroblastoma, cancers of the intestinal tract, and breast cancer (Johnsen et al. 2005; Thiel et al. 2011; Agrawal and Fentiman 2008). The related lipoxygenases (LOXs) add molecular oxygen to arachidonic acid to form the hydro(pero)xyeicosate-traenoic acids (Schneider and Pozzi 2011). Along with cytochrome P450 monooxygenases, these enzymes make up the major pathways for treatment of inflammation (Greene et al. 2011). All three are widely accepted targets for cancer chemoprevention, and as such, they represent yet another link between cancer and inflammation.

Lysyl oxidase (LysOX) is another enzyme implicated in inflammation (Alcudia et al. 2008). This copper-containing extracellular enzyme catalyzes the formation of highly reactive aldehydes from lysine residues in the precursors of collagen and elastin, promoting cross-linking (Siddikuzzaman et al. 2011). Expression of LysOX is regulated by hypoxia-inducible factors (HIFs), and it appears

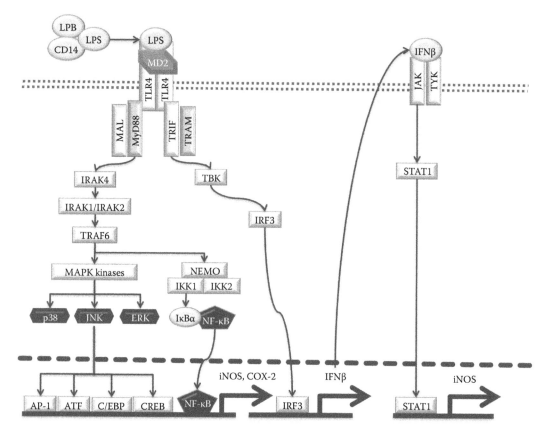

FIGURE 32.1 LPS signaling plays a role in a number of potentially inflammatory pathways, including the expression of iNOS and COX2.

that LysOX plays an important role in hypoxia-induced metastasis by increasing focal adhesion kinase activity (Erler and Giaccia 2006). Although inhibition of LysOX can cause lathyrism, inhibitors may also be useful as anticancer agents (Payne et al. 2007). Other enzyme targets for anti-inflammatory drugs include inosine monophosphate dehydrogenase and p38 pathway kinases (Shu and Nair 2008).

Mitogen-activated protein kinases (MAPKs) are serine/threonine-specific kinases, which respond to extracellular signals, including stress signals and proinflammatory cytokines (Huang et al. 2010). They also play a role in the activation of apoptosis (Miloso et al. 2008). Specifically, p38 MAPKs respond to cellular stresses such as osmotic shock, inflammatory cytokines, lipopolysaccharides (Figure 32.1), ultraviolet light, and growth factors (Cuadrado and Nebreda 2010). c-Jun N-terminal kinases (JNKs) are also responsive to cellular stress signals. These enzymes regulate cellular functions such as cell growth, survival, and apoptosis by controlling the production of several small-molecule nuclear factors (Bogoyevitch 2010). Activation of JNKs will result in increased production of c-Jun, activating transcription factor 2 (ATF2), p53, heat shock factor 1 (HSF1), c-Myc, retinoid X receptor alpha (RXRα), and retinoic acid receptor alpha (RARα) (Dhanasekaran and Reddy 2008). Because the extracellular signal–regulated kinase (ERK) pathway plays a central role in cancer cell migration and development of resistance to apoptosis, inhibitors of these kinases are good candidates for chemopreventive agents (Kim and Choi 2010).

Nitric oxide (NO), the molecular messenger, is synthesized endogenously from arginine by three isoforms of the enzyme NO synthase (Guilford and Pezzuto 2008). Inducible nitric oxide synthase (iNOS) is the isoform most commonly associated with chronic inflammation and tumor production

(Figure 32.1). A consistent relationship between upregulation of iNOS and cancers of the prostate, bladder, ovary, oral cavity, and esophagus has been observed (Singh and Gupta 2011). This suggests the potential use of iNOS inhibitors in chemopreventive strategies. Animal studies also showed the role of iNOS in the promotion of colon carcinogenesis, and the chemopreventive effects of iNOS inhibitors have been shown in preclinical colon cancer models (Rao et al. 1999). The role of iNOS inhibitors as chemopreventive agents has been demonstrated in a primary rat tracheal epithelial transformation system, further predicting their use in chemopreventive strategies (Sharma et al. 2002).

Nonenzymatic targets for anti-inflammatory drugs include TNFα, TNF receptor II (TNFRII), IL-1β, IL-1RA, IL-2, IL-2R, interferon α2 (IFNα2), IFNβ1, IFNγ, histamine 1, cysteinyl leukotriene 1, leukocyte function-associated antigen 1 (LFA-1), cluster of differentiation molecules 11a (CD11a), LFA-3, CD2, very late activation antigen 4 (VLA-4), CD49b, and cytotoxic T lymphocyte antigen-4 immunoglobulin (CTLA4-Ig), among many others.

Another common approach for reduction of inflammation is inhibition of nuclear factor kappa B (NF-κB). TNFα is an activator of NF-κB, an inducible transcription factor that plays an important role in the regulation of apoptosis, cell differentiation, and cell migration (Figure 32.1) (Luqman and Pezzuto 2010). Its activation may promote cell proliferation and further prevent programmed cell death through transcriptional activation of genes that suppress apoptosis (Mayo et al. 2001). As NF-κB is an important regulator in cell fate decisions, such as programmed cell death, proliferation control, and cell invasion, it is critical in tumorigenesis. Inhibition of NF-κB signaling has potential applications for the prevention or treatment of cancer (Dorai and Aggarwal 2004; Schupp et al. 2009). Thus, there are many potential points of intervention capable of blocking the chronic or acute inflammatory response, and it is apparent that even more will be identified in due course.

32.4 ANTI-INFLAMMATORY DRUGS

Several classes of drugs are currently available to treat inflammatory disorders, although adverse side effects are common. Corticosteroids include natural steroid hormones produced by the adrenal cortex, as well as synthetic analogs of these hormones (hydrocortisone-type drugs such as prednisone, acetonides such as budesonide, betamethasone-type compounds like dexamethasone, and corresponding esters) (Maxwell et al. 1994). Glucocorticoids prevent phospholipid release and decrease eosinophil action, among other mechanisms. These drugs, however, can cause Cushing's habitus, hypertension, hyperglycemia, muscular weakness, increased susceptibility to infection, osteoporosis, glaucoma, psychiatric disturbances, and growth arrest (Peppa et al. 2011; Sholter and Armstrong 2000; den Uyl et al. 2011). Long-term use may cause insulin resistance, diabetes mellitus, cataract, anxiety, depression, colitis, ictus, erectile dysfunction, hypogonadism, hypothyroidism, amenorrhea, retinopathy, peptic ulceration, and birth defects (Poetker and Reh 2010). Clearly, safer alternatives are desirable.

Nonsteroidal anti-inflammatory drugs (NSAIDs) act through inhibition of COX2 to decrease prostaglandin biosynthesis, although they are not specific inhibitors. Since COX1 is inhibited, these agents can cause gastrointestinal ulcers, as well as platelet dysfunction (Sostres et al. 2010). For this reason, coxibs (e.g., celecoxib, rofecoxib), which inhibit COX2 with greater specificity, were developed. While these drugs appear both safer and more effective than their predecessors, they can have severe cardiac side effects in some patients (Salvo et al. 2011). Inhibition of prostacyclin formation in the infarcted heart by coxibs, which disrupts the balance of prostacyclin and thromboxane, increases the risk of cardiac complications. In addition, selective inhibitors are quite expensive and do not appear to reduce the risk of renal failure associated with cyclooxygenase inhibition. Thus, there is a continuing need for anti-inflammatory agents that are potent, selective, nontoxic, and abundant (Ward 2008).

Acetylsalicylic acid, or aspirin, is probably the most common and best-known natural anti-inflammatory compound. As early as 400 BC, Hippocrates was using the powdered bark of the willow tree to alleviate pain and fever. It was not until 1897, however, that chemists at Bayer modified salicylic acid to the compound now widely used (Patrono and Rocca 2009). Aspirin functions by inhibiting COX1 and altering the enzymatic activity of COX2 so that it produces lipoxins, which are anti-inflammatory, rather than prostanoids, which are proinflammatory (Katler and Weissmann 1977). In addition, aspirin decouples oxidative phosphorylation in the mitochondria of certain tissues, acting as a buffer and transporting protons. It is also suggested that acetylsalicylic acid may modulate NF-κB, and this in combination with its modulation of COX2 activity suggests that the molecule will be useful as a cancer chemopreventive agent (D'Acquisto and Ianaro 2006; Langley et al. 2011). Although other drugs are now commonly used for the treatment of headache or fever (e.g., acetaminophen and ibuprofen), low-dose aspirin remains in widespread use for the prevention of heart attack and stroke (Dalen 2006).

32.5 ANTI-INFLAMMATORY NATURAL PRODUCTS

Curcumin (**1**, Figure 32.2) is an anti-inflammatory compound that has been extensively studied as a cancer chemopreventive and chemotherapeutic agent. The anti-inflammatory activity of this major component of turmeric (*Curcuma longa*) is well documented in Ayurveda. It has become a molecule of interest for a breadth of beneficial effects (Basnet and Skalko-Basnet 2011). Compound **1** has been touted to guard against Alzheimer's disease, photoageing, melanoma, inflammation-induced obesity, metabolic diseases, radiation-mediated carcinogenesis, inflammatory bowel disease, head and neck squamous cell carcinoma, hematologic malignancies, colorectal cancer, neuroblastoma, hepatocarcinogenesis, ovarian cancer, prostate cancer, and heart disease (Hamaguchi et al. 2010;

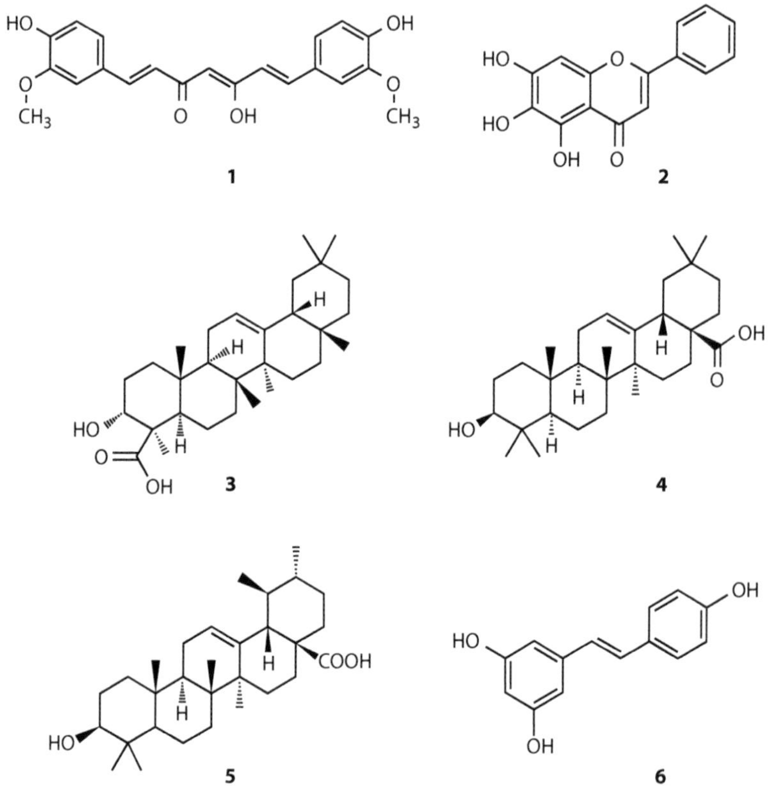

FIGURE 32.2 Structures of several natural product compounds with known anti-inflammatory activity. (1) Curcumin, (2) baicalein, (3) α-boswellic acid, (4) oleanolic acid (5), ursolic acid, and (6) resveratrol.

Heng 2010; Shehzad et al. 2012; Alappat and Awad 2010; Nambiar et al. 2011; Taylor and Leonard 2011; Wilken et al. 2011; Kelkel et al. 2010; Villegas et al. 2008; D'Aguanno et al. 2012; Fujise et al. 2012; Chen et al. 2012; Liu et al. 2011; Wongcharoen and Phrommintikul 2009). In addition, it has been reported to aid recovery from spinal injury (Ormond et al. 2012). Given this wide range of activity, it is not surprising to find that the mechanism of **1** is pleiotropic, and many molecular targets have been reported. Compound **1** has been demonstrated to decrease the expression of or inhibit NF-κB, activator protein 1 (AP-1), early growth response protein 1 (Egr-1), signal transducer and activator of transcription 1 (STAT1), STAT3, STAT5, EpRE, CREB binding protein (CBP), β-catenin, epidermal growth factor receptor (EGFR), human epidermal growth factor receptor 2 (HER2), AKT, Src, Janus kinase 2 (JAK2), tyrosine kinase 2 (TYK2), JNK, protein kinase A (PKA), PKC, VCAM-1, Bcl-2, Bcl-XL, intracellular adhesion molecule 1 (ICAM-1), tissue factor (TF), AR/ARP, ELAM-1, FTPase, urokinase-type plasminogen activator (uPA), xanthine oxidase (XOD), cyclin D1, 5-LOX, COX2, iNOS, MMP-9, TNFα, IL-6, IL-8, IL-12, acetyl coenzyme A acetyltransferase (ACAT), and apoptosis antigen 1 (APO1), while inducing expression or activity of inhibitor of NF-κB (IκB) kinase (IKK), adenosine monophosphate (AMP)–activated protein kinase (AMPK), p53, glutathione S-transferase (GST), and quinone reductase 1 (QR1) (Shanmugam et al. 2011; Zhou et al. 2011; Shehzad et al. 2012). By modulating these and other targets, some evidence suggests that compound **1** inhibits carcinogenesis, inflammation, tumor angiogenesis, and oxidative stress; regulates lipid metabolism; causes cell cycle arrest; and induces apoptosis in cancer cells.

Baicalein (**2**, Figure 32.2) is a major constituent of *Scutellaria baicalensis*, an herb commonly used in traditional Chinese medicine to treat inflammation, hypertension, cardiovascular diseases, and viral and bacterial infections (Li et al. 2011). This compound, a flavone, was found to have significant specific antitumor activity, as well as antioxidant, antithrombotic, anti-inflammatory, antiviral, neuroprotective, and cardioprotective properties (Parajuli et al. 2009; Yuan et al. 2012; Gabor 1986; Chen et al. 2011, 2012; Cui et al. 2010; Huang, Y. et al. 2005; Lee et al. 2011). In a mouse tumor model, oral administration of **2** was shown to inhibit growth of established prostate tumors by approximately 55% (Li-Weber 2009). The compound was also found to induce expression of Bax-1 and p53 in tumor cells, while inhibiting Bcl-2, Bcl-XL, NF-κB, and phosphor-AKT (pAKT). Compound **2** acts through a number of mechanisms, including ROS scavenging; prooxidative activity in cancer cells; inhibition of NF-κB; cell cycle inhibition through reduced levels of cyclin D1, cyclin B1, and cyclin-dependent kinase 1 (CDK1); and induction of apoptosis (Huang et al. 2012; Chi et al. 2012; Kang et al. 2011; Gautam and Jachak 2005). While not as thoroughly studied as **1**, compound **2** shows promise as an anti-inflammatory and cancer chemopreventive compound.

Boswellic acids (such as **3**, Figure 32.2) are found in plants of the genus *Boswellia*, particularly *Boswellia seratta*. These pentacyclic triterpenoids can make up as much as 30% of the resin of the plant. Several boswellic acids have been found to have anti-inflammatory and anticancer activities (Ammon 2006). The primary mechanism of these compounds appears to be inhibition of 5-LOX, but other molecular targets have been identified, including IKKs and topoisomerase I and II (Poeckel and Werz 2006). Acetyl-11-keto-β-boswellic acid was found to inhibit the growth of colorectal tumors and suppress metastasis in mice (Yadav 2012). In addition to inhibition of NF-κB activation, this compound modulated the expression of COX2, Bcl-2, Bcl-xL, cyclin D1, inhibitor of apoptosis 1 (IAP-1), MMP-9, and VEGF. Boswellic acids also inhibit the formation of oxygen radicals (Ammon 2010).

Several other triterpenoids have also demonstrated potent anti-inflammatory activity (Petronelli et al. 2009). Betulinic acid is derived from the bark of one of several plants, most commonly *Betula pubescens* (white birch). It has been demonstrated to have anti-inflammatory, antimalarial, and antiretroviral activity. It also acts as an antitumor agent by inhibiting topoisomerases (Mullauer et al. 2010). Betulinic acid has been reported as a selective inhibitor of melanoma and is known to induce apoptosis in melanoma cells (Liu et al. 2004). Activity of this compound against ovarian cancers, neuroblastoma, and malignant brain tumors has also been reported, as well as antiproliferative effects in the human promyelocytic leukemia cells (HL60), squamous cell carcinoma (SCC25), and SCC9 cell lines (Kessler et al. 2007).

A related compound, oleanolic acid (**4**, Figure 32.2), is found primarily in *Phytolacca americana* (pokeweed) but is also present in garlic. Compound **4** has been demonstrated to have antitumor and antiviral activity, particularly against HIV, and is hepatoprotective (Kuttan et al. 2011). Its activity against cancer cells appears to be due to inhibition of iNOS and COX2 by IFN (Suh et al. 1998). This compound also protects against oxidative stress by potently inducing phase II enzymes (QR1, GST, etc.) (Reisman et al. 2009; Wang et al. 2010).

Ursolic acid (**5**, Figure 32.2) is an isomer of **4** that has demonstrated significant cancer chemo-preventive activity, as well as anti-inflammatory activity (Sultana 2011). This compound is found in a number of plants, many of which are found in the human diet, including apples, bilberries, cranberries, prunes, and several spices (basil, lavender, peppermint, rosemary, oregano, and thyme) (Liu 2005). Compound **5** acts through inhibition of the STAT3 pathway (Pathak et al. 2007). It also downregulates MMP-9 (through the glucocorticoid receptor) and is a weak inhibitor of aromatase (Cha et al. 1996). This compound has been reported to inhibit cancer cell proliferation and to induce apoptosis in cancer cells (Fulda 2010).

Resveratrol (**6**, Figure 32.2) is a naturally occurring polyphenol found in a number of foods, most commonly, grapes and grape products such as red wine. This structurally simple stilbene is pro-duced in response to stress, such as fungal attack, and has a protective function (Bhat and Pezzuto 2002). Compound **6** mediates a plethora of responses, such as regulation of cell cycle progression, induction of apoptosis, inhibition of tumor invasion and angiogenesis, prevention of inflammation, activation of AMPK, scavenging of ROS, and modulation of NF-κB (Calamini et al. 2010). It also inhibits aromatase, induces QR1, and inhibits iNOS. In 1997, **6** was shown by our group to be cancer chemopreventive, blocking dimethylbenz(*a*)anthracene (DMBA)-induced tumorigenesis at all three stages of carcinogenesis: initiation, promotion, and progression (Jang et al. 1997). The same study demonstrated that **6** decreased carrageenan-induced inflammation in rats, based on paw volume (Figure 32.3), presumably through interactions with the arachidonic acid binding site of COX1 or COX2 (Calamini et al. 2010). The compound has been demonstrated to promote apoptosis in cancer cells, protect against viral infections, and even act as a caloric restriction mimetic (Pezzuto 2011). Compound **6** demonstrates activity with numerous targets; several thousand papers have appeared in the literature. This pleiotropic mechanism can be considered an attractive feature of the molecule, since alteration of multiple pathways may counteract drug resistance.

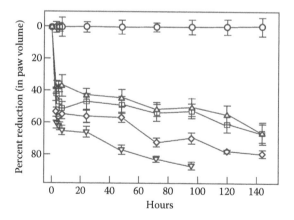

FIGURE 32.3 Effects of resveratrol (square, 3 mg/kg of body weight; diamond, 8 mg/kg); phenylbutazone (triangle); or indomethacin (inverted triangle) on carrageenan-induced inflammation in rats (Jang et al. 1997). Percent reduction (± SD) was obtained by comparing the paw volume in the control group (circle, treated with carrageenan only) with that in the drug-treated group. Dosing was repeated daily for 7 days. "Hours" refers to hours after carrageenan injection. The data for the indomethacin group at 120 and 140 h were not reliable because of the induction of secondary lesions.

32.6 ANTI-INFLAMMATORY LEAD MOLECULES AND SEMISYNTHETIC DERIVATIVES

In addition to these established leads, novel natural products with both anti-inflammatory and anti-cancer potential are continuously being discovered. Further, semisynthetic derivatives, which may prove more potent or selective than the original lead compound, are being developed. This is a promising approach for drug discovery, since it combines the diversity of chemical scaffolds found in nature with target-directed drug design. A brief review of some new natural and semisynthetic anti-inflammatory lead compounds is given below.

A common chemical class displaying anti-inflammatory activity is the alkaloids. Tryptanthrin, isolated from the leaves of *Isatis tinctoria*, has demonstrated potent inhibition of COX2 (half maximal inhibitory concentration $[IC_{50}] = 64$ nM) (Danz et al. 2002). This indoloquinazoline alkaloid was found to inhibit iNOS expression and display anti-inflammatory potential in topical application in humans by reducing the effects of sodium lauryl sulfate (SLS)-induced contact dermatitis (Ishihara et al. 2000; Heinemann et al. 2004). Another alkaloid, rutaecarpine, isolated from fruits of *Evodia rutaecarpa*, suppressed TNFα, IL-4, NO, iNOS, and synthesis of PGE_2, and inhibited COX2, with an IC_{50} value of 0.28 μM (Gautam and Jachak 2005). The compound also exhibited cell cycle arrest, inhibition of cytokine production, and anti-inflammatory activity in carrageenan-induced rat paw edema (Fei et al. 2003; Jeon et al. 2006; Moon et al. 1999). A second alkaloid found in *E. rutaecarpa*, evodiamine, demonstrated similar activity and inhibited NF-κB, with an IC_{50} value of 1.6 μM (Takada et al. 2005). Berberine, found in plants of the genera *Berberis* and *Coptis*, has been shown to inhibit levels of TNFα, IL-1β, IL-6, C-reactive protein, hepatoglobin, NO, iNOS, and COX2 (Vuddanda et al. 2010).

Among fatty acid leads, it has been seen that molecules with greater than 20 carbons tend to be good inhibitors of COX2, while those with fewer than 16 carbons are typically inactive. Among fatty acids with 18 carbons, activity appears to depend on saturation and ether placement (Ringbom et al. 2001). The compounds 13-(*S*)-hydroxy-9,11E-octadecaolienoic acid and (±)-glycerol-1-monolinolate, isolated from the plant *Hernandia ovigera*, have been demonstrated to inhibit COX2 potently and selectively, with IC_{50} values of 0.14 and 0.18 μM, respectively (Jang et al. 2004). Among derivatives of linoleic acid, (±)-10-oxo-*trans*-11-octadecen-13-olide, (±)-13-hydroxy-10-oxo-*trans*-11-octadecenoic acid (13-HOA), and 9-HOA have been found to strongly suppress proinflammatory proteins including COX2, iNOS, TNFα, and IL-6 (Yasuda et al. 2009; Murakami et al. 2005).

Several steroids, including methyl antcinate L, antcin M, and methyl antcinate K, all isolated from *Antrodia salmonea*, have been found to significantly suppress production of NO (Shen et al. 2007). Another steroid, guggulsterol, found in the gum of *Commiphora mukul*, displayed down-regulation of a number of inflammatory mediators, such as IFNγ, IL-12, TNFα, IL-1β, NO, and p38 MAPKs (Manjula et al. 2006). In a clinical study, treatment with *C. mukul* reduced pain and stiffness and improved function for patients with osteoarthritis (Singh et al. 2003). A related compound, (*E*)-guggulsterone, has been shown to inhibit NF-κB activation and downregulate COX2 and MMP-9 (Sarfaraz 2008).

A number of natural terpenoids have displayed anti-inflammatory activity. Diterpenoids isolated from *Croton tonkinensis* and *Isodon excises* were found to potently inhibit NF-κB activation and NO production, with IC_{50} values in the 100 nM range (Gautam and Jachak 2005). A triterpene glycoside isolated from the fruits of *Fomitopsis pinicola* exhibited very potent and selective inhibition of COX2, with an IC_{50} value of 150 nM (Yoshikawa et al. 2005). Two diterpene epoxides from *Tripterygium wilfordii*, triptolide and tripdiolide, demonstrated even more potent COX2 inhibition ($IC_{50} = 30$ nM) and also downregulated iNOS and IL-1β (Ma et al. 2007; Zhou et al. 2012). Another compound from *T. wilfordii*, celastrol, has been shown to downregulate IκBα, IKK, TGF-beta activated kinase 1 (TAK-1), and NF-κB. It appears to increase TNFα-induced apoptosis and inhibits invasion. Clinically, celastrol showed promise as an anti-inflammatory agent against arthritis, lupus, amyotrophic lateral sclerosis, and Alzheimer's disease (Kannaiyan 2011).

Sesquiterpene lactones from *Tanacetum parthenium*, *Magnolia grandiflora*, *Arnica montana*, and other plants have displayed a variety of anti-inflammatory activities, including inhibition of 5-LOX, leukotriene C_4 (LTC$_4$) synthase, NO production, and NF-κB activation (Gautam and Jachak 2005).

In addition to these natural terpenoids, a number of derivatives of the triterpene acids discussed above have been studied. Analogs of **4** and **5** have demonstrated potent inhibition of NO production (Liu 2005). Studies of these analogs demonstrated that the oleanane skeleton is more active than ursane. In ring A, addition of an electron-donating group, such as methoxycarbonyl, carboxyl, or nitrile at C-2, enhanced activity, while the electron-withdrawing hydroxyl, aminocarbonyl, methoxy, chloride, or bromide groups decreased activity. In ring C, nitrile or carboxyl groups in bis(enones) appeared to optimize activity. Analogs of betulinic acid with a cyanoenone functionality in ring A were found to inhibit NO production much more potently than the natural compound, with IC_{50} values in the 20 nM range (Mukherjee et al. 2006).

Anti-inflammatory activity has been reported in a number of natural flavonoids, including luteolin, quercetin, kaempferol, baicalin, wogonin, genistein, naringenin, eriodictyol, hesperetin, panduratin A, gemichalcones A and B, apigenin, diosmetin, fisetin, and pillion (Gautam and Jachak 2005). These compounds modulate a variety of markers, primarily affecting TNFα, MMP-2, MMP-9, NO, IL-4, 15-LOX-1, LOX-L1, PGE$_2$, and β-hexosaminidase. In general, flavones with a planar structure, a double bond between C-2 and C-3, hydroxyl groups at the 5- and 7-positions of the A-ring, and hydroxyl groups at the 3′- and 4′- positions in the B-ring demonstrated the most potent activity. Synthetic derivatives of **2** have increased activity versus NO production (Huang, W.-H. et al. 2005). Analogs of chrysin were found to downregulate expression of COX2 and iNOS, as well as strongly inhibit NO production and COX2 (Cho et al. 2004; Che et al. 2011). Other classes of polyphenolics that have generated lead anti-inflammatory compounds include lignans, phloroglucinols, quinones, phenylpropanoids, diaryl-heptanoids, and stilbenes.

Many stilbene analogs of **6** have been studied (Kondratyuk et al. 2011). Although **6** is active against a very large number of molecular targets, high potency is rarely observed, and rapid and complete metabolism leads to low bioavailability. For these reasons, potent and bioavailable derivatives of **6** are desirable. Certain hydroxylated analogs of **6** have demonstrated both greater potency and increased specificity as inhibitors of COX2 when compared with the parent compound. An analog with three hydroxyl groups on each ring inhibited COX2 with extreme potency (IC_{50} = 1.4 nM) and a selectivity index of 719, greater than that of celecoxib (COX1/COX2 = 546). Since **6** is rapidly metabolized upon ingestion, a study of the sulfate-conjugated metabolites was carried out by our group, but these metabolites were generally less active than **6** itself, and activities of the metabolites decreased as the degree of sulfation increased. Resveratrol-3-sulfate, however, was found to have a greater capacity for QR1 induction, 2, 2-diphenyl-1-picrylhydrazyl (DPPH) radical scavenging, and COX1 inhibition than the parent compound (Hoshino et al. 2010). Recently, a series of thiadiazole analogs of **6** has been studied, and several of these compounds were found to display potent activities (Mayhoub et al. 2012a). In these derivatives, a five-membered heterocycle replaced the stilbene bridge of **6** in order to prevent metabolism to the potentially hepatotoxic *trans*-stilbene oxide. The use of a 3,5-diaryl-1,2,4-thiadiazole scaffold resulted in increased potency and selectivity of compounds as inhibitors of aromatase and NF-κB, and as inducers of QR1, when compared to **6**. The 3- and 4-pyridyl derivatives were found to be the most active against aromatase (Mayhoub et al. 2012b). It was found that thiadiazole *ortho*-dihalogenated derivatives were most active as inducers of QR1, with bromine producing the most potent compound. These analogs were significantly more active and selective than **6**, with CD values in the 100 nM range. The *meta*-methyl or methoxy derivatives showed equal or slightly greater inhibition of NF-κB relative to **6**.

32.7 CONCLUSIONS AND PERSPECTIVE

Given the ever-increasing evidence that inflammation is a common etiological factor in cancer as well as many other diseases, it would appear that effective intervention strategies could be

TABLE 32.1

Natural Product Agents Currently in Clinical Trials for Anti-Inflammatory Activity

Drug	Condition	Stage	Dose	Dosage Frequency	Study Length	Completion	Location	Primary Outcome Measure	Secondary Outcome Measure
Apigenin	Colorectal cancer	Phase II	20 mg apigenin and 20 mg epigallocatechin gallate	QD	3 years	Dec. 2016	Dresden University of Technology, Germany	Recurrence rate of neoplasia	Recurrence-free survival, overall survival, serum flavonoid levels of patients
Boswellic acid	Relapsing remitting multiple sclerosis	Phase II	400–1600 mg	TID	32 weeks	Oct. 2013	Universitätsklinikum Hamburg–Eppendorf, Germany	Mean number of total Gd-enhancing lesions	Number of new active lesions, relapse rate
Curcumin	Colon cancer	Phase I	3–6 g	QD	7 days	Jan. 2013	James Graham Brown Cancer Center, USA	Concentration of curcumin in normal and cancerous tissue	Serum cytokine levels, adverse events
Emodin	Polycystic kidney		100 mg	QD		Sept. 2012	Nanjing University School of Medicine, China	MRI calculated kidney volume, EGFR	End-stage kidney disease (ESRD)
Parthenolide	Contact dermatitis	Phase III	0.003 mg/cm^2	Once	Once	Dec. 2013	Allerderm	Change in frequency and characterization of positive reactions per allergen	Prevalence of late or persistent reactions, irritation, adhesion, subject-reported itching or burning, adverse events
Resveratrol	Chronic subclinical inflammation	Phase III	500 mg	QD	30 days	Mar. 2012	University of Turin, Italy	Circulating concentrations of C-reactive protein	TAS, 4-hydroxynonenal, nitrotyrosine, IL-6, TNF-alpha, eNOS, SOD2, catalase, pentraxin 3

Source: Data provided by the National Library of Medicine, clinicaltrials.gov.

Note: eNOS, endothelial nitric oxide synthase; ESRD, end stage renal disease; Gd, gadolinium; MRI, magnetic resonance imaging; QD, quaque die, once daily; SOD2, superoxide dismutase 2; TAS, total antioxidant status; TID, ter in die, three times daily.

implemented. A few examples of ongoing clinical trials are listed in Table 32.1. However, of the many therapeutic attempts to date, a definitive and predicable clinical outcome is lacking, and frequent adverse side effects are witnessed. In the context of the general population, a question of great interest relates to disease prevention mediated by constituents found in the diet. As described above, many individual compounds have been studied and found to ostensibly function in a beneficial manner, but more careful analysis often reveals issues associated with gastrointestinal absorption or metabolism, or results obtained with in vitro tests that were performed in a manner that is not physiologically relevant. In the context of the human diet, rather than individual components, the question of utmost importance relates to total dietary consumption, and how the sum total of dietary constituents interact and function to control or reduce the inflammatory response. The discovery of novel, potent, selective natural product anti-inflammatory agents and evaluation of the activity of these agents alone and in combination remains of high importance. However, as single agents are found in low concentrations following dietary ingestion, it would be of greatest value to consider any potential response in the broader context of the entire dietary milieu.

It is becoming increasingly clear that the traditional, linear approach to biochemical pathways is insufficient, and we must instead consider signaling networks. As learned from some of the most interesting natural product lead compounds, rather than modulating a single cellular target, pleiotropic mechanisms apply. As such, compounds such as **1** and **6** modulate a variety of molecular targets in multiple pathways. However, these pleiotropic compounds generally lack potency against any single target, so when administered in exceedingly high doses with the intent of preventing disease, it is likely that any therapeutic outcome results from numerous responses that remain largely uncharacterized. Based on this premise, it seems reasonable to combine multiple agents that are more potent but highly selective for a single target. In this way, a pleiotropic therapy with greater potency and efficacy could be rationally engineered. Natural product scaffolds could play a critical role in this process.

REFERENCES

Agrawal, A. and I. S. Fentiman. 2008. NSAIDs and breast cancer: a possible prevention and treatment strategy. *Int J Clin Pract* 62:444–9.

Alappat, L. and A. B. Awad. 2010. Curcumin and obesity: evidence and mechanisms. *Nurt Rev* 68:729–38.

Alcudia, J. F., J. Marinez-Gonzalez, A. Guadall, M. Gonzalez-Diez, L. Badimon, and C. Rodriguez. 2008. Lysyl oxidase and endothelial dysfunction: mechanisms of lysyl oxidase down-regulation by pro-inflammatory cytokines. *Front Biosci* 13:2721–7.

Allavena, P., G. Germano, F. Marchesi, and A. Mantovani. 2011. Chemokines in cancer related inflammation. *Exp Cell Res* 317:664–73.

Ammon, H. P. 2006. Boswellic acids in chronic inflammatory diseases. *Planta Med* 72:1100–16.

Ammon, H. P. 2010. Modulation of the immune system by *Boswellia serrata* extracts and boswellic acids. *Phytomedicine* 17:862–7.

Balkwill, F. and A. Mantovani. 1996. Inflammation and cancer: back to Virchow? *Lancet* 357:539–45.

Balkwill, F. and A. Mantovani. 2010. Cancer and inflammation: implications for pharmacology and therapeutics. *Clin Parmacol Ther* 87:401–6.

Basnet, P. and N. Skalko-Basnet. 2011. Curcumin: an anti-inflammatory molecule from a curry spice on the path to cancer treatment. *Molecules* 16:4567–98.

Bhat, K. P. and J. M. Pezzuto. 2002. Cancer chemopreventive activity of resveratrol. *Ann N Y Acad Sci* 957:210–29.

Bogoyevitch, M. A., K. R. Ngoei, T. T. Zhao, Y. Y. Yeap, and D. C. Ng. 2010. c-Jun N-terminal kinase (JNK) signaling: recent advances and challenges. *Biochim Biophys Acta* 1804:463–75.

Brigati, C., D. M. Noonan, A. Albini, and R. Benelli. 2002. Tumors and inflammatory infiltrates: friends or foes? *Clin Exp Metastasis* 19:247–58.

Calamini, B., K. Ratia, M. G. Malkowski, M. Cuendet, J. M. Pezzuto, B. D. Santarsiero, and A. D. Mesecar. 2010. Pleiotropic mechanisms facilitated by resveratrol and its metabolites. *Biochem J* 429:273–82.

Cha, H. J., S. K. Bae, H. Y. Lee, O. H. Lee, H. Sato, M. Seiki, B. C. Park, and K. W. Kim. 1996. Anti-invasive activity of ursolic acid correlates with the reduced expression of matrix metalloproteinase-9 (MMP-9) in HT1080 human fibrosarcoma cells. *Cancer Res* 56:2281–4.

Che, H., H. Lim, H. P. Kim, and H. Park. 2011. A chrysin analog exhibited strong inhibitory activities against both PGE$_2$ and NO production. *Eur J Med Chem* 46:4657–60.

Chen, J. 2011. Multiple signal pathways in obesity-associated cancer. *Obes Rev* 12:1063–70.

Chen, L., J. Dou, Z. Su, H. Zhou, H. Wang, W. Zhou, Q. Guo, and C. Zhou. 2011. Synergistic activity of baicalein with ribavirin against influenza A (H1N1) virus infections in cell culture and in mice. *Antiviral Res* 91:314–20.

Chen, S. S., A. Michael, and S. A. Butler-Manuel. 2012. Advances in the treatment of ovarian cancer—a potential role of anti-inflammatory phytochemicals. *Discov Med* 13:7–17.

Chi, D. S., T. C. Lin, K. Hall, T. Ha, C. Li, Z. D. Wu, T. Soike, and G. Krishnaswamy. 2012. Enhanced effects of cigarette smoke extract on inflammatory cytokine expression in IL-1β–activated human mast cells were inhibited by baicalein via regulation of the NF-κB pathway. *Clin Mol Allergy* 10:3.

Cho, H., C.-W. Yun, W.-K. Park, J.-Y. Kong, K. S. Kim, Y. Park, S. Lee, and B.-K. Kim. 2004. Modulation of the activity of pro-inflammatory enzymes, COX-2 and iNOS, by chrysin derivatives. *Pharmacol Res* 49:37–43.

Collington, S. J., T. J. Williams, and C. L. Weller. 2011. Mechanisms underlying the localization of mast cells in tissues. *Trends Immunol* 32:478–85.

Cotran, R., V. Kumar, and T. Collins. 1999. *Robbins Pathologic Basis of Disease*. Philadelphia, PA: W.B. Saunders Company.

Coussens, L. M. and Z. Werb. 2002. Inflammation and cancer. *Nature* 420:860–7.

Cuadrado, A. and A. R. Nebreda. 2010. Mechanisms and functions of p38 MAPK signaling. *Biochem J* 429:403–17.

Cui, L., X. Zhang, R. Yang, L. Liu, L. Wang, M. Li, and W. Du. 2010. Baicalein is neuroprotective in rat MCAO model: role of 12/15-lipoxygenase, mitogen activated protein kinase and cytosolic phospholipase A2. *Pharmacol Biochem Behav* 96:469–75.

D'Acquisto, F. and A. Ianaro. 2006. From willow bark to peptides: the ever widening spectrum of NF-kappaB inhibitors. *Curr Opin Pharmacol* 6:387–92.

D'Aguanno, S., I. D'Agnano, M. De Canio, C. Rossi, S. Bernardini, G. Federici, and A. Urbani. 2012. Shotgun proteomics and network analysis of neuroblastoma cell lines treated with curcumin. *Mol Biosyst* 8:1068–77.

Dalen, J. E. 2006. Aspirin to prevent heart attack and stroke: what's the right dose? *Am J Med* 119:198–202.

Danz, H., S. Stoyanova, O. A. Thomet, H. U. Simon, G. Dannhardt, H. Ulbrich, and M. Hamburger. 2002. Inhibitory activity of tryptanthrin on prostaglandin and leukotriene synthesis. *Planta Med* 68:875–80.

Den Uyl, D., I. E. Bultink, and W. F. Lems. 2011. Glucocorticoid-induced osteoporosis. *Clin Exp Rheumatol* 29:593–8.

Demaria, S., E. Pikarsky, M. Karin, L. M. Coussens, Y. C. Chen, E. M. El-Omar, G. Trinchieri, S. M. Dubinett, J. T. Mao, E. Szabo, A. Krieg, G. J. Weiner, B. A. Fox, G. Coukos, E. Wang, R. T. Abraham, M. Carbone, and M. T. Lotze. 2010. Cancer and inflammation: promise for biologic therapy. *J Immunother* 33:335–51.

Dhanasekaran, D. N. and E. P. Reddy. 2008. JNK signaling in apoptosis. *Oncogene* 27:6245–51.

Di Bisceglie, A. M., S. E. Order, J. L. Klein, J. G. Waggoner, M. H. Sjogren, G. Kuo, M. Houghton, Q. L. Choo, and J. H. Hoofnagle. 1991. The role of chronic viral hepatitis in hepatocellular carcinoma in the United States. *Am J Gastroenterol* 86:335–8.

DiPietro, L. A. 1995. Wound healing: the role of the macrophage and other immune cells. *Shock* 4:233–40.

Dorai, T. and B. B. Aggarwal. 2004. Role of chemopreventive agents in cancer therapy. *Cancer Lett* 215:129–40.

Erler, J. T. and A. J. Giaccia. 2006. Lysyl oxidase mediates hypoxic control of metastasis. *Cancer Res* 66:10238–41.

Fei, X. F., B. X. Wang, T. J. Li, S. Tashiro, M. Minami, D. J. Xing, and T. Ikejima. 2003. Evodiamine, a constituent of *Evodiae fructus*, induces anti-proliferating effects in tumor cells. *Cancer Sci* 94:92–8.

Feiken, E., J. Rome, J. Eriksen, and L. R. Lund. 1995. Neutrophils express tumor necrosis factor-alpha during mouse skin wound healing. *J Invest Dermatol* 105:120–3.

Fujise, Y., J. I. Okano, T. Nagahara, R. Abe, R. Imamoto, and Y. Murawaki. 2012. Preventive effect of caffeine and curcumin on hepato-carcinogenesis in diethylnitrosamine-induced rats. *Int J Oncol* 40:1779–88.

Fulda, S. 2010. Modulation of apoptosis by natural products for cancer therapy. *Planta Med* 76:1075–9.

Gabor, M. 1986. Anti-inflammatory and anti-allergic properties of flavonoids. *Prog Clin Biol Res* 213:471–80.

Gardner, A. and R. G. Boles. 2011. Beyond the serotonin hypothesis: mitochondria, inflammation, and neurodegeneration in major depression and affective spectrum disorders. *Prog Neuropsychopharmacol Biol Psychiatry* 35:730–43.

Gautam, R. and S. M. Jachak. 2009. Recent developments in anti-inflammatory natural products. *Med Res Rev* 29:767–820.

Giehl, K., M. Bachem, M. Beil, B. O. Bohm, V. Ellenrieder, S. Fulda, T. M. Gress, K. Holzmann, H. A. Kestler, M. Kornmann, A. Menke, P. Moller, F. Oswald, R. M. Schmid, V. Schmidt, R. Schirmbeck, T. Seufferlein, G. van Wichert, M. Wagner, P. Walther, T. Wirth, and G. Adler. 2011. Inflammation, regeneration, and transformation in the pancreas: results of the Collaborative Research Center 518 (SFB 518) at the University of Ulm. *Pancreas* 40:489–502.

Greene, E. R., S. Huang, C. N. Serhan, and D. Panigrahy. 2011. Regulation of inflammation in cancer by eicosanoids. *Prostaglandins Other Lipid Mediat* 96:27–36.

Guilford, J. M. and J. M. Pezzuto. 2008. Natural products as inhibitors of carcinogenesis. *Expert Opin Investig Drugs* 17:1341–52.

Hamaguchi, T., K. Ono, and M. Yamada. 2010. Curcumin and Alzheimer's disease. *CNS Neurosci Ther* 16:285–97.

Hartman, H., A. Abdulla, D. Awla, B. Lindkvist, B. Jeppsson, L. Thorlacious, and S. Regner. 2012. P-selectin mediates neutrophil rolling and recruitment in acute pancreatitis. *Br J Surg* 99:246–55.

Heinemann, C., S. Schliemann-Willers, C. Oberthur, M. Humburger, and P. Elsner. 2004. Prevention of experimentally induced irritant contact dermatitis by extracts of Isatis tinctoria compared to pure tryptanthrin and its impact on UVB-induced erythema. *Planta Med* 70:385–90.

Heng, M. C. 2010. Curcumin targeted signaling pathways: basis for anti-photoaging and anti-carcinogenic therapy. *Int J Dermatol* 49:608–22.

Hoshino, J., E. J. Park, T. P. Kondratyuk, L. Marler, J. M. Pezzuto, R. B. van Breemen, S. Mo, Y. Li, and M. Cushman. 2010. Selective synthesis and biological evaluation of sulfate-conjugated resveratrol metabolites. *J Med Chem* 53:5033–43.

Huang, P., J. Han, and L. Hui. 2010. MAPK signaling in inflammation-associated cancer development. *Protein Cell* 1:218–26.

Huang, W.-H., A.-R. Lee, P.-Y. Chien, and T.-Z. Chou. 2005. Synthesis of baicalein derivatives as potential anti-aggregatory and anti-inflammatory agents. *J Pharm Pharmacol* 57:219–25.

Huang, W.S., Y. H. Kuo, C. C. Chin, J. Y. Wang, H. R. Yu, J. M. Sheen, S. Y. Tung, C. H. Shen, T. C. Chen, M. L. Sung, H. F. Liang, and H. C. Kuo. 2012. Proteomic analysis of the effects of baicalein on colorectal cancer cells. *Proteomics* 12:810–9.

Huang, Y., S. Y. Tsang, X. Yao, and Z. Y. Chen. 2005. Biological properties of baicalein in cardiovascular system. *Curr Drug Targets Cardiovasc Haematol Disord* 5:177–84.

Hubner, G., M. Brauchle, H. Smola, M. Madlener, R. Fassler, and S. Werner. 1996. Differential regulation of pro-inflammatory cytokines during wound healing in normal and glucocorticoid-treated mice. *Cytokine* 8:548–56.

Hudson, J. D., M. A. Shoaibi, R. Maestro, A. Carnero, G. J. Hannon, and D. H. Beach. 1999. A proinflammatory cytokine inhibits p53 tumor suppressor activity. *J Exp Med* 190:1375–82.

Hume, D. A. 2006. The mononuclear phagocyte system. *Curr Opin Immunol* 18:49–53.

Ishihara, T., K. Kohno, S. Ushio, K. Iwaki, M. Ikeda, and M. Kurimoto. 2000. Tryptantrhin inhibits nitric oxide and prostaglandin E_2 synthesis by murine macrophages. *Eur J Pharmacol* 407:197–204.

Itzkowitz, S. H. and X. Yio. 2004. Inflammation and cancer IV. Colorectal cancer in inflammatory bowel disease: the role of inflammation. *Am J Physiol Gastrointest Liver Physiol* 287:G7–17.

Jang, D. S., M. Cuendet, B.-N. Su, S. Totura, S. Riswan, H. H. S. Fong, J. M. Pezzuto, and A. D. Kinghorn. 2004. Constituents of the seeds of *Hernandia ovigera* with inhibitory activity against cyclooxygenase-2. *Planta Med* 70:893–6.

Jang, M., L. Cai, G. O. Udeani, K. V. Slowing, C. F. Thomas, C. W. Beecher, H. H. Font, N. R. Farnsworth, A. D. Kinghorn, R. G. Mehta, R. C. Moon, and J. M. Pezzuto. 1997. Cancer chemopreventive activity of resveratrol, a natural product derived from grapes. *Science* 275:218–20.

Jeon, T. W., C. H. Jin, S. K. Lee, I. H. Jun, G. H. Kim, D. J. Lee, H. G. Jeong, K. B. Lee, Y. Jahng, and T. C. Jeong. 2006. Immunosuppressive effects of rutaecarpine in female BALB/c mice. *Toxicol Lett* 164:155–66.

Johnsen, J. I., M. Lindskog, F. Ponthan, I. Pettersen, L. Elfman, A. Orrego, B. Sveinbjornsson, and P. Kogner. 2005. NSAIDS in neuroblastoma therapy. *Cancer Lett* 228:195–201.

Johnston, H., H. Boutin, and S. M. Allan. 2011. Assessing the contribution of inflammation in models of Alzheimer's disease. *Biochem Soc Trans* 39:886–90.

Kang, K. A., R. Zhang, M. J. Piao, S. Chae, H. S. Kim, J. H. Park, K. S. Jung, and J. W. Hyun. 2012. Baicalein inhibits oxidative stress-induced cellular damage via antioxidant effects. *Toxicol Ind Health* 28:412–21.

Kannaiyan, R., M. K. Shanmugam, and G. Sethi. 2011. Molecular targets of celastrol derived from Thunder of God Vine: potential role in the treatment of inflammatory disorders and cancer. *Cancer Lett* 303:9–20.

Katler, E. and G. Weissmann. 1977. Steroids, aspirin, and inflammation. *Inflammation* 2:295–307.

Kelkel, M., C. Jacob, M. Dicato, and M. Diederich. 2010. Potential of the dietary antioxidants resveratrol and curcumin in prevention and treatment of hematologic malignancies. *Molecules* 15:7035–74.

Kessler, J. H., F. B. Mullauer, G. M. de Roo, and J. P. Medema. 2007. Broad in vitro efficacy of plant-derived betulinic acid against cell lines derived from the most prevalent human cancer types. *Cancer Lett* 251:132–45.

Kim, E. K. and E. J. Choi. 2010. Pathological roles of MAPK signaling pathways in human diseases. *Biochim Biophys Acta* 1802:396–405.

Kobayashi, Y. 2008. The role of chemokines in neutrophil biology. *Front Biosci* 13:2400–7.

Kondratyuk, T. P., E. J. Park, L. E. Marler, S. Ahn, Y. Yuan, Y. Choi, R. Yu, R. B. van Breemen, B. Sun, J. Hoshino, M. Cushman, K. C. Jermihov, A. D. Mesecar, C. J. Grubbs, and J. M. Pezzuto. 2011. Resveratrol derivatives as promising chemopreventive agents with improved potency and selectivity. *Mol Nutr Food Res* 55:1249–65.

Kusters, J. G., A. H. van Vliet, and E. J. Kuipers. 2006. Pathogenesis of *Heliobacter pylori* infection. *Clin Microbiol Rev* 19:449–90.

Kuttan, G., P. Pratheeshkumar, K. A. Manu, and R. Kuttan. 2011. Inhibition of tumor progression by naturally occurring terpenoids. *Pharm Biol* 49:995–1007.

Langley, R. E., S. Burdett, J. F. Tierney, F. Cafferty, M. K. Parmar, and G. Venning. 2011. Aspirin and cancer: has aspirin been overlooked as an adjuvant therapy? *Br J Cancer* 105:1107–13.

Lee, Y. M., P. Y. Cheng, L. S. Chim, C. W. Kung, S. M. Ka, M. T. Chung, and J. R. Sheu. 2011. Baicalein, an active component of *Scutellaria baicalensis* Georgi, improves cardiac contractile function in endotoxaemic rats via induction of heme oxygenase-1 and suppression of inflammatory responses. *J Ethnopharmacol* 135:179–85.

Li, C., G. Lin, and Z. Zuo. 2011. Pharmacological effects and pharmacokinetic properties of Radix Scutellariae and its bioactive flavones. *Biopharm Drug Dispos* 32:427–45.

Li-Weber, M. 2009. New therapeutic aspects of flavones: the anticancer properties of *Scutellaria* and its main active constituents, wogonin, baicalein, and baicalin. *Cancer Treat Rev* 35:57–68.

Liekens, S., D. Schols, and S. Hatse. 2010. CXCL12–CXCR4 axis in angiogenesis, metastasis and stem cell mobilization. *Curr Pharm Des* 16:3903–20.

Liu, J. 2005. Oleanolic acid and ursolic acid: research perspectives. *J Ethnopharmacol* 100:92–4.

Liu, S., Z. Wang, Z. Hu, X. Zeng, Y. Li, Y. Su, C. Zhang, and Z. Ye. 2011. Anti-tumor activity of curcumin against androgen-independent prostate cancer cells via inhibition of NF-kappaB and AP-1 pathway in vitro. *J Huazhong Univ Sci Technolog Med Sci* 31:530–4.

Liu, W. K., J. C. Ho, F. W. Cheung, B. P. Liu, W. C. Ye, and C. T. Che. 2004. Apoptotic activity of betulinic acid derivatives on murine melanoma B16 cell line. *Eur J Pharmacol* 498:71–8.

Luan, J., R. Shattuck-Brandt, H. Haghnegahdar, J. D. Owen, R. Strieter, M. Burdick, C. Nirodi, D. Beauchamp, K. N. Johnson, and A. Richmond. 1997. Mechanism and biological significance of constitutive expression of MGSA/GRO chemokines in malignant melanoma tumor progression. *J Luekoc Biol* 62:588–97.

Luqman, S. and J. M. Pezzuto. 2010. NFkappaB: a promising target for natural products in cancer chemoprevention. *Phytother Res* 24:949–63.

Ma, J., M. Dey, H. Yang, A. Poulev, R. Pouleva, R. Dorn, P. E. Lipsky, E. J. Kennelly, and I. Raskin. 2007. Antiinflammatory and immunosuppressive compounds from *Tripterygium wifordii*. *Phytochemistry* 68:1172–8.

Maccia, A. and C. Madeddu. 2012. Inflammation and ovarian cancer. *Cytokine* 58:133–47.

Maeda, H. and T. Akaike. 1998. Nitric oxide and oxygen radicals in infection, inflammation, and cancer. *Biochemistry* 63:854–65.

Manabe, I. 2011. Chronic inflammation links cardiovascular, metabolic, and renal diseases. *Circ J* 75:2739–48.

Manjula, N., B. Gayathri, K. S. Vinaykumar, N. P. Shankernarayanan, R. A. Vishwakarma, and A. Balakrishnan. 2006. Inhibition of MAP kinases by crude extract and pure compound isolated from *Commiphora mukul* leads to down regulation of TNF-alpha, IL-1beta and IL-2. *Int Immunopharmacol* 6:122–32.

Maxwell, S. R., R. J. Moots, and M. J. Kendall. 1994. Corticosteroids: do they damage the cardiovascular system? *Postgrad Med J* 70:863–70.

Mayhoub, A. S., L. Marler, T. P. Kondratyuk, E. J. Park, J. M. Pezzuto, and M. Cushman. 2012a. Optimization of the aromatase inhibitory activities of pyridylthiazole analogues of resveratrol. *Bioorg Med Chem* 20:2427–34.

Mayhoub, A. S., L. Marler, T. P. Kondratyuk, E. J. Park, J. M. Pezzuto, and M. Cushman. 2012b. Optimizing thiadiazole analogues of resveratrol versus three chemopreventive targets. *Bioorg Med Chem* 20:510–20.

Mayo, M. W., J. L. Norris, and A. S. Baldwin. 2001. Ras regulation of NF-kappa B and apoptosis. *Methods Enzymol* 333:73–87.

Miller, T. E. and D. W. Watson. 1965. Innate immunity. *Med Clin North Am* 49:1489–1504.

Miloso, M., A. Scuteri, D. Foudah, and G. Tredici. 2008. MAPKs as mediators of cell fate determination: an approach to neurodegenerative diseases. *Curr Med Chem* 15:538–48.

Moon, T. C., M. Murakami, I. Kudo, K. H. Son, H. P. Kim, S. S. Kang, and H. W. Chang. 1999. A new class of COX-2 inhibitor, rutaecarpine from *Evodia rutaecarpa*. *Inflamm Res* 48:621–5.

Mukherjee, R., V. Kumar, S. K. Srivastava, S. K. Agarwal, and A. C. Burman. 2006. Betulinic acid derivatives as anticancer agents: structure activity relationship. *Anticancer Agents Med Chem* 6:271–9.

Mullauer, F. B., J. H. Kessler, and J. P. Medema. 2010. Betulinic acid, a natural compound with potent anticancer effects. *Anticancer Drugs* 21:215–27.

Murakami, A., T. Nishizawa, K. Egawa, T. Kawada, Y. Nishikawa, K. Uenakai, and H. Ohigashi. 2005. New class of linoleic acid metabolites biosynthesized by corn and rice lipoxygenases: suppression of proinflammatory mediator expression via attenuation of MAPK- and Akt-, but not PPARgamma-, dependent pathways in stimulated macrophages. *Biochem Pharmacol* 70:1330–42.

Nambiar, D., P. Rajamani, and R. P. Singh. 2011. Effects of phytochemicals on ionization radiation–mediated carcinogenesis and cancer therapy. *Mutat Res* 728:139–57.

Opdenakker, G. and J. Van Damme. 2004. The countercurrent principle in invasion and metastasis of cancer cells. Recent insights on the roles of chemokines. *Int J Dev Biol* 48:519–27.

Ormond, D. R., H. Peng, R. Zeman, K. Das, R. Murali, and M. Jhanwar-Unival. 2012. Recovery from spinal cord injury using naturally occurring anti-inflammatory compound curcumin. *J Neurosurg Spine* 16:497–503.

Parajuli, P., N. Joshee, A. M. Rimando, S. Mittal, and A. K. Yadav. 2009. In vitro antitumor mechanisms of various *Scutellaria* extracts and constituent flavonoids. *Planta Med* 75:41–8.

Pathak, A. K., M. Bhutani, A. S. Nair, K. S. Ahn, A. Chakraborty, H. Kadara, S. Guha, G. Sethi, and B. B. Aggarwal. 2007. Ursolic acid inhibits STAT3 activation pathway leading to suppression of proliferation and chemosensitization of human multiple myeloma cells. *Mol Cancer Res* 5:943–55.

Patrono, C. and B. Rocca. 2009. Aspirin, 110 years later. *J Thromb Haemost* S1:258–61.

Payne, S. L., M. J. Hendrix, and D. A. Kirschmann. 2007. Paradoxical roles for lysyl oxidases in cancer—a prospect. *J Cell Biochem* 101:1338–54.

Peppa, M., M. Krania, and S. A. Raptis. 2011. Hypertension and other morbidities with Cushing's syndrome associated with corticosteroids: a review. *Integr Blood Press Control* 4:7–16.

Petronelli, A., G. Pannitteri, and U. Testa. 2009. Triterpenoids as new promising anticancer drugs. *Anticancer Drugs* 20:880–92.

Pezzuto, J. M. 2011. The phenomenon of resveratrol: redefining the virtues of promiscuity. *Ann N Y Acad Sci* 1215:123–30.

Phillipson, M. and P. Kubes. 2011. The neutrophil in vascular inflammation. *Nat Med* 17:1381–90.

Poeckel, D. and O. Werz. 2006. Boswellic acids: biological actions and molecular targets. *Curr Med Chem* 13:3359–69.

Poetker, D. M. and D. D. Reh. 2010. A comprehensive review of the adverse effects of systemic corticosteroids. *Otolaryngol Clin North Am* 43:753–68.

Rao, C. V., T. Kawamori, R. Hamid, and B. S. Reddy. 1999. Chemoprevention of colonic aberrant crypt foci by an inducible nitric oxide synthase–selective inhibitor. *Carcinogenesis* 20:641–4.

Reisman, S. A., L. M. Aleksunes, and C. D. Klaassen. 2009. Oleanolic acid activates Nfr2 and protects from acetaminophen hepatotoxicity via Nrf2-dependent and Nrf2-independent processes. *Biochem Pharmacol* 77:1273–82.

Ringbom, T., U. Huss, A. Stenholm, S. Flock, L. Skattebol, P. Perera, and L. Bohlin. 2001. COX-2 inhibitory effects of naturally occurring and modified fatty acids. *J Nat Prod* 64:745–9.

Sadik, C. D., N. D. Kim, and A. D. Luster. 2011. Neutrophils cascading their way to inflammation. *Trends Immunol* 32:452–60.

Salvo, F., A. Fourrier-Reglat, F. Bazin, P. Robinson, N. Riera-Guardia, M. Haag, A. P. Caputi, N. Moore, M. C. Strukenboom, and A. Pariente. 2011. Cardiovascular and gastrointestinal safety of NSAIDs: a systematic review of meta-analyses of randomized clinical trials. *Clin Pharmacol Ther* 89:855–66.

Sarfaraz, S., I. A. Siddiqui, D. N. Syed, F. Afaq, and H. Mukhtar. 2008. Guggulsterone modulates MAPK and NF-kappaB pathways and inhibits skin tumorigenesis in SENCAR mice. *Carcinogenesis* 29:2011–8.

Schiffman, M., P. E. Castle, J. Jeronimo, A. C. Rodriguez, and S. Wacholder. 2007. Human papillomavirus and cervical cancer. *Lancet* 370:890–907.

Schneider, C. and A. Pozzi. 2011. Cyclooxygenases and lipoxygenases in cancer. *Cancer Metastasis Rev* 30:277–94.

Schupp, P. J., C. Kohlert-Schupp, S. Whitefield, A. Engemann, S. Rohde, T. Hermscheidt, J. M. Pezzuto, T. P. Kondratyuk, E. J. Park, L. Marler, B. Rostama, and A. D. Wright. 2009. Cancer chemopreventive and anticancer evaluation of extracts and fractions from marine macro- and microorganisms collected from Twilight Zone waters around Guam. *Nat Prod Commun* 4:1717–28.

Seibert, K., J. Masferrer, Y. Zhang, S. Gregory, G. Olson, S. Hauser, K. Leahy, W. Perkins, and P. Isakson. 1995. Mediation of inflammation by cyclooxygenase-2. *Agents Actions Suppl* 46:41–50.

Shanmugam, M. K., R. Kannaivan, and G. Sethi. 2011. Targeting cell signaling and apoptotic pathways by dietary agents: role in the prevention and treatment of cancer. *Nutr Cancer* 63:161–73.

Sharma, S., B. P. Wilkinson, P. Gao, and V. E. Steele. 2002. Differential activity of NO synthase inhibitors as chemopreventive agents in a primary rat tracheal epithelial cell transformation system. *Neoplasia* 4:332–6.

Shehzad, A., S. Khan, and Y. Sup Lee. 2012. Curcumin molecular targets in obesity and obesity-related cancers. *Future Oncol* 8:179–90.

Shen, C. C., Y. H. Wang, T. T. Chang, L. C. Lin, M. J. Don, Y. C. Hou, K. T. Liou, S. Chang, W. Y. Wang, H. C. Ko, and Y. C. Shen. 2007. Anti-inflammatory ergostanes from the basidiomata of *Antrodia salmonea*. *Planta Med* 73:1208–13.

Sholter, D. E. and P. W. Armstrong. 2000. Adverse effects of corticosteroids on the cardiovascular system. *Can J Cardiol* 16:505–11.

Shu, Q. and V. Nair. 2008. Inosine monophosphate dehydrogenase (IMPDH) as a target in drug discovery. *Med Res Rev* 28:219–32.

Siddikuzzaman, V. M. Grace, and C. Guruvayoorappan. 2011. Lysyl oxidase: a potential target for cancer therapy. *Inflammopharmacology* 19:117–29.

Singh, B. B., L. C. Mishra, S. P. Vinjamury, N. Aquilina, V. J. Singh, and N. Shepard. 2003. The effectiveness of *Commiphora mukul* for osteoarthritis of the knee: an outcomes study. *Altern Ther Health Med* 9:74–9.

Singh, S. and A. K. Gupta. 2011. Nitric oxide: role in tumour biology and iNOS/NO-based anticancer therapies. *Cancer Chemother Pharmacol* 67:1211–24.

Soehnlein, O., L. Lindblom, and C. Weber. 2009. Mechanisms underlying neutrophil-mediated monocyte recruitment. *Blood* 114:4613–23.

Sostres, C., C. J. Gargallo, M. T. Arroyo, and A. Lanas. 2010. Adverse effects of non-steroidal anti-inflammatory drugs (NSAIDs, aspirin and coxibs) on upper gastrointestinal tract. *Best Pract Res Clin Gastroenerol* 24:121–32.

Suh, N., T. Honda, H. J. Finlay, A. Barchowsky, C. Williams, N. E. Benoit, Q. W. Xie, C. Nathan, G. W. Gribble, and M. B. Sporn. 1998. Novel triterpenoids suppress inducible nitric oxide synthase (iNOS) and inducible cyclooxygenase (COX-2) in mouse macrophages. *Cancer Res* 58:717–23.

Sultana, N. 2011. Clinically useful anticancer, antitumor, and antiwrinkle agent, ursolic acid and related derivatives as medicinally important natural product. *J Enzyme Inhib Med Chem* 26:616–42.

Swartzberg, J. 2008. Is inflammation the root of all disease? Wellness Letter. University of California, Berkeley. http://www.wellnessletter.com/html/wl/2008/wlFeatured0108.html#.

Takada, Y., Y. Kobayashi, and B. B. Aggarwal. 2005. Evodiamine abolishes constitutive and inducible NF-kappaB activation by inhibiting IkappaBalpha kinase activation, thereby suppressing NF-kappaB–regulated antiapoptotic and metastatic gene expression, up-regulating apoptosis, and inhibiting invasion. *J Biol Chem* 280:17203–12.

Taylor, R. A. and M. C. Leonard. 2011. Curcumin for inflammatory bowel disease: a review of human studies. *Altern Med Rev* 16:152–6.

Thiel, A., J. Mrena, and A. Ristimaki. 2011. Cyclooxygenase-2 and gastric cancer. *Cancer Metastasis Rev* 30:387–95.

Tracey, K. J. 2007. Physiology and immunology of the cholinergic anti-inflammatory pathway. *J Clin Invest* 117:289–96.

Vandercappellen, J., J. Van Damme, and S. Struyf. 2008. The role of CXC chemokines and their receptors in cancer. *Cancer Lett* 267:226–44.

Vicari, A.P. and C. Caux. 2002. Chemokines in cancer. *Cytokine Growth Factor Rev* 13:143–54.

Villegas, I., S. Sanchez-Fidalgo, and C. Alarcon de la Lastra. 2008. New mechanisms and therapeutic potential of curcumin for colorectal cancer. *Mol Nutr Food Res* 52:1040–61.

Vuddanda, P. R., S. Chakraborty, S. Singh. 2010. Berberine: a potential phytochemical with multispectrum therapeutic activities. *Expert Opin Investig Drugs* 19:1297–307.

Wang, X., X. L. Ye, R. Liu, H. L. Chen, H. Bai, X. Liang, X. D. Zhang, Z. Wang, W. L. Li, and C. X. Hai. 2010. Antioxidant activities of oleanolic acid in vitro: possible role of Nrf2 and MAP kinases. *Chem Biol Interact* 184:328–37.

Ward, S. G. 2008. New drug targets in inflammation: efforts to expand the anti-inflammatory armoury. *Br J Parmacol* 153:S5–6.

Weber, C., A. Schober, and A. Zernecke. 2004. Chemokines: key regulators of mononuclear cell recruitment in atherosclerotic vascular disease. *Arterioscler Thromb Vasc Biol* 24:1997–2008.

Whitcomb, D. C. 2004. Inflammation and cancer V. Chronic pancreatitis and pancreatic cancer. *Am J Physiol Gastrointest Liver Physiol* 287:G315–9.

Wilken, R., M. S. Veena, M. B. Wang, and E. S. Srivatsan. 2011. Curcumin: a review of anti-cancer properties and therapeutic activity in head and neck squamous cell carcinoma. *Mol Cancer* 10:12.

Wongcharoen, W. and A. Phrommintikul. 2009. The protective role of curcumin in cardiovascular diseases. *Int J Cardiol* 133:145–51.

Yadav, V. R., S. Prasad, B. Sung, J. G. Gelovani, S. Guha, S. Krishnan, and B. B. Aggarwal. 2012. Boswellic acid inhibits growth and metastasis of human colorectal cancer in orthotopic mouse model by down-regulating inflammatory, proliferative, invasive and angiogenic biomarkers. *Int J Cancer* 130:2176–84.

Yamanishi, Y., D. L. Boyle, S. Rosengren, D. R. Green, N. J., Zvaifler, and G. S. Firestein. 2002. Regional analysis of p53 mutations in rheumatoid arthritis synovium. *Proc Natl Acad Sci USA* 99:10025–30.

Yasuda, M., T. Nishizawa, H. Ohigashi, T. Tanaka, D. X. Hou, N. H. Colburn, and A. Murakami. 2009. Linoleic acid metabolite suppresses skin inflammation and tumor promotion in mice: possible roles of programmed cell death 4 induction. *Carcinogenesis* 30:1209–16.

Yoshikawa, K., M. Inoue, Y. Mastumoto, C. Sakkakibara, H. Miyataka, H. Mastumoto, and S. Arihara. 2005. Lanostane triterpenoids and triterpene glycosides from the fruit body of *Fomitopsis pinicola* and their inhibitory activity against COX-1 and COX-2. *J Nat Prod* 68:69–73.

Yuan, Y., L. Shuai, S. Chen, L. Huang, S. Qin, and Z. Yang. 2012. Flavonoids and antioxidative enzymes in temperature-challenged roots of *Scutellaria baicalensis* Georgi. *Z Naturforsch* 67:77–85.

Zarbock, A. and K. Ley. 2011. Protein tyrosine kinases in neutrophil activation and recruitment. *Arch Biochem Biophys* 510:112–9.

Zhou, H., C. S. Beevers, and S. Huang. 2011. The targets of curcumin. *Curr Drug Targets* 12:332–47.

Zhou, Z. L., Y. X. Yang, J. Ding, Y. C. Li, and Z. H. Miao. 2012. Triptolide: structural modifications, structure–activity relationships, bioactivities, clinical development and mechanisms. *Nat Prod Rep* 29:457–75.

Zhu, Z., S. Zhong, and Z. Shen. 2011. Targeting the inflammatory pathways to enhance chemotherapy of cancer. *Cancer Biol Ther* 12:95–105.

Index

Page numbers followed f and t indicate figures and tables, respectively.

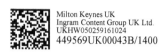

Milton Keynes UK
Ingram Content Group UK Ltd.
UKHW050259161024
449569UK00043B/1400